Clinical Paediatric Dietetics

Clinical Paediatric Dietetics

EDITED BY

Vanessa Shaw

Fourth Edition

WILEY Blackwell

Library of Congress Cataloging-in-Publication Data

Clinical paediatric dietetics / edited by Vanessa Shaw. – Fourth edition.
        p. ; cm.
    Preceded by Clinical paediatric dietetics / edited by Vanessa Shaw and Margaret Lawson. 3rd ed. 2007.
    Includes bibliographical references and index.
    ISBN 978-0-470-65998-4 (cloth)
    I. Shaw, Vanessa, editor.
    [DNLM: 1. Diet Therapy. 2. Child. WS 366]
    RJ53.D53
    615.8′54083–dc23

                                                                            2014007124

A catalogue record for this book is available from the British Library.

Wiley also publishes its books in a variety of electronic formats. Some content that appears in print may not be available in electronic books.

Set in 9.5/11.5pt Palatino by Laserwords Private Limited, Chennai, India
Printed and bound in Singapore by Markono Print Media Pte Ltd

2   2015

Contents

List of Contributors

Eleanor Baldwin BSc, RD
Advanced Dietitian – Adult Refsum's Disease
Chelsea & Westminster Hospital, Fulham Rd,
London SW10 9NH

Jason Beyers BSc, PG Dip Dietetics, RD
Formerly Specialist Paediatric Liver and Critical
Care Dietitian
King's College Hospital, Denmark Hill, London
SE5 9RS

Nicol Clayton BSc, RD
Specialist Paediatric Dietitian – Barth Syndrome
NHS Specialised Services
North Bristol Trust, Southmead Hospital,
Westbury-on-Trym, Bristol BS10 5NB

Zoe Connor MSc, RD
Freelance Paediatric Dietitian and Lecturer
www.zoeconnor.co.uk

Lisa Cooke BSc, MA RD
Head of Paediatric Dietetics
Bristol Royal Hospital for Children, Upper
Maudlin Street, Bristol BS2 8BJ

Marjorie Dixon BSc, RD
Principal Paediatric Dietitian – Metabolic Medicine
Great Ormond Street Hospital for Children NHS
Foundation Trust, Great Ormond Street, London
WC1N 3JH

Jennifer Douglas BSc, BPhEd
PG Dip Dietetics, RD
Formerly Specialist Paediatric Dietitian
Mile End Hospital, London E1 4DG

Georgiana Fitzsimmons BSc, PG Dip Dietetics,
BPhEd, RD
Principal Paediatric Dietitian – Ketogenic Diets
Great Ormond Street Hospital for Children NHS
Foundation Trust, Great Ormond Street, London
WC1N 3JH

Janine Gallagher BSc, PG Dip Dietetics, MSc
Specialist Paediatric Metabolic Dietitian
Royal Manchester Children's Hospital, Central
Manchester Foundation Trust, Oxford Road,
Manchester M13 9WL

Eulalee Green BSc, MSc, RD
Dietitian and Public Health Nutritionist
PO Box 63973, Putney Health, London SW15 9BB

Kate Grimshaw PhD, RD
Research Fellow
University Hospital Southampton NHS
Foundation Trust (UHS), Tremona Road,
Southampton SO16 6YD

Lesley Haynes Dip Dietetics
Formerly Principal Paediatric Dietitian –
Epidermolysis Bullosa
Great Ormond Street Hospital for Children NHS
Foundation Trust, Great Ormond Street, London
WC1N 3JH

David Hopkins BSc, MSc, RD
Specialist Paediatric and Adult Cystic Fibrosis
Dietitian
University Hospital Southampton NHS
Foundation Trust (UHS), Tremona Road,
Southampton SO16 6YD

Leanie Huxham BSc, MNutr, RD
Freelance Paediatric Dietitian
huxham.nutrition@yahoo.co.uk

Tracey Johnson BSc, RD
Senior Specialist Paediatric Dietitian
Birmingham Children's Hospital NHS Trust,
Steelhouse Lane, Birmingham B4 6NH

Alison Johnston BSc, RD
Lead Clinical Specialist Diabetes Dietitian
(Paediatric)
Royal Hospital for Sick Children, Dalnair Street,
Yorkhill, Glasgow G3 8SJ

Caroline King BSc, RD
Specialist Neonatal Dietitian
Hammersmith Hospital, Du Cane Road, London
W12 OHS

Julie Lanigan BSc, PhD, RD
Paediatric Research Dietitian/Clinical Trials
Coordinator
Childhood Nutrition Research Centre, UCL
Institute of Child Health, London WC1N 1EH

Jacqueline Lowdon BSc, MSc, PGCE (FE), RD
Paediatric Dietitian Team Leader
Royal Manchester Children's Hospital, Central
Manchester Foundation Trust, Oxford Road,
Manchester M13 9WL

Anita MacDonald BSc, PhD, RD
Consultant Dietitian in Inherited Metabolic
Disorders, Birmingham Children's Hospital and
Honorary Professor of Paediatric Dietetics,
Plymouth University
Birmingham Children's Hospital NHS Trust,
Steelhouse Lane, Birmingham B4 6NH

Sarah Macdonald BSc, RD
Principal Paediatric Dietitian – Gastroenterology
and Surgery
Great Ormond Street Hospital for Children NHS
Foundation Trust, Great Ormond Street, London
WC1N 3JH

Luise Marino BSc, PG Dip Dietetics, MMed Sci
Nutr, PhD
Chief Paediatric Dietitian
University Hospital Southampton NHS
Foundation Trust (UHS), Tremona Road,
Southampton SO16 6YD

Helen McCarthy BSc, PgCHEP, PhD, RD
Lecturer (Dietetics)
School of Biomedical Sciences, University of
Ulster, Coleraine, Co Londonderry BT52 1SA

Rosan Meyer B Dietetics, MNutr, PhD, RD
Principal Research Dietitian
Great Ormond Street Hospital for Children NHS
Foundation Trust, Great Ormond Street, London
WC1N 3JH

Judy More BSc, RD, RNutr
Freelance Paediatric Dietitian, London
www.child-nutrition.co.uk

Dasha Nicholls MD, MBBS, MRCPsych, FAED
Consultant Child and Adolescent Psychiatrist
Great Ormond Street Hospital for Children NHS
Foundation Trust, Great Ormond Street, London
WCIN 3JH

Graeme O'Connor BSc, PG Dip Dietetics, PhD, RD
Specialist Paediatric Dietitian
Great Ormond Street Hospital for Children NHS
Foundation Trust, Great Ormond Street, London
WC1N 3JH

Carolyn Patchell BSc, RD
Head of Nutrition and Dietetics
Birmingham Children's Hospital NHS Trust,
Steelhouse Lane, Birmingham

Danielle Petersen BSc, MSc, RD
Specialist Paediatric Dietitian
Great Ormond Street Hospital for Children NHS
Foundation Trust, Great Ormond Street, London
WC1N 3JH

Pat Portnoi BSc, RD
Galactosaemia Support Group Dietitian and
Register Coordinator
www.galactosaemia.org

Joanne Louise Price BSc, RD
Chief Paediatric Dietitian – Gastroenterology and
Surgery
Royal Manchester Children's Hospital, Central
Manchester Foundation Trust, Oxford Road,
Manchester M13 9WL

Julie Royle BSc, PG Dip Dietetics
Clinical Specialist Dietitian (Renal) and Team
Leader
Royal Manchester Children's Hospital, Central
Manchester Foundation Trust, Oxford Road,
Manchester M13 9WL

Marian Sewell Dip Dietetics RD
Specialist Paediatric Dietitian
Great Ormond Street Hospital for Children NHS
Foundation Trust, Great Ormond Street, London
WC1N 3JH

Vanessa Shaw MBE, MA, PG Dip Dietetics, RD,
FBDA
Head of Dietetics, Great Ormond Street Hospital
for Children and Honorary Associate Professor of
Paediatric Dietetics,
Plymouth University
Great Ormond Street Hospital for Children NHS
Foundation Trust, Great Ormond Street, London
WC1N 3JH

Melanie Sklar BSc RD
Formerly Principal Paediatric Dietitian –
Epidermolysis Bullosa
Great Ormond Street Hospital for Children NHS
Foundation Trust, Great Ormond Street, London
WC1N 3JH

Zofia Smith BSc, RD
Formerly Community Paediatric Dietitian
St Mary's Hospital, Greenhill Rd, Leeds LS12 3QE

Jacky Stafford BSc, MSc, RD
Great Ormond Street Hospital for Children NHS
Foundation Trust, Great Ormond Street, London
WC1N 3JH

Laura Stewart PhD, RD, RNutr
Paediatric Overweight Service Tayside Team Lead
NHS Tayside, Perth Royal Infirmary, Perth PH1
1NX, and Children's Weight Clinic, Edinburgh

Kate Tavener BSc, PG Dip Dietetics, RD
Specialist Neonatal Dietitian
King's College Hospital, Denmark Hill, London
SE5 9RS

Carina Venter BSc, PG Dip Allergy, PhD, RD
Allergy Specialist Dietitian and Senior Lecturer,
University of Portsmouth
The David Hide Asthma and Allergy Research
Centre, St Mary's Hospital, Newport, Isle of Wight
PO30 5TG

Evelyn Ward BSc, RD
Senior Specialist Paediatric
Oncology/Haematology Dietitian
Leeds Children's Hospital, Leeds General
Infirmary, Leeds LS1 3EX

Ruth Watling BSc, RD
Head of Dietetics
Alder Hey Children's NHS Foundation Trust,
Eaton Road, Liverpool L12 2AP

Fiona White BSc, RD
Lead Specialist Metabolic Dietitian
Royal Manchester Children's Hospital, Central
Manchester Foundation Trust, Oxford Road,
Manchester M13 9WL

Natalie Yerlett BSc, PG Dip Dietetics, RD
Specialist Paediatric Dietitian
Great Ormond Street Hospital for Children NHS
Foundation Trust, Great Ormond Street, London
WC1N 3JH

Preface

The aim of this manual is to provide a very practical approach to the dietary management of children with a wide range of disorders that can benefit from dietary therapy. Interventions range from nutritional support to the diet being the major or sole treatment for particular disorders. The text will be of relevance to professional dietitians, dietetic students and their tutors, paediatricians, paediatric nurses and members of the community health team caring for children who require therapeutic diets. The importance of nutritional support and dietary management in many paediatric conditions is increasingly recognised and is reflected in new text for this edition.

The authors are largely drawn from practising paediatric dietitians around the United Kingdom, with additional contributions from academic research dietitians and a psychiatrist. The need for evidence based practice has demanded a thorough review of the current scientific and medical literature to support clinical practice wherever possible. Where the evidence base is lacking, expert clinical opinion is given.

The major part of the text concentrates on nutritional requirements of sick infants, children and young people in the clinical setting. Normal dietary constituents are used alongside special dietetic products to provide a prescription that will control progression and symptoms of disease whilst maintaining the growth potential of the individual. The section on community based nutrition includes healthy eating throughout infancy, childhood and adolescence, the principles of which underpin many clinical interventions. The distinction between clinical dietetics and nutrition in the community is rather arbitrary and there is of course a continuum between care provided between the acute and community settings.

There has been an expansion of the range of disorders, treatments, guidelines and recommendations described in many chapters, e.g. endocrinology, the ketogenic diet, inherited metabolic disorders, food hypersensitivity and prevention of allergy, eating disorders and neurodisability.

Arranged under headings of disorders rather than type of diet, and with much information presented in tabular form and with worked examples, the manual is easy to use. There are case studies throughout which demonstrate the practical application of the theory.

The most recent information and data has been used in the preparation of this edition, but no guarantee can be given for validity or availability at the time of going to press.

Vanessa Shaw
March 2014

Acknowledgements

I would like to thank a number of dietitians who wrote for the third edition of this book whose work contributed to the following chapters:

Chapter 1 Nutritional Assessment, Dietary Requirements, Feed Supplements: my former co-editor Margaret Lawson

Chapter 5 Nutrition in Critically Ill Children: Katie Elwig

Chapter 9 The Liver and Pancreas: Stephanie France

Chapter 14 Food Hypersensitivity: Kate Grimshaw

Chapter 15 Immunodeficiency Syndromes: Marian Sewell & Vivien Wigg

Chapter 16 Ketogenic Diets: Liz Neal & Gwyneth Magrath

Chapter 20 Lipid Disorders: Patricia Rutherford

Chapter 25 Burns: Claire Gurry

Chapter 28 Children from Ethnic Groups and those following Cultural Diets: Sue Wolfe

Chapter 30 Feeding Children with Neurodisabilities: Sarah Almond, Liz Allott & Kate Hall

Chapter 32 Prevention of Food Allergy: Carina Venter

About the Companion Website

This book is accompanied by a companion website:

www.wiley.com/go/shaw/paediatricdietetics

The website includes:

- Powerpoints of all figures from the book for downloading
- PDFs of all tables from the book for downloading
- PDFs of all chapter references for downloading

Part 1

Principles of Paediatric Dietetics

1 Nutritional Assessment, Dietary Requirements, Feed Supplementation

Vanessa Shaw and Helen McCarthy

Introduction

This text provides a practical approach to the dietary management of a range of paediatric disorders. The therapies outlined in Parts 2 and 3 describe the dietetic interventions and nutritional requirements of the infant, child and young person in a clinical setting, illustrating how normal dietary constituents are used alongside special dietetic products to allow for the continued growth of the child whilst controlling the progression and symptoms of disease. Nutrition for the healthy child and nutritional care in the community is addressed in Part 4.

The following principles are relevant to the treatment of all infants, children and young people and provide the basis for many of the therapies described later in the text.

Assessment of nutritional status

Assessment and monitoring of nutritional status should be included in any dietary regimen, audit procedure or research project where a modified diet has a role. Although the terms are used interchangeably in the literature, nutrition screening is a simple and rapid means of identifying individuals at nutritional risk which can be undertaken by a range of healthcare professionals, whereas nutrition assessment is a more detailed and lengthy means for nutrition experts, i.e. dietitians, to quantify nutritional status.

Nutrition screening

While nutrition screening tools can be used to identify all aspects of malnutrition (excess, deficiency or imbalance in macro and micro nutrients), they are generally used to identify protein energy undernutrition [1]. Despite the recommendations from benchmark standards and national and international guidelines that screening for nutrition risk be an integral component of clinical care for all [2–5], the development of nutrition screening tools for use with children has lagged behind work in the adult world. However, in recent years a number of child specific nutrition screening tools have been developed. Internationally the Nutrition Risk Score (Paris tool), the Subjective Global Nutrition Assessment (SGNA) and the Strongkids tool are available [6–8]. Each of these has strengths and limitations in terms of validity and reliability of the tool, the time taken to complete, and the level of skill required by individuals applying the tool.

Within the UK two child specific tools have been developed: the Screening Tool for the Assessment of

Table 1.1   Child specific screening tools developed and evaluated in the UK.

	STAMP	PYMS
Criteria utilised	Diagnosis Dietary intake Anthropometrics: weight and height centile	Diagnosis Dietary intake Weight loss Anthropometrics: BMI
Scored	High/medium/ low risk	High/medium/ low risk
Criterion validity		
Agreement with full nutritional assessment*	54%	46%
Positive predictive value[†]	55%	47%
Negative predictive value[††]	95%	95%
Training	30 minutes	60 minutes
Used by	Any trained healthcare professional	Registered nurses

STAMP, Screening Tool for the Assessment of Malnutrition in Paediatrics; PYMS, Paediatric Yorkhill Malnutrition Score; BMI, body mass index.
*Children identified as being at nutritional risk by tool and full nutritional assessment.
[†]The proportion of children identified as at risk by the tool who are actually at risk.
[††]The proportion of children identified as not at risk by the tool who are actually not at risk.

Malnutrition in Paediatrics (STAMP) and the Paediatric Yorkhill Malnutrition Score (PYMS) [9, 10]. Both of these tools have been evaluated in practice and comprise a number of elements that are scored to give a final risk score (Table 1.1). The reliability of each of these tools has been published, along with a number of other studies evaluating their use in a variety of clinical settings and conditions [11–13]. The main limitation of these evaluation studies is that they rely on the dietetic assessment of nutritional status as the 'gold standard' and the findings of studies comparing the tools to date have been equivocal. There is an ongoing multicentre Europe-wide study under the auspices of the European Society of Paediatric Gastroenterology, Hepatology and Nutrition (ESPGHAN) to evaluate a range of the tools available. Results have not yet been published, but it is hoped that this will form

the scientific basis for future developments in this area [14].

Nutritional assessment

Nutritional assessment comprises anthropometric, clinical and dietary assessment, all of which should be used to provide as full a picture of the nutritional status of the individual as possible; no one method will give an overall picture of nutritional status. Within these areas there are several assessment techniques, some of which should be used routinely in all centres, whilst others are better suited to specialist clinical areas or research. This chapter provides a brief overview of the common techniques and sources of further information.

Anthropometry

Measurement of weight and height (or length) is critical as the basis for calculating dietary requirements as well as monitoring the effects of dietary intervention. It is important that all measurements are taken using standardised techniques and calibrated equipment. Ideally staff taking measurements should receive some training on how to do this accurately. There are a variety of online resources to support training in anthropometric measurement of children.

Weight
Measurement of weight is an easy and routine procedure that should be done using a calibrated digital scale. Ideally infants should be weighed naked and children wearing just a dry nappy or pants; however, this is often not possible or appropriate. In these situations it is important to record if the infant is weighed wearing a clean dry nappy, and the amount and type of clothing worn by older children. A higher degree of accuracy is required for the assessment of sick children than for routine measurements in the community. Frequent weight monitoring is important for the sick infant or child, and local policies for weighing and measuring hospitalised infants and children should be in place. Recommendations for the routine measurement of healthy infants where there are no concerns about growth are given in Table 1.2 [15]. If there are concerns

Table 1.2 Recommendations for routine measurements for healthy infants and children.

Weight	Length/height	Head circumference
Birth	Birth	Birth or neonatal period
2 months	6–8 weeks if birth weight <2.5 kg or if other cause for concern	6–8 weeks
3 months		
4 months		
8 months		
Additional weights at parent's request; not more frequently than 2 weekly <6 months, monthly 6–12 months 12–15 months	No other routine measurement of length/height	No other routine measurement of head circumference
School entry	School entry	

Source: Adapted from *Health for all Children* [15].

about weight gain that is too slow or too rapid, measurement of weight should be carried out more frequently.

Height
Height or length measurement requires a sta-diometer or length board. Measurement of length using a tape measure is too inaccurate to be of use for longitudinal monitoring of growth, although an approximate length may be useful as a single measure. Under the age of 2 years supine length is measured; standing height is usually measured over this age or whenever the child can stand straight and unsupported. When the method of measurement changes from length to height there is likely to be a drop in stature; this is accounted for in the UK-WHO growth charts (p. 6). Measurement of length is difficult and requires careful positioning of the infant; positioning of the child is also important when measuring standing height. It is recommended to have two observers involved in measuring an infant or young child. It is good practice for sick infants to be measured monthly and older children at clinic appointments or on admission to hospital. Healthy infants should have a length measurement at birth but further routine stature checks are not recommended until the preschool check [15]. Whenever there are concerns

about growth or weight gain a height measurement should be made more often.

Proxy measurements for length/height
In some cases it is difficult to obtain length or height measurements, e.g. in very sick or preterm infants and in older children with scoliosis. A number of proxy measurements can be used which are useful to monitor whether longitudinal growth is progressing in an individual, but there are no recognised centile charts as yet and indices such as body mass index (BMI) cannot be calculated. In younger adults arm span is approximately equivalent to height, but body proportions depend upon age and while there is some evidence that there is a correlation in older children and adolescents, this measurement may be of limited usefulness in children. Ulna length has been demonstrated to act as a good proxy for stature in adults although evidence in children is limited [16]. Measurements of lower leg length or knee–heel length have been used and are a useful proxy for growth [17]. Total leg length is rarely measured outside specialist growth clinics and is calculated as the difference between measured sitting height and standing height. A number of other measures have been used in children with cerebral palsy as a proxy for height (p. 780), but numbers are too small for reference standards to be established [18]. Formulas for calculating stature in children from proxy measurements are available [19].

Head circumference
Head circumference is generally considered a useful measurement in children under the age of 2 years. After this age head growth slows and is a less useful indicator of somatic growth. A number of genetic and acquired conditions, such as cerebral palsy, will affect head growth and measurement of head circumference will not be a useful indicator of nutritional status in these conditions. Head circumference is measured using a narrow, flexible, non-stretch tape. Accuracy is dependent on the skill of the observer and, as such, training and practice in this technique is a requirement.

Supplementary measurements
While the measurement of weight and length or height forms the basis of routine anthropometric assessment, there are a number of supplementary

measurements which can be used. These include the proxy measurements for stature already mentioned and mid upper arm circumference (MUAC). This is a useful measurement in children under the age of 5 years, as MUAC increases fairly rapidly up until this age. Increases in MUAC are less likely to be affected by oedema than body weight; they can also provide a useful method of assessing changes in children with solid tumours and liver disease. There are age related standards for infants and children [19, 20]. Measurement of waist circumference and the index of waist to height can be helpful in the identification and monitoring of overweight and obesity [21–23]. Research has shown links with dyslipidaemias, insulin resistance and blood pressure although the evidence for benefit using waist circumference centiles over BMI centiles is limited [23].

When monitoring interventions, particularly those addressing undernutrition, it is important to determine if changes in weight are due to increases in fat mass or lean muscle mass. In order to fully differentiate between lean and fat, measurement of skinfold thickness (SFT) can be used. This can be unpleasant for young children and is not used as a routine anthropometric measurement in clinical practice, but it can provide valuable data in research studies. The equipment and technique are identical to those used in adults and the measurement is subject to the same high rates of inter-observer and intra-observer error. Reference data for infants and children are available [20] and arm muscle and arm fat area can be calculated. Full details on skinfold measurements and their interpretation has been published elsewhere [19, 24].

Modern technologies can provide information on body composition. Bioelectric impedance analysis is easily undertaken in a clinical setting using foot to foot or hand to foot techniques. However, while studies have reported validity of this method of determining body composition in healthy populations of young children, validity in sick children and infants has yet to be fully established [25, 26]. More invasive technologies for assessing body composition include dual-energy x-ray absorptiometry and air displacement plethysmography. These tend to be restricted to research assessments of body composition and further information can be found elsewhere [19].

Interpreting anthropometric measurements

Anthropometric measurements alone confer limited information on growth, nutritional status and health and require the use of growth reference data and conversion to indices for interpretation.

Growth charts

Measurements should be regularly plotted on a relevant growth chart. In the UK the growth standards are the UK-WHO Growth Charts 0–4 years and the UK Growth Charts 2–18 years [27]. The charts for preschool children incorporate data from the WHO multicentre growth study, a longitudinal study of optimal growth in breast fed singleton births from six countries across the world [28]. Every child in the UK is issued with a growth centile chart as part of the personal child health record that is held by parents and completed by healthcare professionals whenever the child is weighed or measured.

Accuracy is crucial when plotting growth charts, and therefore training is essential as a number of different professionals may be plotting on a single chart and errors could result in the misdiagnosis or non-identification of nutritional and growth problems. When assessing a child in relation to the growth charts a number of factors need to be accounted for including gestational age at birth and parental height. The growth charts give clear guidance on correction for prematurity and the estimation of the child's adult height.

It can be difficult to assess progress or decide upon targets where a measurement falls outside the nine centile lines (<0.4th centile or >99.6th centile). The Neonatal and Infant Close Monitoring growth charts [27] show −3, −4 and −5 standard deviation lines to allow assessment of very small infants up to the age of 2 years. 'Thrive lines' have also been developed to aid interpretation of infants with either slow or rapid weight gain. The 5% thrive lines define the slowest rate of normal weight velocity in healthy infants. If an infant is growing at a rate parallel to or slower than a 5% thrive line, weight gain is abnormally slow. The 95% thrive lines define the most rapid rate of normal weight gain in healthy infants and weight gain that parallels or is faster than the 95% thrive line is abnormally rapid [28]. There are a range of resources available to support training on the plotting and interpretation of growth charts on the Royal College of Paediatrics and Child Health website.

Some medical conditions have a significant effect on growth and where sufficient data exist separate growth charts have been developed, e.g. Down's syndrome, Turner syndrome, sickle cell disease, achondroplasia.

Body mass index

A BMI measurement can be calculated from weight and height measurements: BMI = weight (kg)/height (m^2). This provides an indication of relative fatness or thinness. In children the amount and distribution of body fat is dependent on age and sex. BMI is now routinely used to identify and monitor overweight and obesity in children, on an individual and population basis, in the clinical and research environments [29]. There are limitations, however, to the use of BMI in children:

- It is not recommended in children <2 years of age as during this period BMI changes rapidly and weight gain rather than BMI has been shown to be more indicative of future overweight and obesity [30].
- In chronic undernutrition there is stunting as well as low weight for age and thus undernutrition may be masked by using BMI.
- Although BMI is a relative index of weight to height it does not provide information about body composition; it cannot be used to distinguish between fat mass and lean mass.

Paediatric BMI charts have been developed and can be used to indicate how heavy a child is relevant to its height and age [31]. The UK growth charts have a quick reference guide to estimate BMI centile on the basis of the child's weight and height centiles.

Anthropometric indices and the classification of nutrition status

The World Health Organization (WHO) and research publications frequently report standard deviation (SD) score or z-score for length/height, weight and BMI. This involves converting the measurement or index into a finite proportion of a reference or standard measurement, the calculation giving a numerical score indicating how far away from the 50th centile for age the child's measurements/index falls. For the UK growth charts each centile space equates to 0.67SD; therefore a child on the 2nd centile will have a z-score of −2SD and a child on the 98th centile will have a z-score of +2SD; a measurement that falls exactly on the 50th centile will have a z-score of 0SD. Calculation of z-scores by hand is extremely laborious, but a computer software program is available (www.childgrowthfoundation.org) that will enable calculation of z-scores from height, weight, BMI, gender and age data. The z-score can also used when comparing groups of children when a comparison of the measurements themselves would not be useful.

The WHO defines moderate malnutrition and obesity in children in terms of z-score for weight as −2SD and +2SD respectively [28].

The calculation of height for age, height age and weight for height are useful when assessing nutritional status initially or when monitoring progress in children who are short for their chronological age. Table 1.3 shows examples of calculations for these indices. The Waterlow classification [32] may be of use when assessing children in the UK with severe failure to thrive. An adaptation of the classification is shown in Table 1.4. Calculation of height age is necessary when determining nutrient requirements for children who are much smaller (or larger) than their chronological age.

Clinical assessment

Clinical assessment of the child involves a medical history and a physical examination. The medical history will identify medical, social or environmental factors that may be risk factors for the development of nutritional problems. Such factors may include parental knowledge and finance available for food purchase, underlying disease, treatments, investigations and medications. Clinical signs of poor nutrition, revealed in the physical examination, only appear at a late stage in the development of a deficiency disease and absence of clinical signs should not be taken as indicating that a deficiency is not present.

Table 1.3 Height for age, height age and weight for height.

Worked example: 6-year-old girl with cerebral palsy referred with severe feeding problems

Visit 1	Decimal age = 6.2 years
	Height = 93 cm (<0.4th centile)
	Weight = 10 kg (<0.4th centile)
	50th centile for height for a girl aged 6.2 years = 117 cm
	Height for age = $\frac{93}{117}$ = 79.5% height for age
	Height age is the age at which 93 cm (measured height) falls on 50th centile = 2.7 years
	50th centile for weight for 2.7 years = 14 kg
	Weight for height = $\frac{10}{14}$ = 71% weight for height
Visit 2 (after intervention)	Decimal age = 6.8 years
	Height = 95.5 cm (<0.4th centile)
	Weight = 12 kg (<0.4th centile)
	50th centile for height for a girl aged 6.8 years = 121 cm
	Height for age = $\frac{95.5}{121}$ = 79% height for age
	Height age = 3.1 years
	50th centile for weight for age 3.1 years = 14.5 kg
	Weight for height = $\frac{12}{14.5}$ = 82.7% weight for height

Conclusions: the girl has shown catch-up weight gain. Weight for height has increased from 71% to 83%. She has continued to grow in height, but has not had any catch-up height. Her height continues to be about 79% of that expected for her chronological age

Table 1.4 Classification of malnutrition.

Acute malnutrition (wasting)	Chronic malnutrition (stunting ± wasting)
Weight for height	Height for age
80%–90% standard – grade 1	90%–95% standard – grade 1
70%–80% standard – grade 2	85%–90% standard – grade 2
<70% standard – grade 3	<80% standard – grade 3

Source: Adapted from Waterlow [32].

Table 1.5 Physical signs of nutritional problems.

Assessment	Clinical sign	Possible nutrient(s)
Hair	Thin, sparse	Protein and energy, zinc, copper
	Colour change – 'flag sign'	
	Easily plucked	
Skin	Dry, flaky	Essential fatty acids B vitamins
	Rough, 'sandpaper' texture	Vitamin A
	Petechiae, bruising	Vitamin C
Eyes	Pale conjunctiva	Iron
	Xerosis	Vitamin A
	Keratomalacia	
Lips	Angular stomatitis Cheilosis	B vitamins
Tongue	Colour changes	B vitamins
Teeth	Mottling of enamel	Fluorosis (excess fluoride)
Gums	Spongy, bleed easily	Vitamin C
Face	Thyroid enlargement	Iodine
Nails	Spoon shape, koilonychia	Iron, zinc, copper
Subcutaneous tissue	Oedema Over-hydration	Protein, sodium
	Depleted subcutaneous fat	Energy
Muscles	Wasting	Protein, energy, zinc
Bones	Craniotabes Parietal and frontal bossing Epiphyseal enlargement Beading of ribs	Vitamin D

Typical physical signs associated with poor nutrition which have been described in children in western countries are summarised in Table 1.5. Physical signs represent very general changes and may not be due to nutrient deficiencies alone. Other indications such as poor weight gain and/or low dietary intake are needed in order to reinforce suspicions, and biochemical and haematological tests should be carried out to confirm the diagnosis. These include the analysis of levels of nutrients or nutrient dependent metabolites in body fluids or tissues, or measuring functional impairment of a nutrient dependent metabolic process. The most commonly used tissue for investigation is the blood. Whole blood, plasma, serum or blood cells can be used, depending on the test. Tests may be static, e.g. levels of zinc in plasma, or may be functional, e.g. the measurement of the activity of glutathione peroxidase, a selenium dependent enzyme, as a measure of selenium status.

Although an objective measurement is obtained from a blood test there are a number of factors that can affect the validity of such biochemical or haematological investigations:

- Age specific normal ranges need to be established for the individual centre unless the laboratory participates in a regional or national quality control scheme.
- Recent food intake and time of sampling can affect levels and it may be necessary to take a fasting blood sample for some nutrients.
- Physiological processes such as infection, disease or drugs may alter normal levels.
- Contamination from exogenous materials such as equipment or endogenous sources such as sweat or interstitial fluid is important for nutrients such as trace elements, and care must be taken to choose the correct sampling procedure.

A summary of some biochemical and haematological measurements is given in Table 1.6.

Urine is often used for adult investigations, but many tests require the collection of a 24 hour urine sample and this is difficult in babies and children. The usefulness of a single urine sample for nutritional tests is limited and needs to be compared with a standard metabolite, usually creatinine. However, creatinine excretion itself is age dependent and this needs to be taken into consideration. Stool samples can be useful in determining reasons for malabsorption if suspected. Hair and nails have been used to assess trace element and heavy metal status in populations, but a number of environmental and physiological factors affect levels and these tissues are not routinely used in the UK. Tissues that store certain nutrients, such as the liver and bone, also provide useful materials for investigation, but sampling is too invasive for routine clinical use.

A more detailed overview of clinical assessment can be found elsewhere [19].

Dietary intake

For children over the age of 2 years food intake is assessed in the same way as for adults: using a recall diet history; a quantitative food diary or food record chart at home or on the ward, recorded over a number of days; a weighed food intake over a number of days; or a food frequency questionnaire. These methods are not mutually exclusive and combinations are often used to provide the greatest depth of information. There are benefits and limitations to each of these methods and these are summarised in Table 1.7 [19, 33].

For most clinical purposes an oral history from the usual carers (or from the child if appropriate) will provide sufficient information on which to base recommendations. As well as assessing the range and quantity of foods eaten it is also useful to assess whether the texture and presentation of food is appropriate for the age and developmental level of the child. Estimation of food intake is particularly difficult in infants, as it is not possible to assess accurately the amount of food wasted through, for example, spitting or drooling. Similar difficulties occur in children with physical feeding difficulties and dysphagia. Observation of feeding can be particularly useful in these situations. Recorded intake can often be utilised at annual assessments of children with chronic conditions, in the identification of food related symptoms (allergies and intolerances), or in the assessment of diet related doses of medications such as pancreatic enzymes or insulin. A range of tools are available to assist with the assessment of dietary intake including pictorial portion size guides, computerised dietary analysis programmes and texture descriptors [34]. The adequacy of dietary intake is assessed in relation to the dietary reference values (DRV).

The assessment of milk intake for breast fed infants is difficult and only very general estimations can be made. Historically infants have been test weighed before and after a breast feed to allow the amount of milk consumed to be estimated. This required the use of very accurate scales ($\pm 1-2\,g$) and included all feeds over a 24 hour period as the volume consumed varied throughout the day. Test weighing should be avoided if at all possible as it is disturbing for the infant, engenders anxiety in the mother and is likely to compromise breast feeding. Studies have shown that the volume of breast milk

Table 1.6 Biochemical and haematological tests.

Nutrient	Test	Normal values in children	Comments
Biochemical tests			
Protein	Total plasma protein	55–80 g/L	Low levels reflect long term not acute depletion
	Albumin	30–45 g/L	
	Caeruloplasmin	0.18–0.46 g/L	Low levels indicate acute protein depletion, but are acute phase proteins which increase during infection
	Retinol binding protein	2.6–7.6 g/L	
Thiamin	Erythrocyte transketolase activity coefficient	1–1.15	High activity coefficient (>1.15) indicates thiamin deficiency
Vitamin B_{12}	Plasma B_{12} value	263–1336 pmol/L	Low levels indicate deficiency
Riboflavin	Erythrocyte glutathione reductase activity coefficient	1.0–1.3	High activity coefficient (>1.3) indicates riboflavin deficiency
Vitamin C	Plasma ascorbate level	8.8–124 µmol/L	Low levels indicate deficiency
Vitamin A	Plasma retinol level	0.54–1.56 µmol/L	Low level indicates deficiency
Vitamin D	Plasma 25-hydroxy-colecalciferol level	30–110 nmol/L	Low level indicates deficiency
Vitamin E	Plasma tocopherol level	α-tocopherol 10.9–28.1 µmol/L	Low levels indicate deficiency
Copper	Plasma level	70–140 µmol/L	Low levels indicate deficiency
Selenium	Plasma level	0.76–1.07 µmol/L	Low levels indicate deficiency
	Glutathione peroxidase activity	>1.77 µmol/L	Low levels indicate deficiency
Zinc	Plasma level	10–18 µmol/L	Low levels indicate deficiency
Haematology tests			
Folic acid	Plasma folate	7–48 nmol/L	Low levels indicate deficiency
	Red cell folate	429–1749 nmol/L	Low levels indicate deficiency
Haemoglobin	Whole blood	104–140 g/L	Levels <110 g/L indicate iron deficiency
Red cell distribution width	Whole blood	<16%	High values indicate iron deficiency
Mean corpuscular volume	Whole blood	70–86 fL	Small volume (microcytosis) indicates iron deficiency. Large volume (macrocytosis) indicates folate or B_{12} deficiency
Mean cell haemoglobin	Whole blood	22.7–29.6 pg	Low values indicate iron deficiency
Percentage hypochromic cells	Whole blood	<2.5%	High values (>2.5%) indicate iron deficiency
Zinc protoporphyrin	Red cell	32–102 µmol/mol haem	High levels indicate iron deficiency
Ferritin	Plasma level	5–70 µg/L	Low levels indicate depletion of iron stores. Ferritin is an acute phase protein and increases during infection

Table 1.7 Strengths and limitations of dietary assessment methodologies for individuals.

Method	Strength	Limitation
24 hour recall	Quick and easy Low respondent burden	Relies on memory May not be representative of usual intake
Estimated food diary	Assesses actual usual intake	Respondents must be literate Ability to estimate portion size Longer time-frames increase respondent burden
Weighed food diary	Accurate assessment of actual intake	High respondent burden Respondents must be literate and motivated Setting may not be conducive to weighing (e.g. eating out)
Food frequency questionnaire	Quick Low respondent burden Can identify food consumption patterns: high/ medium/low	Ability to quantify intakes poor

Source: Gibson [19].

Table 1.8 Average weight gain throughout the first year of life.

	Boys (g/week)	**Girls** (g/week)
First 3 months	240	210
Second 3 months	130	120
Third 3 months	80	75
Fourth 3 months	65	60

consumed is approximately 770 mL at 5 weeks and 870 mL at 11 weeks [35]. In general an intake of 850 mL is assumed for infants who are fully breast fed and over the age of 6 weeks. Estimation of nutritional intake in a breast fed infant is further complicated by the varying composition of breast milk [36].

Expected growth in childhood

The 50th centile birth weight for infants in the UK is 3.5 kg for boys and 3.3 kg for girls [37]. Most babies lose weight after birth whilst feeding on full volumes of milk is gradually established. They begin to gain weight between 3 and 5 days of age, with the majority regaining their birth weight by the 10th–14th day of life. The National Institute for Health and Care Excellence (NICE) recommends

that babies are weighed at birth and in the first week of life as part of the overall assessment of their feeding. Thereafter babies should be weighed at 8, 12 and 16 weeks and again at 1 year of age [38].

The average weight gain during the first year of life, using the 50th centile for age of the UK-WHO growth charts [27], is shown in Table 1.8. The increase in length during the first year of life is 24–25 cm. During the second year, the toddler following the 50th centile gains 2.5–2.6 kg in weight and a further 11–12 cm in length. Average weight gain continues at a rate of approximately 2–3 kg per year. Height gain in the second year is 10 cm, steadily declining to 7 cm down to 5 cm per year until the growth spurt at puberty. Puberty in boys usually starts between the ages of 9 and 14 years. Onset of puberty before 9 years of age is considered precocious whilst puberty is delayed if there are no signs by 14 years. For girls, puberty usually begins between 8 and 13 years, with the onset of puberty before 8 years considered to be precocious and puberty not present by 13 years considered to be delayed.

Dietary reference values

The 1991 Department of Health Report on Dietary Reference Values [39] provides information and figures for requirements for a comprehensive range of nutrients and energy. The requirements are termed dietary reference values (DRV) and are for normal healthy populations of infants fed artificial formulas, and for older infants, children and adults consuming food. DRV were not set for breast fed babies as it was considered that human milk provides the necessary amounts of nutrients when fed on demand. In some cases the DRV for infants aged up to 3 months who are formula fed are in excess of those which would be expected to derive from breast milk; this is because of the different bioavailability of some nutrients from breast and artificial formulas.

Table 1.9 Selected dietary reference values, 1991.

	Weight*		Energy (EAR) per day			RNI per day								
						Protein		Sodium		Potassium		Vitamin C	Calcium	Iron
Age	kg	MJ	kJ/kg	kcal	kcal/kg	g	g/kg	mmol	mmol/kg	mmol	mmol/kg	mg	mmol	mg
Males														
0–3 months	5.9	2.28	480–420	545	115–100	12.5	2.1	9	1.5	20	3.4	25	13.1	1.7
4–6	7.7	2.89	400	690	95	12.7	1.6	12	1.6	22	2.8	25	13.1	4.3
7–9	8.9	3.44	400	825	95	13.7	1.5	14	1.6	18	2.0	25	13.1	7.8
10–12	9.8	3.85	400	920	95	14.9	1.5	15	1.5	18	1.8	25	13.1	7.8
1–3 years	12.6	5.15	400	1230	95	14.5	1.1	22	1.7	20	1.6	30	8.8	6.9
4–6	17.8	7.16	380	1715	90	19.7	1.1	30	1.7	28	1.6	30	11.3	6.1
7–10	28.3	8.24	–	1970	–	28.3	–	50	–	50	–	30	13.8	8.7
11–14	43.1	9.27	–	2220	–	42.1	–	70	–	80	–	35	25.0	11.3
15–18	64.5	11.51	–	2755	–	55.2	–	70	–	90	–	40	25.0	11.3
Females														
0–3 months	5.9	2.16	480–420	515	115–100	12.5	2.1	9	1.5	20	3.4	25	13.1	1.7
4–6	7.7	2.69	400	645	95	12.7	1.6	12	1.6	22	2.8	25	13.1	4.3
7–9	8.9	3.20	400	765	95	13.7	1.5	14	1.6	18	2.0	25	13.1	7.8
10–12	9.8	3.61	400	865	95	14.9	1.5	15	1.5	18	1.8	25	13.1	7.8
1–3 years	12.6	4.86	400	1165	95	14.5	1.1	22	1.7	20	1.6	30	8.8	6.9
4–6	17.8	6.46	380	1545	90	19.7	1.1	30	1.7	28	1.6	30	11.3	6.1
7–10	28.3	7.28	–	1740	–	28.3	–	50	–	50	–	30	13.8	8.7
11–14	43.8	7.92	–	1845	–	42.1	–	70	–	80	–	35	20.0	14.8
15–18	55.5	8.83	–	2110	–	45.4	–	70	–	90	–	40	20.0	14.8

EAR, estimated average requirement; RNI, reference nutrient intake.
*Standard weights for age ranges [39].
Source: Department of Health [39]. Reprinted with permission of The Stationery Office.

It is important to remember that these are recommendations for groups, not for individuals; however, they can be used as a basis for estimating suitable intakes for the individual, using the reference nutrient intake (RNI). This level of intake should satisfy the requirements of 97.5% of healthy individuals in a population group. A summary of the 1991 DRV for energy, protein, sodium, potassium, vitamin C, calcium and iron is given in Table 1.9. The DRV for other nutrients may be found in the full report.

The Scientific Advisory Committee on Nutrition (SACN) revised the DRV for energy in 2011 [40] in the light of advancements in the methodology to measure total energy expenditure. This report gives a detailed account of the evidence that SACN used when updating the estimated average requirements (EAR) for energy for infants, children, adolescents and adults in the UK. This has coincided with other revisions of energy requirements by the Food and Agriculture Organization of the United Nations,

World Health Organization and United Nations University (FAO/WHO/UNU) and the Institute of Medicine (IoM) in the USA.

The new EAR for energy have decreased for infants and children under 10 years of age and slightly increased for older children and adults. The new EAR for energy for infants and children are shown in Tables 1.10 and 1.11.

It must be emphasised that these values are for assessing the energy requirements of large groups of people and are not requirements for healthy or sick individuals. Also, when estimating requirements for the individual sick child it is important to calculate energy and nutrient intakes based on actual body weight and not expected body weight. The latter will lead to a proposed intake that is inappropriately high for the child who has an abnormally low body weight. In some instances it may be more appropriate to consider the child's height age rather than chronological age when comparing intakes with the DRV as this is a more

Table 1.10 Estimated average requirements for energy for infants, 2011.

Age (months)	Breast fed kcal (MJ) per kg/day	Breast fed kcal (MJ) per day	Breast milk substitute fed kcal (MJ) per kg/day	Breast milk substitute fed kcal (MJ) per day	Mixed feeding or unknown kcal (MJ) per kg/day	Mixed feeding or unknown kcal (MJ) per day
Boys						
1-2	96 (0.4)	526 (2.2)	120(0.5)	598 (2.5)	120 (0.5)	574 (2.4)
3-4	96 (0.4)	574 (2.4)	96 (0.4)	622 (2.6)	96 (0.4)	598 (2.5)
5-6	72 (0.3)	598 (2.5)	96 (0.4)	646 (2.7)	72 (0.3)	622 (2.6)
7-12	72 (0.3)	694 (2.9)	72 (0.3)	742 (3.1)	72 (0.3)	718 (3.0)
Girls						
1-2	96 (0.4)	478	120 (0.5)	550 (2.3)	120 (0.5)	502 (2.1)
3-4	96 (0.4)	526	96 (0.4)	598 (2.5)	96 (0.40)	550 (2.3)
5-6	72 (0.3)	550	96 (0.4)	622 (2.6)	72 (0.3)	574 (2.4)
7-12	72 (0.3)	646	72 (0.3)	670 (2.8)	72 (0.3)	646 (2.7)

Source: Scientific Advisory Committee on Nutrition [40].

Table 1.11 Estimated average requirement (EAR) for energy for children.

Age (years)	EAR (kcal (MJ) per day)* Boy	EAR (kcal (MJ) per day)* Girls
1	765 (3.2)	717 (3.0)
2	1004 (4.2)	932 (3.9)
3	1171 (4.9)	1076 (4.5)
4	1386 (5.8)	1291 (5.4)
5	1482 (6.2)	1362 (5.7)
6	1577 (6.6)	1482 (6.2)
7	1649 (6.9)	1530 (6.4)
8	1745 (7.3)	1625 (6.8)
9	1840 (7.7)	1721 (7.2)
10	2032 (8.5)	1936 (8.1)
11	2127 (8.9)	2023 (8.5)
12	2247 (9.4)	2103 (8.8)
13	2414 (10.1)	2223 (9.3)
14	2629 (11.0)	2342 (9.8)
15	2820 (11.8)	2390 (10.0)
16	2964 (12.4)	2414 (10.1)
17	3083 (12.9)	2462 (10.3)
18	3155 (13.2)	2462 (10.3)

*Calculated with the median physical activity ratio.
Source: Scientific Advisory Committee on Nutrition [40].

realistic measure of the child's body size and hence nutrient requirement.

In order to make the new EAR for energy more usable in clinical practice, it is suggested that the data given in Tables 1.10 and 1.11 are condensed and summarised (Table 1.12).

The estimated requirements for children with specific disorders are given in the relevant chapters. It is important to remember that requirements are not necessarily increased during illness. Factors to consider when estimating requirements for the individual are: nutritional status prior to onset of the disease; whether the disorder is acute or chronic; is mobility affected; are there any impacts on normal feeding such as dysphagia or reduced appetite; are there increased gastrointestinal losses such as vomiting, diarrhoea; consider any urinary losses; is there an inability to metabolise dietary constituents.

A guide to increased oral and enteral (feeding by tube into the gut) requirements is given in Table 1.13.

Fluid requirements

Preterm and low birthweight infants

Chapter 6 gives a full account of the special requirements of these babies.

The newborn infant over 2.5 kg birthweight

Breast feeding is the most appropriate method of feeding the normal infant and may be suitable for sick infants with a variety of clinical conditions. Demand breast feeding will automatically ensure that the healthy infant gets the right volume of milk and, hence, nutrients. The suck–swallow–breathe sequence that allows the newborn infant to feed orally is usually well developed by 35–37 weeks of gestation. If the infant is too ill or too immature to suckle the mother may express her breast milk;

Table 1.12   Guide to energy requirements in clinical practice.

	Boys			Girls		
Age	Energy (EAR) (kcal/day)	Weight[†]	Energy (EAR)* (kcal/kg/day)	Energy (EAR) (kcal/day)	Weight[†]	Energy (EAR)* (kcal/kg/day)
1–2 months		5.0	96–120		4.7	96–120
3–4		6.7	96		6.1	96
5–6		7.7	72–96		7.0	72–96
7–12		9.0	72		8.3	72
1 years	770	9.6	80	720	9.0	80
2	1000	12.2	82	930	11.5	81
3	1170	14.4	82	1080	13.9	78
4	1390	16.3	85	1290	16.0	81
5	1480	18.6	80	1360	18.2	75
6	1560	21.0	74	1480	21.0	70
7	1650	23.0	71	1530	23.0	67
8	1750	26.0	67	1630	26.0	63
9	1840	29.0	63	1720	29.0	59
10	2030	31.5	64	1940	32.0	61
11	2130	34.5	62	2020	35.9	56
12	2250	38.0	59	2100	40.0	53
13	2410	43.0	56	2220	46.0	48
14	2630	49.0	54	2340	51.0	46
15	2820	55.5	51	2390	53.0	45
16	2970	60.2	49	2410	55.3	44
17	3080	64.0	48	2460	57.0	43
18	3160	66.2	48	2460	57.2	43

1 kcal = 4.18 kJ.
*Depending on method of feeding for infants (see Table 1.10).
[†]Median weight from the UK-WHO growth charts ages 1–4 years [27] and the UK 1990 reference for children aged >4 years [37].

Table 1.13   Guide to increased oral and enteral requirements.

	Infants 0–1 year*	Children
Energy	High: 130–150 kcal (545–630 kJ)/kg/day Very high: 150–180 kcal (630–750 kJ)/kg/day	High: 120% EAR[†] Very high: 150% EAR
Protein	High: 3–4.5 g/kg/day Very high: 6 g/kg/day Very high: 6 g/kg/day	High: 2 g/kg/day* It should be recognised that children may easily eat more than this amount
Sodium	High: 3.0 mmol/kg/day Very high: 4.5 mmol/kg/day A concentration >7.7 mmol Na$^+$/100 mL of infant formula will have an emetic effect	
Potassium	High: 3.0 mmol/kg/day Very high: 4.5 mmol/kg/day	

*Based on actual weight, not expected weight.
[†]May be better to base on height age rather than chronological age in very small children.

Table 1.14 Infant milk formulas and follow-on milks.

Whey based infant formula	Casein based infant formula	Follow-on milks*
Aptamil First Infant Milk	Aptamil Hungry Milk	Aptamil Follow On Milk (Milupa)
Babynat 1	–	Babynat 2 (Vitagermine)
Cow & Gate First Infant Infant Milk	Cow & Gate Infant Milk for Hungrier Babies	Cow & Gate 3 (Cow & Gate)
Hipp First	Hipp Hungry Infant	Hipp Follow on (Hipp UK)
SMA First Infant Milk	SMA Extra Hungry Infant Milk	SMA Follow-on Milk (SMA Nutrition)

*Suitable from 6 months.

expressed breast milk (EBM) may be modified to suit the sick infant's requirements. If EBM is unavailable or inappropriate to feed in certain circumstances (see Chapter 3 Infants under 12 months), infant milk formulas must be used (Table 1.14).

A systematic review of the volumes of breast milk and infant formula taken in early infancy [41] has revealed that formula fed infants have a higher intake than breast fed babies (Table 1.15). Whilst there was variation in the amount of breast milk taken in the first few days of life, on average demand breast fed babies took only 21.5 ± 4.2 mL on day 1, whereas formula fed babies took 170 ± 55.8 mL on day 1. By day 14, the bottle fed babies were still taking a greater volume: 761.8 ± 18 mL vs. 673.6 ± 29 mL in the breast fed babies. Not only did the bottle fed babies take a larger volume, they also had a more energy dense milk: 67 kcal/100 mL vs. 53.6 ± 2.5 kcal/100 mL for colostrum (days 1–5) and 57.7 ± 4.2 kcal/100 mL for transitional milk (days 6–14).

Most babies will need 150–180 mL/kg/day of infant formula until they are 6 months old, although this will vary for the individual baby [42]. Bottle fed babies should be allowed to feed on demand and not be encouraged to 'finish the bottle'. A suggested way to feed these babies is to offer on the first day approximately one seventh of requirements, say 20 mL/kg, divided into eight feeds and fed every 2–3 hours. The volume offered should be gradually increased over the following days to

Table 1.15 Volume of milk taken in the first 2 weeks of life.

Day of life	Breast milk (mL)	Infant formula (mL)
1	21.5 ± 4.2	170.5 ± 55.8
2		265.0 ± 67.7
7	495.3 ± 33.4	
14	673.6 ± 29	761.8 ± 18

Source: Hester et al. [41].

appetite so that newborn babies gradually increase their intake from about 20 mL/kg on the first day of life to around 150 mL/kg by 7–14 days. Breast fed infants will regulate their own intake of milk.

Fluid requirements after the first few weeks

Healthy formula fed infants should be allowed to feed on demand, although parents often wish to get them into a 'routine'. Many infants will take their feeds four hourly, five to six bottles per day at around 4–6 weeks of age, although many will continue to demand feeds more frequently. The infant may start to sleep longer through the night and drop a feed. A fluid intake of around 150 mL/kg should be maintained to provide adequate fluids, energy and nutrients. Infants should not normally be given more than 1200 mL of feed per 24 hours as this may induce vomiting and, in the long term, will lead to an inappropriately high energy intake. Sick infants may need smaller, more frequent feeds than the normal baby and, according to their clinical condition, may have increased or decreased fluid requirements. Breast fed infants will continue to regulate their own intake of milk and feeding pattern.

After the age of 6 months a follow-on milk may be used (Table 1.14). These milks are higher in protein, iron and some other minerals and vitamins than formulas designed to be given from birth and may be useful for infants with a poor intake of solids or who are fluid restricted.

Fluid requirements in older infants and children

Once solids are introduced around the age of 6 months of age the infant's appetite for milk will lessen. Breast milk and infant formulas fed at 150 mL/kg provide 130 mL water/kg. The fluid requirements for older infants aged 7–12 months

Table 1.16 Water content of foods.

Food	Percentage water content
Fruits and vegetables	80–85
Yoghurt and milk puddings	70–80
Rice and pasta	65–80
Fish	70–80
Eggs	65–80
Meat	45–65
Cheese	40–50
Bread	30–45

Source: Grandjean and Campbell [43].

Table 1.17 Daily water requirements for infants and children.

Age	EFSA 2010* [44] Dietary reference values	IoM 2005† [45] Dietary reference intakes
0–6 months	100–190 mL/kg	700 mL
6–12	800–1000 mL	800 mL
12–24	1100–1200 mL	
1–3 years		1300 mL (900 mL from drinks)
2–3	1300 mL	
4–8	1600 mL	1700 mL (1200 mL from drinks)
9–13 (boys)	2100 mL	2400 mL (1800 mL from drinks)
9–13 (girls)	1900 mL	2100 mL (1600 mL from drinks)
14–18 (boys)	2500 mL (adult)	3300 mL
14–18 (girls)	2000 mL (adult)	2300 mL

*Includes water from beverages and food.
†Includes water from beverages, food and drinking water.

decrease to 120 mL/kg, assuming that some water is obtained from solid foods (Table 1.16). At 1 year, the healthy child's thirst will largely determine how much fluid is taken. There are some published fluid requirements for healthy populations (Table 1.17). These are all based on observations of water intakes and urine osmolality, not hydration status.

If all a child's nutrition comes from feed and there is no significant contribution to fluid intake from foods, then fluid requirements may be estimated using an adaptation of the Holliday–Segar formula [46]. This formula was originally designed to calculate fluid requirements for parenteral nutrition and is based on the child's weight, using an average requirement of 100 mL water for each

100 kcal (420 kJ) of energy metabolised. If less energy is required, then less water will be needed. If nutritional requirements are met from a smaller volume of feed, then any extra fluid needed (e.g. if the child is losing more than usual fluid though breathing, sweating, vomiting, diarrhoea, passing dilute urine) may simply be given as water.

Body weight	Estimated fluid requirement
11–20 kg	100 mL/kg for the first 10 kg + 50 mL/kg for the next 10 kg
>20 kg	100 mL/kg for the first 10 kg + 50 mL/kg for the next 10 kg + 25 mL/kg thereafter

Worked example for a child weighing 22 kg

100 mL/kg for the first 10 kg	= 1000 mL
+ 50 mL/kg for the next 10 kg	= 500 mL
+ 25 mL/kg for the final 2 kg	= 50 mL
Total	= 1550 mL
	= 70 mL/kg

Overweight children will need less fluid than the calculated volume as their actual body weight is higher than normal. It would be reasonable to estimate their weight for these calculations as the value on the centile that matches their height centile, e.g.

- 7 year old boy weight with a weight of 35 kg = 99.6th centile: fluid requirements using above formula 1875 mL
- He is 122 cm tall = 50th centile
- Base fluid requirements initially on a body weight of 23 kg = 50th centile, using above formula is 1575 mL
- Monitor fluid status and adjust accordingly. More water may be required, but not necessarily more feed.

For underweight children it is important to calculate their fluid requirement based on their actual weight, not their expected weight for age or height, but as this is lower than normal they will need increased energy and protein density in their feed to achieve catch-up growth.

Supplementing feeds for infants with faltering growth or who are fluid restricted

Supplements may be used to fortify standard infant formulas and special therapeutic formulas to achieve the necessary increase in energy, protein and other nutrients required by some infants. Expressed breast milk can also be fortified using a standard infant formula powder in term babies (Table 1.18) or a breast milk fortifier in preterm infants (p. 92). Care needs to be taken not to present an osmotic load of more than 500 mOsm/kg H_2O to the normal functioning gut; otherwise an osmotic diarrhoea will result. If the infant has malabsorption, an upper limit of 400 mOsm/kg H_2O may be necessary. Infants who are fluid restricted will need to meet their nutritional requirements in a lower volume of feed than usual and the following feed manipulations can be used for these babies.

Concentrating infant formulas

Normally infant formula powders, whether whey and casein based formulas or specialised dietetic products, should be diluted according to the manufacturers' instructions as this provides the correct balance of energy, protein and nutrients when fed at the appropriate volume. However, there are occasions when, to achieve a feed that is denser in energy, protein and other nutrients, it is necessary to concentrate the formula. Most normal baby milks in the UK are made up at a dilution of around 13%. By making the baby milk up at a dilution of 15% (15 g powder per 100 mL water), more nutrition can be given in a given volume of feed, e.g. energy content may be increased from 67 kcal (280 kJ) per 100 mL to 77 kcal (325 kJ) per 100 mL and protein content from 1.3 g/100 mL to 1.5 g/100 mL. Similarly special therapeutic formulas that are usually made up at a dilution of, say, 15% may be concentrated to a 17% dilution. This concentrating of feeds should only be performed as a therapeutic procedure and is not usual practice. The consequence of concentrating feeds is to increase the osmolality. Steele et al. have shown a linear relationship between feed concentration and osmolality so that the osmolality of a concentrated feed can be reliably calculated from the manufacturer's data for normal dilution rather than necessitating the feed to be measured by osmometry in the laboratory [47]. Table 1.18 shows an example of a 15% feed and a 17% feed.

The protein:energy (P:E) ratio of the feed should ideally be kept within the range 7.5%–12% for

Table 1.18 Examples of energy and nutrient dense formulas for infants (per 100 mL).

	Energy kcal	kJ	Protein g	CHO g	Fat g	Na mmol	K mmol	Osmolality mOsm/kg H_2O	P:E ratio
12.7% SMA 1	67	280	1.3	7.3	3.6	0.7	1.7	300	7.6
15% SMA 1	79	330	1.5	8.6	4.3	0.8	2.0	354*	7.6
EBM[†] + 3% SMA 1	85	355	1.6	8.9	4.9	0.8	1.9	–	7.5
17% SMA 1	90	375	1.7	9.8	4.8	0.9	2.3	402*	7.6
SMA High Energy (SMA Nutrition)	91	380	2.0	9.8	4.9	1.0	2.3	387	8.8
Infatrini (Nutricia)	100	420	2.6	10.3	5.4	1.1	2.4	345	10.4
Similac High Energy (Abbott)	100	420	2.6	10.1	5.4	1.1	2.3	333	10.4
17% SMA 1 + Maxijul to 12% CHO + Calogen to 5% fat	100	420	1.7	12.0	5.0	0.9	2.3	–	6.8

P:E, protein:energy. EBM, expressed breast milk.
The Scientific Advisory Committee on Nutrition used an energy density for breast milk of 0.67 kcal/g (2.8 kJ/g) rather than 0.69 kcal/g (2.9 kJ/g) in the revised *Dietary Reference Values for Energy*, 2011 [40].
*Calculated value.
[†]Holland B, Welch AA, Unwin ID et al. *McCance & Widdowson's The Composition of Foods*, 5th edn. Royal Society of Chemistry and Ministry of Agriculture, Fisheries and Food, Cambridge 1991.

infants (i.e. 7.5%–12% energy from protein) and 5%–15% in older children. For accelerated weight gain or catch-up growth [48]:

- weight gain of 10 g/kg/day requires 126 kcal (530 kJ)/kg/day, 2.8 g prot/kg/day, 8.9% P:E
- weight gain of 20 g/kg/day requires 167 kcal (700 kJ)/kg/day, 4.8 g prot/kg/day, 11.5% P:E
- optimal P:E for catch-up height is not determined but is likely to be 11%–12%

In some clinical situations it is not possible to preserve this protein:energy ratio as carbohydrate and fat sources alone may be added to a feed to control deranged blood biochemistry, for example. In these situations it is important to ensure that the infant is receiving at least the RNI for protein.

If infants are to be discharged home on a concentrated feed the recipe may be translated into scoop measures for ease of use. This will mean that more scoops of milk powder will be added to a given volume of water than recommended by the manufacturer. As this is contrary to normal practice the reasons for this deviation should be carefully explained to the parents and communicated to primary healthcare staff.

Nutrient dense ready to feed formulas

Nutrient dense ready to feed formulas are available for hospital use and in the community (Table 1.18). They are nutritionally complete formulas containing more energy, protein and nutrients per 100 mL than standard infant formulas. They are suitable for use from birth and are designed for infants who have increased nutritional requirements or who are fluid restricted. They obviate the need for carers to make up normal infant formulas at concentrations other than the usual one scoop of powder to 30 mL water.

Energy and protein modules

There may be therapeutic circumstances when energy and/or protein supplements need to be added to normal infant formulas or special formulas without necessarily the need to increase the concentration of the base feed. Sometimes a ready to feed formula does not meet the needs of the individual child. Energy and protein modules and their use are described.

Carbohydrate

Carbohydrate provides 4 kcal/g (16 kJ/g). It is preferable to add carbohydrate to a feed in the form of glucose polymer, rather than using monosaccharides or disaccharides, because it exerts a lesser osmotic effect on the gut. Hence, a larger amount can be used per given volume of feed (Table 1.19). Glucose polymers should be added in 1% increments each 24 hours, i.e. 1 g per 100 mL feed per 24 hours. This will allow the concentration at which the infant becomes intolerant (i.e. has loose stools) of the extra carbohydrate to be identified. Tolerance depends on the age of the infant and the maturity and absorptive capacity of the gut. The addition of 2% (2 g per 100 mL) glucose polymer (Super Soluble Maxijul) to infant formulas has been shown to increase the feed osmolality by 31.2 mOsm/kg H_2O [47].

As a guideline the following percentage concentrations of carbohydrate (g total carbohydrate per 100 mL feed) may be tolerated if glucose polymer is introduced slowly:

- 10%–12% carbohydrate concentration in infants under 6 months (i.e. 7 g from formula, 3–5 g added)
- 12%–15% in infants aged 6 months to 1 year
- 15%–20% in toddlers aged 1–2 years
- 20%–30% in older children

If glucose or fructose needs to be added to a feed where there is an intolerance of glucose polymer, an upper limit of tolerance may be reached at a total carbohydrate concentration of 7%–8% in infants and young children.

Fat

Fat provides 9 kcal/g (37 kJ/g). Long chain fat emulsions are favoured over medium chain fat emulsions because they have a lower osmotic effect on the gut and provide a source of essential fatty acids. Medium chain fats are used where there is malabsorption of long chain fat (Table 1.19).

Table 1.19   Energy modules.

Per 100 g	Ingredients*	Energy kcal*	kJ	Na mmol	K mmol	PO$_4$ mmol
Glucose polymers						
Caloreen (Nestle)	Maltodextrin	385	1610	<1.8	<0.3	0
Super Soluble Maxijul (SHS)	Dried glucose syrup	380	1590	0.4	0.04	0.05
Polycal (Nutricia)	Maltodextrin	384	1605	0.1	Trace	0
Vitajoule (Vitaflo)	Dried glucose syrup	380	1590	<0.7	<0.1	0
Fat emulsions						
Calogen[†] (Nutricia)	Canola oil, sunflower oil	450	1880	0.5	0	
Liquigen (Nutricia)	Coconut oil	450	1880	0.65	0	
Combined fat and carbohydrate supplements						
Super Soluble Duocal (Nutricia)	Glucose syrup, canola oil, coconut oil, safflower oil	492	2055	<0.9	<0.1	
MCT Duocal (Nutricia)	Cornstarch, coconut oil, walnut oil, canola oil, palm oil	497	2075	<1.3	<0.5	

*As quoted by manufacturers.
[†]Unflavoured.

Fat emulsions should be added to feeds in 1% increments each 24 hours, so providing an increase of 0.5 g fat per 100 mL per 24 hours. Infants will tolerate a total fat concentration of 5%–6% (i.e. 5–6 g fat per 100 mL feed) if the gut is functioning normally. The addition of 2% long chain fat emulsion (Calogen) to infant formulas has been shown to increase the feed osmolality by only 0.7 mOsm/kg H$_2$O [47]. Children over 1 year of age will tolerate more fat, although concentrations above 7% may induce a feeling of nausea and cause vomiting. Medium chain fat will not be tolerated at such high concentrations and may be the cause of abdominal cramps and osmotic diarrhoea if they are not introduced slowly to the feed.

There are combined carbohydrate and fat supplements using both long and medium chain fats (Table 1.19). Again these must be introduced to feeds in 1% increments to determine the child's tolerance of the product. The addition of 2% of a long chain fat and glucose polymer powder (Super Soluble Duocal) to infant formulas has been shown to increase the feed osmolality by 23.0 mOsm/kg H$_2$O [47].

A schedule for the addition of energy supplements to infant formulas is given in Table 1.20.

Table 1.20   Schedule for the addition of energy supplements to infant formulas.

Day	Energy source added	Additional CHO/fat per 100 mL feed	Energy added per 100 mL (kcal)	(kJ)
1	1% glucose polymer	1 g CHO	4	17
2	2% glucose polymer	2 g CHO	8	33
3	3% glucose polymer	3 g CHO	12	50
4	3% glucose polymer + 1% fat emulsion	3 g CHO 0.5 g fat	17	69
5	3% glucose polymer + 2% fat emulsion	3 g CHO 1 g fat	21	88
6	4% glucose polymer + 2% fat emulsion	4 g CHO 1 g fat	25	105
7	5% glucose polymer + 2% fat emulsion	5 g CHO 1 g fat	29	121
8	5% glucose polymer + 3% fat emulsion	5 g CHO 1.5 g fat	34	140

Table 1.21   Protein modules.

Per 100 g	Type of protein	Energy kcal	kJ	Protein g	CHO g	Fat g	Na mmol	K mmol	Ca mmol	PO$_4$ mmol
Vitapro (Vitaflo)	Whole whey protein	390	1630	75	9.0	6.0	9.6	17.1	9.0	9.2
ProMod (Abbott)	Whole whey protein	426	1780	76	10.2	9.1	16.5	17.5	28.5	18.1
Protifar (Nutricia)	Whole milk protein	380	1590	89	<1.5	2.0	4.3	3.1	33.8	22.6
Pepdite Module 0767 peptides from hydrolysed meat and soya (SHS)		346	1469	86.4	–	–	–	–		
Complete Amino Acid Mix Code 0124 L-amino acids (SHS)		328	1394	82	–	–	–	–		

Table 1.22   Vitamin supplements.

		Healthy Start Children's Vitamin Drops (NHS)	Abidec (Chefaro UK)	Dalivit (LPC)	Ketovite (Paines & Byrne)
		5 drops for all infants from 6 months of age[†]	0.3 mL < 1 year 0.6 mL > 1 year*	0.3 mL < 1 year 0.6 mL > 1 year*	5 mL liquid[+] 3 tablets
Thiamin (B$_1$)	mg	–	0.4	1	3.0
Riboflavin (B$_2$)	mg	–	0.8	0.4	3.0
Pyridoxine (B$_6$)	mg	–	–	0.5	1.0
Nicotinamide	mg	–	8	5	9.9
Pantothenate	mg	–	–	–	3.5
Ascorbic acid (C)	mg	20	40	50	50
Alpha-tocopherol (E)	mg	–	–	–	15
Inositol	mg	–	–	–	150
Biotin	µg	–	–	–	510
Folic acid	µg	–	–	–	750
Acetomenaphthone (K)	mg	–	–	–	1.5
Vitamin A	µg	200	400	1500	750
Vitamin D	µg	7.5	10	10	10
Choline chloride	mg	–	–	–	150
Cyanocobalamin (B$_{12}$)	µg	–	–	–	12.5

*Values relate to 0.6 mL dose.
[†]Unless taking >500 mL infant formula or follow-on milk (see Chapter 27 Vitamin supplements).

Protein

Protein may be added to feeds in the form of whole protein, peptides or amino acids (Table 1.21). Protein supplementation is rarely required without an accompanying increase in energy consumption.

Protein supplements are added to feeds to provide a specific amount of protein per kilogram actual body weight of the child. It is rarely necessary to give intakes >6 g protein/kg; if intakes do approach this value, blood urea levels should be monitored twice weekly to avoid the danger of uraemia developing. Supplements should be added in small increments as they can very quickly and inappropriately increase the child's intake of protein. The osmotic effect of whole protein products will be less than that of peptides, and peptides less than the effect of amino acids.

Vitamin and mineral requirements

Vitamin and mineral requirements for populations of normal children are provided by the DRV [39]. Where no RNI is set, safe levels are given. Some are shown in Table 1.9. In disease states, requirements

Table 1.23   Vitamin and mineral supplements, daily dose.

		Paediatric Seravit Unflavoured powder (SHS)	Forceval Junior Capsule (Alliance)	Forceval Tablet (Alliance)	Fruitivits Soluble Orange flavoured powder (Vitaflo)	Phlexy-Vits Powder and tablet (SHS)
		17 g 6–12 months 17–25 g* 1–7 years	1 capsule >12 years	1 tablet >6 years	6 g 3–10 year	7 g/5 tablets >11 year
Energy	kcal (kJ)	75 (315)	0	9 (38)	2 (8)	0.2[†] (1.4[‡])
CHO	g	18.8	0	0.86	0.5	0.04[†] (0.01[‡])
Protein	g	0	0	0	0.02**	0
Fat	g	0	0	0	0	0.14[‡]
Sodium	mg	<5	0	250	0	8.8[†]
Potassium	mg	<0.8	4	98	0	<1.4[†]
Calcium	mg	640	100	0	800	1000
Phosphorus	mg	430	77	0	500	775
Magnesium	mg	90	30	1	200	300
Iron	mg	17.3	12	5	10	15.1
Zinc	mg	11.5	15	5	10	11.1
Copper	mg	1.2	2	1	1	1.5
Iodine	µg	83	140	75	169	150
Manganese	mg	1.2	3	1.3	1.5	1.5
Molybdenum	µg	88	250	50	68	70
Selenium	µg	34	50	25	41	75
Chromium	µg	34	200	50	41	30
Vitamin A	µg	1050	750	375	500	800
Vitamin D	µg	14	10	5	10	10
Vitamin E	mg	3.7	10	5	9.3	9
Vitamin K	µg	41.5	0	25	60	70
Vitamin C	mg	5.4	60	25	40	50
Thiamin	mg	0.8	1.2	1.5	1.2	1.2
Riboflavin	mg	1.1	1.6	1	1.4	1.4
Niacin	mg	8.8	18	7.5	15	20
Pyridoxine	mg	0.9	2	1	1.7	1.6
Pantothenic acid	mg	4.3	4	2	4.7	5
Vitamin B_{12}	µg	2.2	3	2	2.8	5
Folate	µg	76	400	100	240	700
Biotin	µg	54	100	50	112	150
Inositol	mg	175	0	0	0	0
Choline	mg	87.5	0	0	250	0

*25 g dose.
[†]7 g sachet dose only.
[‡]5 tablet dose only.

for certain vitamins and minerals will be different and are fully described in the dietary management of each clinical condition. The prescribable vitamin and mineral supplements that are most often used in paediatric practice are given in Tables 1.22 and 1.23.

Prescribing products for paediatric use

The majority of specialised formulas, supplements and special dietary foods can be prescribed for specific conditions. The Advisory Committee on Borderline Substances recommends suitable products that can be prescribed for use in the community and defines their indications. Prescriptions from the general practitioner (FP10; GP10 in Scotland) should be marked 'ACBS' to indicate that the prescription complies with recommendations. A list of prescribable items for paediatric use appears in the *BNF (British National Formulary) for Children* under the Borderline Substances Appendix and is also available on line at www.bnf.org. Children under the age of 16 years in the UK are exempt from prescription charges.

Useful links and further reading

Infant and Toddler Forum, Open Book on Growth
https://www.infantandtoddlerforum.org/open-book-on-growth

Royal College of Paediatrics and Child Health, UK-WHO Growth Charts
http://www.rcpch.ac.uk/child-health/research-projects/uk-who-growth-charts/uk-who-growth-charts

Health for all children, Growth charts
http://www.healthforallchildren.com/index.php/shop/category-list/Growth+Charts/0

Gibson RS *Principles of Nutritional Assessment*. Oxford: Oxford University Press, 2005.

Hall DMB, *Elliman D* Health for All Children, 4th edn. Oxford: Oxford University Press, 2003.

2 Provision of Nutrition in a Hospital Setting

Ruth Watling

Introduction

The provision of adequate and appropriate nutrition for infants, children and young people in hospital presents a significant challenge. It must take into account the diverse needs of the paediatric inpatient population in terms of age, development stage, ethnicity and religious beliefs. Furthermore provision of nutrition encompasses the requirements of the nutritionally well, the nutritionally vulnerable and those requiring therapeutic diets. Dietitians will be involved predominantly with the latter two groups but must also act in an expert advisory capacity to those involved with the provision of food to the nutritionally well.

Nutrition care planning

Data on prevalence of undernutrition amongst paediatric inpatients indicate an incidence between 6% and 14% [1]. A child's nutritional status can deteriorate over the course of a hospital admission [2]. In chronic childhood diseases the contribution of frequent and extended admissions combined with the impact of treatment may have a negative effect on nutritional intake and consequently on nutritional status.

The use of a nutrition screening tool should, in theory, provide a simple and rapid means of determining those at risk and those who have specific dietary requirements. From this information a nutritional care pathway for each individual patient can be determined, implemented and monitored. There are a number of paediatric nutrition screening tools available and in a variety of stages of validation [3–5]. There is as yet no universally accepted paediatric nutrition screening tool for the assessment of paediatric inpatients and recent work indicates variable correlation with anthropometric assessment when comparing two of the tools and a need for further validation [6].

Additionally when considering the possible use of a nutrition screening tool for hospital inpatients the enormity of the task should not be underestimated. Between 760 000 and 1.15 million children are admitted annually to UK hospitals with an average length of stay of 2.1 days [7].

In summary, individual nutrition care planning is a prerequisite to optimum nutritional provision but needs to be undertaken in such a way that there is confidence that it can identify the significant numbers who are already malnourished, those who are at risk of becoming so and those with specific requirements, whilst avoiding unnecessary screening of those who are nutritionally well and undergoing a relatively short length of hospital stay.

Condition specific tools, such as the one recently developed for children and young people with

Clinical Paediatric Dietetics, Fourth Edition. Edited by Vanessa Shaw.
© 2015 John Wiley & Sons, Ltd. Published 2015 by John Wiley & Sons, Ltd.
Companion Website: www.wiley.com/go/shaw/paediatricdietetics

cancer (p. 661), may be a more appropriate future strategy to identify nutritional risk amongst paediatric inpatients [8]. Further information about nutrition screening tools may be found in Chapter 1, p. 3.

Nutritionally well inpatients

Provision of nutrition to nutritionally well inpatients should take into account:

- age and developmental stage of the patient
- religious and cultural beliefs
- the need to provide adequate food and fluid to meet normal nutritional requirements within a healthy balanced diet
- food provided should be familiar, tasty and available at the right time for the child; a hospital admission may provide the opportunity to promote aspects of healthier eating to families

Nutritionally well infants

Paediatric inpatient facilities should make every effort to enable mothers to breast feed their infants except for the rare event of a clinical reason to stop breast feeding. Support should include facilities for mothers to feed in comfort, respecting their privacy and dignity; support, facilities and equipment for mothers to express breast milk; safe and hygienic storage of expressed breast milk. Evidence is emerging that breast feeding can be sustained even in infants requiring significant surgical intervention [9].

For infants who are not breast fed and who do not require a specialised infant formula, there should be provision of ready-to-feed (RTF) infant milks. This will minimise the potential infection risks which could result from reconstituting powdered infant milks at ward level and ensure uniform composition. Ideally a selection of both whey and casein dominant milks should be available to meet the personal preference of the family. However, casein dominant RTF formulas are less easily available in UK hospitals and parents can be reassured that their infants' nutritional needs will be adequately met providing the correct volume of any approved infant milk is provided.

For infants from 6 months of age and older appropriate weaning foods should form part of the catering provision.

Nutritionally well children and young people

The food and drinks on offer for nutritionally well children and young people should be designed to meet normal nutritional requirements and promote a healthy balanced diet of familiar foods. Despite a number of initiatives there are no mandatory standards for hospitals in England or Northern Ireland. In Scotland and Wales there are standards in place for caterers to follow which can act as a guide for dietitians to assess the nutritional adequacy of the hospital menu [10, 11]. In the absence of mandatory standards there are good practice guidelines for the hospital menu [12] which include:

- meeting the estimated average requirement (EAR) for energy [13] daily; this can be achieved by provision of energy dense items, by increasing frequency of meals and by providing favourite foods at flexible times throughout the day
- meeting the reference nutrient intake (RNI) for protein [13] daily; this is almost always achieved if the EAR for energy is met
- meeting the RNI for vitamins and minerals over the course of a week
- encouraging a good fluid intake with six to eight drinks daily
- specific nutrients worthy of individual note

  Calcium: 350–500 mL milk should be available to all patients; full fat for under 2 years and semi-skimmed for others

  Vitamin C: 200 mL fruit juice for all and provision of fresh fruit and vegetables

  Iron: inclusion of red meat dishes, iron fortified breakfast cereals, green leafy vegetables and pulses

  Vitamin D: provision of adequate vitamin D in the diet is a challenge; supplementation may be required in long stay patients or those at specific risk of deficiency

The high sodium content of hospital meals has been noted and caterers should be advised to adhere to age specific recommendations [14].

Table 2.1 Food portion sizes for age.

	1–2 years	3–5 years	10+ years	12+ years
Meal pattern	3 small meals and 3 snacks plus milk	3 meals, 2–3 snacks or milk drinks	3 meals, 1–2 snacks or milk drinks	3 meals and 2–3 snacks
Protein sources, e.g. meat, fish, eggs, pulses	20–40 g or 2–4 tablespoons or 1 small item, e.g. fish or chicken goujon, egg	50–80 g or 4–8 tablespoons or 1–3 items depending on size, e.g. 2 fish fingers, 1 egg	90–120 g or 9–10 tablespoons or 1–3 items depending on size	120 g or 10 tablespoons or 2–3 items
Dairy	20 g cheese, 1 small pot yoghurt, 1 cup milk, 5–8 tablespoons custard	20–30 g cheese, 2 small or 1 standard pot yoghurt, 1 glass milk, 8–10 tablespoons custard	30–40 g cheese, 1 standard pot yoghurt, 1 glass milk, bowl of custard	50–60 g cheese, 1–2 standard pots yoghurt, 1 large glass milk, bowl of custard
Bread and other carbohydrates	1/2–1 slice or 1/2–1 item, e.g. crumpet, bagel, 3–5 tablespoons pasta or rice, 1–2 tablespoons potato, 3–5 tablespoons breakfast cereal	1 slice or 1 item, 6–8 tablespoons pasta or rice, 2–3 tablespoons potato, 6–8 tablespoons breakfast cereal or 1–2 Weetabix	2 slices or 2 items, 10–15 tablespoons pasta or rice, 3–4 tablespoons potato, bowl of breakfast cereal or 2 Weetabix	2–3 slices or items, 10–20 tablespoons pasta or rice or 4–6 tablespoons potato, bowl of breakfast cereal or 2–3 Weetabix
Fruit and vegetables Portion sizes to increase with age	5 a day	5 a day	5 a day	5 a day

1 tablespoon = 15 g.

Children in hospital should be provided with breakfast, two main meals and two to three snacks daily. A wide variety of portion sizes will be necessary to ensure that protein and energy requirements are met across the age ranges (Table 2.1). Food should be served in a manner and in an environment that encourages eating. Crockery and cutlery appropriate to the age ranges are required. Menu choices should meet the needs of vegetarians and those with specific cultural or religious beliefs (Chapter 27).

The nutritionally vulnerable and those requiring therapeutic diets

Patients in this group will require some or all of the following during the course of a hospital admission:

- adapted infant milks and specialised formulas
- enteral feeds
- parenteral nutrition (Chapter 4)

- nutrient dense meals
- therapeutic diets

Adapted infant milks and specialised formulas

A designated feed preparation area is required to prepare adapted infant milks, e.g. by thickening or by the addition of nutrients, or to prepare specialised formulas. Patients requiring such feeds are likely to be those at greatest nutritional risk; therefore the highest standards of accuracy are required to ensure the prescribed nutritional content is achieved.

Powdered formulas are a potential medium for bacterial and microbial growth. They are not sterile and have the potential to present an infection risk of *Cronobacter sakazakii* (formerly *Enterobacter sakazakii*) or salmonella species. Therefore hygiene standards in designated feed preparation areas are of paramount importance. The World Health

Organization (WHO) has issued advice for the preparation of powdered formulas for individual infants at home; they are best prepared freshly for each feed [15]. This is not practical for hospitals making large volumes of powdered infant feeds and specialised formulas.

Guidelines for the preparation of adapted infant milks and specialised formulas

In the UK there are no mandatory standards for feed preparation areas in hospital settings. A designated feed making unit is necessary in large hospitals preparing in excess of 15–20 feeds daily, with separate areas for storage, preparation and cleaning. For hospitals and paediatric units preparing less than 15 feeds daily a designated feed preparation room should be sufficient.

Feed preparation must comply with the requirements of the Food Safety Act 1990 [16]. The Paediatric Group of the British Dietetic Association has produced best practice guidelines and, in conjunction with the comprehensive guidelines from the American Dietetic Association, these documents provide essential reference standards for safe, effective and efficient feed making units [17, 18] which are summarised below.

Structural design of feed making areas

The area or unit should be physically isolated from direct patient care with access restricted to authorised personnel. It should be designed to be easily cleaned; prevent the entrance and harbouring of vermin and pests; operated to the highest standards of hygiene. Ideally there should be three separate areas:

- *storage area*: situated adjacent to the feed preparation area, where bulk goods are delivered, unpacked and stored. It should be large enough to accommodate adequate storage racks which are constructed and sited to permit segregation of commodities, stock rotation and effective cleaning. Items must be stored on racks or shelves, not directly on the floor. The temperature should be ambient, not subject to large shifts, and checked daily.
- *feed preparation area*: where very clean conditions prevail and access is only allowed to feed preparation staff who are suitably clothed (see Staffing); entry should be via an anteroom containing a wash-hand basin and storage facilities for outer protective clothing. Bulk storage of items, e.g. large cardboard cartons, is not recommended. There should be sufficient space to allow clean equipment and small quantities of ingredients to be stored, preferably on wheel-mounted stainless steel solid shelving, leaving worktops clear. During the preparation of feeds there should be minimal interruption to ensure standards of accuracy are maintained. If it is necessary for staff to leave the preparation area they must, on re-entry, wash their hands again, according to the correct hand washing procedure.
- *utility area for equipment washing and administrative work*: storage of cleaning materials should be separated from ingredients and equipment and requires a designated clean, dry room or cupboard. A cloakroom with a separate changing room for feed unit staff should be conveniently sited but segregated from the feed-making area. The cloakroom should have a toilet and wash-hand basin with foot or elbow operated taps.

In smaller units there may only be the need for a designated feed making room. Care must be taken to ensure separation of ingredients from prepared feeds. The same standards of preparation apply.

Recommendations for construction of feed units are as follows:

- *walls, floors and ceilings*: hardwearing, impervious and free from cracks and open joints. Smooth surfaces to permit ease of cleaning and coved junctions between floors, walls and ceilings to prevent collection of dust and dirt. Light coloured sheen finish to reflect light and increase illumination.
- *doors in the production area*: self-closing with glass observation panel.
- *windows*: sealed to prevent opening.
- *mechanical ventilation to provide a clean air supply*: with temperature (and preferably humidity) control to give optimum working environment and control bacterial and dust contamination. Steam producing equipment such as dishwashers and pasteurisers should be fitted with a canopy and exhaust fan system to draw off steam and fumes.

- *lighting level*: to allow staff to work cleanly and safely without eye strain, and to expose dirt and dust. Light fixtures flush with wall or ceiling.
- *wash-hand basins*: one provided in each utility and preparation area. Hot and cold water with foot or elbow operated taps. Hand soap and sanitiser as per local policies and single use disposable towels or a hot air hand dryer.
- *water supply*: of potable quality from a rising main. The Department of Health has not advised against the use of tap water in the preparation of feeds. Tap water should be provided from a fixed device such as a gas or electric water boiler to dispense water >80 °C. If sterile water is used it must be heated to >80 °C if it is used in the preparation of powdered formulas.

Large equipment

- Large equipment such as shelving, tables and refrigerators should be castor mounted with wheel brakes to allow easy access for cleaning. Smooth impervious surfaces free from sharp internal corners, which may act as dirt traps, which can be easily cleaned and disinfected, e.g. stainless steel, are recommended.
- Refrigerators which operate at a temperature between 1 and 4 °C; the temperature should be monitored and recorded twice daily.
- Blast chillers to allow rapid cooling of all feeds to below 4 °C within 1 hour of preparation.
- A deep freeze which operates below −18 °C will be necessary if expressed breast milk is to be stored for more than a few hours. Both the refrigerator and freezer should be self-defrosting and have shelves which are easy to clean. An alarm which is activated if the door is left open accidentally or the internal temperature increases is also useful.
- Pasteurisation equipment which is suitable for the range of procedures carried out (see Feed preparation) and which includes a method of monitoring and recording pasteurisation cycles.
- Thermal disinfection of equipment is desirable in a small unit and essential in a large centralised unit. This can be a dishwasher adapted for bottle and equipment washing with a rinse cycle which holds a temperature of 85 °C for 2 minutes. This ensures a surface temperature of 80 °C for 1 minute, which is an effective disinfectant. A drying cycle is useful [19].
- A feed delivery trolley either insulated or with ice packs to ensure feeds remain at <4 °C during delivery to the wards.

Small equipment

- Mixing and measuring equipment including jugs, measures, cutlery and whisks should be made from plastic or stainless steel. They must be easily washed and cleaned.
- Weighing equipment should be easy to clean, easy to use and of the appropriate accuracy for the task.
- Feed bottles are available in glass, polycarbonate or plastic polythene in 50–240 mL sizes. Glass is a hazardous material prone to cracking and chipping; polycarbonate shrinks if autoclaved at temperatures greater than 119 °C and the bottles become scratched or crazed after some time in use. Reusable bottles require washing, sanitising by heat or chemical means; sealing discs or caps need to undergo a similar treatment and are likely to become lost or misshapen with continuous use. Disposable sterile polythene bottles reduce the workload in the unit. The decision to use disposable or reusable bottles is a matter for each individual unit based on cost–benefit analysis and risk analysis of possible contamination from inadequately cleaned bottles. Single use enteral feeding containers will also be required for larger volumes of prepared or decanted RTF formulas.

Staffing

Feed provision is usually required every day of the year and staffing levels should take this fact and the workload into consideration. In large units the dietitian may be managerially responsible for staff and feed preparation. In small areas attached to a ward the supervision and management may be the responsibility of the nursing staff with the dietitian acting in an advisory capacity.

There is no mandatory requirement under the Food Safety Act for formal training but the manager of the unit must ensure that staff are adequately trained in all aspects of food safety as it relates to feed preparation. For additional quality assurance training at Chartered Institute of Environmental

Health (CIEH) Level 2 in food safety, or hazard analysis and critical control points (HACCP), is preferable [20].

Training should cover personal hygiene, prevention of bacterial and foreign matter contamination, preparation procedures, and basic knowledge of the feed composition and clinical indication.

Suitable protective uniforms and footwear are required. A disposable plastic apron should be worn during feed preparation and a disposable head covering should completely cover the hair.

Feed preparation

There are three key components of safe feed preparation. These are appropriate ingredients, safe and accurate preparation and limitation of microbial growth.

- All ingredients received into a feed making area should be of the required standards and specification. Goods received should be checked and stock rotated according to date. Opened tins or packets, e.g. from the patient's home, should not be accepted into the feed making area. If pasteurised cow's milk is used, e.g. to reconstitute powdered supplements, it should be stocked according to its dated shelf-life; if opened any unused milk should be discarded at the end of the working day. Expressed breast milk will require an agreed procedure for storage and use.
- Details of each feed to be prepared should be in a clearly written or printed form including the patient's name, date of birth and hospital number, the weight or volume of each feed ingredient, the total fluid volume, the number and volume of each feed required. All ingredients should be weighed or measured accurately. Prepared feeds should be decanted into the appropriate number and size of bottles and each bottle labelled. The label must include details of the patient's name, ward, feed type, preparation, date and preferably advice to refrigerate and discard after 24 hours.
- Limitation of microbial growth is critical to safe feed provision. The use of boiled water cooled to 70–80 °C for feed preparation reduces the risk of microbial proliferation. Pasteurisation can limit microbial growth and will destroy

Staphylococcus aureus, Enterobacter sp. and *Salmonella* sp., but may be less effective against some potential pathogens, e.g. *Cronobacter sakazakii* is fairly resistant to heat. Two methods of pasteurisation are commonly used:

1 holder method for expressed breast milk where the temperature is raised to 62.5 °C for 30 minutes followed by rapid cooling to <10 °C;
2 flash method for prepared feeds where the temperature is raised to 67.5 °C for 4 minutes followed by rapid cooling to <10 °C.

- Blast chilling is an effective method of limiting microbial growth in prepared feeds by cooling rapidly to <4 °C. Following preparation and pasteurisation or blast chilling feeds should be refrigerated at <4 °C until delivery to the wards. In small units blast chilling or pasteurisation may not be feasible but systems must be in place for rapid cooling and refrigeration of prepared feeds.

Delivery

Feed delivery to wards should be compatible with food safety requirements with feeds being refrigerated at <4 °C. If the preparation unit is some distance from wards this may require a refrigerated or insulated trolley with ice packs.

Cleaning procedures

Sterilisation of small equipment (the destruction of all microorganisms and their spores) is not attainable in a special feeds unit. Sanitation or disinfection of small equipment can be achieved by autoclaving, by a dishwasher or by chemical means.

Autoclaving, although effective, has a number of disadvantages: equipment first has to be washed, dried, packed and sealed; this is costly and time consuming. In addition water condensation forms and remains in feeding bottles, where it can induce bacterial activity.

Thermal disinfection in a dishwasher requires less time and the inclusion of a drying cycle will ensure that all equipment is dry and ready for storage. To achieve thermal disinfection the water in the dishwasher should reach a minimum temperature of 85 °C for 2 minutes.

Chemical disinfection, e.g. hypochlorite, reduces levels of harmful bacteria to acceptable levels and is satisfactory for small (non-metallic) equipment provided recommendations are followed, although heat sanitisation is the preferred method. Disinfection will only be effective if

- the equipment is adequately cleaned; residual organic matter inactivates the chlorine content of the disinfectant;
- the disinfectant is freshly and correctly prepared with all air bubbles removed to ensure the solution comes into contact with all surfaces of the equipment;
- the equipment remains in the disinfectant for the recommended length of time. After disinfection the equipment should be rinsed free of contaminated hypochlorite with clean water. Feed equipment should be covered and used within 24 hours of disinfection. Equipment which is stored for longer than this should be re-disinfected before use.

Quality assurance

The aim of a designated feed making area is to minimise the risk of microbial contamination and proliferation in prepared infant or specialised feeds. Adherence to the published guidelines will support this aim. To ensure satisfactory standards of working practice are maintained a microbiological surveillance policy can be a useful component of quality control. Microbiology personnel can provide useful advice on sampling feeds and the environment for microbial analysis as an additional quality assurance. Any feed production errors or near misses should be reported in line with local incident and risk management procedures.

Procedures and documentation

Clear written procedures are required for every aspect of feed preparation. This includes guidelines for personal hygiene and prevention of cross-infection, procedures for ordering supplies, feed reconstitution, instructions for pasteurisation and blast chilling, cleaning and disinfection, microbiological surveillance, risk management, equipment maintenance and breakdown procedures.

Enteral feeds

Older children and young people who are at risk of malnutrition as a result of underlying disease are often dependent on nutrition support and in hospital will frequently require enteral tube feeding. The increase in the range of sterile RTF products has reduced the need to prepare powdered enteral feeds. A few remain as powdered products and these should be prepared to the same standards as described for infant and specialised formulas.

Care must be taken at ward level to ensure that all prepared feeds are stored in refrigerators at <4°C. The hanging time for feeds that are administered continuously is debatable. The UK National Institute for Health and Care Excellence (NICE) recommends that (non-sterile) reconstituted feeds should hang for no more than 4 hours. However, these are best practice guidelines for the prevention of healthcare associated infections in the community; the guidelines can be adapted for local use in the hospital setting [21]. Sterile RTF enteral formulas may be hung for 24 hours if the administration system (feed reservoir and giving set) is closed.

Food for those at nutritional risk or requiring therapeutic diets

In contrast to food provision in adult hospitals where menu coding is designed to allow patients with specific dietary requirements to choose from the main catering menu, it is preferable in large children's units to have a designated diet kitchen or diet bay. This is supported by the need for attention to detail where food items often have to be weighed very accurately; preparation of prescribed dietary food products which demands special cooking skills to get a good result; prevention of cross-contamination of food allergens. The exception to this is for those with higher than normal requirements for protein and energy where ordinary food from the main menu can be fortified or the provision of extra food at snacks or mealtimes may be sufficient. Consistent use of standard recipes and ingredients in food preparation in the main catering kitchen may render some items from the main menu suitable for therapeutic diets.

Patient groups can provide helpful collaboration in attempts to improve the food on offer to some of the most nutritionally at risk groups in hospitals [22]. For some groups of children specific initiatives have improved their food intake [8].

Staff involved in the preparation of therapeutic diets must be aware of the need for accuracy, appropriate portion size for age, consistency of nutrient content and variety. For those on a therapeutic diet the food provided in hospital is taken as an example of what must be continued at home and must therefore be correct. It is advisable that staff employed to prepare special modified diets have as a minimum qualification City and Guilds 706/2. In-service training of diet cooks should be undertaken by the dietitian, particularly to ensure that staff are kept up to date with changes to dietary treatment. The following points must be considered when providing a therapeutic diet service:

- The dietitian should specify to the caterer the standards of quality and suitability of provisions for use in the diet preparation area. Stocks of specific dietary products such as gluten free and low protein products should be available and those working in the area should be familiar with the use of these products.
- Appropriate equipment for preparation of small quantities of food must be available for the diet cooks. A sturdy industrial liquidiser, small pots and pans and accurate scales are all essential items. Freezer space is also required, as it is useful to keep frozen portions of special items, e.g. vegetable casserole for low protein diets; minimal fat snacks; milk, egg, wheat and soya free baked goods.
- A suitable plating system for diets must be used. Where a bulk catering system is operated individual containers, clearly labelled, are suitable for diet meals. If a plated system is in use the diet meals should be clearly labelled.
- The dietitian should always provide the diet cooks with clear written and verbal instructions for each individual diet being prepared. The written information should include the patient's name, age and ward, the diet required and specific instructions regarding the composition of the diet.
- A diet manual within the diet preparation area should include instructions regarding commonly requested modified diets and appropriate recipes. It is also useful to include details

of any patients on unusual diets if they are likely to be admitted. This manual should be regularly updated.

- To ensure consistency and accuracy and a high quality product, the provision of modified diets should be monitored regularly. The following should all be considered: the quality, freshness and suitability of the provisions; the storage methods; the preparation of raw ingredients; and the presentation to the patient.

Preparation of food for neutropenic patients

Children undergoing bone marrow or peripheral blood stem cell transplantation have periods of severe immunosuppression and neutropenia. Opportunistic infection is a significant cause of morbidity and mortality in immunocompromised patients. Bacterial translocation from the gastrointestinal tract can cause significant infection and in theory can be decreased by reducing the potential sources of bacteria and other pathogens from food. This has been referred to as a low microbial, clean or sterile diet depending on the degree of restriction.

The evidence on the effectiveness of low microbial diets is extremely limited. In an extremely small paediatric study infection rates were similar between two groups randomised to either a neutropenic diet or food safety guidelines diet [23]. In the absence of larger well controlled studies, some have advocated the use of food safety guidelines for neutropenic patients [24]. The need to minimise risk from food borne infection must of course be balanced with the need to support nutritional status in this vulnerable group, with the avoidance of unnecessary restrictions which may impact adversely on nutritional intake.

Current consensus suggests the use of a low microbial diet which avoids the use of raw or lightly cooked foods, reheated foods and foods known to contain higher levels of potential pathogens such as soft cheeses, unpasteurised products, nuts and buffet or deli counter foods. Practice can vary but a summary of common foods to avoid is given in Table 2.2 [25].

In addition strict food hygiene practices must be used in the storage, preparation and service of food

Table 2.2   Suggested foods for a low microbial diet.

Foods to avoid	Alternatives
Meats Raw or undercooked meat and poultry Smoked or cured meats Pâté	Well-cooked meat and poultry Vacuum-packed cold meats such as turkey or ham Tinned meats Pasteurised pâté or paste in tins or jars
Fish Raw, smoked or lightly cooked fish	Well-cooked fish
Eggs Raw or soft-cooked eggs such as homemade mayonnaise, mousses, sauces or meringues	Hard-boiled eggs, shop-bought mayonnaise, mousses, sauces or meringues Other products made with pasteurised eggs
Milk and milk products All unpasteurised dairy products Blue-veined cheese, e.g. stilton Soft ripened cheeses, e.g. brie, camembert, goat's cheese, paneer Probiotics, live, active or bio products such as live yoghurts, probiotic supplements or drinks Soft ice cream	Any pasteurised milk, soya milk, Jersey milk, UHT milk and cheese products Vacuum-packed pasteurised and hard cheeses such as cheddar and edam Processed cheese Pasteurised plain or fruit yoghurts Commercial ice cream individually wrapped portions
Vegetables Unpeeled vegetables including salad items Damaged or overripe vegetables Unpasteurised or freshly squeezed vegetable juices or smoothies	Good quality vegetables that are well cooked or peeled UHT or long life vegetable juices sold in cartons or jars Pasteurised smoothies
Fruit Unpeeled fruit Raw dried fruit such as dates or raisins and products containing these such as muesli Damaged or overripe fruit Unpasteurised or freshly squeezed fruit juices or smoothies	Good quality fruit that is well cooked or peeled UHT or long-life fruit juices sold in cartons or jars Pasteurised smoothies Tinned fruit or cooked dried fruit such as in cake, flapjacks or cereal bars
Herbs and condiments Uncooked herbs, spices and pepper	
Drinks Non-drinking water, bottled mineral or spring water, water from wells, coolers or drinking fountains	Cooled boiled water Sterilised water
Nuts All nuts	
Honey Unpasteurised or 'farm fresh' honey and honeycomb	Pasteurised or heat-treated honey
Miscellaneous Food items from 'pick and mix' or 'buffet' counters Deli counter	Packets should be individually wrapped or portioned on the ward only

Table 2.3 High risk foods.

Raw and undercooked meat, fish or eggs
Soft and blue-veined cheeses
Pâté
Live and bio yoghurts
Take-away foods
Reheated food
Soft whip ice cream
Deli and buffet foods

to neutropenic patients requiring low microbial diets, including

- ensuring that all preparation surfaces and equipment are clean and avoidance of wooden chopping boards and spoons

- thorough hand washing
- use of protective clothing for preparation and service of food
- cooking methods should ensure a core temperature of 70 °C in the final product
- an agreed minimum delay between the food being cooked and eaten

After discharge neutrophil counts will have recovered but there remains a risk and a small number of high risk foods should be avoided, usually for 3–6 months. These foods are outlined in Table 2.3 and food hygiene advice should be emphasised [26].

Part 2

Nutrition Support and Intensive Care

3 Enteral Nutrition

Tracey Johnson

Introduction

Enteral nutrition is the method of supplying nutrients to the gastrointestinal tract. Although enteral nutrition is the term often used to describe nasogastric, gastrostomy and jejunostomy feeding it also includes food and drink taken orally.

Enteral feeding is the preferred method of providing nutrition support to children who have a functioning gastrointestinal tract, with parenteral nutrition reserved for children with severely compromised gut function. It is safer and easier to administer than parenteral nutrition both in hospital and at home and can be adapted to meet the individual requirements of infants and children of all ages.

Some children receive their full nutritional requirements via a nasogastric, gastrostomy or jejunostomy tube, whereas others require nutrition support to supplement poor oral intake or to meet increased nutritional requirements. Enteral feeding may be short term but for many children it can be a long term or even life-long method of feeding. As a result regimens need to be adaptable to ensure each child receives the essential nutrients they require for normal growth and development.

Tube feeding children requires the expert input of a paediatric dietitian who, along with a specialist multidisciplinary team, has the knowledge to use feeds and feeding equipment appropriate for the individual requirements and clinical condition of the patient. Indications for enteral feeding are given in Table 3.1.

Choice of feeds

The choice of feed is dependent on a number of factors:

- age of child
- gut function
- dietary restrictions and specific nutrient requirements
- route of administration
- prescribability and cost

Infants under 12 months

Many infants requiring tube feeding may be given the same feed they would otherwise be taking orally. Children who are breast fed may be able to continue breast milk and there are physiological and psychological advantages to this. Mother's expressed breast milk (EBM) may be given to her own baby or pasteurised donor breast milk may be available. The principal benefits of using breast milk are the presence of immunoglobulins, antimicrobial factors and lipase activity. In addition, there

Table 3.1 Indications for enteral feeding.

Indication	Example
Inability to suck or swallow	Neurological handicap and degenerative disorders Severe developmental delay Trauma Critically ill child requiring ventilation
Anorexia associated with chronic illness	Cystic fibrosis Malignancy Inflammatory bowel disease Liver disease Chronic kidney disease Congenital heart disease Inherited metabolic disorders
Increased requirements	Cystic fibrosis Congenital heart disease Malabsorption syndromes (e.g. short gut syndrome, liver disease) Trauma Severe burns
Congenital anomalies	Tracheo-oesophageal fistula Oesophageal atresia Orofacial malformations
Primary disease management	Crohn's disease Severe gastro-oesophageal reflux Short bowel syndrome Glycogen storage disease Very long chain fatty acid disorders
Refusal to eat	Anorexia nervosa Feeding aversion

is a psychological benefit to the mother if she is able to contribute to the care of her sick child by providing breast milk. These benefits may be outweighed by the possible poorer energy density of EBM, particularly if the fore milk is used which is lower in fat than the hind milk. If the infant fails to gain weight on breast milk alone it can be supplemented with a commercial human milk fortifier (p. 92), or with standard infant formula powder (Table 1.18).

Whether to pasteurise a mother's EBM when it is to be given to her own baby remains a controversial issue. Pasteurisation will destroy some of its nutritional, antimicrobial, probiotic, hormonal and enzymic properties [1–3] but may protect against pathogenic bacterial contamination. Currently there are no national guidelines for pasteurisation of mother's EBM to be fed to her own baby and individual hospitals and units have developed their own local protocols. The evidence for the

transmission of infection via EBM is limited and the role of pasteurisation unclear. This will largely be influenced by the cleanliness of the collection and handling techniques.

Standard infant formulas are suitable for enteral feeding from birth to 12 months of age for those children with normal gut function and normal nutritional requirements. They provide an energy density of 65–70 kcal (270–290 kJ)/100 mL and meet the European Community Infant Formula Regulations [4]. Follow-on milks may also be used after 6 months of age if their higher protein and iron content is thought to be more beneficial to the child. Many infants requiring enteral feeding will have increased nutritional requirements. Nutrient dense infant formulas such as SMA High Energy, Infatrini and Similac High Energy are commercially available and have been shown to promote better growth than standard formulas with added energy supplements (glucose polymer powders and fat emulsions) [5]. Concentrating standard infant formulas achieves a feed that is more nutrient dense and retains an appropriate protein:energy ratio similar to the commercial nutrient dense formulas (p. 17).

Standard infant formulas are based on cow's milk protein, lactose and long chain fat. Infants with impaired gut function who do not tolerate whole protein feeds frequently benefit from the use of hydrolysed protein or amino acid based feeds. Such feeds are hypoallergenic and are free of cow's milk protein and lactose. Many of these formulas also have a proportion of the fat content as medium chain triglycerides which can be beneficial where there is fat malabsorption, e.g. liver disease, short gut syndrome (Table 7.6).

If the specific requirements of an infant cannot be met by a commercial infant formula it is possible to formulate a feed from separate ingredients. These modular feeds allow a choice of protein, fat and carbohydrate and give the flexibility to meet the needs of individual patients. However, they are expensive and time consuming to prepare and there is a greater risk of bacterial contamination and mistakes being made during their preparation. It will take several days to establish a child on a full strength modular feed (Table 7.24). Consequently, modular feeds should only be used if a complete feed is unsuitable and, in the hospital setting, should ideally be prepared in a dedicated special feed preparation area (p. 26).

Children aged 1–12 years (8–45 kg body weight)

Specialist paediatric feeds are available for children 1–12 years of age or who weigh 8–45 kg. Department of Health guidelines [6] indicate that children have differing nutritional requirements according to their age and consequently specifically designed feeds for these age groups are recommended to ensure provision of appropriate levels of protein, micronutrients and electrolytes to optimise growth. Although nutritional profiles of paediatric feeds are designed to meet the specific requirements of children it is still important to assess requirements and intakes for the individual.

Feeds are available for children within three age bands:

- 1–6 years
- 1–10 years
- 7–12 years

All feeds are categorised as Dietary Foods for Special Medical Purposes and must comply with the 1999 EC Directive [7]. Standard paediatric feeds are based on cow's milk protein but are lactose free and provide three levels of energy density: 100 kcal (420 kJ)/100 mL, 120 kcal (500 kJ)/100 mL and 150 kcal (630 kJ)/100 mL. A lower energy feed, 75 kcal (315 kJ)/100 mL, is also available.

Most product ranges are formulated either with or without added fibre. Those with fibre contain a mix of soluble and insoluble fibre. Constipation is common in exclusively tube fed children, particularly those with neurological impairment [8]. A normal diet contains fibre and with an improved knowledge of the role of dietary fibre it is now common practice for children to receive a fibre containing feed as the standard. Studies have shown that the use of fibre enriched feeds reduces the incidence of constipation and laxative use [9, 10].

Children with neurological impairment form the largest single diagnostic group who have long term enteral feeding at home [11]. This group of children frequently has low energy expenditure and, if a standard feed is provided in the necessary volume to meet recommendations for protein and micronutrients, they may show excessive weight gain. The nutritional needs of this group of children are discussed in Chapter 29, p. 778.

The range of paediatric enteral feeds is outlined in Table 3.2.

For children with abnormal gut function, as with infants, feeds based on hydrolysed protein and amino acids are available (Table 7.6) and it is also sometimes necessary to use a modular feed (Table 7.24).

Children over 12 years (>45 kg body weight)

The requirements of children over 12 years of age may still be met by a paediatric feed designed for 7–12 year olds; individual assessment is necessary. Standard adult feeds may also be used and are available with energy densities of 1 kcal (4 kJ)/mL and 1.5 kcal (6 kJ)/mL, with and without fibre. Some adult feeds have a protein content of 6 g/100 mL or more so care should be taken when using such feeds for children, even if they are over 12 years of age, as they may provide an excessively high amount of protein. Intakes of copper, chromium, molybdenum and vitamins E, C, B6 and B12 will also be high. Adult peptide based and elemental feeds can be used for children with impaired gut function and it is also necessary in special circumstances to employ the flexibility of a modular feed.

The choice of feeds suitable for children is given in Table 3.3.

Feed thickeners

Feed thickeners can be a useful dietary intervention for children with gastro-oesophageal reflux. In addition to anti-reflux medication, feed thickeners can help to reduce vomiting and minimise the risk of aspiration. Feed thickeners can also be added to enteral feeds that would otherwise separate out when left to stand (e.g. some modular feeds).

There is a wide range of commercial products that are suitable for thickening enteral feeds (Table 7.26). Thickened feeds may be difficult to give as a bolus via a fine bore nasogastric tube, and syringe feeding or pump feeding may be necessary. It is also important to consider the energy contribution of some of the thickening agents. The thickeners based on modified starch given at a concentration of 3 g/100 mL may result in an increased energy content of more than 10%.

Table 3.2 Paediatric enteral feeds.

		per 100 mL		
	Age/Weight	Energy kcal (kJ)	Protein g	Fibre g
Nutrini Low Energy Multifibre (Nutricia)	1–6 years (8–20 kg)	75 (315)	2.1	0.8
Nutrini (Nutricia)	1–6 years (8–20 kg)	100 (420)	2.8	–
Nutrini Multifibre (Nutricia)	1–6 years (8–20 kg)	100 (420)	2.8	0.8
Paediasure (Abbott)	1–10 years (8–30 kg)	101 (422)	2.8	–
Paediasure Fibre (Abbott)	1–10 years (8–30 kg)	101 (422)	2.9	0.73
Frebini Original (Fresenius)	1–10 years (8–30 kg)	100 (420)	2.5	–
Frebini Original Fibre (Fresenius)	1–10 years (8–30 kg)	100 (420)	2.5	0.75
Clinutren Junior Powder (Nestle)	1–6 years (8–30 kg)	100 (420)	2.97	–
		150 (630)	4.46	–
Frebini Original (Fresenius)	1–10 years (8–30 kg)	100 (420)	2.5	–
Nutrini Multifibre (Nutricia)	1–6 years (8–20 kg)	100 (420)	2.7	0.75
Paediasure Fibre (Abbott)	1–10 years (8–30 kg)	101 (422)	2.9	0.5
Isosource Junior (Novartis)	1–6 years (8–20 kg)	122 (510)	2.7	–
Nutrini Energy (Nutricia)	1–6 years (8–20 kg)	150 (630)	4.1	–
Nutrini Energy Multifibre (Nutricia)	1–6 years (8–20 kg)	150 (630)	4.1	0.8
Paediasure Plus (Abbott)	1–10 years (8–30 kg)	150 (630)	4.2	–
Paediasure Plus Fibre (Abbott)	1–10 years (8–30 kg)	151 (632)	4.2	1.1
Frebini Energy (Fresenius)	1–10 years (8–30 kg)	150 (630)	3.75	–
Frebini Energy Fibre (Fresenius)	1–10 years (8–30 kg)	150 (630)	3.75	1.13
Tentrini (Nutricia)	7–12 years (21–45 kg)	100 (420)	3.3	–
Tentrini Multifibre (Nutricia)	7–12 years (21–45 kg)	100 (420)	3.3	1.1
Tentrini Energy (Nutricia)	7–12 years (21–45 kg)	150 (630)	4.9	–
Tentrini Energy Multifibre (Nutricia)	7–12 years (21–45 kg)	150 (630)	4.9	1.1

Routes of feed administration

Nasogastric feeding

Nasogastric is the most common route for enteral feeding and, unless prolonged enteral nutrition is anticipated, it would usually be the route of choice. However, passing a nasogastric tube can be distressing for both parents and children and careful preparation is beneficial [12]. Frank discussions and a clear explanation of the procedure can help older children, and play therapy with the use of dolls, mannequins [13] and picture books has been shown to alleviate anxieties in the younger age group. Older children, particularly teenagers, are naturally sensitive about their body image and they may be reluctant to start nasogastric feeding. Some children successfully pass their own nasogastric tube at night and remove their tube in the daytime, which can be a successful way of administering supplementary feeds without the embarrassment of a permanent nasogastric tube *in situ*.

Nasogastric feeding is a lifeline for many children, but it is not without its complications. Some of the more serious complications are related to dislodgement, poor placement and migration of tubes. Following a number of deaths, the National Patient Safety Agency published a report suggesting that conventional methods to check tube placement were inaccurate. The common method to aspirate the tube and test with blue litmus paper is not sensitive enough to distinguish between gastric and bronchial secretions; auscultation of air or observation of gastric contents is also considered ineffective. Radiology and testing of gastric aspirate with pH paper are the only acceptable methods of confirming nasogastric tube position [14].

Long term nasogastric feeding in some children can cause inflammation and irritation to the skin where the nasogastric tube is secured to the face. Use of Duoderm or Granuflex placed onto the skin can improve this. Another common problem, particularly with fine bore tubes, is tube blockage. This may result from using the tube to administer

Table 3.3 Choice of feeds for enteral feeding.

	Normal gut function	Impaired gut function
Infants	*Normal energy requirements* Breast milk or standard infant formula *High energy requirements* Breast milk + BMF/standard infant formula Concentrated infant formula Nutrient dense infant formula (e.g. Infatrini, SMA High Energy, Similac High Energy)	Hydrolysed protein formula, e.g. Pepti-Junior (Cow & Gate), Nutramigen Lipil 1, 2 (Mead Johnson) Amino acid infant formula, e.g. Neocate LCP (SHS) Modular feed Infatrini Pepti
1–6 years (8–20/30 kg)	*Normal energy requirements* Standard paediatric enteral feed, e.g. Nutrini (Nutricia), Paedisure (Abbott) ± fibre *High energy requirements* High energy paediatric enteral feed, e.g. Nutrini Energy (Nutricia), Paediasure Plus (Abbott) ± fibre *Low energy requirements* Low energy paediatric feed, e.g. Nutrini Low Energy Multifibre (Nutricia)	Hydrolysed protein formula, e.g. Nutrini Peptisorb (Nutricia), Pepdite 1+ (SHS), Peptamen Junior (Nestle) Amino acid formula, e.g. Neocate Advance (SHS) Modular feed Peptamen Junior Advance (Nestle)
6–12 years (20–45 kg)	*Normal energy requirements* Standard paediatric enteral feed, e.g. Tentrini (Nutricia), Paediasure (Abbott) ± fibre *High energy requirements* High energy paediatric enteral feed, e.g. Tentrini Energy (Nutricia) , Paediasure Plus (Abbott) ± fibre	Hydrolysed protein formula, e.g. Pepdite 1+ (SHS), Peptamen (Nestle) Amino acid formula, e.g. E028/E028 Extra (SHS) Modular feed Peptamen Junior Advance (Nestle)
12+ years (>45 kg)	*Normal energy requirements** Standard adult enteral feed e.g. Nutrison Standard (Nutricia), Osmolite (Abbott) ± fibre *High energy requirements** High energy adult enteral feed Nutrison Energy (Nutricia), Ensure Plus (Abbott), ± fibre	Hydrolysed protein feed, e.g. Peptamen (Nestle), Nutrison Peptisorb (Nutricia) Amino acid feed, e.g. E028/E028 Extra (SHS) Modular feed High energy hydrolysed protein feed, e.g. Perative (Abbott), Vital (Abbott) Peptamen AF (Nestle)

BMF, breast milk fortifier.
*Paediatric feed designed for 6–12 years old may be suitable.

drugs, the use of viscous formulas and inadequate flushing of the tube. Regular flushing of tubes can help to prevent this problem and the use of carbonated liquids can clear and prevent the build-up of feed within the lumen of the tube. It may sometimes be necessary to replace the tube for one with a larger lumen.

Gastrostomy feeding

Gastrostomy is a widely used route of feeding when longer term enteral nutrition is indicated [15]. Gastrostomy feeding is generally well accepted by children as it is more comfortable, obviates the need for frequent tube changes and is cosmetically more acceptable. Indications are not solely for long term feeding; in certain situations gastrostomy feeding is the route of choice. This includes children with congenital abnormalities such as tracheo-oesophageal fistula and oesophageal atresia and children with oesophageal injuries (e.g. following the ingestion of caustic chemicals). It has been suggested that a contraindication for gastrostomy is severe gastro-oesophageal reflux. This can be exacerbated with the introduction of a gastrostomy tube [16] and gastrostomy placement in such children is generally done in combination with a fundoplication (p. 148).

The procedures used to place gastrostomies have significantly evolved over the past decades with endoscopic and laparoscopic techniques now in common use [17] and, more recently, radiological imaging techniques being used. These operations are minimally invasive compared with a gastrostomy performed by open surgery. Percutaneous endoscopic gastrostomy (PEG), radiologically inserted gastrostomy (RIG) and laparoscopic gastrostomy tube placement are completed with a shorter anaesthetic time with fewer complications than an open surgically placed gastrostomy tube. After about 3 months, once the tract is formed, a child can be fitted with a gastrostomy button that sits almost flush against the skin. This is far more discreet than the tubing associated with a conventional gastrostomy catheter and is a popular choice, particularly with teenagers. Primary placement of gastrostomy buttons for feeding tubes is also practised [18]. This intervention often leads to some minor postoperative problems, including gastrostomy site leakage.

Gastrostomy tubes and buttons require less frequent changes than nasogastric tubes. A device secured by a deflatable balloon is easier to change than one secured by an internal bumper bar or disc. If a tube is inadvertently removed it should be replaced within 6–8 hours or the tract will start to close.

The main complications of gastrostomy feeding are wound infection, leakage and excessive granulation tissue around the exit site. Leakage of acidic gastric content can cause severe inflammation and skin irritation and patients and parents should be taught about skin care. Infection may require treatment with topical or systemic antibiotics. There are no evidence based guidelines on the use of prophylactic antibiotics for the insertion of PEG or other gastrostomies in children but adult studies, including a Cochrane review, suggest a single dose of broad spectrum antibiotics before PEG insertion reduces peristomal infections [19–21].

Feeding into the jejunum

Indications for feeding into the jejunum include

- congenital gastrointestinal anomalies
- gastric dysmotility
- severe vomiting resulting in faltering growth
- children at risk of aspiration

When children are fed directly into the jejunum, feed enters the intestine distal to the site of release of pancreatic enzymes and bile. Whole protein feeds may be well tolerated but if malabsorption occurs a trial period of feeding a hydrolysed protein feed is recommended. The stomach normally acts as a reservoir for food or feed, regulating the amount that is delivered into the small intestine. Feed given as a bolus directly into the small intestine can cause abdominal pain, diarrhoea and dumping syndrome (p. 150), resulting from rapid delivery of a hyperosmolar feed into the jejunum. Feeds delivered into the jejunum should therefore always be given slowly by continuous infusion.

Placement of a nasojejunal tube is difficult and maintaining the position of the tube causes numerous problems. The position of the tube can be checked using pH paper. The tube can spontaneously re-site into the stomach or can be inadvertently pulled back; weighted tubes do not seem to be of much value in preventing this [22]. For longer term feeding a surgical jejunostomy tube or a gastrojejunal tube is usually a more successful route for delivering nutrition support.

Complications can include bacterial overgrowth, malabsorption, bowel perforation and tube blockage. Like nasogastric and gastrostomy tubes, jejunostomy tubes need regular flushing to maintain patency and it is recommended that sterile water is always used.

A gastrostomy device with jejunal tube (PEG-J or G-J tube) may be used if access to the stomach and jejunum is required. These devices can be useful in children with delayed gastric emptying or those at risk of aspiration. Feed can be administered via the transgastric jejunal tube and the gastrostomy port can be used for aspiration, decompression or administration of medicines.

The routes of enteral feeding are shown in Fig. 3.1. The advantages and disadvantages of the routes of feed administration are given in Table 3.4.

Orogastric feeding

Orogastric feeding is principally used for feeding neonates where nasal access is not feasible or where breathing would be compromised. The tube is passed via the mouth into the stomach. If all feeds are given via the orogastric tube it can be taped in place, but if the infant is taking some breast or bottle feeds the tube can be passed as required and removed between feeds.

Gastrostomy coupled with oesophagostomy

Following surgery in infants born with tracheo-oesophageal fistula or oesophageal atresia it is not always possible to join the upper and lower ends of the oesophagus in continuity. If a surgical reconnection is delayed to a later date, the child

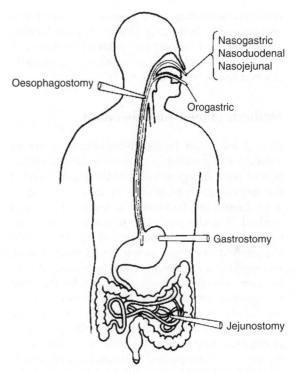

Figure 3.1   Routes of enteral feeding.

Table 3.4   Advantages and disadvantages of various routes of feed administration.

Nasogastric feeds	Gastrostomy feeds	Jejunostomy feeds
Advantages	*Advantages*	*Advantages*
• No surgical procedure required • Placement can be easily taught • Non-invasive	• PEG and RIG tubes can be inserted with a short anaesthetic • No nightly insertion of tube	• No possibility of aspiration • No nightly insertion of tube
Disadvantages	*Disadvantages*	*Disadvantages*
• Nausea • Dislodgement of tube with coughing • Vomiting associated with coughing and reflux • Feeling of satiety • Difficulty in inserting tube • Irritation to the nose and throat • Possibility of aspiration • Visible	• Nausea • Vomiting associated with coughing and reflux • Local infection • Leakage around the exit site causing granuloma formation • Possibility of aspiration • Tube blockage	• Nausea • Tube blockage • Feeling of satiety • Placed under general anaesthesia • Increased risk of nutrient malabsorption • Leakage around the exit site causing granuloma formation • Local infection • Tube dislodgement

PEG, percutaneous endoscopic gastrostomy; RIG, radiologically inserted gastrostomy.
Reprinted with permission of Anita MacDonald.

will receive nutrition via a gastrostomy tube but is encouraged to feed orally to learn normal feeding skills. Any feed or food that is taken orally is collected at an oesophagostomy site and is commonly referred to as a 'sham feed' (p. 145).

Methods of feed administration

Enteral feeds can be given continuously via an enteral feeding pump, or as boluses, or a combination of both. A regimen should be chosen to meet the individual requirements of the child and in most cases it can be tailored to the most practical method of feeding to cause minimum disruption to the child's lifestyle and that of his/her family. Certain situations will dictate a preferred feeding regimen, but a flexible approach to feeding should be taken wherever possible. This enables the child to maintain usual day-to-day activities and for the family to experience minimal disruption to their routines. Flexibility is especially important in children with a need for long term tube feeding who, as time passes, will need a feed that is appropriate to their age and changing nutritional requirements and a regimen that is adaptable as they grow and develop.

Continuous feeding

Generally children will tolerate a slow, continuous infusion of feed better than bolus feeds and this method is sometimes chosen when enteral feeding is first started. Potentially there are fewer problems with intolerance when small feed volumes are infused continuously and there is a smaller time commitment for ward staff and for parents and carers at home. Mobility is affected but is minimised by the use of portable feeding pumps, particularly for children who are on continuous feeding for longer than 12 hours. These portable pumps can be carried by older children as backpacks and for infants can be carried by their parents, carers or attached to a pram or pushchair. Children under 6 years are often too small to carry a heavy backpack, yet cannot be kept still for long periods of continuous feeding. In these children the extra hours of feeding can sometimes be achieved during daytime sleeps and when they are occupied with quieter tasks such as watching television and DVDs.

There are situations where continuous feeding is essential. As previously discussed, feeds given through a nasojejunal tube or a feeding jejunostomy should always be delivered by continuous infusion. Severe gastro-oesophageal reflux can be managed with a slow continuous infusion of feed as an adjunct to anti-reflux medication and positioning. Infants and children with malabsorption will also benefit from a continuous infusion of feed. This will slow transit time and may improve symptoms of diarrhoea, steatorrhoea and abdominal cramps and help to promote weight gain. In children with protracted diarrhoea and short bowel syndrome, continuous enteral feeding with a specialised formula often forms the basis of medical management; continuous tube feeding is also a well established treatment option for children with Crohn's disease to induce remission of disease. Infants and children with glycogen storage disease type I require a frequent supply of dietary glucose to maintain their blood glucose levels within normal limits. A continuous overnight nasogastric infusion of glucose polymer solution or standard feed will maintain blood sugars when children are asleep.

The use of nasogastric tubes for overnight feeding can achieve optimal nutritional intake but may be associated with risks of entanglement and displacement of tubes when infants and children are not closely supervised. There are currently no national guidelines for overnight nasogastric feeding of children but some healthcare professionals no longer advocate or support overnight nasogastric feeding in the community. Development of local policies should involve risk assessments undertaken by the multidisciplinary team and should always consider the medical needs of the individual child.

Intermittent bolus feeding

Bolus tube feeding is successfully used in many children who require enteral feeding both in hospital and at home. Boluses given 3-4 hourly throughout the day via the nasogastric or gastrostomy tube mimics a physiologically normal feeding pattern and can be adapted to fit in with family mealtimes. It is more time consuming than continuous feeding but is the preferred method for many families with children requiring long term feeding as it gives them greater freedom and mobility.

There are situations where bolus feeding is recommended.

- Neonates requiring small volumes may need to be given their feed by hourly bolus as the length of tubing between the reservoir and child creates a 'dead space' holding feed. This can be particularly relevant in infants fed EBM as some fat can be lost by adherence to the sides of the burette and tubing [23].
- Children who have had a surgical anti-reflux procedure are unable to vomit. Large volumes of feed from a continuous infusion can accumulate in the stomach and remain undetected in those who have gastric stasis or poor gastrointestinal motility. This can lead to gastric rupture. Bolus feeding with a gravity feeding pack will prevent over-filling of the stomach as tubes are routinely aspirated before each feed and further feed will be prevented from entering the stomach from the feeding chamber if the stomach is already full.
- Children who frequently try to remove their nasogastric tube risk aspiration if the end of the tube is dislodged into the airways. They will benefit from bolus feeding as they can be constantly supervised during the feed.
- Children with an oesophagostomy who are sham fed should preferably receive bolus feeds to coincide with their oral feeds.
- The continuous delivery of enteral feeds may interfere with the absorption of medications. Bolus feeding will provide periods when medication can be given on an empty stomach to allow optimal absorption.

A schedule of feeding regimens is given in Table 3.5.

Table 3.5   Choosing a suitable feeding regimen.

Regimen	Example
Bolus top-up feeding	*Congenital heart disease* Bottle feeds are not completed due to breathlessness; the remaining feed is topped up via the nasogastric tube
Exclusive bolus feeding	*Long term feeding for children with a neurological handicap* Daytime bolus feeding can allow flexibility and mobility and provide a regimen that can fit in with family mealtimes
	Post-fundoplication Bolus feeding is usually the method of choice for children following a surgical anti-reflux procedure
	Sham feeding Children who are sham fed should receive a bolus feed to coincide with oral feeds
Combination of bolus and continuous feeding	*Chronic illness* Children with anorexia associated with chronic illness may receive a large proportion of their nutrition via a nasogastric or gastrostomy tube. Daytime boluses allow for a normal meal pattern and overnight feeding with a feeding pump reduces the time commitment at night for parents and ward staff
Overnight feeding only	*Supplementary nutrition* Children who require enteral feeding to supplement their poor oral intake or to meet their increased nutritional requirements are usually fed overnight only. This allows the children to maintain a normal daytime eating pattern whilst still providing the nutritional support they require
Continuous feeding only	*Primary disease management* Gastro-oesophageal reflux Malabsorption syndromes (e.g. short gut) Crohn's disease Glycogen storage disease

Enteral feeding equipment

Nasogastric feeding tubes

There is a wide range of paediatric feeding tubes of varying lengths and gauges to meet the requirements of children of all ages. All tubes should conform to British Standards BS 6314 with a male luer connection to avoid connection with intravenous lines and should be radio-opaque to help confirm position. For children, an ideal tube should be of a small gauge with a large internal diameter to make the tube more comfortable and cosmetically acceptable. All tubes will have a syringe adaptor to use for flushing, aspiration or administration of drugs. Some tubes may also have separate side ports.

Polyvinylchloride (PVC) tubes are used for short term enteral feeding. They are for single use only and require changing every week as the tubes stiffen over time and may cause tissue damage. These tubes are least likely to be displaced and so can be used for children who are prone to vomiting.

Fine bore polyurethane or silicone tubes are designed for longer term nasogastric feeding and are very much softer and more comfortable than PVC tubes. Each tube comes with a guidewire or stylet to give the tube rigidity when passed. As a general guide tubes can usually remain *in situ* for 4–6 weeks but manufacturers' instructions regarding usage should always be followed. Unlike PVC tubes which are for single use, these tubes can also be used for overnight feeding and removed during the daytime if storage and cleaning instructions are carefully adhered to.

When passing polyurethane tubes there is a high risk of tracheal intubation in children who have an impaired swallow or who are ventilated. In these children PVC tubes may be preferable despite the need for longer term feeding.

Gastrostomy devices

Gastrostomy devices evolved considerably in the 1990s with an increasing amount of equipment entering the specialised paediatric market. Gastrostomy tubes, whether inserted by an open surgical procedure, PEG or RIG method, are manufactured from pliable biocompatible silicone. PEG and RIG tubes are held in place by a cross bar, plastic disc or bumper that anchors the device to the inside of the stomach wall, preventing inadvertent removal. They require a repeated annual procedure for change of tube, or they can be replaced with a gastrostomy button once the tract has formed. Surgically placed gastrostomy tubes are secured by an inflated balloon which allows easy replacement of the tube. They also have a skin level retention disc preventing migration of the tube. Foley catheters are not ideal but may be used as gastrostomy tubes; they require strapping securely in place, as they have no retention disc and may easily migrate into the duodenum. Children requiring long term gastrostomy feeding will usually elect to have their tube replaced by a gastrostomy button once a tract has been established. These devices are secured within the stomach by an inflated balloon facilitating removal and replacement.

Enteral feeding pumps

Choice of feeding pumps will depend on the requirements of individual hospitals and individual children but there are a number of features that are either essential or desirable:

- occlusion and low battery alarms
- easy to operate
- durable
- tamper proof
- easy to clean
- low noise
- small and lightweight if designed to be portable
- long battery life if designed to be portable
- accurate flow rate setting (5%–10%)
- small flow rate increments (1 mL/hour preferable)
- option of bolus feeding
- good servicing backup

Feed reservoirs

Many sterile ready to feed paediatric formulas are now ready to hang (RTH) and come in pre-filled plastic bottles or flexible packs that can be connected directly to the giving set. This reduces the need for decanting and the consequent risk of bacterial contamination. If using a closed RTH system, the feed reservoir and giving set can be used for up to 24 hours and then discarded.

If it is necessary to decant a feed into a reservoir there are many different flexible and rigid containers on the market for this purpose. Generally children require smaller reservoirs than adults do, especially when using a portable system. Infants requiring small volumes of feed may have their feed decanted into a burette which has a small capacity; this is principally for hospital use.

Bacterial contamination is common [24, 25] so if there is a need to decant feeds this should always be done in a clean environment. Sterilising and re-using feed reservoirs potentially leads to contamination and is not recommended.

The length of time a feed can safely be left 'hanging' varies. While sterile RTH feeds may be delivered over a period of up to 24 hours, local policy will determine the hanging time for reconstituted feeds. Hanging time is much shorter and is generally no longer than 4–6 hours in the hospital setting.

Home enteral feeding

When a decision is made to commence enteral feeding at home it is important that the parents/carers undergo a training programme that will teach them to look after all aspects of feeding and equipment. Correct procedures and adherence to safety are paramount and help and supervision must be given to familiarise the parents with the necessary techniques prior to hospital discharge [26]. Pictorial teaching aids may be used to help families for whom English is not their first language and those unable to read and follow written guidelines [27]. It is essential to identify and liaise with community teams who will be sharing care when a child is discharged; they will have a key role in supporting the child and family. Whilst it is essential that the child receives adequate nutrition the enteral feeding regimen should be planned to fit in as much as possible with the family's lifestyle.

Home enteral feeding companies can supply both feeds and feeding equipment directly to the patient's home. With more companies providing a home delivery service the market has become competitive; they may insist on the use of their own brand of equipment and feeds so it is important to ensure the child gets a suitable pump and feed that have been prescribed based on clinical need.

The National Institute for Health and Care Excellence (NICE) gives recommendations for infection control during enteral feeding in the community [28]. These include guidelines for education of patients, their carers and healthcare personnel; preparation, storage and administration of feeds; care of feeding devices. They recommend that prepackaged ready to use feeds should be used in preference to feeds requiring decanting, reconstitution or dilution, and that reconstituted feeds when used should be administered over a maximum 4 hour period. They acknowledge that the recommendations need to be adapted and incorporated into local practice guidelines.

The social and emotional aspects of tube feeding are often overlooked. Studies have shown that families experience frequent problems with enteral feeding at home related to sleep disturbance, tube dislodgement, tube blockage and difficulties with home delivery of feed and equipment [29, 30]. Dietitians and community nurses need to explore solutions to the common problems associated with overnight feeding. Regular review is necessary in long term patients to continue to identify and minimise problems.

Enteral feeds are prescribed by the general practitioner although the costs for disposable equipment may be funded by a number of different agencies. These include hospital, community and dietetic budgets.

Feed administration and tolerance

The way in which a feed is administered ultimately depends on the clinical condition of the individual child and there are no set rules for starting enteral feeds. Neonates may need to be started on just 1 mL/hour infusion rates whereas older children may tolerate rates of 100 mL/hour. In most cases feeds can be started at full strength with the volume being gradually increased in stages either at an increased infusion rate or as a larger bolus.

Gastrointestinal symptoms are the most common complications of enteral feeding but with the wide choice of feeds, administration techniques and enteral feeding devices it should be possible to minimise gastrointestinal symptoms. Some causes of feed intolerance and their resolution are given in Table 3.6.

Table 3.6 Feed intolerance.

Symptom	Cause	Solution
Diarrhoea	Unsuitable choice of feed in children with impaired gut function	Change to hydrolysed formula or modular feed
	Fast infusion rate	Slow infusion rate and increase as tolerated to provide required nutritional intake
	Intolerance of bolus feeds	Frequent, smaller feeds or change feeding regimen to continuous infusion
	High feed osmolarity	Build up strength of feeds and deliver by continuous infusion
	Contamination of feed	Use sterile commercially produced feeds wherever possible and prepare other feeds in clean environments
	Drugs (e.g. antibiotics, laxatives)	Consider drugs as a cause of diarrhoea before feed is stopped or reduced
Nausea and vomiting	Fast infusion rate	Slowly increase rate of feed infusion or give over a longer period of time
	Slow gastric emptying	Correct positioning and prokinetic drugs
	Psychological factors	Address behavioural feeding issues
	Constipation	Maintain regular bowel motions with adequate fluid intakes, fibre containing feeds and laxatives
	Medicines given at the same time as feeds	Allow time between giving medicines and giving feeds or stop continuous feed for a short time when medicines are given
Regurgitation and aspiration	Gastro-oesophageal reflux	Correct positioning, anti-reflux drugs, feed thickener, fundoplication
	Dislodged tubes	Secure tube adequately and test position of tube regularly
	Fast infusion rate	Slow infusion rate
	Intolerance of bolus feeds	Smaller, more frequent feeds or continuous infusion

Monitoring children on enteral feeds

Children who are commenced on enteral feeds require monitoring and review. There are at present no standards for the monitoring of children on long term enteral feeding at home in the UK.

At the initiation of enteral feeding, goals must be set with respect to the aim of the nutritional intervention, e.g. an improvement in nutritional status, control of symptoms, palliative care, and the expected growth of the child, taking into account their underlying clinical disorder. Regular follow up is required to monitor both short term and longer term progress. Anthropometry, blood tests and control of any symptoms should all be included in the monitoring procedure. As children gain weight and get older their requirements change and follow up is essential to ensure they continue to receive adequate nutrition. Although enteral feeds are formulated to be nutritionally

complete it is wise to check nutritional status with blood tests, particularly if tube feeding is the sole source of nutrition [31]. Routine checks of albumin, electrolytes and haemoglobin are useful as well as assessment of micronutrient status. Blood tests can also be helpful in assessing response to nutritional therapy, e.g. monitoring of inflammatory markers in children with active Crohn's disease. Both hospital and community staff have a role to play in monitoring a child's progress and helping the family cope with tube feeding at home. The needs of a young infant are quite different from those of a toddler or teenager and the individual needs of each child should be considered at different stages of their development.

Regular follow up can be important for the family as well as the child. Home enteral feeding has a big impact on family life, resulting in both psychological and practical problems which should be addressed regularly. Good communication between the family, hospital and community teams is essential and the family must be given a contact for professional help in the case of any emergency.

Another important aspect of follow up is the encouragement to maintain oral feeding skills. Children who miss out on early experiences of taste and texture are much more likely to develop feeding problems [32]. Offering a small amount of food gives children the chance to use the lips and tongue and develop their oromotor skills whilst experiencing a range of tastes. This is particularly important around the time of weaning when children are often more willing to accept different foods. Studies have also shown that in long term tube fed children even tactile stimulation of the face and mouth alone can help re-establish oral feeding [33].

Useful links

PINNT: Patients on Intravenous and Nasogastric Nutrition Therapy (PINNT) is a support group for patients receiving parenteral or enteral nutrition with a sub-group HALF PINNT for children. The group promotes public awareness and encourages contact between patients receiving similar treatment. As well as providing general support the group provides assistance with claiming benefits and can provide members with portable equipment for holidays.

PINNT
PO Box 3126, Christchurch, Dorset, BH23 2XS, UK
www.pinnt.com

4 Parenteral Nutrition

Joanne Louise Price

Introduction

Although parenteral nutrition (PN) in a paediatric patient was first described in 1944 [1], it first became available for general use in the 1960s. Problems with infusion of high concentration hyperosmolar carbohydrate solutions into peripheral veins meant that severe phlebitis limited the length of time PN could be used. However, in 1968 Wilmore and Dudrick [2] and Dudrick *et al.* [3] described the provision of intravenous nutrients to an infant via a central venous catheter. Since that time intravenous lipids have been developed, improving energy density in iso-osmolar solutions. The 1970s saw the development of crystalline amino acid solutions, reducing the risk of anaphylaxis.

PN is now an established therapy, to which many patients of all ages owe their lives. It has transformed the outcome for many previously fatal conditions including feeding preterm infants and postsurgical neonates with short bowel syndrome [4].

The composition of PN continues to be researched, developed and refined. As with many lifesaving procedures PN is not without its risks and it is associated with fatal complications (Table 4.1). PN should therefore not be used casually, but in a disciplined and organised manner in carefully selected patients [5, 6]. Paediatric PN should be prescribed only where there is an experienced multidisciplinary team of doctors, dietitians, pharmacists and nurses contributing to the provision and monitoring of the PN therapy, preferably in an experienced paediatric centre.

Nutrition support teams

It is generally agreed that paediatric parenteral feeding requires considerable clinical, pharmaceutical and nursing skills, with many centres now following the principle of a multidisciplinary nutrition support team (NST) facilitating treatment with PN [6, 7]. However, a report from the National Confidential Enquiry into Patient Outcome and Death (NCEPOD) of a case based observational peer review of PN clinical practice in England, Wales and Northern Ireland found wide variability in practice [8]. Seventy children and 264 neonates in 74 hospitals (as well as 877 adults) were surveyed. Good practice, defined as 'a standard that the reviewer would accept from themselves and their trainees in their institution' was found in only 24% of those neonates surveyed. Areas of concern raised included delayed commencement of PN, inconsistent nutrient provision and inconsistent monitoring and review.

Clinical Paediatric Dietetics, Fourth Edition. Edited by Vanessa Shaw.
© 2015 John Wiley & Sons, Ltd. Published 2015 by John Wiley & Sons, Ltd.
Companion Website: www.wiley.com/go/shaw/paediatricdietetics

Table 4.1   Some complications of parenteral nutrition.

Gut related	Solution related	Line related
Villous atrophy	Over/under delivery of nutrients	Sepsis
Decreased digestive enzyme activity	Hyperglycaemia	Catheter occlusion
Cholestasis	Hyperlipidaemia	Accidental line removal
Bacterial overgrowth/bacterial translocation	Micronutrient toxicity	Site infection
Fluid/electrolyte imbalance	Toxic effects of non-nutrient components	
Metabolic bone disease	of solutions	
	Growth failure	
	Refeeding syndrome	
	Cholestasis	
	Metabolic bone disease	

NCEPOD stated that it would be valuable to develop a team approach to parenteral nutritional support, recognising that this should be a multidisciplinary exercise with sharing of expertise. The report also recommends that a large scale national audit of PN care in children in the UK should be undertaken to determine the quality of PN care in this group of patients.

Good interdisciplinary communication is paramount if patient care is to be of the highest standard. Improvement in outcome of PN has been demonstrated where a multidisciplinary NST is involved [7, 9–12]. Core members of the team and their roles:

- paediatric consultant – often a paediatric gastroenterologist oversees patient care
- paediatric surgeon – inserts feeding lines and advises regarding surgical management as required; many PN dependent children have a surgical diagnosis and will be under the overall care of a paediatric surgeon
- paediatric dietitian – see below
- medical specialist paediatric registrar – advises on prescription of PN and many other aspects of care
- PN pharmacist – responsible for production and checking of solutions, advises regarding prescription when necessary
- PN nurse – trains carers and staff, coordinates patient care
- biochemist – advises on monitoring and interpretation of blood biochemistry and appropriate biochemical tests.

The NST produces protocols and procedures and organises audit and reviews of the PN service; it may be monitored by the hospital's nutrition steering committee.

Other key members of the NST to include as required are psychologists, speech and language therapists, play specialists. These have a particularly important role with children undergoing long term PN.

The role of the dietitian in paediatric parenteral nutrition

As a key member of the NST [12, 13] the dietitian ensures the child's nutritional requirements are met in order to maintain adequate growth and development. There is also a role in the development of the child's oral feeding skills. The dietitian will:

- set targets for enteral and parenteral feeding and devise a feeding plan
- monitor that correct volumes of prescribed enteral feeds/PN are received
- calculate total nutrient intake and compare with the individual's requirements
- use appropriate centile charts to plot the child's height, weight and head circumference. It is imperative that inadequate growth is recognised and discussed with the NST at the earliest opportunity
- advise regarding suitable adjustments to feeding regimens to enhance intake and absorption and if necessary advise on changes to feeds in cases of malabsorption or feed intolerance
- review the nutritional biochemistry and contribute to the discussion and decision making with regard to nutrient intakes and adjustments to the PN

The NST usually reviews the child's progress at least weekly, with daily reviews by some specialties as necessary. In centres where NSTs have been established, reported benefits include a reduction in mechanical line problems, reduced sepsis, fewer metabolic complications, shorter courses of PN (due to faster transition to appropriate enteral formulas) and savings on the cost of providing PN [9–11].

Learning points

- *PN usage is increasing and practice varies widely across the UK*
- *Research on some components of PN (e.g. lipids) is proliferating rapidly*
- *Nutrition support teams improve outcomes in PN patients*
- *Dietitians have a key role within the NST in ensuring adequate delivery of nutrients*

Indications for parenteral nutrition in children

Indications for PN are given in Table 4.2. This is not an exhaustive list. PN is a hazardous and expensive form of nutritional support in children and is indicated only where enteral nutrition cannot prevent or reverse growth failure. The timing and duration of PN is dependent upon the child's nutritional reserves, expected duration of starvation and severity of illness. PN is normally built up over 2–4 days and therefore it is neither reasonable nor clinically indicated to routinely prescribe PN for less than 5 days [14]. Some long term patients will require PN for a number of years, sometimes into adulthood.

Considerations in paediatric parenteral nutrition

Enteral nutrition

PN is associated with many complications and for this reason it is widely accepted that enteral nutrition should always be given where possible. If the gut works, it should be used, even if only minimal feeds are tolerated [15]. Absence of luminal nutrients has been associated with atrophic changes in the gut mucosa and it is well recognised that enteral feeding is the single most effective way of preventing many gut related complications.

Nutritionally insignificant volumes of enteral nutrition have been found to have a trophic effect on the gut, encouraging intestinal adaptation, and have been linked to enhanced gut motility, decreased incidence of PN induced cholestasis and decreased bacterial translocation [16, 17, 18]. After gastrointestinal surgery, particularly that resulting in short bowel syndrome, intraluminal nutrients and luminal substrates are essential for optimal intestinal adaptation [19]. Initiation of enteral feeding is strongly recommended early in the postoperative period.

Breast milk or standard infant formulas are indicated unless there has been previous evidence of malabsorption or feed intolerance. Short frequent breast feeds or small boluses of expressed breast

Table 4.2 Indications for parenteral nutrition in children.

Intestinal failure	Other common indications	Patients requiring additional nutrition support
Short bowel syndrome	Functional immaturity in preterm infants	Trauma, burns
Surgical and gastrointestinal abnormalities, e.g. gastroschisis, intestinal atresia	Chemotherapy (leading to acute intestinal failure)	Chronic kidney disease
Necrotising enterocolitis	Pancreatitis	Liver disease
Protracted diarrhoea	Chronic aspiration due to gastro-oesophageal reflux	Malignant disease
Malabsorption syndromes		
Inflammatory bowel disease		
Chronic pseudo-obstruction		

milk or infant formula, as little as 1–2 mL/hour, are beneficial. If there are signs of malabsorption a hydrolysed protein feed, which is also lactose free and has a proportion of its fat as medium chain triglycerides, may be indicated, e.g. Pregestimil Lipil, Pepti-Junior. It may be advantageous to deliver the feed continuously via an enteral feeding pump to aid absorption. (More detailed management of intestinal failure is discussed in Chapter 8.)

Growth

Malnutrition in children results in impaired growth and development. All children on PN should be weighed and measured regularly and the measurements recorded and plotted on appropriate centile charts to ensure appropriate growth is maintained.

Nutritional requirements and demands vary considerably with age and size, with critical periods in infancy and puberty when growth is fastest. The majority of brain growth occurs in the last trimester of pregnancy and the first 2 years of life. Extra special care should be taken to avoid malnutrition and biochemical abnormalities at this time as poor nutrition during these critical periods not only results in slowing and stunting of growth but may permanently affect neurological development [20, 21].

Infants are at considerable risk due to their limited energy reserves and the commencement of PN in a small infant who cannot tolerate enteral feeds is a matter of urgency. A preterm infant weighing 1 kg has only 1% body fat and may survive for only 4 days if starved [22].

Equally adolescents are at significant risk of not achieving their growth potential if nutrient requirements are not met at the onset of and during puberty.

Cholestasis and liver disease

The prevalence of PN associated liver disease (PNALD) is much greater in children than in adults. It has been reported that up to 65% of infants on PN develop abnormal liver function tests within 2–3 weeks of starting PN [23, 24]. The pathogenesis of PNALD is not completely understood. The aetiology is thought to be multifactorial and can progress to cirrhosis and end stage liver

failure in some cases [25]. The early introduction of enteral feeding is the most important measure that can be taken to help reduce the risk of cholestasis [6, 26].

In preterm neonates enteral feeding may be delayed or withheld in order to help prevent necrotising enterocolitis (NEC); this has been an area of much debate. A recent Cochrane analysis found that delaying enteral feeds increased length of stay, prolonged use of PN and increased the incidence of cholestasis [27]. Results of a UK multicentre trial (ADEPT) concluded that 'Early introduction of enteral feeds in growth-restricted preterm infants results in earlier achievement of full enteral feeding and does not appear to increase the risk of NEC' [28]. Therefore enteral feeding should be introduced as early as possible, even in preterm infants. Recent American guidelines recommend that all preterm babies over 1000 g are commenced on minimal feeds by the second day of life [29].

As well as lack of enteral feeds, PNALD is associated with intrauterine growth retardation, prematurity, immature enterohepatic circulation, underlying disease, number of infections/septic episodes, number of surgical procedures and number of blood transfusions [30, 31]. PN solutions themselves may have a role to play in the development of liver disease; lipid emulsions have been implicated [32] and overfeeding of glucose has been associated with hepatic steatosis [25]. High risk for PNALD is also associated with PN dependency from a young age, very short bowel and predicted prolonged PN.

Cyclical, rather than continuous, PN (p. 64) and cycling of lipid in particular (and sometimes restricting lipid to certain nights of the week) may afford some protection to the liver and is common practice in patients on long term PN, particularly those who have PN at home. This usually involves giving the PN over a shorter period allowing some hours off. There are obvious implications to energy intake and tolerance of solutions and these need to be monitored carefully. Due to the implications on growth, particularly where lipid is restricted, cycling should only be used in long term stable patients who have an experienced NST looking after them. Cases of PNALD which do not improve should be referred to a supraregional liver unit for assessment at the earliest opportunity. Other measures taken to prevent or reverse PNALD include the use of ursodeoxycholic acid, a synthetic bile acid, and treatment of bacterial overgrowth caused by intestinal stasis. This will help to prevent recurrent sepsis from translocation of bacteria across the gastrointestinal wall.

Learning points – Prevention of PNALD

- *Early enteral feeding even if only minimal*
- *Oral feeding if possible*
- *Avoidance of line sepsis by rigorous line care*
- *Prompt treatment of sepsis*
- *Cyclical PN – particularly lipid*
- *Use of ursodeoxycholic acid*
- *Use of lipid solutions containing ω3 PUFA (Table 4.5)*

PN related bone disease

Children on long term PN can develop a type of bone disease resembling rickets. The aetiology is multifactorial and may be related to physical inactivity, underlying disease, disordered vitamin D metabolism, hypercalcuria, raised alkaline phosphatase and hypophosphataemia.

Regular biochemical monitoring including measurements of urinary calcium, plasma calcium, plasma phosphorus, plasma parathyroid hormone, vitamin D concentrations and serum alkaline phosphatase activity along with dual-energy x-ray absorptiometry scanning is recommended to evaluate these children [13, 33]. Referral to an endocrine/metabolic specialist may be necessary in cases of concern.

Oral hypersensitivity

Oral hypersensitivity occurs when the oral route is not used for feeding for lengthy periods of time. Lack of stimulation together with unpleasant oral procedures/experiences such as intubations, suction, vomiting, choking may lead to long term feeding problems. Steps to prevent oral feeding aversion will help progress onto enteral feeding and subsequent reduction in PN.

Early involvement of a specialist speech and language therapist to advise regarding oral

desensitisation is recommended, particularly in cases of refusal to feed or distress during feeding. A play specialist can work with children around oral desensitisation using messy play and play involving food. In addition to these specialist techniques early and sustained oral feeding when safe to do so, use of dummies (pacifiers), sips and tastes should always be employed (where safe to do so) to maintain oral function, especially in infancy.

Learning points – PN in children

- *Continuing growth with key stages of development*
- *Immature liver and bowel*
- *Inefficient enzyme production*
- *Susceptibility to PNALD*
- *Immature immune system, increased susceptibility to infection*
- *Vulnerable to central venous line infection*
- *High risk of cross-contamination due to inability to self-care*
- *Oral feeding often not established, aversion common*
- *Delayed weaning from PN due to inability to feed orally*

Nutrient requirements and solutions

Recommended requirements vary and tend to be based on clinical experience [6, 8, 20, 34, 35]. The European Society of Paediatric Gastroenterology, Hepatology and Nutrition (ESPGHAN) guidelines [13] are the most recent with regard to paediatric PN at the time of writing.

Fluid and electrolytes

Age, size, fluid balance, the environment and clinical conditions are all factors affecting fluid requirements. Recommendations are given in Table 4.3. Cardiac impairment, renal disease and respiratory insufficiency are examples of conditions that may limit fluid volumes, whereas high fluid losses due to diarrhoea, high output fistula/stoma and fever may all increase fluid needs.

Table 4.3 Summary of parenteral fluid and electrolyte requirements for children.

Age/weight	Fluid (mL/kg/day)	Na (mmol/kg/day)	K (mmol/kg/day)
<1500 g	140–180	2.0–3.0	1.0–2.0
>1500 g	140–160	3.0–5.0	1.0–3.0
Preterm to 2 months	140–160	2.0–5.0	1.5–5.0
2 months to 1 year	120–180	2.0–3.0	1.0–3.0
1–2 years	80–150	1.0–3.0	1.0–3.0
3–5 years	80–100	1.0–3.0	1.0–3.0
6–12 years	60–80	1.0–3.0	1.0–3.0
13–18 years	50–70	1.0–3.0	1.0–3.0

Source: Adapted from [13].

Also additional fluid may be needed if radiant heaters/phototherapy are used.

Infants have immature organ systems and require high volumes of fluid in order to excrete electrolytes sufficiently. Young children are physiologically unable to concentrate urine and conserve fluid as effectively as adults. Maximum urine concentrations are 550 mOsm/L in preterm infants and 700 mOsm/L in term infants compared with 1200 mOsm/L in adults [36]. Electrolyte requirements are often higher, but dehydration and metabolic acidosis can occur if these are given without adequate fluid. Care should always be taken that fluid requirements are met.

Electrolyte requirements vary with age, clinical condition and blood biochemistry. Electrolyte solutions are usually added to PN in response to each individual child's blood biochemistry.

Due to very tight homeostatic mechanisms, sodium depletion is not always reflected in blood biochemistry. Sodium depletion can be a direct cause of poor growth. Monitoring of urinary sodium excretion to assess total body sodium is useful especially in cases of high sodium losses such as high output fistula or cystic fibrosis. A low (<20 mmol/L) urinary sodium concentration indicates the need for increased enteral/parenteral sodium provision.

The available fluid volume for PN may influence the choice of nutrient solutions and the route of delivery. Some of the available fluid for PN may be taken up by medications. If concentrated PN solutions are needed to provide adequate nutrition (due to fluid restrictions), then the peripheral route for delivering the solutions may be contraindicated as there is a risk that they will cause thrombophlebitis. Children who are severely fluid restricted will only receive adequate nutrition if the necessarily concentrated PN is delivered via a central venous catheter.

Macronutrients

Recommendations for macronutrient intakes are summarised in Table 4.4.

Energy

Diet induced thermogenesis reflects the amount of energy needed for food digestion and absorption and usually accounts for about 10% of daily energy needs. Generally parenteral energy requirements are around 10% less than enteral requirements for this reason.

If energy intakes are inadequate protein accretion falls and dietary/intravenous protein will be metabolised for energy. The child may become catabolic using body tissue protein stores for fuel. This results in linear growth failure. Adequate energy intake will promote weight gain, but will not always promote linear growth in the absence of adequate protein.

Many well infants and children will achieve their expected growth rate if the energy intakes shown in Table 4.4 are provided. An appropriate gain in weight for the age, sex and size of the individual child, taking the clinical condition into consideration, is likely to indicate that the prescription is adequate.

In the disease state these requirements will vary and research suggests that actual energy requirements for many children are less than originally thought [37]. It is recommended that energy intakes should be adapted for those disease states found to increase resting energy expenditure, e.g. head injury, burn injury, pulmonary and cardiac disease [13]. Also extremely low birthweight neonates requiring ventilation have been found to have significantly increased rates of energy expenditure [38]. Uncomplicated surgery does not significantly increase energy requirements [39, 40]. In critically ill children energy requirements vary from day to day [41]. The very sick child may not have significantly increased resting energy expenditure as

Table 4.4 Summary of recommended daily intakes of macronutrients from PN.

Energy		Amino acids		Lipid		CHO	
Age	(kcal/kg)	Age	(g/kg)	Age	(g/kg)	Weight (kg)	(g/kg)
Prem	110–120	Prem	1.5–4	Prem	3–4	Up to 3	Up to 18
0–1 years	90–100	Term	1.5–3	Infants	3–4	3–10	16–18
1–7 years	75–90	2 months to 3 years	1.0–2.5			10–15	12–14
7–12 years	60–75					15–20	10–12
						20–30	<12
12–18 years	30–60	3–18 years	1.0–2.0	Older children	2–3	>30	<10

Prem, preterm; CHO, carbohydrate. 1 kcal = 4.18 kJ.
Source: Adapted from [13].

the catabolic process inhibits growth [42]. Recommendations specifically relating to neonates can be found elsewhere [13, 43, 44].

Whichever estimate of energy requirement is used for an individual child it is essential to monitor closely to ensure appropriate growth is achieved without adverse biochemical consequences.

Lipid

Lipid preparations provide a concentrated source of energy in an isotonic solution: 2 kcal (8 kJ)/mL in a 20% lipid solution compared with only 0.8 kcal (3 kJ)/mL in a 20% carbohydrate solution. When the fluid volume is limited, maximum energy intake can only be achieved via a *central* venous catheter by using dextrose and fat mixtures. Lipid emulsions normally contribute 25%–40% of non-protein energy. However, lipid emulsion via a *peripheral* vein can help provide sufficient energy for growth, avoiding the complications associated with central venous access, and it may prolong the life of peripheral lines in infants [45].

Intravenous lipid particles in solution resemble endogenously produced chylomicrons in terms of size and are hydrolysed by lipoprotein lipase. Intravenous lipids provide essential fatty acids (EFAs) and improve net nitrogen balance compared with glucose alone as a source of non-protein energy [25]. Current ESPGHAN guidelines [13] make no specific recommendation about the type of lipid used but suggest that a minimum *linoleic acid* intake of 0.25 g/kg/day should be given to preterm infants and 0.1 g/kg/day to term infants and older children to prevent EFA deficiency. In premature infants, due to low stores, EFA deficiency can occur within 72 hours of birth [46].

Intravenous lipid emulsions available in the UK that are considered safe for use in paediatric PN are given in Table 4.5. All solutions contain glycerol and phospholipids and are available as 10% and 20% emulsions.

Higher concentration emulsions are advantageous where there is fluid restriction and also deliver less phospholipid per gram of triglyceride, leading to more normal plasma phospholipids and cholesterol levels [47]. In children it is recommended that 20% or higher concentrations of lipid emulsions are used due to the higher phospholipids:triglyceride ratio found in 10% emulsions [13].

Lipid emulsions currently used are either based on long chain triglycerides (LCT) or long chain and medium chain triglycerides (MCT) mixed together. Both LCT and MCT/LCT solutions are considered safe to use in paediatrics.

Soya oil emulsions have been available for many years and are the most commonly used. There have been some concerns over the effect of the highly polyunsaturated, unphysiological fatty acid supply from soybean oil. The development of PNALD seems to be associated with the composition of the soybean oil based lipid emulsion, possibly as a result of the pro-inflammatory metabolites of ω6 fatty acids. There is mounting evidence that the ω6 polyunsaturated fatty acids (PUFA) most prevalent in soybean oil may in part have a role in the onset of liver injury [32].

Olive oil emulsions may produce more physiological levels of linoleic and oleic acid and better antioxidant status [48]. However, there is currently not enough evidence to recommend one particular solution above another.

Table 4.5 20% lipid emulsions*.

Name	Manufacturer	Composition	TG (g/L)	Energy (kcal/mL)	Soya oil (g/L)	Olive oil (g/L)	Fish oil (g/L)	MCT (g/L)	α-tocopherol (mg/L)
Intralipid	Fresenius Kabi	Soya	200	2	200	0	0	0	240
ClinOleic	Baxter	80% olive 20% soya	200	2	40	160	0	0	No data
Lipofundin MCT/LCT	B Braun	50% soya 50% coconut	200	2	100	0	0	100	170 ± 40
SMOF	Fresenius Kabi	30% soya 30% coconut 25% olive 15% fish	200	2	60	50	30	60	169–225
Lipidem	B Braun	40% soya 50% coconut 10% fish	200	2	80	0	20	100	190 ± 30
Omegaven[†]	Fresenius Kabi	100% fish	200	2	0	0	200	0	130–296

TG, triglycerides; MCT, medium chain triglycerides; LCT, long chain triglycerides. 1 kcal = 1.48 kJ.
*Some 10% emulsions are available but are not recommended due to the high phospholipid/triglycerides ratio [13].
[†]Omegaven is to be used as a supplement, not a complete source of lipid.

Coconut oil emulsions (MCT) have the advantage of carnitine independent uptake by the mitochondria and therefore have a more rapid clearance from the plasma after infusion. Solutions with 50% MCT have been used in paediatric PN for many years. MCT solutions contain approximately 50% less EFAs than LCT solutions alone, yet measured plasma EFAs and their derivatives (linoleic and alpha linolenic acid) were similar compared with LCT solutions [49–51].

Fish oil emulsions contain a significant amount of ω3 PUFA. A number of paediatric reports have cited improvements in liver function tests and a drop in conjugated bilirubin and reversal of PNALD when patients were switched from soybean based lipid solutions to fish oil containing solutions [52–55]. There is an emulsion of fish oil alone (Omegaven) which may be used temporarily as mono therapy, but due to risks of EFA deficiency it cannot be recommended for long term use and is used as a 'rescue therapy' in PNALD [56].

SMOF (Fresenius Kabi) will provide just 30% and Lipedem (BBraun) 40% of EFAs contained in Intralipid due to the relatively lower soya oil content of these solutions. This is still adequate at normal volumes but may quickly become inadequate if lipid intake is restricted. To date there has been no published multicentre randomised control trial to assess the long term physiological effects of fish oil solutions. There are also reports that

fibrosis seen on liver biopsy may persist despite the improved liver function tests [57, 58]. As such these lipid solutions are recommended for compassionate use in carefully selected individuals and those at high risk of PNALD [56, 59] (p. 185).

Serum lipid levels should be monitored to ensure adequate clearance and hence utilisation. Clearance of lipids from the plasma is limited by the rate of activity of lipoprotein lipase. The amount of fat infused should be adapted to the lipid oxidation capacity, approximately 3–4 g/kg/day [5, 13]. Hyperlipidaemia will result if the enzyme is saturated by excessive doses of fat or by rapid infusion [60]. Gradually increasing the volume of the lipid emulsion by 1 g/kg/day over 3–4 days and maintaining a steady rate of infusion helps prevent possible hypertriglyceridaemia. Tolerance of lipid emulsions has been found to be improved if given continuously in preterm infants [61] although it is usual practice to give 4 hours off the infusion per 24 hours to allow all administered fat to clear the circulation before the next infusion begins. Serum lipids should be monitored as the volume of fat given increases and should always be taken 4 hours after the infusion is completed. Peak levels of triglyceride and free fatty acids normally occur towards the end of the infusion, returning to fasting levels 2–4 hours later. Once they are stable, weekly monitoring is likely to be sufficient.

In malnourished children, it is good practice to assess baseline serum lipids prior to starting PN as children who have failed to thrive or lost weight due to suboptimal intake frequently have raised triglyceride levels that return to normal when sufficient energy is provided. Restricting lipid, and therefore energy, would not be beneficial in this case. A reduced lipid dose may be indicated for children with a marked risk of hyperlipidaemia, e.g. low birth weight infants, sepsis, catabolism [13].

EFA deficiency can be prevented with as little as 0.5–1.0 g/kg total lipid/day [13, 62], although suboptimal energy intake will be the limiting factor. As discussed above, reduction in lipid intake may improve abnormal liver function; however, this cannot be sustained over a long period due to suboptimal energy provision and a long term effect on growth.

If reducing intake for any reason including treating PNALD the source of lipid is an important consideration; as discussed, not all solutions contain equivalent long chain triglyceride levels and subsequently vary in their EFA content (see above).

Some intravenous medication may be given in fat emulsions, e.g. the sedative propofol or the antifungal amphotericin. Consideration should be made of the fat (and therefore energy) content of this.

Learning points – lipid solutions

- *Soya, MCT, fish and olive oil solutions are available, research ongoing*
- *10% solutions not recommended in paediatric PN due to high ratio of phospholipids to triglycerides*
- *20% solutions most widely available ≡ 200 g TG/1000 mL (20 kcal/100 mL)*
- *Lipids should provide 25%–40% of non-protein energy*
- *0.5 g–1 g/kg/day LCT required to prevent EFA deficiency*
- *Solutions containing lower LCT levels will be lower in EFAs*

α-tocopherol

α-tocopherol is the most important lipid soluble antioxidant; it helps prevent tissue damage by free radicals produced from peroxidation of the PUFA within parenteral lipid solutions [63].

Most parenteral lipid solutions have α-tocopherol present in adequate amounts for this reason (Table 4.5).

Amino acids

Crystalline L-amino acid solutions are used as the nitrogen source for PN. Despite routine use of PN, surprisingly few clinical efficacy data are available to guide total or specific amino acid dosing in paediatric (and adult) patients.

Commercially available mixed amino acid formulations provide both essential and non-essential amino acids. All provide the nine essential amino acids (histidine, isoleucine, leucine, lysine, methionine, phenylalanine, threonine, tryptophan and valine). They also contain varying amounts of classically non-essential amino acids that may become conditionally essential under certain circumstances. In children arginine, cysteine, glycine, proline, taurine and tyrosine may be conditionally essential [13].

The products designed for use in infants and children are Vaminolact, which is based on breast milk amino acid profile, and Primene, which is based on the profile of cord blood (Table 4.6). The ideal amino acid profile for PN solutions for infants and children is still unclear. A solution which contains insufficient quantities of essential amino acids will inhibit protein synthesis and may limit growth [64].

Estimates of protein requirements are often based on 10%–20% of the total energy intake (Table 4.4). All nitrogen can be converted to energy (via the Krebs cycle) and where inadequate energy is provided (from fat and carbohydrate) the child may become hypoproteinaemic as nitrogen is used for energy. The child subsequently will not grow. Sufficient energy intake is 30–40 kcal (125–165 kJ)/g protein or 250 kcal (1.05 MJ)/g nitrogen [65], although in preterm infants this ratio may indeed be less: 150–200 kcal (630–835 kJ)/g nitrogen [43].

Guidelines [13] are based on amounts required to maintain nitrogen balance and growth. Whilst it is difficult to assess if nitrogen provision is adequate it is generally agreed that inadequate nitrogen intake is reflected by a low plasma urea level and poor linear growth. (A high plasma urea level is more likely to be attributable to dehydration than over-provision of nitrogen.)

Table 4.6 Amino acid solutions.

Name	Manufacturer	Total AA (g/L)	Cysteine (g/L)	Tyrosine (g/L)	Taurine (g/L)	Comment
Aminoplasmal (10%)	B Braun	100	0	0.4	0	For children >2 years
Primene (10%)	Baxter	100	1.89	0.45	0.6	For neonatal and infant PN
Vamin 9 Glucose	Fresenius Kabi	70	1.4	0.5	0	Contains glucose 100 g/L
Vaminolact	Fresenius Kabi	65	1.0	0.5	0.3	For neonatal and infant PN

AA, amino acids.

Learning points – amino acid solutions

- *Based on cord blood or breast milk amino acid profiles so not necessarily the ideal profile for growing children*
- *Aim to provide 10%–20% of energy from protein*
- *Protein in PN normally expressed as nitrogen (N) or amino acids (AA)*
- *$1 g N \equiv 7.5 g AA \equiv 6.25 g P$*
- *In order to ensure efficient protein utilisation and tissue accretion sufficient energy should be given alongside nitrogen $\equiv 250 kcal/g N$*
- *Low plasma urea levels, particularly in preterm infants, may indicate inadequate nitrogen provision*

Glutamine

Endogenous biosynthesis of glutamine may be insufficient for tissue needs in states of metabolic stress. Trials in adults have suggested that glutamine supplementation improves clinical outcomes in critically ill adults [66]. It has been suggested that glutamine supplementation may benefit preterm infants, particularly very low birth weight infants. However, a systematic review concluded that glutamine supplementation does not have a statistically significant effect on mortality, invasive infection, necrotising enterocolitis, time to achieve full enteral nutrition or duration of hospital stay [67]. Currently is no evidence for the routine supplementation of glutamine in preterm infants and there is no evidence for its routine use in paediatric PN.

Carnitine

Carnitine is a nitrogen based compound and plays a role in the beta-oxidation of long chain fatty acids which it transports across the mitochondrial membrane in the form of carnitine esters. Carnitine is present in breast milk and formula feeds but current PN formulations do not contain it. Carnitine can usually be synthesised in the liver from lysine and methionine and the ability to synthesise it is age dependent [68]. Non-supplemented parenterally fed infants have very low tissue carnitine levels [69]. Relative carnitine deficiency may impair fatty acid oxidation. However, a Cochrane review has failed to find evidence to support the routine supplementation of parenterally fed neonates with carnitine [70] and further studies in this group are required. It is recommended that carnitine supplementation should be considered on an individual basis in infants on exclusive PN for more than 4 weeks [13].

Carbohydrate

The major source of non-protein calories in PN is D-glucose (dextrose). Carbohydrate normally provides 60%–70% of the total non-protein energy intake. Glucose is an essential fuel for infants and is the most important substrate for brain cell metabolism; a continuous supply is essential for normal neurological function. Excessive intravenous glucose administration can lead to hyperglycaemia, hepatic steatosis, excessive carbon dioxide production, EFA deficiency (in the absence of lipid) and impaired protein metabolism [25]. Insulin resistance may occur in some situations, e.g. steroid use, very low birth weight, sepsis, trauma and stress. Glucose infusion rates may need to be reduced in order to prevent hyperglycaemia. In critically ill adults it is accepted practice to use insulin infusions to manage hyperglycaemia; in children this has not been sufficiently researched and should only be considered when reduction of glucose infusion has failed [13].

Glucose should be administered gradually, increasing over 3–4 days to maximum infusion rates. Rates of glucose oxidation vary significantly with age and clinical status. It is recommended in term neonates and children up to 2 years of age that glucose intake should not exceed 18 g/kg/day [13,71]. Infusion rates exceeding glucose oxidative capacity result in conversion of carbohydrate to fatty acids and can consume up to 15% of the available energy from carbohydrate [72].

In cyclical PN the maximal rate of glucose infusion may exceed glucose oxidation rate. The maximal infusion rate should not exceed 1.2 g/kg/hour (20 mg/kg/min) [13].

Learning points – parenteral carbohydrate

- *Should make up 60%–70% of the non-protein energy provision*
- *Maximum infusion of 18 g/kg/day should not be exceeded*
- *Maximum delivery rates of 1.2 g/kg/hour should not be exceeded*
- *Solutions given cyclically should be ramped up and down during the initial and final 2 hours of the infusion to prevent hyperglycaemia and hypoglycaemia (Table 4.10)*

Micronutrients

A summary of reasonable intakes of micronutrients for paediatric PN can be found in Tables 4.7 and 4.8. These are guidelines and should be used in conjunction with the document from which they are taken [13]. Requirements for intravenous vitamins in infants and children remain unclear. The last major publication on parenteral vitamin requirements in children was in 1988 [73]. A Cochrane review [74] in premature (<32 weeks' gestation) infants found an association between supply of vitamin A and a reduction in death or oxygen requirement at 1 month of age and of oxygen requirement at 38 weeks post-menstrual age. Current knowledge is based on the historical use of available vitamin and mineral solutions and the apparent lack of deficiencies/complications associated with this. Optimal requirements in children have not been determined and there has been little published research on this topic in the last 20 years.

Following the guidelines currently in use appears to maintain blood levels within acceptable ranges for infants and children and is based on expert opinion [5,13,73,75]. The amount of intravenous vitamins given is usually recommended to

Table 4.7 Vitamin solutions.

Vitamin	Water soluble	Fat soluble	Suggested reasonable intakes, adapted from [13]	
	Solvito (Fresenius Kabi) per vial (10 mL)	Vitlipid Infant* (Fresenius Kabi) per vial (10 mL)	Infants (kg/day)	Children (dose/day)
Dose	1 mL/kg	10 mL/day		
Vitamin A (µg)	0	690	150–300	150
Vitamin D (µg)	0	10 (400 IU)	0.8 (32 IU)	10 (400 IU)
Vitamin E (mg)	0	7.9	2.8–3.5	7.0
Vitamin K (µg)	0	200	10	200
Thiamin B$_1$ (mg)	2.5	0	0.35–0.5	1.2
Riboflavin B$_2$ (mg)	3.6	0	0.15–0.2	1.4
Pyridoxine B$_6$ (mg)	4.0	0	0.15–0.2	1.0
Cobalamin B$_{12}$ (µg)	5.0	0	0.3	1.0
Vitamin C (mg)	100	0	15–25	80
Niacin (mg)	40	0	4.0–6.8	17
Pantothenic acid (mg)	15	0	1.0–2.0	5.0
Biotin (µg)	60	0	5.0–8.0	20
Folic acid (µg)	400	0	56	140

No upper limits are given; care must be taken to avoid over-delivery of individual nutrients. Where nutrient mixtures are used manufacturers' guidelines should be followed.
*In 10% Intralipid.

Table 4.8 Recommended intakes of trace elements and solutions.

Trace element (Atomic mass)	Requirement (ESPGHAN 2005) [13]	Paediatric (<40 kg)			Adult	
		Peditrace (Fresenius Kabi) (µg/1 mL)	Peditrace (Fresenius Kabi) (µmol/1 mL)	Tracutil (B Braun) (µmol/1 mL)	Decan (Baxter) (µmol/1 mL)	Additrace (Fresenius Kabi) (µmol/1 mL)
Iron (55.845) Not necessary in short term PN (<3 weeks duration) Monitor carefully to avoid toxicity (see text)	Preterm: up to 200 µg/kg/day (3.58 µmol/kg/day) Infant and child: 50–100 µg/kg/day (0.895–1.76 µmol/kg/day)	0	0	3.5	0.45	2.0
Zinc (65.39) Preterm infants and children with thermal injuries may have increased requirements	Preterm: 450–500 µg/kg/day (6.9–7.6 µmol/kg/day) Infant <3 months: 250 µg/kg/day (3.8 µmol/kg/day) Infant >3 months: 100 µg/kg/day (1.52 µmol/kg/day) Child: 50 µg/kg/day (max 5 mg/day) (0.76–1.52 µmol/kg/day) (max 76.5 µmol/day)	250	3.82	5.0	3.8	10
Copper (63.54) Requirements may increase with high gastrointestinal losses or thermal injuries Toxicity risk in cholestasis	20 µg/kg/day (0.315 µmol/kg/day)	20	0.315	1.2	0.19	2.0
Manganese (24.305) In toxicity CNS deposition of manganese can occur without symptoms Monitor regularly	1 µg/kg/day (max 50 µg/day) (0.029 µmol/kg/day) (max 2.06 µmol/day)	1	0.0182	1.0	0.091	0.5
Chromium (51.99) A contaminant – not usually added to PN	0.2 µg/kg/day (max 5 µg/kg/day) (max 0.004 µmol/kg/day) 0.096 µmol/day)	0	0	0.02	0.007	0.02
Selenium (78.96)	2–3 µg/kg/day (0.03–0.04 µmol/kg/day)	2	0.0253	0.03	0.022	0.04
Iodine (126.90) Optimal dose unclear	1 µg/day (0.008 µmol/kg/day)	1	0.0079	0.1	0.0003	0.1
Fluoride (18.99)		57	3.0	0.3	1.9	5.0
Molybdenum (95.94)	Preterm: 1 µg/kg/day (0.01 µmol/kg/day) Infant and child: 0.25 µg/kg/day (max 5 µg/day) (0.003 µmol/kg/day) (max 0.05 µmol/day)	0	0	0.01	0.0065	0.02

Where upper limits are not given care must be taken to avoid over-delivery of individual nutrients. Where nutrient mixtures are used manufacturers' guidelines should be followed. PN, parenteral nutrition; CNS, central nervous system.
Source: Adapted from [13].

Table 4.9 Suggested intakes of parenteral calcium, phosphorus and magnesium.

Age	Ca mg (mmol)/ kg	P mg (mmol)/ kg	Mg mg (mmol)/ kg
0–6 months	32 (0.8)	14 (0.5)	5.0 (0.2)
7–12 months	20 (0.5)	15 (0.5)	4.2 (0.2)
1–13 years	11 (0.2)	6 (0.2)	2.4 (0.1)
14–18 years	7 (0.2)	6 (0.2)	2.4 (0.1)

Where upper limits are not given care must be taken to avoid over-delivery of individual nutrients. Where nutrient mixtures are used manufacturers' guidelines should be followed.
Source: Adapted from [13].

be higher than that given enterally. This is to allow for losses of the vitamins by adsorption onto the PN bag and giving set or biodegradation due to light exposure, thus reducing the available intake. Vitamin A is most affected by these problems [76]. Addition of the vitamins to the lipid bag and protecting lipids from direct sunlight is the best method of preserving the vitamin concentration. Artificial light has little effect on the stability of the vitamins [13]. Table 4.7 shows the commercially available vitamin solutions for preterm infants and neonates, none of which fully meets current neonatal guidelines [13,44]. Daily administration is recommended with the exception of vitamin K which may be given weekly [13].

Considerations should be made in cholestatic patients with obstructive jaundice as they can accumulate copper and manganese (normally excreted in bile) [77]. Renal patients may not be able to excrete selenium, molybdenum, zinc and chromium [71]. High fluid losses result in greater losses of magnesium and zinc.

Calcium, phosphorus and magnesium are usually added as individual solutions and the suggested intakes are listed in Table 4.9.

Individual preparations of some (not all) trace elements are available where there is a particular need to exclude or increase doses of single trace elements. In cases where there is an apparent overload or deficiency action should be taken after discussion with members of the NST.

Iron

Current commercially available paediatric mineral solutions do not contain iron (Table 4.8).

Intravenous iron supplementation is controversial due to the risk of adverse side effects [78]. Parenterally administered iron bypasses the normal homeostatic mechanism of the intestine and excess iron may lead to iron overload syndrome. Iron enhances the risk of Gram-negative septicaemia [79] and also has powerful oxidative properties; it may therefore increase demand for antioxidants. Monitoring of serum ferritin and reduction/removal of iron supplementation, if levels become too high, is recommended [13]. Ferritin is a poor measure of deficiency as growing children and adolescents use most of the iron supplied almost immediately to accrete tissue and red blood cells so they rarely have any significant iron stores. Although iron reserves should be adequate to supply red cell production for 3–5 months (much less in preterm infants) iron deficiency has been found to develop much sooner. However, this is very much dependent upon the underlying condition and the degree of blood loss interoperatively.

Iron deficiency may lead to increased blood manganese levels [80]. In the absence of iron, manganese binds to transferrin [81] and iron deficiency upregulates both iron and manganese absorption from the intestine [80].

When required iron preparations may be added to the intravenous solution, but this must be done with care due to its poor solubility and risk of anaphylaxis; additional iron is usually given by week 3 of receiving PN. Top-up blood transfusions may be given, when required, if oral or intravenous supplementation fails [13].

> **Learning points – iron**
>
> • *Iron is not present in commercially available paediatric intravenous mineral solutions*
> • *Iron should be added if PN is long term (>3 weeks)*
> • *Iron status should be monitored to avoid toxicity/deficiency*

An example PN prescription is given in Table 4.10.

Administration of parenteral nutrition

A more detailed account of the techniques of PN administration is available in other publications

Table 4.10   Example of a paediatric parenteral nutrition prescription.

1-year-old boy with short bowel syndrome; weight 7 kg, length 70 cm. He has a central venous catheter to provide his full requirements from PN. He requires some extra fluid due to high stool output

Energy requirement = 90 kcal/kg/day (375 Kj/Kg/day)
Nitrogen requirement = 0.36 g N/kg/day (2.25 g protein/kg/day)
Fluid requirement = 120 mL/kg

Solution	Dose (mL)	Energy (kcal)	Carbohydrate (g)	Lipid (g)	Nitrogen (g)
Glucose (20%)	415	332 (1.39 MJ)	83		
Intralipid (20%)	120	240 (1.0 MJ)		24	
Vaminolact	275	66 (0.27 MJ)			2.55
Vitlipid Infant*	10	10 (0.04 MJ)		1	
Solivito	7				
Peditrace	7				
Total	827	648 (2.7 MJ)	83	25	2.55
Per kg	118	92.6 (0.38 MJ) including energy from protein	11.9	3.6	0.36

*10% lipid.
Electrolytes, calcium, phosphorus and iron need to be added in recommended doses.

Rates of infusion

The above is a typical PN content sheet and is supplied with the PN solutions; it is not a prescription. PN is prescribed by writing the rates of 'Aqueous' and 'Lipid' solutions on an intravenous (IV) prescription chart

The rates are usually specified/recommended by pharmacy and are calculated as follows:

Aqueous solution (Vaminolact and 20% glucose and trace elements; could also include water, electrolytes, calcium and phosphate and any IV drugs given in the aqueous phase of the PN)

In this example volumes are calculated as follows:

Total 415 + 275 + 7 = 697 mL = 29 mL/hour given for 24 hours

Lipid solution (Intralipid and vitamins; could also include any IV drugs given in the lipid phase of the PN)

In this example volumes are calculated as follows:

Total = 120 + 10 + 7 = 137 mL = 6.9 mL/hour given for 20 hours

Lipid solution is usually given over 20 hours to allow time off for clearance of lipid from the blood prior to blood sampling

When the boy becomes more stable some enteral feeds are given. PN infusion rates are increased to give some hours off PN:

PN given over	Aqueous phase (mL/hour)	Lipid phase (mL/hour)
20 hours	34.9	6.9
18 hours	38.7	7.6
16 hours	43.6	8.6

Rates of infusion of glucose solution must be calculated and ideally should not exceed the maximum glucose oxidation rate of 1.2 g/kg/hour.
The PN in this example provides 83 g glucose per 24 hours = 5.2 g glucose per hour if given for 16 hours.
At a weight of 7 kg = 0.74 g glucose/kg/hour, this is within the recommended rate.

(continued overleaf)

Table 4.10   *(continued)*

Tapering or 'ramping' PN up and down

If PN is being given at higher rates it is recommended that it is tapered up and down over the first and final 2–3 hours of infusion. This will steadily increase and reduce the glucose infusion in order to avoid hypoglycaemia and hyperglycaemia. For example:

	Aqueous phase (mL/hour)	Lipid phase (mL/hour)
PN to be given over	20 × 1 hour	3.9 × 1 hour
a total of 14 hours	38.5 × 1 hour	7.6 × 1 hour
with a ramping up	58 × 10 hour	11.4 × 10 hour
and down for the	38.8 × 1 hour	7.6 × 1 hour
first and final 2	20 × 1 hour	3.9 × 1 hour
hours of the infusion	Total = 697 mL	Total = 137 mL

Rate of infusion of glucose solution: PN provides 83 g glucose per 24 hours. For 10 hours this PN prescription will deliver 6.9 g glucose per hour

At a weight of 7 kg = 0.98 g glucose/kg/hour, this is within the recommended rate

[4, 13]. PN may be infused via a peripheral vein or a central venous catheter. Each route has advantages and disadvantages [82]. For the purpose of providing PN, it is necessary to differentiate peripheral from central venous access.

Peripheral lines

A needle or short catheter is placed into a subcutaneous vein to gain peripheral access. Peripheral lines are rarely associated with septicaemia. They are useful in short term PN (7–10 days' duration) when the fluid allowance is not restricted and the concentration of PN solutions is <600 mOsm/L, and when venous access is good. They are often used in neonates. One major disadvantage is the risk of thrombophlebitis caused by the hypertonic solutions used. The maximum concentration of glucose solution that should be used with these lines is 12%. Infiltration is also a common problem: the peripheral line may penetrate the surrounding tissues resulting in leaking of the infusion. This leakage is known as extravasation and if undetected can cause tissue necrosis and severe scarring. Line sites must be inspected frequently to avoid this. Lines that fail must be re-sited quickly to avoid the risks of hypoglycaemia and suboptimal nutritional intake.

Central venous catheters

A central venous catheter (CVC), e.g. a Broviac or Hickman catheter, is one which is tunnelled beneath the skin and inserted into the superior or inferior vena cava or outside the right atrium via a subclavian vein. It can be inserted either surgically or percutaneously. It is made of silicone which helps decrease sepsis rates and inhibits fibrin production and is therefore less likely to block. It has a Dacron cuff planted subcutaneously which serves to fix the line in place and also inhibits the migration of microorganisms from the skin.

The maximum concentration of glucose solution that can be given via a CVC is 25%. The line can remain *in situ* for months. The major disadvantages of a CVC are the risks associated with insertion and catheter care. Complications include sepsis, occlusion, infection of the line site and accidental removal. Loss of venous access can be a life limiting factor in PN dependent children, e.g. those with intestinal failure. It is therefore imperative that these lines are cared for. The more frequently a line is accessed the greater the risk of infection. Only PN or fluid (not drugs) should be given via a single lumen catheter [6, 82].

For the taking of blood samples or the administration of blood products or medication separate venous access should be organised. In the case of home PN where monitoring is less frequent the line may be accessed as long as it is done aseptically. Multiple lumen catheters are usually inserted when frequent intravenous drug therapy is required as well as PN and where the child is critically unwell, e.g. bone marrow transplants or intensive care. The rate of infection of these catheters is higher compared with single lumen catheters [83] and this is probably a reflection of more frequent catheter manipulation.

Accidental damage to, or removal of, the catheter is common. Young children will chew and pull their catheter, given the opportunity, and it is important that nursing staff and parents carefully loop and tape the catheter securely to the skin. It is then best practice to cover with a vest and other clothing to keep the line out of reach.

Learning points – central venous catheter (CVC)

- *Hickman or Broviac catheters, also known as central lines*
- *Maximum glucose concentration in a CVC = 25% (12% in a peripheral line)*
- *CVC can stay in for years if well cared for*
- *CVC is high risk as a route of infection and source of sepsis*
- *Central venous access or lack of it is a life limiting factor for children with intestinal failure*

Portacath

A portacath is a totally implantable device, which requires needle sticking for vascular access. It has limited value for PN but is useful for vascular access for frequent medications, e.g. prophylactic antibiotics in cystic fibrosis.

Delivery methods

PN can be delivered by a variety of systems. Infants and children usually have a system in which amino acids and dextrose are mixed and delivered over 24 hours. The fat emulsion is delivered from a separate container but mixes with the amino acid and dextrose solution as close as possible to the peripheral or central line. All the components are compounded in a specialist pharmacy unit under

aseptic conditions in an isolator. Computer based programs are available for use by specialist pharmacists to ensure that the nutrient content of the bag is appropriate for the child's age, condition and biochemistry. They also help to ensure that solution stability is assessed and drug–nutrient interactions avoided [84].

Compounded PN is supplied from the manufacturing pharmacy in a premixed collapsible bag with an opaque cover to protect nutrients in the solution from photodegradation. When low rates of infusion are prescribed and the solution remains in the burette for long periods, light protective sets may also be used although these have limited effectiveness and are most useful if solutions are exposed to direct sunlight rather than artificial light [13]. Home PN is often given during the night thus reducing the risk of photodegradation further. Manufacturers' guidelines advise on stability, dosage and administration.

'All in one' mixes (containing amino acids and dextrose with and without lipid) are available. They are used more commonly in adults. Products that can be used in children >2 years are Oliclinomel (Baxter) and Kabiven (Fresenius Kabi).

There are two solutions (Table 4.11) which can be used from birth (whether preterm or term) to 2 years: Babiven (Fresenius Kabi) and Numeta (Baxter). These products do not contain vitamins or complete mineral profiles; these must be added to the bag before it is infused. Babiven does not contain lipid which must also be given separately. Standard solutions such as these may be useful in order to increase the capacity of a busy aseptic pharmacy unit and decrease preparation time [85]. They may also help avoid some areas of risk previously identified such as delayed PN commencement where the pharmacy capacity or ordering may delay the provision of PN. They may also avoid inadequacy in delivery of solutions as prescribing errors are minimised when 'all in one' bags are used at 'standard' rates.

The stability of 'all in one' PN depends on the stability of the premixed nutrient solutions. The formulations cannot be varied greatly; therefore they are not suitable for unstable patients or those with unusually low or high requirements. As the mixing of the lipid and aqueous solutions shortens the shelf life of the PN some solutions come in separate

Table 4.11 Standard paediatric parenteral nutrition bags.

Numeta G13% (preterm) (Baxter)

	Activated 2 Chamber (no lipid)	Activated 3 Chamber (with lipid)
mL/kg/day	102.3	127.9
Amino acids g/kg/day	4.0	4.0
Glucose g/kg/day	17.1	17.1
Lipid g/kg/day	0	3.2

Numeta G16% (term to 2 years) (Baxter)

	Activated 2 Chamber (no lipid)	Activated 3 Chamber (with lipid)
mL/kg/day	72.3	96.2
Amino acids g/kg/day	2.5	2.5
Glucose g/kg/day	14.9	14.9
Lipid g/kg/day	0	3.0

Babiven Maintenance (Fresenius Kabi) No Lipid

mL/kg/day	100	120
Amino acids (N) g/kg/day	2.6 (0.37)	3.1 (0.44)
Glucose g/kg/day	11.1	13.3
Lipid g/kg/day	0	0

Babiven Term (Fresenius Kabi) No lipid

mL/kg/day	100	135
Amino acids (N) g/kg/day	2.19 (0.31)	2.96 (0.42)
Glucose g/kg/day	11.1	15
Lipid g/kg/day	0	0

N, nitrogen.

chambers which can be rolled together and mixed just before use.

Best practice demands that children should have individually prepared PN as 'all in one' solutions may not contain sufficient calcium, phosphate and other electrolytes. They are safe for use in short term PN; however, close monitoring of biochemistry is necessary.

Equipment

A steady flow rate should be maintained when infusing PN. Hyperglycaemia and hyperlipidaemia will result if infusions are delivered too quickly. If the line blocks or the infusion stops suddenly, hypoglycaemia may occur [6]. Volumetric pumps are sufficiently accurate for use in children; these deliver measured volumes via a cassette with a syringe mechanism ensuring accuracy. Syringe pumps are used instead of volumetric pumps when small volumes are required. These have a linear drive mechanism and can be set to deliver as little as 0.5 mL/hour. Filters are needed to remove any potential bacterial or fungal contaminant and

prevent air embolism and entry of particulate matter. It is considered good practice to filter PN solutions with a pore size of

- 0.22 microns for amino acid and dextrose solutions. This safely removes bacteria, endotoxins, air and particles (this is not used for lipid solutions as the pore size is too small for lipid to pass through)
- 1.2 microns for 'all in one' bags and lipids. This safely removes candida, air and particles (the pore size is large enough for the lipid to pass through). It is not a sterilising filter as it will not remove bacteria.

Cyclical parenteral nutrition

This refers to the intermittent administration of intravenous fluids with a regular break in each 24 hour period. There may be advantages in terms of changes in insulin/glucagon balance and decreased lipogenesis; time off to allow for physical activity; and reduction in the risk of development of liver disease [86].

Infusion rates are usually built up gradually over a period of days or weeks. Often patients on long term PN will have infusion rates increased to enable them to have the prescribed volume of solutions delivered overnight only, leaving them free from PN during the day. However, this is very much dependent upon the age of the child, e.g. infants, particularly preterm infants, have very low glycogen stores and need an almost constant supply of glucose; any breaks in PN require close monitoring to avoid hypoglycaemia. With increased rates of delivery, there is a risk of hyperglycaemia on commencement of PN and a risk of rebound hypoglycaemia on cessation of PN. For this reason it is recommended that infusion tapering may be warranted, particularly in children <2–3 years old to limit risk [87]. Rates are ramped up and down over the initial and final 2–3 hours of PN (Table 4.10).

Weaning off parenteral nutrition

In order to wean the child from PN, i.e. reduce the amount of PN given; it is essential that some degree of enteral nutrition is maintained. The concentration and rate of delivery of enteral feed will be gradually increased depending on tolerance and growth parameters. If fluid restriction is not a major issue, once enteral feeds or diet provide at least 25% of the total nutritional requirements a corresponding reduction can be made to the PN prescription. Once 50% of requirements are met enterally the PN can be decreased to 50%, with a further decrease to 25% once the enteral route meets 75% of requirements. When more than 75% of requirements are achieved by enteral nutrition the PN could be stopped in most cases [88]. These reductions are dependent upon satisfactory growth and development of the child. Weaning from PN may take a few days where it has been used for nutritional support in the short term, e.g. following acute surgery, or be very gradual over months and sometimes years where it has been used for long term support, such as in short bowel syndrome whilst waiting for gut adaptation. If the PN is provided as separate lipid and aqueous (carbohydrate and amino acid) solutions it is important to decrease each solution proportionally in order to maintain an adequate energy:nitrogen ratio.

If fluid restriction is a complicating factor and the weaning off period is prolonged the PN should be made up as concentrated as possible (depending upon the route of administration and the solutions used). Thereafter the PN will usually need to be decreased by each millilitre that the enteral nutrition is increased (although a greater fluid volume is usually tolerated via the enteral route than the parenteral route due to losses from the gut). Care and attention to actual intake must be employed in these cases to ensure maximum nutrition is achieved, as enteral feeds are often less concentrated than PN. This is especially important in infancy or for malnourished children.

Home parenteral nutrition

Although the majority of patients discontinue PN it is recommended that PN at home be considered for any patient likely to be dependent on PN for more than 3 months [89]. Home parenteral nutrition (HPN) improves quality of life for these patients and their families due to obvious psychosocial benefits. It is also associated with lower risks of catheter infection and a decreased risk of PNALD [90] and reduces the cost of caring for these children during long hospital admissions.

The demand for HPN services for children has risen over the past 20 years. Due to better understanding and management of complications long term survival rates on PN have improved. Published surveys show a fourfold increase in patients registered on HPN since 1993 [89]. Short bowel syndrome was the most common diagnosis with an increase from 27% to 63% of cases [89]. It is widely recognised among expert practitioners in this field that a national strategy is needed to manage this expanding group of patients with chronic intestinal failure.

Patients on HPN should be managed by a specialist centre with significant expertise in this area [91]. Dedicated specialist nurses must train parents and carers in preparation for discharge, with community services supporting the family by providing equipment and a suitable environment for the administration of PN in the home. Home assessments must be undertaken and, if necessary, re-housing or structural changes to housing must be made. Manufacturers of PN solutions usually provide homecare packages which may be funded by local health purchasers; contracts are often agreed on a case need basis.

5 Nutrition in Critically Ill Children

Rosan Meyer and Luise Marino

Introduction

Data from the Paediatric Intensive Care Audit Network in the UK indicate that only 1.1%–7.7% of children are admitted to a paediatric intensive care unit (PICU), with the majority of those children (47%) being below 1 year of age [1]. Nutritional management of critically ill children (CIC) is therefore a very specialist and challenging area in paediatric practice. In addition to minimising the effects of starvation associated with suboptimal nutrition and preventing nutritional deficiencies and excesses, its goal is to sustain organ function and prevent dysfunction of the cardiovascular, respiratory and immune systems until the acute-phase inflammatory response resolves (Table 5.1) [2]. Both undernutrition and overnutrition have the potential to compromise this goal and significantly complicate and increase the length of hospital stay [3–5]. Overfeeding can lead to increased carbon dioxide production, resulting in difficulties with weaning from mechanical ventilator support, fatty liver, as well as diarrhoea associated with electrolyte imbalances and other well documented metabolic and physiological complications [6]. Underfeeding, however, is a more common occurrence in PICUs that has not improved over the last 30 years, in spite of great medical advances.

Pollack *et al.* [3] found in 1981 that 16%–20% of critically ill children develop significant, acute protein energy malnutrition (PEM) within 48 hours of admission to a PICU; in 2006, Hulst *et al.* found that 24% of children have PEM [7]. An even higher prevalence of moderate severe malnutrition was found by Delgado *et al.* [8] in 2008, with 53% of the children suffering from PEM. This has a significant effect on muscle strength [9], it reduces wound healing due to altered immunity and increases rates of sepsis [7]. Ensuring optimal nutritional support in critically ill children is therefore crucial.

Inflammatory and metabolic responses that impact on nutritional requirements

Endocrine and inflammatory response

A knowledge of metabolic changes and fuel utilisation during physiological stress can assist dietitians in commencing nutritional support at the appropriate time and suggesting a suitable feeding route and feed composition.

Critical illness is characterised by a cascade of endocrine and metabolic reactions, affecting all major organs (Fig. 5.1). The reaction of the body to physiological stress changes over time. The acute

Table 5.1 The effect of critical illness on the major organs.

Gastrointestinal system	Cardiovascular system	Respiratory system	Renal system
• Gastroparesis (motility affected due to medication, e.g. morphine, inotropic agents and antibiotics, as well as the disease process itself) [12] • Impaired digestive enzyme secretion • Cholestasis [18] • Impaired lipid metabolism due to affected liver function [18] • Increased intestinal permeability [12] • Poor gut perfusion [12]	• Tachycardia • High cardiac output [18] • Fluid shift from the intracellular to the extracellular compartments [103]	• Respiratory deterioration leading to artificial ventilation [18]	• Renal impairment may occur during critical illness and may be as severe as acute renal failure requiring haemofiltration [10]

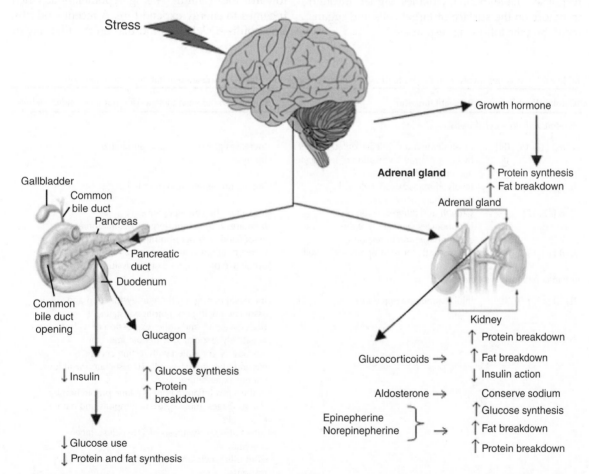

Figure 5.1 Endocrine and metabolic cascade in critically ill children [13, 14, 18, 114]. Source: Adapted from Krause MV, Mahan LK, Arlin M Physiological stress: trauma, sepsis, burns and surgery. In: *Krause's Food, Nutrition and Diet Therapy*, 10th edn. Philadelphia: WB Saunders Company, 2002, p. 492. Reprinted with permission of Elsevier.

phase response can be divided into the ebb phase and flow phase. The ebb phase is characterised by the body's attempt to maintain normal perfusion and mobilisation of stress hormones; the flow phase is the dynamic state of acute injury and affects substrate (protein, carbohydrate and fat) metabolism. The final phase, the anabolic phase, is characterised by the slow re-accumulation of protein and body fat after the metabolic response to injury subsides [10–12].

During critical illness immune cells, e.g. macrophages, lymphocytes and neutrophils, regulate the inflammatory response through the release of cytokines [in particular interleukins (IL) such as IL-1, IL-6, IL-8, IL-10 and tumour necrosis factor α (TNFα)] and chemokines such as heat shock protein 70. All are important mediators of the stress response (Table 5.2). Cytokines signal through receptors on the surface of target cells and organs mediating the following responses:

- upregulation or downregulation of gene expression influencing wound healing and immunocompetence
- release of counter-regulatory hormones
- cell to cell signalling orchestrating the inflammatory response which affects substrate metabolism [13–15].

Energy metabolism

There has been significant debate over the last 10 years about the impact of acute illness on energy metabolism in children, which differs from that seen in adults. Some older studies have suggested a hypermetabolic state during the acute phase of illness [16]; however, new evidence points towards more children being hypometabolic when it comes to energy expenditure. A recent study by Briassoulis et al. [17] found that on the first day of

Table 5.2   Cytokines involved in the acute phase of injury and possible effects on substrate metabolism and nutrition.

Cytokines	Relevant function	Interaction between metabolism, nutrition and cytokines
Pro-inflammatory cytokines		
TNFα [13, 15, 104]	Pro-inflammatory; release of leucocytes by bone marrow; activation of leucocytes and endothelial cells	Increases glucose transport and impacts on muscle lipolysis
IL-1 [13, 17]	Involved in pyrexia; T-cell and macrophage activation	Impact on hepatic and muscle lipogenesis
IL-6 [13, 17]	Growth and differentiation of lymphocytes; activation of the acute-phase protein response	Impact on hepatic lipogenesis Increases during multi-organ dysfunction and associated with poor nutritional status
IL-8 [13, 15]	Chemotactic for neutrophils and T-cells	Concentrations during the first 24 hours are predictive of worsening organ dysfunction
Anti-inflammatory cytokine		
IL-10 [15, 17]	Inhibits immune function	Increases during multi-organ dysfunction and associated with poor nutritional status Both excessive and under expression of IL-10 is negatively associated with outcome Negatively correlated with resting energy expenditure: increase in IL-10 associated with lower energy expenditure Inhibits pro-inflammatory cytokine production by macrophages, monocytes, neutrophils and natural killer cells Attenuates the synthesis of TNF cell surface receptions Controlling cytokine regulating the inflammatory response

IL, interleukin; TNF, tumour necrosis factor.

admission 48.6% of children were hypometabolic (<90% of predicted basal metabolic rate, BMR), 40.5% were normometabolic (90%–110% of predicted BMR) and 10.8% were hypermetabolic (>110% of predicted BMR). A hypermetabolic pattern only emerged after 2 weeks of admission in 60% of children. This unique pattern of metabolism may be explained by a multitude of factors, including the physiological response to stress, improved medical treatment as well as the unique nature of fuel utilisation in critically ill children (Tables 5.2 and 5.3) [11, 12, 18, 19].

In addition to the factors listed in Table 5.3 authors have speculated that during the acute phase growth does not take place and this energy is diverted into the recovery processes [19, 20]. This hypothesis is supported by the data from Hulst et al. [21] who found that insulin-like growth factor 1 (an anabolic hormone) remained low until day 4 of PICU admission and T3 levels remained below normal at days 4 and 6 in 88% and 89% of the older children, respectively. Although more research needs to take place before specific guidelines on energy expenditure can be published, it is clear that substrate metabolism varies greatly during admission and that during the early phase of illness hypometabolism is usual, whereas in the later phase of illness hypermetabolism predominates. This needs to be taken into account when calculating energy requirements and choosing feeds for these patients, which may require changes being made to prescribed energy intake during the course of a PICU stay.

Substrate utilisation

Several studies have focused on the relation between CIC's metabolic state, their nutritional intake, substrate utilisation and nitrogen balance. In a similar way to critically ill adults the stress response and the severity of disease are characterised by protein catabolism. In contrast to adults, fat is the preferred fuel in children and is readily oxidised. Conversely carbohydrates are poorly utilised during critical illness. Gluconeogenesis is also a characteristic of paediatric critical illness and muscle mass is rapidly depleted of amino acids, such as glutamine, which are utilised in de novo glucose production [22, 23]. Maximal glucose oxidation occurs at a glucose intake of 5 mg/kg/min. If intake exceeds 8 mg/kg/min lipogenesis takes place, leading to an increase in triglyceride levels, fat deposition in the liver and an increase in fat instead of lean body mass [18]. It is therefore important to ensure that carbohydrate intake in CIC is monitored, especially if parenteral nutrition (PN) is used.

Mechanism for muscle wasting

Sepsis associated muscle wasting is well described in the adult intensive care unit (ICU), although the prevalence is not known in children. Causative factors include sepsis, muscle disuse, fasting, cancer, cardiac failure and renal dysfunction. In ICU there is often prolonged bed rest or immobilisation, use

Table 5.3 Factors that influence energy expenditure.

Factor	Influence on energy expenditure
Sedation [105]	↓ Energy expenditure (reduced brain activity)
Muscle relaxants [20, 105]	↓ Energy expenditure but not of clinical significance
Ventilation (with humidified air) [20]	↓ Energy expenditure, reduces the workload of breathing as well as heat loss in fully ventilated children, but where ventilatory support is minimal may not have impact
Thermoneutral environment [19]	↓ Insensible losses, therefore lowers energy expenditure
Pyrexia [106]	↑ Energy expenditure (8%–12% increase in energy expenditure per 1°C above normal)
Paracetamol/NSAIS [106]	↓ Energy expenditure as blunts response to fever; clinical relevance questionable
Severity of disease [20]	Inconclusive evidence
Diagnosis [19, 20]	No difference in energy expenditure in different diagnoses
Severity of disease [20]	No significant difference in energy expenditure
Movement/activity [42]	↑ Energy expenditure

NSAIS, non-steroidal anti-inflammatories.

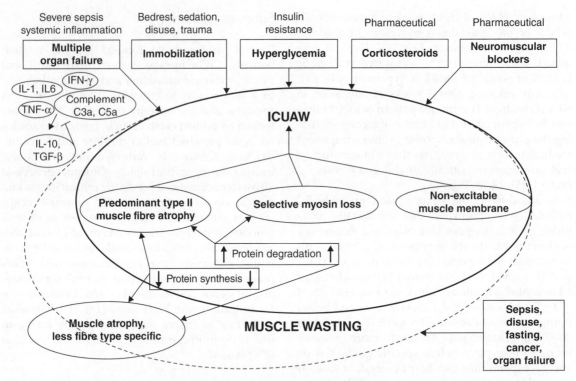

Figure 5.2   Risk factors for muscle wasting and ICU associated wasting from Schefold *et al.* with permission [24]. ICUAW, intensive care unit acquired weakness. Reprinted with permission of Springer.

of sedatives and neuromuscular blockades, acute or chronic organ dysfunction, medication using steroids [24] and increased levels of cytokines, e.g. IL-6, IL-10, TNFα (which are associated with muscle degradation), amongst other factors [15, 24] (Fig. 5.2).

There is often an imbalance between anabolism and catabolism with protein turnover outstripping protein synthesis leading to a net loss of muscle mass which occurs as a result of *de novo* gluconeogenesis [22, 24]. Muscle wasting and ICU induced myopathy has not been described in children and it may be that the pathophysiology of paediatric critical illness does not result in this phenomenon. However, as a significant number of children admitted to PICU develop malnutrition it is likely that muscle wasting also occurs in children.

Nutritional assessment

Growth failure is common amongst children admitted to PICU. It is therefore imperative to classify the type of growth impairment (i.e. wasting, stunting or faltering growth) to enable a targeted nutritional care plan. Malnutrition in this population is multifactorial and may be illness and non-illness related and it is important to identify the contributors (Fig. 5.3). The multifactorial nature of malnutrition in this population makes nutritional assessment particularly challenging [25].

Anthropometry, biochemical markers, clinical and dietary review form part of the nutritional assessment in CIC [26]. This process, however, is notoriously difficult due to a multitude of factors including oedema, ascites and severity of disease, which often makes it challenging to obtain an accurate body weight. In addition, the emotional impact of having a child in the PICU frequently makes the diet history from the carers unreliable.

A recent UK study found that only 20.5% of CIC had an accurate admission weight documented [27] so it is quite common practice to estimate their weight. In the past the Advanced Paediatric Life Support formula [(age + 4) × 2] was used [28]; however, Luscombe *et al.* [27, 29] found

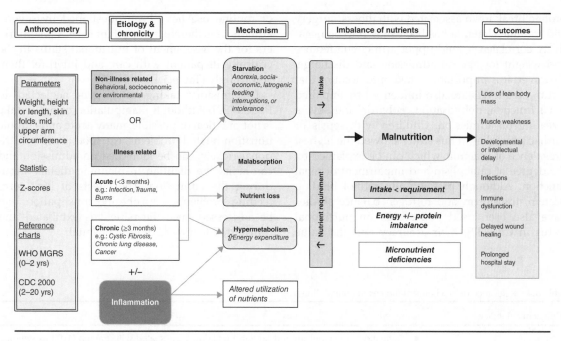

Figure 5.3   Aetiology of illness and non-illness related malnutrition in CIC [25] (Reprinted with permission of Sage).

that this formula underestimates the weight significantly and that a new formula [weight = 3(age) + 7] allows for a more safe and accurate estimation. A formula, however, can never replace an accurate weight measurement, as it is used not only in the assessment of nutritional status and for calculating nutritional requirements but also for estimating fluid requirements and medication doses. Transfer and hospital notes as well as the child's personal health record (red/blue book) may have a recent accurate weight (often height and head circumference as well), which may be useful. It is important that available accurate weight, height and head circumference is plotted on an appropriate growth chart [26, 30].

The use of both triceps skin fold thickness and mid upper arm circumference has been documented in this population. Although the mid upper arm circumference is less affected by oedema, both measurements have limited use in children with a short PICU stay (4–5 days); however, they should be considered for children who remain in the PICU for a longer period of time (>1 week). They are most helpful when followed over time and measured by the same trained person [26, 30]. Hulst *et al.* [26] studied the feasibility of routinely performing

nutritional assessments using non-invasive methods in CIC. It was found that anthropometry was reliably obtained within 24 hours of admission in 56%–91% of patients. Unfortunately the more seriously ill patients were those where measurements were less feasible, but who might have benefited the most from having them done. Recently, Vermilyea *et al.* [31] have proposed the use of a subjective global nutritional assessment (SGNA) tool, specifically designed for PICUs. That study found that, although not predictive of outcome, the SGNA was valid and strongly correlated with standard anthropometrical measurements. Although this does not replace an accurate measurement, healthcare professionals may consider this in those children where measurements are not feasible.

Most laboratory markers of nutritional status are affected by the acute inflammatory response, renal impairment and fluid shifts. The prevalence of hypomagnesaemia (20%), hypertriglyceridaemia (25%), uraemia (30%) and hypoalbuminaemia (52%) was reported in a study in CIC [32]. Except for uraemia, no significant associations between the biochemical parameters and anthropometric measurements were found. Serum urea levels can indicate the degree of catabolic stress and levels of protein breakdown associated with illness, surgery and trauma. Uraemia has been shown to be negatively correlated to mid upper arm circumference and weight for age on admission and discharge. However, it is important to take into account that serum urea levels are also influenced by impaired renal function, dehydration, polyuria and severe sweating on admission. Children with sepsis or cardiac anomalies in this study showed the highest prevalence of uraemia, which can be explained by the degree of catabolism and impairment of renal function. Although pre-albumin, retinol binding protein, transferrin and nitrogen balance studies have also been used in research on nutritional status in CIC [32], their accuracy and the value

of routine use have been questioned by several authors. It is therefore important to select biomarkers for the assessment of nutritional status in the critically ill patient with care and interpret them accordingly (Table 5.4).

Diet history taking often gets neglected in PICUs [30]. Although manipulation of oral intake is not practical or possible, many acute and chronic nutrition related problems, e.g. food allergy, nutritional rickets, can be identified on admission and can assist the dietitian in planning dietary input during the admission. The effects of long term feeding problems, e.g. obesity, constipation, can be addressed once the patient is extubated and transferred to a ward or local hospital.

Table 5.4 Relevance of biochemical indices in critical illness.

Biochemical indices	Comment
Serum urea	• Indication of catabolism and protein breakdown associated with trauma [107] as well as impaired renal function, dehydration, polyuria or severe sweating which will impact on fluid management [32] • Although there is a link between muscle mass and urea, it is not a reliable marker to assess nutritional support
Glucose	• There is currently a great deal of interest in the use of tight glycaemic control in critically ill children. There is no clear guidance on this topic from a nutritional perspective, however [108] • It is important to monitor glucose levels, in particular in children on IV preparations and those with PN (p. 52) [109]
Albumin	• Levels are likely to be low especially in those receiving IV saline • Albumin is not a good marker of nutritional status due to a long half-life and is more a marker of inflammation, intravascular/extravascular fluid shifts and catabolism [32, 107]
C-reactive protein (CRP)	• Is used as an index of the acute phase response and is usually measured serially • Serum pre-albumin and CRP are inversely related, e.g. serum pre-albumin levels decrease and CRP levels increase in proportion to the severity of illness, returning to normal (<5 mg/dL) once the illness has resolved • In infants a value of <2 mg/dL is associated with a return of anabolism with a concomitant rise in pre-albumin levels [2]
Magnesium/calcium	• Hypomagnesaemia is commonly found in CIC [110] • It is strongly associated with hypokalaemia and hypocalcaemia
Phosphorus	• Hypophosphataemia (in up to 61% of CIC) [11, 22], selenium, zinc [90] and manganese are also commonly found in critical illnesses [32]
Lactate	• Lactic acidosis is common in CIC and reflects hypoperfusion, including diabetic ketoacidosis, septic shock and cardiogenic shock • Lactic acidosis, base excess and a strong anion gap are associated with increased risk of mortality • A level of >2 mg/dL may be used as a crude proxy for cell function and a resolution of lactic acidosis is correlated with survival [111]

IV, intravenous; PN, parenteral; CIC, critically ill children.

Nutritional requirements

Energy requirements

Several predictive equations have been used and studied in the paediatric critical care setting to calculate energy requirements. They include Harris–Benedict [33], World Health Organization [34], Talbot [33], Schofield [35], PICU regression equations and Meyer et al.'s [36] prediction equation. A number of studies have confirmed the inaccuracy of these equations and more recently Meyer et al. [36] found that 75% of patients had a predicted energy expenditure that differed by 26%–29.6% from the measured energy expenditure, independently of which formula was used [19, 37]. Only 25% of patients had a predicted energy expenditure within <10% variation using the different formulas, concurring with a recent systematic review of predictive equations for ventilated adults which indicated that only 28% of patients had their energy expenditure predicted within 10% of measured requirements [38]. Most of the prediction equations, except for the formulas by Meyer et al. [36] and White et al. [39], require the addition of stress and activity factors, which have been based mainly on adult data and are dependent on the subjective opinion of a dietitian or clinician [34, 40].

Most authors have found that the actual energy expenditure is closer to the resting energy expenditure. These studies are summarised in Table 5.5.

The Schofield equation is used most commonly in the UK and also in 55% of European PICUs [41], with some evidence of reasonable correlation with ventilated CIC. The gold standard for measuring energy expenditure is indirect calorimetry. In the absence of this, BMR, calculated by Schofield using the formula which requires an accurate weight with or without additional activity factor of 0%–20%, may be used (Table 5.6). The use of a physical activity factor is described by van der Kuip et al. [42]. After 1 week of admission, energy requirements should be re-calculated. Patients admitted for more than 2 weeks will need to have their energy expenditure reassessed and may also benefit from indirect calorimetry, if available. Although current guidelines [2] recommend the routine use of indirect calorimetry there is a considerable cost related to running and maintaining them [43–46]. It is important to use only validated metabolic carts, which at the moment are limited to the Deltatrac II (GE Healthcare) for paediatric intensive care.

Protein requirements

Although there are no specific guidelines on protein requirements in ventilated CIC, research has shown that patients with an adequate energy and protein intake have a positive nitrogen balance, unlike patients who are underfed. Nitrogen (N) balance correlates with feeding to total measured energy expenditure and providing sufficient nitrogen [47]. Agus and Jaksic [48] suggest that the critically ill infant and child should receive 2–3 g/kg and 1.5 g/kg of protein, respectively, and in severely stressed states may require even more (≥3 g/kg). The 2009 American Society for Parenteral and Enteral Nutrition guidelines for CIC recommend the following protein intakes: 0–2 years, 2–3 g/kg/day; 2–13 years, 1.5–2 g/kg/day; and 13–18 years, 1.5 g/kg/day [2]. Disease specific protein recommendations, e.g. renal failure, cystic fibrosis, also provide useful guidelines for children in PICUs.

Table 5.5 Mean energy expenditure (published studies since 2000).

Publication	Number of children enrolled	Diagnosis	Mean energy expenditure
Taylor et al. [19]	57	Mainly liver disease, some head injury and other disorders	37.2 kcal/kg (155 kJ/kg)
Martinez et al. [112]	43	Post surgery, liver transplant, medical disorders	47 kcal/kg (196 kJ/kg)
De Wit et al. [113]	21	Post cardiac surgery	67.8 kcal/kg (283 kJ/kg)
Botran et al. [61]	46	Post surgery and medical patients	48.8 kcal/kg (204 kJ/kg)
Meyer et al. [36]	175	Respiratory, surgical, sepsis, liver and cardiac	44.6 kcal/kg (186 kJ/kg)

Table 5.6 Predictive equations for calculating basal metabolic rate (BMR) in critically ill children.

Name of equation	Equation (kcal/24 hours)
Schofield (if accurate weight is available)	*Males* <3 years: $(59.512 \times W) - 30.4$ 3–10 years: $(22.7 \times W) + 504.3$ 10–18 years: $(17.5 \times W) + 651$ *Females* <3 years: $(58.317 \times W) - 31.1$ 3–10 years: $(22.706 \times W) + 485.9$ 10–18 years: $(13.384 \times W) + 692.6$
Schofield (if an accurate weight and height is available)	*Males* <3 years: $(0.167 \times W) + (1517.4 \times H) - 616.6$ 3–10 years: $(19.59 \times W) + (130.3 \times H) + 414.9$ 10–18 years: $(16.25 \times W) + (137.2 \times H) + 515.5$ *Females* <3 years: $(16.252 \times W) + (1023.3 \times H) - 413.5$ 3–10 years: $(16.969 \times W) + (161.8 \times H) + 371.2$ 10–18 years: $(8.365 \times W) + (465 \times H) + 200.0$

W, weight (kg); H, height (m).

Vitamins and minerals

Vitamin and trace mineral metabolism in critically ill and postoperative paediatric patients is not a well researched area. As a result no specific recommendations exist for ventilated patients in PICUs. The pharmacological use of vitamins and trace minerals in paediatric illness is controversial due to reports of toxicity [49]. When energy and fluid requirements are met by commercial enteral tube feeds, CIC should receive sufficient vitamins and minerals to meet the reference nutrient intake for both. However, many patients require additional supplementation, depending on diagnosis and treatment modality, e.g. premature infants, haemofiltration. This should be done under supervision and monitored with blood biochemistry.

Nutrition care plans in PICU outcomes

Defining energy and protein requirements is integral to any part of a nutrition care plan [50]. In addition, there is a growing focus on clinical outcomes as part of the nutrition care pathway [51]. A large multicentred retrospective study in CIC investigated whether early documentation of nutrition care plans had any effect on daily energy intake and route of nutrition support: 47.7% had energy requirements documented in the medical notes and these patients had significantly higher total daily energy intake and were more likely to be fed enterally during the first 4 days of admission to a PICU compared with those without a nutrition care plan [50]. In another large international prospective study increased intake of energy and protein, in adults, was associated with better clinical outcomes [52]. As a result, the Intensive Care Society has published minimum standards for intensive care units [53] which recommend that a dietitian is part of an intensive care multidisciplinary team contributing to improved delivery of nutrition support to all ICU patients.

Nutritional management

When to commence nutrition support

Traditionally nutrition support has been withheld in children in PICUs until metabolic and cardiopulmonary stability has been established. However, many units have changed their protocols and guidelines to include nutritional support at an earlier stage.

The concept of early feeding has mainly been developed in adult surgical patients. In paediatric practice most authors agree to the definition of 'early enteral nutrition' as the initiation of enteral feed within 24–48 hours of PICU admission. Others describe patients receiving immediate feeding, but unfortunately this term does not come with a clear definition [10, 54].

Four main hypotheses could justify the use of early feed in CIC:

- fasting has a deleterious effect on these patients
- energy supply plays an important role in the promotion of energy metabolism
- the delivery of nutrients is important for gut maintenance
- specific nutrients provide support for organ and system functions

Several studies have been published showing a delay in commencement of nutrition support ranging from 2 to 3 days after admission to the PICU [55]. The prevalence of significant PEM within 48 hours of admission therefore comes as no surprise. Early enteral nutrition (within 12 hours of admission) has been successfully used by numerous PICUs in children with a variety of diagnoses (in the absence of any bowel sounds) and has resulted in an improved nitrogen balance [54, 56]. In fact, Meyer *et al.* [57] showed that commencing enteral nutrition support within 5 hours of admission is possible and safe, if enteral feeding protocols are used.

The combination of decreased blood flow to the gut and interactions with drugs can lead to a reduction of nutrient absorption and gastric motility, failure of gastric acid secretion and increase in intestinal permeability and bacterial translocation [12]. Early enteral nutrition support may reverse these effects by reducing catabolism, promoting wound healing and most probably decreasing the frequency of clinical sepsis.

Route of feeding

Although it is an acknowledged fact that using the enteral route is more physiological and beneficial to the CIC, the debate of enteral versus PN in critical care has changed its focus to the delivery of nutrients in the most effective and safe way, using the most appropriate route for the individual patient [56].

Standard protocols have been shown to be useful in improving the time taken to initiate feeding as well as the progression to full feeds [54, 58, 59]. Enteral feeding protocols guide medical and nursing staff through the choice of tube feeds, the feeding rates depending on the child's age and weight, as well as guidelines for the continuous monitoring process.

Nasogastric versus nasojejunal feeding

Nasogastric feeding (NG) is most widely used and is usually safe and well tolerated in CIC [2]. However, gastric delivery of enteral feed may be poorly tolerated due to disordered gastric motility which may lead to aspiration. In addition, the use of gastric residual volume as a marker of tolerance of NG feeding has a poor evidence base and is often

blamed for inadequate delivery of feed [60, 61]. Horn *et al.* [62] defined delayed gastric emptying in CIC as >5 mL/kg gastric residuals every 4 hours. Although this provides some guidance, this is still an arbitrary volume and may still lead to feeds being inappropriately stopped. Therefore interest has focused on postpyloric feeding. Nasojejunal (NJ) feeding has been shown by several centres to be safe and effective in this subset of patients, enabling adequate delivery of energy in a shorter period of time in the majority of patients and so reducing the problems had PN been used: hyperglycaemia, hypertriglyceridaemia and hepatic dysfunction [63–65]. However, in cyanotic patients it is important to note a risk in the development of necrotising enterocolitis with enteral feeding; therefore additional care in the monitoring of haemodynamic status is warranted when NJ feeds are given to this subgroup of patients [66]. Many units avoid postpyloric feeding as NJ tubes are extremely difficult to place and become dislodged very easily [65]. Several blind (non-radiological guided) bed-side techniques have been successfully developed using weighted or unweighted polyurethane NG tubes with hydrophilic guide wires. Meyer *et al.* [64] have shown that, with continuous training and audit, a blind placement technique can be maintained at 96% success rate.

Continuous feeds versus bolus feeding

Both continuous as well as bolus feeding have been used in paediatric critical care. The pros and cons of both are well studied in the neonatal and adult setting [67, 68], but in paediatrics individual units have their preferred practice. Although bolus feeding is more physiological difficulties with monitoring the tolerance, as well as the additional nursing input, has led to many PICUs preferring continuous feeding. On the other hand continuous feeding has been shown to delay gastric emptying in adult ICUs [69] and reduce gallbladder contraction [70]. Horn *et al.*, however, showed that gastric residual volumes did not differ between children on bolus or continuous feeds [56]. In the absence of substantial clinical evidence, the consensus is that adequate delivery of nutrition support should be the main goal in feeding CIC and should not be hampered by the feeding route. A case study of a child admitted to a PICU is given in Table 5.7.

Table 5.7   Case study: a child admitted to the paediatric intensive care unit.

A 13-month-old boy with meningococcal sepsis was admitted to the paediatric intensive care unit. He received fluid resuscitation and after 5 hours of admission the doctors deemed him haemodynamically stable so he can commence enteral nutrition. He is fully sedated (including muscle relaxants) and ventilated, requiring adrenalin.

Anthropometry

weight: 11.2 kg

length: no recent length available

Biochemistry

Electrolytes are all within normal range, but in order to achieve this he is receiving potassium and magnesium corrections. Albumin is low, urea is increased, creatinine is increased.

Clinical

Necrotic areas in all extremities: fingers and toes. Necrotic areas on the face as well.

Diet history

Parents report that he usually eats well at home and consumes 500–600 mL of full fat cow's milk, has red meat twice per week and otherwise has fish or chicken.

Nutritional requirements

Activity: physiotherapy twice per day; he is turned four times per day and is not fully ventilated.

Energy requirements $= (59.512 \times 11.2) - 30.4$
$$= 564.72 + 10\%$$
$$= 636\,\text{kcal}\ (2.66\,\text{MJ})$$

Protein requirements 2–3 g/kg/day: 22.4–33.6 g/day

Enteral feed: 1 kcal/mL feed with a multifibre mix

Feeding route: trial NG. Likelihood of having gastroparesis is high (adrenalin, shock) and may therefore require NJ.

Monitoring

Ideally CIC should have their nutrition monitored daily. The clinical situation can change rapidly and may impact on nutritional requirements. Nutrition is also impacted by the following:

- *Fluid volume restriction* – the main barrier to adequate nutrition delivery. The dietitian needs to establish whether such strict fluid restriction is required in the light of inadequate nutrient delivery and to change the enteral feed (if necessary); also to negotiate whether drugs running in intravenous (IV) fluids can be made more concentrated, thus liberating volume for feeding [71].
- *Procedural interruptions* – can account for 11%–57% of total interruptions affecting up to 62% of patients [60]. The most common interruptions arise from surgery, radiological procedures, attempts at extubation and the administration of medication. Often feeding rates are not increased to compensate for time lost during the interruption making it

challenging to achieve nutrition goals, with the resultant large energy and protein deficits negatively impacting on weight [4, 71].
- *Interruption due to gastrointestinal intolerance* – especially where there is vomiting, diarrhoea, large gastric residuals and abdominal distension which may occur in up to 57% of patients [71].
- *Mechanical problems* – such as NJ tube dislodgement, NG blockage [71].

The dietitian's role is critical to improving nutrient delivery and ensuring protocols and procedures are in place to allow for optimal nutritional support [72]. Table 5.8 shows how often aspects of nutrition support need to be monitored.

Complications

Refeeding syndrome

As the prevalence of malnutrition within the PICU population is high, the risk for refeeding syndrome should be considered. When enteral nutrition or PN

Table 5.8 Monitoring frequency in paediatric intensive care unit.

	Daily	2–3 times per week	Once per week
Anthropometry		×*	×*
Biochemistry	×		
Recalculation of nutrient requirements			×
Evaluation of delivery of feed	×		

*Frequency of anthropometry depends on the age of the child. Infant will require weight twice per week. Teenager will require weight once per week.

is commenced in children who have not received optimal nutritional support for some time, e.g. ≥3 days, it is important to ensure that there is a multidisciplinary approach to determine the risk of refeeding syndrome in addition to an appropriate management strategy regarding electrolyte replacement, vitamin supplementation and energy and/or protein restriction [73–75]. Figure 5.4 provides a management outline on refeeding syndrome in PICUs [76].

Future research and unanswered questions

Immunonutrition

The use of immune enhancing enteral feeding formulas is well known in adult intensive care. In addition to the normal macronutrients and micronutrients, these feeds contain a mixture of omega-3 and omega-6 fatty acids (which have pro- and anti-inflammatory properties); additional arginine and/or glutamine (which become conditionally essential amino acids during increased physiological stress); and increased levels of the antioxidants selenium and β-carotene [77].

Although these enteral feeding formulas have all the ingredients to improve outcome, results in the adult population have been conflicting. A meta-analysis of 15 studies of immune enhancing diets in critically ill patients after trauma, sepsis or major surgery showed that enteral immunonutrition decreased the incidence of infection, number of ventilator days and length of hospital stay, but had no effect on stay in the ICU [77]. More recent multicentre randomised studies have shown

conflicting results with higher mortality rates in the immunonutrition group among patients with severe sepsis or septic shock [78, 79].

The only documentation of an immune enhancing enteral feeding formula being used in the paediatric critical care setting is by Briassoulis et al. who used an adult feed as there was no available paediatric formula [73]. Preliminary results showed that the immune enhancing formula achieved a positive nitrogen balance by day 5, but was associated with an exacerbated metabolic response in a stressed state compared with the control group [80].

This area of paediatric critical care nutrition is still very new and the limited evidence does not yet support routine use of immune enhancing feeds or supplementation because of possible deleterious effects. Until such data are available specifically for CIC, the following ad hoc additions to feeds or future immune enhancing feeds should be used with caution.

Glutamine

Glutamine is the most abundant free amino acid in the body and blood glutamine levels reflect the balance between synthesis, release and consumption by all types of cells [23]. It serves as a metabolic intermediate, providing carbon and nitrogen for the de novo synthesis of other amino acids, nucleic acids, fatty acids and proteins [81]. The primary source of glutamine is skeletal muscle, which during times of stress is an active net exporter of free glutamine [22]. The main functions of glutamine within the cell include

- nitrogen transport
- maintenance of the cellular redox state through glutathione
- metabolic intermediate
- source of energy [22]

In addition to this glutamine has been shown to increase the expression of heat shock protein 70 (HSP70), which is part of a family of proteins involved in cell protection [82]. Supplementation in glutamine depleted adults shows increasing HSP70 production with improved clinical outcomes and influence on survival [83, 84]. However, in critically ill septic adults supraphysiological levels of glutamine increased the risk of mortality [85].

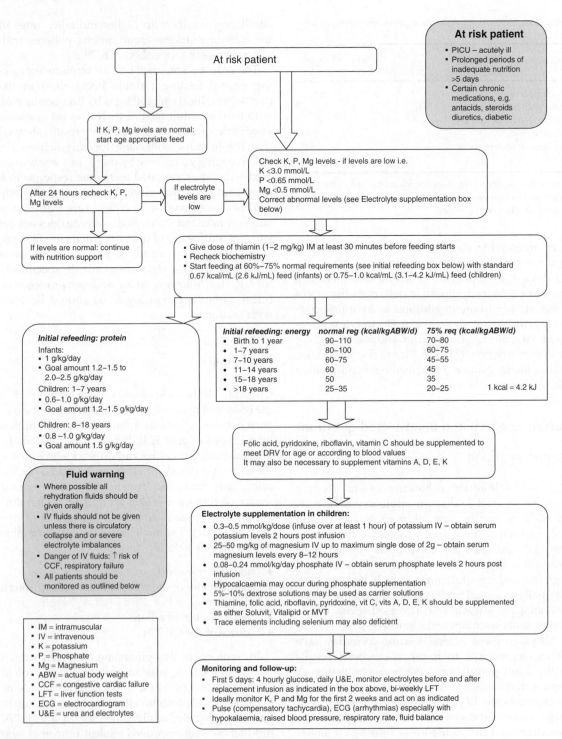

Figure 5.4   Management of refeeding syndrome in the paediatric intensive care unit.

A UK study investigating glutamine levels in CIC reported early significant glutamine depletion compared with convalescent levels [86]. There were inverse correlations with the number of days spent in the PICU and on mechanical ventilation, lactate and C-reactive protein (CRP) suggesting that, as with adults, low glutamine levels are associated with disease severity [87]. In addition there were significant positive correlations between plasma HSP70 levels and length of PICU stay, duration of mechanical ventilation, severity of disease (PRISM), lactate and CRP, which have been described separately in paediatric and adult critical illness [84, 88].

There is a paucity of research in CIC and results have been inconsistent, with glutamine supplementation failing to show any benefit in infants with gastrointestinal disease requiring surgery, but the converse has been shown in burns, acute diarrhoea and mucositis in stem cell transplants [83, 89]. However, there are numerous methodological issues with earlier studies which may have impacted on the results, e.g. use of L-glutamine versus stable dipeptide [90], suboptimal delivery of essential amino acids and the number of days it took to achieve goal rate of delivery. Intravenous glutamine supplementation appears to have the most benefit, making glutamine available for immune cells and other rapidly dividing cells [23, 24]. At present, due to the converse result regarding the benefits of glutamine in critical illness, there is insufficient evidence to recommend the routine use of glutamine supplementation in CIC.

Zinc

Zinc is an essential trace element which is required for the function of numerous enzymes and transcriptional factors. Zinc homeostasis maintains immune function, oxidative stress response, neurocognitive function and promotes growth and development [91]. During critical illness investigators have found the expression of numerous genes that either require zinc and or have a role in regulating zinc homeostasis [92]. CIC have been found to have significantly lower plasma zinc levels in the first few days of their illness which is correlated with markers of inflammation (IL-6 and CRP levels). Persistently low plasma concentrations were also associated with the severity (and number) of

organ(s) dysfunction [91] and increased mortality rate in septic shock [92]. What is not known is whether the low plasma levels are a result of a protective mechanism relative to zinc redistribution to decrease the level of inflammation, similar to infection related hypoferraemia [49] – laboratory studies suggest that some bacteria use zinc as a mechanism for adherence – or whether higher levels of zinc increase the ability of immune cells to fight infections [93]. Further studies are required to determine whether or not oral zinc supplementation ameliorates the low plasma levels seen in critical illness. Also is this micronutrient beneficial to CIC (and/or subgroups), as seen in children with acute diarrhoeal disease and pneumonia?

Selenium

Selenium is an essential trace element with antioxidant and immunological functions. Selenium has been shown to inhibit the expression of proinflammatory genes, downregulating the inflammatory response. Decreased selenium levels are found in adults with systemic inflammatory response syndrome and multi-organ failure [94]. High doses of selenium given as IV infusion selenite (1000–1600 µg) has shown to be well tolerated, significantly increasing selenium levels with resultant lower incidence of hospital acquired ventilator associated pneumonia; to reduce infection risk; and to decrease mortality in patients with severe sepsis or septic shock [94, 95]. Selenium given enterally as a feed constituent has not been shown to be as effective, although the dose delivered was significantly lower at 300 µg. There are no studies considering the efficacy of selenium in CIC.

The paediatric Critical Illness Stress-induced Immune Suppression (CRISIS) trial is currently considering the effect of an enterally administered whey protein supplemented with trace zinc, selenium and glutamine. These results are awaited with interest and may change practice in relation to glutamine, zinc and selenium supplementation [96].

Vitamin D

There are a number of disease conditions in the general population which are associated with vitamin D deficiency. There are numerous reports of low vitamin D levels in CIC, which are associated with a greater severity of illness [97], although the causality and the impact of vitamin D on outcomes during critical illness remain unclear [98].

Probiotics

A probiotic is a live microbial feed supplement which beneficially affects the host by improving its intestinal microbial balance [99]. Altering enteric flora is a concept gaining popularity throughout the world and the use of probiotic bacteria in PICUs is developing too. Intestinal permeability is increased during critical illness particularly after burns, major trauma and sepsis. In addition bacterial translocation has been demonstrated in patients with bowel obstruction. The administration of some probiotic strains has been associated with a reduction in bacterial translocation and intestinal inflammation [100].

In critically ill patients, the main concern remains the possibility of septicaemia related to the provision of live bacteria to patients that are relatively immunocompromised. Although there are some studies showing not only their beneficial effects but also their safe use in critical care [101], Boyle et al. [102] hint towards caution in the extreme premature infant and those that are immunocompromised [89], in particular where the permeability of the gastrointestinal tract has been impaired. Because of the paucity of information regarding the mechanisms through which probiotics act, appropriate administrative regimens and probiotic interactions, further investigation is needed in these areas.

Part 3

Clinical Dietetics

6 Preterm Infants

Caroline King and Kate Tavener

Introduction

A preterm infant is one born before 37 weeks completed gestation. An infant born <2500 g is termed low birthweight regardless of gestation, <1500 g very low birthweight (VLBW) and those <1000 g extremely low birthweight (ELBW). Categorisation of infants born smaller than expected is more contentious; however, they are often divided into small for gestational age (SGA) and/or intrauterine growth restricted (IUGR). Classification of SGA infants is usually defined as <9th percentile for weight at birth (depending on source of definition) and they constitute a heterogeneous group, i.e. those destined to be born small due to genetic influences and those who are IUGR. The former group tends to be proportionally small. Those who are IUGR will have a similarly low birthweight but may show head and/or length sparing depending on the timing of intrauterine nutrient restriction. These infants are at high risk of both perinatal and later problems [1]. This chapter will deal predominantly with the nutritional needs of preterm infants.

The early nutritional management of preterm infants may be vital to their later outcome, but can be hampered by an immature or dysfunctional gastrointestinal tract and poor tolerance of parenteral and enteral nutrition.

Small term infants in general are mature with respect to oromotor function and can usually grow well if allowed breast or standard infant formula *ad lib*. Only where comorbidities exist may small term infants need specialised nutritional input. It is not recommended that these infants are given any formula designed for preterm infants as there may be adverse outcomes [2, 3].

Nutritional requirements

Preterm infants have limited stores of many nutrients as accretion occurs predominantly in the last trimester [4]. They are poorly equipped to withstand inadequate nutrition; theoretically endogenous reserves in a 1000 g infant are only sufficient for 4 days if unfed [5]. In addition, the gastrointestinal system is immature; thus it is generally accepted that most infants of <30 weeks' gestation will need some parenteral nutrition (PN) while enteral feeds are gradually increased to ensure an adequate nutritional intake. The most recent comprehensive reviews and recommendations for enteral and parenteral nutritional requirements

Table 6.1 Recommended enteral and parenteral nutrient intakes for very low birthweight infants.

Nutrient (per kg per day)	Tsang et al. [7] enteral	Agostoni et al. [8] (ESPGHAN) enteral	Term infant RNI (1991)* enteral	Tsang et al. [7] parenteral
Energy	110–130 kcal (460–545kJ)	110–135 (460–565kJ)	115–100 (480–420kJ)	90–100 (375–420kJ)
Protein (g)	–	–	2.1	–
Protein (g), <1000 g body weight	3.8–4.4	4.0–4.5	N/S	N/S
Protein (g), 1000–1500 g body weight	3.4–4.2	3.5–4.0	N/S	3.2–3.8
Carbohydrate (g)	7–17	11.6–13.2	N/S	9.7–15
Fat (g)	5.3–7.2	4.8–6.6 (<40% MCT)	N/S	3.0–4.0
DHA (mg)	≥18	12–30	N/S	≥11
AA (mg)	≥24	18–42	N/S	≥14
Sodium (mmol)	3.0–5.0	3.0–5.0	1.5	3.0–5.0
Phosphate (mmol)	1.9–4.5	1.9–2.8	2.2	1.5–1.9
Iron (mg)	2–4	2–3	0.3	0.1–0.2
Calcium (mmol)	2.5–5.5	3.0–3.5	2.2	1.5–2.0
Zinc (mg)	1.0–3.0	1.1–2.0	0.7	0.4
Selenium (µg)	1.3–4.5	5–10	1.7	1.5–4.5
Folic acid (µg)	25–50	35–100	8.5	56
Vitamin A (µg)	212–454	400–1000	59	212–454
Vitamin D (µg/day)[†]	10	20–25	8.5	1–4
Vitamin E (mg)	4–8	2.2–11	0.37	1.9–2.3

DHA, docosahexaenoic acid; AA, arachidonic acid; RNI, reference nutrient intakes.

Agostoni et al. recommendations are for stable growing preterm infants up to a weight of 1800 g; no recommendations are made for infants <1000 g except for protein. Tsang et al. recommendations presented are for stable growing VLBW infants from 1000 to 1500 g; no recommendations are given for infants over 1500 g.

*Estimated average requirement for energy and reference nutrient intake for 0–3 months (Department of Health Report on Health and Social Subjects No. 41. *Dietary Reference Values for Food. Energy and Nutrition for the United Kingdom*. London: The Stationery Office, 1991).

[†]Vitamin D is per day not per kg. 1 µg vitamin A = 3.33 IU. 1 µg vitamin D = 40 IU. N/S = not specified.

are those of Tsang et al. [7] and Agostoni et al. [8] (Table 6.1). The interested reader is advised to refer to these publications for further information. There is also a review of recommendations for preterm infant formulas which although published in 2002 has some useful background information [6].

Precise requirements for infants born between 1800 g and 2500 g are not given in these publications. This has led to varying interpretations of the weight cut-offs for feeding preterm formulas or fortifying breast milk. Higher nutrient density feeds are not routinely recommended for term SGA infants so gestational age as well as birthweight should dictate local feeding policy. In practice most infants born <2000 g and <34 completed weeks will benefit from the higher nutrient intakes recommended by Tsang et al. [7] and Agostoni et al. [8].

At the time of going to print a new text containing nutrient recommendations for preterm infants has been published by Koletzko et al. and readers are also encouraged to refer to this publication. A brief review shows very few significant changes but the background discussion will be of great interest to anyone involved in preterm nutriiton Ref: Koletzko, B., Poindexter, B., Uauy, R. (2014) Nutritional Care of Preterm Infants. Scientific Basis and Practical Guidelines.

Interpretation of requirements

Caution must be exercised when interpreting recommendations for requirements for two reasons. First, the evidence base for nutrient requirements in preterm infants is not robust with very few randomised controlled trials (RCTs) having been undertaken, particularly in VLBW or ELBW infants. Recommendations for requirements are compiled from a variety of data sources including fetal tissue analysis, placental transfer studies, cohort studies, case reports of deficiency or toxicity, breast milk composition and a few RCTs of controlled intake. Much of the data for infants <1000 g is extrapolated. Second, preterm infants are a heterogeneous group and requirements are highly variable depending on post conceptional age (inversely related), accumulated nutrient deficit (prenatally and postnatally), body composition and variations in resting energy expenditure. In addition, as with other recommendations for requirements, these are for whole populations rather than individuals.

Recommended nutrient intakes are typically greater for enterally fed compared with parenterally fed infants, and greater for preterm compared with term. The following provides further information regarding certain key nutrients. Requirements refer to those via the enteral route unless specified.

Fluid

During the initial phase of adaptation to extrauterine life, fluid management is complicated as there is a delicate balance between matching high transcutaneous losses and avoiding fluid overload due to renal immaturity (although the former should be minimised by appropriate nursing techniques). Very sick preterm infants are often fluid restricted but nutritional intakes should always be optimised within the fluid allowed and restrictions lifted as soon as clinical condition permits. Recommendations from Agostoni et al. [8] suggest 135 mL/kg/day is the minimum requirement with an upper reasonable limit of 200 mL/kg/day. Between 150 and 180 mL/kg/day is likely to meet enteral requirements if feeding fortified human milk, and the lower end of the range if preterm formula is given.

Energy

Recommended energy intakes vary according to the baby's birthweight and postnatal age but are generally higher than term requirements [7]. There may be variations in resting energy expenditure with requirements potentially reduced in very sick, ventilated infants and increased in infants with increased respiratory effort. Some IUGR babies may have increased needs to facilitate catch-up growth but this will vary between individuals and can only be established by monitoring progress and adjusting intakes accordingly. Optimising body composition is essential and excessive energy intake may lead to excessive fat deposition. However, severity of illness rather than diet appears to be most closely linked to increased abdominal adiposity [9]. It is recommended that >100 kcal (420 kJ)/kg/day is generally appropriate for enteral formula feeding as long as adequate protein, 3.0–3.6 g/100 kcal (420 kJ), is provided [8]. There are currently only three preterm formulas that meet this requirement: Aptamil Preterm, Nutriprem 1 and Hydrolysed Nutriprem. Monitoring linear growth as a proxy for lean mass accretion is recommended.

Protein

Current recommendations for protein requirements assume an accumulated nutrient deficit due to an inability to provide full requirements during sickness and periods of fluid restriction and are therefore significantly higher than term requirements. Both Tsang et al. [7] and Agostoni et al. [8] have revised recommendations upwards compared with previous recommendations. Individual requirements will vary according to post conceptional age and degree of nutrient deficit. A requirement of 4 g/kg/day protein can be met with 180–200 mL/kg/day of fortified breast milk, 160 mL/kg/day Nutriprem 1 or 180 mL/kg/day SMA Gold Prem 1.

The benefits of early provision of amino acids (AA) in PN for preterm infants is generally well accepted; however, the amount required initially is the subject of debate. A recent RCT looked at 3.5 vs. 2.4 g AA/kg from day 1 and found equal nitrogen retention but more abnormal blood results in the 3.5 g AA/kg group [10]. They also found better nitrogen retention if lipid was given on day 1 at around 2 g/kg. Another RCT showed that achieving 4 g AA/kg within the first 3 days led to improved head growth after 4 weeks [11]; in this study both groups received 1.8 g AA/kg for the first 2–3 days. In an observational study Poindexter et al. [12] found that the provision of early AA to ELBW infants (≥3 g/kg/day at ≤5 days of life) resulted in improved weight, length and head circumference at 36 weeks post conceptional age although there was no difference between groups at 18 months and no difference in neurodevelopmental outcome. Further research is required before firm conclusions can be drawn about the benefits of early, high protein provision and outcome.

Fat

Fat absorption can vary between individuals but the more immature the infant the higher the risk for malabsorption due to low bile salt pools [13] and reduced pancreatic lipase levels [14]. Despite this, the fat component of both enteral and parenteral nutrition is crucial to attain the high energy requirements of preterm infants and to provide essential fatty acids. Feeding with non heat treated breast milk has the advantage of an endogenous lipase (bile salt stimulated lipase) which ensures optimum fat absorption [15].

For many years studies have investigated the theory that enteral medium chain triglycerides (MCT) lead to improved fat absorption. However, a systematic review found no consistent advantage [16]. Agostoni et al [8] recommend that fat in the form of MCT should not exceed 40% of the total fat content of preterm formulas. Preterm formulas currently contain SMA Gold Prem 1 12.5% fat as MCT; Nutriprem 1, Hydrolysed Nutriprem and Aptamil Preterm 18% fat as MCT.

It has been recommended that the long chain polyunsaturated (LCP) derivatives of linoleic and α-linolenic acids, namely arachidonic and docosa-hexaenoic acids, are provided in the diet of preterm infants [7,8]. However, controversy remains concerning their role with recent reviews concluding that there were few significant benefits although no evidence of harm [17,18]. Outcomes with respect to neurodevelopment have been inconsistent which may be due to genetic variations between individuals in their ability to manufacture LCPs from precursors [19]. There also appears to be risk of greater adiposity and blood pressure for preterm

girls supplemented with LCP [19]. Conversely, recent research suggests that girls may show positive effects of LCP supplementation with respect to neurodevelopment [20]. Conclusions are made difficult by the heterogeneity of studies and they also generally include only mature and healthy preterm infants. Despite this, all current preterm formulas are supplemented with LCP whereas the standard lipid emulsions used for parenteral feeding are not.

Enteral requirements for fat are in the range 4.8–6.6 g/kg/day [8]. Parenterally most infants will tolerate 3 g/kg/day of lipid, although extremely premature or very low birthweight infants may develop hypertriglyceridaemia at this level of administration and caution should be exercised. A healthy preterm infant will probably tolerate and grow well on 3.5 g/kg/day lipid. Preterm infants, particularly those born VLBW and ELBW, will develop essential fatty acid deficiency very rapidly without an exogenous supply. This can be obtained from as little as 0.5 g/kg/day of one of the current parenteral lipid emulsions [21].

Carbohydrate

Lactase activity is present from 10 to 12 weeks' gestation and approaches levels expected at term at 36 weeks' gestation. Exposure to lactose may help to induce intestinal lactase activity. In practice, lactose malabsorption is rarely seen.

A large range of oligosaccharides are present in breast milk, being highest in colostrum and decreasing with the duration of lactation. They may help to protect against gut problems, both by encouraging growth of a beneficial intestinal flora and by inhibiting binding of pathogens. They may improve feed tolerance and reduce stool viscosity [22]; however, a recent review of the literature by the European Society of Paediatric Gastroenterology, Hepatology and Nutrition (ESPGHAN) states that more research is required before firm conclusions about their benefits can be drawn [23]. Oligosaccharides are currently added to Aptamil Preterm and Nutriprem 1 feeds.

Tolerance to carbohydrate load in PN needs close monitoring, especially in the sick or extremely preterm infant. Most preterm infants require 15 g/kg/day glucose in order to meet requirements and limits for glucose oxidation are approximately

18 g/kg/day, above which net lipogenesis occurs [24]. Limits for glucose administration peripherally are approximately 10%–12% concentration.

Calcium, phosphorus and vitamin D

The homeostasis of calcium, phosphorus and magnesium is fundamental to the development of bone and this in turn is regulated by factors including hormones and vitamin D. Metabolic bone disease of prematurity is a recognised morbidity. Causes include an inadequate supply of nutrients (calcium, phosphorus, vitamin D), prolonged PN, immobilisation and medications. Immobilisation stimulates bone reabsorption whilst steroids (occasionally still used to treat chronic lung disease) reduce calcium absorption, increase urinary losses and have a direct effect on bone. Diuretics and methylxanthines such as caffeine, used to optimise respiratory status, increase renal calcium excretion. Premature infants are also born with poor reserves of calcium, phosphorus and vitamin D and have a high requirement in order to optimise bone mineralisation. Infants born IUGR or SGA are also more likely to show signs of osteopenia due to poor placental supply.

The recommendations provided by Tsang et al. [7] and Agostoni et al. [8] for calcium and phosphate are similar; however, vitamin D recommendations from Agostoni et al. are significantly higher. They argue that since the prevalence of maternal vitamin D deficiency is high, supplementation with 800–1000 IU (20–25 µg) per day is required to achieve optimal serum levels of 25-hydroxyvitamin D. There is no evidence that this higher amount of vitamin D is beneficial and there is some evidence that these higher levels will be excessive for some infants [25]. However, babies of mothers with documented vitamin D deficiency will benefit from the higher levels as the placental supply will have been compromised. This will need to be given as a supplement as current breast milk fortifiers and preterm formulas do not contain sufficient vitamin D to match this recommendation. The ratio between calcium and phosphorus is also important for adequate bone mineralisation and Agostoni et al. recommend an enteral Ca:P ratio of 1.5–2.0.

In PN solutions, stability of these nutrients is a limiting factor as calcium and phosphate can bind and precipitate, although the introduction of organic phosphate salts has led to improved solubility and allows greater amounts to be given. The ideal Ca:P ratio should be no less than 1:1 in PN solutions [26].

Iron

At birth there is an abrupt reduction in erythropoiesis leading to early anaemia of prematurity which is not affected by iron supplementation. Preterm iron stores are low and infants may also lose significant volumes of blood through phlebotomy. Iron, in excess, is toxic and therefore supplementation needs to be carefully weighed up against potential overload. Babies receiving regular blood transfusions may benefit from delayed iron supplementation.

Preterm infants will become iron deplete by 8 weeks without supplementation [27]. Current recommendations are that supplements should commence between 2 and 8 weeks of age (earlier in ELBW infants) as either a supplemented formula or medicinal iron at a dose of 2–4 mg/kg/day [7]. These recommendations can easily be met by adequate volumes of currently available preterm infant formulas. Breast milk fortifiers in the UK and PN solutions do not provide iron and therefore supplementation will be required if these are used.

Conditionally essential nutrients

Beta-carotene, nucleotides and inositol are present in human milk and are often added to preterm infant formulas and breast milk fortifiers; however, there is currently no evidence of benefit in the preterm population.

Parenteral nutrition

PN has become the cornerstone of neonatal nutritional care in the very preterm infant, without which many infants would not survive. PN is required when adequate nutrients to sustain growth and development cannot be provided via the enteral route. PN should therefore be considered in infants

• born <30 weeks' gestation

- with congenital gastrointestinal abnormalities, e.g. exomphalos, gastroschisis
- with gastrointestinal dysfunction, e.g. feeding intolerance, necrotising enterocolitis (NEC), short bowel syndrome
- who are at high risk of developing NEC (p. 100) and require prolonged minimal enteral nutrition

PN can usually be started safely and effectively within the first few hours of birth in the preterm infant [10, 28]. Solutions used are the same as those for term infants; however, quantities provided vary in order to meet their nutritional needs. An example of a suitable parenteral feeding regimen for a preterm infant is given in Table 6.2 and a case study is presented in Table 6.3.

Monitoring

Monitoring PN administration in preterm infants is imperative. A suggested guide for frequency of monitoring is given in Table 6.4. More frequent monitoring may be required according to the clinical condition of the infant.

Parenteral nutrition related complications

Some of the smallest and sickest infants tolerate PN the least, whilst they also have the greatest nutritional needs; managing the complications of PN administration whilst optimising nutrition is therefore a significant challenge in this patient group.

Hyperglycaemia

This is common in small preterm infants and results from impaired glucose homeostasis which may be aggravated by over zealous carbohydrate provision via PN solutions or unwittingly administering excess glucose in the form of intravenous drugs and flushes. Often this is temporary, lasting only a few days, but can significantly affect total energy provision if the glucose infusion rate is lowered. Insulin can be used cautiously in these cases in order to optimise nutrient provision, but glucose infusions >8 mg/kg/min should be avoided in very preterm infants as this may lead to excessive fat deposition (see Carbohydrate).

Hypertriglyceridaemia

ELBW, SGA and septic infants have lower lipoprotein lipase activity and therefore struggle with lipid clearance, often leading to hypertriglyceridaemia. The significance of this is unclear, but based on the limited evidence available the most recent recommendations suggest that triglyceride levels >250 mg/dL (2.8 mmol/L) should be avoided [26].

Table 6.2 Example parenteral feeding regimen for a preterm infant.

Nutrient (per kg per day)	Day 1	Day 2	Day 3, fluid limited	Day 3, standard PN
Volume (mL/kg/day)	60	90	120	150
Protein (g)	1.5	2.2	2.8	3.5
Nitrogen (g)	0.24	0.35	0.46	0.56
Glucose (g)	6.7	9.5	12.2	15
Lipid (g)	1.5	2	3	3.5
Sodium (mmol)	Variable*	Variable*	2.4	3.0
Potassium (mmol)	0.9	1.3	1.6	2.0
Phosphate (mmol)	0.7	0.95	1.2	1.5
Calcium (mmol)	0.7	0.95	1.2	1.5
Magnesium (mmol)	0.09	0.13	0.15	0.2
Solivito (mL/kg/day)	1.0	1.0	1.0	1.0
Vitlipid Infant (mL/kg/day)	4.0	4.0	4.0	4.0
Peditrace (mL/kg/day)	1.0	1.0	1.0	1.0
Total energy (kcal/kg/day)	48	67	90	109

PN, parenteral nutrition.

*Supplementation is usually delayed until a postnatal fluid loss has been demonstrated over the first few days.

Table 6.3 Case study: preterm infant on parenteral nutrition.

Baby girl, born at 27⁺³/40, birthweight 890 g (25th centile). Maternal premature rupture of membranes with maternal antenatal steroids given

Day	Narrative	Biochemistry	Nutritional intervention
1	Continuous positive airways pressure (CPAP) commenced Umbilical line inserted for fluid administration	NA	Standard bag of parenteral nutrition (PN) commenced at 60 mL/kg/day* providing 1.5 g protein†/kg/day, 6.7 g/kg/day glucose, total 48 kcal (200 kJ)/kg/day Lipid infused separately at 1.5 g/kg/day 15 mL/kg/day maternal expressed breast milk (MEBM) + donor breast milk (DBM) as bolus feeds
2	NA	NA	PN increased to 90 mL/kg/day* 30 mL/kg/day MEBM + DBM as bolus feeds
3	NA	NA	PN increased to 120 mL/kg/day* PN provides 3.5 g protein/kg/day, 15 g glucose/kg/day, 3.5 g lipid/kg/day, total 109 kcal (455 kJ)/kg/day 50 mL/kg/day MEBM as bolus feeds
5	Increased oxygen requirements Sepsis Intubated and ventilated Insulin started	Blood sugar levels increase to 9–11 mmol/L	PN kept at 120 mL/kg/day Feeds reduced to 15 mL/kg/day MEBM as bolus feeds
7	Worsening sepsis High nasogastric aspirate volumes Total fluids restricted to 100 mL/kg/day as intravenous fluids	Blood sugar levels remain >9 mmol/L Triglyceride levels raised at 4.5 mmol/L	Nil by mouth PN infusion rate reduced to 100 mL/kg/day giving glucose load of 12.5 g/kg/day Lipid reduced to 1 g/kg/day due to raised blood sugars and raised serum triglycerides
9	Nasogastric aspirates reducing	NA	20 mL/kg/day MEBM restarted as bolus feed
12	Chest improving Total fluids liberalised to 120 mL/kg/day Insulin stopped Weight = 920 g (9th centile)	Blood sugar levels normalising at 5–7 mmol/L	PN increased to provide 3.5 g/kg/day protein, 15 g glucose/kg/day, 3.5 g lipid/kg/day, total 109 kcal (455 kJ)/kg/day Feeds increased by 20 mL/kg/day
14	Extubated back to CPAP Total fluids = 150 mL/kg/day	NA	80 mL/kg/day MEBM, continues increasing by 20 mL/kg/day PN maintained at 70 mL/kg/day
16	NA	NA	120 mL/kg/day MEBM as bolus feed PN stopped Enteral feeds continue to increase up to 180 mL/kg/day in 20–30 mL/kg/day increments

NA, not available;
*Intravenous infusion with electrolytes also given as needed depending on serum biochemistry.
†Protein × 1.12 = amino acids.

Table 6.4   Guide for monitoring parenteral nutrition (PN).

	Urea and electrolytes	Liver function tests	Calcium	Phosphate	Magnesium	Triglycerides	Conjugated bilirubin	Trace elements (selenium, zinc, copper, manganese)
First 2 weeks of PN or unstable infant	Daily	Daily	Daily	Daily	Weekly	Weekly	Weekly	–
>2 weeks PN and stable infant	Twice weekly	Twice weekly	Twice weekly	Twice weekly	Weekly	Weekly	Weekly	Monthly once on PN >3 weeks

Reducing, rather than stopping, lipid infusions is advised in order to prevent essential fatty acid deficiency [21].

Parenteral nutrition associated liver disease

Preterm infants are particularly vulnerable to parenteral nutrition associated liver disease (PNALD) due to functional and anatomical immaturity of the liver. PNALD development is associated with increased length of time on PN, sepsis, lack of enteral feeding, overfeeding and low birthweight [29]. Practices that may limit its severity or development include

- limiting carbohydrate infusion to <18 g/kg/day
- introducing and maintaining at least minimal enteral nutrition
- alternative lipid emulsions

There is currently increasing evidence to suggest that the type of lipid emulsion used may play a role in the development of PNALD. Lipid emulsions containing ω3 LCP, such as SMOF (soya, MCT, olive and fish oils), have been developed and early studies suggest that they may be of benefit in ameliorating the development of PNALD or even reversal of cholestasis in long term PN use in children [30]. Evidence for using SMOF in preterm infants is limited, but has been demonstrated to be safe in the short term and to improve serum fatty acid levels [31]. Long term data are needed on growth as studies have demonstrated slower growth when preterm formulas supplemented with LCP contained docosahexaenoic acid (an ω3 LCP) without sufficient arachidonic acid [32,33]. Due to the current lack of RCTs with sufficient follow-up, such lipid emulsions should not currently be used routinely in preterm infants.

Significant PNALD leads to reduced bile flow resulting in fat malabsorption and poor weight gain. Enteral formulas containing MCT, such as Pepti-Junior and Pregestimil, may be of benefit. If the infant is feeding breast milk the use of these formulas should be clearly justified and they need to be introduced cautiously in infants at high risk of NEC. Maintaining a proportion of the enteral nutrition (25%–30%) as breast milk may help with tolerance and deliver the immunological benefits of breast milk over formula. As with all term formulas, the use of MCT based formulas will not meet the nutritional needs of the preterm infant. They should therefore be used strictly as clinically indicated and stopped as soon as liver function improves. In order to optimise nutritional status these formulas should ideally be given at a minimum of 180–200 mL/kg/day and should be concentrated up to 15% (15 g powder in 100 mL water) or 1 scoop powder to every 25 mL water. Extra vitamins, particularly fat soluble vitamins, should also be administered.

Prescribing practice

PN should ideally be prescribed by an experienced neonatal pharmacist alongside a neonatologist and neonatal dietitian. Input from other sources including specialist nutrition nurses, gastroenterologists, hepatologists and surgeons may also be helpful. A recent national enquiry into prescribing practice in the UK found significant variability [34]. Optimising nutritional content and facilitating early PN are clear areas for improvement. Standard bags have been shown to improve rates of early PN administration and improve nutritional intake and costs

[35, 36]. Infants who are well and stable will typically tolerate and grow if given adequate volumes of a standard PN bag.

Benefits of standard bags include

- availability from first day of life
- consistency of nutritional care
- cost
- accuracy – the end product is tested

Limitations of standard bags include

- inflexibility in supply of electrolytes
- nutritionally adequate only if full volume provided

Minimal enteral nutrition

Structural development of the gut *in utero* initially commences outside the body of the fetus. At 8–12 weeks' gestation the primitive gut rotates and returns into the abdominal cavity. Villi develop from around 12 weeks' gestation and they mature from approximately 22 weeks. Functional maturation occurs somewhat later with enzymes being produced from around 8 weeks' gestation and increasing in production from around 25 weeks. Motor function also begins to develop around 25 weeks' gestation so that structure and most function is in place around this time [37]. However, immature motor function is likely to be the most common cause of enteral feed intolerance in the VLBW infant.

A lack of enteral nutrition leads to risk of gut atrophy and impairs gut development. Minimal enteral feeding (also known as 'non nutritive feeding', 'trophic feeding' or 'gut priming') is the process by which small volumes of milk (12–24 mL/kg/day) are provided enterally for up to 7 days to facilitate gut adaptation rather than for nutritive gain. It is believed that these small amounts of milk can promote intestinal maturation and prevent or reverse the mucosal changes seen during starvation.

When to start

It is generally accepted that enteral feeds should be commenced as early as possible in the stable, low risk preterm infant [38, 39] and evidence is accumulating to suggest that it is also safe to introduce feeds early in the higher risk infant [40, 41]. There is no evidence that delaying enteral feeds (>5–7 days) in VLBW infants reduces the risk of NEC [42]. Evidence also suggests that the severity of NEC is greatest if an infant has never received enteral feeds before diagnosis [43], which also supports the practice of introducing early enteral feeds. The ADEPT trial [41] investigated the effect of enteral feeding on NEC in high risk growth restricted preterm infants with abnormal antenatal Doppler. The authors concluded that early feeding (within 24–48 hours of birth) in this group of infants led to a reduced time to full enteral feeds compared with late feeding (within 120–144 hours of birth) without an increased risk of NEC. However, it is important to note that infants with abnormal antenatal Doppler who were born at <29 weeks' gestation in this study were approximately four times more likely to develop NEC irrespective of whether they were fed early or late. This group of infants may therefore benefit from a more prolonged period of minimal enteral nutrition and slower advancement of feeds [44].

What to give

See Enteral nutrition.

How to progress

A recent Cochrane review [45] comparing slow (15–20 mL/kg/day) versus rapid (30–35 mL/kg/day) advancements of feeds concluded that there was no significant difference in risk of NEC, but that the slow group took longer to regain birthweight and to establish full enteral feeds. It should be noted, however, that this review did not include high risk infants including those who were ELBW or who were growth restricted. In practice, evidence suggests that caution should be exercised when increasing feeds in high risk infants and continual review of the literature is recommended [39]. An extended period of trophic feeding (5–7 days) followed by cautious increases in feeds at a limit of 20 mL/kg/day is recommended in this patient group. Evidence in lower risk infants indicates increases of 30 mL/kg/day are considered safe [44]. Evidence also suggests that the number of days to full feeds are reduced in VLBW infants if fed 2 hourly compared with 3 hourly [46].

Enteral nutrition

Breast milk

The freshly expressed breast milk (EBM) from a preterm baby's own mother is considered the optimal enteral feed [47]. Much of the evidence is gathered from studies other than RCTs as it is impossible to randomise a baby to receive their mother's own milk. No RCTs were found for inclusion in a Cochrane review [48]. Where there have been RCTs including the use of breast milk they have involved randomising babies to donor breast milk or formula when their mother chose not to provide breast milk. When NEC was examined separately it was found that breast milk in the form of donor breast milk did significantly reduce risk [49]. There are a large number of observational studies to support mother's own freshly EBM as the milk of choice for preterm babies. Several studies confirm association with mother's EBM and lower risk of NEC [50–52]. There may also be long term neurodevelopmental advantages [53–56].

Breast milk may be nutritionally adequate in many respects for babies >33 weeks' gestation when fed in sufficient volumes (up to 220 mL/kg/day in well infants) although vitamin and mineral supplements will be needed (Table 6.5). However, in infants <33 weeks many nutrients will be limiting from the start of feeding, e.g. phosphorus, sodium and most vitamins, particularly the fat soluble ones; or become limiting after 2–3 weeks of feeding, e.g. protein, calcium and zinc.

Preterm breast milk during the first 2–3 weeks of lactation usually has higher protein levels than later on [57, 58]. Protein fortification will eventually be needed for babies <33 weeks. Some units start this routinely while others wait until there are signs that additional protein is needed [59] (see Serum biochemistry, and Table 6.5). A commercial multinutrient breast milk fortifier (BMF) has many advantages over the addition of nutrients as separate supplements, e.g. reduced risk of excessively high osmolality, reduced risk of errors in administration and reduced nursing time. Those currently available in the UK are Nutriprem and SMA breast milk fortifiers. Typical composition of a BMF is given in Table 6.6.

A systematic review concluded that BMFs promote short term growth, and that despite lack of longer term outcome data it was unlikely that further trials would be carried out with an unfortified breast milk group [60]. The BMFs available in the UK provide nutrients sufficiently close to current recommendations [8]; however, they do not contain iron so a separate supplement is necessary. Table 6.7 compares fortified breast milk with the guidelines.

Despite concerns around increased osmolality and bacterial growth with the use of BMF the evidence does not support this [61], and there is little evidence to suggest a link with NEC [62]. Unfortunately the latter paper perpetuated a misconception that there is evidence that a fortifier based on human milk protein has been shown to reduce the risk of NEC [63]. However, it is advisable to add BMF to the minimum amount of milk possible and to feed this before fortifying any more to avoid prolonged storage and any potential consequent disruption of immunological components, which has not yet been quantified. All feeds should be handled and stored according to current guidelines to avoid contamination [64].

Strategies are needed to ensure that mothers of preterm babies are able to produce milk in time for their baby's first feed and, if planning to breast feed on discharge, to provide sufficient quantities to support the volume their baby will need longer term [65]. Table 6.8 shows a sample check list which can be used to ensure mothers are given appropriate support and information at the relevant times. Another useful resource is the booklet produced by the UK based charity for sick and preterm babies, BLISS; see the website for the most recent publications.

If mothers are advised to express 8–10 times per day including once at night, and to fully empty the breast of all the fat rich hind milk, they should produce milk of sufficient energy content to preclude the need for energy supplementation. However, human milk is prone to fat loss and should be handled carefully to avoid this. If it is felt that more energy is required it may be useful for the baby to be preferentially fed hind milk [66]. Supplementation of human milk with energy alone is not advised unless there is a very strong suspicion that

Table 6.5 Case study: preterm infant on enteral nutrition.

Baby boy, born at 27/40, birthweight 800 g (9th centile). Spontaneous rupture of membranes, maternal antenatal steroids given

Day	Narrative	Biochemistry (mmol/L)	Nutritional intervention
1	Mother visited by member of neonatal unit staff within 6 hours of delivery and provision of her breast milk (BM) discussed; she is happy to express Advised on breast massage and hand expressing	NA	Parenteral nutrition (PN) started 6 hours postnatally At 12 hours old 0.5 mL colostrum used for mouth care
2	Mother and father have long visits to baby Mother encouraged to express after visiting	Sodium 136 Phosphorus 1.9 Urea 8	PN given at 150 mL/kg and proportionally decreased once baby on 20 mL/kg BM BM increased 10–20 mL/kg/day depending on tolerance
3	Meconium passed and yellow seedy stools appear Maternal milk production >10 mL at each expression so instruction in mechanical expression given	NA	PN volume decreased as BM increased
5	Enteral feed well tolerated, minimal aspirates and bowels open 1–2 times per day Maternal lactation checked: 200 mL/day and increasing	Sodium 133 Phosphorus 1.5 Urea 6	PN decreased to 30 mL/kg BM 120 mL/kg Supplements started: sodium 2 mmol/kg and phosphorus 1 mmol/day
7	Enteral feed tolerance as above Parents having skin to skin cuddles with baby Cotside expressing encouraged	NA	PN stopped BM 140 mL/kg and increasing by 10–15 mL twice a day to max 180 mL/kg Multivitamin supplement containing 400 IU vitamin D and 5000 IU vitamin A started*
10	Maternal lactation checked: <600 mL/day Further advice on expressing given	NA	BM 180 mL/kg
13	Maternal lactation improving with increase to 8–10 expressions per day, including at night	Sodium 135 Phosphorus 2 Urea 3	BM 180 mL/kg To remain on same supplements
17	The need for breast milk fortifier (BMF) discussed with parents and its use explained	NA	BM 180 mL/kg Sodium and phosphorus supplements kept the same BMF started† Multivitamin supplement stopped once on full strength BMF
20	Baby now 32 weeks and beginning to nuzzle at breast during skin to skin contact; will begin first attempts at suckling over next week Mother reports largest volumes of milk expressed after skin to skin contact	Sodium 137 Phosphorus 2.4 Urea 2.2	BM 180 mL/kg + BMF Sodium and phosphorus supplements stopped Iron supplement written up to start the next day

NA, not available.

*Some units will also give folic acid and vitamin E but evidence for benefit during the short period between stopping PN and starting BMF is lacking.

†Could be half strength for 24 hours or full strength straight away; there is no consensus.

Table 6.6 Typical composition of a multinutrient breast milk fortifier.

Protein (whole or hydrolysed)
Calcium
Phosphorus
Sodium
Fat soluble vitamins including vitamin E
Water soluble vitamins including folic acid
Trace elements, e.g. zinc, selenium, copper, magnesium, iodine, manganese
Some contain iron (but not those available in the UK)

only more energy is needed as the protein:energy ratio in the milk may be reduced to an unacceptably low level.

If mother's own milk is not available or there is a delay in obtaining it, donor breast milk is the alternative feed of choice to initiate enteral feeding as it is associated with a reduced risk of NEC [48]. There are guidelines from the National Institute for Health and Care Excellence (NICE) for the processing and handling of donor milk in the UK [67]. All donor milk in the UK is pasteurised to ensure microbiological safety with the preservation of as many immunological components as possible.

However, this leads to denaturation of the bile salt stimulated lipase with subsequent lower fat absorption; therefore to achieve optimal growth babies are usually graded onto preterm formula once full feed volumes are established, if mother's milk remains unavailable [68]. Although not all units have a milk bank, any baby in the UK can have access to donor breast milk; it can be purchased from many of the established milk banks and delivered to the requesting unit. Further information is available on the UK Association for Milk Banking (UKAMB) website (www.ukamb.org).

Preterm formulas

For those babies <2000 g birthweight and <35 weeks' gestation who do not have access to human milk, either mother's own or donor, a preterm formula is the feed of choice. However, if they are at high risk of NEC donor milk is advisable if there is no mother's own milk. If there is no option but formula feeding, there is evidence that preterm rather than term formula reduces risk of later poor developmental outcome, particularly in boys [53]. Where mother's milk supply is inadequate and there is

Table 6.7 Nutrients in fortified breast milk compared with guidelines.

Nutrient per kg	100 mL/kg mature BM*	180 mL/kg mature BM	180 mL/kg mature BM + SMA BMF full strength	180 mL/kg mature BM + Nutriprem BMF full strength	Agostoni et al. 2010 [8]	Tsang et al. 2005 [7]
Energy (kcal)	69	124	150[†]	153[†]	110–135	110–130
	(290 kJ)	(520 kJ)	(630 kJ)	(640 kJ)	(420–565 kJ)	(420–545 kJ)
Protein (g)	1	1.8	3.6	4	3.5–4.5	3.4–4.4
Sodium (mg)	15	27	59	92	69–115	69–115
Phosphorus (mg)	15	27	110	95	60–90	60–140
Iron (mg)	0.07	0.1	0.1	0.1	2–3	2–4
Calcium (mg)	34	61	223	180	120–140	100–220
Zinc (mg)	0.3	0.5	1	1.6	1.1–2.0	1.0–3.0
Selenium (µg)	1	1.8	1.8	5	5–10	1.3–4.5
Iodine (µg)	7	13	13	33	11–55	10–60
Folic acid (µg)	5	9	63	63	35–100	25–50
Vitamin A (µg)	58	104	590	520	400–1000	212–454
Vitamin D (µg)	0.04	0.07	14	9	20–25 [‡]	10 [‡]
Vitamin E (mg)	0.34	0.6	6	5.3	2.2–11	6–12

BM, breast milk; BMF, breast milk fortifier. 1 µg vitamin A = 3.33 IU. 1 µg vitamin D = 40 IU.
*Holland B, Welch AA, Unwin ID *et al. McCance & Widdowson's The Composition of Foods*, 5th edn. Royal Society of Chemistry and Ministry of Agriculture, Fisheries and Food, 1991.
[†]Does not take account of high risk of fat loss on handling.
[‡]Expressed as per day not per kg.

Table 6.8 Lactation and breast feeding check list (adapted from Imperial College Healthcare NHS Trust Division of Neonatology). Neonatal Unit – Baby Feeding Check List. ·

1. To be completed within _6 hours_ of admission: During visit to mother by a staff member:	TICK WHEN ACHIEVED/ CIRCLE AS APPROPRIATE	PRINT NAME & INITIAL	DATE AND TIME
Interpreter required	Y / N		
Ask feeding intention and record here:	❑		
Discuss the importance of colostrum as first feed and breast milk for the preterm baby with respect to the following • Reduced risk of Infection • Improved development • Improved gut tolerance • Reduced risk of NEC For mother; reduced risk of breast and ovarian cancer, osteoporosis.	❑		
Breast milk expressing pack given and explained	❑		
Advise watching Small Wonders DVD films:			
Film 3. First hours	❑		
Film 4. Expressing breastmilk	❑		
Advise mother to start expressing now even if on medication. (Prescribed/ non prescribed/ herbal). Safety concerns can be checked before milk is given to baby. Ask pharmacist if unsure	❑		
Advise on the detrimental effects of alcohol and smoking on lactation	❑		
If baby is a candidate, get verbal consent for donor breast milk from mother. Obtained by.. (Name)	Y/N		
Is there a reason why feed at 6 hrs is not appropriate in this baby? If not give feed. Reason:..	Y / N		
Is the baby likely to feed at the breast within _6 hours_ of delivery? If yes move to section 7	Y / N		
6 hours post-delivery: Call to midwife to check mother has expressed – in this hospital or one mother is in. Name of midwife discussed with	❑		
2. Within the first 24 hrs: during mother's first visit to the unit:			
Highlight hygiene practice in relation to breast milk expressing and skin to skin contact including regular bathing / showering	❑		
Importance of skin to skin contact with baby explained and check the mother has watched the film on the Small Wonders DVD: Film 5. Holding your baby	❑		
Breast massage and hand expressing observed and breast milk expressing log offered	❑ Log taken Y/N		
Benefits of using colostrum and breastmilk for mouth cares explained	❑		
Importance of frequent milk expression explained i.e. 8-10 times in 24 hr (including once at night between 2 and 4am)	❑		
Benefits of non-nutritive sucking explained (calming, maximising CPAP, sucking practice during tube feeds) _(parent leaflet on shared drive)_	❑		
If mother unable to visit the unit within 24 hours go down to visit her to complete this section or if in another hospital phone her midwife to check expression has commenced	❑		
Check mother is taking vitamin D (10ug or 400IU per day)	❑		
3.Day 2- 4			
Safe collection and storage of expressed breast milk explained, including guide to minimise contamination	❑		
Offer mother manual pump and demonstrate use when milk comes in	❑		
Use of electric breast pump demonstrated and breast milk expressing log reoffered	❑ Log taken Y/N		
4. Day 5			
Check that milk has come in and the volume of expressed breast milk is increasing? If not, give support	❑		
Record volume expressed in last 24 hours here Document support given _if needed_:..	Volume = mls		

(_continued overleaf_)

Table 6.8   *(continued)*

5. Day 10			
Check that production has increased and milk is being stored in the freezer (750mls in 24hrs is optimal). If not, give support	❑		
Record volume expressed in last 24 hours here Document support given *if needed*:..	Volume= mls		
6. Day 14			
Discussion regarding the possible need for breast milk fortifier to meet a preterm baby's additional requirements (see guideline)	❑ N/A		
If appropriate advice has been given and followed by the mother but milk yield is not increasing, is she taking domperidone? Date started?...	Y / N		
Check frequently that mother's milk supply is being maintained. If not offer support early			
7. Stable and ready to feed			
Support the mother to watch the film on the Small Wonders DVD: Film 7. Feeding independently	❑		
Importance of mother's availability for breastfeeding and rooming in discussed with support for any potential obstacles considered?	❑		
Breast feeding observed, baby's position and attachment has been supported and signs of milk transfer explained	❑		
Disadvantages explained re introduction of bottles before breast feeding is fully established (different technique, undermines confidence in breast feeding success)	❑		
Consent for bottles given if necessary and developmentally supportive feeding demonstrated	❑		

low risk of NEC, preterm formula can be used to supplement the baby's requirements. It is not advisable to mix and store human milk with formula for prolonged periods, although mixing just before feeding may help tolerance of the formula [69]. Some work suggests that hydrolysed protein formulas lead to shorter gastrointestinal transit times compared with whole protein [70] and might be preferable. This has resulted in reduced time taken to reach full feeds in one trial [71], although giving breast milk led to the largest cumulative feeding volume when compared with either milk formulas [72]. Hydrolysed Nutriprem is a new hydrolysed protein formula designed to meet the needs of the preterm infant. It may be indicated in certain infants who are not tolerating a standard preterm formula and who are not candidates for donor milk. However, human milk has been found to be consistently better tolerated than formula be it whole or hydrolysed protein and where gut problems are suspected human milk would always be the feed of choice.

Preterm formulas are highly specialised feeds designed to meet the increased nutritional needs of preterm infants without exceeding volume tolerance; their composition is based on major published recommendations [7,8]. If their composition is altered in any way this should be compared with these recommendations to ensure compliance with the guidelines. Those available in the UK are Nutriprem 1 and Aptamil Preterm (with similar composition) SMA Gold Prem 1 and Hydrolysed Nutriprem.

There is a wide variation in practice as to the age and weight at which feeding with preterm formula is stopped. A suggested range is 2000–2500 g body weight or discharge from the neonatal unit, whichever is sooner. Using the upper weight limit may shorten time to achieve catch-up growth and allow infants to achieve their required nutrient intakes without having to take very large feed volumes [73]. Babies can then be given a post discharge formula (see Post discharge nutrition). It is important to remember that each baby must be assessed to decide on the optimum formula and this should not be arbitrarily based on age or weight alone.

Method of enteral feeding

Due to an immature suck–swallow–breathe pattern, preterm infants usually require at least a proportion of their feed by tube until around 35 weeks' gestation, some for longer. Methods of enteral feeding differ markedly around the world [59]. There are advantages and disadvantages to both bolus and continuous gastric tube feeding with a systematic review unable to give a firm recommendation of one method over the other [74]. Bolus feeding has been associated with less feed intolerance [75] but may lead to a deterioration in respiratory function (due to gastric distension) in very compromised infants compared with continuous feeds [76]. Continuous feeding of human milk can lead to excessive fat loss due to adherence to tubing [77] and risk of sedimentation of added minerals. Transpyloric feeding is not recommended for routine use due to adverse outcomes in preterm infants [78].

Transition to oral feeding

For some infants, particularly those who have been very unwell, the transition to oral feeding, either to breast or bottle, can be difficult [65]. Despite inherent problems there has been an increase in babies leaving the neonatal unit breast feeding, even the most preterm, and this has been facilitated through many different approaches including early evidence based support for lactation; promotion of skin to skin contact between baby and mother; encouraging mothers to 'room in' on the unit [65]. If a mother has chosen to breast feed, the baby can start early feeding attempts as soon as they show cues during skin to skin contact. However, full nutritive oral feeding is usually not attained until at least 35 weeks and later in some infants [65]. Totally demand breast feeding may not be possible even at 35 weeks as the baby may still have immature sleep patterns and therefore need to be woken to ensure at least eight breast feeds per 24 hours. Some neonatal units discharge babies on tube feeds with support to facilitate breast feeding and weaning off the tube at home.

Babies who develop chronic lung disease, have neurological impairment, gastro-oesophageal reflux disease or other long term health problems can find the transition to full oral feedings particularly challenging and the input of a speech and language therapist is recommended.

Nutritional assessment

The appropriateness and adequacy of nutritional management can be assessed through both serum biochemistry and growth.

Serum biochemistry

Protein status is difficult to assess whereas adequacy of protein intake in the short term can be approximately assessed via measurement of serum urea levels. In healthy preterm infants, after the first 2–3 weeks, serum urea is likely to fall to <1.6 mmol/L when intake of human milk protein is <3 g/kg/day [79]. Since a protein intake of 3.5–4 g/kg/day is desirable, a sufficient intake is probably indicated by maintaining serum urea levels >2.0 mmol/L. Dehydration, renal and hepatic dysfunction, sepsis, steroid therapy and insufficient non-protein energy can all raise serum urea levels despite protein intake being <3 g/kg/day and should be taken into account; so in some circumstances it may be appropriate to increase protein intake despite there being a urea level >2.0 mmol/L.

Calcium and phosphorus are essential for bone health; phosphorus is also needed for soft tissue deposition. Serum phosphorus levels vary more than calcium levels, but both are very useful to assess needs. It is recommended that supplements are titrated to keep serum calcium and phosphorus within normal levels. A supplement of 0.5 mmol phosphorus twice daily has been shown to be a good starting point should serum levels drop <1.8 mmol/L [80]. Alkaline phosphatase is a marker of both bone formation and reabsorption. Sudden very large increases in serum levels may indicate a fracture or be due to increasing levels of the liver iso enzyme during an acute phase reaction. Levels that gradually increase with time but stay below the upper normal range usually reflect bone activity during growth and are not a concern.

Trace elements are most important to monitor during PN (see Table 4.8), e.g. manganese and copper which can build up to excessive levels in the liver when bile flow is reduced. During prolonged renal dysfunction selenium and molybdenum levels may accumulate so it may be advisable to assess these in this circumstance.

Other parameters to check are haemoglobin and sodium. Sodium depletion has been associated with poor growth [81]. Preterm babies have higher requirements for sodium than term babies due to renal immaturity whereby they are unable to conserve sodium initially and can quickly become hyponatraemic. If they are on sodium wasting diuretics they are also at risk of depletion due to higher renal losses.

Growth

A healthy preterm baby's growth rate rapidly responds to both poor nutrition and nutritional rehabilitation. Accurate weight measurement is essential in the neonatal unit as it gives important information about fluid balance as well as changes in body mass. Head circumference is also routinely measured as it can alert to abnormal brain growth after certain insults as well as contributing to growth monitoring. Length measurement is carried out less frequently due to the high risk of inaccurate measurements using inappropriate equipment. A simple measure is now available to take the length of preterm babies, both in incubators and in cots (the Leicester Incubator Measure available from Harlow Printing, hfac4@harlowprinting.co.uk, Fig. 6.1). It is accurate if used according to a protocol and by two observers and has been shown to lead to minimal disturbance of the baby [82]. The value of length measurements is that they reflect growth of the skeleton and therefore body mass, including lean mass as well as adipose tissue, and are not affected by fluid balance changes. It is

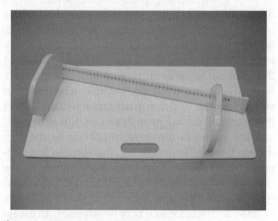

Figure 6.1 Leicester Incubator Measure.

becoming apparent that preterm babies are often more stunted than wasted by the time they are discharged from the neonatal unit, but this can only be evaluated if length measurements are routinely carried out [83, 84].

Weekly measurements of length and head circumference are sufficient to give information on growth. Weighing may be carried out twice a week initially and during acute episodes to estimate fluid balance; thereafter weekly should be sufficient to monitor growth.

These anthropometric measurements can be plotted on a growth chart for preterm babies, the UK Neonatal and Infant Close Monitoring Chart, available from Harlow Printing (www.growthcharts .rcpch.ac.uk for further information and training materials). This chart is based on cross-sectional data on size at different gestational ages at birth and does not necessarily represent how babies at different gestational ages should grow. There are data showing postnatal growth of babies in North America [85] which are based on a cohort of babies from 1994. Similar data from UK babies has been published [86]; there are some striking similarities with the North American cohort of 1994 with both showing an initial loss of weight then tracking along a lower centile.

All preterm babies experience a reduction in extracellular fluid which is usually demonstrated by a weight loss in the first few days after delivery and it is debatable whether this fluid should be regained. They should rapidly catch up to their birth centile or not. The perceived benefit or detriment of catch up growth is still being debated. There is a move toward ensuring satisfactory growth early on so that less catch up growth is needed later on. In general it is acceptable for a baby to drop 1 or 2 weight centiles in the first few days and then grow along the new centile. Babies who are born growth restricted may cross centiles upwards even when fed according to standard preterm nutritional recommendations.

Rather than considering gains in weight, length and head circumference in isolation it is useful to look at patterns of growth on a centile chart. There will be no loss of head circumference or length *per se*, but there may be a lag phase before these consistently follow a particular centile. It is difficult to quickly establish when growth is failing unless weight, length and head circumference are all considered together as babies may show weight faltering that is mainly due to loss of fluid rather than other tissue. Where there are concerns about growth a wide range of possible causes need to be evaluated alongside nutrition (Table 6.9).

A lag in resumption of weight gain after preterm delivery has been associated with perceived accumulated deficits of energy [87]; however, a drawback of this study was the assumption that babies have full protein and energy requirements immediately from birth, whereas Tsang *et al.* [7] acknowledge that this is unlikely and give lower values for requirements in the early postnatal period.

Feeding issues in special conditions

Necrotising enterocolitis

Concerns regarding the introduction of enteral feeds to the preterm gut relate to the risk of NEC and this must be balanced against the risks of not feeding. NEC is a potentially life threatening condition leading to acute inflammation of the bowel. Severity can range from low grade mucosal damage to bowel perforation and it predominantly affects preterm infants. In severe cases infants present with acute abdominal distension, feed intolerance, bloody stools and sepsis. Incidence is highly variable between units, but it affects approximately 5% of preterm infants <33 weeks' gestation [88] and can have devastating consequences. The aetiology is multifactorial and not well understood; however, the majority of affected infants have received enteral feeds. It appears to be triggered by a combination of one or all of the following factors: prematurity, hypoxia leading to gut ischaemia, gut bacterial overgrowth, sepsis, feeding of formula milk and rapid advancement of enteral feeds. High risks for NEC include

- <28 weeks' gestation
- <1000 g birthweight
- IUGR (birthweight <2nd centile)
- abnormal antenatal Doppler (absent or reversed)
- circulatory redistribution leading to potentially altered blood flow to the gut, e.g. infants with hypoxic ischaemic encephalopathy or cardiac anomaly such as patent ductus arteriosus

- congenital gastrointestinal abnormalities, e.g. gastroschisis
- unstable, ventilated and hypotensive infants
- altered gut microflora

Treatment is bowel rest and PN with slow regrading of enteral feeds, ideally onto human milk (p. 91). A small number of infants may require surgical management and gut resection. Severe NEC is associated with a poor neurodevelopmental outcome [89] and high morbidity and mortality rates (20%–25% in NEC stage II and above). Standardised feeding protocols appear to reduce the incidence of NEC [90]. The use of probiotics in the prevention of NEC has received increasing attention recently [91]; however, this remains controversial.

Feed intolerance

Feed intolerance is extremely common in the very preterm infant and may occur independently of NEC. The more immature the infant the higher the risk of feed intolerance with SGA, birth asphyxia and morphine administration also increasing the risk.

Definition of feed intolerance is difficult and the volume of gastric residuals and bile stained aspirate alone may not be sufficient reasons to withhold feeds. The latter may often be due to immature gut motility leading to periodic antiperistalsis [37]. In addition stimulation of bile flow may, in theory, help reduce risk of cholestasis. Although feed intolerance is almost unavoidable in some babies, giving human milk will reduce the risk [92, 93]. For babies where human milk is not available a formula containing prebiotics may help. Slow intragastric infusions of milk over 2 hours with 1 hour breaks may promote faster gastric emptying than rapid bolus feeds [94].

In order to avoid prolonged PN in babies with severe feed intolerance pharmaceutical agents have been tried. One of the most common used is erythromycin (a motilin agonist); however, maximum effectiveness may be limited to those >32 weeks [95]. In addition there are concerns around its effect on the gut flora despite being used in submicrobial doses [96].

Table 6.9 Possible causes of poor growth in preterm infants.

Causes	Remedies

Inadequate nutrient input	• See below regarding breast milk fat
	• Optimise volume of parenteral nutrition and enteral feeding
	• Ensure timely breast milk fortification
	• Caution is required when adding energy supplements alone
	  ○ To feeds of demand feeding infants
	  ○ To term formula or mature breast milk

Immature digestion and absorption	• Vomiting or diarrhoea – treat root cause • When MEBM unavailable and infant on DBM, consider introduction of preterm formula in infants at low risk of NEC • No benefit has been found in the use of medium chain triglycerides
Fluid restriction	• Ensure that fluid restriction is clinically necessary and negotiate a liberalisation of fluid input as soon as feasible
Inadequate sodium replacement	• After early postnatal diuresis has occurred, monitor serum sodium levels and supplement when necessary • Monitor serum sodium levels carefully during sodium wasting diuretic therapy
Breast milk fat	• Evaluate milk expression technique – ensure MER and breast emptying • Ensure 8–10 expressions per day • Ensure all steps taken to avoid loss of fat on handling, e.g. avoid decanting cold breast milk and leaving fat residues in bottles • If continuous feeding ensure syringe tilted upwards to deliver fat first • Consider the creamatocrit technique • Consider preferential feeding of hind milk
Postnatal steroids	• Additional energy supplements are not recommended as risks excessive adiposity • Additional protein is not recommended as baby will be catabolic • Ensure liberalisation of nutritional input after steroids are finished to allow catch-up growth
Renal/metabolic Inactivity	• Excess mineral loss due to renal immaturity – monitor biochemistry and supplement accordingly • Metabolic acidosis needs prompt treatment as it interferes with protein synthesis • Not currently recommended but if further evidence shows benefit and no harm try gentle, passive exercise
Suspected increase energy expenditure	
1. Respiratory or cardiac disease	• Trial of high energy density feeding, e.g. glucose polymer added to formula or preferential hind milk feeding for babies being tube fed breast milk • Monitor protein adequacy to ensure that protein insufficiency is not masked by increased adipose deposition, e.g. serum urea taking into account hydration, drug use, renal and hepatic function • Discontinue after trial period if no improvement (usually 1 week)
2. Other causes	• Ensure that the infant is kept in a thermo neutral environment • Ensure that methylxanthine levels are not excessive • Ensure infant is nursed to minimise energy expenditure

MEBM, mother's expressed breast milk; DBM, donor breast milk; NEC, necrotising enterocolitis; MER, milk ejection reflex.

Chronic lung disease

Chronic lung disease (CLD) was first described following the survival of mechanically ventilated preterm babies. It appears that this condition is now on the decline due to several factors including more widespread use of prenatal steroids to help accelerate maturation of the baby's lungs; postnatal surfactant administered directly into the baby's lungs to improve compliance; and, more recently, more rapid transfer from mechanical intratracheal ventilation to nasal continuous positive airway pressure (CPAP). It is now only the most immature and compromised at birth who develop this disease.

There is evidence for some increase in energy requirements with CLD; however, this is probably restricted to babies with severe forms of the disease [97]. Most babies today have a milder form of CLD and grow well without routine energy supplementation.

Post discharge nutrition

All mothers are encouraged to continue breast feeding for as long as they wish after discharge from hospital. Babies who are exclusively or predominantly breast fed will need a multivitamin preparation containing vitamin D which should continue as long as breast milk is the main drink. An iron supplement is also needed until around 1 year of age but may be stopped earlier if there is sufficient iron in the diet. The practice of giving a single dose of iron daily throughout the first year (e.g. 5.5 mg/day) allows the baby to gradually grow out of the dose per kilogram so that when the supplement is finally stopped it is a relatively small dose, as the diet becomes the predominant source of iron.

Babies who are breast fed post discharge are at risk of slower growth [98]. This often leads to the introduction of formula; however, the continued use of BMF has been investigated. A Cochrane review concluded that giving BMF after leaving hospital led to continued improved growth at 12 months but only one small study was available for inclusion at the time [99].

It has been common practice to stop BMF in all babies once feeding fully from the breast and the feeding tube has been removed. Recent studies have now been published reporting on the administration of BMF after discharge, which led to improved growth without compromising length of breast feeding [100–102]. Risk of later allergy was not found to be increased [103] and there appears to be a neurodevelopmental advantage [104]. The studies involved adding BMF to breast milk in the normal dilution (or slightly more concentrated) and giving to babies by bottle or cup; approximately half the dose was given compared with the amount used when the babies were inpatients. The intervention continued for 12–16 weeks corrected age. The authors' practice has been different: each sachet is dissolved in a small amount of breast milk and given via a teat or syringe just before a breast feed, the aim being to avoid introducing a bottle where possible and risk any interference with breast feeding. There is an argument that BMF could be given at half the usual dose to gradually reduce the nutritional concentration, as happens when changing from preterm to post discharge formula (PDF). This approach has not been investigated in clinical trials but has been used in various units and anecdotally it has been found not to interfere with breast feeding, which has been voiced as a concern [105]. BMF is currently not prescribable in the community in the UK and depends on the individual neonatal unit to supply it.

As healthy preterm babies reach term their feeding skills improve and mature allowing them to take large enough volumes to satisfy energy and possibly protein needs, precluding the need for BMF. Therefore BMF could be stopped at around 1–2 weeks' corrected age, but more evidence is needed to see if there are advantages in administration up to 12 weeks' corrected age. If a baby is discharged on BMF at half the dose they would normally have received in hospital, they will need an iron supplement and a half dose of multivitamin preparation containing vitamin D, increasing to a full dose once the BMF is stopped if exclusive breast feeding is continued.

For babies who leave hospital on formula feeds, or who need top-ups while breast feeding, PDFs are available on prescription. Their nutritional composition falls between preterm and term formulas and there is no need for vitamin or mineral supplementation. They were developed following observations that preterm infants demanded up to 300 mL/kg/day of term formula post discharge

[73] which parents reported to be a difficult feeding schedule. Subsequent work looking at the long term benefits of PDF on growth and development remains equivocal [98, 105, 106]. It is of interest to note that one of the trials included in the Cochrane review reported results contrary to all other studies in that the group receiving PDF grew more slowly than the group receiving term formula and this skewed the overall conclusion of the review [107]. High energy formulas designed for term infants are not recommended for preterm babies post discharge as they have lower nutrient density per kilocalorie (kilojoule) compared with PDF, so as babies tend to feed to energy requirements they are at risk of having a lower nutrient intake.

There are two brands of PDF available on prescription in the UK: Nutriprem 2 and SMA Gold Prem 2. These formulas are prescribable to 6 months' corrected age which may benefit those who have accrued the greatest nutritional deficit while on the neonatal unit; for others their use up to 3 months' corrected age is probably sufficient [106, 108]. Although PDFs are currently prescribable for low birthweight term as well as preterm infants there is no evidence that they are of any benefit for small term infants [2].

After PDF is stopped a term formula can be used up to 12–18 months of age. Iron status should be adequately maintained without supplementation [109], although some infants with limited dietary intakes may still need extra iron. When unmodified cow's milk is given at 12–18 months instead of formula or breast milk the toddler should be started on Healthy Start Children's Vitamin Drops as per Department of Health guidelines (see Table 1.22).

Weaning onto solids

Introduction of solids is not recommended before 6 months for the general population; however, these UK government guidelines are not intended for special groups such as preterm babies [110]. There are no national guidelines for preterm babies; however, a consensus statement is available from the British Association of Perinatal Medicine [111]. This statement is backed up by a review of the available literature [112]. In summary it is recommended that babies are considered for weaning between 5 and 8 months' uncorrected age and that they should be at least 3 months' corrected age to allow for sufficient

motor development. The decision as to the actual time of weaning is based on observing each individual baby. Table 6.10 shows some suggested cues for weaning. These recommendations have been incorporated into a practical guideline for parents produced by BLISS [113].

Table 6.10 Cues for weaning healthy preterm babies.

Positioning

- has some head control and a stable head position with or without support
- can be supported easily in a sitting position on a lap, bouncy or high chair
- caution should be taken when starting to wean babies who cannot be assisted to achieve the above skills

Behaviours

- alert and appears ready for a new type of feeding
- showing an interest in others eating

Oral skills

- can breast, bottle or cup feed efficiently. This is desirable although some babies who are not managing milk feeds efficiently can still be tried with weaning foods. A specialist speech and language assessment should be initiated for such babies
- has started to bring their hands to their mouth and explore fingers and/or toys with their mouth
- is demonstrating a 'munching' or up down jaw movement when mouthing non-food items
- absence of tongue protrusion during feeding was advocated in the 2004 UK Department of Health Report: Weaning and the Weaning Diet; however, the group noted that tongue protrusion disappears gradually with time and maturity, and should not deter weaning if other cues are present

Some factors have been used in the past but are now not recommended

- that a certain target weight is reached
- demanding feeds more frequently as this will often be a growth spurt and should be managed initially by offering more milk

Some factors may only develop once weaning has begun; their absence should not prevent a baby's progression with weaning

- managing to clear the spoon with their lips; this skill develops with experience
- presence of teeth, as they are not essential for chewing

Taken from: *Joint Consensus Statement on Weaning Preterm Babies* [111].

There are fears that the recommended age for weaning is too early; these are centred around immature gastrointestinal and renal systems; increased risk of allergy; potential for passive over-feeding; risk of reduced nutritional intake. All these factors are addressed in a review article [112] and, with the exception of reduced nutritional intake, there is no evidence for any detrimental effects. On the other hand preterm infants seem to have a higher prevalence of behavioural feeding problems [114]. This may be due to the introduction of solids (particularly lumps) being delayed beyond a critical period for their acceptance. Direct evidence for this is lacking, but case studies [115] and other observational data indicate a link [116]. Once weaning has started it should proceed according to normal guidelines with particular attention being paid to ensuring appropriate nutrient dense foods.

Useful links

BLISS – The charity for babies born too small, too soon, too sick
www.bliss.org.uk
British Association of Perinatal Medicine
www.bapm.org

Best Beginnings – Working to give every baby in the UK the healthiest start in life
www.bestbeginnings.org.uk

7 Gastroenterology

Sarah Macdonald

Introduction

Gastroenterology is one of the most interesting and challenging areas in paediatric dietetics. The medical conditions encountered are diverse and require an understanding of normal gastrointestinal (GI) function before correct dietetic advice can be given. Problems as varied as diarrhoea, constipation and GI dysmotility can affect normal intake and absorption of nutrients. Manipulation of feeds and diet is often the primary treatment for the underlying condition and carers need careful explanation of the principles of the feed and diet prescribed.

Nutritional requirements

Nutritional requirements vary according to the underlying disorder. Normal requirements for most nutrients will suffice for GI disorders that do not result in malabsorption, with additional energy and protein required for catch-up growth.

When malabsorption is present requirements for all nutrients are raised to allow for stool losses particularly fluid, energy, protein and electrolytes. Most infants will have high to very high requirements. Table 7.1 can be used as a guide for requirements for infants with malabsorption who are fed enterally and are based on actual rather than expected weight. For all the clinical conditions described the assessment and monitoring of the child's nutritional status is paramount. Anthropometric measurements should be plotted serially on appropriate growth charts. In conditions resulting in malabsorption, or in those requiring a very restrictive diet, iron indices, trace elements, vitamins (particularly fat soluble vitamins and B_{12}) and urinary sodium levels should be monitored with additional supplements prescribed as necessary.

Acute diarrhoea – fluid and dietary therapy

Acute diarrhoea remains one of the leading causes of childhood morbidity and mortality in developing nations, with an estimated 5–18 million deaths attributed to this cause each year. In industrial nations the mortality rate is much lower. Infants and children are particularly vulnerable to the effects of acute diarrhoea because of their greater relative fluid requirements and their susceptibility to faecal-oral agents.

The causative mechanisms in the GI tract are

- increased secretion
- decreased absorption

Clinical Paediatric Dietetics, Fourth Edition. Edited by Vanessa Shaw.
© 2015 John Wiley & Sons, Ltd. Published 2015 by John Wiley & Sons, Ltd.
Companion Website: www.wiley.com/go/shaw/paediatricdietetics

Table 7.1 Suggested requirements for infants with malabsorption, per day.

Energy	High	130–150 kcal/kg (540–630 kJ/kg)
	Very high	150–220 kcal/kg (630–900 kJ/kg)
Protein	High	3–4 g/kg
	Very high	Maximum 6 g/kg
Sodium	High	3.0 mmol/kg
Potassium	Very high	4.5 mmol/kg
Fluid	High	180–220 mL/kg

Often these coexist to produce an increased fluid load that exceeds the colonic absorptive capacity, resulting in diarrhoea. Both viral and bacterial pathogens can affect the gut in this way. Diarrhoea and vomiting can also be due to other infections (such as urinary tract infections), food hypersensitivity or surgical causes which should be considered on presentation.

Transport of glucose and amino acids is an active process and requires the presence of a sodium gradient across the brush border membrane maintained by the Na^+-K^+ ATPase pump. The movement of water in the gut is a passive event driven by the movement of solute. The regulation of electrolyte transport is controlled by several mediators and inhibition of these pathways results in poor absorption and active chloride secretion into the gut.

In infective diarrhoea the decreased absorption seen is not necessarily due to reduced villous size. With increased cell loss immature epithelial cells replace fully differentiated, mature absorptive cells. These cells demonstrate defective electrolyte and nutrient transport and functional impairment may be severe. This situation is worsened by cycles of fasting and starvation commonly seen in infants and children with acute diarrhoea in developing countries.

Acute gastroenteritis is defined as a decrease in stool consistency (loose or liquid) and/or an increase in the frequency of bowel actions with or without fever or vomiting. The diarrhoea should not last longer than 14 days. In Europe the incidence ranges from 0.5 to 1.9 episodes per child per year in children younger than 3 years, with rotavirus being the most frequent infective agent [1].

Oral rehydration solutions

Oral rehydration therapy is used to correct dehydration and maintain hydration. The sodium–glucose coupled transport mechanism stimulates water and electrolyte transport. This process is preserved in acute diarrhoeal disorders and first line therapy for managing acute gastroenteritis in children should utilise this mechanism. If the child cannot drink sufficiently then a nasogastric tube should be passed to ensure that the oral rehydration solution (ORS) can be given. Enteral rehydration is associated with significantly fewer major adverse events and a shorter hospital stay compared with intravenous (IV) therapy and is successful in most children [1].

Specific recommendations for the composition of ORS for European children were published by the European Society of Paediatric Gastroenterology, Hepatology and Nutrition (ESPGHAN) in 1992 [2]:

- carbohydrate should be present as either glucose or glucose polymer at concentrations between 74 and 111 mmol/L
- ORS should contain 60 mmol/L sodium, compared with 75 mmol/L recommended by the World Health Organization (WHO) and United Nations Children's Fund (UNICEF) in developing countries, to minimise the risk of hypernatraemia
- potassium should be added to replace stool losses
- osmolality should be low (200–250 mOsm/kg H_2O) to ensure optimal water absorption

Systematic reviews have confirmed that this is still the best composition of ORS to use in children admitted to hospital with diarrhoea [3]. However, there may be some advantage in using polymer based ORS for all cause diarrhoea and in diarrhoea caused by cholera [4]. The ORS available in the UK are summarised in Table 7.2.

Feeding during acute diarrhoea

For many years it was common practice to stop feeds during diarrhoeal episodes. It was thought that decreased lactase activity, chiefly associated with rotavirus gastroenteritis, would cause lactose malabsorption if milk feeds were introduced too early and that food proteins could be

Table 7.2   Oral rehydration solutions (mmol/L).

	Na$^+$	K$^+$	Cl$^-$	CHO
Dioralyte* (Sanofi-Aventis)	60	20	60	90 (glucose)
Electrolade* (Actavis)	50	20	40	111 (glucose)
Dioralyte Relief* (Sanofi-Aventis)	60	20	50	30 g (rice starch)
WHO formulation Oral Rehydration Salts	75	20	65	75 (glucose)

Flavoured preparations are not suitable for young infants.
*Reconstitute 1 sachet with 200 mL water.

transported across an impaired mucosal barrier and cause sensitisation [5]. Consequently bottle fed infants with gastroenteritis were fed ORS alone for 24 hours followed by the introduction of dilute feeds. This advice resulted in a reduced nutritional intake at a time when requirements were increased due to infection [6].

A meta-analysis of randomised clinical trials published in 1994 showed that the routine dilution of milk feeds and use of lactose free formula was not justified in the treatment of infants and children with acute diarrhoea [7]. A multicentre European study showed that the complete resumption of a child's normal feeding after 4 hours of rehydration with ORS led to a significantly greater weight gain during hospitalisation and did not result in worsening or prolonged symptoms [8]. A recent meta-analysis has shown the same outcome [9]. This is especially important in developing countries where children may already be malnourished.

ESPGHAN has published recommendations that management of gastroenteritis should consist of oral rehydration with a low osmolar ORS for 4 hours (100 mL/kg over 4–6 hours in moderately dehydrated patients), followed by resumption of normal feeding [10]. Formula dilution and gradual reintroduction of feeding is not indicated. Supplementing the usual feeds with ORS (10 mL/kg/ liquid stool) can prevent further dehydration. Breast feeding should be continued at all times with supplementation of ORS.

Use of lactose free formula

There is no evidence to support the use of reduced lactose or cow's milk protein free formulas in

Table 7.3   Low lactose, cow's milk protein based formulas.

Galactomin 17 (Scientific Hospital Supplies)
Enfamil O-Lac (Mead Johnson)
SMA LF (SMA Nutrition)

For lactose content see Table 18.9.

infants and children with acute diarrhoea, even if the infective agent is rotavirus. A very small minority of patients who show signs of feed intolerance (defined as worsening of diarrhoea with acidic stools containing >0.5% reducing substances) may need the temporary use of a low lactose formula (Table 7.3). These have been shown to support normal growth in infancy [11].

Congenital chloride losing diarrhoea

This is a selective defect in intestinal chloride transport in the ileum and colon which is inherited as an autosomal recessive trait. Lifelong secretory diarrhoea occurs with high chloride concentrations. It has been reported in most populations including the UK; however, it is most commonly seen in Finland, the Arabian Gulf and Poland [12].

In the past it generally resulted in severe lethal dehydration. Watery diarrhoea is present from birth but often goes unnoticed as the fluid in the nappy is thought to be urine. Dehydration occurs rapidly followed by disturbances in electrolyte concentration causing hypokalemia and hypochloraemia with mild metabolic alkalosis.

Treatment

As the intestinal defect cannot be corrected treatment requires replacement of the diarrhoeal losses of chloride, sodium and water. Initially this may need to be given IV but this should gradually be changed to the oral route. Insufficient salt substitution causes chronic dehydration, salt depletion and activation of the renin-aldosterone system which may lead to chronic kidney disease. Dietary manipulation is not required in this disorder other than to ensure a normal intake for age in conjunction with the prescribed electrolyte and fluid therapy.

Food allergy in gastroenterology

It is thought that the relatively high incidence of adverse reactions to food proteins seen in infancy is the result of immaturity of local and systemic immune systems, often in association with increased gut permeability to large molecules. Allergic sensitisation involves a failure to develop oral tolerance, an immunologic response induced by tolerogenic food proteins in contact with the gut associated lymphoid tissue. One common cause of this is the postenteritis syndrome where a loss of barrier function and the breakdown of normal immune tolerance follows an enteric infection. Deficiency of immunoglobulin A (IgA), which is involved in the immune defence of mucosal surfaces, is a common associated finding in allergic infants.

Food allergy may broadly be classified as either antibody mediated, e.g. IgE mediated (immediate GI hypersensitivity and oral allergy syndrome), or cell mediated, e.g. T cell mediated (dietary protein enteropathy, protein induced enterocolitis and proctitis) [13,14]. In some patients both mechanisms can coexist (eosinophilic oesophagitis and gastroenteritis). Pathological inflammatory changes can be seen in the GI tract. Cells and mediators of the immune system such as eosinophils (a type of white blood cell) and lymphocytes can be found in biopsies of inflamed sites. Allergic reactions can affect GI secretion, absorption (with or without mucosal damage) and motility. Interactions between the allergic cells and the mucosal nervous system are important in mediating alterations in secretion and motility. Both IL-5 (a Th2 produced cytokine) and the chemokine eotaxin play a role in allergic responses that can present as delayed gastric emptying, gastro-oesophageal reflux and constipation [15]. GI conditions caused by allergic reactions to dietary proteins are summarised in Table 7.4. Often in the clinical setting dietary manipulations are used to treat symptoms before any formal investigations are carried out. An algorithm of suggested management is given in Fig. 7.1.

Although the most common foods to cause GI food allergy problems are cow's milk, egg, wheat and soya, any food ingested could be allergenic [16,17]. The current tests available (skin prick tests, patch tests and specific IgE) are of limited use in identifying food allergens causing GI disease. The prescribed exclusion diet is usually based on an underlying first degree family history of atopy (hay fever/allergic rhinitis, asthma, eczema), allergies and organ specific autoimmunity combined with

Table 7.4 Gastrointestinal disorders that can be caused by allergy to dietary proteins.

Oral allergy syndrome
Eosinophilic oesophagitis
Eosinophilic gastroenteropathy
Food protein induced enterocolitis syndrome (FPIES)
Eosinophilic colitis
Enteropathy
Proctocolitis
Constipation

the age at presentation of symptoms and food intake at that time. Sometimes a number of dietary manipulations need to be tried before the correct dietary restriction for the individual is achieved. In the presence of multiple food allergies a few foods diet (p. 314) or exclusive use of a hypoallergenic feed may be needed with subsequent single food introductions to identify the causative food allergens.

Exclusion diets are difficult to manage at home and are expensive. Selection of suitable patients is important. Use of anti-allergic or anti-inflammatory drugs as a therapeutic alternative to dietary restriction should be considered in situations where the family will not cope with a strict exclusion diet.

When multiple foods are excluded from the diet it is important to sequentially challenge the excluded foods (p. 315) to identify those the child is reacting to in order to avoid over-restricting the diet.

Non-IgE mediated gastrointestinal hypersensitivities

Eosinophilic gastrointestinal diseases

Eosinophils are customary inhabitants and key effector cells of the innate immune system within the GI tract. They protect against parasitic infections, the rate of which has decreased markedly in the developed world. It is thought that hypersensitivity reactions to allergens may now be the driving force for recruitment and activation of gut eosinophils. When activated they release multiple cytotoxic agents and immunomodulatory cytokines resulting in local inflammation and tissue damage [18].

Eosinophilic gastrointestinal diseases (EGID) are a heterogeneous group of diseases (eosinophilic

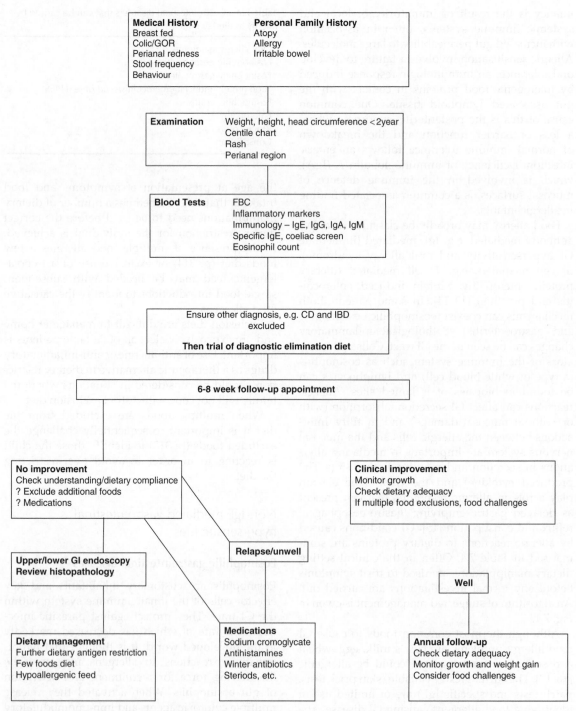

Figure 7.1   Suggested management of food allergy in gastroenterology. CD, coeliac disease; FBC, full blood count; GI, gastrointestinal; GOR, gastro-oesophageal reflux; IBD, inflammatory bowel disease; Ig, immunoglobulin.

oesophagitis, eosinophilic gastroenteritis, eosino-philic colitis) characterised by GI symptoms and increased eosinophils in the absence of other causes. Apart from eosinophilic oesophagitis the diagnosis of these disorders is unclear due to the uncertainty as to the normal number of eosinophils seen in different parts of the GI tract and their distribution within the mucosa [19].The latter may differ with geographical environment.

EGID are classified based on the location of the inflammatory response, even though their symptoms, prognosis and treatment vary considerably. In view of the close relationship between food allergies and some EGID, controlling antigen exposure is one of the most widely used strategies. In one study 80% of patients with EGID were found to have coexisting atopy and anaphylaxis to foods was present in a significant number [20].

Eosinophilic oesophagitis

This is the most common and best described of the EGID and is seen in both children and adults. It is a chronic immune/antigen mediated disease characterised clinically with symptoms related to oesophageal dysfunction and histologically by eosinophil predominant inflammation. There are high rates of concurrent asthma, allergic rhinitis, eczema and food allergy/anaphylaxis. It is more common in boys. Young children typically present with symptoms of gastro-oesophageal disease (GORD), food refusal or growth faltering whilst adolescents tend to present with dysphagia [21]. Complications include food impaction, oesophageal stricture formation and perforation. Serum IgE and skin prick tests for immediate type food allergy are warranted to identify comorbid food induced allergic disease, but these tests alone are not sufficient to make the diagnosis of food allergy driven eosinophilic oesophagitis. First line therapies must include the use of protein pump inhibitors, as oesophageal eosinophilia can be secondary to GORD. If symptoms fail to improve then dietary therapy should be tried as sole treatment or in conjunction with topical swallowed corticosteroids (steroids that are usually inhaled but are taken orally) [22].

Dietary therapy has been shown to be an effective treatment when assessing the histopathology of patients and three different regimens have been used. Complete amino acid based feeds have been shown to induce remission in 96% of patients, the majority of whom needed a nasogastric tube to complete the treatment; the trial of feeds is followed by an extended period of food reintroductions to identify specific allergens [23]. Dietary restrictions based on allergy testing or the exclusion of the most likely food antigens have also been used. The former was successful in 69% of patients [24].The latter (excluding cow's milk, soy, wheat, egg, peanut and seafood) has demonstrated a 74% success rate [25]. A recent retrospective case series of patients treated with one of these three elimination diets showed the greatest efficacy with complete amino acid based (elemental) feeds with 96% remission. Empirical removal of the most common allergens from the diet was as successful as a directed diet based on skin prick tests and patch testing alone (remission rates of 81% and 65%); however, the treatment chosen was not randomised and depended on negotiations with the family [26].

Consensus recommendations suggest that the specific therapy prescribed should take into account the family lifestyle, adherence to therapy and resources [22, 27]. Multiple food exclusions are difficult for the family to manage and expose the child to the dangers of dietary inadequacy, so careful monitoring is required with amino acid based supplemental feeds or vitamin and mineral supplements as needed. Once the disease is in remission foods should be reintroduced sequentially with careful monitoring so that only the foods the child is allergic to continue to be excluded. In one study cow's milk was found to be the most common allergen followed by wheat, egg and soy [28].

Eosinophilic gastroenteritis

Eosinophilic gastroenteritis is a chronic inflammatory disorder of the GI tract characterised by eosinophil accumulation in the mucosa or in deeper layers of the GI wall. Symptoms often mimic those of inflammatory bowel disease or irritable bowel syndrome. Under healthy conditions the stomach and the small intestine show detectable baseline numbers of eosinophils but their number is increased in eosinophilic gastroenteritis. Symptoms vary according to the site affected and include pain, dysmotility, nausea, vomiting, diarrhoea, blood loss, malabsorption, protein losing enteropathy and faltering growth [29].

There are no consensus guidelines on which to base therapies due to the rarity of this diagnosis and depends on whether associated food allergy and food allergens can be confirmed. Four food exclusion diets (milk, egg, wheat and soya free), few foods diets or exclusive elemental (amino acid based) enteral feeds can be tried [30]. If there is a limited response to these therapies then medical treatment is unavoidable [31].

Eosinophilic colitis
Primary eosinophilic colitis (EC), also known as allergic colitis of infancy or dietary protein induced proctocolitis, is thought to be non-IgE based (with skin prick tests usually negative).The exact immunological mechanism is not fully understood. This disease entity is predominantly a disorder of infants younger than 3 years. The classical presentation is of blood streaked stools in an otherwise healthy infant; however, it can also be seen in older children and adolescents where it may present with abdominal pain, anorexia and weight loss. Endoscopic findings include increased eosinophils and lymphonodular hyperplasia. Elimination of the causal protein is usually followed by resolution of symptoms [32]. In EC the most common causal protein is cow's milk and, as a large number of infants with this disorder are breast fed, this necessitates a maternal exclusion diet [30]. In one series of 95 breast fed infants with EC dietary exclusions were successful in 89% of cases. Of the remainder, seven responded to an extensively hydrolysed protein formula (EHF) and the remaining 4 (all of whom had eczema) needed an amino acid based formula (AAF) [33]. Prognosis of EC that develops in infancy is good; however, for young adults the natural history is that of a more chronic disease [34].

Food protein induced enterocolitis syndrome

Food protein induced enterocolitis syndrome (FPIES) is also a non-IgE mediated food hypersensitivity characterised by GI symptoms and a systemic inflammatory response in young infants. This can be chronic when the food is eaten regularly or acute when the causative food is ingested intermittently. Due to the atypical presentation and lack of diagnostic tests FPIES is often misdiagnosed initially and surgical, septic or viral causes investigated. Vomiting is the main feature in all cases with 75% of infants appearing acutely ill and 15%–20%

developing hypotension. Local inflammation has been demonstrated on biopsy and it is thought that this leads to increased gut permeability and fluid shifts resulting in emesis, diarrhoea and lethargy.

The most common allergens are cow's milk, soy and rice although a wide array of other foods have been implicated. Proposed diagnostic criteria are symptoms occurring before 9 months of age; repeated exposure to causative foods elicits GI symptoms without an alternative (including IgE mediated) cause; removal of specific foods results in symptom resolution; re-exposure elicits symptoms within 4 hours. Infants frequently react to more than one food [35]. In an American review where cow's milk was the causative food, 90% of the patients had recovered by the age of 3 years. No concomitant reaction to soy was detected in this population [36]. In a similar Australian review a wider range of trigger foods were identified (rice, soy, cow's milk, meats, vegetables and fruits, oats and fish). They also found high rates of resolution for the two most common food triggers before the age of 3 years. Children frequently experienced multiple episodes of FPIES before the correct diagnosis was made [37].

Exclusion of cow's milk protein

Cow's milk is the most common food to cause a reaction in infants and the incidence of cow's milk protein allergy reported in developed countries is between 1.9% and 4.9% with 32%–60% cases developing GI symptoms [38]; 0.5% of breast fed infants are reported to be food allergic or intolerant, reacting to exogenous food proteins secreted into the mother's milk. When an alternative infant formula is tried it is necessary to persist with this formula for a reasonable length of time, observing symptoms carefully before abandoning it in favour of a different feed. Delayed reactions to dietary proteins can occur several days after their ingestion.

Prognosis is good with remission in approximately 80% of children by 4 years of age with some evidence that children with delayed reactions become tolerant faster than those with immediate reactions [38].

Alternative infant formulas

It is vital that an infant is given a nutritionally complete milk substitute to replace a cow's milk protein based formula. In breast fed infants the mother's diet needs to be modified by the removal of cow's milk and any other foods allergenic to the infant. Care needs to be taken to ensure that the maternal diet continues to include adequate amounts of calcium, vitamin D, energy, protein and fluid. It has been found that breast fed infants can be sensitised to multiple allergens including egg, soy, wheat and fish [39]. ESPGHAN recommends that the dietary trial should be continued for up to 14 days if delayed GI reactions are suspected. If there is no improvement then the child should be further evaluated. If multiple food allergies are suspected then an AAF or EHF can be tried. The mother should be encouraged to express her milk whilst the clinical response to the hypoallergenic feed is evaluated [40].

Mammalian milks

Mammalian milk is not suitable to be used as an infant feed without modification due to its high renal solute load and inadequate vitamin and mineral content. The proteins in goat's and sheep's milks share antigenic cross-reactivity with cow's milk proteins [38, 41]. Infant formulas based on goat's milk are not recommended for use in GI food intolerances [42].

Soy protein based formulas

A soy protein based formula was used for the first time in 1929 to feed infants with cow's milk protein allergy. Today these feeds are based on soy protein isolate supplemented with L-methionine to give a suitable amino acid profile for infants. They are lactose free with glucose polymer as the most common source of carbohydrate. The fat is a mixture of vegetable oils that provide long chain fatty acids, including essential fatty acids. Feeding modern soy formulas to infants is associated with normal growth, protein status and bone mineralisation [43].

However, in the UK the use of soy formulas in infants under the age of 6 months has been advised against by the Chief Medical Officer, unless there is a specific medical indication, due to their high phytoestrogen content [44]. There appears to be less risk to the infant after 6 months of age as the amount of isoflavones per kilogram body weight is reduced as dependence on formula as a source of nutrition decreases. The infant's potentially vulnerable organ systems are likely to have matured by that age. The Committee on Toxicity of Chemicals in Food, Consumer Products and the Environment is reviewing more recent research in this area.

Soy protein has a very large molecular weight and after digestion can generate a large number of potential allergens. IgE mediated soy allergy is common, affecting 0.4% children in the USA [45]. Severe GI reactions to soy protein formula have been described for more than 30 years and include enteropathy, enterocolitis and proctitis. In FPIES caused by cow's milk protein 30%–64% had concomitant soy induced enterocolitis which responded to the use of EHF. It is suggested that an intestinal mucosa damaged by cow's milk protein allows increased uptake and increased immunological reaction to soy protein. A reported 60% of infants with cow's milk protein induced enterocolitis are equally sensitive to soy [46]. The American Academy of Pediatrics state that soy formulas are not recommended in the management of cow's milk protein enteropathy or enterocolitis; however, most children can resume soy protein consumption safely after 5 years of age [43]. EPSGHAN concludes that the use of EHF (or AAF if the hydrolysate is not tolerated) should be preferred to soy protein feeds and the latter should not be used before the age of 6 months. If soy formulas are used for therapeutic use after the age of 6 months due to their lower cost and better acceptance, tolerance to soy protein should first be established by clinical challenge [46].

Older infants with documented IgE mediated allergy to cow's milk protein can do well on soy protein based formula [47–49]. In other GI manifestations of possible cow's milk allergy, such as constipation, soy feeds can be tried. In one of the first papers looking at cow's milk allergy and chronic constipation 68% of the children responded to soy milk. Soy formula has the benefit of being at least half the cost of EHF and is much more palatable. Prospective studies looking at the incidence of soy allergy in patients with GI conditions are required. Soy infant formulas available in the UK are summarised in Table 7.5.

Feeds based on protein hydrolysates

Infants with cow's milk allergy and proven or suspected soy intolerance need an alternative formula. The allergenicity or antigenicity of a particular protein is a function of the amino acid sequences

Table 7.5 Composition of soy infant formulas, per 100 mL.

	Dilution (%)	Energy (kcal)	(kJ)	CHO (g)	Protein (g)	Fat (g)	Osmolality (mOsm/kg H$_2$O)
InfaSoy (Cow & Gate)	12.8	66	275	7	1.6	3.5	150
Wysoy (SMA Nutrition)	13.2	67	280	6.9	1.8	3.6	204

present and the configuration of the molecule. An epitope is the area of a peptide chain capable of stimulating antibody production. During the manufacture of a hydrolysate the protein is denatured by heat treatment and hydrolysed by proteolytic enzymes leaving small peptides and free amino acids. The enzymes are then inactivated by heat and, along with residual large peptides, are removed by filtration [50].

The proteins used to make a hydrolysate vary and production methods also differ between manufacturers. The profile of peptide chain lengths between different feeds will not be identical, even when the initial protein is the same.

Potential problems with hydrolysate formulas
Despite the rigorous conditions employed in the manufacture of these feeds there are still potential sequential epitopes present that can be 'recognised' by sensitive infants. Extensively hydrolysed protein based feeds vary considerably in their molecular weight profile and hence in their residual allergenic activity (Table 14.7). Feeds with peptides >1500 Da have been demonstrated to have residual allergenic activity [51, 52]. The degree of hydrolysis does not predict the immunogenic or the allergenic effects in the recipient infant. It has been recommended that dietary products for treatment of cow's milk protein allergy in infants should be tolerated by at least 90% of infants with documented cow's milk allergy [42]. In instances where an infant is not malnourished and fails to tolerate one EHF, a second EHF from a different protein source can be tried.

Table 7.6 shows the composition of EHF available in the UK. Feed choice may be influenced by

- palatability, which is affected by the presence of bitter peptides. This is particularly important in infants older than 3 months of age

- coexisting fat malabsorption, where a feed with some of the fat as medium chain triglycerides (MCT) may be indicated
- cost, some hydrolysates being twice as expensive as others
- religion and culture, where parents do not wish their children to be given products derived from pork

Introduction of hydrolysate formulas
Hydrolysed protein formulas should be introduced slowly to infants with severe GI symptoms as they have a higher osmolality than normal infant formulas. Feeds containing a high percentage of MCT should also be introduced gradually to ensure tolerance. If the diarrhoea is very severe then it may be necessary to introduce quarter strength feeds, grading up to full strength feeds over 4 days. If severe diarrhoea is present in an older infant it is preferable to stop all solids while a new feed is being introduced to assess tolerance.

In an outpatient setting, where symptoms may be less severe, full strength formula can usually be introduced from the outset. In infants older than 6 months there may be an advantage in initially mixing 1 part EHF to 3 parts their usual formula to slowly introduce the new taste and encourage acceptance, increasing the proportion of EHF over the next 3 days. Milk shake flavourings at 2%–4% concentration (2–4 g per 100 mL) can also be used in this age group if sucrose is not contraindicated.

If an infant refuses to drink the EHF a nasogastric tube needs to be passed to ensure adequate volumes are taken. Where faltering growth coexists, feeds can be fortified in the usual manner by increasing formula concentration or the judicial use of carbohydrate and fat supplements [53] (see Table 1.18). All changes should be made slowly to ensure they are tolerated.

Table 7.6 Extensively hydrolysed infant formulas, per 100 mL.

	Dilution (%)	Energy (kcal)	Energy (kJ)	CHO (g)*	Protein (g)	Fat (g)†	Na (mmol)	K (mmol)	Osmolality (mOsm/kg H₂O)
Casein									
Nutramigen Lipil 1 (Mead Johnson)	13.6	68	280	7.5	1.9	3.4	1.4	2.1	280
Nutramigen Lipil 2‡ (Mead Johnson)	14.6	68	285	8.6 17% fructose	1.7	2.9	1.1	2.1	340
Pregestimil Lipil (Mead Johnson)	13.5	68	280	6.9	1.9	3.8 (55%)	1.3	1.9	280
Similac Alimentum (Abbott)	12.9	68	283	6.6 22% sucrose	1.9	3.8 (33%)	1.3	1.8	274
Whey									
Pepti-Junior (Cow & Gate)	12.8	66	275	6.8 trace lactose	1.8	3.5 (50%)	0.8	1.7	210
Aptamil Pepti 1 (Milupa)	13.6	67	280	7.1 37% lactose	1.6	3.1	0.9	1.9	280
Aptamil Pepti 2‡ (Milupa)	14.3	68	285	8 36% lactose	1.6	3.1	1.1	2.0	290
Althera (Vitaflo)	13.2	67	280	7.3 52% lactose	1.7	3.4	0.8	1.8	335
Infatrini Peptisorb§ (Nutricia)	–	100	420	10.3 trace lactose	2.6	5.4 (50%)	1.4	2.8	350
Pork and soya collagen									
Pepdite (SHS)	15	71	297	7.8	2.1	3.5 (5%)	1.5	1.5	237
MCT Pepdite (SHS)	15	68	286	8.8	2.0	2.7 (75%)	1.5	1.5	290

SHS, Scientific Hospital Supplies.
*Carbohydrate is present as glucose polymers unless otherwise stated.
†Figures in parentheses indicate the percentage of fat present as medium chain triglycerides (MCT).
‡Suitable from 6 months of age.
§Liquid feed, designed for infants <9 kg body weight requiring a nutrient dense feed. Not suitable for cow's milk allergy.

Pepti-Junior, Aptamil Pepti 1 and Althera have sodium contents similar to standard infant formula which may be insufficient for an infant with increased stool losses. Low urinary sodium concentation (<50 mmol/L) alongside a normal plasma sodium concentration may indicate sodium depletion and supplementation with sodium chloride may be required.

Amino acid based infant formulas
Only pure amino acid mixtures are considered to be non-allergenic as there are no peptide chains present to act as epitopes. In infants who fail to tolerate an EHF this is the next logical step, so long as there is not a coexisting fat or carbohydrate intolerance. In these situations a modular feeding approach should be used (see Table 7.24). There are

Table 7.7   Infant formulas based on amino acids, per 100 mL.

	Dilution (%)	Energy (kcal)	(kJ)	CHO (g)	Protein (g)	Fat (g)	Na (mmol)	K (mmol)	Osmolality (mOsm/kg H$_2$O)
Neocate LCP (SHS)	13.8	67	279	7.2	1.8	3.4 (4% MCT)	1.1	1.8	340
Nutramigen AA (Mead Johnson)	13.6	68	286	7.0	1.9	3.6 (3% MCT)	1.4	1.9	348
Alfamino (SMA)	13.8	69	291	7.9	1.8	3.4 (25% MCT)	1.1	2.0	360

three infant AAFs available in the UK: Alfamino, Neocate LCP and Nutramigen AA and Alfamino (Table 7.7). Neocate Spoon, which contains highly refined rice starch as a thickener, can be offered as a nutrient dense hypoallergenic weaning food if required.

First line treatment with, EHF or AAF

At present there is a paucity of evidence on which to base this decision in GI food allergy. The World Allergy Organisation (DRACMA) report reviewed the few randomised studies comparing AAF with EHF (both whey and casein based) in IgE mediated allergy and could not identify a net benefit of substituting cow's milk with AAF over EHF. They recognise that the response to feeds in non-IgE mediated cow's milk allergy may be different and plan to address this in future updates [38]. The DRACMA guidelines have been summarised in Table 14.8. ESPGHAN continues to recommend EHF as first line treatment over AAF; however, AAF may be considered as first line therapy in infants with severe enteropathy indicated by hypoproteinaemia and faltering growth. The incidence of infants reacting to EHF is estimated to be <10%; however, this may be higher in infants with enteropathy or multiple food allergies [40]. One retrospective study found that up to 30% of food allergic infants, many with delayed reactions to foods, were intolerant of EHF [17]. Intolerances to hydrolysate formulas resulting in GI disturbances have been described [52].

There is a difference in cost between EHF and AAF with the latter being more than twice as expensive. The Health Improvement Network has shown that EHF was the most effective option in the treatment of cow's milk allergy, using data from primary care organisations. There were no significant differences in clinical outcomes between the two types of feed [54]. Differences in prescribing patterns can be

seen in a single geographical area which shows that current guidelines are not being followed [55]. There is an urgent need for a prospective randomised controlled trial looking at the risk of intolerance of EHF in GI allergy.

Introduction of solids

Weaning should take place at the recommended age of around 6 months and not before 17 weeks. It is important to ensure that food offered is free of cow's milk protein. Other dietary proteins that are most commonly implicated and may therefore need to be excluded include egg, soy and wheat. In very sensitive infants it may be wise to introduce new foods singly (p. 315).

Milk free diet

It is important that carers of infants requiring a cow's milk protein free feed are given appropriate advice to enable them to exclude cow's milk from solids. EU law (Directive 2003/89/EC, November 2005) regarding labelling of ingredients now means that products containing milk must be clearly identifiable. Exceptions include foods that are not prepacked such as bread from a bakery. Many manufacturers will now print an allergy statement on their packaging but, as this is not compulsory, parents should always be advised to check ingredients. Avoiding foods labelled with 'may contain' should be taken seriously in IgE mediated allergy but these foods do not generally need to be avoided by children with GI food allergy. Parents need clear advice about this due to the increasing number of foods carrying this label (p. 322). For foods manufactured outside the EU it is still necessary to teach families the following ingredients which indicate the presence of cow's milk in a manufactured food: casein, hydrolysed caseinates, whey,

Table 7.8 Milk free diet.

Foods permitted	Foods to be excluded	Check ingredients
Milk substitute Vegetable oils Custard made with milk substitute, sorbet	All mammalian milks, cheese, yoghurt, fromage frais, ice cream, butter	Margarines
Meat, fish, eggs, pulses		Sausages, pies, foods in batter or breadcrumbs Baked beans
All grains, dry pasta, flour Most breads, most breakfast cereals	Pasta with cheese or milk sauce, milk bread, nan bread Cream cakes, chocolate cakes	Tinned pasta Bought cakes or biscuits
Fruit and vegetables		Instant mashed potato
Plain crisps, nuts		Flavoured crisps
Sugar, jam, jelly Marmite	Milk chocolate, toffee	Plain chocolate Ketchup, salad dressings, soups
Milk shake syrups and powder Pop, juice, squash	Malted milk drinks	

hydrolysed whey, lactose, milk solids, non-fat milk solids, butter fat. Milk free dietary information is summarised in Table 7.8.

Exclusion of soy protein

In conditions where soy intolerance is present in addition to cow's milk protein allergy, foods containing soy and milk protein should be excluded from the diet (Tables 7.8 and 7.9). Vegetable or soy oils and soya lecithin are normally tolerated by individuals sensitive to soy protein and should not need to be excluded from the diet except in severely affected individuals [56, 57].

Milk, egg, wheat and soy exclusion diets

In conditions where a simple exclusion diet has not worked or where there is a diet history suggestive of multiple food intolerances this dietary regimen may be tried. Soy, eggs and wheat are covered by EU law (Directive 2003/89/EC, November 2005) and must be clearly labelled on all prepacked

Table 7.9 Foods containing soya protein.

All soy based products including tofu, tempeh and soy sauce
Texturised vegetable proteins
Breads, biscuits and cakes containing soy flour
Baby foods containing soy protein
Soy margarines

foods. Families need a lot of help and information about commercial foods to enable them to adhere to this regimen. Suitable wheat free products that are available via the Advisory Committee on Borderline Substances (ACBS) cannot be prescribed for wheat allergy and a separate letter to the GP requesting help is often required. Many of these products will contain milk, egg or soya so families need help to identify suitable substitutes. For foods manufactured outside the EU it is still necessary to teach families the following ingredients which indicate the presence of egg, wheat and soya in manufactured foods: egg albumin, wheat flour, wheat starch/bran, edible starch, modified starch, hydrolysed wheat protein, rusk, batter, breadcrumbs, thickener (unless specified as being made from another cereal), soy protein isolate, soya grits, tofu, hydrolysed/spun/textured vegetable protein, miso, tempeh (Tables 7.10 and 14.6).

Suitable feeds for older children

A suitable infant formula should be continued for as long as is nutritionally indicated in children on an exclusion diet and is preferable under the age of 2 years [38]. In situations where a large percentage of the child's nutrition comes from a formula either it will need fortification to meet nutritional requirements or a feed designed for older children should be used. If an infant formula is modified

Table 7.10   Milk, egg, wheat and soya free diet.

Foods permitted	Foods to be excluded	Check ingredients
Milk substitute Vegetable oils	All mammalian milks and products, soya milks and soy products, shredded suet Eggs	Margarines
All meat, poultry, fish, shellfish (fresh or frozen), pulses	Meat or fish dishes with pastry, breadcrumbs or batter Tofu, tempeh, soy beans, Quorn	Sausages, beef and vegetarian burgers, hot dogs, ready meals
Rice, rice noodles or pasta, maize, corn pasta, cornflour, tapioca, sago, arrowroot, buckwheat, barley, oats, gram flour, potato flour, rye, ground almonds, carob, teff, amaranth, millet	Wheat, rye and soya flour, spelt flour, wheat bran or germ, semolina, couscous, tabouleh, pancakes, batter, pizza, stuffing mixes, ordinary pasta, e.g. spaghetti	Gluten free bread, cakes, biscuits, pasta Oatcakes
Breakfast cereals made from rice, corn and oats, rice and corn cakes	Wheat based breakfast cereals Bread, crispbreads, crackers, chapatti, croissants, biscuits, cake	Poppadoms
Jelly, plain custard powder, rice, tapioca or sago pudding (made with milk substitute)	Pies, pastries, mousse, trifle, cheesecake, instant desserts	Sorbet, blancmange powders
Fruit and vegetables	Potato croquettes	Vegetables in dressing, e.g. coleslaw, potato waffles, instant mashed potato
Plain crisps		Flavoured potato crisps
Marmite, Bovril	Ordinary mayonnaise, salad creams, soy sauce	Stock cubes, gravy mixes, soups, sauces
Sugar, jam, honey, syrup, plain fruit lollies, milk shake syrup and powder, cocoa	Chocolate spread, lemon curd, milk chocolate, instant milk drinks	Plain chocolate, jelly sweets, marshmallows, baking powder, drinking chocolate, malted drinks

care needs to be taken to ensure an appropriate protein to energy ratio. Rather than addition of energy supplements it is often preferable to concentrate the feed. This should be done slowly and taking into account individual tolerance [53]. Most feeds in Table 7.11 have been designed to meet the requirements of older children requiring hypoallergenic feeds. Adult feeds based on soy or hydrolysed protein should be used with care in older children and may require modification or vitamin and mineral supplementation. Not all the feeds are categorised as EHF and care needs to be taken when selecting a feed for cow's milk allergy.

In children over the age of 2 years consuming a balanced diet and tolerating soy protein, supermarket 'adult' liquid soy milks can be given as an alternative to cow's milk. Those with added calcium and vitamins help to ensure nutritional adequacy. For children intolerant of soy and cow's

milk, there are alternative drinks made from proteins as diverse as oat, nut and coconut. Many brands of rice drinks are available but these are not recommended for children under the age of 5 years due to concerns about their arsenic content (Food Standards Agency, 2009). All these products are available in supermarkets and health food shops and can be useful as a social replacement for cow's milk. Although fortified with calcium and vitamins, calcium supplements may still need to be given if the reference nutrient intake (RNI) is to be achieved [58]. All children under the age of 5 years should be given a vitamin D supplement if consuming less than 500 mL infant formula per day. Most of these drinks contain very little protein so the diet must be checked to ensure that high protein foods are eaten twice a day.

Calcium intakes below recommended intakes have been identified in a number of children

Table 7.11 Hydrolysate and amino acid based feeds for older children, per 100 mL.

	Dilution (%)	Energy (kcal)	(kJ)	CHO* (g)	Protein (g)	Fat[†] (g)	Na (mmol)	K (mmol)	Osmolality (mOsm/kg H_2O)
Hydrolysate feeds									
Pepdite 1+ (SHS)	23	100	420	13	3.1	3.9 (35)	2.1	3	465
MCT Pepdite 1+ (SHS)	20	91	380	11.8	2.8	3.6 (75)	1.8	2.6	460
Peptamen Junior~ (Nestle)[‡]	22	100	420	13.8	3	3.8 (60)	2.9	3.5	310
Nutrini Peptisorb (Nutricia)[§]	–	100	420	13.7 trace lactose	2.8	3.9 (35)	2.6	2.8	345
Paediasure Peptide~ (Abbott)[§]	–	100	420	13.0	3.0	4 (50)	3.0	3.9	320
Amino acid feeds									
Neocate Advance[¶] (unflavoured) (SHS)	25	100	420	14.6	2.5	3.5	2.6 (35)	3.0	610
Neocate Active[¶**] (SHS)	21	100	420	11.3	2.8	4.8	1.3	2.1	510
Elemental 028 Extra[¶††] (unflavoured) (SHS)	20	89	374	11.8	2.5	3.5 (35)	2.7	2.4	502
Emsogen[¶†‡‡~] (unflavoured) (SHS)	20	88	370	12	2.5	3.3 (83)	2.6	2.4	539

SHS, Scientific Hospital Supplies.

*All present as glucose polymer.

[†]Figures in parentheses show percentage fat present as MCT.

[‡]Also available as a liquid feed.

[§]Liquid feed.

[¶] Flavoured versions also available.

**Nutritional supplement rather than complete feed.

[††]Use with caution for children between 1 and 5 years.

[‡‡]Patients who are receiving a significant proportion of their nutrition from Emsogen may need to supplement their intake of α-linolenic acid to meet UK DRV 1991 guidelines [58].

~Protein is not extensively hydrolysed.

who are limiting cow's milk in their diet, which may affect bone density [59]. A study in Norway showed that children aged between 31 and 37 months following milk free diets had significantly lower intakes of energy, fat, protein, calcium, riboflavin and niacin than age matched controls. Careful monitoring of dietary adequacy and supplementation with calcium and vitamins if needed is required [60]. Suitable calcium supplements may be found in Table 18.11.

Coeliac disease

Coeliac disease (CD) is an immune mediated systemic disorder characterised by a variable combination of gluten dependent clinical manifestations, specific antibodies and enteropathy [61]. There are at least two prerequisites for developing CD: a genetic predisposition (associated with HLA molecules DQ2 and DQ8 found in at least 98% of patients) and ingestion of gluten. More than one member of a family may be affected. The prevalence of CD in the UK is estimated to be 1 in 100 although only 10%–15% of people are clinically diagnosed [62]. There is considerable variation in the age of onset and in the mode of presentation, with patients being diagnosed well into adulthood as the disease may be atypical or clinically silent in apparently healthy people. Such patients run the risk of long term complications such as osteoporosis and infertility. Undiagnosed CD is associated with an increased risk of non-Hodgkin's and Hodgkin's lymphoma and small bowel cancer, but overall rates are low. It is recommended that children with non-specific GI symptoms such as iron deficiency anaemia, chronic diarrhoea and prolonged fatigue; asymptomatic children with a known increased risk of CD such as type 1 diabetes mellitus, autoimmune thyroid disease and Down's syndrome; and first degree relatives have serological testing for the condition. This is well summarised in the recent guidelines from the National Institute for Health and Care Excellence (NICE) [62]. Children can present with an elevated or normal body mass index at diagnosis [63].

CD is an immunological disorder with local and systemic production of autoantibodies against structural proteins of the small intestine mucosa and other organs, in association with a specific pattern of cell mediated damage in the small intestine. CD-specific antibody tests measure IgA tissue transglutaminase (tTG) and IgA anti-endomysial antibodies (EMA) (the same antibody measured by different methods). These antibodies may not be raised in IgA deficient individuals so IgA should always be measured at the same time. Children should be consuming sufficient gluten in their diet at the time of testing. Previously the gold standard for diagnosis was a small intestinal biopsy demonstrating mucosal damage followed by a clinical response to gluten withdrawal. ESPGHAN now recommends that if tTG results measured by a qualified laboratory are >10 times the upper normal limit, the likelihood of CD is high and additional laboratory tests (EMA, HLA) can be taken to make the diagnosis without duodenal biopsy. In other cases, e.g. tTG raised but <10 times the upper limit of normal, a small bowel biopsy is still recommended to diagnose the condition. The histology should be interpreted using the Marsh grading system [64]. A similar approach is

likely to be adopted by the British Society of Paediatric Gastroenterology, Hepatology and Nutrition (BSPGHAN).

Treatment

Currently the only treatment for CD is the exclusion of all dietary sources of gluten, a protein found in wheat, rye and barley. Gluten can be divided into four subclasses: gliadin, glutenins, albumins and globulins. In wheat the injurious constituent is the prolamin fraction of α-gliadin. The equivalent in rye is secalin and in barley hordein. Enzymatic degradation studies have suggested that the damaging fraction is an acidic polypeptide with a molecular weight <1500 Da.

Gluten free diet

All possible sources of wheat, rye and barley need to be excluded from the gluten free (GF) diet which needs to be followed for life (Table 7.12). This excludes a number of staple foods such as bread, pasta, biscuits and cakes; parents need support and help in finding suitable substitutes which the child will eat. Wheat flour is commonly used in processed foods as a binding agent, filler or carrier for flavourings and spices. Patients should be advised that kamut and spelt (ancient forms of wheat) and triticale (a cross between wheat and rye) are gluten containing cereals and should be excluded. Tests using a more sensitive analysis method have shown that some breakfast cereals containing malt flavourings derived from barley exceed the accepted threshold allowed by the international Codex Standard and are no longer considered suitable for inclusion in the gluten free diet. Parents and children with CD need to be taught to identify sources of the offending cereals in lists of food ingredients. Food labelling legislation (Directive 2003/89/EC, November 2005) means that all foods containing gluten or wheat must be clearly labelled; exemptions to ingredient listing of compound ingredients have largely been abolished. Incorporating an allergy box on the label of manufactured foods is not compulsory and so it is important that ingredient lists on labels are checked. Ingredients made from a gluten containing grain which is processed to remove all the gluten are exempt from the above labelling;

Table 7.12   Gluten free diet.

Foods permitted	Foods to avoid	Check ingredients
Milk, butter, cream, cheese		Cheese spreads, yoghurts, custard
Meat, fish, eggs, pulses	Products with pastry, thickened gravies and sauces, breadcrumbs, batter	Sausages, tinned meats
Rice, corn (maize), buckwheat, millet, tapioca, soya, gram flour, arrowroot	Wheat, rye, barley, bread, crumpets, cakes, biscuits, crackers, chapattis, nan bread, pasta, noodles, semolina, couscous	Oats*
Special gluten free flours, breads, biscuits and pasta	Wheat based cereals, e.g. Weetabix, Shredded Wheat	Corn and rice based cereals
Vegetables, potato, fruit and nuts	Potato croquettes	Flavoured potato crisps, dry roasted nuts
Sugar, jam, honey, some chocolates	Liquorice	Filled chocolates, boiled sweets
Tea, coffee, drinking chocolate, fizzy drinks, juice, squash	Malted milk drinks, e.g. Horlicks and Ovaltine Barley water, beer	

*Exclusion may be necessary.

however, sometimes manufacturers still state the grain source in the ingredient list. Parents should be reassured that glucose syrups derived from wheat or barley and wheat based maltodextrins are safe to include in the gluten free diet.

Children tend to be the highest consumers of savoury snack foods and processed foods that need to be excluded from this diet. The *Food and Drink Directory* produced annually by Coeliac UK, updated monthly on their website using data from supermarkets and manufacturers, is an important resource for all coeliacs. An increased variety of permitted foods will improve patient compliance. Young children should be taught to check with parents before eating foods outside the home or foods offered by siblings or friends. Where possible food should be prepared that is suitable for the whole family so that the child is not excluded from eating the family meal. The importance of cross-contamination in the home should be explained with toasters, bread boards, pots of butter and jam all being potential sources of gluten. Children's parties are a source of concern to parents and the child with CD should be sent with suitable foods of their own to eat.

Dietary adherence is important to avoid potential long term complications. In addition quality of life (QoL) has been found to be lower in children who do not adhere strictly to the GF diet; more physical problems, a higher burden of illness and more problems in leisure time were reported compared with adolescents who were compliant with the diet [65].

Commercially produced gluten free foods

A large number of proprietary GF foods are available and the standards for these are governed by the Codex Alimentarius Commission [66], established by the Food and Agriculture Organization of the United Nations (FAO) and the World Health Organization (WHO) to provide international food standards, guidelines and codes of practice to ensure the safety and quality of the international food trade. Until 2012 the standard was set to include foods containing <200 mg/kg gluten. It became recognised that this limit was too high for most coeliacs and from 2012 only manufactured foods that comply with the International Gluten Free Standard of <20 mg/kg gluten can be labelled as gluten free and be safely included in the GF diet. Foods specially processed to reduce their gluten content to 20–100 mg/kg may be labelled as 'very low gluten' in the UK; however, at the time of writing these are not being marketed in the UK. These foods might cause problems for those with a greater sensitivity to gluten. Finally, the term 'no gluten containing ingredients' is used when a food has not undergone testing to guarantee a safe level but is made from gluten free ingredients under good conditions with controls on cross-contamination. A number of staple food items have been passed as prescribable for patients with CD by ACBS, while more 'luxury' items such as fruit cakes can be purchased via pharmacies or health food shops. Many supermarkets are now producing their own ranges of GF foods.

A prescribing guide has been produced by BSPGHAN defining the minimum monthly GF food prescription requirements for children and adults with CD in the UK [67]. There is a limited availability of GF foods in some shops in the UK and these have been found to cost much more (76%–518% more expensive) than their gluten containing counterparts [68]. Dietary compliance is enhanced by the ease with which patients can obtain suitable amounts of GF foods on prescription. A complete list of prescribable GF foods can be found in the *British National Formulary* or in Coeliac UK's *Food and Drink Directory*. Products vary and patients should be encouraged to try different food items. Some of the larger companies will send newly diagnosed patients trial packs of their own products on application. At the time of writing there is considerable debate in the primary care sector around the prescribing of these food items due to budgetary constraints. Coeliac UK continues to lobby for GF staple items to remain on prescription and the British Dietetic Association has produced a policy statement backing this stance [69].

Oats

The inclusion of oats in the GF diet remains controversial; benefits include providing a source of soluble fibre as well as adding variety and increasing food choice. It is unclear whether the prolamin in oats, avenin, contains the amino acid sequences that trigger the histological changes in the small intestinal mucosa. The quantity of avenin in oats is much less than the prolamins in other cereals; thus a larger quantity of the product may be required to produce an effect. Problems with early studies to determine the effect of oats in the diet included small patient numbers, insensitive functional tests and small intestinal biopsies that were often difficult to interpret [70]. Two papers purport to show the safety of oats when ingested

by adults and children with CD. The adult data showed no harm at 5 years, yet a significant number (33%) of the original subjects did not include oats in their diet during the follow-up period [71]. The randomised double blind paediatric study had a high number of withdrawals in both the group that ate oats (26%) and those whose diet remained free of oats (11%). At the end of the study the children consuming oats were taking smaller amounts than prescribed which, in some, may have resulted in too little avenin to cause an effect [72]. Two systematic reviews have concluded that oats can be symptomatically tolerated by most patients with CD; however, the long term effects of a diet containing oats remain unknown [73, 74].

A further complicating factor is that oats can be contaminated with wheat at various stages of production: in fields, transportation, storage, milling and processing. Care should therefore be taken to avoid contaminated sources. Coeliac UK recommends that the introduction of oats should be considered on an individual patient basis. The author's current practice is to initially advise avoidance of oats at the start of the GF diet but to review this at a later date once the patient is responding to the diet. Oat products are now included in an appendix to Coeliac UK's annual food list.

Bone health

One of the main complications of CD in adults is reduced bone mineral density (BMD) leading to osteoporosis. It is unclear if this is due to calcium malabsorption for prolonged periods prior to diagnosis. One study found that whilst the bone mineral content of coeliac children was significantly lower than control subjects at diagnosis, after 1 year on a GF diet it had returned to normal. The calcium intake of the children was not assessed during this time [75]. Another longitudinal study found that, although there was an improvement after 1–2 years on the GF diet, BMD scores were still lower than expected for the normal population [76]; BMD has also been found to be lower in children with CD with poor dietary adherence [77]. Suboptimal vitamin D and K status may contribute to the increased risk for poor bone health in childhood CD and careful consideration should be given to supplementation with these vitamins at the time of diagnosis [78]. Although there are no formal recommendations it would appear sensible to ensure that children's intake is at least equal to the RNI for calcium for their age [58]. Some GF products are fortified with calcium.

Coeliac UK

This is an independent registered charity which all parents of children with CD should be encouraged to join. The society acts as an invaluable resource on all aspects of management of the GF diet, including topics as diverse as eating out to travelling abroad, and now produces travel sheets with specific information on nearly 40 countries. It also produces many helpful publications. Membership is free for the first 6 months and then costs £20 per year for the carers of a child with CD (www.coeliac.org.uk).

Gluten challenge

Gluten challenge is only necessary when there is some doubt at the time of initial diagnosis. This should always be preceded by HLA typing and assessment of mucosal histology and should be avoided in children under the age of 5 years and during the adolescent growth spurt, where possible [64]. For challenge purposes gluten can be introduced into the diet in two forms: either as gluten powder that can be mixed in foods such as yoghurt; or as gluten containing foods. Both need to be given daily in sufficient amounts to ensure an adequate challenge [79]:

- 10 g gluten per day in young children
- 10–15 g per day in older children

2–3 g gluten is found in one medium slice of bread, two rusks or digestive biscuits, four tablespoons of cooked pasta or one Weetabix. Parents are often anxious that the inclusion of normal foods in the diet will make returning to the GF diet difficult if the diagnosis of CD is confirmed. Reassurance is required and an explanation of the procedure to the child is very important in ensuring its success.

Associated food intolerances

Although a secondary disaccharidase deficiency can be demonstrated at the time of diagnosis it is rarely necessary to exclude lactose from the diet of a child newly diagnosed with CD. However, some infants seem to have cow's milk protein hypersensitivity and benefit from a temporary dietary exclusion in addition to avoidance of gluten. They should be rechallenged with cow's milk 2–3 months after the commencement of the GF diet.

Carbohydrate intolerances

Sugar malabsorption increases the osmotic load of GI fluid, draws water into the small intestine and stimulates peristalsis, resulting in pain, bloating, abdominal distension and diarrhoea. The severity depends on the quantity of ingested carbohydrate (CHO), the metabolic activity of colonic bacteria (which is reduced after antibiotic therapy) and the absorptive capacity of the colon for water and short chain fatty acids.

The infant is at a disadvantage compared with the adult as the small intestine is shorter and the reserve capacity of the colon to absorb luminal fluids is reduced. Because of a faster gut transit time there is less time for alternative paths of CHO digestion to be effective. The undigested sugar is either excreted unchanged or is fermented by bacteria in the colon to short chain fatty acids and lactic acid.

When suspecting CHO intolerance a careful diet history, which includes the timing of introduction of sugars into the diet and the onset of symptoms, can aid in the diagnosis of these disorders.

Disaccharidase deficiencies: congenital sucrase-isomaltase deficiency

In the brush border of the small intestine there are four disaccharidase enzymes with the highest level of activity occurring in the jejunum (Table 7.13). Deficiencies of these enzymes can be primary in nature, due to a congenital enzyme defect, or secondary to some other GI insult.

Congenital sucrase-isomaltase deficiency (CSID) is an autosomal recessively inherited disease which is a rare, but frequently misdiagnosed, cause of chronic diarrhoea in infants and children. It results in a deficiency in the ability to hydrolyse sucrose, maltose, short 1–4 linked glucose oligomers, branched (1–6 linked) α-limit dextrins and starch. The current gold standard method of diagnosis is measuring the intestinal disaccharidase activity in

Table 7.13 Brush border enzyme activity in the small intestine.

Enzyme	Substrate	Product
Sucrase-isomaltase (accounts for 80% maltase activity)	Sucrose α1–6 glucosidic bonds in starch molecule (approximately 25%) Isomaltose Maltose Maltotriose	Glucose Fructose
Maltase-glucoamylase (accounts for 20% maltase activity)	Maltose Maltotriose Starch	Glucose
Lactase	Lactose	Glucose Galactose
Trehelase	Trehalose	Glucose

small bowel biopsy specimens which show normal morphology.

Patients with CSID have different phenotypes and enzymatic activities which range from mild reduction of sucrase activity to complete absence. Isomaltase is the only enzyme to possess the α1–6 glucosidic activity needed to cleave the linkages present in the branch points of the α-limit dextrins found in high concentrations in amylopectin [80]. Although considered rare, the prevalence of CSID may have been underestimated and it is likely that the disease remains undiagnosed in numerous patients with a history of chronic diarrhoea, some of whom are diagnosed with CSID as adults. The SI gene has been identified and more than 25 mutations discovered which raises the possibility of genetic screening in the future. Current estimates of the prevalence of CSID in the North American and European populations range from 1 in 500 to 1 in 2000 among non-Hispanic Caucasians [81].

Whilst being breast fed or given a normal infant formula (where the sugar is lactose) the infant remains asymptomatic and thrives. The introduction into the diet of starch or sucrose in weaning foods, or a change in formula to one containing sucrose or starch (sucrose is added to the EHF Similac Alimentum and starch is found in prethickened formulas) initiates symptoms. The clinical presentation of CSID is very variable. Chronic watery diarrhoea and faltering growth are common findings in infants and toddlers. A

delay in the diagnosis may be related to the empirical institution of a low sucrose diet by parents, which controls symptoms. Some children attain relatively normal growth with chronic symptoms of intermittent diarrhoea, bloating and abdominal cramps before diagnosis. In older children such symptoms may result in the diagnosis of irritable bowel syndrome.

Treatment

In the first year of life treatment usually requires the elimination of sucrose from the diet. Starch is excluded initially and then increased to tolerance (Table 7.14). The lactose in normal infant formula, breast milk and mammalian milks is tolerated. Such a diet is very restrictive and care needs to be taken to ensure an adequate energy and vitamin intake. It may be beneficial to continue an infant formula after 1 year of age. For infants requiring a high energy feed SMA High Energy would be suitable as the CHO is lactose; however, the higher energy feeds Similac High Energy and Infatrini are contraindicated as these contain 5 g per 100 mL maltodextrin/galacto-oligosaccharides. Oral nutritional supplements (sip feeds) for older children should not be prescribed as these all contain sucrose as a sweetener. Fructose and glucose can be used in food and low calorie drinks to provide extra

Table 7.14 Low sucrose, low starch solids (<1 g per 100 g).

Protein	Meat, poultry, egg*, fish
Fats	Margarine, butter, lard, vegetable oils
Vegetables	Most vegetables *except* potato, plantain, yam, sweet potato, parsnip, carrots, peas, onion, sweetcorn, beetroot, okra, beans and lentils [83]
Fruits	Initially use fruits <1 g sucrose per 100 g fruit (Table 7.15) Most fruits contain negligible amounts of starch
Milk	Breast milk, infant formula (free of glucose polymer and sucrose) Cow's milk, unsweetened natural yoghurt, cream
Others	Marmite, Bovril, vinegar, salt, pepper, herbs, spices, 1–2 teaspoons of tomato purée can be used in cooking, gelatine, essences and food colourings, sugar free jelly, sugar free drinks, fructose, glucose

*Soft eggs should not be given to babies <1 year of age.

energy. In addition butter, margarine and oils can be added to savoury foods. All medications should be sucrose free; Ketovite liquid and tablets are a suitable complete CHO free vitamin supplement.

Once the infant or child is symptom free the tolerance for the excluded CHO should be tested by slowly increasing dietary intake; if the capacity to absorb CHO is exceeded this will cause osmotic diarrhoea or a recurrence of abdominal symptoms. Reducing the CHO to the previously tolerated level will result in normal stool production. With increasing age the tolerance of starch and the lower sucrose containing foods should improve until, by the age of 2–3 years, the restriction of starch may no longer be needed.

An international support group based in the USA tracks children with CSID and provides further information on this disorder: www.csidinfo.com. It has followed 7433 individuals and has identified five different phenotypes who can tolerate varying amounts of starch in the diet [82].

The sucrose content of fruits is shown in Table 7.15. Fruits containing higher amounts of sucrose can be added to the diet according to tolerance [84]. If children have problems tolerating starch in reasonable quantities, soy flour can be used in recipes to replace wheat flour as it only contains 15 g starch per 100 g compared with 75 g per 100 g in wheat flour. Parents need reassurance that occasional dietary indiscretions will not cause long term problems.

Newly diagnosed older children should initially be advised to avoid dietary sources of sucrose only. Advice should be given about alternative sweeteners that are suitable. The following have been found to be tolerated: crystalline glucose, dextrose, corn syrup, crystalline fructose. None of the phenotypes identified by the CSID Parent Support Group could tolerate hydrogenated glucose syrup, galactose/maltose/malt sugar, acesulfame K, maltitol and brown rice syrup. If avoidance of sucrose does not lead to a prompt improvement in symptoms then the starch content of the diet should be reduced, particularly those foods with a high amylopectin content such as wheat and potatoes. Glucose tablets may be included in the diet.

Enzyme substitution therapy

Sacrosidase, a liquid preparation containing high concentrations of yeast derived invertase (sucrase), has been used with good results and is available on a named patient basis (Sucraid, BS Orphan Ltd, www.bsorphan.com). It is stable if refrigerated and tasteless when mixed with water. This formulation has been shown to be resistant to acidic pH. Degradation by intragastric pepsin is buffered by taking the enzyme with protein foods. Unlike human intestinal sucrase-isomaltase, it has no activity on oligosaccharides containing 1–6 glucosyl bonds.

A controlled, double blind trial of sacrosidase in 14 patients with CSID showing symptoms of diarrhoea, abdominal cramps and bloating were prevented or ameliorated in patients consuming a sucrose containing diet. The recommended dose is 1 mL with each meal in patients weighing <15 kg, and 2 mL for those weighing >15 kg. This allows the consumption of a more normal diet by children with CSID and decreases the high incidence of chronic GI complaints seen in this condition [85, 86].

It is suggested that the product is introduced when the child's tolerance of sucrose is known. Doses should be split, with half the dose given at the start and the other half midway through the meal to maximise the enzyme's activity. Data from 229 patients using Sucraid showed that 65% of patients were able to consume either a normal or mildly restricted diet. However, 27% still needed to maintain a strict sucrose restriction with some level of starch restriction to maintain acceptable suppression of their GI symptoms. The addition of enzymes to enhance maltase and glycoamylase activity in the future may help these patients to cope with the continued problem of starch malabsorption [81].

Table 7.15 Sucrose content of some common fruits (per 100 g edible portion) [83].

<1 g sucrose	<3 g sucrose	<5 g sucrose
Avocado, bilberries, blackberries, blackcurrants, cherries, cooking apples, damsons, dates, gooseberries, grapes, lemons, loganberries, lychees, melon (Cantaloupe, honeydew), pears, raisins, raspberries, redcurrants, rhubarb, strawberries, sultanas	Galia melon, grapefruit, kiwi fruit, passion fruit, plums, watermelon	Apples, apricots, oranges, clementines, satsumas

Disaccharidase deficiencies: lactase deficiency

Congenital lactase deficiency is very rare, the largest group of patients being found in Finland. Severe diarrhoea starts during the first days of life, resulting in dehydration and malnutrition, and resolves when either breast milk or normal formula are ceased and a lactose free formula is given (Table 7.3).

Primary adult type lactase deficiency is found in approximately 70% of the world's population. Lactase levels are normal during infancy but decline to about 5%–10% of the level at birth during childhood and adolescence. These population groups are common in East and South East Asia, tropical Africa and Native Americans and Australians. The age of onset of symptoms varies but is generally about 3 years or later, and only if a diet containing lactose is offered. In the majority of Europeans lactase levels remain high and this pattern of a declining tolerance of lactose with age is not seen.

In other ethnic groups with this problem a moderate reduction of dietary lactose will be sufficient, using either lactose reduced milks available from the supermarket or milk substitutes based on soya, oats and rice milks. It is important to ensure that children meet their requirements for calcium [87].

Disaccharidase deficiencies: secondary disaccharidase deficiency

Carbohydrate malabsorption can result from secondary damage to the GI mucosa. This can present at any age, with onset of symptoms occurring shortly after the primary injury, for instance in cow's milk protein enteropathy, rotavirus infection, Crohn's disease, short gut syndrome and immunodeficiency syndromes.

Lactase deficiency is the most common secondary enzyme deficiency to be seen, probably because it has a lower activity than the other intestinal enzymes and is produced on the distal end of the villous tip which is more susceptible to damage. However, a secondary sucrase-isomaltase deficiency can also occur.

Treatment

Treatment is to eliminate the offending CHO and treat the primary disorder causing the mucosal damage. Clinical course depends on the underlying disease but studies in infants with rotavirus infections have shown an incidence of 30%–50% lactose intolerance which recovers 2–4 weeks after the infection.

Infants requiring a lactose free formula and diet can use either lactose free, cow's milk protein based formula (Table 7.3) or soy formula if older than 6 months (Table 7.5). A milk free diet (Table 7.8) is necessary although mature cheese can be included. Medications need to be checked as these can contain lactose as a bulking agent.

Monosaccharide malabsorption: glucose-galactose malabsorption

This is an extremely rare congenital disorder resulting from a selective defect in the intestinal glucose and galactose/sodium co-transport system in the brush border membrane. Glucose, galactose, lactose, sucrose, glucose polymers and starch are all contraindicated in this disorder. It presents in the neonatal period with the onset of severe watery, acidic diarrhoea leading to dehydration and metabolic acidosis. It is a heterogeneous condition in its expression and older children seem to have considerable variation in their tolerance of the offending carbohydrates.

Treatment

Initial IV rehydration is required. The use of ORS, all of which are glucose or starch based, is contraindicated. A fructose based complete infant formula, Galactomin 19, should be introduced slowly, initially as quarter and half strength formula with IV carbohydrate and electrolyte support to avoid metabolic acidosis (Table 7.16).

Once the infant is established on feeds and gaining weight, it is important to discuss with the child's doctor a suitable protocol for oral rehydration should the child become unwell. Plain water or a 2%–4% fructose solution can be given, but this does not have the same effect on water absorption as ORS. In severe infectious diarrhoea the infant may need IV fluids.

Fructose is available on prescription for this condition and can be used to sweeten foods for older children and as an additional energy source. It is important to ensure that all medicines are CHO free.

Table 7.16   Composition of Galactomin 19 per 100 mL.

	Dilution (%)	Energy (kcal)	Energy (kJ)	Protein (g)	CHO (g)	Fat (g)	Na (mmol)	K (mmol)	Osmolality (mOsm/kg H_2O)
Galactomin 19 (Scientific Hospital Supplies)	12.9	69	288	1.9	6.4	4.0	0.9	1.5	407

First weaning solids should contain minimal amounts of starch, sucrose, lactose and glucose (Table 7.17). Manufactured baby foods are not suitable and it is necessary for weaning solids to be prepared at home. All foods should be cooked without salt and initially blended to a very smooth texture. To save time parents can prepare foods in advance and freeze in clean ice cube trays. Recipes are available from the author for egg custard sweetened with fructose and for fructose meringues.

With increasing age children gradually begin to absorb more of the offending CHO due to colonic salvage. The foods in Table 7.18 are grouped to allow a gradual increase in the amount of glucose and galactose in the diet. These lists can be used as a guide by parents. Small amounts of new foods can be introduced cautiously and increased as tolerated. Too much of these foods will exceed the individual's tolerance and cause diarrhoea. In this situation the child should return to the diet previously well tolerated and food introductions tried again a few months later.

Infants and children are very dependent on Galactomin 19 to meet their requirements for energy and parents should be encouraged to continue this formula for as long as possible. It can also be useful for older children entering adolescence who find it difficult to meet their increased energy requirements from eating a low starch diet. If sufficient formula is taken a vitamin supplement should not be needed.

Fat malabsorption

Intestinal lymphangiectasia

Intestinal lymphangiectasia is a congenital, acquired or inherited disorder characterised by dilated enteric lymphatic vessels which rupture and leak lymphatic fluid into the gut, leading to protein loss. The presentation is variable but diarrhoea, hypoproteinaemic oedema and decreased levels of immunoglobulins are commonly seen. Peripheral lymphoedema of the limbs is reported in 22% of cases. Failure to thrive can also be a significant problem. Children usually present in the first 2 years of life although cases diagnosed as late as 15 years of age are documented [88]. The diagnosis is definitively established by a small intestinal biopsy demonstrating the characteristic lymphatic abnormality although, as the lesion is a patchy one, negative biopsy does not exclude the diagnosis [89]. Techniques that allow visualisation of the small intestine, such as video capsule endoscopy or double balloon enteroscopy, may be required to diagnose this disorder [90].

Table 7.17   Foods allowed in children with glucose-galactose malabsorption (<1 g glucose and galactose per 100 g)*.

Protein	Meat, poultry, egg[†], fish
Fats	Margarine, butter, lard, vegetable oils
Vegetables	Ackee (canned), asparagus, bamboo shoots, beansprouts (canned only), broccoli, celery, cucumber, endive, fennel, globe artichoke, lettuce, marrow, mushrooms, spinach, spring greens, steamed tofu, watercress, preserved vine leaves
Fruits	Avocado pear, rhubarb, lemon juice
Milk Substitute	Galactomin 19 Formula
Others	Marmite, Bovril, vinegar, salt, pepper, herbs, spices, 1–2 teaspoons of tomato purée can be used in cooking, gelatine, essences and food colourings, sugar free jelly, sugar free drinks, fructose

*The lists of foods have been compiled calculating the amount of glucose and galactose as g starch + g glucose + g lactose + 0.5g sucrose [83].

[†]Soft eggs should not be given to babies under 1 year of age.

Table 7.18   Glucose and galactose content of foods (per 100 g edible portion) [83].

1–2 g glucose + galactose	2–3 g glucose + galactose	3–5 g glucose + galactose
Protein		
Quorn, all 'hard' cheeses, cream cheese, brie, camembert		
Vegetables		
Aubergine, beans – french and runner, brussels sprouts, cabbage, cauliflower, celeriac, courgettes, gherkins (pickled), leeks, okra, onions (boiled), green peppers, radish, spring onions, swede, tomatoes (including tinned), turnip	Carrots	Sugar snap peas, butternut squash, mange tout
Fruits		
Gooseberries, redcurrants	Apples – cooking (sweetened with fructose or artificial sweetener), blackberries, loganberries, melon (all types), pears, raspberries, strawberries	Apricots, blackcurrants, cherries, clementines, peaches, pineapple, grapefruit, nectarines, oranges, satsumas, tangerines
Other		
Ordinary mayonnaise (retail) – not reduced calorie	Double cream	Whipping cream

Treatment

Treatment is by diet unless the lesion is localised enough to allow surgical excision of the involved part of the intestine. A reduced long chain triglyceride (LCT) diet is needed to control symptoms. This reduces the volume of intestinal lymphatic fluid and the pressure within the lacteals. It has been recommended that the amount of LCT should be restricted to 5–10 g/day [89]. A very high protein intake may also be needed to maintain plasma levels of albumin. Intakes of protein as high as 6 g protein/kg/day with sufficient energy to ensure its proper utilisation have been suggested, although these guidelines are not evidence based. If the intestinal leakage can be stopped by reducing the lymphatic flow then such a high intake of protein should not be required. Enteric protein loss can be monitored by measuring faecal α1-antitrypsin levels. MCT can be used as an energy source and to increase the palatability of the diet as these are absorbed directly into the portal system and not via the lymphatics. Supportive parenteral nutrition (PN) may also be needed [91].

Papers reviewing nutritional treatments in this condition have shown that 63%–85% of paediatric cases having dietary intervention showed improvement in clinical symptoms and laboratory parameters. The exact composition of the diet in terms of fat and protein content is not reported [92, 93]. Suitable feeds in infancy and early childhood are Monogen or Caprilon (Table 7.19). Caprilon provides appreciably more LCT. If additional protein needs to be given to maintain plasma albumin levels, this can be added to a complete feed, e.g. Vitapro. The fat and electrolyte content of these products should be calculated in addition to the quantities supplied by the feed.

Minimal fat diet

Minimal fat weaning solids should initially be introduced and gradually expanded aiming to keep the total LCT intake <10 g/day, certainly in the first 2 years of life. Details of minimal fat diets are given elsewhere (p. 298). Attention needs to be given to protein intake and extra very low fat, high protein foods may be included.

As the problem is lifelong it is necessary to continue dietary restrictions, certainly until the end of the pubertal growth spurt, although maintaining such a low intake of fat becomes increasingly difficult as the child becomes older. There is no information about the degree of fat restriction required in older children and some relaxation of the diet should be possible so long as symptoms

Table 7.19 Composition of minimal fat, cow's milk protein based infant formulas, per 100 mL.

	Dilution (%)	Energy (kcal)	Energy (kJ)	Protein (g)	CHO (g)	Fat (g)	Na (mmol)(mmol)	K (mmol)(mmol)	Osmolality (mOsm/kg H$_2$O)
Monogen (SHS)	17.5	74	310	2.2	12.0	1.9 (80% MCT)	1.5	1.6	280
Caprilon (SHS)	12.7	66	277	1.5	7.0*	3.6 (75% MCT)	0.9	1.7	233

SHS, Scientific Hospital Supplies.
*12% lactose.

are controlled and growth is adequate. Minimal fat or fat free nutritional supplements such as Build Up made with skimmed milk or Paediasure Plus Juce, Ensure Plus Juce and Fortijuce are useful to ensure adequate protein intake in older children (Table 11.3).

As the dietary restrictions are long term it is particularly important to ensure that the recommended amounts of essential fatty acids (EFA) are included in the diet once the volume of complete infant formula is reduced. Walnut oil provides the most concentrated source of EFA and can be given as a measured amount as a daily dietary supplement. Recommended amounts would be at least 0.1 mL per 56 kcal (235 kJ) provided from foods and drinks not supplemented with EFA (see Table 19.4); however, there are no data as to how well this is absorbed in this disorder. It may be prudent to give double the normal amount of walnut oil as a divided dose mixed with food or as a medicine. This needs to be included in the daily fat allowance.

Fat soluble vitamin supplements (A, D, E) to meet at least the RNI for age should be given separately. If the above oral nutritional supplements are used they are fortified with these vitamins so separate supplementation may not be required. Blood levels should be monitored at outpatient clinics. A 4-year-old girl presenting with tetany caused by hypocalcaemia due to vitamin D deficiency has been described [94].

Neonatal enteropathies and protracted diarrhoea

The causes of protracted diarrhoea in the first few months of life are mostly post infectious and food allergic enteropathies. Rare, and usually early onset, congenital enterocyte disorders include microvillous inclusion disease, tufting enteropathy (intestinal epithelial dysplasia) and autoimmune enteropathy [95]. Congenital glucose-galactose malabsorption, congenital chloride losing diarrhoea and congenital sodium losing diarrhoea will also manifest from birth but villus morphology is normal in these babies.

Microvillous inclusion disease (MVID) is a congenital enterocyte defect that requires PN for fluid and nutritional maintenance. Unusually it does not manifest *in utero* with hydramnios (as a result of intrauterine diarrhoea), but becomes apparent most commonly in the first few post natal days. A late onset presentation is also recognised. MVID is almost invariably fatal without PN support. Early onset syndromes are characterised by secretory diarrhoea (typically 200–250 mL/kg/day) and intolerance of any oral nutrition. The management of the PN is difficult with frequent complications of acute dehydration and metabolic imbalance. Trace mineral deficiencies have been reported so it is important to carefully monitor nutritional parameters [96]. Trophic feeds should be offered so long as the resulting osmotic diarrhoea does not further complicate fluid balance. Many babies in this group have early onset cholestatic liver disease. A case series of three infants with MVID and cholestasis showed improvement with the substitution of conventional IV lipid sources with a fish oil based lipid emulsion [97].

A later onset form of MVID has been described in a few patients who appear to have a better prognosis with one reported case weaning off PN. Small bowel transplantation is the only curative treatment in the early onset form of the disease; however, the decision and timing should be carefully assessed due to recent improvements in PN management. A case series of 24 patients, detailing the complexity of managing these patients, has been published [98].

Children with tufting enteropathy have a more favourable outcome. The disorder is thought to be related to abnormal enterocyte development and/or differentiation; there is a higher prevalence in areas with a high degree of consanguinity and in patients of Arabic origin [99]. Infants require PN support, but there appears to be a range of severity in these disorders with some children becoming less dependent on, and even stopping, PN as they progress through childhood [100]. The enteral management of tufting enteropathy is limited to the exclusion of major food allergens if there is concurrent inflammation in gut biopsies.

Autoimmune enteropathies are characterised by persistent villous atrophy, resistance to bowel rest and evidence of antigut autoantibodies. Treatment with immunosuppression is usually required. Patients do not respond to dietary modification and some will require PN [101, 102]. Where there is evidence of an underlying primary immunodeficiency haematopoietic stem cell transplantation might be considered (p. 340). IPEX syndrome is an x-linked syndrome systemic form of autoimmune enteropathy presenting with villous atrophy, endocrinopathy, dermatitis and other autoimmune phenomena.

Modular feeds for intractable diarrhoea and short bowel syndrome

Intractable diarrhoea can be defined as chronic diarrhoea in the absence of bacterial pathogens of greater than 2 weeks' duration, together with failure to gain weight. Some infants with severe enteropathy or short bowel syndrome fail to respond to feed manipulation using protein hydrolysate or AAF, as previously described, and a modular feed becomes the feed of choice [103]. This allows individual manipulation of ingredients resulting in a tailormade feed for a child. Careful assessment and monitoring is important to prevent nutritional deficiencies and to evaluate the response to feed manipulation. The grading of stools using the Bristol stool chart is important to help assess the response to feed alterations [104].The use of modular feeds can also assist in the diagnosis of the underlying problem. Theories as to why modular feeds work include

- the omission of a feed ingredient which is poorly tolerated

- the very slow mode of introduction which allows time for gut adaptation to take place
- the delay in adding fat to the feed (traditionally the last ingredient to be added) which may alter the inflammatory response in the gut

None of these theories has been proved but clinical experience has demonstrated the approach can be effective.

Feed ingredients

Some of the possible choices of feed ingredients and their advantages and disadvantages are listed in Tables 7.20–7.23. Before starting there needs to be a discussion with the medical staff regarding the appropriate feed composition for the individual baby and to establish good medical support for the dietitian managing the baby's nutrition. The aim is to produce a feed that is well tolerated and meets the infant's nutritional requirements. The following parameters need to be considered:

- total energy content and appropriate energy ratio from fat and carbohydrate
- protein, both type used and quantity
- essential fatty acid intake
- full vitamin and mineral supplementation, including trace elements
- suitable electrolyte concentrations
- feed osmolality

Practical details

- Accurate feed calculation and measurement of ingredients is required to make the necessary small daily feed alterations. Scoop measurements are not accurate enough and ingredients should be weighed on electronic scales.
- Infants with protracted diarrhoea or short bowel syndrome will tolerate frequent small bolus feeds given one to two hourly, or continuous feeds via a nasogastric tube, better than larger bolus feeds.
- Attention needs to be given to the combination of ingredients as these will affect the feed osmolality. The smaller the molecular size the greater the osmotic effect. Most hospital chemical pathology laboratories will analyse feed osmolality on request.

Table 7.20 Protein sources for use in modular feeds.

	Protein type	Suggested dilution (g/100 mL)*	Protein equivalent (g/100 mL)	ACBS prescribable	Comments
Hydrolysed Whey Protein/ Maltodextrin Mixture (SHS)	Hydrolysed whey	4	2	N	At this dilution: 1.5 g glucose polymer 0.8 mmol Na + 0.6 mmol K
Pepdite Module (Code 0767) (SHS)	Hydrolysed pork and soya	2.5	2.2	N	At this dilution: 1 mmol Na + 0.4 mmol K
Complete Amino Acid Mix (Code 0124) (SHS)	L-amino acids	2.5	2.0	N	Amino acids increase feed osmolality No electrolytes

ACBS, Advisory Committee on Borderline Substances; SHS, Scientific Hospital Supplies.
*This is a suggested dilution only. Quantities can be varied according to the desired protein intake, age of child and feed tolerance.

Table 7.21 Carbohydrate sources for use in modular feeds.

	Suggested concentration (g/100 mL)	ACBS prescribable	Comments
Glucose polymer,* e.g. Maxijul (SHS), Polycal (Nutricia), Vitajoule (Vitaflo)	10–12	Y	Carbohydrate of choice as has the lowest osmolality
Glucose	7–8	Y	Use when glucose polymer intolerance is present A combination of the two monosaccharides can be used to utilise two transport mechanisms
Fructose	7–8	Y	Monosaccharides will increase final feed osmolality

ACBS, Advisory Committee on Borderline Substances; SHS, Scientific Hospital Supplies.
*Intolerance to glucose polymers has been documented in the literature. This may be due to a deficiency of pancreatic amylase or of the disaccharidase glucoamylase. Monosaccharides become the carbohydrates of choice in this situation. It may be possible to use sucrose as an alternative carbohydrate.

Table 7.22 Fat sources for use in modular feeds.

	Suggested concentration (g/100 mL*)	Comments
Calogen (canola, sunflower oil emulsion) (SHS)	6–10	Contains linoleic acid (C18:2) + α-linolenic acid (C18:3)
Liquigen (coconut, palm kernel oil emulsion) (SHS)	4–8	MCT increases feed osmolality Does not contain EFA
Vegetable oils, e.g. olive, sunflower[†]	3-5	Not water miscible. An emulsion can be prepared by mixing 50 mL oil with 50 mL water and liquidising with 1–2 g gum acacia

SHS, Scientific Hospital Supplies; MCT, medium chain triglycerides; EFA, essential fatty acids.
*The amount of fat used will depend on tolerance.
[†]These ingredients are not Advisory Committee on Borderline Substances listed.

Table 7.23 Vitamin and mineral supplements for modular feeds.

Paediatric Seravit (Scientific Hospital Supplies)	Contains glucose polymer which may be contraindicated. Does not contain electrolytes (p. 21)
Phlexy-vits (Scientific Hospital Supplies)	Designed for children >11 years. Reduced dose to be given for younger children. May need additional vitamins and minerals prescribed separately according to requirements. Does not contain electrolytes (p. 21)
Ketovite (Paines and Byrne)	Sugar free complete vitamin supplement. Does not contain any minerals or electrolytes (p. 20)

- Infants requiring a modular feeding approach will have high requirements for all nutrients.
- Paediatric Seravit used in conjunction with a fat emulsion, such as Calogen or Liquigen, causes the fat to separate out. For feeds given as a continuous infusion it is recommended that these products are administered separately.
- There is no carbohydrate free complete vitamin and mineral supplement for infants in the UK. If intolerance of glucose/glucose polymer is suspected then Paediatric Seravit cannot be used. Phlexy-Vits could be used in small quantities with specific nutrients added according to individual requirements. Ketovite liquid and tablets are a sugar free complete vitamin supplement.

Introduction of modular feeds

Depending on the clinical situation feeds are often introduced very slowly and the concentration of the individual components is gradually increased (Table 7.24). Occasionally, if an infant is already taking a full strength complete feed such as Neocate LCP and the necessary dietary change is to use a modular feed with, say, a different fat source (in this case MCT instead of the LCT found in Neocate LCP) then the full strength modular feed can be introduced more rapidly.

- Before starting a modular feed it is necessary to assess the infant's symptoms and current nutritional support. If PN is not available feeds should be introduced rapidly to prevent long periods of inadequate nutrition.

- In the absence of IV glucose the carbohydrate content of the feed should never be less than 4 g/100 mL because of the risk of hypoglycaemia. A higher percentage of energy from fat than from carbohydrate may result in excessive ketone production.
- An example of the slow introduction of an amino acid based modular feed (Tables 7.24 and 7.25) can be applied to other protein sources. Suggested incremental changes can take place every 24 hours. If well tolerated this process can be accelerated.
- The infant's response to each change of feed should be assessed daily before making any further alterations. Where possible making more than one change at a time should be avoided.
- Feed changes should be avoided during intercurrent infections as these tend to worsen GI symptoms and make it difficult to assess feed tolerance.

Preparing and teaching for home

After a period of time on a modular feed a nutritionally complete feed should be tried again to see if this is now tolerated. The formula nearest in composition to the modular feed should be chosen and challenged slowly, either by substituting one or two small feeds or by regrading over 4 days, starting with a quarter strength complete feed mixed with three-quarters strength modular feed. If this is not possible or the complete feed is not tolerated, the aim should be to simplify feed ingredients as much as possible in readiness for discharge home. Many preparation errors in the home environment have been noted including poor recipe adherence, incorrect use of measuring equipment and errors in ingredient measurement [105].

- Electronic scales should be used that measure in 1 g increments. If this is not possible to arrange at home, ingredients need to be converted into scoop measurements, using the minimum number of different scoops possible to avoid confusion.
- Syringes need to be supplied for accurate measurement of electrolyte solutions.
- A 24 hour recipe should be given to reduce inaccuracies in feed reconstitution, paying due care to issues of hygiene and refrigeration of feed until it is used. It is important to demonstrate

Table 7.24   Example of slow introduction of a modular feed based on Complete Amino Acid Mix.

Time	Complete Amino Acid Mix	NaCl and KCl	Glucose polymer, e.g. Maxijul	Fat, e.g. Liquigen*	Volume
Days 1–3	½ strength increasing to full strength	Full strength	4%	Nil	As prescribed†
Days 4–9	Full strength	Full strength	Increase in 1% increments daily to total of 10%	Nil	No change
Days 10–15	Full strength	Full strength	10%	Add in 1% increments to 6%	No change
Day 16+	Full strength	Full strength	10%	6%	Increase volume

A vitamin and mineral supplement such as Paediatric Seravit is required to make a complete feed. This should be administered separately if the feed contains a fat emulsion and is being fed continuously.
*Liquigen does not contain essential fatty acids. Walnut oil must be given separately (see Table 19.4).
†If the child is having total parenteral nutrition 10–20 mL/kg/day of feed should be given until a full energy feed is established, after which the feed volume can be increased in 2–5 mL/kg daily increments and the parenteral nutrition reduced in tandem.

Table 7.25   Example of a full strength modular feed using Complete Amino Acid Mix, per 100 mL.

	Energy		Protein	CHO	Fat	Na	K
	(kcal)	(kJ)	(g)	(g)	(g)	(mmol)	(mmol)
2.5 g Complete Amino Acids	8	34	2	–	–	–	–
10 g Maxijul	38	160	–	9.5	–	–	–
6 mL Liquigen	27	113	–	–	3	0.1	–
1.4 mL NaCl (1 mmol/mL)	–	–	–	–	–	1.4	–
0.8 mL KCl (2 mmol/mL)	–	–	–	–	–	–	1.6
Final feed per 100 mL	73	307	2	9.5	3.0	1.5	1.6

the method for making the feed to the infant's carers on at least one occasion before discharge.

- A laminated recipe and wipe off pen for home is useful so that parents can tick off ingredients as they are added.
- Not all the suggested ingredients for modular feeds are ACBS listed. A separate letter to the child's general practitioner will be needed to arrange a supply of the product. A supply of these items may need to be given from the hospital.

Introduction of solids

Where possible solids should be introduced after the infant or child is established on a nutritionally complete feed. The restrictions imposed will depend on the underlying diagnosis. If this is not practical then two or three items should be chosen and these should be allowed daily without variation. Often it is necessary to introduce food items singly to determine tolerance of different foods.

Inflammatory bowel disease

Crohn's disease

Crohn's disease (CrD) is caused by a chronic transmural inflammatory process that may affect any part of the GI tract from the mouth to the anus. It is an extremely heterogeneous disorder with great anatomical and histological diversity. The small intestine is involved in 90% of cases. The aggressive inflammatory process can cause fibrosis of the small bowel, stricture formation and ulceration leading to fistula formation. The aetiology of CrD is not yet fully understood but is thought to be the response to environmental triggers such as infection, drugs or other agents in genetically susceptible individuals. Mutations of one gene (CARD15/NOD2) have been associated with small intestinal CrD in white populations and link innate immunity with the gut bacterial flora [106].

The presentation of CrD in children depends largely on the location and extent of the inflammation. In most cases it is insidious in onset with non specific GI symptoms and growth failure often leading to an initially incorrect diagnosis [107]. It can also be associated with other inflammatory conditions affecting the joints, skin and eyes. The gold standard for the diagnosis of inflammatory bowel disease (IBD) remains endoscopy with biopsy. Methods of assessing small bowel involvement include contrast radiology, magnetic resonance imaging, ultrasound and wireless capsule endoscopy [108]. The appropriate organisation and delivery of services are an integral part of good care. Management remains a team approach with many centres now employing specialist nursing staff to enhance the care of the children [109].

Nutritional problems

Over time the disease causes nausea, anorexia and malabsorption. The mean energy intake of patients with active CrD has been found to be up to 420 kcal (1.75 MJ)/day lower than in age matched controls [110]. The energy and protein deficit is reflected as weight loss (occurring in over 80% children) and a decreased height velocity. Growth failure occurs in 15%–40% children with CrD. In addition to a reduced oral intake, the pro-inflammatory cytokines are increased in CrD and have been shown to adversely affect growth [111, 112]. Specific nutrient deficiencies such as calcium, magnesium, zinc, iron, folate, B_{12} and fat soluble vitamins are common findings at diagnosis with antioxidant trace elements and vitamins being consistently reported at suboptimal concentrations [113]. As some of these levels are affected by the acute phase response in inflammatory conditions the true significance of the findings is not understood; however, there is good evidence that IBD patients experience increased oxidative

stress [114]. During periods of active inflammation there is often enteric leakage of protein resulting in hypoalbuminaemia. Accompanying this is retarded bone mineralisation and development and delayed puberty [115]. At present there are no specific recommendations for bone health in children with IBD but the interpretation of bone mineral density should be adjusted according to the child's bone age as it is known that these patients have delayed skeletal maturation [116].

Treatment

CrD is a chronic and as yet incurable disease and its management requires a combination of nutritional support, judicious use of drugs and appropriate surgery. The primary aim of treatment for IBD is to induce and maintain remission, prevent adverse longer term outcomes such as stricture and fistula formation, and normalise growth and development. A systematic review of the medical treatments of paediatric IBD highlighted a paucity of trials of high methodological quality [117]. There are consensus based British clinical guidelines for the management of IBD [106]. Medical treatments have been defined as first line (exclusive liquid diet/exclusive enteral nutrition or corticosteroids) followed by maintenance therapy as second line treatment (azathioprine or 6-mercaptopurine). For persistent disease third line therapy is with anti-tumour necrosis factor monoclonal antibodies such as infliximab. Surgery is recommended for local complications such as strictures.

Enteral feeds as primary therapy

Exclusive enteral nutrition (EEN) as a treatment for active CrD was identified in the 1970s and involves the administration of a liquid diet for a defined period, with the concomitant exclusion of food. Since then many trials (mostly of poor methodological quality) have been completed with the aim of establishing its efficacy as a primary therapy. These have compared enteral feeds with corticosteroids, and the effectiveness of different types of feed (elemental, hydrolysate and polymeric). There has been no trial of EEN against placebo.

A Cochrane review concluded that steroids were more effective than EEN in inducing remission in active CrD, although the latter was effective in inducing disease remission in a significant number of patients. Confounding factors include that these were all adult studies and nasogastric tubes were not used in patients unable to complete the enteral feeds orally which affected the results on an intention to treat basis. The protein composition (including the addition of glutamine) did not influence the effectiveness of EEN. A non-significant trend was seen favouring feeds with a very low fat and very low LCT content with the recommendation that larger trials are needed to explore this further [118]. Two less rigorous systematic reviews of paediatric trials suggested that nutritional treatment and steroids were equally effective in children [119, 120]. Since these were published a paediatric randomised controlled trial (RCT) has demonstrated similar efficacy between a polymeric and elemental (amino acid based) feed [121].

The mechanism by which EEN exerts a therapeutic effect is still not understood. The anti-inflammatory effect of EEN is recognised and precedes nutritional restitution [122]. Fat could potentially affect the production of pro- or anti-inflammatory mediators. EEN is known to induce mucosal healing in the affected GI tract whilst corticosteroids do not do so [123]. This is now the aim of treatment modalities in CrD and so offers another benefit of using EEN. EEN has also been shown to result in an improved QoL [124].

Modulen IBD and Alicalm are feeds designed specifically for patients with CrD. The former has demonstrated immunomodulatory effects purportedly due to the presence of transforming growth factor-β, an anti-inflammatory cytokine present in casein. The latter is an energy dense (1.35 kcal/mL, 5.6 kJ/mL) polymeric feed with 50% fat present as MCT and thus a low LCT content which may increase its efficacy. There are no published trials to date comparing these feeds against standard paediatric polymeric feeds. It should be noted that Nutrison Standard has been demonstrated to be effective as a treatment in one paediatric study [125].

Most paediatric centres use EEN as a primary therapy despite the increased cost compared with steroids and the potential difficulty following the treatment prescribed. As children with CrD are often chronically malnourished enteral feeds are important for nutritional repletion. Feeds are also preferable as a first line treatment because of the deleterious effect of steroids on growth with one study demonstrating that the use of steroids in puberty resulted in lower adult height [126, 127]. There is currently only low quality evidence to confirm the benefits of feeds on growth in children [111].

Protocol for enteral feeding in CrD

A survey of centres in the UK, Europe, the USA and Asia-Pacific showed wide variations in EEN protocols used throughout the world; 93% used polymeric formulas, with flavourings commonly added to enhance acceptability [128]. Polymeric feeds have the advantage of being more palatable and cheaper than the elemental alternatives. One centre found that use of the former significantly decreased the need for nasogastric tubes in their patients, and this did not affect adherence to the EEN regimens prescribed [129]. Elemental feeds should be used in individuals where cow's milk allergy is suspected.

A randomised paediatric study compared children having EEN with children who received 50% of their requirements from feeds and were allowed to eat normally (partial enteral nutrition, PEN). On analysis nutritional parameters improved equally in both groups; however, blood indices of inflammation failed to improve in the PEN group, showing that significant amounts of food affects the anti-inflammatory response to enteral feeds [130]. The effect of allowing small amounts of food whilst having 100% nutritional requirements from feeds has never been examined.

Regardless of the type of feed the following protocol can be applied.

- Feeds should be gradually introduced over 3–5 days depending on symptoms. In severely malnourished patients there is a risk of refeeding syndrome and daily biochemical monitoring with appropriate electrolyte and mineral supplementation should be instituted until the patient has reached their target nutritional intake and is metabolically stable.
- The enteral feed should provide complete nutrition for a 6–8 week period. There are no data to advise the best length of time for administration of EEN and this is the consensus of UK centres.
- If the feed is well tolerated but the child has difficulty managing the volume, the concentration of powdered feeds may be increased to lower the volume of enteral feed required.

- Clear fluids, boiled sweets and chewing gum are allowed orally by some centres to improve compliance. There is no evidence to inform best practice.
- All solid food should be stopped for the duration of the treatment.

As patients with CrD are generally adolescents they find this particularly difficult and require a high degree of support and motivation to complete the treatment. Despite this feeds are well tolerated by most patients and the full 6 weeks is usually adhered to. If the patients are sure that they will be able to manage orally, feeds can be introduced at home. If a nasogastric feeding regimen is required this is best started as an inpatient.

Once the feed choice and prescribed volumes have been decided the aim is to give as much control to the patient as possible. Feeds should be tried orally with different flavourings to enhance compliance; the daily volume required must be explained carefully so that it is understood that the prescribed volume must be completed every day. If the patient chooses to have a tube they are taught to pass this each night and remove it in the morning to cause minimum inconvenience to their daily routine. Some patients choose to drink the full volume even of hydrolysate feeds; others opt for a combination approach (a percentage orally and the remainder via the tube); some opt for solely nocturnal nasogastric feeds.

Nutritional requirements and monitoring

Most studies have failed to show increased basal energy requirements in patients with CrD unless the patient has a fever [131,132]. One study confirmed that measured resting energy expenditure (REE) in children with Crohn's disease fed with PN correlated well with the predicted REE using FAO/WHO/UNU equations and was not increased [133]. However, a prospective study showed that the median energy intake of enterally fed children with CrD was 117.5% of estimated average requirement (EAR) for energy for age [134].

The initial aim should be to provide 100%–120% EAR for age for energy and the RNI for protein from the full feed, checking that all vitamins and minerals are present in amounts at least equivalent to the RNI [58]. Children are allowed to take a larger feed volume than prescribed if they are still hungry.

They should be weighed weekly and monitored by telephone contact. A follow-up appointment should be arranged 2–3 weeks after discharge to ensure that the patient is responding to treatment and that weight gain is being achieved.

Introduction of foods and discontinuation of feeds

There is no agreement about the best methods of food introduction to patients completing a period of enteral feeds. In the UK two main centres have published data with conflicting results, both at a time when elemental feeds were routinely used. The East Anglian study found that a large number of patients were food intolerant, the most common foods cited as causing problems being corn, wheat, yeast, egg, potato, rye, tea and coffee [135]. This trial has been criticised as patients only completed 2 weeks of an elemental diet before foods were introduced which would not have been long enough to allow for full disease remission. This approach has been modified and a reduced allergen, low fat, low fibre diet devised to be introduced at the end of the 2–3 week period of enteral feeds with subsequent food reintroductions [136].

The group at Northwick Park Hospital introduced foods singly over 5 day periods after 4–8 weeks on exclusive enteral feeds. Food sensitivities could only be identified in 7% of the patients by double blind challenge. Most importantly, there was no significant difference in the duration of remission between patients who did or did not identify food sensitivities [137].

Beattie and Walker-Smith concluded that neither study confirmed that intolerance to foodstuffs is seen in CrD and that no particular foods are known to exacerbate symptoms in a large group of patients [138].

Until there is further evidence it would appear prudent to reduce feed volume over a period of 2–4 weeks and gradually introduce a normal diet, ensuring that continued weight gain is maintained. Many centres exclude high fibre foods in the initial stages. Atopic patients requiring an elemental feed should be advised to exclude suspected food allergens, ensuring an adequate energy and calcium intake. Patients with a tight stricture in the ileum may require a low fibre diet to control symptoms until the stricture is surgically removed.

Long term outcome in Crohn's disease

Some patients require continued nutritional support by nasogastric tube, gastrostomy or orally if appetite remains poor. It has also been reported that continued use of supplementary feeds in addition to a normal diet is associated with prolonged periods of disease remission. A Cochrane review identified two adult randomised controlled trials that suggest that supplementary enteral nutrition may maintain disease remission [139]; however, this is not current UK practice.

A pilot study looking at QoL in a small group of children with apparently stable disease showed the impact of CrD. Difficulties in taking holidays, staying at friends' houses and inability to engage in school sports (due to lack of energy or presence of a stoma) were reported as well as frequently missing school [140]. A more recent study identified that children had a lower QoL in the first 6 months post diagnosis compared with children diagnosed for longer than 6 months [141]. Support from the multidisciplinary team and patient support groups help families overcome these difficulties.

Orofacial granulomatosis

Orofacial granulomatosis (OFG) is a condition where there are granulomas in the orofacial region in the absence of any recognised systemic condition. Clinical features vary with lip swelling and skin lesions commonly seen. OFG and oral CrD may be on the same disease spectrum and some patients appear to respond to the exclusion of certain items from their diet [142]. A systematic review of the literature identified common hypersensitivities to benzoic acid, benzoates, cinnamaldehyde, cinnamon and chocolate. EEN, using an AAF, followed by single food introductions to identify specific dietary triggers may also be successful [143]. Advice sheets for professionals working with children with this diagnosis can be obtained from the King's College London website www.kcl.ac.uk.

Ulcerative colitis

Like CrD, ulcerative colitis (UC) is a chronic, relapsing, inflammatory disease of the intestine which is confined to the colonic and rectal mucosa. Childhood onset UC has a worse disease course compared with that in adults with a 30%–40% colectomy rate at 10 years, compared with 20% in adults. It also has an unknown aetiology with evidence for an inherited predisposition to the disease alongside other, possibly environmental, factors.

Drug therapy is used to induce and maintain disease remission. There is no evidence to support the use of enteral nutrition as a primary therapy in UC. The nutritional problems found in UC are not as severe as in CrD because of the lack of involvement of the small intestine [115]. Height velocity is usually normal unless there is excessive steroid use. As patients with IBD are at risk of vitamin D deficiency it is recommended that this is routinely measured and supplemented when appropriate. Nutritional support is needed if there is growth failure or weight loss and this can be given as a high energy diet and oral nutritional supplements [106, 144].

Transition

Transition should be an integral part of any IBD service, preferably with joint clinics held between adult and paediatric gastroenterology teams which young people can attend for as long as is appropriate. Guidelines endorsed by BSPGHAN are available from the Crohn's in Childhood Research Association and the National Association for Colitis and Crohn's Disease [106].

Disorders of altered gut motility

Gastro-oesophageal reflux

Gastro-oesophageal reflux (GOR) is defined as the passage of gastric contents into the oesophagus, with or without regurgitation and vomiting. It is a normal physiological process that occurs several times a day in healthy infants, children and adults. Most episodes of GOR in healthy individuals occur after meals, last <3 minutes and cause few or no symptoms [145]. Approximately 50% of infants regurgitate at least once a day and, in the majority of children, this can be considered as an uncomplicated self-limiting condition which spontaneously resolves by 12–15 months of age. This is due to the lengthening of the oesophagus and the development of the gastro-oesophageal sphincter.

More severe forms of this problem are found when an infant with regurgitation does not respond to simple treatment and develops gastro-oesophageal reflux disease (GORD). Acid induced lesions of the oesophagus and oesophagitis develop and are associated with other troublesome symptoms such as faltering growth, haematemesis, respiratory symptoms, apnoea, irritability, feeding disorders and iron deficiency anaemia. GORD is a common finding in infants with neurological problems, obesity, oesophageal atresia and cystic fibrosis. Consensus guidelines to define GORD in the paediatric population have been published but there is a recognition that further research in this area is needed [146].

Diagnosis of GORD in infants and toddlers is complicated by the fact that there is no symptom or group of symptoms that is diagnostic or predicts response to therapy. Investigations used include oesophageal pH monitoring, impedance studies and endoscopy with biopsy [145].

Treatment

Parental reassurance is very important and may preclude the need for any other measures in physiological GOR. However, recurrent symptoms of inconsolable crying or irritability, feeding or sleeping difficulties, persistent regurgitation or vomiting leads to unnecessary parental distress, recurrent medical consultations and may need further treatment.

Positioning
Postural treatment of infants has been demonstrated to help and a prone elevated position at 30° is the most successful in reducing GOR [147]. It is no longer possible to recommend this as several studies have shown an increased risk of sudden infant death syndrome in the prone sleeping position. A more practical approach is to avoid positions that exacerbate the situation. Young infants tend to slump when placed in a seat, which increases pressure on the stomach and makes the reflux worse. It is better to place them in a seat that reclines or to lie them down.

Feeding
The infant must not be overfed and should be offered an age appropriate volume of milk. Small volume, frequent feeds may also be beneficial by reducing gastric distension, e.g. 150 mL of formula/kg/day as 6–7 feeds [148]. In practice frequent feeds may be difficult for parents to manage and reduced feed volumes may cause distress in a hungry baby.

Commercial antiregurgitation (AR) formulas and feed thickeners decrease visible regurgitation episodes [145, 149, 150]. Two studies have demonstrated that AR formulas (containing pre-gelatinised cornstarch) decreased GOR episodes as measured by oesophageal pH monitoring [150, 151]. Although the actual number of reflux episodes may not decrease with AR formulas, the reduction in regurgitation may improve QoL for caregivers; it should be noted that the allergenicity of commercial thickening agents is uncertain [145].

Enfamil AR and SMA Staydown are nutritionally complete pre-thickened infant formulas based on cow's milk protein, available on prescription. Enfamil AR contains a high amylopectin, pre-gelatinised rice starch and SMA Staydown contains pre-cooked cornstarch. The manufacturers' instructions should be followed when reconstituting these feeds. They thicken on contact with the acid pH of the stomach. Aptamil AR and Cow & Gate anti-reflux are formulated with carob bean gum which thickens on mixing. The EC Scientific Committee for Food has accepted the addition of starch to a maximum of 2 g/100 mL in infant formula.

A variety of feed thickeners are available on prescription, based either on locust bean gum or modified maize starch (Table 7.26). Instant Carobel can cause, in a minority of infants, the passage of frequent loose stools; however, it has the flexibility of being able to be mixed as a gel and fed from a spoon before breast feeds.

Where there is faltering growth a maize based thickener can be used to provide extra energy. These products are classified as 'not suitable for children under 1 year except in cases of failure to thrive'. Their use in infants should be under the supervision of a healthcare professional. The lowest amount of thickener recommended should be added initially and the amount gradually increased to the maximum level if there is no resolution of symptoms. Feeding through a teat with a slightly

Table 7.26 Feed thickeners.

	Thickening agent	Suggested dilution (g/100 mL)	Added energy per 100 mL (kcal)	(kJ)
Instant Carobel (Cow & Gate)	Locust bean gum	1–3	3–8	13–33
Thick and Easy (Fresenius Kabi)*	Pre-cooked			
Thixo-D (Sutherland)*	maize starch	1–3	4–12	17–50
Vitaquick (Vitaflo)*				
Multi-thick (Abbott)*				
Nutilis Powder (Nutricia)*				
Resource ThickenUp (Nestle)*				

*Only prescribable for <1 year in cases of failure to thrive.

larger hole, or a variable flow teat, is recommended. Ordinary cornflour can also be used as a thickening agent for infant feeds but has the inconvenience of requiring cooking. This should be done in approximately half the volume of water required for the final feed recipe and cooled before the formula powder is added. Such feeds generally require sieving before use.

Aptamil Comfort and Cow & Gate Comfort are thickened infant formulas made from partially hydrolysed whey protein with reduced lactose content that contain prebiotic oligosaccharides. SMA Comfort is similarly made from partially hydrolysed whey protein with reduced lactose levels. These feeds are designed for bottle fed babies with minor digestive problems.

Food allergy
Symptoms of GORD, particularly in infants, may be indistinguishable from those of food allergy [146]. 30%–40% of infants with GOR resistant to treatment have cow's milk allergy, with symptoms significantly improving on a cow's milk protein free diet [152,153]. Although the mechanism is still poorly understood, Borrelli *et al.* suggest that foregut dysmotility is affected by neuro-immune interactions induced by food allergens [154]. In food sensitive patients cow's milk has been shown to cause gastric dysrhythmia and delayed gastric emptying which may exacerbate GOR and induce reflex vomiting [155]. When GOR fails to respond to simple treatment, a therapeutic change of formula to EHF or AAF can be tried for 2–4 weeks followed by rechallenge if symptoms have improved. Breast fed infants should have a trial of maternal cow's milk and egg exclusion [145].

Medical treatment
The major pharmacological agents used for treating GORD in children are gastric acid buffering agents, mucosal surface barriers and gastric antisecretory agents. Acid suppressant agents are the mainstay of treatment for all patients except for those with very infrequent symptoms. H_2 receptor antagonists such as ranitidine and proton pump inhibitors such as omeprazole reduce gastric acid secretion. At present it is felt that there is insufficient evidence of clinical efficacy to justify the routine use of prokinetic agents such as domperidone for GORD [145].

In extreme cases that do not respond to the above treatments, surgery may be needed to correct the problem. A fundoplication which wraps the fundus of the stomach around the lower oesophageal sphincter creates an artificial valve and prevents GOR (p. 148). A gastrostomy is usually inserted for venting gas from the stomach and, occasionally, for feeding purposes. There is considerable morbidity associated with this operation.

Feeding problems in GOR

Feeding difficulties are common in this disorder and are characterised by food refusal, distress during feeding, poor appetite and negative feeding experiences by the mother [156]. Infants with GOR are significantly more demanding and difficult to feed and have been found to ingest significantly less energy than matched infants without GOR [157]. These problems often persist after medical or surgical treatment.

Where there are severe feeding problems it may be necessary to instigate nasogastric or gastrostomy tube feeding to ensure an adequate nutritional intake [145]. Wherever possible an oral intake, however small, should be maintained to minimise later feeding problems. The child's feed should be administered as oral or bolus day feeds with continuous feeds overnight at a slow rate to avoid feed aspiration. The feed volume may need to be reduced below that recommended for age to ensure tolerance, with feeds fortified in the usual way to ensure adequate nutrition for catch-up growth. If using a fine bore nasogastric tube to administer bolus feeds, thickening agents should be kept to the minimum concentration recommended to prevent the tube blocking and an inappropriate length of time being taken to administer the feed. There is no evidence that reduced fat feeds promote gastric emptying and reduce GOR in these infants [158]. Transpyloric feeding can be tried where GORD continues to be a problem; however, one study showed that reflux can still occur during feeding times, and aspiration events and reflux related hospitalisations are still possible [159].

The requirement for tube feeding can continue for prolonged periods of time, as long as 36 months [160]. Parents of infants with feeding problems secondary to GOR need a great deal of support. Optimal management should employ a multidisciplinary feeding disorder team including a psychologist with experience of children with these problems, a paediatrician, a dietitian and a speech and language therapist.

Functional gastrointestinal disorders

Functional gastrointestinal disorders are a heterogeneous group of symptom based conditions which cannot be explained on an organic basis. The aetiology of these conditions is unknown and they are usually classified according to their predominant presenting symptoms in children of different ages [161, 162]. They include functional dyspepsia, functional abdominal pain, cyclical vomiting syndrome and irritable bowel syndrome. In adults it has been demonstrated that a diet low in fermentable oligosaccharides, disaccharides, monosaccharides and polyols (FODMAP) can be beneficial in treating the symptoms of IBS [163]. At present there are no data on the use of the diet in children and great care would be needed to ensure nutritional adequacy.

Functional constipation

Constipation is a symptom rather than a disease and can be caused by anatomical, physiological or histopathological abnormalities. Functional constipation is not related to any of these and is thought to be most often due to the intentional or subconscious withholding of stool after a precipitating acute event. Peak incidence occurs at the time of toilet training with an increased prevalence in boys. Constipation has been found to account for 3% of visits to general paediatric outpatient clinics and 10%–25% of visits to a paediatric gastroenterologist [162].

Average stool frequency has been estimated to be four stools per day in the first week of life, two per day at 1 year of age, decreasing to the adult pattern of between three per day and three per week by the age of 4 years. Within these patterns there is a great variation. The Paris Consensus on Childhood Constipation Terminology (PACCT) Group [164] defined chronic constipation as the occurrence of two or more of the following characteristics during the last 8 weeks:

- less than three bowel movements per week
- more than one episode of faecal incontinence per week
- large stools in the rectum or palpable on abdominal examination
- passing of stools so large they obstruct the toilet
- retentive posturing and withholding behaviour
- painful defaecation

In idiopathic constipation prolonged stretching of the anal walls associated with chronic faecal retention leads to an atonic and desensitised rectum. This perpetuates the problem as large volumes of faeces must be present to initiate the call to pass a stool. Faecal incontinence (previously described as encopresis or soiling) is mostly as a result of chronic faecal retention and rarely occurs before the age of 3 years.

One longitudinal study of children enrolled at the age of 5 years or older found that 60% of children were successfully treated at 1 year [165]. However, despite therapy constipation was still present in 30% of children after puberty, contradicting the general belief that childhood constipation gradually disappears by the teenage years.

Information and support should be tailored according to the child's response to treatment with ongoing support from health professionals including school nurses and support groups. If constipation does not respond to initial treatment within 3 months the child should be referred to a practitioner with expertise in the problem [166].

Treatment

The 2010 NICE guidelines emphasise that dietary interventions alone should not be used as first line treatment. Constipation should be treated with laxatives and a combination of age appropriate behavioural interventions. Treatment should involve disimpaction, if needed, followed by maintenance therapy. Movicol Paediatric Plain (Norgine) containing polyethylene glycol '3350' with electrolytes should be first line treatment with a stimulant laxative (senna, docusate sodium, bisacodyl, sodium picosulfate) added as required [166].

Dietary fibre can be classified into water soluble and insoluble forms. The former includes pectins, fructo-oligosaccharides (FOS), gums and mucilages that are fermented by colonic bacteria to produce short chain fatty acids. This has been shown to increase stool water content and volume. Insoluble fibre mainly acts as a bulking agent in the stool by trapping water in the intestinal tract and acting like a sponge. Both soften and enlarge the stool and reduce GI transit times.

Surveys have shown that constipated children often eat considerably less fibre than their non-constipated counterparts. Even when advised to increase their fibre intake by a physician the fibre intake was only half the amount of the control population. It appears that families can only make the necessary changes with specific dietary counselling [167, 168]. Behavioural intervention can significantly increase dietary fibre intake at 3 months, but this increase is not sustained at 6 months and 1 year [169], confirming the difficulties initiating and maintaining high fibre diets in children. Children with chronic constipation have been shown to have lower energy intakes and a higher incidence of anorexia. It is difficult to know if this existed previously and predisposed to the condition or whether it is caused by early satiety secondary to constipation [170].

There are currently no UK guidelines for appropriate fibre intakes in children. In the USA recommendations are for children older than 2 years to consume daily a minimum number of grams of dietary fibre equal to their age in years plus 5 g/day, e.g. a 4-year-old should have a minimum of 4 + 5 = 9 g fibre/day [171]. In infancy and childhood it is important to ensure that adequate fluids are taken. As a guide children should have 6–8 drinks a day preferably as water or juice and including any milk. For children who continue to drink insufficient amounts foods with a high fluid intake should be encouraged such as ice lollies, jelly and sauces. Fruit, vegetables and salad have a high fluid content as well as being desirable because of their fibre content.

In babies the addition of carbohydrate to feeds can induce an osmotic softening of the stool, but is not to be encouraged as a general public health message. Once solids are introduced these should include fruit and vegetables, with wholegrain cereals being introduced after the age of 6 months. Bran should not be used in infancy and with caution in older children.

No randomised controlled trial has shown an effect on stools in constipated children of any of the above dietary measures. The fact that constipation is uncommon in societies which consume a high fibre diet has been used to justify this treatment. A double blind randomised control trial (DBRCT) studying the effects of infant cereal supplemented with FOS in normal infants showed that this resulted in more frequent and softer stools [172]. Another DBRCT using glucomannan as a water soluble fibre supplement in the diet of children aged 4 or older with chronic constipation showed a beneficial outcome whilst cocoa husk supplementation has been found to be helpful, particularly in children with slow colonic transit times [173, 174]. There are currently no confirmed positive effects of the use of probiotics in constipation.

Food allergy

In a select group of children with constipation who fail to respond to conventional treatment, cow's milk protein (CMP) free diets have been shown to be beneficial [175]. Motility studies in these patients have indicated that the delay in faecal passage is a consequence of stool retention in the rectum and not of a generalised motility disorder [176]. It has therefore been proposed that all children with chronic constipation who fail to respond to normal treatment as outlined above should be considered for a trial of CMP free diet (Table 7.8), especially if they are atopic [177]. One study showed that, of 52 patients with chronic constipation, 58% had an eosinophilic proctitis caused by an underlying food allergy. This was confirmed by double blind food challenges. The majority of children were intolerant of CMP; however, six patients had multiple food intolerances identified by the use of a few foods diet [178]. A systematic review concluded that the available evidence does support a causal link between CMP and functional constipation in some children [179].

Gut motility disorders

Integration of the digestive, absorptive and motor functions of the gut is required for the assimilation of nutrients. In the mature and adult gut, motor functions are organised into particular patterns of contractile activity that have several control mechanisms.

After swallowing, a bolus of milk or food is propelled down the oesophagus by peristalsis; this action differs from the motility of the rest of the intestine in that it can be induced voluntarily. The lower oesophageal sphincter relaxes to allow food or fluid to pass into the stomach which acts as a reservoir and also initiates digestion. It has a contractile action that grinds food to 1–2 mm particle size. Gastric emptying can be modulated by feed components via hormonal secretion.

In the small intestine, motor activity is effected by smooth muscle contraction which is controlled by myogenic, neural and chemical factors. In the fasting state the gut has a contractile activity (the migrating motor complex) that keeps the luminal bacteria in the colon. Abnormalities of this phasic activity can result in bacterial overgrowth of the small intestine and malabsorption. Post prandial activity is initiated by hormones and food eaten to produce peristalsis in the gut, relaxation of the muscle coats below and contraction above the bolus of food through the intestine. Disturbances in this coordinated system can occur at all levels.

Toddler diarrhoea

Toddler diarrhoea, also known as chronic non-specific diarrhoea, is the most frequent cause of chronic diarrhoea in children between the ages of 1 and 5 years of age. Symptoms include frequent watery stools containing undigested foodstuffs in a child who is otherwise well and thriving. It is a disease of exclusion and treatable causes such as post-enteritis syndrome, infections, CD and IBD should be considered. Despite the children generally presenting in a good nutritional state, parental anxiety is high. The diarrhoea ceases spontaneously, generally between 2 and 4 years of age [180].

Proposed mechanisms

A primary problem has still not been identified. Children with this disorder are known to have a rapid gut transit time and intestinal motility is generally thought to be abnormal, although it is unsure whether this is due to a reduced colonic transit time or a disturbance of small intestinal motility.

Carbohydrate malabsorption, particularly of fructose, has been extensively investigated in this disorder. Fructose is known to be slowly absorbed in the small intestine and is often present in large amounts in fruit juice. Young children have an increased amount of fruit squash and fruit juices over water for their drinks [181]. Apple juice particularly has been implicated in causing toddler diarrhoea; studies have been completed using hydrogen breath tests to measure carbohydrate malabsorption. What seems to be evident is that non-absorbable monosaccharides and oligosaccharides, such as galacturonic acid, are produced by enzymatic treatment of the fruit pulp in clear fruit juices, including apple, grape and bilberry juices. It is thought that these may cause problems in sensitive individuals, rather than fructose [182].

Treatment

All sources agree that parental reassurance is of primary importance. The role of diet in this disorder is controversial [183]. Advice is needed to correct any dietary idiosyncrasies. Excessive fluid intake, particularly of fruit juices and squash, should be discouraged. Fibre intake has frequently been reduced by parents in an attempt to normalise stools, therefore increasing this to normal levels should be recommended. The intake of fat may have been reduced, either due to the excessive consumption of high carbohydrate fruit drinks or for health reasons, and should be increased to 35%–40% of total dietary energy. Often parents try excluding foods from the child's diet, mistakenly believing the problems to be due to food intolerance. Once the diagnosis is established these foods should be reintroduced.

Chronic idiopathic pseudo-obstruction disorder

This term embraces a heterogeneous group of disorders that cause severe intestinal dysmotility with recurrent symptoms of intestinal obstruction in the absence of mechanical occlusion. Gut transit time is generally in excess of 96 hours. Primary chronic idiopathic pseudo-obstruction disorder (CIPO) is classified into three main groups: neuropathic, mesenchymopathic and myopathic depending on the predominant involvement of enteric neurons, interstitial cells of Cajal and smooth muscle. The urinary tract may also be involved [184, 185]. The alterations of smooth muscle contractile function lead to abnormal intestinal tract peristalsis. It is an extremely rare disorder with a high morbidity and mortality. QoL has been shown to be poorer than a peer group with reductions in school attendance and pain being a common finding. Parents' QoL is affected by having to be vigilant in assessing their child's fluid balance and the need to follow complicated and time consuming nutritional support protocols [186]. The management goals are to improve GI motor activity where possible, relieve symptoms and restore nutrition and hydration.

Nutritional support is vital for these children. In one series of 44 patients, 72% required PN for a relatively long period of time, seven children dying of PN related complications with a further 10 remaining dependent on long term home PN [187]. In a second series of 105 children only 18 were able to be enterally fed through their illness and 11 patients died [188].

It is possible to achieve full enteral nutrition in some patients, but it needs to be started slowly with a gradual decrease in PN volume as the enteral nutrition is increased. Particular attention needs to be paid to fluid and electrolyte requirements. Many children have an ileostomy fashioned to decompress the gut. The loss of sodium rich effluent through the stoma can result in high sodium requirements (up to 10 mmol/kg/day). Enteral feed can be pooled in the intestine for a prolonged period of time before passing through the stoma, resulting in a lack of appreciation of the relatively high fluid requirements of these children. In certain children (especially those with a migrating motor complex) jejunal feeding may be successful if a trial of gastric feeds has failed [189].

Nutritional treatment
The following suggestions for the nutritional management of these patients have proved beneficial; however, there is no evidence base to support these practices. Oral intake is influenced by the extent of GI disease. Children with gastroparesis are more likely to have difficulty with oral intake than those with predominantly small bowel involvement [190].

- Liquids are easier for the dysmotile gut to process than highly textured foods. The aim should be to give full requirements from a feed or PN, or a combination of the two, to minimise intake of solids.
- Enteral feeds are more likely to be tolerated as a continuous infusion than as bolus feeds.
- The feed constituents may influence gastric emptying:
  ○ whey dominant and whey hydrolysate feeds have been found to empty more rapidly from the stomach than casein dominant feeds in neurologically impaired children [191, 192]
  ○ whey hydrolysate feed has been shown to improve gastric emptying in healthy infants with GOR compared with casein dominant or soy formula [193]
  ○ osmolality and carbohydrate content of the feed may decrease gastric emptying [194]
  ○ the author's current practice is to use whey hydrolysate feeds in children with CIPO
  ○ further studies are needed to compare the relative gastric emptying of whole protein, hydrolysate and amino acid based feeds in this population group
- Care should be taken to ensure that enteral feeds are made as cleanly as possible to prevent the introduction of microorganisms into the gut, which could contribute to bacterial overgrowth. In older children the use of sterile feeds is preferable.
- Fluid balance and sodium requirements should be accurately assessed and supplements given

as needed. When unwell, children often need additional IV fluids to prevent dehydration.

• Where solids are taken these should be low in fibre so as not to cause obstruction and to minimise intestinal gas formation. Semisolid or bite-dissolvable consistencies such as purées, mashed potato and puffed rice cereal will be more easily digested. High fat foods should be avoided in order to limit the delay in GI transit.

The child's weight measurements are not always accurate due to distended loops of gut pooling large quantities of fluid. Weight should be used in conjunction with other anthropometric measurements such as mid-arm circumference or skinfold thickness to assess nutritional status.

Where there are life threatening complications of PN such as loss of IV access or end stage liver disease, or an intolerable QoL, multivisceral transplantation is an option. One centre has reported 77% survival at 2 years post transplantation [195, 196].

Use of probiotics in gastrointestinal diseases

Although there is much interest in this area due to the potential influence of gut microbiota in a number of GI diseases, no recommendations can currently be made. A World Allergy Organization paper concludes that they do not have an established role in the prevention or treatment of allergy and that supplementation remains empirical [197]. Efficacy of the use of probiotics in paediatric UC trials has been demonstrated for VSL#3 (Ferring Pharmaceuticals) [144].

Further reading and useful links

Guandalini S *Textbook of Pediatric Gastroenterology and Nutrition*. London: Taylor & Francis, 2004.

Beattie M et al. *Oxford Specialist Handbooks in Paediatrics*. Paediatric Gastroenterology, Hepatology and Nutrition, 2009.

Resource

Dietitians working in paediatric gastroenterology in the UK are encouraged to join the Associate Members group of the British Society for Paediatric Gastroenterology, Hepatology and Nutrition (BSPGHAN), www.bspghan.org.uk.

Crohn's in Childhood Research Association (CICRA)
www.cicra.org

Crohn's and Colitis UK
www.nacc.org.uk

Digestive Diseases Foundation
www.digestivesdisorders.org.uk

Living with Reflux
www.livingwithreflux.org

Promoting Continence & Product Awareness
www.promocon.co.uk

Childhood Constipation
www.childhoodconstipation.com

Education and Resources for Improving Childhood Continence (ERIC)
www.eric.org.uk

Coeliac UK
www.coeliac.org.uk

Allergy UK
www.allergyuk.org

Families Affected by Eosinophilic Disorders (FABED)
www.fabed.co.uk

Parents Own (generic family support group for parents of children with GI disorders)
www.parentsown.co.uk

Little Leakers (for children with intestinal lymphangiectasia)
www.littleleakers.com

Congenital Sucrase-Isomaltase Deficiency (CSID) parent support group
www.csidinfo.com

Half PINNT (for children on intravenous and nasogastric feeding)
www.pinnt.com

8

Surgery in the Gastrointestinal Tract

Danielle Petersen, Vanessa Shaw and Tracey Johnson

Congenital Malformations

Danielle Petersen and Vanessa Shaw

Introduction

There are a number of congenital malformations that require surgery during the neonatal period. These malformations affect the oesophagus, stomach, and small and large intestines. The type of feed and the method by which it is given will be governed by the area of gut affected, the surgery performed to correct the defect and the condition of the remaining gut.

Oesophageal atresia and tracheo-oesophageal fistula

Oesophageal atresia (OA) has a prevalence of 1 in 2500 to 1 in 4500 births [1, 2]. The oesophagus ends blindly in a pouch, resulting in a non-continuous route from the mouth to the stomach. At birth infants are unable to swallow saliva and are noted to have excessive salivation. Aspiration of this saliva causes choking and cyanotic attacks.

Eighty-six per cent of infants with OA also have a distal tracheo-oesophageal fistula (TOF) where the proximal end of the distal oesophagus is confluent with the trachea [2] (Fig. 8.1). In this case any reflux of stomach contents will enter the trachea and hence the lungs. Isolated 'pure' OA, where there is no fistulous connection with the trachea, occurs in 7% of infants and the rarer presentation of a tracheo-oesophageal fistula without OA ('H' fistula) occurs in 4%. The aetiology of OA is unknown and different environmental factors have been suggested to play a role [2].

OA is associated with other anomalies, associations or syndromes in about 50% of cases. Pedersen *et al.* [1] conducted a population based study using data from a large European database for the surveillance of congenital anomalies over 20 years: 1222 cases of OA were identified. The most common associated anomalies in these infants were congenital heart defects (29.4%), urinary tract anomalies (16.4%), other gastrointestinal

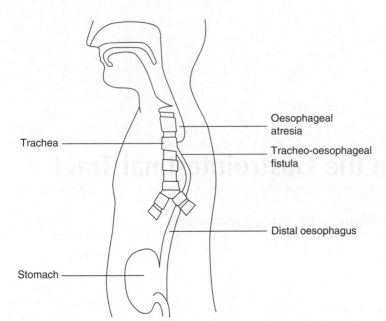

Trachea

Oesophageal
atresia

Tracheo-oesophageal
fistula

Distal oesophagus

Stomach

Figure 8.1 Oesophageal atresia and
tracheo-oesophageal fistula.

anomalies (15.5%) and limb anomalies (13.1%).
VACTERL association (vertebral, anorectal, cardiac, tracheo-oesophageal, renal and limb defects)
occurred in 9.6% of the infants and CHARGE
syndrome (coloboma, heart defects, choanal atresia, retarded growth and development, genital
hypoplasia and ear abnormalities) in 1% of infants.
Similar incidences are found in reports from other
authors [2–4]. Over the last 50 years the mortality
rate of infants with OA has decreased dramatically
due to improvements in surgical, anaesthetic and
neonatal care. Infants with a birth weight greater
than 1500 g and with no major cardiac problems
should have a near 100% survival rate. In those
infants with a very low birth weight (<1500 g) or a
major cardiac anomaly the survival rate is reduced
to 82%, and in those with a very low birth weight
and a major cardiac problem the survival rate is
50% [5, 6].

Following diagnosis, the upper pouch should be
suctioned using a Replogle tube to reduce the risk
of aspiration. The tube also helps increase the size
of the pouch at the blind end of the upper oesophagus. Treatment of OA, whether associated with TOF
or not, is undertaken as soon as possible after birth.
It involves the repair of the oesophagus by anasto-
mosing the upper and lower ends, after closing any
TOF if present, so that both the oesophagus and trachea are separate and continuous. Until the lesion is

corrected surgically, the infant cannot be fed orally.
Depending on the length of the gap and the surgical
management, either enteral or parenteral nutrition
(PN) (p. 50) will be commenced [5].

Feeding the baby with oesophageal atresia and trachea-oesophageal atresia

A primary anastomosis is performed when the
distance between the proximal and distal ends of
the oesophagus is short enough for the two to be
joined in one procedure. This is possible in the
majority of patients, especially when a distal fistula
is present. Most surgeons pass a trans-anastomotic
tube (TAT) which allows gastric decompression
in the early postoperative period and a route for
nasogastric feeding.

Feeds are often started 48–72 hours after corrective surgery and may be given orally once the
infant is swallowing saliva [2]. Ideally, breast feeding should be initiated or expressed breast milk
(EBM) given. If this is not possible then a standard
infant formula is used. Puntis *et al.* [7] found that
50% of infants undergoing a primary anastomosis
were breast fed for a median period of 3 months.
If a chest drain has been inserted postoperatively,
nasogastric feeding via the TAT may be prolonged
for 7 days or so until contrast studies show that the
oesophagus is intact.

A study by Patel *et al.* [8] reviewed a 12 year period of a more simplified management of OA with TOF where chest drains, TAT and contrast studies were not routinely used. Seventeen infants were managed without a TAT and 23 with a TAT. The time to establishment of full oral feeding was 2–8 (average 3.9) days in the infants without a TAT, and 2–12 (average 5.9) days in those with a TAT. They concluded that sizeable minorities of infants do not require a TAT and that early introduction of oral feeds in this group is not associated with an increased risk of complications, such as developing strictures.

In some babies, the distance between the upper and lower ends of the oesophagus exceeds more than 3 vertebrae; this is termed 'long gap OA'. An anastomosis between the upper and lower ends of the oesophagus is not possible and a delayed primary repair is required. The optimal surgical repair for babies with long gap OA remains controversial and there is no clear consensus, with practice differing between centres [5,9]. In these infants the following interventions are suggested.

- Primary repair could be delayed for up to 12 weeks whilst maintaining suction to the upper pouch with a double lumen Replogle tube and feeding via a gastrostomy, allowing the gap to gradually shorten. Regular monitoring of the gap would be carried out and a repair attempted when the two ends can be approximated or overlap. If a TOF is present, it must be disconnected and the defect in the trachea closed before feeding can commence.
- Alternatively, tension can be applied to the oesophageal ends over a period of 6–10 days and a primary anastomosis is then performed.
- Another alternative is that the oesophagus is temporarily abandoned and a cervical oesophagostomy may be formed to allow the infant to swallow saliva and a gastrostomy placed for feeding [2]. In these infants the oesophagus is left for 3–6 months before attempting to join the upper and lower ends. Although cervical oesophagostomy prevents growth in the upper pouch of the oesophagus, the lower pouch hypertrophies and shortens the distance between the two ends.

If radiological studies show that it is still not possible to join the two ends of the oesophagus, the infant may be considered for an oesophageal substitution procedure. Feeding infants undergoing a delayed or staged repair presents more of a challenge than primary anastomosis.

The gastrostomy feed will be either EBM or infant formula and should be given at the same volume and frequency as the infant would receive had they been fed orally. Infants with cervical oesophagostomies should start sham feeding as soon as possible, which will allow the infant to experience normal oral behaviour. To facilitate normal development and coordination, the sham feed should be of the same volume as the gastrostomy feed, and the feed should be of the same duration and frequency so that the baby learns to associate sucking with hunger and satiety. Ideally the feed that is offered with sham feeding should have the

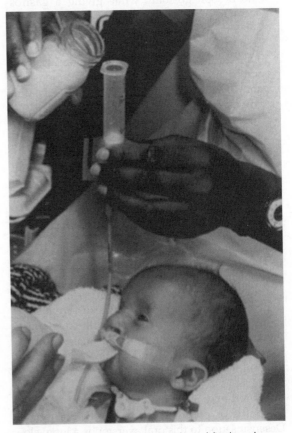

Figure 8.2 Infant with tracheo-oesophageal fistula and cervical oesophagostomy receiving oral sham feeds whilst being fed via a gastrostomy tube. The infant also has a tracheostomy and cleft palate and takes oral feeds from a Rosti bottle.

same taste as that being put down the gastrostomy so that there is no refusal of feeds on the grounds of taste once the infant has an intact gut later. However, it is now more common practice for mothers who wish to give their babies breast milk to express their milk so that this can be given via the gastrostomy and the infant would be given infant formula by mouth for the sham feed. The sham feed seeps out of the oesophagostomy, along with saliva, and is usually managed by wrapping a towel or other absorbent material around the infant's neck (Fig. 8.2). Puntis *et al.* [7] reported that 38% of infants with oesophagostomies were breast fed for a median duration of 2.5 months. There are, however, problems with sham feeding.

- It is difficult to coordinate holding the baby, feeding from a bottle and mopping up feed from the oesophagostomy while giving a gastrostomy feed. This event may defeat nursing staff let alone the mother coping single-handedly at home.
- One-third of infants with oesophageal atresia suffer from cardiovascular complications and may need ventilating, making sham feeding impossible.
- Infants may tire quickly and not be able to suck for long enough to take the same volume orally as is going through the gastrostomy.
- Many infants have small stomachs and initially require small volumes of gastrostomy feed frequently, e.g. 2 hourly, making it difficult to coordinate sham with gastrostomy feeding. However, this problem rapidly corrects itself when the feed volume is increased.

There is no route for sham feeding if an oesophagostomy has not been formed as part of the initial corrective surgical procedure. Infants deprived of oral feedings for the first weeks to months of life can experience difficulty in establishing sucking. This should not be a major problem if oral feeding is established within 2–3 months of life, but if oral feeding is delayed any longer than this it is associated with gagging and vomiting; the infant may avert its head at the very sight of the bottle or push out the teat with the tongue. Desensitisation to this oral aversion is a long, slow process. It is important to remember that feeding is not just a process of providing nutrition; infants are very alert at feeding time and develop cognitive and motor abilities while feeding.

Infants with oesophageal atresia with or without TOF can grow well on breast milk and normal infant formulas, if an adequate volume of feed is taken. If there is a problem with weight gain, feeds can be concentrated and supplemented or commercial nutrient dense formulas may be indicated (Table 1.18).

Feeding the older baby and toddler

In order to promote normal development, these babies should be weaned at the appropriate age of around 6 months. When the primary repair is performed soon after birth without complications, feeding is initiated early and normal feeding progression should be achieved. However, in infants with long gap OA, the primary anastomosis is most often delayed and these infants often experience feeding difficulties. It has been observed that weaning in infants that have undergone a primary anastomosis occurs around 6 months of age and the introduction of lumpy solids is delayed until 12 months of age [7]. If the infant is sham fed, weaning solids should also be sham fed if the oesophagus has not yet been joined up. There has been controversy in the past over what should go down the gastrostomy tube at this stage. A nutritionally adequate feed must be given in preference to weaning solids. In order to get strained weaning foods of the right consistency to go down the tube, they have to be watered down, thereby diluting their energy and nutrient content. If this practice is continued in the long term, failure to thrive could occur. In the study published by Spitz *et al.* [4] in 1987, of 148 children with OA, 27% of the patients were below the third centile for height and weight at 6 months and 5 years of age. A contribution to this could well have been the practice of inappropriate solids being administered down gastrostomy tubes, as was common practice at that time. A review in 2006 of 15 children with OA and TOF who had primary repair at birth found that all were between the 50th and 75th percentile of expected growth at 12 years of age [10]. A more recent review in 2012 of 57 children with OA and TOF found that 9% of patients were underweight and 16% were overweight, according to weight/height z scores [11].

If gagging is experienced when sham weaning solids are introduced, oral intake may be reduced to just tastes of food rather than giving large amounts in order to dispel the association between solid food and gagging. Foods need to be moist, and fibrous foods should be avoided. Fluid should be given at mealtimes to help the food go down. Both mother and child need to build up confidence about eating. Until joined up, sham feeding of age appropriate foods should continue orally with nutritionally adequate feeds via the gastrostomy. If the child does not have an oesophagostomy, enteral feeds should be given via the gastrostomy to promote normal growth. Standard infant formulas and high energy formulas (SMA High Energy, Infatrini or Similac High Energy) may safely be used up to the age of 1 year or so, but will need to be replaced by a more nutritionally adequate feed such as Paediasure, Nutrini or Frebini to maintain good growth in the older child (Table 3.2).

Oesophageal substitution procedures

There are various methods of correcting a long gap OA: gastric transposition, growth by traction, colonic interposition and jejunal interposition. Of these, the optimal technique remains controversial. However, there is consensus that the native oesophagus should be used wherever possible [9].

Colonic interposition involves removing a piece of the colon and transposing it into the chest between the oesophagus above and the stomach below. The advantages are that the required length of the graft is available and the diameter of the lumen of the transposed colon is appropriate for joining to the oesophagus. The disadvantages of this procedure are that the blood supply to the colon is poor; the transposed colon does not have very good peristaltic function to propel food down to the stomach; with time the transposed colon may lose its muscular activity; there is a high incidence of leakage around the anastomosis and the development of strictures.

In **gastric transposition** the whole stomach is mobilised and moved into the chest. The proximal end of the oesophagus is joined to the top of the stomach in the neck. The blood supply is excellent and the rate of both leakage and strictures is low. A review of gastric transposition by Spitz [12] in 192 children (138 had OA) showed that in over 90% of patients the outcome was considered good to excellent in terms of absence of swallowing

difficulties or other gastrointestinal symptoms. There was a 4.6% mortality and 12% leak rate, with 20% of patients needing anastomotic dilatation for strictures. The procedure does have its disadvantages: poor gastric emptying; due to the bulk of the stomach being in the chest it reduces respiratory capacity; gastro-oesophageal reflux (GOR) can be a problem and dumping can occur (p. 150).

Foker *et al.* [13] reported outcomes in 70 infants with OA, with or without TOF, who underwent primary repair of their OA. Ten of these infants had long gaps of 5.0–6.8 cm of which four could not be pulled together initially and had traction sutures placed in the upper and lower segments. There were no surgery related deaths, but 11% mortality later in life. No discernible anastomotic leaks were recorded and one late recurrent TOF occurred; 46% of infants had significant GOR (34% of whom required a Nissen fundoplication) and 30% of patients needed dilatations due to anastomotic strictures. These symptoms were more common in infants with longer gaps. All patients over 2 years of age were reported to be eating satisfactorily or excellently and 93% of the children were eating like their siblings.

Ron *et al.* [9] conducted a survey of current practices of 88 paediatric surgeons based in the UK and abroad. The results showed that gastric transposition (48%) was the most preferred technique for long gap OA when primary anastomosis was not possible, and 94% of surgeons who used it were satisfied with it. Growth by traction was preferred by 39% of the surgeons, followed by colonic interposition by 8% and jejunal interposition by 5%.

Feeding post oesophageal substitution

The oesophagostomy, if present, is closed at the time of the oesophageal substitution. A feeding jejunostomy may be formed as a route for enteral nutrition while the child is sedated post surgery for gastric transposition, as the pre-existing gastrostomy can no longer be used. Gastrostomy feeding can continue if colonic or jejunal interposition has been performed. Oral nutrition is introduced as soon as possible, but supplementary overnight gastrostomy/jejunostomy feeds may be indicated until an adequate intake is taken by mouth. Oesophageal replacement procedures have their problems when feeding recommences as indicated above. The advantage of the gastric transposition is that there is only one anastomosis in the gastrointestinal tract, but the stomach is now sited in a much smaller place in the thorax than it usually occupies in the abdomen. The volume of feed or meals that can be taken comfortably may be greatly reduced, imposing a feeding regimen of little and often. The problem with colon interposition is that two areas of the gut have undergone surgery and anastomosis. Over time the transplanted colon makes a rather 'baggy' oesophagus because of the nature of its musculature, and the repaired oesophagus may not have normal peristaltic function. The colon may suffer temporary dysfunction because of surgical trauma and malabsorption may ensue, necessitating a change to a hydrolysed protein feed (Table 7.6). The end result of these surgical interventions may be oesophageal continuity, but not necessarily normal oesophageal function.

Problems with oesophageal function following repair

Gastro-oesophageal reflux is common following repair, with a reported incidence of 30%–45% [5, 11, 14, 15]. It may respond to medical management, e.g. thickening fluids (Table 7.26), positioning the baby appropriately after feeding or the administration of drugs such as metoclopromide and domperidone. These are dopamine receptor antagonists which stimulate gastric emptying and small intestinal transit, and enhance the strength of oesophageal sphincter contraction. H_2 receptor antagonists such as ranitidine may be administered to reduce gastric acid output so that the reflux does less damage to the oesophageal mucosa. If GOR is severe and unresolved by these methods, surgical correction may be required by performing a fundoplication.

There are various anti-reflux operations, e.g. Nissen, Thal and Belsey. The choice depends on what the surgeon believes to be the best procedure for the individual child. The Nissen fundoplication is the most common and involves mobilising the fundus of the stomach and wrapping it around the lower oesophagus, thus fashioning a valve at the junction of the oesophagus and stomach. Between 30% and 39% of children undergoing repair for OA have significant GOR, leading to life threatening aspiration of feed, and require such anti-reflux

surgery [11, 15]. Together with children with neurological dysfunction, infants and children who have a repaired OA and TOF comprise the majority of patients requiring such procedures.

The anti-reflux surgery is not without its postoperative complications. Whilst preventing reflux into the oesophagus, the fundoplication may also stop the child from burping, and gas bloat can be very uncomfortable in the stomach. Parents need to be taught to 'wind' their child through the gastrostomy tube. Although the child should not be able to vomit, they often experience severe retching which is very distressing for both child and parent, but this usually disappears after a few weeks or months. Fundoplication can also cause dumping (p. 150). Occasionally the valve created by the procedure weakens with time (usually a number of years, but sometimes after a few months) and GOR returns. If this cannot be managed medically the Nissen has to be 're-done'.

The change from receiving full nutrition from a gastrostomy/jejunostomy feed to maintaining an adequate intake orally is slow and there is often a long period where the child needs supplementary tube feeds while learning to eat normally. Prior to being joined up, the child has not experienced the sensation of a bolus of food passing the entire length of the oesophagus. Although the child may have been exposed to sham feeding, this method of feeding does not always lead to successful swallowing. Therefore, many children panic when offered any food other than in liquid form and the establishment of normal feeding has to proceed through stages of gradually altering the consistency of foods, from purées to finely minced and mashed foods and then to the normal diet.

After repair, whether the child has undergone a primary repair in the first few days of life, a delayed repair or a staged procedure, a circular scar will form where the upper and lower segments of the oesophagus are sutured together. With perfect healing the scar will have the same diameter as the oesophagus and will grow with the child. However, if the gap between the upper and lower pouch is >2.5 cm the two ends of the oesophagus will have been stretched to meet and the repair will be put under tension. This tension is thought to increase the risk of an anastomotic stricture developing. Other factors which have been suggested to influence stricture formation include a reduced blood supply in the lower oesophagus following repair, the type of suture material used and the suture pattern employed [5]. Legrand *et al.* [11] reported that of 57 patients with OA and TOF, 46% presented with anastomotic stenosis which required dilatation. These strictures prevent the normal passage of food with bread, meat, poultry, apple and raw vegetables being the foods most often cited as getting stuck.

If there is reflux of stomach contents up into the oesophagus, the acid will inflame the healing scar which may also lead to stricture formation. The presence of an oesophageal stricture has been reported in 52% of patients with GOR as opposed to 22% of patients with no reflux [16]. Children with these problems will often show difficulty in feeding and a reluctance to swallow; they will choke and splutter. Strictures require repeated dilatations to soften the scar tissue and allow the easier passage of solid food. The oesophagus may also go into spasm at the site of the anastomosis and particular foods like mince and peas may get stuck.

The frightening experience of repeated choking leads to fraught mealtimes that both parents and children come to dread. One-third of parents of babies with primary repair in Puntis *et al.*'s [7] study reported problems with choking or coughing, 17% with vomiting and 20% with feed refusal at feeding times at least twice a day in the first year of life. A similar frequency was seen in children after closure of the oesophagostomy. The introduction of solids in these delayed repair children was significantly later than in both controls and children with primary repair, with solid foods being introduced at 12 months and lumpy foods as late as 18 months. It is often easier for parents to abandon the feeding of solids and go back to a completely liquid diet. If this is not supervised, the diet can quickly become nutritionally inadequate.

Children often become bored with food; if foods are liquidised to stop them getting stuck in the throat, there is the danger that every meal will end up looking like the same brown unappetising mush. This can be improved by liquidising the foods separately so that tastes and colours can be distinguished. Mealtimes can become very antisocial; choking and vomiting are common at meals and children may need hefty pats on the back to dislodge food that has become stuck. Eating can be a very slow process for the child, as foods have to be thoroughly chewed before swallowing can be attempted. Parents understandably feel inhibited about eating out of the home, which curtails the social experience of the

child. It is often difficult for parents and carers to understand the problems with swallowing following repair of OA and force feeding the child may be a temptation.

Adequate nutrition can usually be achieved with small frequent meals that are energy dense, and the provision of fluids at mealtimes to help wash down the food. Such are the problems associated with eating that families need help, advice and encouragement from all professionals with appropriate experience, including dietitians, speech and language therapists and clinical psychologists as well as the medical and nursing professions. The Tracheo-Oesophageal Fistula Support Group (TOFS) is a self-help organisation where carers of these children can share their experiences and offer advice.

Dysphagia may remain a problem for many years after repair, but improves with time. Half of the children in Puntis *et al.*'s [7] study experienced feeding difficulties at the age of 7 years. Anderson *et al.* [17] looked at the long term follow-up of children undergoing either colon interposition or gastric transposition to see if one method of oesophageal replacement had an advantage over the other. Most of the children fell at or below the 10th percentile for height and weight, half needed to eat slowly and to avoid certain meats, and dysphagia was rare. There was no apparent difference between the two groups. Davenport *et al.* [18] studied the long term effects of gastric transposition in 17 children who had undergone the procedure more than 5 years previously. They concluded that gastric transposition is compatible with life and allowed satisfactory growth and nutrition for the majority of subjects. They suggested that all children should have oral iron supplementation after the procedure to correct or prevent any defect in iron absorption since low ferritin levels were found in all children tested; one-third were anaemic. Iron absorption is facilitated by the presence of acid in the stomach, and the high incidence of hypochlorhydria seen in some adults after gastric transposition suggests this as a mechanism for defective iron absorption.

Outcome

Chetcuti *et al.* [19] interviewed 125 adults born with OA with or without TOF before 1969 to see how their congenital disease had affected their quality of life (QoL). Dysphagia and symptoms of GOR were present in over half the adults, but most enjoyed a normal diet, provided they drank fluids with their meals. Their social achievements and failures matched those of the rest of the population. Legrand *et al.* [11] studied 81 patients with OA and TOF who were treated in their institution from 1989 to 1998. In 2008, 57 of these patients returned for nutritional status, digestive and respiratory symptoms and QoL assessments. The mean age was 13.3 years; 61% had dysphagia and 35% GOR disease, with only 19% of patients having no digestive symptoms. Their QoL was good but was lower than in healthy controls and was lower in patients born prematurely, with symptoms of GOR disease and a barky cough. The association between complaints of dysphagia and GOR disease, oesophageal function and QoL was also investigated in 25 adults who had previously undergone correction of OA [14]: 48% reported complaints of dysphagia; 33% of GOR. Manometry showed low oesophageal contractions in 20% of patients and pH measurements showed pathological reflux in 14%. Patients reporting dysphagia more often had disturbed motility and appeared affected by these symptoms in their QoL. No association was found between QoL and GOR complaints. The authors' hypothesis was that this may be because these patients had grown up with these symptoms and had got used to them.

Dumping syndrome

Following oesophageal replacement

Dumping syndrome is often seen in infants and young children following gastric transposition and is most probably due to rapid gastric emptying [20]. Ravelli *et al.* [21] studied gastric emptying in 12 children who had undergone gastric transposition using electrical impedance tomography. Gastric emptying was normal in one patient, delayed in seven and accelerated in four. Like the repaired oesophagus, the transposed stomach does not behave normally. The stomach retains its function as a reservoir but its emptying is extremely irregular. Spitz [20] found that the dumping experienced in the early postoperative period was short lived, although it lasted for as long as 6 months in some children and recurred periodically in one child. Michaud *et al.* [22] reported two children

who underwent primary repair of their OA and presented a few months later with dumping syndrome. Neither child had undergone anti-reflux surgery nor had known precipitating factors. They suggested that dumping syndrome can occur after primary anastomosis of OA without anti-reflux surgery and it should be considered in children with OA when they present with gastrointestinal symptoms, faltering growth or refusal to eat.

Following Nissen fundoplication

Dumping can also occur in children following Nissen fundoplication for severe GOR. Pacilli *et al.* [23] measured gastric emptying in eight children before and after laparoscopic Nissen fundoplication. Their results showed that gastric emptying was accelerated in all but one patient and concluded that gastric emptying for liquids is accelerated following Nissen fundoplication. When gastric emptying is accelerated, the result is that hyperosmolar foodstuffs leave the stomach very rapidly and hence draw large quantities of fluid into the small bowel. This produces the 'early' symptoms of distension, discomfort, nausea, retching, tachycardia, pallor, sweating and dizziness. This may be associated with hyperglycaemia. 'Late' symptoms may occur from 1 to 4 hours later as a result of hypoglycaemia and may be indistinguishable from early symptoms [24].

Dietary interventions

There are no large studies on children with dumping syndrome and most of the published papers are case histories; all report it as difficult to treat. Various dietary interventions have been tried to overcome the symptoms of dumping but no one treatment is recommended. The aim is to avoid swings in blood sugar levels. Some children respond to a combination of treatments. In summary these are

- giving small frequent meals [20, 24]
- taking fluids separately from solid foods [20, 25]
- avoiding a high glucose intake [20, 25]
- adding uncooked cornstarch to feeds at a concentration of 3.5%–7% [22] or 50 g/L of feed [26]
- adding pectin to the diet: 5–10 g (<12 years) or 10–15 g (>12 years) divided into six doses [25]

- administering continuous feeds with added fat (both long chain and medium chain fats are used) or small frequent meals enriched with fat [26–28]

Borovoy *et al.* [29] described eight children with dumping syndrome fed by gastrostomy and found that uncooked cornstarch controlled glucose shifts, resolved most of the symptoms, allowed bolus feedings and enhanced weight gain. A guideline for the administration of uncooked cornstarch could be taken from the treatment of glycogen storage disease (p. 549).

Duodenal atresia

Duodenal atresia is a cause of congenital intestinal obstruction and occurs in about 1 in 10 000 births [30]. In most cases the atresia occurs below the ampulla of Vater. A plain x-ray demonstrates the typical 'double-bubble' of the dilated stomach and duodenum proximal and distal to the atresia. Duodenal atresia most often presents as bilious vomiting, with secreted bile unable to pass down the intestine. Less common presentations include faltering growth, abdominal distension secondary to gastric dilatation, aspiration and delayed passing of meconium. The obstruction is corrected by cutting the blind end of the duodenum and connecting it to the lower intestine. There are other anomalies associated with this atresia: Down's syndrome, structural cardiac defects, tracheo-oesophageal fistula, imperforate anus and malrotation occur in over 50% of infants with duodenal atresia [31,32]. Mortality is related to the severity of the associated anomalies and the prognosis for this condition has significantly increased since the early 1970s. Mooney *et al.* [33] reported an improvement in survival from 72% in 1973 to 100% in 1983. Burjonrappa *et al.* [31] reported a 100% survival rate in a recent review of 59 duodenal atresia infants born between 1983 and 2008. Choudhry *et al.* [32] reported a 96% survival rate in 61 duodenal atresia infants born between 1995 and 2004.

PN is used routinely to feed these infants in the first days of life (p. 50). Once the amount of bile aspirate decreases (indicating that the lower gut is patent) and bowel sounds return, enteral feeding can be commenced; PN is then titrated down as enteral feeds are increased. A TAT may be passed post surgery to help in the delivery of feeds. In a study of 17 babies undergoing upper gastrointestinal surgery (10 with duodenal atresia, six with malrotation and one with jejunal atresia) enteral feeding was started via transgastric transanastomotic feeding jejunostomy tubes by day 2 post surgery in 14 cases; the authors concluded that this method of feeding was well tolerated and preferable to PN [34].

Breast feeding should be possible within a week of surgery. If bottle fed, EBM or standard infant formula should be given and, if administered correctly, should provide adequate nutrition. If weight gain is poor, the usual methods of feed fortification can be used (Table 1.18). These same feeds should be used if enteral feeding needs to be continued.

Feeding problems post surgery

The feeding problems following repair of duodenal atresia are usually associated with the motility of the duodenum. *In utero*, the duodenum proximal to the atresia is stretched because ingested material cannot get past the atretic area of gut. The musculature may not function properly once the obstruction is removed, resulting in a baggy proximal duodenum. The infant may feed normally, but milk will accumulate in the lax duodenum rather than continuing its passage down the gut. This can result in large vomits, up to 200 mL at a time. Feeds need to be small and frequent to overcome this problem.

If GOR is present, feeds can be thickened and the baby should be positioned correctly after feeding. As the gut grows and matures with the infant, problems should resolve so that the older child will feed normally.

Hirschsprung's disease

Hirschsprung's disease, also known as congenital megacolon or aganglionic megacolon, is an anomaly where there is a total absence of ganglion cells in the affected part of the large intestine resulting in a loss of peristalsis. It has an incidence of 1 in 5000 infants with a higher incidence in boys than girls (4:1). In 75% of cases the rectosigmoid colon is involved and in 8% there is total colonic involvement [35]. Presentation occurs before 3 months of age in the majority and 80% of cases present by 1 year of age. The aganglionic parts of the colon cannot pass faeces; therefore some affected neonates present with complete intestinal obstruction, bilious vomiting and profound abdominal distension, with a delayed passage of meconium. Other infants present with constipation, abdominal distension, vomiting, diarrhoea and poor growth after the neonatal period. Surgery aims to clear the obstruction by fashioning a colostomy as the initial procedure. When appropriate, the stoma is closed, the non-functioning segment of colon is removed, and a pull-through procedure is performed which connects the functioning bowel to the anus. In some cases the pull-through can be done as a primary procedure.

Some children present later with intractable constipation alternating with diarrhoea which may be treated symptomatically with a high fibre diet. Constipation may also persist in children despite successful surgery. Jarvi et al. [36] recently assessed bowel function and gastrointestinal QoL among 92 adults with previous operated Hirschsprung's disease. These patients reported increased incidence of inability to hold back defaecation (40% vs. 17% in controls), faecal soiling (48% vs. 22%), constipation (30% vs. 9%) and social problems related to bowel function (29% vs. 11%). Gastrointestinal QoL, however, was only slightly lower in the Hirschsprung's group than the control group.

In long segment Hirschsprung's disease there is small intestinal involvement; resection of aganglionic bowel will be necessary, leaving the infant with a shortened length of bowel. The dietary management is as described for short bowel syndrome (p. 155).

Abdominal wall defects

Exomphalos and gastroschisis are not abnormalities of the gastrointestinal tract but are abdominal wall defects involving the exposure of the infant's intestine to the outside world.

Exomphalos

The incidence of exomphalos is 1 in 3000 births [37]. There is a risk of associated malformations and chromosomal abnormalities in babies with exomphalos. An exomphalos can be small or large and occurs when the lateral folds of the abdominal wall fail to meet *in utero*, resulting in incomplete closure of the abdominal wall and herniation of the midgut. Not only bowel but also solid viscera like the liver, spleen, ovaries or testes may be exposed, contained in a translucent membrane composed of amnion and peritoneum. Emergency surgery is necessary as fluids and body heat are crucially lost through the exposed intestines. If the exomphalos is small, there can be a primary closure: the bowel is placed back inside the abdomen, the abdominal wall is then closed and a navel is fashioned. If the exomphalos is too large for this procedure, a staged repair is performed. The exposed intestines and other organs are covered with a prosthetic mesh sac ('silo') to protect them. The silo is suspended above the child and is tightened regularly as the intestine gradually moves back into the abdominal cavity by gravity. The abdomen is then closed and a navel fashioned.

Gastroschisis

The incidence of gastroschisis is 4.4 in 10 000 births in Britain (2004), showing an increasing incidence compared with 1994 when the incidence was 2.5 in 10 000 births [38]. This increasing incidence has been seen in other countries and has been associated with lower maternal age; it is thought to be associated with tobacco smoking and recreational drugs around the time of conception.

In gastroschisis, a rupture of the umbilical cord *in utero* in early pregnancy allows the intestine to escape outside the abdominal wall; in this case, unlike in exomphalos, the intestine has no covering membrane. Surgical strategies for gastroschisis have evolved but with limited evidence and no consensus between experts. The techniques for closing the defect consist of primary or staged and operative or non-operative techniques. A recent study across all 28 surgical units in the UK and Ireland indicated that operative primary closure and staged closure after placing a preformed silo around the exposed intestines were the most commonly used techniques for simple gastroschisis. The development of preformed silos in the early 1990s has changed the management of gastroschisis as they can be placed without the need for a general anaesthetic and surgery on the first day of life. The defect is reduced by the silo and the abdomen is later closed either with operative or non-operative techniques [39, 40]. Bradnock et al.

[40] found that infants managed with preformed silos took on average 5 days longer to reach full enteral feeding compared with those managed with primary closure. Other outcome measures for both groups were similar.

Feeding the infant with abdominal wall defects

The pressure of the silo or the closed abdominal wall forces the intestine back into the abdomen, but this continual pressure may upset its normal function and the gut may suffer a prolonged paralytic ileus. Most of these infants will need PN (p. 50) for several weeks or months before bowel function returns and the use of PN is of major importance in the survival of these infants [41].

Adam *et al.* [42] found that delayed closure of the abdomen in exomphalos leads to more readily established enteral feeding. However, Sauter *et al.* [43] found no difference in the time taken to establish enteral feeding in infants with gastroschisis and exomphalos whether they underwent primary repair or a staged procedure. Kitchanan *et al.* [44] found that neonates with gastroschisis had significant delays in reaching full enteral feeds compared with those with exomphalos (24 days vs. 8 days) and required prolonged support with PN (23 days vs. 6 days). The age at which the infant with gastroschisis is first given enteral feeds affects the length of stay in hospital and the duration of PN; each day delay in starting enteral feeds was associated with an increase hospital stay of 1.05 days and increased PN duration of 1.06 days. Median day of first enteral feeds was day 8 post surgery (range 3–40 days) [45]. A more recent follow-up study of 301 infants [40] found that infants with complex gastroschisis (bowel perforation, necrosis or atresia) required PN for an average of 51 days, compared with infants with simple gastroschisis (intact, uncompromised, continuous bowel) who required PN for an average of 23 days. Mean length of stay was 84 days for complex gastroschisis and 36 days for simple gastroschisis.

Enteral feeding is considered when bowel sounds return and nasogastric aspirate has decreased. Expressed breast milk or infant formula is usually tolerated if given as small frequent boluses or as a continuous feed. Large boluses are not tolerated as the intestinal tract is under constant pressure and cannot accommodate a large amount

of fluid at once. If the baby can be handled normally and does not need to be nursed flat, breast feeding is possible. In one study 70% of babies were breast fed on discharge, 28% were bottle fed and 2% were on solids (median hospital stay 24 days, range 6–419 days) [45]. If there is malabsorption, then a hydrolysed protein feed is indicated (Table 7.6). Infants with gastroschisis may have persistent intestinal dysmotility.

Exomphalos and gastroschisis were fatal abnormalities prior to the 1970s. The advent of PN and temporary prosthetic sacs, or silos, which allow delayed abdominal closure has allowed the good survival rates seen today [46].

Outcome

A 10 year review of neonatal outcome of gastroschisis (21 infants) and exomphalos (five infants) published in 2000 shows survival rates of 91% and 100% respectively [44]. Henrich *et al.* [47] followed up 22 survivors of gastroschisis and 15 of exomphalos who were treated between 1994 and 2004. Developmental delays were rapidly made up after treatment and 75% of these children had no gastrointestinal problems, or suffered from these rarely. Most children were of normal weight and height, with physical and intellectual development delay in a third. Congenital abnormalities (limited to the gastrointestinal tract) were shown in 28% of children with gastroschisis; 81% with exomphalos showed further abnormalities. The initial gastrointestinal problems and developmental delays were most often made up during the first 2 years of life and, except for those with severe defects, the children had good QoL scores.

van Eijck *et al.* [48] studied long term outcomes and QoL in 111 patients with exomphalos (89 minor and 22 major) treated between 1971 and 2004. Fifty one per cent of patients had associated congenital anomalies and 20% of the 111 patients died within the first 8 years of life. Of the surviving patients older than 18 years, 21 (19 minor and two major exomphalos) completed a QoL questionnaire which indicated a good to very good QoL in both groups compared with controls.

Follow up of 23 survivors of gastroschisis born between 1972 and 1984 found that, despite experiencing intrauterine growth retardation, children with uncomplicated gastroschisis eventually achieved relatively normal growth and most babies surviving infancy after repair of gastroschisis could expect to become healthy adults [49]. A more recent study of 301 infants with gastroschisis showed a 96% survival rate after the first year of life [40].

Intestinal atresia occurs in 10%–20% of babies with gastroschisis and they may also develop intestinal necrosis, which may lead to short bowel syndrome. The management of this is described below.

Short Bowel Syndrome

Tracey Johnson

Introduction

Short bowel syndrome (SBS) is a collection of disorders where a loss of intestinal length has occurred that compromises the ability to digest and absorb nutrients. Short bowel syndrome in children may occur at any age, but the majority of cases result following extensive bowel resection in the early neonatal period. Resection may be required in infants born with congenital abnormalities, e.g. gastroschisis, bowel atresias and malrotation, or in infants who develop necrotising enterocolitis. In older children SBS may result from extensive resection following volvulus, trauma, intestinal malignancy or Crohn's disease. Even in the absence of resection children may have conditions leading to a 'functional short bowel' including long segment Hirschsprung's disease, gastroschisis without resection and radiation enteritis.

After an extensive bowel resection there are many factors determining outcome. All these factors will have a bearing on the management of the individual patient.

Infants are born with a small bowel length of 250 cm ± 40 cm [50]. Loss of intestinal length results in loss of surface area for absorption and loss of digestive enzymes and transport carrier proteins, leading to malabsorption. In general, loss of up to 50% of small bowel can be tolerated without any major nutritional problems and clinical features of SBS usually result when more than 75% of the small intestine has been resected. Although it is important, the length of remaining bowel is not the only factor determining outcome; the quality of the remaining gut, the site of resection, presence or

Table 8.1   Absorptive functions of the jejunum and the ileum.

Jejunum	Ileum
Glucose	Vitamin B_{12}
Disaccharides	Bile salts
Protein	Fluid
Fat	Electrolytes
Calcium	
Magnesium	
Iron	
Water soluble vitamins	
thiamin	
riboflavin	
pyridoxine	
folic acid	
ascorbic acid	
Fat soluble vitamins	
vitamin A	
vitamin D	

absence of the ileo-caecal valve (ICV), the primary diagnosis and any ensuing complications will also influence the prognosis.

The key to survival after an extensive small bowel resection is the ability of the remaining bowel to adapt and take over the functions of the resected segment of bowel. Adaptation begins within 24–48 hours after resection. The remaining small bowel hypertrophies increasing the surface area and the absorptive function. The absorptive functions of the jejunum and ileum are given in Table 8.1.

Despite the jejunum being the site of absorption of the majority of nutrients, loss of jejunum is tolerated better than ileal resection. The reasons for this are as follows.

- The ileum has a greater capacity for adaptation than the jejunum. The ileum can adapt and compensate for the absorptive functions of the jejunum, but the jejunum does not have the same potential for adaptation and cannot develop the specialist functions of the ileum, namely bile salt and vitamin B_{12} absorption.

- Transit time in the ileum is slower than in the jejunum, allowing luminal contents to be in contact with the mucosa for longer periods of time.
- The ileum has the capacity to absorb fluid and nutrients against an osmotic gradient leading to favourable absorption compared with the jejunum.

Presence or absence of the ICV also has an important part to play in determining outcome in patients with SBS. The valve slows transit time, which increases the duration of contact of luminal nutrients with the mucosal surface and minimises fluid and electrolyte losses. It also serves as a barrier to prevent bacterial overgrowth which can interfere with nutrient and fluid absorption.

Residual disease may worsen the prognosis of infants following small bowel resection, e.g. after resection for necrotising enterocolitis the remaining bowel may not be of good quality. This may affect function and reduce the potential for adaptation. A diagnosis of gastroschisis may be associated with intestinal dysmotility resulting in poor feed tolerance even in infants with a good length of bowel.

Dependence on PN appears to be most governed by the remaining intestinal length and absence of the ICV. This was recognised by Wilmore in 1972 [51] and has since been confirmed by other studies [52–54].

Nutritional support

The aims of management are to maintain nutritional status, facilitate adaptation of the remaining bowel, control diarrhoea and minimise complications. Nutritional therapy needs to be tailored to the individual child and is ideally managed by a multidisciplinary nutrition team comprising a paediatric gastroenterologist, dietitian, pharmacist, specialist nurse and biochemist.

The development of PN is the most significant factor in the improved survival of children with SBS. PN assures adequate balanced nutrition to maintain hydration and nutritional status (p. 50)

and allows time for intestinal adaptation to occur. Although PN provides essential fluid and energy, prolonged exclusive PN can lead to complications so it is important to give PN in the longer term as nutritional support rather than as the total source of nutrition.

Enteral feeds may not be nutritionally insignificant, but they are nevertheless very important and should be commenced as soon as post-surgical ileus has resolved. Intraluminal nutrients are the single most important factor in promoting intestinal adaptation in SBS [55]. Enteral feeds:

- promote pancreatic secretions, hormones and bile
- are an important factor in preventing intestinal failure related liver disease [56]
- may also help to prevent bacterial translocation [57]

Although children with SBS may require PN for long periods there is potential for progression to full enteral nutrition. Figure 8.3 illustrates the progression from parenteral to enteral nutrition. Managing this transition is challenging as progression can be both prolonged and unpredictable. Initially oral rehydration solutions (Table 7.2) may be used, changing to a feed as tolerated. As feeds are increased PN can be reduced with the ultimate aim of independence from PN. The process may take months or even years to complete and can involve changing feeds and trials of trophic factors (p. 157).

The ability to advance enteral feeds results from the process of intestinal adaptation. There are various strategies that can help this process. As already discussed it is important to put some feed into the bowel and if the distal bowel is not in continuity this should include feeding stoma effluent into a distal mucous fistula to maintain function.

Choice of feed

The choice of nutrients may be important. Complex nutrients, especially long chain triglycerides (LCT), stimulate adaptation better than simple nutrients, the hypothesis being that the more work the bowel has to do to digest a nutrient, the greater the stimulus to adapt [58]. There is no consensus regarding the best formula for infants with SBS. Two systematic reviews of nutritional therapies in paediatric SBS showed the evidence was limited

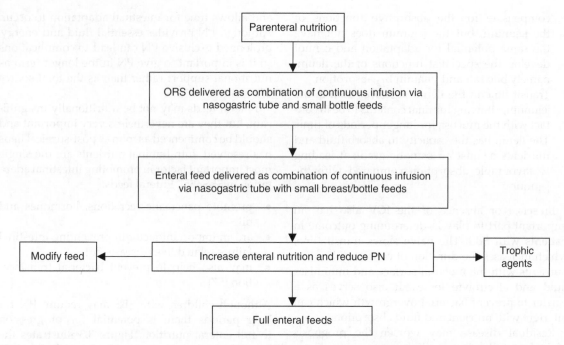

Figure 8.3   Progression from parenteral to enteral nutrition. ORS, oral rehydration solution; PN, parenteral nutrition.

and of poor quality [59, 60]. There is a lack of randomised trials and most human data on the nutritional management of SBS are derived from retrospective analysis of case series. As a result, in individual centres, practices depend more on years of personal experience than on research.

Protein

Infants with SBS might be expected to benefit from an extensively hydrolysed protein feed because of the insufficient luminal surface area for digestion and absorption, but protein digestion and absorption is completed in the upper small gut and is generally not a significant problem in SBS. There is probably little absorptive benefit from using amino acids or hydrolysed protein feeds [61] and complex proteins may in fact be superior in stimulating adaptation. However, cow's milk protein intolerance can occur in surgical neonates and has also been reported in SBS so there may be a role for extensively hydrolysed or amino acid based feeds when inflammation is present [62]. Children with SBS, especially young infants, may have a risk of secondary non-IgE mediated intestinal allergic disease. Secondary protein intolerance is a common phenomenon after mucosal injury [63] and

increased permeability to food antigens in SBS may lead to an enteropathy or inflammatory colitis [64].

Fat

A similar compromise is needed when considering dietary fat. LCT has the greatest potential for stimulating adaptation, is a source of long chain polyunsaturated fatty acids and essential fatty acids and has a lower osmolarity than medium chain triglycerides (MCT). However, many children with SBS have significant fat malabsorption and feeds with a high content of LCT may result in steatorrhoea. In contrast MCT is water soluble and therefore efficiently absorbed. The disadvantage of MCT is its higher osmolarity and experimental evidence has shown that formulas containing MCT stimulate less intestinal adaptation than those containing LCT [65]. A mixture of LCT and MCT, to combine the physiological advantage of MCT and the positive effects of gut adaptation from LCT, may be the best compromise.

Carbohydrate

Carbohydrate has the greatest intraluminal osmotic effect, but potentially can be well absorbed as brush border enzyme activity can be induced according to the composition of the feed. Feeds containing sucrose will induce sucrase and those containing glucose polymer will induce isomaltase [66]. The exception to this is lactose.

Monosaccharides need no digestion but have a higher osmotic load than polysaccharides. Just as with protein and fat, it can be suspected that polysaccharides may stimulate intestinal adaptation better than monosaccharides. Intact starch can also be fermented to short chain fatty acids in the colon, stimulating sodium and water absorption and providing a primary energy source for the colonocytes.

Breast milk

Breast milk may not seem the ideal feed as it contains whole protein and lactose; however, it is associated with good gastrointestinal tolerance. As well as the psychological benefits for the mother of using breast milk it contains high levels of IgA, nucleotides and leucocytes. Glutamine, LCT and growth hormone in breast milk may play a role in intestinal adaptation and there may also be benefits associated with protective colonic bacteria. Importantly, studies have shown that the use of breast milk correlates highly with a shorter duration of PN and that highly specialised formulas confer no advantage over breast feeding [67]. It is the practice in most centres managing infants with SBS to use mother's EBM in the initial stages of feeding.

Formula feeding

It is important to have a flexible approach to feeding and knowledge of gut anatomy and physiology allows informed decisions about nutritional management to be made. In the absence of EBM, or when there is intolerance of EBM, the most appropriate feed to try would be a protein hydrolysate feed with approximately 50% of the fat as MCT. Suitable feeds would be Pepti-Junior and Pregestimil Lipil (Table 7.6).

As feed volumes are advanced malabsorption frequently occurs. It is helpful then to formulate a feed to suit the individual child with a choice of ingredients not predetermined by the composition of a commercial formula. A modular feeding

system allows this flexibility giving a choice of protein, fat and carbohydrate so that ingredients can be manipulated individually to find a feed composition that is tolerated. Modular feeds can be successfully used in the management of children with SBS leading to improved absorption, advancement of enteral feeds and ultimate independence from PN [68].

Tables 7.20, 7.21, 7.22 show some of the components that may be used in a modular feed. The protein source can be a whole protein, hydrolysed protein or amino acids. The carbohydrate source may be polysaccharides, disaccharides (sucrose, lactose) or monosaccharides and in practice a combination of carbohydrate sources may be beneficial so as not to saturate the capacity of a single brush border enzyme. The ratio of LCT:MCT can also be manipulated to tolerance. Electrolytes and micronutrients are added to make the feed nutritionally complete (Table 7.23). An example modular feed is shown in Table 7.25.

Establishing a modular feed involves systematic stepwise changes to feed concentration and volume. Careful description of volume and consistency of stools needs to be documented and serial analysis of stool or stoma fluid for reducing sugars, pH and fat is crucial to make informed decisions about feed composition.

Trophic factors

There are few studies conducted in infants and children regarding trophic factors and, like other aspects of managing SBS, more controlled studies are required to justify their widespread use. Their current use is based on trial and error but, as a non-invasive inexpensive intervention, a trial of pectin or glutamine may be useful.

Pectin is a water soluble fibre. In animal experiments pectin has been shown to slow gastric emptying, slow transit through the small bowel and enhance adaptation. Following fermentation to short chain fatty acids by colonic bacteria pectin may also improve colonic absorptive function [69–72]. Slower transit allows a longer nutrient contact time with the intestinal mucosa and in children with a preserved colon pectin may also stimulate water and sodium absorption [73]. A dose of 1 g/100 mL feed has been suggested [74].

Partially hydrolysed guar gum has also been shown to reduce stool frequency in children with SBS when added to enteral feeds and solids [75].

Glutamine (available as Adamin G) is considered to be an important energy source for rapidly dividing cells such as the cells of the intestinal mucosa. The benefit is unclear but glutamine supplements may enhance adaptation, have an anabolic effect on body tissues and improve enterocyte glucose absorption [76, 77]. The ideal dose is unclear but animal studies suggest that increasing the glutamine content of feeds to 25% total amino acids may enhance adaptation [74].

Continuous tube feeding

Infants and children with SBS frequently tolerate continuous enteral feeds better than oral bottle or enteral bolus feeds. A slow infusion of feed allows constant saturation of brush border enzymes and carrier proteins leading to improved absorption. Luminal nutrients are the single most important stimulus for adaptation so maximising the time during which nutrients are in contact with the intestine will optimise the potential for adaptation.

Oral feeding

Continuous feeding allows for maximum nutrient absorption, but infants need to learn to suck, swallow and chew. Small intermittent breast or bottle feeds should be initiated to maintain oral feeding skills and to lessen the likelihood of feeding difficulties commonly seen in children who are tube fed for extended periods [78]. Oral feeding will also stimulate gall bladder contraction and gastrointestinal secretions and perhaps therefore contribute to a reduced risk of intestinal failure associated liver disease.

Solids should be introduced at the appropriate time around 6 months of age. There is no consensus on the type of solids offered, but it seems sensible when infants are receiving a special formula that they are cow's milk protein and lactose free. There is no evidence to support the avoidance of other foods such as egg, gluten, wheat or disaccharides but in individual cases it may be necessary to exclude other foods if intolerance is suspected.

Pharmocological agents

H₂ receptor antagonists and proton pump inhibitors

Gastric hypersecretion frequently occurs after massive bowel resection. This will increase gastric aspirates and stool and stoma output, but more importantly can impair absorption by inactivation of pancreatic enzymes. Treatment with drugs such as ranitidine and omeprazole is frequently required. Gastric hypersecretion is a transient phase and treatment with these drugs should cease once hypersecretion has resolved; it is important to restore an acid environment in the stomach to inhibit the growth of microorganisms.

Anti-diarrhoeal agents

Loperamide can be used to slow transit time and control diarrhoea.

Cholestyramine

Resection of the terminal ileum can result in bile salt malabsorption. Bile salts are conjugated to bile acids by colonic bacteria leading to diarrhoea. Cholestyramine may help to bind the bile salts.

Growth hormone

Growth hormone has been used to promote intestinal autonomy in SBS but there is little evidence to support its use to improve weaning from PN. Reduced dependence on PN has been shown in some patients but further evaluation is required [77, 79].

Short bowel syndrome in older children

Intestinal adaptation begins 24–48 hours after resection and can continue for up to 3 years. As children get older their feeds need to be reviewed regularly. Feeds need to be age appropriate and always given at the maximum level of tolerance. Children often have voracious appetites, particularly after PN is stopped, and will consume vast amounts of food to compensate for malabsorption. For this reason overnight tube feeds are often continued to provide additional nutritional support.

Weaning from parenteral nutrition

The transition to full enteral nutrition may take many months or years to complete, but many children with SBS can eventually be weaned from PN. It is important to always provide the maximum amount of enteral nutrition and minimum amount of PN whilst maintaining hydration and nutritional status. This requires careful adjustment as advancing enteral nutrition too quickly will result in malabsorption and osmotic diarrhoea. In this circumstance feeds can be reduced to tolerance and attempts made to advance again in subsequent days and weeks. Failure to attempt to advance feeds may lead to longer dependence on PN with the risk of associated complications.

As feed tolerance improves PN can usually be reduced. Initially the number of hours on PN and the volume infused are reduced and, with time, it is usually possible to reduce the number of nights children receive their PN. Careful monitoring is required during the period of transition both to ensure optimal growth and to prevent micronutrient deficiencies.

Complications

Intestinal failure associated liver disease

PN has improved the outcome for children with SBS but paradoxically it is associated with many potentially fatal complications. These complications include intestinal failure associated liver disease (IFALD) which is seen in 40%–60% of children on long term PN [80]. The cause of liver disease in children on PN is multifactorial with risk factors including prematurity [81], nutrient excess, bacterial infection [82], failure to tolerate enteral feeds [83] and failure to establish continuity of the gut. Prevention and management of IFALD involves aggressive use of enteral nutrition, prevention of line sepsis, the use of ursodeoxycholic acid and 'cycling' of PN to reduce the number of hours, or days, that a child receives PN (p. 51). There has been recent interest in the use of novel

intravenous lipid sources containing fish oil to treat IFALD. There are no randomised controlled trials looking at these lipid sources (SMOF lipid, Omegaven) but several case series report reversal of cholestasis and suggest a potential benefit in preventing and treating IFALD in young children [59, 84–86].

Small bowel bacterial overgrowth and D-lactic acidosis

Small bowel bacterial overgrowth (SBBOG) occurs commonly in SBS. It results from anatomical and physiological changes associated with the condition where there is dilatation of the small bowel associated with the adaptation process and changes in motility. Patients with SBBOG typically develop symptoms of nausea, bloating, vomiting and diarrhoea resulting from nutrient malabsorption and an increased number and/or type of bacteria in the small intestine [87]. It can be controlled with antibiotics which are frequently given in 'cycles'.

D-lactic acidosis presents as a severe metabolic acidosis with neurological manifestations that can include slurred speech, ataxia, irritability and drowsiness. In patients with SBS carbohydrates can reach the colon in undigested or partially digested form and are fermented there to produce organic acids. This results in a progressive decrease in intraluminal pH, which favours the overgrowth of acid resistant bacteria such as *Lactobacillus acidophilus*. These bacteria produce D-lactate which is poorly metabolised in humans. Antibiotic treatment can resolve the acidosis by treating the bacterial overgrowth, but it may also be necessary to modify the type and/or amount of carbohydrate in the diet.

Monitoring

Monitoring is an important part of the management of children with SBS receiving PN and is even more important as they are weaned from PN. As previously mentioned assessment of stool output is crucial to monitor feed tolerance. This is the best indicator to assess the potential to increase enteral feeds and reduce PN.

Serial anthropometric measurements are useful to evaluate nutritional status and track progress.

These should include not just weight and length but head circumference, mid upper arm circumference and skinfold measurements.

Nutritional bloods are also needed. Micronutrients may be poorly absorbed and deficiencies are commonly seen in children who are weaning from PN and in those who are exclusively enterally fed. The most common deficiencies seen are fat soluble vitamins, calcium, magnesium, zinc, iron and selenium. Oral supplements should be started to avoid clinical signs of deficiency.

Vitamin B_{12} receptors are restricted to the terminal ileum and if this has been resected children will require lifelong injections of B_{12} to prevent deficiency. Regular monitoring is needed to assess the appropriate time for commencement of vitamin B_{12}.

Sodium depletion can also occur in children with either high stoma output or watery diarrhoea and is a common cause of poor weight gain. Urinary electrolytes are a good indicator of sodium status and should be measured regularly, aiming to maintain a urinary sodium concentration >20 mmol/L and a sodium:potassium ratio of approximately 2:1.

Home parenteral nutrition

Many children with SBS can eventually be weaned from PN. However, if PN is required for extended periods of time it is appropriate to continue the treatment in the home environment and there is good evidence that catheter sepsis is reduced when children are discharged home [88].

Surgery

A number of surgical interventions have been tried to alter intestinal transit and promote adaptation in children with SBS. These include plication of the intestine and bowel lengthening procedures [89, 90]. Some children who develop end stage liver disease as a result of IFALD, but have the potential to eventually achieve independence from PN, may benefit from isolated liver transplantation [91]. Small bowel transplantation has developed over the past 20 years to become a life saving option for children with SBS who develop the complications of intestinal failure. For children with an extremely short bowel, permanent intestinal failure is almost inevitable. Long term PN remains the treatment of choice for this group, but intestinal transplantation may be indicated for those children who develop irreversible liver disease or impaired venous access. Advances in surgical techniques and immunosuppression have improved the outcome of intestinal transplantation, but the survival rate does not yet justify transplantation for children who can be safely managed on parenteral nutrition [92].

Useful links

TOFS (Tracheo-Oesophageal Fistula Support Group)
St George's Centre, 91 Victoria Road, Netherfield, Nottingham NG4 2NN
www.tofs.org.uk

GEEPS (Gastroschisis, Exomphalos, Extrophies Parents Support)
www.geeps.co.uk

9 The Liver and Pancreas

Jason Beyers

The Liver

Introduction

Liver disease in children differs greatly from that in adults. Klein *et al.* have summarised the differences [1]:

- liver disease in paediatric patients is rare
- the causes of disease are more diverse
- there is a greater prevalence of inherited metabolic disorders, biliary tract disease, primary infections and autoimmune disorders
- the higher anabolic needs for growth plus high levels of malabsorption and the catabolic effects of liver disease may result in more nutritional deficiencies

The nutritional management of an infant or child will depend on whether the liver disease is acute, chronic or metabolic. Potential problems warranting nutritional attention occur when there is a disturbance in the usual metabolic functions of the liver. These include glucose homeostasis, protein synthesis, bile salt production, lipid metabolism and vitamin storage. Dietary therapy is usually aimed at managing the consequences of these disturbances (Fig. 9.1).

Screening and investigations

In the UK, newborn screening is performed in the first week of life using the newborn screening collection card. The number of conditions tested for varies between regions, but includes phenylketonuria, cystic fibrosis and medium chain acyl-CoA dehydrogenase deficiency. Many countries outside the UK use this test for a wider range of conditions.

An infant presenting with conjugated hyperbilirubinaemia (CHB) or a suspected inherited metabolic disorder (IMD) requires a referral to a specialist liver centre. A full range of laboratory screening tests are undertaken to investigate potential liver pathology and up to 150 laboratory tests within the first 24 hours of admission may be initiated (Table 9.1). Additional functional laboratory tests (including biopsy) may also be ordered.

Clinical Paediatric Dietetics, Fourth Edition. Edited by Vanessa Shaw.
© 2015 John Wiley & Sons, Ltd. Published 2015 by John Wiley & Sons, Ltd.
Companion Website: www.wiley.com/go/shaw/paediatricdietetics

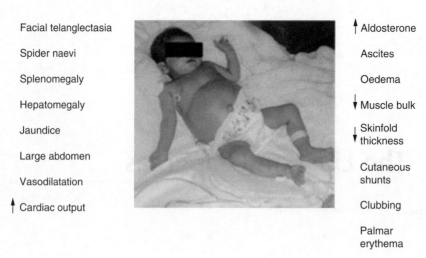

Facial telanglectasia

Spider naevi

Splenomegaly

Hepatomegaly

Jaundice

Large abdomen

Vasodilatation

↑ Cardiac output

↑ Aldosterone

Ascites

Oedema

↓ Muscle bulk

↓ Skinfold thickness

Cutaneous shunts

Clubbing

Palmar erythema

Figure 9.1   Liver disease in children.

Table 9.1   Core conjugated hyperbilirubinaemia work up tests for a patient less than 6 months old.

Haematology	Biochemistry	Virology	Immunology	Other tests	Functional tests
INR	Creatine kinase	Hepatitis markers	Anti tissue transglutaminase	Gal-1-PUT	Liver ultrasound
Reticulocyte count	Alpha-1-antitrypsin phenotype	Lymphadenopathy/ Glandular fever screen	Antineutrophil cytoplasmic antibody	Vitamin D	Liver biopsy
Full blood count	Alpha feto protein	Viral & microbiology serology: CMV IgM, toxoplasma & EBV, HIV (needs consent)		Vitamin E	Anteroposterior spine x-ray
Direct antiglobulin test	Bilirubin (conjugated)		Auto antibodies	Vitamin A	
Group and screen	Lactate (plasma)		Immunoglobulins	Amino acids (urine)	Skeletal survey
	Lipid profile			Bile acids (urine)	Eye examination (Alagille's syndrome)
	Biochemistry				
	ALT				
	Renal/Liver/Bone/Urea				

INR international normalised ratio
ALT alanine transaminase
CMV cytomegalovirus
IgM immunoglobulin M
EBV Epstein-Barr virus
HIV human immunodeficiency virus
Gal-1-PUT galactose-1-phosphate uridyl transferase

Biochemistry

Preliminary biochemical tests help identify possible causes of liver disease (Table 9.1) and these test results identify further necessary investigations. Due to the high number of potential causes of liver disease a variety of tests are required to determine the likely diagnosis, e.g. patients presenting with neonatal jaundice will require biochemical tests and a possible ultrasound, whereas a patient who presents with suspected biliary atresia will require more additional invasive procedures including liver biopsy or exploratory laparotomy.

Nutritional assessment

Patients with liver disease require regular nutritional assessment. The frequency of assessment is determined by the stage and severity of liver disease. Acute, acute on chronic and end stage liver disease (ESLD) assessment are highly variable and are discussed below. After liver transplantation progress is monitored closely over the ensuing weeks and constant reassessment is required until full oral feeding is established. By 6 months post liver transplant the majority of children are taking a normal diet.

Children with acute on chronic or advanced ESLD require regular anthropometric measurements for weight, length, head circumference (if < 2 years), mid upper arm circumference (MUAC) and triceps skinfold. Care is needed when assessing weight, which can be affected by organomegaly, oedema and ascites [2]. The plotting of length/height can indicate chronic malnutrition over longer time periods [3] but is often confounded by inter-observer error. Some liver conditions (e.g. Alagille's syndrome, progressive familial intrahepatic cholestasis (PFIC) and α_1-antitrypsin deficiency) predispose the child to short stature, with length often falling well below the 0.4th centile. Serial measurement of head circumference for children < 2 years is an excellent long term measure of nutritional status. MUAC is used as an indicator of muscle and subcutaneous adipose tissue and has the advantage of not being greatly affected by fluid shifts. It is useful as a short term measure of nutritional status [4]; MUAC centiles are available for infants < 5 years of age [5]. Triceps skinfold measurement can be helpful to determine medium to long term nutrition status [6–8]. The use of total body potassium depicts diminishing cell body mass in ESLD patients and is three times more predictive than anthropometry alone [9]. However, it is costly and labour intensive so is not routine practice in most institutions [10].

The severity of malnutrition does not always correlate with measurable biochemical markers such as liver function tests or vitamin and mineral status [11] and many other measures are not useful malnutrition markers in liver disease [12].

Assessment should also include signs of any self-imposed dietary restrictions (particularly for children with Alagille's or PFIC), early satiety and clinical signs of malnutrition or vitamin deficiencies. It is important to consider any nutrition related problems such as nausea, vomiting, diarrhoea, anorexia or severe itching (e.g. pruritis).

Vitamins and minerals

Fat soluble vitamin deficiencies are a feature of cholestatic and chronic liver disease (CLD). All infants and children with cholestatic liver disease require additional fat soluble vitamins [13] (Table 9.2). Cholestyramine is prescribed to increase gall bladder contraction and this impairs absorption of fat soluble vitamins. Monitoring is essential and additional oral vitamin doses should be given and adjusted accordingly. In severe malabsorption, adequate levels become difficult to achieve and vitamins may need to be given as intramuscular injections.

There is limited research regarding water soluble vitamin supplementation. Due to an altered hepatic metabolism, twice the recommended daily allowance for water soluble vitamins has been recommended in CLD [14]. In adequately nourished patients, oral nutritional supplements given to achieve energy requirements will indirectly increase micronutrient intake, possibly alleviating the need to supplement with water soluble vitamins and minerals. However, in cases of faltering growth it would be prudent to monitor levels and supplement as needed. Increased mineral requirements may include iron if bleeding has been a problem; zinc if vitamin A deficiency occurs; and calcium and phosphate if rickets is diagnosed. Selenium deficiency is associated with essential fatty acid (EFA) deficiency.

Acute liver failure

Acute liver failure (ALF) in children was first described in 1996 by Bhaduri and Mieli-Vergani [15] as a heterogeneous and multi-systemic disorder in which severe impairment of liver function, with or without encephalopathy, occurs in association with hepatocellular necrosis in a patient with no recognisable underlying CLD.

Infants tend to present with symptoms of biliary tract disorders that can progress to a chronic

Table 9.2 Practice guide for vitamin supplementation (King's College Hospital, London).

Vitamin	Product	Age	Daily oral dose
Multi vitamins (A, B group, C & D)	**Abidec/Dalivit drops** (given with α-tocopheryl acetate, see below)	Birth-1 year > 1 year	0.6 mL 1.2 mL
	Forceval capsule	> 12 years	1 capsule
Vitamin E	**α-tocopheryl acetate** (vit E deficiency with cholestasis and severe liver disease)	1 month-12 years	10 mg/kg initially (up to 200 mg daily)
Vitamin D	**Alfacalcidol oral drops 2 μg/mL** (prevention of vit D deficiency in cholestatic liver diseases)	1 month-12 years (<20 kg)	15-30 ng/kg (maximum up to 500 ng)
	or **Colecalciferol 3000 IU/mL**	1-6 months 6 months-12 years 12-18 years	3 000 IU 6 000 IU 10 000 IU
Vitamin K	**Menadiol tablets** (water soluble Vit K tablet preparation for oral supplementation as liver patients have problems with fat malabsorption)	Infants Children	1 mg 5-10 mg

condition. Acute presentations are usually due to poisoning, or as a result of an IMD. An acute presentation in an older child may be due to hepatitis infection, ingestion of a toxic substance or to decompensation of an underlying CLD which has been 'silently' progressing over time. Examples include Wilson's disease or autoimmune liver disease.

Causes of ALF

- infective, e.g. hepatitis A, B or C, cytomegalovirus
- IMD including haemochromatosis, galactosaemia, tyrosinaemia
- toxins/drugs, e.g. parenteral nutrition, chemotherapy or paracetamol overdose
- irradiation, e.g. radiotherapy
- ischaemic, e.g. Budd–Chiari syndrome
- infiltrative such as leukaemia
- autoimmune, e.g. autoimmune hepatitis, autoimmune sclerosing cholangitis
- trauma from abuse, a fall from a horse or bicycle, or a seat belt laceration caused by a road traffic accident

All patients presenting with symptoms of ALF are suspected to have an IMD, which are most commonly seen in neonates and young infants. Clinical presentations are varied and require specific dietary treatment. Prevention of hypoglycaemia is the primary aim (see emergency regimen, Table 9.6) as the risk of prolonged or frequent bouts can accelerate irreversible liver or neurological damage. Dietary manipulation of macronutrients is managed according to routine monitoring of blood glucose levels and specific serum laboratory tests until a diagnosis is confirmed. Often, until a diagnosis is made macronutrient provision is advised by the metabolic team, who review blood results daily and advise on upper limits (particularly in disorders of protein metabolism). Once a diagnosis is made lifelong dietary management will be required (Chapters 17–19) unless the child has a condition that can be alleviated by liver transplantation.

Examples of symptoms associated with ALF according to age at presentation and the suspected IMD are listed in Table 9.3.

The Paediatric Acute Liver Failure (PALF) study group (http://www.palfstudy.org) reports that a cause for ALF is not determined in 47% of patients and that death or liver transplantation occurs in up to 45% [16]. At the author's institution approximately 10%–20% of children with ALF will receive a liver transplant with a 1 year survival rate of 60%–75%.

Table 9.3   Common clinical symptoms at first presentation of acute liver failure in patients with suspected genetic defects.

Age group	Common symptoms	Possible disease according to age of presentation	Age of onset
Neonate	Hypoglycaemia, jaundice, poor feeding, vomiting, diarrhoea, lethargy, sepsis, lactic acidosis, haemolysis, hypotonia, seizures, liver failure	Neonatal iron storage disease Inborn error of bile acid synthesis	24-48 hr
		Alpha-1-antitrypsin deficiency Niemann-Pick type C	Neonate
		Galactosaemia Tyrosinaemia Glycogen storage disease	Neonate - infant
Infant	Hypoglycaemia, jaundice, faltering growth, vomiting, hepatosplenomegaly, deranged LFT, chronic liver disease, fever, cataracts	Fructosaemia Cystic fibrosis PFIC 1, PFIC 2 Alpha-1-antitrypsin deficiency Alagille's syndrome PFIC3	Infant Child
Child	Hepatomegaly, faltering growth, developmental delay, short stature	Wilson's disease* Autoimmune hepatitis*	Adolescent

*Acute presentation with symptoms relating to acute liver failure may be due to an undiagnosed chronic condition, e.g. Wilsons disease or autoimmune hepatitis
LFT liver function test
PFIC progressive familial intrahepatic cholestasis

Diagnosis of ALF

Fulminant hepatic failure often results in severe impairment of hepatic function or significant hepatocyte death in the absence of pre-existing liver disease with or without encephalopathy. In infants and young children the early stages of encephalopathy may be unrecognisable, in which case an escalating international normalised ratio (INR) along with an increasing activated partial thromboplastin time (APPT) and uncontrolled coagulopathy indicates a positive diagnosis. If a diagnosis of fulminant hepatic failure is strictly adhered to, a problem arises. It is difficult to distinguish between disease that is actually acute and that which is (undiagnosed) chronic disease, manifesting as acute. The two conditions can appear the same. A thorough investigation of all possible causes is necessary.

If onset is dramatic there is a possibility of the critical life threatening complication of cerebral oedema, requiring patients to be treated in the paediatric intensive care unit. If the child survives, liver function can return to near normal. However, increasing levels of bilirubin, INR and APPT, despite declining aspartate transaminase levels (which at this stage often indicates an accumulation of hepatocyte necrosis) suggest poor prognosis (Table 9.4). At the author's institution some patients are offered alginate hepatocyte bead transplantation and are placed on the liver transplant waiting list. Ultimately patients with a poor prognosis are placed on the super urgent liver transplant list.

Table 9.4 illustrates the biochemical profiles of two different presentations of acute liver failure seen in a 2½-year-old boy and a 10-year-old girl. These examples show the blood biochemistry results in the days prior to orthotopic liver transplantation (OLT) and at 1 week post OLT, when there is a return to normal (or near normal) levels.

Nutritional requirements in ALF

If presentation is rapid, infants and children are often well nourished, so management is based

Table 9.4 Examples of biochemistry results pre and post orthotopic liver transplantation.

| | 2½ year old male with unknown aetiology | | | | | 10 year old female unknown aetiology | | | | |
	Day 1	Day 2	Day 3	1 week post OLT	Range	Day 1	Day 3	Day 5	1 week post OLT	Range
Albumin	31	25	24	46	35–55 g/L	30	26	26	35	35-50 g/L
Bilirubin	330	300	344	38	<20 mmol/L	268	291	327	47	3-20 mmol/L
AST *	1140	328	474	80	<77 IU/L	1513	894	469	100	7-36 IU/L
GGT	35	32	34	76	<55 IU/L	66	55	55	218	1-55 IU/L
ALP	315	312	350	106	<291 IU/L	830	783	802	138	156-386 IU/L
ALT	1763	944	750	–	<55 IU/L	1931	–	940	–	1-55 IU/L
INR	3.04	7.6	8.75	1.10	<1.2 (ratio)	2.76	4.60	3.40	1.18	< 1.2 (ratio)
APPT	1.590	2.060	2.230	0.970	<1.150 (ratio)	1.51	1.60	1.65	1.02	0.85-1.15 (ratio)
Ammonia	122	–	140	–	<50 mmol/L	108	126	164	–	12-50 mmol/L

*A declining AST indicates hepatocellular necrosis
OLT orthotopic liver transplantation
AST aspartate transaminase
GGT gamma glutamyl transferase
ALP alkaline phosphatase
ALT alanine transaminase
INR international normalised ratio
APPT activated partial thromboplastin time

on preventing hypoglycaemia and maintaining nutritional status until there is some clinical improvement (Table 9.5).

Dietetic management of ALF

The dietetic management of ALF lacks consensus [18]. Hypoglycaemia is present in 40% of patients with ALF due to increased plasma insulin levels secondary to reduced glucose uptake and gluconeogenesis [19]. Current practice is to provide maximum nutritional support during the diagnostic workup by avoiding hypoglycaemia and the build-up of toxic byproducts of metabolism. It is difficult to determine the diagnosis, particularly in infants, as IMD can be responsible and the liver may be sufficiently damaged to produce secondary biochemical abnormalities [20].

Older children and adolescents are less likely to have an undiagnosed IMD, with the exception of Wilson's disease. A standard enteral formula may be given to these patients and if fluid restriction is no barrier nutritional requirements will be rapidly met.

Glucose management

In the presence of hypoglycaemia without a diagnosis, or if continuous feeding cannot achieve normoglycaemia, a continuous intravenous (IV) dextrose infusion is started. If there is no evidence of dehydration a two-thirds fluid restriction is imposed to avoid cerebral oedema. Sufficient energy must be given to avoid catabolism and its associated endogenous production of ammonia by delivering a glucose infusion rate according to age and weight (Table 9.6). The aim of treatment initially is to meet the glucose oxidation rate to prevent protein/fat catabolism.

Usually a diagnosis of galactosaemia or tyrosinaemia is excluded quickly. Other conditions are likely to be ruled out from the clinical presentation. Following the use of the emergency regimen a suitable special formula can be used for the suspected condition, with little indication for the use of a modular feed. It is essential to meet basal protein and energy requirements as soon as possible to prevent catabolism to preserve muscle and fat stores. In the majority of cases a standard infant formula feed can be used and titrated against the

Table 9.5 Nutritional requirements in acute liver failure.

Energy

All ages (IMD ruled out)

    120-150% EAR [17]

Intensive care (intubated, sedated & $^2/_3$ fluid restriction)

    use predictive energy equation without stress factors (e.g. Schofield, WHO, p. 74)

Intensive care (extubated, no fluid restriction)

    use predictive energy equation with appropriate stress factors or use EAR

Glucose

All ages

    If normoglycaemic meet age appropriate requirements

    If hypoglycaemic meet glucose oxidation rates (monitor blood glucose levels)

Intensive care

    meet glucose oxidation rate (monitor blood glucose levels)

    may need to add glucose polymer (NB lactose free and fructose free source of carbohydrate)

    may need to commence intravenous dextrose (emergency regimen Table 9.6)

Protein

All ages

    100-120 % RNI (excessive amounts should be avoided)

Intensive care

    if no IMD maximise according to age appropriate requirements

    if IMD not ruled out may need to avoid until metabolic team advises safe upper limit

    may need to avoid specific amino acids if IMD suspected

    start at 0.8-1.0 g/kg/day and increase to upper allowable limit according to metabolic team recommendations

    if severe acute liver failure may need to limit to 1.5 g/kg/day

Fat

All ages

    if no IMD suspected meet age appropriate requirements

    if IMD suspected maximise according to metabolic team recommendations

    if cholestatic use age appropriate MCT formula

IMD inherited metabolic disorder
EAR estimated average requirement
MCT medium chain triglyceride
RNI reference nutrient intake

Table 9.6 Emergency regimen.

Emergency regimen (ER)

On presentation an IMD may be suspected so an ER should be started as soon as possible as IV dextrose (and saline) with additional potassium if the child is having diuretic therapy. Enteral feeding should be started by adding glucose polymer (i.e. a lactose and fructose free source of carbohydrate) to either oral rehydration solution or water. Additional sodium/potassium supplements are necessary. The child should be fed continuously over 24 hours.

Guidelines for glucose requirements are:

infants: 8-9 mg/kg/min (11.5-13 g/kg/day)
toddlers and children: 7 mg/kg/min (10 g/kg/day)
adolescents: 4 mg/kg/min (6 g/kg/day)

Steps to take when initiating an ER

The amount of glucose given should be increased slowly according to tolerance
Depending on the type of venous access and fluid allowance either 10%, 15% or 20% dextrose can be used
In rare cases dextrose concentrations greater than 25% have been used to prevent hypoglycaemia
e.g. an infant, weight = 3.5 kg, fluid restriction = 67 mL/kg/day (i.e. $^2/_3$ fluid restriction*) requiring 8 mg/kg/min glucose infusion will need:

8.4 mL/hr (or 57.6 mL/kg) of 20% dextrose via a central vein to meet glucose oxidation rate***
Infants can tolerate up to 18 g glucose/kg/day, i.e. 12.5 mg/kg/min
Initially, blood glucose monitoring should be hourly then increased to 4 hourly once stable
Target serum blood glucose levels should be between 4-8 mmol/L

*At the authors institution 100 mL/kg/day (or 4 mL/kg/minute) is a standard paediatric intensive care fluid allowance for children who are ventilated and sedated. A $^2/_3$ fluid restriction equates to 67 mL/kg/day. If there is a high risk of cerebral oedema a maximum fluid allowance 67 mL/kg is imposed in children <1 year of age or $^2/_3$ normal age appropriate fluid requirements for children >1 year.
**Dextrose concentrations greater than 10% will require central venous access to avoid the risk of thrombophlebitis.
***At a 67 mL/kg fluid restriction, 57 mL/kg may not be available for dextrose as IV medications take precedence. IV medications are deducted from the total available IV fluid allowance before nutrition or maintenance fluids are added. A higher dextrose concentration at a lower volume may be required to meet the glucose infusion rate.
IMD inherited metabolic disorder
ER emergency regimen
IV intravenous

IV dextrose over 24–48 hours to maintain blood glucose levels. In cases where fluid restriction is upheld, a glucose polymer may need to be added to the standard feed to provide sufficient glucose. In some institutions a modular feed is designed to provide complete nutrition (p. 184).

Addition of protein

In the presence of encephalopathy it is important not to over-restrict protein and severe prolonged protein restriction is no longer practised as it could result in increased endogenous ammonia production from protein catabolism. However, a child with a suspected IMD of protein is initially protein restricted. With guidance from the metabolic team, complete protein requirements would be reintroduced within 24–48 hours. Further investigation by the metabolic team can provide an upper tolerable limit of the offending amino acid without increasing toxic byproducts. In practice a standard infant formula is used to provide up to the first 1 g/kg protein with the addition of a glucose polymer to meet the glucose oxidation rate. Infants should be given minimum protein requirements to meet the lower reference nutrient intake.

In cases where a modular feed is required protein should be added as soon as possible. If galactosaemia has not yet been excluded Essential Amino Acid Mix is a suitable lactose free source of protein. If tyrosinaemia has not been excluded, and depending on plasma amino acid levels, TYR Anamix can be given (the feed being based on a tyrosine free amino acid mix). The practice of using a methionine free formula has been replaced by the medication 2-(2-nitro-4-fluoro-methylbenzoyl)-1,3-cyclohexanedione, which prevents the toxic build-up of succinyl acetone that can damage the liver.

Addition of fat

If a modular feed is used it will require the addition of fat to meet energy requirements. Fat in the form of long chain triglycerides (LCT), e.g. Calogen, or medium chain triglyceride (MCT) fat emulsions, e.g Liquigen, can be added as the condition of the child is monitored. Increments of 1 g fat/kg/day are recommended. If LCT fats are limited to <10% of total fat intake, small quantities of walnut oil (p. 601) may be needed to provide EFAs.

Vitamins and minerals

Many children will have adequate nutritional status during the acute phase and will probably receive adequate nutrition once they are established on a standard formula. In those who require a modular feed the addition of a complete vitamin and mineral supplement, such as Paediatric Seravit, is needed.

Feeding issues

In the majority of paediatric ALF cases medical treatment can result in full recovery. In children with advanced ALF nutrition support will be managed in the intensive care unit and adjustments to ventilation, sedation and fluid allowance will be needed. Often the rate at which any feed can be given is severely limited due to fluid restriction, with the majority of fluid volume taken up by IV medications and infusions. Continuous pump feeding together with concentrating the infant formula or adding glucose polymer is often required to avoid hypoglycaemia. In older children a 1.5–2 kcal (6–8 kJ)/mL formula may be required to meet energy demands. If hypoglycaemia is not corrected, partial or full IV dextrose infusion is required to meet glucose oxidation rates (Table 9.6). If renal filtration is commenced the fluid allowance may be liberalised to achieve an adequate feed rate.

In younger children after transplantation, surgery is performed to reroute the biliary ducts directly to the small bowel (i.e. a new Roux loop is formed) and a compulsory 5 day period of nil by mouth is usually imposed until the surgeons are satisfied that the risk of small bowel perforation is avoided. Parenteral nutrition (PN) is not usually given during this period unless nutritional status prior to OLT is very poor or, because of complications, the surgical team estimate that enteral feeding is unlikely to commence after 5 days. Older children can receive a duct-to-duct procedure, which does not involve rerouting of the biliary ducts to the small bowel, and feeding can usually commence within 24 hours.

The nutritional management of infants receiving liver transplantation due to ALF involves close nutritional monitoring for the first year. Some of these patients experience complications post liver transplant prolonging their progression to oral intake. In rare cases home enteral nutrition support may be required until appropriate weaning and adequate growth is achieved. Older children who have received a liver transplant for ALF tend to progress well on a normal diet once they get over the initial surgical insult. If normal growth is restored within the first year the need for specialist dietetic intervention diminishes.

A case study to show the management of a young child with ALF is given in Table 9.7.

Chronic liver disease

There are many causes CLD. Time of presentation can range from infancy through to adolescence; the chance of requiring liver transplantation increases with advancing age and liver disease progression. Children are at risk of malnutrition due to failing to meet the demands of growth. Post transplantation morbidity and mortality was strongly linked to advancing malnutrition status in a review at the author's institution. Common factors contributing to malnutrition in ESLD are listed in Table 9.8.

Nutritional requirements

Nutritional requirements in CLD are given in Table 9.9. The dietary management of disorders that lead to CLD are given below.

Disorders presenting in infancy

- inherited metabolic disorders, e.g. glycogen storage disease, urea cycle defect
- infections, e.g. hepatitis
- biliary malformations, e.g. biliary atresia, choledocal cysts
- vascular lesions, e.g. hepatocellular carcinoma, haemangioma
- toxic and nutritional disorders
- cryptogenic disorders, e.g. cirrhosis or hepatitis

Jaundice

Jaundice is a condition that causes the infant or child to appear yellow in complexion and in the whites of their eyes; it is classified as either conjugated or unconjugated. Unconjugated jaundice is characterised clinically by a jaundiced appearance without bilirubin in the urine. This may be physiological in the newborn due to an increase of bilirubin production, decreased bilirubin clearance or a combination of both. Treatment does not usually require dietetic intervention. Conjugated jaundice occurs when the total serum bilirubin is raised and the conjugated fraction is >20% of the total bilirubin (normally <5%). This needs further investigation and usually requires dietetic management. Conjugated bilirubin is made water soluble by the addition of glucuronide in the liver and enters the bile. If bile flow from the liver is reduced the stools will lack pigment. In this case the (conjugated) bilirubin glucuronide passes into the serum and is then excreted as dark urine.

Infantile conjugated hyperbilirubinaemia

Infantile CHB is the most common presentation for an infant with hepatobiliary disease. The majority of newborn infants seen in specialist liver centres present with CHB. This type of jaundice represents significant hepatobiliary disease and is described as cholestatic liver disease. The bile flow from the liver into the gut is limited and fat emulsification and digestion is reduced. This leads to malabsorption of fat, fat soluble vitamins and some minerals. Steatorrhoea, growth failure and rickets are common clinical consequences [21, 22]. Galactosaemia needs to be excluded as a diagnosis. Dietetic management of CHB is summarised in Table 9.10. Most of the possible diagnoses for CHB are given below.

Common liver diseases in infants and young children and dietetic management

Neonatal hepatitis

The cause of neonatal hepatitis is unknown. Severity varies and rarely results in cirrhosis. Usually bile flow resolves with time, but in a majority of these cases fat malabsorption is treated with formulas

Table 9.7   Case study - acute liver failure, unknown aetiology, suspected viral hepatitis.

Admission: 2 year 9 month old male twin, previously well and healthy Wt = 15.5 kg (83rd centile) MUAC = 17.2 cm (89th centile)

Presentation history: Deranged liver function, coagulopathy and INR of 6.0 with acute liver failure, grade 1-2 encephalopathy, jaundice, pale stools, dark urine, lethargy, loss of appetite, abdomen soft, no organomegaly

Impression: Post viral hepatic failure with encephalopathy and neutropenia

Acute interventions: Admitted to PICU, intubated and sedated, $^2/_3$ fluid restriction on 10% IV dextrose. Target glucose infusion rate = 7 mg/kg/min

Clinical concerns: Blood glucose = 3.3 mmol/L. Bilirubin remained excessive, INR rapidly increased along with a declining AST indicating hepatocellular death. Albumin declined indicating worsening synthetic liver function. Required super urgent liver transplantation.

Biochemistry *(grey arrow depicting the time of liver transplant)*

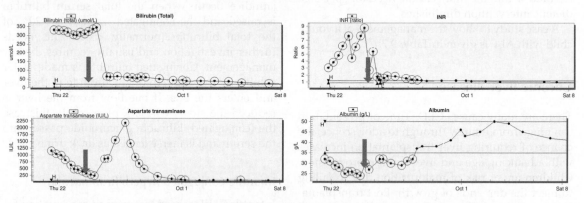

Nutrition management in PICU prior to transplant

Day 1: Blood glucose levels (BM) were 3.3-4.1 mmol/L on $^2/_3$ fluid restriction of 60 mL/kg. This comprised 43 mL/kg intravenous (IV) 10% dextrose and 17 mL/kg of IV medications in a 5% dextrose solution.

- 10% dextrose @ 43 mL/kg provides 4.8 mg/kg/min glucose plus 0.6 mg/kg/min from IV medications in 5% dextrose = a total of 5.4 mg/kg/min glucose infusion rate
- Due to limited fluid availability and BM predominantly less than 4 mmol/L, 12.5% IV dextrose was used = 6 mg/kg/min
- The dextrose in IV medications was increased to 10%, bringing the total glucose infusion rate to 7.2 mg/kg/min
- Energy requirements = basal metabolic rate (BMR) 58 kcal/kg

Day 2: BM 4.7-5.4 mmol/L

Aim to commence trophic nasogastric (NG) feeding, but due to limited volume to provide sufficient exogenous glucose to meet glucose needs and likely liver transplantation within 48 hours, enteral feeding was not initiated.

Day 3: Received liver transplant during the early hours of the morning. Returned to PICU intubated and sedated.

Nutrition interventions post transplant - *no special formula required*

Days 1-5: NBM due to new Roux loop. IV fluids met full fluid requirements. Extubated on day 2.

Day 5: Weight = 14.7 kg (69th centile) MUAC = 16.3 cm (70th centile). Started NG feeding @10 mL/hr using a standard formula and increased feed rate 10 mL/hr every 6 hours. Target non ambulatory feed rate = 52 mL/hr which provided 80 kcal (335 kJ)/kg (EAR) + 2.2 g/kg protein. Pre surgical weight of 15.5 kg was used.

Day 6: Transferred to high dependency unit on continuous NG feeding.

Day 7: Chyle seen in abdominal drain fluid. Laboratory testing revealed chyle leak secondary to chylous ascites. Changed to high medium chain triglyceride (80% MCT) formula.

Day 8: Started oral sips of fat free fluids and started low long chain triglyceride (LCT) diet.

Day 10: Transferred to liver ward. NG feeding stopped during daytime hours to allow appetite for solid food. Continued overnight NG feeding.

Days 12-14: Weight = 14.7 kg (67th centile) MUAC = 16.5 cm (75th centile). Chylous ascites resolved on day 14, NG tube removed. Started two oral nutritional supplement drinks (1.5 kcal, 6 kJ/mL) per day.

(continued overleaf)

Table 9.7   (continued)

Week 3: Weight = 15.1 kg (74th centile) MUAC = 16.8 cm (81st centile). Energy supplements continued.

Week 4: Weight = 15.4 kg (78th centile) MUAC = 17.2 cm (88th centile). Refused oral supplements but replaced these with high protein/energy snacks. Discharged to local hospital. Aim was to continue to provide up to 120% of EAR for energy over the next 3-6 months depending on growth and to monitor for excessive weight gain due to steroids.

3 month follow up at liver outpatient clinic: Weight = 16.0 kg (82nd centile) MUAC = 17.6 cm (92nd centile). Management unchanged.

6 month follow up at liver outpatient clinic: Weight = 16.7 kg (83rd centile) MUAC = 18.3 cm (96th centile). Had nonspecific unwell episodes which were related to sero-conversion of CMV. Symptoms resolved. 1 year follow up planned.

1 year post liver transplantation: Weight = 16.0 kg (53rd centile) MUAC = 17.6 cm (87th centile). Developed post transplant proliferative disorder (PTLD). Received bone marrow transplant at local hospital. Nutrition managed by dietitian at local hospital. Oral intake and weight reported to have improved.

MUAC mid upper arm circumference **INR** international normalised ratio **AST** aspartate transaminase **PICU** paediatric intensive care unit **NBM** nil by mouth **EAR** estimated average requirement

Table 9.8   Potential causes of malnutrition in chronic liver disease.

Physical complications	Inadequate intake, anorexia, nausea, vomiting, irritability	• early satiety as a result of tense ascites, enlarged liver/spleen • behavioural feeding problems • hospitalisation related depression • unpalatable diet/feeds
Malabsorption	Impaired nutrient digestion and absorption	• bile salt deficiency • pancreatic insufficiency • portal hypertension related enteropathy • malnutrition related villous atrophy
Hypermetabolic effects	Increased nutritional requirements	• hypermetabolism (during stress such as infection) • accelerated protein breakdown • insufficient protein synthesis during fasting
Medication effects	Volume displacement, lethargy, timing of medication interfering with meal times	• early satiety • tiredness, prolonged sleeping • nausea, vomiting

Table 9.9   Nutritional requirements for chronic liver disease.

Acute on chronic liver disease with cholestasis

Energy	infants 100-150 kcal (420-630 kJ)/kg/d depending on level of malabsorption children 100-120% EAR
Protein	10-12% TE
Fat	1-4 g/kg of which 30-70% as MCT (dependent upon diagnosis)

Chronic liver disease

	Energy	**Protein**	**Fat**
Infants (0-1 year)	100-150 kcal (420-630 kJ)/kg/day	1-4 g/kg (10-12% TE)	meet EAR - if
Children (pre school)	130-150% EAR	3-6 g/kg	cholestasis use
Children (school age)	100-130% EAR	3-5 g/kg	high MCT formula
ESLD all ages	150% EAR	up to 4 g/kg	or supplement

EAR estimated average requirement [17] **MCT** medium chain triglycerides **TE** total energy **ESLD** end stage liver disease

Table 9.10 Summary of dietetic management for infantile conjugated hyperbilirubinaemia/cholestatic jaundice.

1. Is galactosaemia suspected?
   - **No**, change formula to MCT formula with or without breast feeds
   - **Yes**, change to lactose free formula without breast feeds

2. Is galactosaemia diagnosed?
   - **No**, remain on an MCT formula (some breast feeding can also be reintroduced)
   - **Yes**, change to suitable lactose free formula

3. Is infant breast fed?
   - **No**, use 150-180 mL/kg MCT formula
   - **Yes**, give 100-120 mL/kg MCT formula and the remaining 50-80 mL/kg as breast milk. Feeding regimens include:
     - giving MCT formula at the beginning of feeding then topping up with breast feed
     - breast feeding for every 3rd feed
     - breast feeding overnight and MCT formula during the day

4. Is cholestasis is resolving?
   - **No,** remain on above regimen
   - **Yes**, give breast feeds or a suitable infant formula

5. Are blood sugar levels maintained?
   - **No**, consider adding glucose polymer initially up to 3% concentration, minimum 3 hourly feeds day and night, may need 2 hourly or continuous feeding if necessary
   - Beware the addition of energy supplements reduces the ratios of protein and EFA to energy unless adequately supplied from solids
   - **Yes**, continue management

6. Is there faltering growth with an adequate feed volume?
   - **No**, consider NG feeding
   - **Yes**, consider concentrating feeds

7. At weaning
   - encourage normal weaning from around six months
   - encourage rapid progression in food textures if possible
   - add MCT formula when making up dried baby foods instead of water or cow's milk
   - alternatively add household foods (cream, butter, cheese) and/or glucose polymer or fat supplement to increase energy content of puréed home cooked or commercial baby foods

7. Continue to review and monitor

MCT medium chain triglyceride **EFA** essential fatty acids

containing a high percentage of MCT until bile flow and adequate growth resume. Suitable formulas with a high MCT content are given in Table 9.11.

Dietetic management

Depends on corrected age and nutritional needs

Premature neonatal infants who are still inpatients:

  breast milk with added breast milk fortifier can be used up to corrected age for term
  some MCT formula may be required in order to optimise weight gain and growth
  exclusive breast feeding or a preterm or high energy formula

After discharge from hospital:

  jaundice/cholestasis continues – as per Table 9.10
  jaundice cleared – exclusive breast feeding at 180 mL/kg
  faltering growth – use a high energy formula

Galactosaemia

In some countries galactosaemia is tested on the Guthrie card at birth. However, if this is not available the measurement of the infant's blood galactose-1-phosphate uridyl transferase (Gal-1-PUT) level is tested and is the current gold standard (p. 529). However, if the infant has not been fed galactose recently or has received a blood transfusion within 6 weeks of testing a false result can occur, in which case both parents will need to be screened. Common clinical presentations are jaundice, poor feeding, lethargy, hypoglycaemia and *Escherichia coli* sepsis [23].

Dietetic management

While awaiting Gal-1-PUT result to exclude galactosaemia:

  a lactose free formula high in MCT, e.g. Pregestimil Lipil, MCT Pepdite, should be started and breast feeding discontinued (mothers should be encouraged to express their breast milk)

If the test is positive for galactosaemia:

  a soya formula, e.g InfaSoy, Wysoy, should be started; a formula high in MCT is no longer required;
  weaned children will require a lifelong low lactose diet

Table 9.11   Formulas and supplements high in medium chain triglycerides per 100 mL.

	% MCT	Energy kcal (kJ)	CHO g	Protein g	Fat g	Linoleic acid mg	α-linolenic acid mg	EFA ratio	Osmolality mOsm/kg H20	Dilution %
Powdered formulas										
Caprilon (SHS)*	75	66 (275)	7.0	1.5	3.6	5.6	0.8	7.5	233	12.7
Heparon Junior (SHS)	49	86 (360)	11.6	2.9	3.6	8.2	1.2	6.8	310	18.0
Generaid Plus (SHS)	32	102 (425)	13.6	2.4	4.2	3.7	1.0	4	390	22.0
Pregestimil Lipil (Mead Johnson)*	55	68 (285)	6.9	1.89	3.8	10.1	0.6	16.8	330	13.5
Pepti-Junior (Cow & Gate)*	50	66 (275)	6.8	1.8	3.5	12.8	0.2	64	210	12.8
MCT Pepdite (SHS)*	75	68 (285)	8.8	2.0	2.7	5.1	0.8	6.4	290	15.0
Monogen (SHS)*	80	74 (310)	12	2.0	2.1	1	0.2	4.6	280	17.0
Peptamen Junior (Nestle)	60	100 (420)	13.8	3.0	3.85	–	–	–	260	22.0
Emsogen (SHS)**	83	88 (370)	12	2.5	3.3	3.4	0.1	48	580	20.0
Ready to feed formulas										
Peptamen Junior Liquid (Nestle)	60	100 (420)	13.2	3.0	4.0	–	–	–	319	–
Peptamen Junior Advance (Nestle)	61	150 (630)	18	4.5	6.6	–	–	–	380	–
Nutrison MCT (Nutricia)***	61	100 (420)	12.6	5.0	3.3	5.3	0.7	7.6	265	–
Nutrison Peptisorb (Nutricia)***	50	100 (420)	17.6	4.0	1.7	–	–	–	455	–
Paediasure Peptide (Abbott)	50	100 (420)	13.0	3.0	4.0	–	–	–	272	–
Energy modules										
Liquigen (SHS)	98	450 (1880)	0	0	50	0	0	0	10	–
MCT oil (SHS)	99	855 (3575)	0	0	95	0	0	0	–	–
Calogen (SHS)	0	450 (1880)	0.1	0	50	24	4.7	5	360	–
Duocal (SHS)	35	123 (515)	18.1	0	5.6	4.4	1.1	4	196	25.0****
Liquid Duocal (SHS)	28	166 (695)	23.7	0	7.9	15.7	0.2	68	400	–
MCT Duocal (SHS)	75	165 (690)	24	0	7.7	6.3	0.9	7	427	33.0****
Liquid Maxijul	0	247 (1030)	61.9	0	0	0	0	0	1400	

*Infant formulas
**Formulas not suitable for children <5years old
***Formulas not suitable for children <7 years old
****Suggested dilution
MCT medium chain triglyceride
EFA essential fatty acids
SHS Scientific Hospital Supplies

Biliary atresia

Biliary atresia (BA) is defined as the complete inability to excrete bile due to obstruction, destruction or absence of the extrahepatic bile ducts which leads to bile stasis in the liver with progressive inflammation and fibrosis.

BA is a rare progressive disease occurring in 1 in 9000–16 000 births [24] but is the most frequent hepatic cause of death and requirement for transplantation [25]. At least 50% of children with this condition are likely to receive liver transplants in the first 2 years of life [26] with a further 20%–30% likely to require a transplant later in life [27]. Up to two-thirds of BA survivors who have not received liver transplantation may develop portal hypertension, but maintain adequate growth [28].

Bile drainage can be restored by the Kasai operation which involves bypassing the blocked ducts. It should be performed as soon as possible after birth. Native liver survival rate and jaundice clearance is reported to be improved when the Kasai procedure is performed earlier than 60 days, with outcomes showing better results the earlier Kasai is performed (i.e. before 30, 45 or 60 days of life) [29]. A late Kasai operation, i.e. after 60 days of age, is associated with poor prognosis [30]. Prior to the use of formulas containing a high proportion of fat

Table 9.12   Summary of dietetic management for symptoms of chronic liver disease.

Fat malabsorption

Bottle or NG feeding

- ○ 100-120 mL/kg MCT formula (30-70% MCT formula) + 30-80 mL/kg EBM or breast feeding to provide LCT
- ○ Ideally 20-50% of remainder of fat intake should be as LCT
- ○ May need to supplement with walnut oil (1-2g per 100 kcal/420 kJ) (p. 601)

Toddlers or children

- ○ Normal solids with MCT formula or oral nutritional supplements

Hypoglycaemia

Optimise feed volume

- ○ 150-180 mL/kg

Give more frequent feeds

- ○ Infants - 3 hourly or 2 hourly breast or bottle feeding
- ○ Children - regular carbohydrate meals and snacks with a low glycaemic index
- ○ In some children >2 years uncooked corn starch (UCCS) may be useful (p. 549)
- ○ Consider NG continuous feeding if necessary

Increase carbohydrate content of feeds using a glucose polymer

- ○ Initially 1-3% concentration, may gradually increase to a maximum of 6% concentration, but monitor protein:energy ratio
- ○ Beware of rebound hypoglycaemia due to large amounts of glucose

NG continuous feeding if necessary
If uncontrolled with continuous feeding use emergency regimen (Table 9.6)

Faltering growth

Ensure adequate intake
Concentrate feeds

- ○ Infants - increase by 2% concentration in a step wise fashion e.g. 15%, then 17%*
- ○ Children - concentrate up to 1.5 kcal (6 kJ)/mL or use a 1.5 kcal (6 kJ/mL) ready to feed formula

Advise protein and energy dense meals/snacks
Ensure an adequate protein:energy ratio, i.e. 2.5g protein/100 kcal (420 kJ) or 10%
Add energy supplement if protein:energy ratio maintained from solids
Use higher protein feed or supplements, or a high BCAA formula, e.g. Heparon Junior, Generaid Plus
Consider NG feeding, overnight feeding if possible
Consider continuous feeds for enhanced absorption

Table 9.12   (*continued*)

Ascites

Change to frequent, smaller, nutrient dense meals and snacks
Consider NG boluses or continuous feeding
Concentrate feed or use a high energy formula if fluid restricted
Limit sodium intake in feeds and avoid salty foods
Older children, use high energy oral nutritional supplements between meals

Portal hypertension and malabsorption

Initiate nutrition support
Consider hydrolysed protein feeds (p. 113)
Consider continuous feeds rather than bolus feeds
Assess the need for pancreatic enzyme replacement therapy (p. 236)
Consider parenteral nutrition preferably in addition to enteral nutrition

Encephalopathy

Initiate emergency regimen if necessary to meet glucose oxidation rate
Initiate NG feeding as soon as possible
Ensure adequate energy intake
Initially aim to provide a minimum protein intake of 1.0 g/kg protein
Maximise protein intake as soon as possible to prevent catabolism
Concentrate feeds and add energy supplements

---

*Most infant formulas can be safely concentrated up to 20%, but will require close monitoring, However, Heparon Junior can be safely concentrated up to 25% (1.2 kcal, 5 kJ/mL)
NG nasogastric **MCT** medium chain triglyceride **EBM** expressed breast milk **LCT** long chain triglyceride **BCAA** branched chain amino acids

as MCT, the majority of children did not survive post Kasai [31].

Despite having the Kasai procedure a large proportion of children will require liver transplantation at some point in the future. In these patients a focus on the nutritional management is extremely important as studies have shown that improvement of nutritional status in the pre transplant period may improve outcomes after transplantation [24, 28]. These patients require close monitoring and are likely to benefit from early aggressive nutrition support to maximise growth and nutrition status in preparation for liver transplant.

Dietetic management

As shown in Tables 9.10, 9.11 and 9.12
If there is faltering growth increase concentration of MCT
    formula further*

4–6 months after Kasai:

wean onto solids as per standard weaning guidelines
if remains jaundiced or bilirubin remains high continue
    MCT formula
if jaundice cleared and bilirubin near or within normal
    range change to standard infant formula
if jaundice cleared and bilirubin near normal but faltering
    growth change to high energy formula

* Infants on a standard concentration MCT formula are not
    likely to grow adequately. The concentration of the MCT
    formula can be increased initially by approximately 2%
    and then an additional 2%–3% if required [32]

α_1-antitrypsin deficiency

The exact physiological role of α_1-antitrypsin
remains unknown. The liver disease is thought to
be secondary to the uninhibited action of proteases,
which are critical in the inflammatory response
(although the explanation is unlikely to be as simple as this). The severity of this condition, degree
of liver involvement and nutritional management
vary significantly. The genetic deficiency of the
glycoprotein α_1-antitrypsin can cause varying
degrees of liver disease in infancy and can present
with cholestasis. In a landmark prospective study
33 127 of 200 000 screened newborn infants (1 in
1575) exhibited α_1-antitrypsin deficiency. Within
this group, 11% had severe liver disease and 4%
had mild liver disease.

Dietetic management

Some children require no nutritional intervention and are
    clinically well
Severely affected children (who may come to transplanta-
    tion before the age of 1 year):

    see Table 9.12 for summary of dietetic management of
        chronic liver disease

Alagille's syndrome

This syndrome is a genetic autosomal recessive condition and can present as a spectrum of disorders
including intrahepatic biliary hypoplasia (paucity
of the intrahepatic bile ducts), cardiovascular, skeletal, facial and ocular abnormalities. Some infants
are affected worse than others. It is a rare condition
that is typically diagnosed in 7% of all neonatal
cholestasis cases [34]. Chronic cholestasis predominates clinically [35] although some have cyanotic
heart disease as their main problem. Conjugated
hyperbilirubinaemia presents followed by pruritus
and finally, if severely affected, xanthelasma which
usually appears by 2 years of age. Alagille's syndrome is possibly the most challenging condition
in terms of nutritional management.

Frequent problems include poor growth,
appalling appetite (fussy eating), pancreatic insufficiency and malabsorption, vomiting, severe itching
thought to be exacerbated by improved nutrition,
renal acidosis. Indeed malnutrition and severe
itching may be the main indications for transplantation, provided that the associated heart disease is
not a compounding factor.

Dietetic management

Faltering growth without symptoms of chronic liver disease:

    if poor oral intake persists start nasogastric feeding
    if requires long term enteral nutrition support, and in the
        absence of organomegaly and portal hypertension,
        gastrostomy feeding should be considered
    in children severely affected with xanthelasma there is
        no evidence to restrict saturated fats

Faltering growth with advancing liver disease:

    see Table 9.12 for summary of dietetic management of
        chronic liver disease

Haemangioma

Haemangiomas are benign vascular tumours of
the liver which fall into two categories: those that
undergo spontaneous regression by thrombosis
and scarring; and those that grow rapidly. Initially, spontaneous regression is awaited. If large
in size, the tumours are supplied by wide blood
vessels taking a large proportion of the cardiac
output, resulting in immediate medical treatment
to decrease blood pressure, increase cardiac output
and reduce the risk of fluid overload. In young
infants where cardiac failure develops, hepatic
artery ligation is essential to cut off the blood
supply to the tumour. If surgical intervention is

not curative, or in some cases ligation cannot be performed, the child may require liver transplantation. These cases are dramatic and present with a huge liver, worsening cardiac function and may struggle to meet nutritional requirements.

Dietetic management

Small haemangioma:

nutrition intervention is often not required at all

Large haemangioma:

likely to be placed on fluid restriction

newborn infants who are breast fed will need fortified breast milk (fortifier or infant formula)

if not breast fed use a standard high energy/protein formula

in severe cases continuous nasogastric feeding will be required

---

Inspissated bile syndrome

Inspissated bile syndrome is conjugated jaundice caused by a plug of thick bile blocking the bile duct and hence affecting bile flow. Resolution may occur naturally with time, or with the help of ursodeoxycholic acid (enhancing bile flow), or under percutaneous transhepatic cholangiography (PTC), or in rare cases it requires surgical excision. The syndrome often occurs in infants who have been nil by mouth, e.g. after surgery and long courses of PN.

Dietetic management

Infants with significant conjugated jaundice:

MCT-containing formula may be necessary until PTC

Choledochal cyst

Choledochal cysts are dilatations of all or part of the extrahepatic biliary tract. They may occur in infants (and can be detected *in utero*) and children. They may remain undiagnosed for years. Ursodeoxycholic acid will improve bile flow and may enable a small cyst to disappear requiring no further treatment. However, cysts often require surgical removal. Indeed some are so large and invasive that the extrahepatic bile ducts have to be removed and

a Kasai procedure is performed. Post surgery, any required catch-up growth should occur quickly, negating further nutritional intervention.

Dietetic management

Infants or children with significant conjugated jaundice or fat malabsorption:

MCT-containing formula may be necessary

Those requiring a Kasai procedure:

Infants – see for Kasai procedure (p. 175)

Children – age appropriate diet (sometimes MCT supplementation required)

Cystic fibrosis

Cystic fibrosis (Chapter 11) can present in the newborn as CHB and should be picked up on screening on the Guthrie card.

Dietetic management when presenting with liver complications

Faltering growth:

Most children will tolerate a 1.5 or 2 kcal (6 or 8 kJ)/mL age appropriate formula

If there is malabsorption or portal hypertension a peptide or amino acid feed, e.g. Pepti-Junior for infants, Peptamen Junior or Emsogen for older children, may be beneficial

The feed may be concentrated into small volumes and fed overnight. Hyperosmolar feeds tend to be well tolerated in children with cystic fibrosis

---

Progressive familial intrahepatic cholestasis

PFIC is a group of liver diseases involving membrane transport proteins required for the formation of bile. Growth is a major problem and most children have short stature and reduced muscle and fat mass. Fat malabsorption and diarrhoea remain a significant problem, even after surgical interventions. Cholestyramine has been used to treat the diarrhoea with some success, by binding the bile acids. However, fat and vitamin malabsorption is an associated side effect. There are three types as shown in Table 9.13.

Table 9.13   Types of progressive familial intrahepatic cholestasis.

	PFIC 1 *Familial intrahepatic cholestasis (FIC 1 or Byler's disease)*	PFIC 2 *Bile salt export pump (BSEP) deficiency*	PFIC 3 *Multi drug resistance 3 (MDR3) disease*
Average age of presentation	3 months	early neonatal to 3 months	3 ½ years (range 8 months to 20 years)
Disease progression	progresses quickly to cirrhosis in the first year of life	aggressive course towards end stage liver disease and a higher incidence of hepatocarcinoma	slow progression of cirrhosis and liver disease
Symptoms and management	pruritis is a significant complication that develops usually requires internal ileal exclusion	early neonatal cholestasis pruritis is a significant complication that develops usually treated with external biliary diversion	pruritis not as severe in most cases
Biochemical or functional hallmarks	low levels of GGT a subgroup have pancreatic insufficiency and require pancreatic enzyme replacement	low levels of GGT	elevated GGT normal bilirubin low concentrations of phospholipids in bile
Effect on hepatocyte	affects apical membranes, colon, intestine, pancreas	affects canicular membrane of the hepatocyte	affects canicular membrane of the hepatocyte

PFIC progressive familial intrahepatic cholestasis
GGT γ-glutamyl transpeptidase
Pruritis severe itching due to bile acids near the skin surface

Pruritis is a major symptom, out of proportion to the level of jaundice. Internal ileal exclusion or external biliary diversion surgery may remove 30%–50% of bile to alleviate the itching. Because the severity of the condition is so diverse, surgery may be ineffective and transplantation the last option to improve symptoms. However, in PFIC 1 the defective gene may be expressed in other organs and liver transplantation is questionable. More research is needed in this disease.

Dietetic management

Problems frequently seen in children with PFIC
Fat malabsorption is considerable:

- those with poor bile flow have a greater need for MCT fat
- in some bile flow is high but the bile quality is poor so require MCT formula
- if on medication to bind bile acids MCT fat and fat soluble vitamin supplementation is required

Diarrhoea:

- may benefit from hydrolysed protein formula with high MCT fat

Scratching:

- itching causes general irritation and distraction from eating
- gastrostomy tubes easily become dislodged

Nutrition support:

- gastrostomy tube feeding is commonly used but risk of being dislodged due to scratching
- long term nasogastric support may require gastrostomy insertion
- gastrostomies are more often considered in children with PFIC 1 and 2

Cirrhosis

Cirrhosis represents the end stage of any CLD. The chronic disease may initiate a repetitive sequence of cell injury and repair. The consequence of this is that cyclical necrosis and fibrogenesis can lead to irreversible damage superimposed onto the original disease process [36]. The liver can compensate for the damage such that the cirrhosis is asymptomatic. Decompensated cirrhosis occurs when damage within the liver causes blood flow to be impaired, resulting in symptoms such as portal hypertension, ascites and varices (Table 9.12).

Common chronic liver disease symptoms that can necessitate dietetic intervention

Chronic liver disease often manifests as a range of common symptoms shared by different types of liver disease and can be grouped into the complications below. These symptoms are either the direct result of disordered metabolism or a physiological manifestation of liver disease [37]. Dietetic management is described in Table 9.12.

Fat malabsorption

The absence or shortage of bile results in malabsorption of LCT from the gastrointestinal tract. Infants lose a large proportion of their energy intake through fat malabsoption. If left untreated it can result in faltering growth, fat soluble vitamin deficiency and EFA deficiency. However, to ensure an energy dense diet is given, fat should not be restricted. Many cholestatic infants compensate for the loss of energy through fat malabsorption by consuming high volumes of breast milk or infant formula. Intakes can be more than twice normal fluid requirements. The exclusive use of formulas very high in MCT may increase the risk of EFA deficiency. However, most MCT formulas contain 20%–50% of their total fat content as LCT (Table 9.11). If a child is requires a very low LCT diet (<20% of the total fat) in the long term, e.g. in chylous ascites, then EFA monitoring and supplementation may be required. However, the duration of low LCT diet for chylous ascites is typically 1–2 weeks and EFA deficiency is unlikely for this duration.

Pancreatic enzyme insufficiency

Some types of liver disease, including Alagille's syndrome, progressive intrahepatic cholestasis and choledochal cysts, may be accompanied by pancreatic enzyme deficiency which aggravates malabsorption. Since bile salts are required to activate pancreatic lipase a functional deficiency may be present in cholestasis. The finding of a low stool elastase may support a deficiency. In this case, pancreatic enzymes should be started and continued if a clinical benefit is seen. It is unwise to use doses above 10 000 units lipase/kg/day [38].

Hypoglycaemia

The liver is essential for glucose homeostasis. It stores glycogen and, during fasting, mobilises glucose. Infants and children with liver disease commonly become hypoglycaemic due to impairment of this function. Muscle glycogen homeostasis is also disrupted in liver disease. As with ALF an acute on chronic presentation may require an emergency regimen (see Table 9.6) to control blood sugars while a feeding regimen is established. It may be necessary to provide a continuous overnight feed, or evening doses of uncooked cornstarch (p. 549) to ensure blood glucose is maintained throughout the night. In some infants care is needed not to give too much glucose so as to cause hyperinsulinaemia. Dietetic management is described in Table 9.12.

Faltering growth

In decompensated liver disease faltering growth is very common as a result of increased energy requirements [39, 40]. A diet high in energy and protein is encouraged, but in many infants and children appetite is poor and utilisation of nutrients is compromised [41]. Children with some conditions (e.g. Alagille's syndrome, PFIC 1 and 2, α_1-antitrypsin deficiency) are small for their age and it is a struggle to achieve adequate growth velocity. In the majority appetite is poor, possibly requiring nasogastric (NG) bolus feeding during the day or continuous overnight feeding. Formulas supplemented with the branched chain amino acids (BCAA) leucine, valine and isoleucine have been used with some success with improved nutritional status [42] and reduction in the complications of liver disease [43, 44]. Supplementation with BCAA has been shown to increase protein synthesis and nitrogen balance and correct amino acid imbalances [42, 45].

The possible reasons for the beneficial effects of BCAA are as follows.

- They may help to promote protein synthesis. Unlike other amino acids they are metabolised in the muscle and therefore are available for protein synthesis even when there is poor hepatic function.

- They may be used to help meet energy requirements. Leucine, as a ketogenic acid, may be used preferentially as an energy substrate while valine and isoleucine are diverted towards gluconeogenesis [46]. The result is preservation of precious reserves of fat and lean body mass.
- They may promote liver regeneration by activating the synthesis of hepatocyte growth factor [47] and may improve immune function by enhancing the phagocytic function of neutrophils [48].

Dietetic management is described in Table 9.12.

Ascites and hepatomegaly

The most profound effect on nutrition status from ascites and hepatomegaly is the physical impact on loss of appetite and early satiety due to abdominal discomfort and reduced gastric capacity. Ascites is a feature of decompensated liver disease and is managed with sodium and fluid restriction. Diuretics are used in preference to restricting fluids to allow an adequate nutritional intake; however, resistant ascites may warrant a fluid restriction of 60%–80% of normal requirements. In extreme cases it may be that the child self-restricts fluid intake to a greater extent than that imposed. Failure to achieve diuretic management may require therapeutic paracentesis [49], which often results in immediate improvement of appetite secondary to the reduction of intra-abdominal pressure on the stomach. The discouragement of salty foods (p. 248) may help to reduce thirst. A rigid sodium restriction is not recommended, is difficult to impose in children and often results in a corresponding reduction in appetite and energy intake and should therefore be avoided.

Portal hypertension

Cirrhosis can obstruct blood flow to the liver causing portal hypertension and an associated enteropathy and malabsorption. This condition is secondary to increased pressure in the mesenteric venous system, i.e. oedema of the mucosa of the small intestine. The exact degree of portal hypertension and extent of malabsorption remains unknown, and the liver disease itself can contribute to intestinal losses [50]. Oesophageal varices, splenomegaly and thrombocytopenia are clinical and biochemical features of portal hypertension and can accelerate the need for liver transplantation if uncontrolled.

Oesophageal varices

The presence of varices is not normally a contraindication to NG tube feeding, or to continuing oral intake. Occasionally in ESLD, the huge varices that frequently bleed mean that NG tube placement may be contraindicated and PN may be needed. Clear fluids and progression onto a soft diet are introduced 16–24 hours after sclerotherapy/oesophageal banding.

Chronic encephalopathy

Severe prolonged restriction of dietary protein in CLD is no longer an accepted method for treating encephalopathy and can contribute to faltering growth [51]. Almost half of the body's ammonia is endogenously produced by gut flora and is primarily managed with medical interventions (e.g. sodium benzoate may permit tolerance of a higher protein intake). The degree of encephalopathy must be assessed to determine the level of restriction. In the child with ESLD a protein restriction of 1–2 g/kg/day can have deleterious effects on nutritional status and is likely to lead to muscle catabolism and ultimately ammoniogenesis. Sufficient energy from other macronutrients needs to be supplied with close consideration to protein:energy ratio to prevent protein breakdown. In practice protein should contribute between 7.5% and 12% for infants and 5%–15% for older children (p. 000). The use of BCAA has not proven to be efficacious [52].

A case study to show the management of a baby with CLD is given in Table 9.14.

Common presentations of liver disease in older children

- Inherited disorders, e.g. cystic fibrosis, Wilson's disease
- Infections and inflammatory conditions, e.g. sclerosing cholangitis, autoimmune hepatitis

Table 9.14 Case study - chronic liver disease.

Admission: 8 week old female with conjugated hyperbilirubinaemia, dark urine and pale stools. Wt = 3.75 kg (3^(rd) centile)
Presentation history: Excessive bottle feeding on breast milk and standard infant formula = 260 mL/kg/day. Galactosaemia ruled out
Impression: Possible biliary atresia, presented at 40 days old
Dietetic interventions: Changed to high MCT formula + up to $^1/_3$ fluid as breast milk (total intake = 150-180 mL/kg) while awaiting ultrasound scan
Ultrasound results: Biliary atresia confirmed and Kasai operation booked 5 days after admission (grey arrow)

Biochemistry

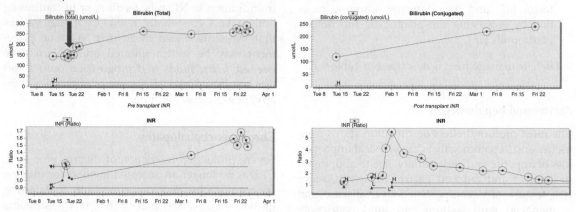

Day 1- 5: Post Kasai procedure, NBM, on IV fluids
Day 5: Commenced on 2 hourly Dioralyte up to 120 mL/kg and then started on 2 hourly feeds of a high MCT formula
Day 6-8: Feed volume gradually increased to 150 mL/kg = 100 kcal (420 kJ)/kg + 2.2 g/kg protein via NG tube or bottle
Day 8-10: Bottle fed 150 mL/kg MCT formula and the remainder (approximately 30 mL/kg) given as breast milk
Day 10: Commenced 15% concentrated MCT formula = 79 kcal (330 kJ)/100 mL. Discharged home with advice to call the liver team weekly to discuss progress and provide a weight

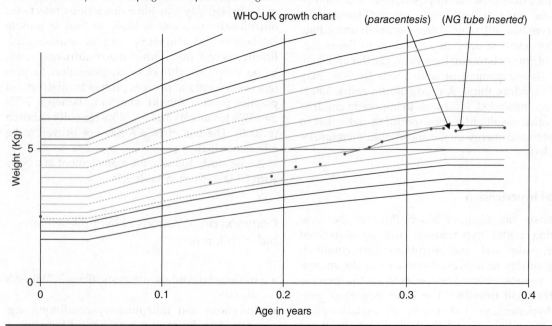

(continued overleaf)

Table 9.14   *(continued)*

Second admission 8 weeks after discharge: Readmitted with increased abdomen size, not clearing jaundice and two week history of feeding on high volumes of up to 200 mL/kg (might have been related to steroid medications). On admission was only taking 100 mL/kg. Further investigations showed ascites and splenomegaly with increasing HARI. No significant oesophageal varices. Required ascites drainage *(paracentesis)*. Weight increased secondary to increasing abdominal girth. Faltering growth indicated by static MUAC.

Day 1: Wt = 5.78 kg (23rd centile) MUAC = 11.0 cm (1st centile). Feeding regimen: 150 mL/kg of 15% concentrated MCT formula via a bottle and breast milk in addition

Day 2-3: Not managing full feed volume so NG tube inserted to provide top up feeds

Day 4-7: Kasai procedure deemed a failure as had worsening liver function (e.g. INR, CHB) and portal hypertension. Liver transplant assessment completed. Was managing 100 mL/kg via bottle but was requiring overnight NG feeding to meet requirements. Formula increased to 17% concentration

Day 8: Wt = 5.8 kg (22nd centile) MUAC = 10.8 cm (0.4th centile). Discharged from hospital on daytime bottle feeding and overnight NG feeding providing 150 mL/kg 17% MCT formula = 133 kcal (555 kJ)/kg + 3.6 g/kg protein. Mum also continued to breast feed occasionally

1 week post discharge: Telephone review Wt = 5.8 kg (15th centile), static growth. Only having 130 mL/kg. Advised to increase to 150 mL/kg.

2 weeks post discharge: Telephone review Wt = 5.8 kg, static, abdominal girth increased by 2 cm, appetite poor due to early satiety. Unable to increase feed volume above 130 mL/kg. Arranged to see at consultant outpatient appointment same week.

Consultant liver clinic: Wt = 5.8 kg (12th centile), MUAC 10.3 cm (0.1st centile). Rapid progression of end stage liver failure. Formula changed to 18% concentration Heparon Junior (low sodium, high MCT, with BCAA). Commenced top up NG feeds during the day in addition to overnight feeds if unable to manage full volume of 150 mL/kg.

1 week follow up at outpatient clinic: Wt = 5.82 kg (10th centile) MUAC = 10.2 cm (0.1st centile). Poor oral feeding tolerance due to organomegaly and ascites. Formula concentration increased to 22.5%, aiming for 150 mL/kg. Recommended to commence on solids.

Received living related liver transplant: 3 months after initial presentation

MCT medium chain triglyceride **INR** international normalised ratio **NBM** nil by mouth **IV** intravenous **NG** nasogastric **HARI** hepatic artery resistance index **MUAC** mid upper arm circumference **CHB** conjugated hyperbilirubinaemia **BCAA** branched chain amino acids

- Biliary malformations such as choledochal cyst
- Toxic disorders, e.g. copper toxicity from Wilson's disease
- Malnutrition, lifestyle disorders, e.g. non-alcoholic fatty liver disease (NAFLD), non-alcoholic steatohepatitis
- Cryptogenic disorders including malnutrition

Autoimmune hepatitis

Children who present with autoimmune hepatitis are typically older and have good nutrition status. Remission is achieved in 80% of children with prednisolone in combination with azathioprine [53] and rarely necessitates dietetic intervention, unless associated with inflammatory bowel disease. Presenting symptoms which may need dietetic input range from faltering growth and malabsorption to obesity aggravated by steroid therapy. Some of

these children will need liver transplantation due to failure to prevent progression to CLD secondary to cirrhosis. Martin *et al.* report the 5 year survival rate to be 86% [54].

Wilson's disease

Wilson's disease is an IMD resulting in defective copper metabolism. It leads to an accumulation of copper in the liver, brain, kidney and cornea. Accumulation can take years and hence presentation is delayed. Oral chelating agents, e.g. penicillamine, bind dietary copper and have negated the need for a strict low copper diet although avoiding foods with a high copper content is sensible. In advanced disease, or acute onset, liver transplant may be the only option due to the poisonous nature of copper.

Dietetic management

If the child is at high risk of non-compliance with chelating medications, dietary copper restriction is recommended

Foods containing high levels of copper:

Offal, particularly liver; animals/fish eaten whole (which contain the liver, e.g. shellfish)

Foods containing moderate levels of copper, but not typically eaten in quantities to warrant a restriction:

Mushrooms
Cocoa, chocolate
Chocolate milk, energy drinks [55]

Cystic fibrosis related liver disease

Liver disease is a known complication of cystic fibrosis although only a small proportion will develop liver failure. Significant portal hypertension and associated malnutrition are a characteristic of severe cystic fibrosis related liver disease (CFRLD). Jaundice is rarely seen. Liver function tests are not reliable markers for disease severity. Assessment and treatment needs to take into account:

- the use of body mass index (BMI) in the nutritional assessment of patients with CF is not useful due to ascites and organomegaly; anthropometry of the upper arm is more reliable
- an increase in malabsorption with progressive liver disease in CF is most likely to be as a result of portal hypertension enteropathy; increases in pancreatic enzyme replacement therapy above 10 000 units lipase/kg are thus unlikely to be helpful
- large volumes of feeds are not tolerated well due to organomegaly and ascites
- restrictions in sodium may not be needed as requirements are greater in CF

Dietetic management

Nutritional failure is common in advanced CFRLD:

provide nutritional support aiming for 150% estimated average requirement for energy for age

oral nutritional supplements and overnight tube feeding is common

overnight nasogastric feeding can improve nutritional status prior to transplantation

---

Liver tumours

Tumours rapidly infiltrate the liver whether benign or malignant. Medical management includes the use of steroids and chemotherapy to reduce the tumour size. Resection may then be possible allowing the liver to regenerate; otherwise transplant may be the only option and is regarded as a successful treatment in those without extrahepatic disease [56]. Nutritional support and monitoring is required throughout the course of treatment.

Bone marrow transplantation – immune deficiency disorders

Immune deficiency causing liver destruction has led to a need for bone marrow transplantation followed by liver transplantation, in some cases. The main nutritional complications include severe vomiting and diarrhoea, requiring nutritional support in the form of enteral nutrition and PN throughout the critical course of treatment.

Additional factors to consider when assessing a child with liver disease are given in Table 9.15.

Non-alcoholic fatty liver disease and non-alcoholic steatohepatitis

Non-alcoholic fatty liver disease (NAFLD) is reported to be the most common cause of liver disease in children. It encompasses a range of aetiologies from mild fatty infiltration of the liver and mild inflammation, advancing to hepatocellular fibrosis with portal inflammation, i.e. non-alcoholic steatohepatitis, which leads to cirrhosis and eventually end stage liver failure [57]. It can present in children as young as 2 years of age, but is typically diagnosed around age 12 years in children who are obese and are ≥95th centile for BMI for age and sex. It is 40% more common in obese boys.

NAFLD can arise from a host of conditions ranging from systemic, genetic-metabolic or rare hereditary genetic disorders, to hepatotoxic drugs [58]. It is overtly linked as a manifestation of obesity and its associated metabolic syndrome effects of insulin resistance, dyslipidaemia (particularly raised serum triglycerides), altered adipocytokines and increasing visceral fatness [59–61]. An increasing central adiposity measured by waist circumference in already obese children has been

Table 9.15   Additional factors to consider when assessing a child with chronic liver disease.

Organomegaly and the hepatic artery resistance index (HARI) can be assessed on ultrasound scan
An increase in liver size suggests worsening disease
An increase in spleen size can indicate worsening portal hypertension
A HARI of 0.8-1.0 indicates sufficiently reduced arterial blood flow through the liver, contributing to worsening hypotension
A repeated HARI >1 denotes reverse blood flow through the artery and indicates severe damage, potentially warranting transplant

INR
A measure of prothrombin time or blood clotting can suggest poor synthetic liver function
If the INR is repeatedly >2 it can indicate transplantation is imminent

Repeatedly low albumin
Low levels denote worsening liver function in chronic liver disease

Worsening LFT
Indicate declining synthetic function of the liver, particularly a declining AST with elevated INR/APPT

Ongoing jaundice
Pale stools with dark urine suggest a high level of CHB
Significant cholestatic liver disease will usually result in cirrhosis
Cirrhosis may still occur in the absence or improvement of jaundice as hepatocyte damage can continue

Fat malabsorption
Pale stools indicate fat malabsorption due to lack of pigment from bilirubin
High volume and regular intake with faltering growth supports energy loss from fat malabsorption
Can still occur in some conditions, e.g. PFIC, where the bilirubin level is not significantly elevated and is due to the inability to produce bile salts, hence an inability to emulsify and digest fat, but without the presence of significant jaundice. In these cases the diagnosis is an important consideration alongside the symptoms

All the above parameters can be temporarily worse in acute on chronic disease or infection

INR international normalised ratio **LFT** liver function tests **AST** Aspartate transaminase **APPT** activated partial thromboplastin time **CHB** conjugated hyperbilirubinaemia **PFIC** progressive familial intrahepatic cholestasis

shown to predict an odds ratio of 1.4 for diagnosing liver steatosis [62].

Children with NAFLD are reported to have higher levels of depression compared with obese controls [63]. They have been shown to consume a higher proportion of total fat, higher saturated fat, lower polyunsaturated fats, lower carbohydrates and lower fibre and antioxidants compared with controls [64,65]. Treatment aims are to correct metabolic disturbances by reversing insulin resistance, reduce visceral fatness, and reduce oxidative stress and inflammation [66]. The Cochrane Collaboration review, 2011 [67], concludes that there are some beneficial effects for patients with NAFLD from weight reduction via diet and exercise, but evidence is sparse and requires well controlled randomised trials. One study investigating a 10 week structured lifestyle programme which restricted energy intake and involved daily exercise showed a reduction in liver fatness and improved insulin resistance [68]. These improvements were maintained for a quarter of participants at 1 year follow-up. Participants who reverted to their pre intervention BMI were again at a high risk of morbidity from NAFLD. Evidence for other treatment options including metformin, vitamin E and anti-inflammatory fats [69] or orlistat [67] have thus far produced equivocal results.

Dietetic management

Reverse metabolic syndrome:
    energy restricted diet
    incorporate regular physical activity
It may also be beneficial to:
    increase ω3 polyunsaturated fats and decrease saturated
        fat intake
    include foods rich in antioxidants

Nutrition support in liver disease

Enteral nutrition

Nasogastric tube feeding

NG feeding improves body composition in paediatric liver disease [70]. Fine bore polyurethane/silicone tubes are well tolerated and associated with low risk of variceal haemorrhage [71]. Feeds may be administered as boluses, top-up feeds, continuous feeding or overnight feeding via a pump (Table 9.16). Overnight feeds are particularly useful in addition to the usual daytime eating and allow the child freedom to choose foods without the pressure of having to meet full requirements from food during the day. In some areas in the UK overnight continuous NG feeding in the home is not supported by community teams, making it difficult to achieve adequate energy intake.

Gastrostomy feeding

The placement of gastrostomies is contraindicated in liver disease if the child has ascites, significant organomegaly or portal hypotension. It may also create potential problems with access to the abdominal cavity (due to adhesions) during liver transplantation. Variceal formation at the gastrostomy stoma site also poses a risk. The enlarged liver/spleen is at greater risk of being punctured if undergoing endoscopic placement for gastrostomy. However, gastrostomies have been successfully placed in exceptional circumstances (Alagille's syndrome, IMD or cystic fibrosis) when portal hypertension is not advanced [72].

Modular feeds

In circumstances where commercial formulas cannot meet the specific demands of nutrition therapy, modular feed can be used. Oral feeding with a modular feed is challenging due to poor palatability, but can work well for patients receiving NG feeding. Some specialist centres offer modular feeds that are designed to specifically allow flexibility in energy and protein content, MCT:LCT ratio, electrolyte concentration and fluid volume. Vitamin and mineral supplementation is necessary. If concentrated slowly a modular feed can be given at a density of 2 kcal (8 kJ)/L if nutritional requirements are high or fluid tolerance is low. An example of a suitable modular feed is given in Table 9.17. Care is needed when teaching parents to prepare feeds at home, particularly when more than two ingredients are used. Parents need to ensure that they have an adequate supply of each ingredient and the correct equipment to prepare the modular feed.

Parenteral nutrition

PN can be safely used in children with CLD. However, all attempts to provide full enteral nutrition must be made. Depending on treatment goals, commencement of PN can be used in children with advanced ESLD who are listed to receive a liver transplant in the near future (e.g. living related liver transplant). In these children the risk of PN exacerbating liver disease is outweighed by improvement of nutritional status prior to, and after, liver transplantation [27]. The nutrition support team plays an important role in optimising PN and promoting enteral nutrition support at the earliest possible indication [73].

Depending on the institution's PN policy, children with liver disease <10 years of age or weighing <30 kg will require bespoke PN prescriptions. At the author's institution all children weighing <20 kg receive individualised PN prescriptions.

Table 9.16 Factors to consider when deciding on mode of nasogastric feeding.

Indication for nasogastric feeding
Continuous feeding
• Malabsorption, e.g portal hypertension, organomegaly, PFIC, Alagille's syndrome
• Hypoglycaemia, e.g glycogen storage disease, ALF, hyperinsulinaemia, end stage CLD
• Poor day time oral intake, e.g. anorexia or early satiety due to organomegaly/ascites
Bolus feeding
• Infants - not able to commence breast feeding or bottle feeding
• Children - oral aversion, increased energy demands beyond a regular oral intake
• When continuous overnight feeding is not an option

PFIC progressive familial intrahepatic cholestasis **ALF** acute liver failure **CLD** chronic liver disease

Table 9.17 Example of a modular feed for liver disease.

		Energy		Protein	Fat	%	CHO	Sodium	Potassium	Calcium
		(kcal)	(kJ)	(g)	(g)	MCT	(g)	(mmol)	(mmol)	(mmol)
25 g	Vitapro (Vitaflo)	95	390	19	1.5		1.9	2.5	4.5	2.5
125 g	Maxijul (SHS)	475	2019				119	1.1	0.2	
25 mL	Calogen (SHS)	113	463		12.5			0.1		
40 mL	Liquigen (SHS)	180	740		20	97		0.5		
14 g	Paediatric Seravit (SHS)	42	179				10.5	0.1		9.0
0.8 mL	30% Sodium chloride (50 mmol in 10 mL)							4.0		
5 mL	Potassium chloride (20 mmol in 10 mL)								10.0	
Sterile water up to a total of 900 mL										
Total		**905**	**3791**	**19**	**34**		**131.4**	**8.3**	**14.7**	**11.5**
Per 100 mL		**101**	**421**	**2.1**	**3.8**	**59**	**14.6**	**0.9**	**1.6**	**1.3**

Premixed PN solutions pose challenges in meeting electrolyte requirements (particularly calcium, magnesium and phosphate) and risk affecting the stability of the fat emulsion. Careful consideration not to exceed macronutrient requirements in children with liver disease is needed to prevent unnecessary hepatic damage. A reduction or elimination of some or all trace elements may be indicated, particularly manganese, as it is toxic to hepatocytes and may accumulate in the brain. However, most modern PN preparations no longer contain high levels of trace elements such as manganese.

Parenteral nutrition associated liver disease and cholestasis

Cholestasis with increasing serum bilirubin levels and raised serum liver enzymes are the hallmarks of parenteral nutrition associated liver disease (PNALD) in neonatal and term infants [74]. The exact pathogenesis of PNALD remains unknown, but the aetiology is multifactorial [75]. PNALD is most pronounced in premature infants and children with short bowel syndrome [76], neonates who are small for gestational age with cholestasis, or those who have gastrointestinal surgery within the first 14 days of life [77] (pp. 88, 159). Prolonged periods of nil by mouth and starvation contribute significantly to PNALD due to decreased bile flow, decreased gastric secretions and poor gastric motility. In children with non-adapted gut or irreversible intestinal disease the presence of PNALD

will accelerate the need for liver and possibly small bowel transplantation [78].

Historically, PN lipid emulsions were predominantly soy or safflower based (high in ω6 content and low levels of vitamin E) which were given in higher quantities (3–4 g/kg lipid or >30% of total energy intake). These lipid solutions are regarded as pro-inflammatory and have been shown to contribute to PNALD in children [79] (p. 51). Modern lipid solutions containing ω3 lipids have emerged in recent years reducing the incidence of PN cholestasis. These are either 100% fish oil ω3 (e.g. Omegaven) given as part of the lipid formulation or are part of a complete lipid formulation of 30% soybean oil, 30% MCT, 25% olive oil and 15% fish oil (e.g. SMOF lipid). These formulations have been shown to reduce PN related cholestasis in children [79–82]. It has become routine practice at the author's institution to use ω3-containing lipid solutions in all paediatric liver disease patients.

Liver transplantation

Liver transplantation in children is technically more challenging than in adults. In children under 2 years of age the donor liver is usually split or cut down to size, using part of the left lobe. The United Network for Organ Sharing (UNOS) [83] database investigating 5 year survival rates in 570 liver transplant recipients weighing <5 kg at time of transplantation demonstrated higher mortality and graft loss compared with children weighing >5 kg.

However, increased use of living related donors, improved skill of the surgeon, improvements in intensive care and refined immunosuppression methods have improved survivor and graft loss rates in children under 2 years of age to 76% and 63% respectively.

Liver transplantation can be a cure for many metabolic diseases, e.g. Crigler Najjar syndrome type 1, carbomyl phosphate synthase deficiency and ornithine transcarbamylase deficiency. It has also been used in other conditions, e.g. propionic acidaemia and methylmalonic acidaemia, where there is also extrahepatic enzyme expression and hence liver transplantation is not completely curative. In these situations the timing and type of transplant are important considerations. The long term prognosis for many of these children is not known [84], however, and liver transplantation should be evaluated on an individual basis. The long term outcomes from paediatric liver transplantation are much improved over the past 10 years. Patient and graft survival rates in patients with hereditary tyrosinaemia type 1 are similar to other non-metabolic survival figures [85].

In conditions where there is a pre-existing dietary protein restriction, nutritional management usually requires PN immediately after surgery. This is to maintain adequate carbohydrate, lipid and protein supply to avoid catabolism postoperatively. The aim, while establishing the success of the grafted liver, is to gradually build up protein intake to ensure production of toxic metabolites (e.g. ammonia, organic acids) is kept to a minimum. In many cases 1–1.5 g/kg/day protein within the first 48–72 hours after transplant is well tolerated depending on the underlying condition.

Enteral feeding with a standard formula is commenced and titrated against PN. Protein restriction is no longer required in urea cycle defects; however, it may be necessary in those where the defect is not completely corrected. Patients are often reported to continue to self-restrict protein intake following transplantation [86]. Due to the vast heterogeneity of this group it is difficult to provide specific dietary guidelines and patients will need to be treated on an individual basis. In some cases lean body mass:fat mass ratio due to lifelong protein restriction is very low, posing increased postoperative risk, e.g. poor gastrointestinal wall integrity, increased risk of perforation or poor glycaemic control secondary to high level of visceral fatness. Predicting energy requirements in these patients is very challenging and they are often lower than the normal estimated average requirement for age.

Nutritional support pre liver transplantation

As decompensation occurs, appropriate growth and nutrition status become increasingly difficult to maintain in the child with CLD. A decline in nutritional status despite maximal nutritional support often highlights the need for transplantation. Malnutrition adversely affects the outcome of liver transplantation [87] and improving nutritional status prior to transplant can help to reduce complications [88]. Once the child is considered for listing for transplant a detailed nutritional assessment is necessary. Waiting time on the transplant list is unpredictable and depends on the potential recipient's severity of disease, disease type and blood type [89]. The advancement of living related liver transplantation can reduce time on the waiting list with earlier transplantation and improved outcomes due to more aggressive pre transplantation nutrition support and reduced rates of rejection.

Nutritional support post liver transplantation

It is estimated that 80%–90% of liver transplanted children who have had a new Roux loop formation will tolerate enteral feeding within 24 hours of transplantation, but that 10%–20% will be at increased risk of severe postoperative gastrointestinal complications. For this reason these patients at the author's institution remain nil by mouth (NBM) for five days before commencing trophic feeding. Older children may receive a liver that has an intact bile duct which can be surgically joined to their native bile duct, avoiding the need for an extended NBM period. Once enteral nutrition can be started an age appropriate standard or energy dense formula is introduced gradually over a 24–48 hour period. In some older children full nutritional requirements can be achieved orally without tube feeding after transplantation. Transplanted children who have had gastrointestinal complications during transplantation (e.g. perforation of the bowel) are likely to be NBM for >5 days and should be considered for PN.

The clearing of long standing jaundice, reduction in abdominal pressure and the introduction of high dose steroids (as antirejection treatment) can play an important role in promoting good appetite. In infants, taste acceptance can improve dramatically post transplantation, possibly due to the use of more palatable formulas and an increased willingness to eat. In older infants and children, where an oral intake was established prior to transplant, a normal diet for age is expected within 6 months post liver transplant [90], but is often sooner. It can be surprising how many children begin to eat well, including those previously reliant on tube feeding. The difficulty for some children is that taste can be adversely altered by medications (e.g. tacrolimus), and can delay acceptance of food. In this group NG tube feeding is extremely common, particularly in infants with pre-established oral aversion, and may be needed for an extended period after transplantation. During periods of sepsis or rejection bile flow may temporarily become limited, necessitating a return to an MCT formula.

Monitoring and follow up

Infants and younger children who are not fully weaned onto solids or who had significant nutrition support prior to transplantation are at higher risk of oral aversion and may require referral to a specialist feeding clinic. If eating well prior to discharge, normal eating patterns should be restored within 6 months and dietetic management is often shared between the specialist liver dietitian in an outpatient setting and the local or community dietitian. Depending on post-transplant recovery, fortnightly or monthly weights should be taken and any concerns discussed with specialist liver dietitians. Older children usually pose fewer challenges where there has been a previously established oral intake. However, pre-transplant obesity (BMI >95th centile for age and sex) has been associated with post-transplant obesity [91]. Obese patients were 10 times as likely, and severely obese were 14 times as likely, to be obese 1 year after transplantation compared with healthy weight individuals pre transplant. Steroids may play a significant role in promoting obesity but evidence suggests that obesity in children at the time of liver transplant has an associated decreased survival risk [92].

Complications after liver transplant

Chylous ascites

Chylous ascites may develop as a result of damage to lymph vessels during transplant surgery, due to retroperitoneal dissection of the lymph glands. The leaking chyle has a milky appearance in the abdominal drain fluids and can resolve spontaneously. A low LCT diet (ideally <20% total fat as LCT) will be required for 1–2 weeks (p. 298). Formulas with LCT content <20% total fat can also be used (Table 9.11). After this time a normal diet or standard formula is restarted if no chyle is seen (where an abdominal drain is *in situ*) or triglyceride levels are normal.

Immunosuppression

The commonly used antirejection medication tacrolimus (and to a lesser extent cyclosporin) can present nutritional challenges. Tacrolimus is preferentially used but can be nephrotoxic or contraindicated by cardiac complications. The pharmacokinetics of tacrolimus are affected by the presence of food in the gut; therefore consistency with giving medication and ensuring that the same sequence of timing of meals and taking the medication at the same time of day is needed.

Both cyclosporin and tacrolimus lower serum magnesium levels. Magnesium needs to be monitored and supplementation may be required (as much as 0.5–1.0 mmol/kg/day orally). Once serum tacrolimus levels are consistently within the therapeutic range the need for magnesium supplementation generally resolves at around 6 weeks post transplantation. Magnesium supplements are typically not well tolerated initially, causing diarrhoea; protein bound magnesium is better tolerated. Grapefruit (including juice), pomegranate and blood oranges need to be avoided as they may induce toxicity.

Safe food handling is necessary (p. 30) and must be practised lifelong due to immunosuppression.

Infection

Infection is the most common cause of post transplantation mortality and morbidity. Intestinal perforation is a post transplantation risk, requiring complete gut rest, and PN may be needed. Infection rates are higher in recipients with low weight (<5 kg) and less than 1 year of age [83].

Epstein–Barr virus (EBV), cytomegalovirus (CMV) and herpes simplex virus are the primary viral infections that may lead to delayed enteral nutrition support. A majority of paediatric liver recipients are seronegative to EBV and CMV and often receive a liver from donors who are seropositive for these viruses. Gastrointestinal perforation and bleeding are severe consequences of EBV and CMV infection. Depending on the virus, medical management is successful in the majority of cases. However, if unsuccessful, and in the case of EBV infection, post-transplant lymphoproliferative disorder (PTLD) can result. Treatment for advanced PTLD includes chemotherapy and radiotherapy, further exacerbating poor nutritional status, delaying growth and significantly increasing mortality risk.

Rejection

At the author's institution acute rejection occurs in approximately 50% of transplant recipients and is treated with a short course of high dose steroids. If the child has commenced oral nutrition prior to steroid treatment, appetite can be enhanced as a positive side effect of steroids. Chronic rejection occurs in smaller numbers (5%–10%) and is often treated with adjustments to immunosuppression, but if unsuccessful retransplantation is a possibility. Progressive cholestasis may require MCT supplementation to displace LCT fat intake prior to retransplantation.

Donor size mismatching

The nutritional management of small sized recipients can be a challenge in the immediate period post transplantation. The sheer bulk of a large piece of liver can occupy much of the intra-abdominal cavity which can delay abdominal closure. The associated risks of an open abdomen, such as slower weaning off ventilation, an increased risk of gut ischaemia, portal hypertension and friable gut integrity, can all delay transition onto enteral feeding.

These children are at higher risk of being NBM for more than 5 days, increasing the risk of gut bacterial translocation, decreased bile flow and subsequent compromised graft hepatic function. Without tolerance to trophic feeding the risk of gastrointestinal perforation is high, necessitating close monitoring for abdominal sepsis. Trophic feeding should be initiated and if PN is indicated careful management is required in this group to avoid PNALD (p. 51).

Transition to adult care

The process for transition to an adult liver service commences at pre transition clinic between the ages of 12 and 16 years, before attending transition clinic from 16 to 18 years of age. Many paediatric liver transplant children have concerns about leaving their paediatric service with the perception that the adult service is less caring and will provide a lower quality of service [93]. The result is decreased adherence after transfer to adult services [94].

The challenges young people and their families face will differ depending on a number of factors, e.g. chronic versus acute diseases. Young people will have had a huge variety of experiences by the time they reach 18 years. Some will have been unwell from birth and then well since transplantation. Others may have presented in later childhood, received a chronic course of medical treatment and then had a transplant in adolescence. Non-adherence to medications and appointments post-transplant is more prevalent in adolescents than young children; it has been reported to be >50% in adolescents [95]. This should be considered when setting nutritional goals.

Adolescents are reported to feel vulnerable around their peers at a time when they are looking for acceptance. They find it difficult to plan due to the unpredictable time of adolescent life and may not have a clear view of the future [96]. These factors impact on how they feel about their future appointments and their perceived severity of illness.

To manage these challenges a clear pathway from paediatric through to adult services is recommended and should be structured around chronological age with built-in flexibility. Early preparation and a proactive approach to transitioning are essential. Patient education needs to be consistent and ongoing and the communication between staff of both paediatric and adult services needs to be seamless [97]. Institutions should provide a pre-transition clinic which takes place in the adult service [98–100].

The Pancreas

Introduction

The pancreas is involved in three primary functions associated with digestion and regulation of macronutrients: production of bicarbonate fluid to neutralise gastric acid in the duodenum; synthesis and secretion of digestive enzymes; and production of hormones to regulate nutrient use and storage. Pancreatitis is the result of inflammation within the parenchyma of the pancreas. Acute pancreatitis can be regarded as an event that can fully resolve, whereas chronic pancreatitis is the result of irreversible damage to the anatomy and function of the pancreas. The incidence of pancreatitis in children is reported to have increased in recent years and is attributed to key factors such as changes in trends in pancreatic aetiologies; increased referral to specialist centres; and improved methods for diagnosis [101]. Diagnostic criteria have been reclassified ensuring that pancreatitis is more accurately defined [102] as shown in Table 9.18.

A retrospective review investigating what we have learned about acute pancreatitis in children [103] showed that aetiologies of pancreatitis differ not only between paediatric and adult populations but also in subcategories within the paediatric population, i.e. age bands of 0–2 years, 3–10 years and 11–20 years (in the UK a diagnosis must be made by the age of 16 years). In this review biliary (i.e. gallstones, sludge), drugs and idiopathic aetiologies are listed as the main causes for acute pancreatitis across all age groups. Inherited metabolic disorders feature in the 0–2 year age group only. Significant differences in acute pancreatitis symptoms according to age bands are seen in the 0–2 year age group, i.e. a lower incidence of abdominal pain, epigastric pain and nausea/vomiting. Children <2 years of age also have an increased length of hospital stay, higher number of referrals to a specialist gastroenterologist and are managed with enteral or parenteral nutrition in higher proportions than children >2 years. Chronic pancreatitis is more prominent in older children.

Table 9.18 Diagnostic criteria for pancreatitis.

Type of pancreatitis	Diagnostic criteria
Acute	*Requires at least 2 of 3 criteria*: • lipase/amylase greater than three times the upper normal limit • epigastric/abdominal pain • imaging, e.g. MRI/ERCP indicating acute pancreatitis
Acute-recurrent	*Requires 2 distinct episodes of acute pancreatitis and*: • complete resolution of pain for more than 1 month between episodes • or complete normalisation of serum amylase/lipase between episodes
Chronic	*Requires at least 1 of 3 criteria*: • abdominal pain • exocrine or endocrine pancreatic insufficiency and suggestive pancreatic imaging findings • surgical or pancreatic biopsy showing histopathalogical features of chronic pancreatitis

MRI magnetic resonance imaging
ERCP endoscopic retrograde cholangiopancreatography

Diagnosis and severity of pancreatitis

Causes for pancreatitis in children differ from those of adults due to lifestyle factors such as alcohol, smoking and chronic obesity, which have not been introduced or had time to manifest in younger children. However, biliary pancreatitis in young children is almost exclusively caused by aetiologies such as biliary sludge, long common channel syndrome, choledochal cysts or autoimmune pancreatitis. However, by the time older children present with biliary pancreatitis obesity has been found to be an independent risk factor for pancreatitis caused by gallstones [104]. Acquired disorders, such as trauma causing injury to the liver and pancreas, are seen in 10%–40% of studies investigating children with acute pancreatitis [101]. Abdominal trauma may be as a result of child abuse, injury from handle bars on bicycles and seat belts in road traffic accidents, or sporting injuries from ball games, contact sports or even horse riding.

Nutritional management

Studies investigating nutrition interventions for pancreatitis have been based on adult populations [105] so extrapolating nutritional recommendations to the paediatric population must be undertaken with caution. The recommendations below serve as a guideline based on adult evidence and current consensus from the author's institution.

Nutrition support should be implemented in any pancreatitis patient regardless of disease severity if anticipated to be NBM for >5–7 days. However, each patient requires individualised assessment, particularly in acute pancreatitis which can present initially with mildly elevated serum markers and low levels of pain, but can worsen rapidly due to surgical interventions or the natural course of the disease. Nutrition support is particularly important in acute pancreatitis caused by trauma. Not only has the pancreas suffered an injury causing inflammation, tearing or splitting, but the duodenum also receives insult causing delays in achieving enteral nutrition support goals. The result can be a loss of lean mass and significant weight loss beyond that already anticipated due to the nature of the catabolic and hypermetabolic state seen in pancreatic injury. In addition the sporadic nature of procedural fasting due to surgical interventions may worsen any energy deficit. Optimal nutrition is essential but cannot fully prevent loss of lean tissue mass in patients who are in near cachectic states. It is important to consider implementing PN early when enteral feeding is unsuccessful. Ideally nutrition support will provide optimal energy and micronutrient intake to reduce the effects of catabolism and will be in place when the anabolic flux returns.

The use of very low fat diets in children with acute or chronic pancreatitis needs further investigation. A reduction in pancreatic enzyme secretion (lipase) is the primary reason for recommending a low fat diet. There is currently no sound evidence

in paediatric patients on the efficacy of very low fat diets or the upper tolerable limit as a treatment for pancreatitis. In patients who have reported abdominal pain, a standard polymeric formula (40% of total energy from fat) fed into the jejunum is usually well tolerated. Low fat diets can increase the likelihood of weight loss as fat is such a significant source of energy. This is particularly problematic in children with chronic pancreatitis who are at risk of faltering growth. A dietary fat intake that is within normal healthy dietary recommendations, and not excessive at any one meal, should be recommended.

Acute pancreatitis

Often children present with abdominal pain that has been persistent for a number of days leading up to admission to hospital. Repeated abdominal pain and or nausea/vomiting upon eating deter the child from eating and create anxiety around food. Parents report that they notice their child withdrawing from mealtimes. The child has typically lost weight upon admission (often up to 10% body weight) and is reluctant to eat.

Short term nutrition management for acute pancreatitis in children is poorly understood and has not been researched. Short term complications of severe acute pancreatitis may result in multi-organ dysfunction (liver, lung, kidney) or shock, and may need to be managed in the high dependency or intensive care unit. Intravenous fluid resuscitation and enteral nutrition, usually via nasojejunal (NJ) tube, within the first 24–48 hours have been recommended in adults with severe pancreatitis [101, 106]. However, a systematic review (one cohort study and three randomised controlled trials) comparing NG with NJ feeding in adults demonstrated that there were no additional disadvantages to using NG feeding in severe acute pancreatitis [107]. Furthermore, exacerbation of abdominal pain occurred in only 4% with 79.3% of patients reaching full gastric feeding tolerance according to visual analogue score and continuation of an oral diet without relapse.

The UK guidelines for management of acute pancreatitis in adults suggest that NG feeding is likely to be tolerated in up to 80% of patients [108]. In mild-moderate pancreatitis NG feeding has been tolerated well when commenced within

Table 9.19   Dietetic management of pancreatitis.

Acute pancreatitis

Early nutrition support is recommended in acute pancreatitis:
 In some patients IV fluids will be started and nutrition support initiated after 48 hours
 Consider starting NG feeding within 24 hours if possible
 Continuous enteral nutrition is preferred over bolus feeding
 If likely to be NBM >5 days commence PN

If serum amylase/lipase increasing or if pain persists or increases:
 Consider NJ feeding
 MCT/peptide based feed may be beneficial if a polymeric feed is not tolerated
 For patients with biliary associated complications consider MCT peptide based feed

If no resolution of pain:
 PN should be initiated
 PN fat emulsions are generally well tolerated if no current or previous history of hyperlipidaemia

Surgical interventions:
 If an ERCP is performed nutrition is likely to be restarted within 24-48 hours
 If more invasive surgery, such as the Puestow procedure (a side-to-side anastomosis of the pancreatic duct to the jejunum),
 the child will require NBM for 5 days

Considerations for younger children:
 Younger children are more likely to rely on enteral nutrition support rather than oral intake
 The threshold to initiate nutrition support due to NBM or prolonged poor oral intake should be much lower than in older
 children

Considerations for older children:
 Oral diet should be first line nutrition unless clinical presentation requires aggressive nutrition support
 Enteral nutrition support is generally not needed unless complications develop and unable to commence an oral diet within
 48-72 hours

Acute-recurrent pancreatitis

For acute presentation - see Acute pancreatitis

Young child:
 If unlikely to commence oral diet within 48-72 hours commence enteral feeding as per acute
 pancreatitis

Older children:
 Aim to resume oral diet within 48-72 hours
 If poor oral intake consider overnight enteral feeding support
 May require oral nutritional supplements to meet energy demands
 To follow a healthy diet and not to consume foods high in fat (NB a low fat diet is not necessary)

Chronic pancreatitis

Inpatient:
 Resume normal oral diet within 72 hours
 If unable to tolerate oral diet see interventions for Acute pancreatitis

Outpatient:
 To follow a healthy diet and not to consume foods high in fat (NB a low fat diet is not necessary)
 If significant weight loss commence high energy diet and dietary supplements if indicated
 If abdominal pain start NG or NJ feeding support
 If pain free for 72 hours restart oral diet and change to continuous overnight tube feeding
 Aim to resume full oral diet while giving overnight tube feeding
 If tolerates oral diet may need to continue high energy diet with low fat food choices

IV intravenous **NG** nasogastric **NBM** nil by mouth **PN** parenteral nutrition **NJ** nasojejunal **MCT** medium chain triglyceride

Table 9.20   Case study - pancreatitis.

Admission: 15 year old male. Wt = 52.3 kg (34th centile) Ht = 160.5 cm (12th centile) BMI = 20.3 (20th centile). Fell off bike onto handlebars which poked into abdomen, vomited once, then vomited upon eating meal at home with significant abdominal pain

Presentation history: Active and physically fit with good nutrition status prior to accident

Impression: CT showed tear in tail of pancreas. MRI showed swelling with fluid around the tail of pancreas. Acute pancreatitis secondary to abdominal trauma

Acute interventions: IV fluids and standard analgesia given at local hospital prior to transfer. Surgeons recommended transfer back to local hospital if amylase fell below 300 IU/L. Or, if amylase and abdominal pain increased then surgeons would perform ERCP

Biochemistry

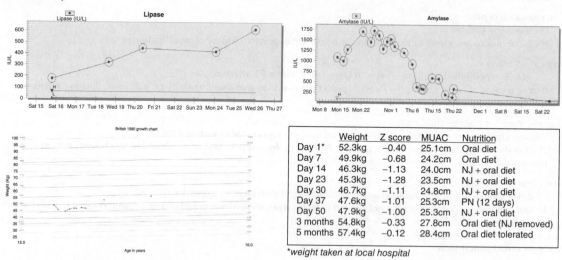

	Weight	Z score	MUAC	Nutrition
Day 1*	52.3kg	−0.40	25.1cm	Oral diet
Day 7	49.9kg	−0.68	24.2cm	Oral diet
Day 14	46.3kg	−1.13	24.0cm	NJ + oral diet
Day 23	45.3kg	−1.28	23.5cm	NJ + oral diet
Day 30	46.7kg	−1.11	24.8cm	NJ + oral diet
Day 37	47.6kg	−1.01	25.3cm	PN (12 days)
Day 50	47.9kg	−1.00	25.3cm	NJ + oral diet
3 months	54.8kg	−0.33	27.8cm	Oral diet (NJ removed)
5 months	57.4kg	−0.12	28.4cm	Oral diet tolerated

weight taken at local hospital

Day 1-2: Low level of abdominal pain and non tender abdomen. A normal healthy diet was recommended with avoidance of high fat options

Day 3-7: Parents wanted to follow a severely restricted fat diet after looking on the internet. Amylase was increasing. Advised to have a normal diet, but with avoidance of very high fat foods.

Day 7-10: Was eating 50-60% of meals, but refusing hospital food. Amylase increasing, no pain reported on standard analgesia. Patient avoiding all foods containing fat and consuming sugar free drinks and low nutrient dense foods. Educated again on sensible food choices including non diet drink options and encouraged parents to bring foods from home

Day 10-14: Abdominal pain absent although amylase was 1400 IU/L. Surgeons recommended discharge due to lack of pain and symptoms and that the patient might eat better at home. Sent home on a trial of 1-2 oral nutritional supplements per day. Follow up appointment with local hospital dietitian arranged

1 week post discharge: Readmitted with severe abdominal pain and weight loss of 1.0 kg since discharge (a total of 13% weight loss in 3 weeks). Patient did not follow a sensible diet and chose meals known to be high in fat. Amylase >1700 IU/L. Team and family decision to commence NJ feeding for 15 hours per day whilst an inpatient and to move to overnight feeding once commenced oral diet.

Day 1: Received pancreatic stenting to tail of pancreas but NJ tube not placed

Day 2: NJ tube booked for insertion

Day 3: NJ feeding tolerated well. Discussed discharge plans with local home enteral tube feeding team. Aim to commence snack foods once tolerating feeding for 48 hours without additional pain or vomiting

Day5-7: Weight gain = 1400 g, MUAC increased 1.3 cm. Started oral diet. Patient admitted having high fat foods (nuggets, chips, pizza and crisps) over the weekend and subsequently had increased pain and vomiting. NJ feeding continued but made NBM until pain resolved. Feeds increased to 1600 mL/day = 2400 kcal (10MJ) + 96 g protein/day

(continued overleaf)

Table 9.20   *(continued)*

Day 7-10: Restarted low fat diet and NJ feeding continued
Day 10-14: NJ feeding reduced to 1000 mL overnight on day 12. Was making sensible food choices from the menu
Day 15: Weight increased by 900g since admission, MUAC increased by 7mm. Vomiting and increased pain. Pancreatic collection increased from 7 mL to 21 mL. Pancreatic stent remained *in situ*. NJ feeding stopped and PN commenced using a standard premix PN solution providing 2000 mL, 2320 kcal (9.7MJ), 81g protein/day
Day 22: NJ feeding restarted at 5 mL/hr with a plan of increasing by 10 mL/hr depending on pain. Target rate = 67 mL/hr using 1.5 kcal (6 kJ)/mL polymeric feed = 1600 mL = 2400 kcal (10MJ) + 96g protein/day. PN was titrated once the feed rate was at 15 mL/hour
Day 27: Static weight and MUAC. PN stopped. NJ feeding hours reduced to 16 hours/day to allow time off the feeding pump
Day 28: Reported pain upon increasing feed rate. Feed rate reduced to 20 mL/hr continuous NJ feeding and made NBM. Aim to gradually increase the rate to 67 mL/hr for 24 hours.
Day 30: Handed over to local dietitian in preparation for transfer to local hospital. Feed rate increased to allow for a longer feeding break
Day 33: Discharged on 20 hours feeding @80 mL/hr = 1600 mL = 2400 kcal (10MJ) + 96g protein/day via NJ tube

3 months post injury: Regained weight and increased MUAC on exclusive NJ feeding which provided 1600 mL = 2400 kcal (10MJ) + 96g protein/day. Advised not to start oral diet until review at outpatient clinic, but patient had hunger pains and chose to eat a week before his appointment with no pain or vomiting related to pancreatitis. Good weight gain. Recommended to reduce NJ feeding to 800 mL/day and to follow a sensible diet with the avoidance of foods which were very high in fat. The aim was to eventually remove the NJ tube if continued to eat well with no pain

5 months post injury: Selecting healthy food choices. No pain reported since retried oral diet 2 months previously

BMI body mass index **CT** computed tomography **MRI** magnetic resonance imaging **ERCP** Endoscopic retrograde cholangiopancreatography **NJ** nasogastric **MUAC** mid upper arm circumgerence **NBM** nil by mouth **PN** parenteral nutrition

the first 8 hours after admission and demonstrated improved pain scores, decreased analgesia requirements and reduced time to commence oral diet compared with patients placed on an NBM regimen [109]. However, there is no classification for mild or severe acute pancreatitis in children; caution is warranted when attempting to decide on the severity of acute pancreatitis in children as the condition can change so rapidly. Careful assessment of the individual presentation is necessary when following the dietetic recommendations below.

Standard polymeric feeds are usually well tolerated unless the pancreatitis has a biliary cause, in which case a feed high in MCT can be used. The theory of pancreatic rest is historical and shown by four recent randomised controlled trials [110–113] to provide no additional benefit, whether using a stimulatory (NG) or non-stimulatory (NBM, PN or NJ) method of feeding. In addition, the risk of gut translocation due to prolonged periods of NBM may exacerbate pancreatic infection risk [114].

Common problems in acute pancreatitis management in children are:

- paediatric patients exhibit a wider variety of aetiologies than adults

- malnutrition occurs more quickly in young children
- young children require earlier implementation of nutrition support compared with older children
- an assessment of nutritional status and growth history is essential
- less severe presentations can rapidly become severe
- each presentation requires individualised nutrition intervention due to heterogeneity of acute pancreatitis

Acute–recurrent pancreatitis

Approximately 15%–35% of children who have acute pancreatitis will develop recurrent pancreatitis, with the number of recurrences ranging from two to three episodes [101]. Recurrent pancreatitis is more commonly seen in older children with biliary abnormalities, metabolic disorders (namely hypertriglyceridaemia), autoimmune and idiopathic and hereditary pancreatitis [115]. There are no significant data in children describing the transition point when recurrent pancreatitis develops into chronic pancreatitis.

Chronic pancreatitis

In children, chronic pancreatitis is most commonly associated with genetic, hereditary or idiopathic conditions. It initially presents as acute pancreatitis manifesting into recurring episodes before progressing to irreversible morphological changes and fibrosis as a result of recurrent or chronic inflammatory processes. A North American study based on a cohort of patients with longstanding pancreatitis found that the average age at initial presentation was 7.2 years, 20% required pain medication and 40% required pancreatic enzyme replacement therapy [116]. They reported a clinically significant

lower quality of life and higher level of fatigue score compared with healthy children.

Common problems in chronic pancreatitis management in children are:

- faltering growth secondary to increased energy expenditure
- malnutrition due to food avoidance, chronic abdominal pain, nausea and vomiting
- patients with biliary involvement may require MCT and additional fat soluble vitamins
- insulin therapy due to pancreatic islet cell destruction to manage diabetes mellitus
- enteric coated pancreatic enzymes may be required

The dietetic management of pancreatitis is summarised in Table 9.19. A case study of an adolescent with pancreatitis is described in Table 9.20.

10

Endocrinology

Alison Johnston and Jacqueline Lowdon

Diabetes Mellitus

Alison Johnston

Introduction

Type 1 diabetes is a disease of insulin deficiency due to autoimmune destruction of the pancreatic islet β cells which make the hormone insulin. It accounts for over 90% of diabetes in the under 25 years age group.

The incidence of type 1 diabetes in children and young people within Europe is increasing significantly. The Scottish incidence of type 1 diabetes by 10 year age bands per 100 000 population during 2007–2010 for children <10 years was 26, and for those aged 10–19 years was 43 [1]. The prevalence of diabetes in children and young people aged 0–17 years in England in 2007 was 207 per 100 000 [2]. It is predicted that between 2005 and 2020 prevalent cases younger than 15 years in Europe will rise by 70% [3].

Other types of diabetes do occur in young people: advances in molecular science mean that monogenetic forms of the condition are being identified; diabetes secondary to pancreatic disease is increasingly recognised (e.g. as in cystic fibrosis); and type 2 and other insulin resistance syndromes are on the increase [4].

Evidence based publications outline nutritional recommendations for people with diabetes; there are many of these including:

- the National Institute of Care Excellence's document *Type 1 Diabetes Diagnosis and Management of Type 1 Diabetes in Children and Young People* [5]
- the Scottish Intercollegiate Guidelines Network, *SIGN 116 Management of Diabetes, A National Clinical Guideline* [6]

Clinical Paediatric Dietetics, Fourth Edition. Edited by Vanessa Shaw.
© 2015 John Wiley & Sons, Ltd. Published 2015 by John Wiley & Sons, Ltd.
Companion Website: www.wiley.com/go/shaw/paediatricdietetics

- the American Diabetes Association Position Statement *Evidence-based nutrition principles and recommendations for the treatment and prevention of diabetes and related complications* [7]
- Diabetes UK's *Evidence-based Nutrition Guidelines for the Prevention and Management of Diabetes* [8]
- more specifically for children, the International Society of Paediatric and Adolescent Diabetes (ISPAD) clinical practice guidelines *Nutritional management in children and adolescents with diabetes* [9] (which have been adopted by Diabetes UK)

There are no recent published dietary guidelines for children and young people with type 1 diabetes in the UK. Extensive literature searches carried out for the compilation of the guidelines highlight that the evidence for specific paediatric diabetes dietary management and education is limited and more scientific research is required. However, there is robust evidence for the nutritional requirements of children. Dietary recommendations for children with diabetes are based on the assumption that they have the same nutritional requirements as those who do not [10], and therefore healthy eating principles apply. There is also no debate about the vital role of nutritional management in diabetes care or that carbohydrate is the main dietetic consideration for glycaemic control. This chapter reflects current recommendations.

It is recommended that children and young people with type 1 diabetes attend a specialist children's clinic and are cared for by an appropriately trained paediatric multidisciplinary diabetes team providing ongoing integrated education and support [11]. This team should include a paediatrician, diabetes nurse specialists and a paediatric dietitian; children and young people should have access to psychological services and social workers in addition to services offered in primary care. The team should work collaboratively with the child and their family to optimise diabetes control, whilst enabling them to manage their diabetes day to day and reduce the risk of complications. To be most successful, dietary guidance and education must be tailored to individual clinical, social, psychological, cultural and economic needs and dietitians should convert the scientific knowledge about food into practical, feasible advice.

The parents of a child who is diagnosed with a chronic disease (including a newly diagnosed diabetic child) are initially shocked and traumatised. Parents can also feel a sense of guilt: they may feel that their child has developed diabetes because they have permitted him or her to eat sweets excessively and should be reassured that this is not the case. Since the cause of diabetes is partly genetic, parents can feel guilty about passing on 'bad genes', a feeling exacerbated if there is a family history.

An effective, family-based dietary education programme which is going to result in the modification of a child's eating habits can only begin properly when parents are allowed to grieve and come to terms with the diagnosis of diabetes in their child. It is vital to develop a rapport with the family so that a high quality of consistent dietetic care can be provided. Frequent and short teaching sessions are preferable, with the entire family if appropriate. Group sessions offering structured education provide an alternative method and further research is required to evaluate the most effective way for healthcare professionals to educate children [5]. Many families have fears about what their child will be allowed to eat and drink which must be allayed. Conducting the teaching sessions in the family's own home has many advantages: less disruption, familiar surroundings, the child's usual food and exercise pattern is maintained, first-hand knowledge of the domestic set-up and the session may become more learner centred. The disadvantages are that these sessions are costly in terms of travelling time and resources. A room organised and furnished as a teaching environment, away from the clinical setting, may prove to be a useful compromise.

The field of paediatric diabetes has changed markedly with the increasing incidence of type 1 and non-type 1, children being diagnosed at a younger age, the advent of analogue insulins, improved technology (such as insulin pumps and continuous glucose monitoring systems (p. 571) and intuitive blood glucose meters) and scrutiny of the effectiveness of methods of diabetes education. There has never been a time when the importance of strict glycaemic control has been so prominent and accentuated with the families. The dietitian has a vital role to play in the interdisciplinary team to optimise glycaemic control and quality of life.

Aims of dietetic management

The aims of dietetic management are the following.

- *To meet the child's nutritional requirements and to inculcate good dietary habits for good health.* Children with diabetes have the same basic nutritional needs as their non-diabetic counterparts. It can be emphasised that the recommended eating plan is 'healthy eating' for the entire family. Eating a balanced breakfast, lunch, dinner and bedtime snack (with sensible mid-morning and mid-afternoon snacks if necessary or desired) will provide a healthy diet and offers a platform for regular blood glucose testing.

- *To contribute towards optimising blood sugar levels and hence HbA1c (glycosylated haemoglobin) results <58 mmol/mol avoiding swings between hyperglycaemia and hypoglycaemia.* Before basal bolus therapy and insulin pumps were the predominant models for insulin therapy, it was vital to distribute carbohydrate through the day to counter the inevitable periods of hyperinsulinaemia. While matching insulin to food is now much better, it remains important to consider how the insulin and food will interact. A preprandial blood glucose of 4–6 mmol/L is ideal; however, a target of obtaining 80% of the blood sugars in the range 4–8 mmol/L is probably more realistic. It is imperative to aim to maintain blood glucose concentrations close to the normal range to decrease the frequency and severity of long term microvascular and cardiovascular complications [12]. Recurrent episodes of hypoglycaemia are undesirable, particularly in young children where the developing brain may be particularly susceptible.

- *To ensure dietary modifications allow normal growth and development.* Dietary energy should be sufficient for growth, allow for variable exercise patterns and should not provoke obesity but maintain a healthy body mass index (BMI). Growth should be plotted at regular intervals using recommended height and weight centile charts. Growth velocity charts and BMI are useful for anticipating the onset of obesity or stunting. Growth can be a useful indicator of diabetes control, as poor physical development may be a consequence of inadequate diabetes management. Obesity is less of a problem in children with diabetes than in adults with diabetes, but if children do gain weight disproportionately to their height, suitable dietetic advice should be given at a very early stage.

- *For the diet to contribute to minimising the development of diabetic complications* such as cardiovascular and microvascular disease.

- *To prevent and treat acute complications of diabetes,* e.g. hypoglycaemia and hyperglycaemia and also to aid the management of diabetes during exercise and periods of illness.

- *To provide a tailor-made eating plan* which takes into consideration the psychological, cultural, social and emotional implications of food.

Dietary recommendations

Energy intake

The recommended distribution of total daily energy intake [13] is outlined in Table 10.1. It should be recognised that in children the energy distribution between carbohydrate, fat and protein will differ depending on age: breast fed infants will obtain approximately 55% energy from fat, 5% from protein and 40% from carbohydrate, whereas a 5-year-old may derive 35% energy from fat, 15% from protein and 50% from carbohydrate. Traditional dietary guidelines have emphasised only the carbohydrate component. Present day practice adopts a more holistic dietary approach. In addition

Table 10.1 Recommended distribution of total daily energy intake.

Nutrient	Distribution
Total carbohydrate	45%–60% of energy intake
Sucrose	Up to 10% of daily energy intake, provided it is eaten in the context of a healthy diet
Total fat	<35% of energy intake
Saturated and transunsaturated fat	<10% of energy intake
n-6 polyunsaturated fat	<10% of energy intake
Cis-mono-unsaturated fat	10%–20% of energy intake
Protein*	10%–15%

*Recommendation from NICE guidelines [5].

the energy content of the diet should be tailored to the individual. This is of major importance in order to minimise the risk of chronic degenerative disease such as obesity and coronary heart disease.

Considerations about energy intake and body weight

The following need to be considered.

- At the time of diagnosis many children have suffered catabolic weight loss resulting in subsequent increased appetite and calorie intake [14]. This settles when their appropriate weight has been restored, usually within 1–4 weeks.
- Regular dietary review should encompass monitoring growth and revising advice to accommodate changes in age and lifestyle, nutritional requirement and insulin therapy. The review should include consistent advice about the prevention and treatment of hypoglycaemia to avoid over-treatment. The insulin regimen should be examined and if necessary adjusted to minimise hypoglycaemia and the need for large calorific snacks.
- Prevention of children and young people becoming overweight and obese is paramount and advice should be given about suitable portion sizes, eating healthy meals regularly, exercise and self-control.
- Withholding food in an effort to control blood glucose or make children eat when they are not hungry should be discouraged [15] as it may have a detrimental effect on growth and development. Furthermore it can make children resent having diabetes and they may perceive food differently because of these practices. Necessary adjustments should be made to insulin doses instead.
- Throughout puberty energy requirements increase significantly as do insulin requirements.
- In childhood the prevalence of obesity is increasing rapidly [16] due to excessive calorie intake and lack of physical activity. In addition for children with diabetes over-insulinisation, snacking and excess energy intake to avoid or treat hypoglycaemia can be contributing factors.
- Motivational interviewing can be used with older children when dealing with weight management.

- Maintaining a static weight in children who are overweight or obese whilst they are still growing taller is a success as they are in effect slimming down. This can be a more realistic and achievable target than actual weight loss. A growth centile chart should be used with the child and their family to show progress.
- Unexpected weight loss must be investigated and can be a sign of coeliac disease, insulin omission or an eating disorder.

Carbohydrate

Children and adolescents with diabetes are recommended to eat the same amount of carbohydrate as children eating a healthy diet who do not have the condition and carbohydrate remains a fundamental factor in optimising diabetes control. The type and amount have an effect on postprandial blood glucose levels.

The total amount of carbohydrate eaten in meals and snacks has a significantly greater effect on glycaemia than the source or type [16]. The recommended total energy intake from carbohydrate is 45%–60%.

Sources of carbohydrate from healthy foods should be encouraged such as wholegrain breads and cereals, peas, beans, lentils, fruit, vegetables and low fat dairy products. The Department of Health (now through the Food Standards Agency) recommends the consumption of five portions of fruit and vegetables per day [17].

Glycaemic index

The glycaemic index (GI) is a measure of the glycaemic response when consuming a particular food. It estimates how much each gram of available carbohydrate in a food consumed will raise the blood glucose level relative to the consumption of glucose or bread. Current validated methods use glucose as the reference food which has a GI of 100. Low GI ($\leq$55) foods will release glucose slowly into the blood stream and will result in a lower postprandial glucose peak. Medium GI foods are classified as those with a GI of 56–69. High GI foods ($\geq$70) cause a rapid rise in the blood glucose and can be useful to treat hypoglycaemia.

A number of factors affect the glycaemic response to food including the composition and amount of carbohydrate, the effect of cooking or processing, the ripeness of fruit and vegetables, physical entrapment of the starch molecules and other meal components such as fat and protein (fat and protein lower GI). The glycaemic response from a food differs from one person to another and in the same individual from day to day and is dependent on blood glucose levels and insulin resistance. The diet for a child with diabetes should not be based solely on the GI ranking of foods. GI can provide a useful guide to the effect a food will have on the glycaemic response but will not necessarily result in a nutritionally balanced diet. It should be borne in mind that the total amount of carbohydrate eaten is more significant, in terms of blood glucose response, than the type of carbohydrate eaten. Some foods considered to be relatively 'unhealthy' such as chocolate cake and ice cream have a low GI and other foods commonly included in a 'healthy diet' such as brown bread, baked potato and rice have a high GI.

Including low GI foods instead of higher GI foods in the diet may reduce postprandial peaks in glucose and HbA1c [18, 19]. Table 10.2 gives ideas of how to increase low GI foods in the diet.

The GI does not take into account the amount of carbohydrate actually consumed. A related measure, the glycaemic load, takes this into consideration by multiplying the glycaemic index of the particular food by the carbohydrate content of the actual serving. However, the practicality of families calculating glycaemic load is questionable.

Sucrose

Avoidance of sugar and sugary foods was the main feature of dietary advice for many decades. More recently it has been shown that sucrose can provide up to 10% of the total daily energy intake without a detrimental effect on blood glucose control and conversely total abstinence of all sucrose containing foods may have a negative psychological impact and is not necessary. Sucrose has a similar glycaemic effect to isocaloric amounts of starch [20]. This information should be used in the context of a healthy diet and sugary drinks should be avoided (unless treating hypoglycaemia) as they may cause hyperglycaemia.

Fibre

Dietary fibre is an integral part of any healthy diet. The UK recommendations for fibre in childhood are imprecise and dated. The UK recommended dietary values for children state that fibre intake should be proportionately lower than that of adults, related to body size and that children <2 years of age should not be given fibre rich foods at the expense of energy rich foods [10]. There is no real evidence to substantiate the concern that a high fibre diet may lead to growth retardation and malabsorption of minerals; a higher fibre diet that reduces energy intake may be beneficial with the increasing incidence of obesity in children [21]. In the USA the recommendation is 2.8–3.4 g fibre/MJ (240 kcal) for children >1 year [22]. Soluble fibre in legumes, vegetables and fruit can aid reduction of lipid levels [23] and fruit pectin may improve protection against cardiovascular disease [24].

Many children eat a low fibre diet prior to diagnosis and gradual changes to increase fibre intake are necessary to minimise colic, flatulence and abdominal distension. Children can easily include a number of high fibre foods in their diet, e.g. wholemeal bread and pasta, high fibre breakfast cereals, baked beans and high fibre baked goods. A significant proportion of children do not achieve the recommended intake of five portions of fruit and vegetables per day but will eat at least one portion of fruit each day; many do not like vegetables, but will take them when included in soups and stews. Often raw vegetables will be taken in preference to those that are cooked. Many children will eat pulses in the form of baked beans, peas, sweetcorn, kidney beans or lentil soup.

Table 10.2 Increasing low glycaemic index foods in the diet.

Basmati rice instead of white or brown rice

Pasta and noodles instead of white rice or mashed potatoes

Sweet potato or new boiled potato instead of baked or mashed potato

Plenty of fruit and vegetables, lentils and beans

Granary or rye bread instead of white or wholemeal bread

Porridge, Special K and muesli instead of cornflakes and rice crispies

Fruit, low fat yoghurt and popcorn for snacks

Fat

Fat is necessary in children's diets to provide adequate energy, fat soluble vitamins and essential fatty acids. The recommended amount of fat is 30%–35% of the total daily energy intake and studies have found that children with diabetes exceed the recommendations [25]. Detailed recommendations regarding the composition of the fat in the diet can be found in the ISPAD guidelines [9] and for many children the emphasis can be simply placed on reducing fat intake in general. The following advice can be given to reduce dietary fat:

- take grilled and oven baked foods in preference to fried foods
- cut off visible fat on meat
- eat fish and poultry instead of red meat
- cut down on the quantity of crisps eaten to 2–3 bags per week (often a compromise of a maximum of one bag per day has to be conceded); use reduced fat crisp varieties
- have reduced fat cheeses or varieties that are lower in fat (cottage cheese is not popular with children, so it is more realistic to limit the amount of high fat cheese and encourage lower fat varieties such as Edam or half fat hard cheese)
- use semi-skimmed milk over 2 years of age and semi-skimmed or skimmed milk in the over 5s, provided appetite is good and an adequate energy intake can be maintained
- choose fruit for snacks instead of biscuits or crisps

It is advisable for children to eat oily fish once or twice per week. Families should be informed of the importance of healthy eating in reducing the risk of cardiovascular disease, including advice about types and amounts of fat in the diet. People with diabetes are prone to dyslipidaemia so attention to dietary fat intake is as important as good metabolic control.

Protein

Children with diabetes should have protein intakes no higher than those taken by other children and should not exceed 15% of energy intake. In the diets of most children, protein provides 15% of dietary energy, although actual requirements are considerably lower than this [10].

Salt

The daily recommended maximum amount of salt children should eat [26] depends on age: 1–3 years, 2 g salt; 4–6 years, 3 g salt; 7–10 years, 5 g salt; 11 years and over, 6 g salt. This should be adhered to in order to reduce the risks of developing hypertension. An excess of salty foods should be avoided and only a little salt added in cooking if necessary. No salt should be added at the table.

Low sugar and diabetic products

Diet and low calorie drinks are valuable in the diet of a child with diabetes. Sugary squashes and fizzy drinks should be avoided completely (except when used to treat hypoglycaemia). Diet drinks sweetened with artificial sweeteners provide an alternative, whilst water is better still. Other low sugar and diet products marketed for the general population can also be useful, for instance reduced sugar jams, fruit canned in natural juice, low sugar desserts. Diabetic products, however, have no place in the diet for the child with diabetes. They are expensive and can be unpalatable and high in fat. In addition they may contain sorbitol or other sugar alcohols that have a laxative effect. The child should be encouraged to regard the diet as one of 'sensible eating' and not one which relies on the need to eat different or 'special' foods.

Sweeteners

Sweeteners are substances used to sweeten food. Sucrose (table sugar) can be eaten in moderation. Fructose has no advantage over sucrose in terms of taste as a sweetener, it contains as many calories and gives less satisfactory results in baking. Although it does not require insulin for its metabolism it has a glucose-sparing effect in the body and causes a rise in blood glucose if large quantities are taken.

Artificial and intense sweeteners

Polyols (sorbitol, xylitol, isomalt, maltitol, mannitol) do not increase blood glucose levels as much as sucrose or fructose. They are often added to foods such as diabetic chocolate and biscuits. Polyols have similar energy (or slightly lower) value to carbohydrate and are nutritive sweeteners. They are poorly absorbed and can cause osmotic diarrhoea, particularly in children, who have a lower body mass than that of the adult for whom the products are designed.

Non-nutritive sweeteners can be useful in drinks and desserts and to sprinkle on breakfast cereals. They are energy free, do not contribute to dental caries, are intensely sweet and do not affect blood glucose levels. In the UK five non-nutritive sweeteners are available: saccharin, aspartame, acesulfame K, cyclamate and sucralose. Many people find that saccharin has a bitter aftertaste. Aspartame, which many find more palatable, has a limited use because sweetening power is lost when it is subjected to prolonged heating. Acesulfame K is heat resistant and without aftertaste. Sucralose is 600 times as sweet as sucrose; it is stable under heat and can be used in cooking and baking and many find the taste palatable. These sweeteners are used in low sugar, diet or 'light' products to improve sweetness and taste.

Education

Dietary education should be a lifelong process commencing at the point of diagnosis. It is important to give the family ongoing practical dietary advice which is age related and the child should be involved, with age appropriate education, at every stage. The information should be delivered at a rate which considers the social, intellectual and cultural background of the child and builds on the family's level of knowledge and understanding, taking into account their literacy and numeracy. Verbal instructions should be reinforced with appropriate written information and other resources should be used where possible, e.g. DVD, websites (see Further reading).

There is a lack of evidence to recommend a qualitative or quantitative approach as the most effective method of dietary education [6]. A qualitative approach teaches healthy eating along with the concept that carbohydrate is the component of food that increases the blood glucose level and the diet plan does not necessitate measuring or estimating carbohydrate amounts. Regular healthy eating and food with low glycaemic index is encouraged, with carbohydrate eaten at each meal and snack.

In practice it is agreed that carbohydrate counting is a necessary skill required to support intensive insulin therapy whether it be basal bolus or pump therapy. Carbohydrate counting can be challenging for those with limited mathematical ability but most families can do so to a greater or lesser extent.

There are two methods of managing the diabetes diet using carbohydrate counting: consistent carbohydrate intake and using insulin to carbohydrate ratios.

Consistent carbohydrate intake

The child or young person is recommended a set amount of carbohydrate to eat distributed at each meal and snack time following dietary review, agreement with the family and bearing in mind the action of insulin and the weight and height of the individual. The carbohydrate is counted using lists of portions of food that contain 10 g of carbohydrate and by calculating the carbohydrate content of food using the nutrition information on the product's label. The daily amount of carbohydrate that an individual has been suggested should be regularly reviewed (ideally 4 monthly but not less than once per year) to ensure that it is apt. The child and their family learn to adjust insulin doses depending on the patterns of blood glucose readings to achieve target blood glucose levels.

Insulin to carbohydrate ratios

Insulin to carbohydrate ratio necessitates a more advanced level of teaching, understanding, monitoring and support to be successful. It involves calculating the ratio of rapid acting insulin to carbohydrate for each meal. The carbohydrate content of the meal is calculated and the appropriate amount of insulin administered. Adjustments can be made to the bolus dose of insulin allowing for exercise about to be undertaken and additional insulin given as a 'correction dose' if the blood glucose is above the target range. This liberates the child or young person from having to have consistent amounts of carbohydrate at each meal. However, reasonable regularity in mealtimes and eating routines are nevertheless important for optimal glycaemic control. The ratios must be calculated for each individual and for each mealtime and are determined by the child's insulin requirement, duration of diabetes, sex, pubertal status and the time of day. The ratios can be calculated by carrying out 'paired readings', which is checking a preprandial blood glucose level and rechecking 90–120 minutes after the meal. If the preprandial and postprandial readings are the same (±2 mmol/L) then the dose of rapid acting insulin matches the amount of carbohydrate eaten.

Checklist

A checklist of dietary teaching that outlines topics to be covered with the family, which are dated and signed off on completion by the person conducting the education session, is worthwhile. This not only aids record keeping but also informs the entire diabetes team about the stage of dietary education a particular family has reached. A checklist for education is given in Table 10.3. An easily accessible, succinct record of any one to one or group teaching sessions that a child or young person and their family attended can be useful.

Table 10.3   Topics for education checklist.

Introduction to diabetes and food

Basic principles of the diet

Food groups and healthy eating

Foods which contain carbohydrate

How to count carbohydrate

How to work out the carbohydrate content of a portion of food using the nutrition information on a label

Signs, symptoms and treatment of hypoglycaemia

Eating out

Exercise

Dealing with diabetes at school

Illness

Using insulin to carbohydrate ratios

Methods and tools

Education is essential to provide knowledge and skills to enable self-management and optimise glycaemic control and cardiovascular outcomes. Ongoing education is vital particularly because as a child grows he/she takes on more responsibility and becomes more independent. Proficiency is required in selecting the correct method and approach because if it is too difficult it may lead to failure or confusion and if too dogmatic it may cause the family to feel guilty and distressed [27, 28].

There is no consensus on the most appropriate methods or tools for education. There is recognition, however, that structured education based on sound educational principles and problem solving plays a key role in effective self-management and children and adolescents should have access to such programmes [6, 11, 29, 30].

Dose Adjustment for Normal Eating [31] (DAFNE) is a comprehensive structured education programme for adults, using basal bolus insulin and insulin to carbohydrate ratios. The principles of this programme have been modified to suit teenagers. Kids in Control of Food [32, 33] (KICk-OFF), based on DAFNE, has been subject to a national clinical trial and audited.

Hypoglycaemia

Hypoglycaemia is the most common acute complication of the treatment of diabetes in children. The recommended lower target for blood glucose levels in children and adults with insulin treated diabetes is 3.9 mmol/L [34] although there is no universally agreed definition. In clinical practice hypoglycaemia in children is generally defined as a blood glucose level <4 mmol/L as it provides families with a figure that is easy to remember; action should be taken in the interest of avoiding moderate or severe hypoglycaemia.

Causes of hypoglycaemia include:

- insufficient carbohydrate eaten, or being late for or missing a meal or snack. If on a basal bolus insulin regimen or an insulin pump the cause can be overestimation of carbohydrate intake or incorrect insulin to carbohydrate ratios

- exercise, without additional carbohydrate or reduction in insulin dose
- too much insulin or dose given at the wrong time
- food not absorbed, e.g. vomiting and diarrhoea
- alcohol

Whatever the exact reason, hypoglycaemia in diabetes is always about relative hyperinsulinaemia (relative to the insulin level in the non-diabetic state).

The symptoms and signs of autonomic (andrenergic) activation (e.g. shaking, pounding heart, pallor, cold sweatiness) and/or neurological dysfunction (neuroglycopenia) (e.g. difficulty concentrating, disturbed vision and hearing, slurred speech, dizziness and in severe episodes loss of consciousness and seizure) can be experienced during hypoglycaemic episodes. Children can also have behavioural changes and mood swings including irritability, erratic behaviour, becoming upset and tearful. There are also non-specific symptoms such as hunger, headache, tiredness and nausea though these may be present when the blood glucose level is high. Children often find it difficult to describe their own symptoms, but might experience shaky or wobbly legs or a 'funny' feeling.

Hypoglycaemia is frequently categorised as mild, moderate or severe depending on symptoms and the ability of the individual to treat the 'hypo' themselves. Younger children will nearly always need to be treated by an adult and there are no important clinical reasons to distinguish between mild and moderate hypoglycaemia. If the hypo is moderate the child may be unaware of it, but appears to be confused and uncooperative. In severe hypoglycaemia the child is unconscious and may be fitting. Regular episodes of even mild hypoglycaemia indicate that the diet and insulin and perhaps exercise are out of balance and that a review of diabetes management is necessary. The possibility of surreptitious extra insulin administration should also be considered.

If hypoglycaemia is suspected the blood glucose should be tested to confirm it. Hypoglycaemia should be treated as soon as possible. Treatment depends on the severity of the hypo and the aim is to restore the blood glucose level to 5.6 mmol/L [35] (euglycaemia).

Extrapolation from adult studies shows that 0.3 g/kg of glucose in the form of glucose tablets will raise the blood glucose by 2.5–3.6 mol/L [36] in children. For example approximately 10 g of carbohydrate will be required to treat hypoglycaemia for a 30 kg child. The amount of carbohydrate required to restore euglycaemia will depend on the weight of the child, type of insulin therapy and time since its administration, recent activity and starting blood glucose. The type of carbohydrate is significant. Glucose is the preferred carbohydrate for the immediate treatment of hypoglycaemia as it does not require digestion or metabolism. Chocolate, milk and sweets containing fat should not be used to treat hypoglycaemia as the fat will cause the blood glucose to rise slowly. Twice the amount of carbohydrate from fructose (in the form of fruit juice) was needed compared with that from glucose tablets to raise blood glucose by similar amounts [37]. Sucrose and milk also require greater amounts to provide the same rise in blood glucose.

It is advised that a remedy for hypoglycaemia is available at all times, but for some children the temptation of carrying sweets is too great. It can be useful to view the hypo remedy as a 'treatment' and carry glucose tablets or a glucose drink.

Mild hypoglycaemia

In practical terms, mild hypoglycaemia should be treated:

- with 10 g of carbohydrate, e.g. glucose tablets such as 3 Dextro Energy tablets or 2.5 Gluco Tabs, or 60 mL of glucose drink such as Lucozade Original
- wait 10–15 minutes and then recheck the blood glucose level
- if it is >4 mmol/L the usual meal or snack should be eaten if it is due or 10 g of starchy carbohydrate, such as an apple, should be taken to maintain blood glucose levels until the next meal
- if the blood glucose is <4 mmol/L another 10 g of fast acting carbohydrate should be taken and the process repeated until the blood glucose is >4 mmol/L
- some diabetes services across the UK also include jelly beans, cola drinks and fruit juice in the list of suitable hypo remedies

Moderate hypoglycaemia

At the stage of moderate hypoglycaemia:

- the child will need help to take a sugary drink or food
- the treatment is the same as that for mild hypoglycaemia
- Glucogel, Dextrogel or Rapilose (prescribable tubes of rapidly absorbed glucose gel) can be most useful. Each tube contains 10 g of carbohydrate that can be squeezed into the mouth if the child is uncooperative
- this should be followed up with starchy carbohydrate once the child has recovered
- if there is any concern about ability to swallow then oral remedies should not be attempted because of the risk of choking

Severe hypoglycaemia

- Most centres advise that parents and carers keep an emergency supply of a GlucaGen HypoKit for severe hypoglycaemia.
- This is a glucagon injection to use at home if the child is unconscious or fitting or if the parents are unable to resolve hypoglycaemic symptoms by other means.

Recommending an eating plan

A dietary assessment is essential on diagnosis so that the child's normal intake and meal pattern can be ascertained. The carbohydrate or energy allowance and distribution can then be tailored to the home situation. Providing the child is not overweight, the usual energy intake prior to the onset of diabetic symptoms can be used as a basis for deciding the diet.

Recommendations for particular insulin regimens

Recommendations for dietary management must take into consideration the child's current insulin regimen.

Single dose

A single daily dose of intermediate or long acting analogue insulin injection regimen is outdated and seldom used. It necessitates a rigid set amount of carbohydrate to be eaten at regular intervals as three meals and three snacks throughout the day to reduce the risk of hypoglycaemia and hyperglycaemia.

Twice daily injections

Two injections each day of mixed rapid or short acting and intermediate acting insulins (one before breakfast and one before the evening meal) require regular fixed amounts of carbohydrate throughout the day to reduce the risk of hypoglycaemia and hyperglycaemia. This regimen is seldom used with children in the UK now as intensified insulin therapy is preferred, i.e. basal bolus regimens and pump therapy. Carbohydrate in excess of 50–60 g given at any one time may produce an inappropriately raised postprandial blood sugar when using mixed insulins. A meal pattern of three meals and three snacks each day is appropriate for most children, although very young children and adolescents may need more snacks. Carbohydrate should be distributed throughout the day taking account of the peak periods of insulin action.

Split evening insulin

A split evening regimen involves having three injections per day: a mixed (rapid or short and intermediate acting) insulin before breakfast; a rapid or short acting insulin with the evening meal; and an intermediate or long acting dose given either with the evening meal or before bed. The advice for twice daily insulin applies during the day but this system allows more flexibility with the amount of carbohydrate eaten at the evening mealtime. The amount of rapid or short acting insulin can be proportionally adjusted to suit the quantity of carbohydrate eaten. The advantage of such a regimen is that there is no need for a lunchtime injection at school, but good glucose control is unlikely to be achieved without adherence to regular and consistent amounts of carbohydrate day to day.

Basal bolus

Basal bolus therapy uses four or more injections per day. The basal or background insulin is given as intermediate or long acting insulin once or twice daily and boluses of rapid or short acting insulin are given before meals or snacks containing more than 10–20 g of carbohydrate. Some centres advocate giving boluses even with very small snacks, although many consider it impractical to expect a child to inject for all meals and snacks and therefore 20 g is often used as a limit above which a bolus should be given.

It is preferable to inject bolus doses prior to a meal to optimise glycaemic control by reducing the postprandial rise in glucose and lessening the possibility of an injection being forgotten. In the case of toddlers or young children, where it is difficult to assess how much they will eat, a compromise is to give a postprandial injection. Apart from using a pump, this method of giving insulin offers the most flexible way to eat as there is no need to adhere to rigid meal and snack times as rapid or short acting insulin is injected with food. The amounts of carbohydrate at meals can be varied and appropriate adjustments made to bolus doses using insulin to carbohydrate ratios. Another benefit of using rapid acting insulin prior to meals is that due to its short duration of action snacks between meals are not always necessary. This is useful for those trying to lose weight or for those who dislike eating snacks. Bedtime snacks, however, are often necessary to reduce the risk of nocturnal hypoglycaemia.

Paediatric diabetes services throughout the UK employ a variety of approaches to establish the insulin to carbohydrate ratio (ICR) for meals and managing snacks. ICR must be calculated for the individual child and for each meal. One method is to initially suggest fixed amounts of carbohydrate for the three meals in the day based on diet history or recall. Snacks of 10–20 g are suggested and not normally covered by bolus insulin. Basal insulin may be given once or twice daily and these doses are titrated to those required by the child. Some centres work out the ICR by examining the amount of insulin given with the meal and the blood glucose result of the test done at the following meal (or bedtime snack in the case of the dinner ICR). In others the family is asked to do an '8-point profile'. This profile is blood glucose testing before breakfast, lunch, evening meal and bedtime snack, 90 or 120 minutes post main meals and at 3 am. The pre meal blood glucose tests will indicate the appropriateness of the basal insulin and the post meal tests the effectiveness of the rapid acting insulin. The insulin dose is deemed correct for the amount of carbohydrate if the blood glucose reading pre meal is the same as that checked 90 or 120 minutes after the meal ($\pm$2 mmol/L). Once the rapid acting doses are adjusted to match the carbohydrate ICR can be established. For example if 4 units of insulin is required for a 40 g carbohydrate breakfast the ICR is 1u:10 g; if 3 units of insulin are required for a 60 g carbohydrate lunch the ICR is 0.5u:10 g.

Another way of stating the same ratio is in terms of the number of grams of carbohydrate which will match one unit of insulin. For example, an ICR of 0.5u:10 g can be expressed as 20 g:1u. Many insulin pumps and some blood glucose meters have in-built 'bolus calculators' to assist with the calculations and these normally use this grams per unit system.

Once the ICRs have been established the child can eat to appetite (within the context of a healthy diet) at mealtimes and inject with the suitable amount of rapid acting insulin. If snacks containing more than 10–20 g are desired a bolus of rapid acting insulin can be taken. Many teenagers will want to eat a bedtime snack that is more than 20 g of carbohydrate.

Frequently, different ICRs are required at the three mealtimes and normally breakfast requires more insulin per 10 g of carbohydrate compared with other times in the day because of insulin resistance from hormones such as cortisol and growth hormone. It is necessary to regularly check, by blood glucose testing and using the 8-point profile, that the ICR is adequate as children's insulin requirements change as time goes on.

Insulin pumps

Insulin pumps, or continuous subcutaneous insulin infusion, offer the most freedom. The pump delivers a fixed or variable basal dose continuously throughout the day and bolus doses are administered each time carbohydrate is eaten. As no injection is required, it is advised to give a bolus with every snack, even very small ones.

As with basal bolus therapy the ability to count carbohydrate is paramount when using a pump. Accurate carbohydrate counting and ensuring that the individual's ICR is correct for each time block in the day will contribute towards an optimal HbA1c result. Pumps also incorporate sophisticated calculators that assist in, for example, avoiding 'stacking' of insulin doses on top of each other.

Most pumps now have the ability to deliver the bolus in various ways. A straightforward single dose may be given but it is also possible to deliver the bolus over a prolonged period of time (sometimes known as a 'square wave') or have part of the bolus delivered immediately and the remainder over a period of time (sometimes known as a 'dual wave'). This allows the bolus to be delivered to match the postprandial glucose excursion of the meal (dependent on the glycaemic index or fat content of the meal). A square wave is useful if the meal is going to be eaten over a prolonged period of time such as at a family celebration. If a child has an irregular eating pattern and it cannot be guaranteed that they will finish their meal the square wave will deliver the bolus over a period of time, perhaps an hour, and will be cancelled if necessary if the food has not all been eaten. It is also possible to deliver several small bolus doses if they eat little and often. This makes a pump ideal for infants and toddlers. A dual wave is effective for high fat foods that are carbohydrate dense such as pizza and creamy pasta dishes [38–40].

Studies in healthy subjects [41] and in those with diabetes revealed that food containing mainly carbohydrates causes a rapid and short glucose rise, whereas protein and fat containing meals result in a milder but prolonged increase in blood glucose levels. There is evidence emerging that meal related insulin dosing based on fat and protein counting, in addition to carbohydrate counting, reduces postprandial glucose levels [42]. Some centres across Europe are using carbohydrate plus fat and protein counting with normal, dual and square wave boluses and where prolonged boluses are utilised the duration is dependent on the amount of fat and protein in the meal. The more protein and fat the longer the duration of the bolus. The fat and protein counting algorithm used by Pańkowska et al. [43] has been adopted by some centres. Further studies are required to investigate translating findings from pump therapy to multiple injection therapy. Questions remain about how this can be implemented in practice.

The families have to experiment with different foods and bolus methods using blood glucose monitoring as their guide to get the best use of their pump's features.

Exercise

Insulin, carbohydrate and exercise are the three fundamental influencing factors in blood glucose control. The many benefits of exercise, including weight control and reduced cardiovascular risk, far outweigh the potential risks of hypoglycaemia and hyperglycaemia associated with exercise. Families need dietary education about exercise management to contribute towards optimising control, providing adequate nutrition and, for older and competitive youngsters, optimising performance.

Exercise has the effect of lowering blood glucose levels by increasing the non-insulin dependent uptake of glucose by cells and increasing insulin sensitivity. During exercise, in type 1 diabetes, the pancreas does not control insulin levels and there may be impaired glucose counter regulation; as a consequence, hypoglycaemia frequently occurs during exercise or afterwards.

Children can have variable blood glucose outcomes as a result of additional activity. Levels can be maintained if the insulin doses are suitably adjusted and the intake of carbohydrate is sufficient. Hypoglycaemia can result due to excessive insulin, prolonged exercise without consuming additional carbohydrate, or moderate intensity aerobic exercise. Hyperglycaemia can be a consequence of a lack of insulin before and throughout the activity, the emotional reaction to competing or excitement causing an adrenalin surge, eating or drinking too much carbohydrate, an increase in adrenalin response due to brief, sporadic bouts of intense anaerobic exercise or after exercise when glucose production exceeds utilisation. Table 10.4 shows the factors associated with the effect of exercise on blood glucose levels.

Table 10.4 Factors associated with the effect of exercise on blood glucose levels.

Duration and intensity of the exercise

Type of activity (aerobic or anaerobic)

Metabolic control (there is a probability of ketosis developing if blood glucose levels are high and insulin levels are insufficient)

Type and timing of insulin doses

Type and timing of carbohydrate consumed

Absorption of insulin

Competitive nature of the sport (adrenalin will increase the blood glucose level)

Timing of the activity

It can be easier to manage diabetes using a pump or a basal bolus regimen with children and young people who are extremely active and are involved in competitive sports.

Practical advice is key and families must learn to manage exercise by experimenting, regularly checking blood glucose levels and building on their experiences. A detailed log of carbohydrate intake, insulin doses and intensity and duration of activity can aid the family and the diabetes team in observing cause and effect of the various factors on the blood glucose. Accordingly changes can be instigated to improve the management of blood glucose control and exercise. Children should not exercise if the blood glucose is >14 mmol/L and they have ketonuria or ketonaemia. Extra insulin should be taken and the situation rectified before exercise is undertaken.

Dietary advice for exercise:

- Most periods of exercise or activity lasting more than 30 minutes will necessitate some adjustment to carbohydrate intake and or insulin.
- The type of activity, the weight of the child and the level of circulating insulin will determine how much carbohydrate will be necessary to avoid hypoglycaemia.
- Additional carbohydrate may be required before, during and after exercise; eating carbohydrate afterwards helps to replace hepatic and muscle glycogen stores.
- For younger children their energy expenditure is so variable from day to day and hour to hour

that it is more practical, in most instances, to cover additional activity with extra carbohydrate. Often exercise can be easily dealt with by giving a snack of 10–20 g of carbohydrate as fruit, dried fruit, fruit juice, a cereal bar or bread. This can also be a time to allow a 'fun size' bar of chocolate; the fat slows down the absorption of the sugar and makes it more suited for longer lasting activities such as swimming or long walks.

- An isotonic drink containing 6% simple sugar such as glucose, fructose or sucrose is ideal if additional carbohydrate is required for short duration exercise. This is preferable to more concentrated juices and carbonated sugary drinks that may cause stomach ache and delay gastric absorption [44]. Many swimmers choose to drink this as the bottle can be left at the edge of the pool and sips easily taken throughout the session.
- Adolescents may require up to 1.0–1.5 g carbohydrate/kg/hour for moderate to intense exercise [45].
- Older children involved in strenuous exercise over a long period should have a balanced meal with protein, fat and carbohydrate 3–4 hours beforehand to maximise the endogenous energy stores and permit time for digestion. Up to an hour before the activity a carbohydrate drink (1–2 g carbohydrate/kg) may be taken to increase energy stores and provide fluid for hydration; this will boost glycogen stores [44].
- For some older children additional pre-exercise carbohydrate may necessitate bolus insulin if the exercise is high intensity or strenuous or anaerobic [46]. Hyperglycaemia and poor performance can be caused by insufficient insulin.
- Fluid intake should be adequate as dehydration can impair performance.
- Following moderate or intense exercise carbohydrate stores must be replenished to lower the risk of hypoglycaemia, as insulin sensitivity remains raised for several hours.
- High intensity, brief, anaerobic exercise such as sprinting may not need carbohydrate beforehand but may result in a fall in blood glucose afterwards. In this case it is preferable to prevent hypoglycaemia by taking additional carbohydrate after the sport.

- Activities of a longer duration such as swimming, cycling, jogging, football may require additional carbohydrate before, during and afterwards.
- To minimise post exercise hypoglycaemia low GI foods, a reduction in basal insulin and a lower than usual bolus dose with the post exercise meal can be helpful.
- A remedy to treat hypoglycaemia must be carried at all times or be close by whilst exercising and it is advisable to also have some form of 'diabetes identification'.
- Adults supervising children with diabetes including teachers, coaches, activity holiday staff should all be aware of the possibility of hypoglycaemia and know how to treat it.
- Hypoglycaemia can occur several hours after exercise (up to 24 hours) due to increased insulin sensitivity. Additional carbohydrate and/or a reduction in insulin may be required to prevent this. The risk of post exercise nocturnal hypoglycaemia is high and extra carbohydrate eaten at bedtime can reduce this threat.

The 'Exercise in children and adolescents with diabetes' [47] ISPAD guideline provides evidence based recommendations for people with diabetes.

Illness

Children often do not wish to eat during periods of illness and infection. Blood glucose levels are likely to be high at these times, so it is important that insulin therapy is continued. It is easier to manage diabetes during illness when a child is on a basal bolus regimen or on an insulin pump as additional insulin can be readily and safely given (with proper instruction and education) to prevent ketones developing or rid the body of them. For those on insulin twice or three times per day, a change in the insulin regimen to several doses of rapid acting insulin may be advised. Carbohydrate intake must not be cut to control the blood glucose level and is essential to prevent the body using fat reserves as a source of fuel with consequent ketone production. Blood glucose should be controlled by the insulin therapy using correction doses as recommended by the diabetes team.

If the usual diet is refused it is not essential to completely replace all the carbohydrate. A realistic aim is to give 70%–80% of the normal intake. Small frequent doses of rapidly absorbed carbohydrate, preferably as a liquid, are often best tolerated. Water and/or low calorie/sugar free drinks should be encouraged to prevent dehydration. Diarrhoea and vomiting illnesses can cause blood glucose to fall. At this time insulin should never be stopped (to prevent ketosis) but doses may be reduced and carbohydrate given as sugary drinks such as Lucozade or flat cola drinks.

Parents should always contact their diabetes team if concerned about their child's condition. During recovery the child should return gradually to foods normally eaten.

Diet throughout childhood

Regular and continued dietetic input is essential in order that the dietary advice is appropriate for the child's continuing and changing needs and lifestyle. Throughout childhood the dietitian should be involved in the diabetes education of the child and his/her carers, including nursery and school staff.

Babies

Adequate nutrition to promote growth is of major importance during the early months of life. Infants with diabetes should have their carbohydrate intake based on requirement for milk feeds, which are the principal source of nutrition. If at the time of diagnosis the infant is breast fed the mother should be encouraged to continue. However, many mothers are anxious about hypoglycaemia if they are uncertain of the amount being consumed at each feed and will need reassurance. Whether breast or bottle fed, a baby's fluid requirement is 150–200 mL/kg/day; 150 mL breast or infant formula contains approximately 10 g carbohydrate. Providing growth and development is normal, the daily carbohydrate intake can be based on the baby's usual feeding pattern with the insulin dose adjusted accordingly. As with all infants, breast milk or infant formula should be the milk of choice until the child is 12 months old.

An insulin pump is the delivery method of choice for babies and many children under 5 as their varying insulin requirements can be met more easily and unpredictable eating patterns dealt with.

Basal bolus insulin therapy is an alternative. Breast fed infants can be given a bolus of insulin before or after each feed. For bottle fed babies the amount of carbohydrate in the formula feed can be calculated, insulin to carbohydrate ratios can be established and the appropriate amount of insulin matching the feed delivered by a pump or insulin pen. In some instances diluted insulin is necessary if the total daily requirement is small.

Weaning

Weaning advice for the general population applies to infants with diabetes. Most term infants need no nutrition other than breast milk or formula milk until 6 months (26 weeks) of age. Weaning can start around this time. Non-carbohydrate foods may be used initially (e.g. 1–2 teaspoons puréed vegetables) as these will not alter the carbohydrate intake. This allows the baby to become accustomed to the different taste and texture of solids without any anxiety being generated by food refusal. Once the baby has become familiar with spoon feeding, carbohydrate containing foods such as baby rice and rusk may be introduced. Water and dilute low sugar squashes can be given as an additional drink. Weaning is an anxious time for any parent and this anxiety is heightened if a dietary modification has to be observed. Tension about food must be relieved as a baby may refuse solids completely if the mother is fussing or worrying.

The Department of Health recommendations for vitamin supplements for infants and young children [48] also apply to the child with diabetes. The first year of life is the period of most rapid growth. Dietary intake is constantly changing due to the child's progression through normal feeding and developmental milestones. It is essential that the dietitian is in frequent contact with the family to offer advice.

Hypoglycaemia is a real fear for parents and can be hard to recognise in babies. It may only be noted when parents are routinely checking blood sugars. Advice should be given on how to recognise and treat symptoms. Extra milk, with or without additional sugar, or glucose polymer, Ribena or sweetened fruit juice may be used. Usually 10 g carbohydrate given as 150 mL baby milk or 75 mL baby milk plus one teaspoon (5 g) of glucose polymer is sufficient to treat hypoglycaemia. Nocturnal hypoglycaemia is a concern; milk and a cereal can be given before the baby settles for the night if (s)he is no longer having night feeds and blood glucose levels are dropping overnight.

Toddlers

After 1 year of age the child can drink cow's milk and from 2 years semi-skimmed milk can be introduced as long as the child is taking a nutritionally adequate diet. Fully skimmed milk or 1% fat milk, however, contains too little fat (and hence energy) for the under 5s and is not usually recommended. The introduction of skimmed milk over the age of 5 is a useful way to reduce the overall fat content of the diet. There is little fibre in the diets of children in their first year of life, but this can gradually increase. Some forms of fibre such as Weetabix, raisins, bananas and baked beans are popular with children; vegetables and wholemeal bread need to be encouraged.

Small children do not understand the importance of their diet, so parents and health professionals must be flexible and compromise as much as is practical. Erratic eating patterns are common in children between 2 and 4 years of age. Rigid mealtimes and snacks often do not work and well presented finger foods can be offered throughout the day. Most families manage to cope with the 'food refusal syndrome' without being manipulated, but the toddler with diabetes poses a real problem; with hypoglycaemia always a possibility, food refusal can become a powerful weapon. Parents are torn between maintaining good glycaemic control with the accompanying risk of hypoglycaemia, and allowing the blood sugars to be a little raised. Advice should be given not to force feed, nor to offer numerous alternatives, and to avoid fuss around mealtimes. The child's falling blood glucose causing hunger and a desire to eat can be relied upon. In a small minority of cases toddlers' food refusal can be a persistent and unremitting problem causing parents enormous worry about hypos. If the child is not on an insulin pump, one practical solution is to allow the child to eat meals with no fuss and when the meal is over to give an appropriate dose of rapid acting insulin analogue to cover the amount of food consumed.

Some young children with diabetes complain of incessant hunger. This may occur if control is poor and glucose is being lost in the urine or if the child is using food as a means to seek attention. Measurements of height, weight and dietary intake should be done regularly to reassure parents that adequate nutrition is being maintained.

Toddlerhood can prove to be a challenging stage when it is often difficult to achieve good glycaemic control and the families need plenty of support from their diabetes team.

Schoolchildren

While at school the teacher becomes one of the child's main carers and must know about the condition and in particular how to recognise and treat hypoglycaemia. There are governmental acts across the UK that place requirements on education authorities to support children in schools and nurseries with conditions such as diabetes [49–51]. Concern has been raised amongst a number of schools about managing diabetes since the advent of pump therapy and increasing numbers of children on basal bolus therapy requiring 'medical' intervention at school. However, liaison with diabetes teams and information shared with the school resolves these worries and the child's diabetes can be cared for capably at school. Diabetes UK provides information about managing diabetes at school and on school trips. Moreover many diabetes teams have their own literature and information available on websites. This information should be given to each child's teacher. The dietitian and/or the diabetes nurse specialist may offer to visit the school to provide advice.

Children with diabetes are advised to carry a hypo remedy (glucose tablets) at all times. The teacher should be equipped with glucose tablets and/or a glucose drink in case of hypoglycaemia. Teachers of physical education should be aware of the need for extra carbohydrate before exercise and to check that children are carrying extra carbohydrate during periods of prolonged exercise.

School lunches can, but should not, present a problem; it is not always possible for children to go home and they may prefer to have school lunch with their friends. Older children with a good grasp of their diet can choose their own meal and the cafeteria-style canteen allows a flexible choice of food. The organisation and provision of school meals can vary from area to area; it is not desirable for the child to have a 'special diet' away from friends or at a different time from them. A normal main course should be suitable, with the dessert or pudding being replaced by fresh fruit or diet yoghurt. Discussion with the school cooks as well as teachers should help smooth problems. Advice can be given to parents about suitable packed lunches. Some local authorities provide information about the carbohydrate content of portions of foods available at school lunches; all authorities should be encouraged to do so.

Children frequently eat sweets in the school playground and it is tempting for a child with diabetes to eat sweets also. Other less sweet snacks such as fruit, bread, low sugar cereal bars, raisins, yoghurt and sugar free chewing gum should be suggested as alternatives. The best attitude is to use positive reinforcement when the child is doing well and to recommend that the best time for sweets is prior to exercise or after a main meal. If habitual bingeing is causing a problem the services of a child psychologist may be needed; bingeing suggests underlying stress.

Adolescents

As in other age groups, height and weight monitoring is important for early recognition of weight loss or disproportionate weight gain. Poor growth may be a sign of delayed puberty, coeliac or thyroid disease, omission of insulin, disordered eating or poor diabetes control. Excessive weight gain requires a careful examination of insulin dosage, dietary intake and physical activity. Occasionally, simply cutting out crisps and fried foods and exercising can achieve weight control. The amount of carbohydrate in the diet should only be reduced after very careful examination of the diet as a whole, as this may cause an increase in consumption of fat and protein. In order to get the message across, it is useful to point out the energy content of some of the carbohydrate portions, e.g. one packet of crisps provides 10 g carbohydrate and 150 kcal (630 kJ); one apple also contains 10 g carbohydrate but only 50 kcal (210 kJ).

Teenagers soon become aware of the fact that poor control can result in weight loss. A number will omit insulin as a method of weight control. The benefits of weight loss achieved by healthy lifestyle (eating and exercise) should be reinforced and the risks associated with poor control, acute and chronic, outlined. Some teenagers, both male and female, can have a distorted view of their weight. Eating disorders can present just as in the non-diabetic population with bingeing, anorexia nervosa and bulimia. Diabetes is a condition which makes weight control possible without the avoidance of food. Diabetes may increase the risks of eating disorders in children and young people, particularly in young women, as there is a greater focus on food, on weight (weighing people at each clinic visit, rapid weight gain with insulin) and a fear of hypoglycaemia often coupled with low self-esteem. Young people suffering from an eating disorder need careful monitoring and intervention by the diabetes team and the psychiatrist/psychologist.

Adolescence is a time of physical, social and emotional change. Teenagers with diabetes may not want to be different from their peers, worrying about gaining acceptance whilst fighting for independence with parents. Education about diet and re-education is important at this stage as an assumption can be made that because someone has had diabetes for a long time they know all about it when in fact it was the parents who learned about the condition. Support from the diabetes team whilst young people learn to manage their own diabetes is crucial during this period.

Snacking and eating out in the evening is common and advice about how to manage this is needed. Advice about alcohol and its hypoglycaemic effect will be necessary for teenagers, as it is known that many youngsters imbibe before they reach the legal age to do so. Alcohol is dangerous in excess as it suppresses gluconeogenesis and may induce prolonged hypoglycaemia in young people with diabetes. Carbohydrate should be eaten before, during and after alcohol intake especially if exercise is performed during or after drinking, e.g. dancing. Awareness of the alcohol content of drinks particularly targeted at young people should be raised.

Arrangements for transition of care to adult services varies widely across the UK but there should always be good communication between the paediatric and adult dietitians to ensure continuity of care.

Parties and eating out

Parties are highlights in a child's life and advice is required to ensure that children with diabetes can enjoy the party as much as everyone else. They can eat most of the party fare and it is important to ensure that sufficient carbohydrate is eaten to compensate for extra activity and excitement. The host can help by providing low calorie drinks for everyone. Parties can involve sleepovers and advice should be discussed about food intake, timing of insulin doses and managing additional activity.

Many fast food eating places and restaurants publish the carbohydrate content of their foods in leaflets and on websites. Children should be educated about their diet as soon as possible so that they are able to manage it independently, with support from parents as necessary. All children are different, but most children from the age of about 8 should be actively encouraged to have a full understanding of their diet. Parents may need encouragement gradually to hand over responsibility of treatment to the child.

Travel

Travel should pose no problems with a little extra planning. Carbohydrate foods, e.g. sandwiches, fruit or biscuits, should be carried to cover inevitable delays, as should a hypo remedy. More food is required on activity holidays and usually a reduction in the insulin dose (of around 20%) too to prevent hypoglycaemia. When holidaying abroad advice should be given on practical issues related to long distance travel, e.g. when best to eat and inject insulin whilst travelling across time zones, how to avoid food poisoning and as always the children should wear some form of identification, e.g. SOS Talisman or Medicalert.

Non type 1 diabetes

Paediatric diabetes dietitians are more frequently being faced with the dietary management of children with non type 1 diabetes as the incidence is increasing.

Type 2 diabetes

There is little evidence regarding the dietary recommendations for children with type 2 diabetes and therefore advice suggested is derived from treatment of overweight and obese children, children with type 1 diabetes and adults with type 2 diabetes. The aims of dietary management are

- to achieve optimal blood glucose levels and normal HbA1c
- to prevent further weight gain in those with BMI on the 85th–95th percentile
- weight loss for those with BMI >95th percentile with normal linear growth [52, 53]
- to deal with comorbidities such as hypertension and dyslipidaemia

Most children with type 2 diabetes are overweight and dietary intervention aims to achieve weight loss or keep weight static with normal linear growth. Often the whole family is overweight and to teach and counsel the entire family about calorie reduction and increasing energy expenditure may be beneficial, rather than concentrating solely on the child or young person. There is some evidence that substitution of low GI foods for high GI foods may help with weight, lipid levels and control of appetite [54, 55].

Dietary management should incorporate:

- *Cutting out sugary soft or fizzy drinks and fruit juices completely.* This single dietary change can make the most significant change and result in weight loss. These drinks can be replaced with water, diet drinks and sugar free beverages.
- *Healthy eating advice for the whole family* with guidance about regular eating and avoiding the use of sweet foods as a reward or token of affection. Meals should ideally be eaten as part of a family routine, eaten in one place

(preferably at a table) and with no distraction such as watching television, reading or playing. High fat and high calorie foods should be limited in the home. Education and instruction about reading nutrition information on food labels should be given to help the family when making food choices whilst shopping.

- *Advice about exercising portion control* within the family and that food should not be eaten out of a tin or packet but should be served on a plate or bowl.
- *Keeping food diaries* as this can raise awareness or food issues and help monitor progress.
- *Positive reinforcement should be given for success,* no matter how small, such as no or minimal weight gain, eating less of a high calorie food; it is seldom useful to criticise failure.

A number of children with type 2 diabetes are on oral medication and or insulin therapy. Those on insulin should have detailed education about carbohydrate counting and hypoglycaemia.

Diabetes secondary to pancreatic disease

Cystic fibrosis related diabetes (p. 239) is due to insulin deficiency but insulin resistance during acute illness and medication may also contribute to impaired glucose tolerance and diabetes. Blood glucose levels should be controlled, as high levels will promote catabolism and affect response to infection. It has been documented that early initiation of insulin therapy may have value for growth, weight and pulmonary function [56, 57]. Insulin doses and types may need to be adjusted when nutritional supplements, overnight or continuous enteral feeding are being used and during times of acute infection. Dose adjustment should take priority over dietary restriction.

Dietary management includes:

- ensuring sufficient calorie and intake to meet the individual's requirements
- avoiding sugary drinks
- advice about the effect of carbohydrate on blood glucose levels and matching insulin dose with ingested carbohydrate.

Regular healthy eating advice may be sufficient; however, carbohydrate counting and use of insulin to carbohydrate ratios may also be necessary.

Diabetes secondary to medication

Some drugs, such as high dose steroids, can cause transient hyperglycaemia for the duration of the prescription and others, such as tacrolimus and cyclosporin, may cause islet cell destruction and the diabetes is permanent (p. 663). In oncology protocols some chemotherapy drugs induce diabetes which coincides with the cyclical nature of the chemotherapy. Following transplantation such as renal transplantation (p. 271), diabetes most commonly occurs with the use of high dose steroids and tacrolimus. Dietary management depends on how the diabetes is medically managed. In some instances instruction about avoiding sugary drinks and foods and healthy eating is sufficient. Other children are commenced on daily long acting analogue insulin and require additional information about eating regularly, having a bedtime snack and hypoglycaemia. Basal bolus or insulin pump therapy can also be initiated and the advice is similar to that given to those with type 1 diabetes.

Coeliac disease

Coeliac disease occurs in 10% of children with diabetes [58]. It is associated with poor growth, delayed puberty, nutritional deficiencies and hypoglycaemia; however, the presence of coeliac disease can often be asymptomatic. A gluten free diet must be incorporated into the diabetes eating plan as it is the only treatment for coeliac disease. It is understandable that many of the children who develop coeliac disease do not adhere to the gluten free diet [59] but should be encouraged to do so. Commonly these children are upset about having two conditions which require dietary modification and they may benefit from referral to the psychologist attached to the diabetes team to discuss the dual diagnosis. Advice should be given about the gluten free diet, gluten free products and the nutritional adequacy of the diet especially for iron, calcium, vitamin D, fibre and vitamin B intake (p. 117). Children with diabetes and coeliac disease should have frequent reviews by a paediatric dietitian with experience in both fields. Vitamin D and iron status should be checked regularly.

Dietary review

There should be an initial dietary teaching package for newly diagnosed children and young people with diabetes and they should have the opportunity to see a dietitian at each outpatient appointment; they should have access by telephone for advice at all times. As a minimum there should be an annual dietetic review. More frequent consultations are required in situations such as a change of insulin regimen, an excessive weight gain or loss, or where there is a need for further dietary education, e.g. poor knowledge or advice about diet and exercise, activity holidays, dyslipidaemia, comorbidities such as coeliac disease.

Summary

The dietetic care of children and young people is multifaceted and must be ongoing. Youngsters with diabetes should have an optimal quality of life in which a suitably tailored eating plan is an essential part. The dietitian has a unique role to play in the multidisciplinary team in the management of childhood diabetes and the education of the child and the family. They can offer support and reassurance along with dietetic expertise. Nutritional assessment and support must be an integral part of initial and continuing education programmes. Diabetes control and compliance can be less than ideal but this does not detract from the importance of balanced nutrition in this serious chronic disease.

Further reading and information

Food for Life, book of dietary information by Alison Johnston and Anne Morrice. Available from GGC Children's Diabetes Service, Royal Hospital for Sick Children, Glasgow G3 8SJ, and on website http://www.childdiabetes-scotland.org/ggc

Supporting Children and Young People with Diabetes in Education by Alison Johnston and Nicola Thomson. Available from GGC Children's Diabetes Service, Royal Hospital for Sick Children, Glasgow G3 8SJ, and on website http://www.childdiabetes-scotland.org/ggc

Patient Held Record, a diabetes manual by Ian Craigie and Fiona Lamb. Available from GGC Children's Diabetes Service, Royal Hospital for Sick Children, Glasgow G3 8SJ, and on website http://www.childdiabetes-scotland.org/ggc

ISPAD Clinical Practice Consensus Guidelines 2009 Compendium available at www.ispad.org

Ives Diabetes Exercise and Sports Association (www.diabetes-exercise.org), an international organisation that provides guidance and networking between beginners, health professionals and experienced athletes with diabetes

www.runsweet.com, a website which shares knowledge on how to manage diabetes with different sports and exercises

Useful addresses

Diabetes UK
Central Office, Macleod House, 10 Parkway, London NW1 7AA
Tel: 020 7424 1000
www.diabetes.org.uk

Congenital Hyperinsulinism

Jacqueline Lowdon

Introduction

Congenital hyperinsulinism (CHI) is the most common cause of severe, persistent hypoglycaemia in newborn babies and children [60]. It is a clinically heterogeneous disorder characterised by severe recurrent hypoglycaemia associated with elevated serum insulin, C-peptide and pro insulin levels that are inappropriately high for the concentration of blood glucose.

Clinical presentation

CHI can be associated with several well defined clinical conditions such as uncontrolled maternal diabetes, perinatal asphyxia and Beckwith–Wiedemann syndrome, which all manifest with transient hyperinsulinism [61–63]. However, the focus here is on persistent hypoglycaemia so these conditions will not be covered.

Most infants with CHI present during the first few days of life, others during the first year. Very rarely, some older children may present with hypoglycaemic symptoms. The first clinical indications of CHI can include non-specific features of hypoglycaemia such as floppiness, jitteriness, poor feeding and lethargy [64]. If left untreated, CHI can lead to permanent neurological damage, or coma and death, secondary to severe hypoglycaemia [64–66]. Some infants with hyperinsulinism might present with macrosomia [67].

Hyperinsulinism in infancy can be clinically very heterogeneous, ranging from a severe life threatening disease to very mild clinical symptoms which may be difficult to recognise. Some of the most difficult to manage are those infants of normal or low birth weight, including preterm infants [64].

Incidence

Estimated incidence is 1 in 50 000 live births in western Europe [68, 69] with the highest incidence rate of 1 in 2500 births found in countries with high rates of consanguinity [70].

Early referral to a specialist centre

Due to the challenges of managing infants with CHI, early transfer to a specialist centre is recommended [71]. There are two centres in the UK: the Northern Congenital Hyperinsulinism (NORCHI) service which is a joint service between the Royal Manchester Children's Hospital and the Alder Hey

Table 10.5 Criteria for diagnostic indicators for hyperinsulinism.

- Glucose requirement >8 mg/kg/min to maintain blood glucose >2.6 mmol/L (normal requirement 4–6 mg/kg/min)
- Laboratory blood glucose level <2.6 mmol/L
- Detectable insulin at time of hypoglycaemia with elevated C-peptide
- Inappropriately low levels of blood free fatty acids and ketone bodies at the time of hypoglycaemia

Table 10.6 Intermediary metabolites and hormones measured at the point of hypoglycaemia.

Blood	Urine
Glucose	Ketone bodies
Lactate/pyruvate	Reducing substances
Ketone bodies	Organic acids
Free fatty acids	
Amino acids	
Ammonia	
Total/free carnitine	
Acyl-carnitine profile	
Insulin/C-peptide	
Cortisol	

Children's Hospital, Liverpool; and Great Ormond Street Hospital for Children, London. Paediatric dietitians may have initial contact with a new CHI infant and thereafter have shared care with the specialist centre dietitians.

Figure 10.1 outlines the admission management pathway for a new CHI patient to the Royal Manchester Children's Hospital.

Establishing diagnosis

There is a well established consensus for the primary and secondary diagnostic indicators for hyperinsulinism (HI) [71] shown in Table 10.5. Blood taken at the time of hypoglycaemia must be assayed for the substances listed in Table 10.6.

Genetics and pathogenesis of CHI subtypes

The clinical heterogeneity of CHI includes a variable age of onset, degree of severity and

sensitivity to medical treatment. Two distinct histopathological types have been described [65, 72, 73]. Most exhibit diffuse involvement of the beta cells throughout the pancreas (diffuse HI), while some cases have focal adenomatous hyperplasia (focal HI). With focal HI a distinct area of the pancreas is involved, while the rest of the pancreas is histologically and functionally normal.

Genetic heterogeneity has also been described with over 40 different mutations [74] in seven different genes being detected in patients with CHI so far. Both autosomal recessive and dominant inheritance has been described [75] with the majority being recessively inherited [74].

In 30%–50% of patients there are abnormalities in either genes controlling intracellular metabolic pathways or membrane cation transport [76]. Most cases of CHI are caused by genetic mutations that result in an abnormal formation or function of K_{ATP} channels [77]. Consequently the beta cells secrete insulin even when blood glucose levels are low. The K_{ATP} channels are controlled by two genes: the sulphonylurea receptor gene (SUR1 now known as ABCC8) [78] and the inward-rectifying potassium channel gene (KiR6.2 now known as KCNJ11) [79].

Most cases of CHI due to K_{ATP} channel defects are recessively inherited. K_{ATP}-HI can result in diffuse or focal disease, depending on which parent the mutation is inherited from. Heterozygous mutation on the paternal allele can cause focal disease. Within the focal lesion there is selective deletion of maternal copy.

Other CHI cases are caused by mutations in the main enzymes involved in glucose metabolism [77], the beta cell enzymes glucokinase (GK-HI) and glutamate dehydrogenase (GDH-HI). Genetic mutations in genes coding for the GDH and GK enzymes are dominantly inherited and result in diffuse disease [77].

Although a number of gene mutations have been associated with CHI, the commonest mutations causing CHI are in the K_{ATP} channel genes. Rapid K_{ATP} channel gene mutation testing has significantly improved the investigation and management of CHI [80].

Testing for mutations in ABCC8 and KCNJ11 and identification of parental origin is useful in assessing the likelihood of focal and diffuse HI early in the treatment. Further, ^{18}F-DOPA positron emission tomography (PET) CT scan imaging

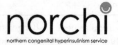

New CHI admission Management Pathway

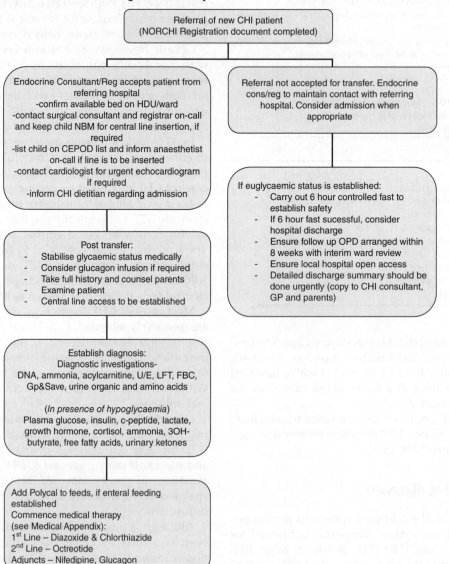

Figure 10.1   New CHI patient admission management pathway. Reprinted with permission of Royal Manchester Children's Hospital.

of the pancreas in select cases, e.g. those with paternal heterozygous mutations or no identifiable mutation, is critical to the diagnosis of focal HI [81–84]. The purpose of this scan is to determine whether there is a focal lesion within the pancreas that would be responsive to surgical resection. All children who have a CHI genotype consistent with possible focal disease should be considered for this scan. The scan should also be given to infants where no genetic mutations have been found but who remain on treatment for their CHI [85]. In the UK the scan is only available at the two specialist centres.

Management of CHI

Management aims are:

- prevention of hypoglycaemic brain damage, allowing for normal psychomotor development
- establishment of normal feeding regimen appropriate for the age of the infant/child – volume, frequency, type
- ensuring normal and safe tolerance to fasting that is appropriate for age, without developing hypoglycaemia
- maintenance of family unit and quality of life [71]
- optimal growth

Effective management is essential for a good outcome. Neuroglycopenia occurs with associated hypoketosis when blood glucose levels are below the normal range of 3.5–6.0 mmol/L. A high degree of psychomotor or developmental delay has been reported in up to 44% of cases, with epilepsy in up to 25% of cases [86] including infantile spasms occurring in a number of individuals [80]. Most recent data suggest persisting learning difficulties in 29% of patients [87].

Medical treatment

Initial stabilisation

The objectives of medical management are [71]

- stabilisation of blood glucose concentrations above 3.5 mmol/L
- establishment of a feeding regimen that is acceptable to the family without compromising

the safety of the child, achieving normal blood glucose concentrations during a reasonable length of fast.

If high glucose infusion rates are required (>20 mg/kg/minute) [71], the insertion of a central venous catheter may be required for intravenous (IV) dextrose and/or IV glucagon; this may need to be considered even if the requirement for glucose is less.

A normal hepatic glucose production rate in a full term newborn infant is 4–6 mg/kg/minute [88]. However, in CHI the requirement is much higher, sometimes as high as 25 mg/kg/minute. It is important to estimate the glucose requirement to maintain euglycaemia and increased glucose requirement can be an important diagnostic step. The glucose requirement will continue to be a fundamental feature requiring careful and regular assessment in order to prevent severe hypoglycaemia, symptomatic and asymptomatic.

To calculate glucose requirement for IV fluids:

$$\frac{\% \text{ dextrose infused} \times \text{mL/hour}}{\text{weight (kg)} \times 6} = \text{mg/kg/minute}$$

fluid rate (mL/hour)

$$= \frac{\text{CHO requirement (mg/kg/minute)} \times \text{weight (kg)} \times 6}{\% \text{ dextrose}}$$

(CHO, carbohydrate)

Once blood glucose has stabilised on IV dextrose, enteral feeds can be commenced.

Dietetic management

To calculate glucose requirement for enteral feeds:

total CHO (g) × 1000 (mg) ÷ weight (kg)

÷ 24 (hours) ÷ 60 (minutes) = mg/kg/ min

This calculation is for a 24 hour period.

The above formula can only be a rough guide for estimating the glucose requirement for maintaining euglycaemia as there may be factors influencing the absorption of feeds. Euglycaemia may be achieved with the provision of adequate carbohydrate and regular feeding. It may be necessary to give feeds via a nasogastric tube if inadequate amounts are taken orally. A gastrostomy may be required if poor feeding continues.

Feeds need to be given very frequently such as 2 hourly initially, aiming for 3 hourly and, if possible, 4 hourly closer to the time of discharge home from hospital. However, it is crucial that this longer spacing of feeds is tried in hospital first to ensure tolerance and acceptable blood glucose levels. Some infants may require continuous overnight feeding to achieve stable blood glucose levels. During the day, feed may be given as a bolus gravity drip feed or via a pump over 30–60 minutes depending on tolerance.

If the regimen consists of a combination of day-time bolus feeds and overnight continuous feeds, a bolus feed may need to be given soon after the overnight feed stops as the blood glucose level can drop quite quickly after the continuous feeding period. This is similar to the situation prior to the start of the overnight feed, which should be started soon after the last bolus feed of the day.

Glucose polymers, such as Polycal, Maxijul or Vitajoule, can be added to the feed to increase carbohydrate intake. The glucose polymer should be added in small amounts and increased as required and tolerated. Care needs to be taken, however, as increasing the osmotic load can predispose to the onset of necrotising enterocolitis, particularly in preterm infants (p. 100). Care also needs to be taken to ensure that the optimal protein:energy ratio is maintained (p. 18).

Depending on requirements for carbohydrate, energy, energy:protein ratio and fluid it may be more effective to use a high energy feed, e.g. Infatrini, Similac High Energy, SMA High Energy, or standard infant formulas can be concentrated (p. 17).

Uncooked corn starch therapy is usually not advised under the age of 2 years due to the immaturity of intestinal amylase, which may not make it effective. However, it may be a good treatment in older children (p. 549).

Pharmacological agents (e.g. diazoxide) can be given to try to decrease insulin secretion, with a view to normalising carbohydrate intake [71]. In practice, a combination of drug therapy and carbohydrate modification is commenced soon after diagnosis and will continue to be required while the child remains hyperinsulinaemic. A balance is required between the carbohydrate modification and drug therapy, with their attendant side effects.

Long term feeding difficulties

Children with CHI often develop long term feeding difficulties. The pathophysiology is yet to be determined, but one of the reasons thought to contribute to this is foregut dysmotility [89]. Infants often show poor suck and swallow with intolerance of large feed volumes. Feeding difficulties are likely to be due to a combination of dysmotility induced by excess insulin secretion, abnormal gastrointestinal peptide secretion and adverse effects of medical treatment with diazoxide and octreotide. Long term tube feeding and the use of IV fluids without oral feeding may hinder the process of learning to feed by mouth. The infant should be encouraged to feed orally as soon as possible and referral to a speech and language therapist for early intervention is recommended.

Gastro-oesophageal reflux (GOR) with retching and vomiting is common. Anti-reflux medications may need to be given (p. 137). Some patients may benefit from a thickened formula (p. 136) taking into account the CHO content of the thickening agent and adjusting the amount of glucose polymer accordingly. For some, a change in feed to a hydrolysed protein formula may be beneficial (p. 113). Amino acid based formulas, however, are absorbed too quickly creating difficulties with maintaining blood glucose levels. A fundoplication may be required for those with severe GOR (p. 150).

For some children, excessive weight gain can become a problem. This is associated with forced tube feeding to prevent hypoglycaemia. Forced tube feeding can also contribute to suppressing the appetite and preventing the child from developing the desire to eat, so contributing to feeding difficulties.

Blood glucose monitoring

Figure 10.2 outlines the management for blood glucose monitoring at the Royal Manchester Children's Hospital. Parents need to be taught how to measure and interpret finger/heel prick blood glucose levels, using a handheld device, prior to going home. The specialist nurse and/or ward

Flow Chart for the management of Blood Glucose (BG) Monitoring in Children with Hyperinsulinism on IV fluids only

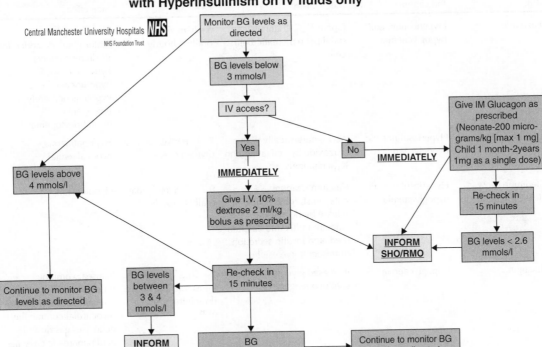

Figure 10.2   Blood glucose monitoring in CHI. Reprinted with permission of Royal Manchester Children's Hospital.

nursing staff should help with this. Blood glucose testing will normally be done prior to every feed and at other times when clinically indicated. This is very individual and parents need to be advised what is suitable for their child.

The parents need to be provided with an emergency regimen and a recipe for a 20% glucose polymer solution (20 g in 100 mL water) to be used if the child becomes acutely unwell and blood glucose levels are 2.6–4.0 mmol/L, assuming the child is conscious and able to swallow.

Pharmacological treatment

A summary of the drugs used in CHI are given in Table 10.7 [90]. Along with CHO supplementation, recommended initial drug treatments are oral diazoxide and chlorothiazide, which must be given together. Second line drugs are generally given when these drugs are ineffective, especially if glucose IV infusion remains essential. In

practice, however, they are often commenced if hypoglycaemia management is poor. They are given via injection or infusion.

Surgical treatment

Surgical treatment needs to be considered if medical management fails. Consensus opinion [71] has been that children should proceed to surgery sooner rather than later. However, more recent consensus is to try and preserve the pancreas by medical treatment as far as possible [90].

Focal lesionectomy should be considered if a solitary focus in the pancreas has been identified by PET CT scanning. In diffuse HI, the goal should be to ensure euglycaemia with medical treatment. However, if medical therapy fails to achieve satisfactory glucose levels, subtotal pancreatectomy (i.e. approximately 95% pancreas removed) may have to be considered. There is a high incidence of pancreatic endocrine and

Table 10.7 Pharmacological treatment.

Drug	Indications	Mechanism	Dose	Side effects
Diazoxide	Hyperinsulinaemic hypoglycaemia	Opens K_{ATP} channels and stabilises pancreatic beta cells	5–20 mg/kg/day orally 8 hourly	Fluid retention (chlorothiazide added for its diuretic effects), hypertrichosis, hyperuricaemia, hypotension, rarely leucopenia, thrombocytopenia
Chlorothiazide	Hyperinsulinaemic hypoglycaemia	Acts synergistically with diazoxide by activating non K_{ATP} channels	7–10 mg/kg/day in 2 divided doses	Hyponatraemia, hypokalaemia
Nifedipine (slow release preparation)	Hyperinsulinaemic hypoglycaemia	Calcium channel antagonist, inhibits insulin release by decreasing calcium influx and calcium mediated insulin secretion from secretory vesicles	0.25–2.5 mg/kg/day orally 8 hourly	Hypotension
Glucagon	Hypoglycaemia	Increased glycogenolysis/gluconeogenesis	1–10 µg/kg/hour IV infusion, 1 mg bolus dose intramuscular or IV	Nausea, vomiting, increases growth hormone concentrations, increases myocardial contractility, decreases gastric acid/pancreatic enzymes
Octreotide	Hyperinsulinaemic hypoglycaemia	Activates G protein coupled rectifier K channel	5–20 µg/kg/day IV or subcutaneous infusion	Suppression of growth hormone, steatorrhoea, cholelithiasis, abdominal distension, hair loss, hepatitis

IV, intravenous.

exocrine insufficiency after subtotal pancreatectomy. This is in contrast with focal lesionectomy for children with focal disease where, in most instances, a majority of normal pancreatic tissue can be conserved.

Postoperative management

Glucose intolerance

Infants often become hyperglycaemic in the immediate postoperative period. Sliding scale insulin will often be required with a small dextrose requirement [71]. This requirement for insulin usually lessens early on in the postoperative period. The optimal result, of course, is to be able to cease all medical treatment. Those with focal

disease have the better outcome [91] and cure from hypoglycaemia is achieved without the risk of long term diabetes.

Diabetes

After a 95% subtotal pancreatectomy the risk of developing secondary diabetes mellitus is high [92, 93]. However, unlike in children with type 1 diabetes, there appears to be a resistance to diabetic ketoacidosis and hyperketonaemia [94]. Usually an intermediate acting insulin or a mix of short and long acting insulin is the preferred treatment option, along with dietary manipulation [71]. As yet, it is not known if these children will go on to develop the same diabetic complications, and to the same extent, as children with type 1 diabetes mellitus.

Pancreatic exocrine insufficiency

In children undergoing subtotal pancreatectomy, the diagnosis of impaired pancreatic exocrine function is carried out by measurement of faecal elastase. Pancreatic enzyme replacement therapy (PERT) will be required in those with decreased levels (p. 223). If the child is being tube fed, it may be necessary to use a feed with a high level of medium chain triglyceride fat if there is difficulty in achieving good absorption, even with the use of PERT. An example of this is a child who is primarily tube fed or who is nil by mouth and unable to take PERT orally.

Chylothorax

Chylothorax is a possible complication post surgery. It can be treated conservatively using a minimal long chain triglyceride diet or feed, for as long as is required (p. 294).

Further hypoglycaemia

In diffuse disease, even after 95% subtotal pancreatectomy, there is a small risk that some children will remain hypoglycaemic. This may be due to excess insulin secretion from the remnant pancreatic tissue. If hypoglycaemia persists after focal lesionectomy, the possibility of inadequate resection of the focal lesion or an ectopic lesion should be considered. For some children with diffuse HI there may be an initial period of good control, with worsening glycaemic status developing weeks or months later. While the cause for this is not fully clear, it is assumed that regeneration or regrowth of pancreatic remnant tissue may be partially responsible. Table 10.8 summarises the features of diffuse and focal disease post resection.

Psychosocial aspects

With its relentless treatment and the ever present risk of severe hypoglycaemia and its potential for hypoglycaemic brain damage, managing CHI can place an unbearable load on families. Skilled and

Table 10.8 Features of diffuse and focal disease post resection.

Diffuse disease	Focal disease
Small risk of hypoglycaemia remains	Usually cured of hypoglycaemia after a partial pancreatectomy
Postoperative risk of diabetes	No increased risk of diabetes
May require pancreatic enzyme replacement therapy postoperatively	No increased risk of fat malabsorption

experienced psychological and social support is essential.

Acknowledgements

With thanks to the CHI team at Royal Manchester Children's Hospital for their comments, particularly Dr I. Banerjee and Dr R. Padidela, Specialist CHI Nurse Lindsey Rigby and dietetic colleague Lynette Forsyth.

Useful addresses

The website for families of children with hyperinsulinism

> http://www.sur1.org

Congenital Hyperinsulinism International

> http://congenitalhi.org/

UK CHI Support Group Website:

> http://www.hi-fund.org/www.hi-fund.org
> Tel: 07974 973621
> Email: matthewammo@hotmail.com

Children's Hyperinsulinism UK Facebook Discussion

> http://www.facebook.com/groups /137059853012784/

Follow CHI on Twitter

> https://twitter.com/HIFundUK

11

Cystic Fibrosis

Carolyn Patchell

Introduction

Cystic fibrosis (CF) is the most common recessively inherited life limiting disease in the UK. Incidence rates are around 1 in 2500 live births and approximately 1 in 25 of the population is a carrier for the disease [1]. There are approximately 9000 patients currently in the UK [2]. CF mostly affects Caucasian populations; however, there are a significant number of cases amongst families from the Indian subcontinent and the Middle East. It is rare in Chinese, South East Asian and African-Caribbean ethnic groups.

The outlook for patients with CF has steadily improved over the years as a result of early diagnosis; more aggressive treatment; agreed standards of care which define assessment, monitoring, detection and treatment of complications; and the recommendation that care is delivered in specialist centres by a multidisciplinary team of trained health professionals experienced in the management of the condition [3]. The proportion of adults with CF has increased dramatically and currently stands at 56% of the CF population [2]. Median survival is 41.4 years and is predicted to be 50 years of age for infants born in 2000 [4].

CF is caused by a mutation of the cystic fibrosis transmembrane conductance regulator gene (CFTR). This results in dysfunction in the regulation of salt and water across the cell membranes of secretory epithelial cells and in thickened secretions in all organs with epithelial cells; hence CF is a multi-organ condition. Approximately 1500 different genetic mutations have been identified. The most common genotype which accounts for around 52% of cases is homozygote ΔF508, with F508 plus one other genotype accounting for approximately 39% of cases. Class I, II and III mutations are the most severe giving rise to more typical presentations of CF. Class IV and V mutations give rise to milder or atypical CF.

The clinical consequences include

- recurrent respiratory infection, inflammation, bronchial damage, bronchiectasis resulting ultimately in respiratory failure
- exocrine pancreatic dysfunction with approximately 85% of patients suffering from insufficiency in pancreatic enzyme production, malabsorption and, if not adequately controlled, malnutrition
- bowel obstruction with approximately 15% of infants suffering from meconium ileus at birth, and recurrent bowel blockages in older patients due to distal intestinal obstruction syndrome
- impaired glucose tolerance or CF related diabetes

- liver disease and portal hypertension
- reduced bone mineral density
- gut motility problems
- infertility in most males
- CF arthropathy
- behavioural and psychological problems as a result of severe life limiting disease

Diagnosis

Newborn screening for CF was introduced across the UK in October 2007. All infants born since this date are offered screening for CF on day 5 of life. There are best practice guidelines defining the protocol for screening and diagnosis, and guidelines for management of infants picked up through screening [5, 6]. The majority of CF diagnoses are made through this programme and should be confirmed by sweat test and/or genetic mutation analysis by 4 weeks of age. Early diagnosis through newborn screening has been shown to confer significant benefits, especially in terms of growth and nutrition [7, 8].

The majority of cases picked up through screening have typical CF; however, the nature of the screening programme will result in some cases where diagnosis is uncertain because of anomalies in the genotype, phenotype or sweat test result. These cases should still be managed in a CF specialist centre.

Some cases of CF will not be picked up through the screening programme, either because they were born before October 2007, were born outside of the UK, or missed the screening process. A clinical diagnosis will be made in these patients, confirmed through sweat test and genetic mutation analysis.

Clinical features

Chronic respiratory disease

The lungs are normal at birth but may become affected early in life [5, 6]. Due to the abnormal secretions there is obstruction of the small airways, with secondary infection and inflammation. Recurrent infection with organisms such as *Staphylococcus aureus*, *Haemophilus influenzae* and *Pseudomonas* sp. leads to damage of the bronchial wall, bronchiectasis and abscess formation.

The major objective of chest treatment is to prevent infection, remove secretions and thereby delay the rate of lung damage and maintain respiratory function. This is done by:

- regular surveillance of secretions and prompt and aggressive treatment of infection with antibiotic therapy, either oral, aerosol or intravenous
- oral prophylactic antibiotic therapy in younger children
- regular chest physiotherapy to aid removal of bronchial secretions
- use of bronchodilators and oral steroids to open the airways and reduce inflammation
- encouragement of an active lifestyle and physical exercise

Gastrointestinal symptoms

Pancreatic insufficiency

Pancreatic insufficiency (PI) is the most common gastrointestinal defect in CF affecting approximately 95% of patients in northern Europe [9]. Approximately 92% of infants will be pancreatic insufficient by the age of 12 months [10], although the introduction of newborn screening and early identification of patients with milder mutations may result in the proportion of patients with known pancreatic sufficiency increasing in the future.

PI develops when more than 90% of acinar function is lost. Damage begins *in utero* and there is ongoing destruction of acini and replacement with fibrous and fatty tissue. Consequently the secretion of digestive enzymes and bicarbonate is reduced or absent, resulting in malabsorption of fat, protein, bile, fat soluble vitamins and vitamin B_{12}. Treatment is with the use of pancreatic enzyme replacement therapy (PERT).

Diagnosis of PI is made by faecal elastase measurement. In the 10%–15% who are defined as having normal pancreatic function at diagnosis, enzyme secretion may be diminished. However, it may be sufficient for digestion of nutrients without the need for PERT [11]. A proportion of those with normal faecal elastase will go on to develop PI; faecal elastase should be rechecked periodically and if symptoms of malabsorption develop.

Meconium ileus

Meconium ileus is the presenting feature in up to 25% of infants with CF. It becomes apparent within the first days of life and often before the result of newborn screening is available. It is caused by a blockage of the terminal ileum with thick meconium and develops *in utero*. Management of meconium ileus may be conservative; however, some patients will require surgical intervention, with or without intestinal resection and stoma formation.

Distal intestinal obstruction syndrome

Distal intestinal obstruction syndrome (DIOS) is a common complication in CF and estimates suggest a prevalence of 5–12 episodes per 1000 patients per year in children [12]. It is characterised by frequent abdominal pain, accompanied by complete or partial intestinal obstruction. Faecal material and mucus gathers in the distal ileum and there is often a palpable mass in the right lower abdomen.

DIOS is more common in older patients, in those with PI (although it can be seen in pancreatic sufficient patients) and in those who have had previous gastrointestinal surgery. It usually responds to medical management including rehydration combined with stool softening laxatives or gut lavage. In extreme cases surgical intervention may be necessary.

Gastro-oesophageal reflux

Gastro-oesophageal reflux (GOR) has been reported in approximately 20% of infants with CF [13], although in a review of screened infants at one UK centre incidence was as high as 43% [14]. The mechanisms are unclear; however, it is considered to be mainly due to inappropriate relaxation of the gastro-oesophageal sphincter. GOR is most prevalent in young children with CF and improves with age. GOR may result in poor weight gain, feeding disturbances, abdominal pain, and respiratory symptoms including wheeze and reflex bronchospasm. Treatment includes thickening feeds and the use of anti-reflux medication [15].

Abdominal pain

Abdominal pain has been reported in approximately 30% of patients [16]. It is particularly common in children with poorly controlled malabsorption or constipation, but may be due to other disorders including intussusception, appendicitis, Crohn's disease and cow's milk protein enteropathy. Abdominal pain may negatively impact on nutritional intake and nutritional status.

Other gastrointestinal problems

Other problems include rectal prolapse, acute pancreatitis, coeliac disease and Crohn's disease.

Other clinical problems

CF related diabetes

CF related diabetes (CFRD) is the most common comorbidity affecting approximately 19% of adolescents and up to 50% of adults [17]. The prevalence is increasing with the increased survival of people with CF. It is a distinct type of diabetes with features of both type 1 and type 2 diabetes. There is progressive fibrous and fatty infiltration of the exocrine pancreas resulting in destruction of the islet cells, leading to loss of endocrine cells and reduced insulin production. In addition there may be insulin resistance.

The development of CFRD is often gradual, preceded by worsening of nutritional status and decline in lung function. Regular screening and prompt treatment is essential to prevent clinical deterioration. The development of CFRD has a negative impact on growth in adolescents [18] and on nutritional status, respiratory function and survival [17, 19–21]. It is more common in females than males [22–24].

Treatment aims are to eradicate hyperglycaemia and to maintain good nutrition and lung function. Clinical improvement and reversal of decline in pulmonary function and nutritional status has been documented when the diabetes is treated with insulin [25, 26].

Diagnosis and screening
Annual screening for CFRD is recommended through random blood glucose level monitoring; in some situations detailed assessment may be required in between annual reviews. The incidence of CFRD increases after 10 years of age by approximately 5% annually.

International consensus is yet to be established; however, UK CF Trust and American Diabetes Association guidance [27, 28] recommends that all patients over the age of 12 years should be screened annually by performing a standard oral glucose tolerance test (OGTT, T0, T120 75 g). A diabetic OGTT does not necessarily mean that the individual has CFRD, but shows that at the time of the assessment the patient had abnormal handling of glucose which may revert to normal. The result of the OGTT should be considered alongside the clinical picture at the time. An abnormal OGTT or impaired OGTT indicates a higher risk for developing CFRD. HbA1c is not considered sensitive enough for detecting CFRD, possibly because hyperglycaemia may be transient or because red blood cell turnover is elevated due to chronic inflammation in CF.

Assessment of glycaemic control in between annual assessments should be considered in the following circumstances:

- symptoms of hyperglycaemia or hypoglycaemia
- unexplained decline in nutritional status
- unexplained decline in lung function
- on commencement of continuous enteral feeding; mid and immediate post feeding blood glucose levels should be measured and repeated monthly at home
- during infective exacerbations or corticosteroid use

Possible action to be taken on the results of routine OGTT are given in Table 11.1.

Whilst OGTT remains the gold standard for the diagnosis of CFRD, continuous glucose monitoring is increasingly being used to aid diagnosis and

Table 11.1 Possible action to be taken on the results of routine oral glucose tolerance test (OGTT).

OGTT result	Action
Normal OGTT	Repeat in 1 year
Impaired OGTT	Repeat in 1 year or sooner if clinical parameters worsen
Diabetes OGTT without symptoms	Home blood glucose monitoring. If normal repeat in 6 months
Diabetes OGTT with symptoms	Start treatment

treatment [29–31]. Dobson et al. [32] describe a 'pre diabetic phase' in the development of CFRD which may be clinically significant. This phase may present up to 4 years prior to diagnosis of CFRD using OGTT, and is characterised by deterioration in lung function, poor growth and weight gain. This raises concern regarding the sensitivity of the standard OGTT as a diagnostic tool and a continuous glucose monitoring system (CGMS) may be more sensitive in detecting this early stage [33, 34].

CGMS may be particularly useful for patients receiving overnight enteral nutrition, when the overnight glucose loading may predispose to nocturnal hyperglycaemia and home monitoring may be practically difficult.

Medical management and treatment
Patients should be referred to a diabetologist, ideally one who has an interest in CF and works alongside the CF team, seeing patients where possible in joint CF/diabetes clinics.

Insulin is the mainstay of treatment of CFRD [28, 35] and the aim of treatment is to eradicate symptoms of hyperglycaemia, maintain nutritional status and pulmonary function, and reduce the risk of long term microvascular complications. Insulin has a potent anabolic effect which may be of additional benefit for children and young people with growth and nutritional difficulties.

Optimal control may be difficult to achieve in the adolescent age group due to difficulties with compliance, variable food intake, exercise and growth. Insulin regimens need regular review and adjustment and should be individualised to take into account the eating habits and lifestyle of the child or adolescent. Once or twice daily mixed insulin injections may be used; however, better control may be obtained with multiple daily injections of short acting insulin given with meals. The advantage of this is that the dose may be adjusted for differing intake of food. Multiple daily injections, however, increase the burden of treatment and carry a risk of hypoglycaemia. Recent uncontrolled trials suggest that once daily injections of intermediate or long acting insulin improve weight and lung function and are useful in CFRD and early insulin deficiency [36].

Experience in the use of insulin pumps for the treatment of CFRD is in its infancy; however, initial studies suggest improvements in blood glucose control, body weight and lean body mass [37].

Cystic fibrosis associated liver disease

Approximately 5%–10% of patients develop multi-lobular cirrhosis during the first decade of life. Most patients later develop signs of portal hypertension with complications such as variceal bleeding. Liver failure develops later usually in adult life, but is not inevitable. Cystic fibrosis associated liver disease (CFLD) is associated with more severe CF phenotypes [38].

Annual screening for liver disease is important to detect pre symptomatic signs; the bile acid ursodeoxycholic acid, which may halt progression of liver disease, should be commenced. Liver disease should be considered if the patient has two of the following: persistently abnormal liver function tests, abnormal physical examination or abnormal liver ultrasound. A liver biopsy should be performed if there is doubt over the diagnosis. Patients should have annual assessment of liver function.

The development of liver disease has a negative impact on nutritional status [38], often as a result of worsening fat absorption, and aggressive nutritional management is important to reverse this trend [39]. Liver transplantation remains the only option for those who develop end stage liver disease and is considered to be effective, initially stabilising the decline in pulmonary function which is a feature of the development of CFLD. One year survival post transplant is estimated at 92.3% and 84.1% after 5 years [40]. Studies suggest, however, that nutritional status does not improve post liver transplant and pre transplant body mass index (BMI) does not alter survival [41].

Bone disease

Reduced bone mineral density (BMD) was first described in CF in 1979, but the full extent of the problem was not apparent until the 1990s when detailed studies were performed. Patients may develop low BMD through either osteoporosis or vitamin D deficiency osteomalacia. Studies suggest that BMD is normal in well nourished CF children with well preserved lung function, but many patients fail to gain bone mass normally and/or experience premature bone loss in adolescence or early adult life; 23.5% of adults are reported to have osteoporosis [42] and up to 38% of patients assessed in one centre demonstrated evidence of reduced bone mineral mass [43]. The premature bone loss is preceded by reduced peak bone mass accrual in adolescence [44, 45].

The aetiology of low BMD is multifactorial and major risk factors include [46, 47]

- overall disease severity, including links to FEV1 (forced expiratory volume in 1 second)
- the frequency and duration of intravenous antibiotic therapy
- corticosteroid use
- exercise tolerance and levels of physical activity
- DF508 genotype
- CFRD
- delayed puberty

Peak growth velocity is associated with high bone mass accrual. In healthy populations, peak bone mass accrual occurs at 11.7 years in girls and 13.4 years in boys. Puberty may be delayed in CF and this is associated with a reduction in bone age and delay in peak height velocity by 9–14 months [48].

There are also nutritional factors:

- nutritional status and lean body mass
- vitamin D status may result in impaired bone mineralisation and increased loss
- vitamin K deficiency may contribute by altering the balance of bone formation and resorption
- calcium intake

Diagnosis of low BMD

CF Trust guidelines [45] recommend that BMD should be measured in the lumbar spine from around 10 years of age. These scans (DXA scans) should ideally be done in a centre with a clinical team experienced in performing and interpreting bone densitometry in children. DXA scans should be repeated every 1–5 years; serial measurements will allow for identification of peak bone mass and this may influence treatment options if premature bone loss occurs.

Recommendations to optimise bone health

Low BMD in adults has its origins in childhood and factors to optimise bone health should be considered in paediatric care. Dietary factors play a significant role and it is important that patients are regularly reviewed by an experienced paediatric dietitian with the aim of achieving normal weight, height, body composition, optimal vitamin D and K status and adequate calcium intake.

Weight bearing physical exercise should be encouraged. Children and adolescents should be encouraged to exercise for 20–30 minutes three times per week and exercises should include high impact weight bearing exercises.

Glucocorticosteroid use should be minimised and CF pulmonary exacerbations should be promptly treated to minimise the systemic inflammatory effect on bone. Pubertal delay should be recognised and treated.

Malnutrition in cystic fibrosis

The malnutrition seen in CF is multifactorial and is determined by three main features: energy loss, increased energy expenditure and anorexia.

Energy loss

Pancreatic insufficiency in the majority of patients with CF results in pancreatic exocrine secretions containing fewer enzymes and bicarbonate; pancreatic secretions have a lower pH and are a smaller volume than in those with pancreatic sufficiency. The consequence, when untreated, is foul smelling frequent loose stools. Malabsorption of fat and nitrogen is severe in untreated patients; however, carbohydrate malabsorption is minimal. Malabsorption can be controlled with the use of PERT although, even when treated, many patients still have a degree of fat malabsorption. Estimates suggest that stool energy losses account for up to 11% of gross energy intake [49].

Pancreatic bicarbonate deficiency results in reduced buffering of gastric acid in the duodenum, resulting in decreased efficiency of pancreatic enzymes. Mucosal ion transport abnormalities affect water and electrolyte transport and there may be impaired mucosal uptake of nutrients. Altered motility may affect intestinal transit time and impact on absorption of nutrients.

Energy losses may be further exacerbated by previous gastrointestinal surgery for meconium ileus which may result in shortening of the bowel, strictures at the site of anastomoses, malrotation and adhesions. Energy may be lost due to vomiting following coughing and GOR. Untreated CFRD will cause energy loss through glycosuria. CFLD may increase malabsorption.

Increased energy expenditure

Many investigators describe an increase in resting energy expenditure (REE) in patients with CF, with a large range of requirements. Impaired lung function significantly increases REE and can double REE above that of controls [50]. Increased REE is closely associated with declining pulmonary function and subclinical infection [51–54].

Continuous injury to the lungs leads to progressive fibrosis and airway obstruction, with increased work of breathing. Data are conflicting on total energy expenditure, with evidence that patients with moderate lung impairment adapt to increased REE by reducing activity levels, thereby maintaining their energy expenditure levels [55]. The variability in energy requirements between patients emphasises the need for individual assessment.

Anorexia and low energy intakes

Poor dietary intake can contribute to malnutrition in children with CF. Appetite is often reduced during pulmonary exacerbations. This leads to a familiar pattern of weight gain between exacerbations and weight loss during, thus impairing long term nutritional status. Dietary assessments in CF children demonstrate that energy intake is higher than in controls, but rarely exceeds 111% [56–58].

Behavioural feeding difficulties and poor child–parent interactions at mealtimes can be a problem and mealtimes are often reported to be a time of conflict. Abnormal eating behaviours include excessively long mealtimes, delay tactics, food refusal and spitting out food [59,60].

Benefits of good nutrition

There has been evidence of strong links between improved nutritional status and survival for over 30 years. A study compared patients in two North American clinics: one treated patients with the low fat diet which was the gold standard treatment at the time; the other clinic treated patients with a high fat diet. Those receiving the high fat diet were found to be taller and heavier and to have improved survival [61]. The improvement in nutritional status was considered to be the main difference for the increased survival seen between the two clinics.

Other studies have shown the effect of nutrition on prognosis. Growth failure and wasting are both independent prognostic indicators in survival. Patients with height <5th percentile at 5 years of age have a significantly increased risk of death; this increase persists at 7 years of age [62]. Patients with ideal body weight >85% have a better prognosis at 5 years of age than those with body weight <85% [63]. Good nutritional status is also positively correlated with lung function [64]. Malnutrition results in poor height growth, impaired respiratory muscle function, immunological impairment and increased susceptibility to infection [65, 66].

Assessment of growth and nutritional status

Regular and accurate nutritional assessment is vital so that decline in nutritional status is picked up and treated promptly. European [50], UK [67] and North American guidelines [68] give guidance on frequency and methods of assessment and interpretation of results.

Weight, height and head circumference

Sequential measurements of height and weight (and head circumference in children <2 years of age) should be carried out at every clinic visit so that malnutrition is prevented or at least detected early and interventions are put in place promptly. Measurements should be carried out by appropriately trained staff following national and local guidelines and plotted on appropriate centile charts so that comparison may be made with standards [69].

Delayed puberty in adolescents with CF should be taken into account when interpreting growth as there may be an overestimation of malnutrition, as height velocity slows prior to the pubertal growth spurt. Assessment and consideration of pubertal stage is therefore important when considering nutritional status in this age group [67, 68].

Body mass index

BMI is a measure of body fatness or thinness and is a calculation of weight (kg) ÷ height (m)^2. There are BMI centile charts for age and sex (UK 1990 data). Care should be taken in the interpretation of BMI, as inaccurate assessments can be made in children whose height has been impacted by chronic malnutrition or delayed puberty. An expert consensus group of the Royal College of Paediatrics and Child Health (2009) recommended that BMI be used in children as a measure of thinness or fatness in children over 2 years of age, when height can be measured accurately [70]. For children <2 years, when height/length is more difficult to measure, BMI measurements should be interpreted with caution and used in combination with other measures. BMI centile may pick up nutritional failure in children >2 years of age more accurately than height for age percentile, weight for age percentile and percentage ideal body weight [71].

Percentage weight for age, height for age and percentage weight for height

Percentage weight for height (%wt/ht) is often used in CF centres as a measure of nutritional status and is calculated by weight (kg) × 100/weight (kg) equivalent to current height centile.

Serial measurements of %wt/age and %ht/age are also useful to track progress of individual patients. %wt/ht, like BMI, assesses weight in proportion to height, but does not assess stunting or the impact of delayed puberty. Serial measurements of %wt/age and %ht/age must be considered together. Although the calculation is simple to do, a high degree of inaccuracy has been reported in clinical practice [72]. Since no single method provides an accurate assessment of nutritional status, a variety of the above measures should be used, and any changes over time used to inform nutritional management.

Skinfold thickness and mid upper arm circumference

Measurement of skinfold thickness uses subcutaneous fat to determine total body fatness; however, reliability of this as a proxy for body fatness is poor [73] so skinfold thickness measurements are not used routinely in clinical practice.

Mid upper arm circumference gives an estimation of lean body mass and may be a useful measure of nutritional status in patients with significant organomegaly or fluid retention, as may be seen in patients with advanced CFLD. There are normal data to compare individual patient data against so that trends can be monitored [74].

Bone age and bone mineral density

Bone age should be assessed in any child with stunting (%ht/age <90%, or height <0.4th centile) or with pubertal delay.

Bone mineral density should be measured in a specialist CF centre in all children >10 years of age and repeated every 1–5 years, depending on the degree of reduced BMD observed.

Definitions of growth failure

Consensus reports and UK CF Trust guidelines define malnutrition in children and young people up to the age of 18 years as follows.

Children <5 years of age:

- wt/ht <85%
- weight loss or plateau in weight over two clinic visits (maximum interval 4 months)

Children 5–18 years of age:

- wt/ht <85%
- weight loss or plateau in weight over two clinic visits (maximum interval 6 months)

Aims of nutritional management

The aims of nutritional management are that children with CF are appropriately nourished, with normal weight, height, body composition, pubertal development, normal feeding behaviour; and have optimal vitamin, mineral, antioxidant and essential fatty acid status.

Nutritional requirements

Nutritional requirements are increased in CF as a result of the demands of progressive pulmonary disease, plus malabsorption of fat and protein in pancreatic insufficient patients. Crude estimates suggest that patients require 120%–150% of the estimated energy requirement for age and sex [51, 52].

The heterogeneity of CF patients, including the presence of respiratory infection, extent of chronic pulmonary disease, nutritional status and presence of comorbidities, makes it difficult to give universal recommendations for energy requirements. For this reason, it is essential that each patient's nutritional status is closely monitored and adjustments made to energy intake in response to progress.

Some children will grow normally by consuming no more than the estimated energy requirement for energy while others with more advanced disease, or during respiratory exacerbations, will need considerably more. In patients exhibiting poor growth or weight gain, a useful guide is for the current intake to be assessed by an experienced paediatric dietitian and an increase in energy of between 20%–30% recommended, followed by monitoring and further adjustment as necessary.

International consensus recommends that patients have access to a CF specialist dietitian at every outpatient review, annual assessment and inpatient admission [3]; and that nutritional status and growth are constantly monitored, with a staged nutritional intervention approach as shown in Table 11.2, depending on nutritional status [67].

Table 11.2 Criteria for different stages of nutritional intervention.

	<5 years	5–8 years
Normal nutritional status: preventative counselling	Weight/height 90%–110%	Weight/height 90%–110%
Active intervention: consider supplements	Weight/height 85%–89% or weight loss over 4 months or plateau in weight for over 6 months	Weight/height 85%–89% or weight loss over 6 months or plateau in weight for over 6 months
Aggressive nutritional support	Supplements tried and either weight/height <85% or weight falling 2 centile spaces	Supplements tried and either weight/height <85% or weight falling 2 centile spaces

Preventative counselling

Preventative counselling is recommended for all patients regardless of nutritional and clinical status. The diet should be assessed and advice given to ensure adequate energy, protein, vitamin and mineral intake to meet the patient's individual requirements based on their changing clinical needs. It is important that a good routine is established and a wide variety of foods is given; and attention should be paid to the psychological, social, behavioural and developmental aspects of feeding. Parents should be encouraged to adopt normal feeding routines and advice should be given to minimise the development of poor feeding behaviours.

Increased energy intake from normal diet

If weight gain is suboptimal, advice should be given to maximise intake from a normal diet by increasing the energy density of foods and encouraging mid meal snacks. A high fat diet is usually recommended. Advice should be given to substitute low fat foods, eaten by the family, with high fat alternatives such as full fat yoghurt, full fat milk and cheese. This allows the child to eat a similar diet to the rest of the family but to achieve a higher energy intake. With the increasing longevity of patients with CF it seems prudent to encourage the use of mono-unsaturated and polyunsaturated fats where possible; these fats can be used in spreads and cooking oils.

Refined carbohydrate intake may also be increased as this will increase energy intake without increasing the bulk of the diet significantly. Snacks should be encouraged between meals, but these should be age appropriate in size and timed such that they do not reduce the intake of energy at main mealtimes. Care should be taken to ensure that a good routine is maintained, that snack foods do not substitute meals and that the overall quality of the diet is maintained.

The increased public awareness of healthy eating may result in the need to explain the reasons for a seemingly 'unhealthy' diet to others who care for the child with CF, e.g. school, nursery, child minder and extended family members. Many schools have healthy eating policies which discourage the consumption of snacks between meals and, with the family's consent, the school should be approached to request that snacks are given.

Oral supplementation

Oral nutritional supplements may be useful if wt/ht is 85%–89%; there has been no weight gain for 4 months in children under 5 years of age, or 6 months in children over 5 years of age; there has been a plateau in weight for 4–6 months, despite maximising energy intake from a normal diet.

A wide range of supplements are available and are approved for prescription by ACBS (Advisory Committee on Borderline Substances) (Table 11.3). The type and quantity should be prescribed for the individual depending on age, preferences and nutritional requirements. They should be used to supplement a normal diet and care should be given over the quantity and timing to ensure that they do not replace meals.

A UK multicentre longitudinal study has shown that their use can promote weight gain [75] and improve protein and energy intakes [76,77], although a Cochrane review of trials assessing the efficacy of oral supplements in CF reported an increase in energy intake in those taking supplements, but no difference in nutritional or growth factors was observed. The conclusion was that dietary counselling was sufficient to manage the diet of moderately malnourished children and that randomised controlled trials should look at the use of oral supplements for acute weight loss and for long term use in adult patients [78].

The use of supplements in the management of patients with CF is therefore controversial, but these products are frequently used in clinical practice and their use should be considered if there are ongoing nutritional concerns despite maximising dietary intake from food.

Enteral nutrition

Enteral feeding should be considered if dietary counselling and oral nutritional supplements have failed to prevent or reverse nutritional decline and the child has wt/ht <85%; or weight falling by 2 centile positions.

Early discussion about enteral feeding is important so that the patient and family understand the need for this should other methods of nutrition support fail. The decision to start enteral feeding should be made in consideration of other factors and a global nutritional and clinical assessment may prompt the introduction of feeding sooner, or

Table 11.3 Useful dietary supplements in cystic fibrosis suitable for children aged 1–16 years.

	Energy (kcal)	(kJ)	Protein (g)	Fibre (g)
Fortified milk shakes (per 100 mL)				
Ensure	100	420	4.0	–
Fresubin	100	420	3.8	–
Paediasure	100	420	2.8	–
Paediasure Fibre	100	420	2.8	0.5
Fortini	150	630	3.4	–
Fortini Multi Fibre	150	630	3.4	1.5
Fortini Smoothie	150	630	3.4	1.4
Fortisip	150	630	6.0	–
Fortisip Multi Fibre	150	630	6.0	2.3
Fortisip Yogurt Style	150	630	6.0	200 mg
Frebini Energy Fibre	150	630	3.8	1.1
Paediasure Plus	150	630	4.2	–
Paediasure Plus Fibre	150	630	4.2	1.1
Resource Junior	150	630	3.0	–
Fortified 'juice' drinks (per 100 mL)				
Ensure Plus Juce	150	630	4.8	–
Fortijuce	150	630	4.0	–
Fresubin Jucy	150	630	4.0	–
Paediasure Plus Juce	150	630	4.2	–
Fortified semi-solid supplements (per 100 g)				
Ensure Plus Crème	137	570	5.68	–
Fortisip Fruit Dessert	133	560	7.0	2.6
Fortini Creamy Fruit	150	630	3.5	1.9
Resource Dessert Energy	160	670	4.8	–
Glucose polymer powders (per 100 g)				
Caloreen	390	1630	–	–
Polycal	384	1605	–	–
Super Soluble Maxijul	380	1590	–	–
Vitajoule	380	1590	–	–
Glucose polymer drinks (per 100 mL)				
Liquid Polycal	247	1030	–	–
Liquid Maxijul	200	840	–	–
Fat supplements (per 100 mL)				
Calogen	450	1880	–	–
Fat and carbohydrate (per 100 mL)				
Duocal Liquid	166	695	–	–
Protein, fat and carbohydrate (per 100 mL)				
Enshake	450	1880	8.4	–
Pro-Cal Shot	334	1395	6.7	–
Scandishake	500	2090	4.7	–

Table 11.4 Criteria for starting enteral feeding in cystic fibrosis.

Objective criterion	Subjective criterion
Previous weight history	Psychosocial implications
Rate of weight loss	Emotional acceptance
Control of malabsorption	Patient and/or carer workload
Respiratory function	
Frequency of respiratory exacerbation	
Clinical disease severity	
Transplant status	
Liver disease	
Diabetic status	

delay it. Some factors to take into consideration are listed in Table 11.4 [79].

Enteral tube feeding has been shown to improve weight gain and nutritional status in CF patients [80, 81] and to have a positive impact on respiratory function [82–84], and early intervention is shown to have the greatest impact in terms of improvements in height for age and BMI [85]. Feeding may be by nasogastric tube or gastrostomy tube. Concerns may be raised about body image, especially in the adolescent age group; however, positive outcomes in terms of improved quality of life have been reported [86].

Feeds are usually given overnight and oral diet is encouraged in the daytime. The timing of the enteral feeding should be adjusted to fit in with family lifestyle. Compliance may be improved if there is some flexibility in terms of the number of nights of feeding to be given, with the option of one or two nights per week without feeding to allow for social activities to continue. There are few published data or randomised controlled studies looking at routes of feed administration or type of feed used in CF. A survey of dietitians in the USA demonstrated a wide range in practice [87] and the need to develop evidence based clinical guidelines for children with CF.

Routes of feeding

Nasogastric feeding

Nasogastric (NG) feeding is often considered as a short term option to support weight gain during respiratory exacerbations, or as a trial prior to gastrostomy insertion. The choice of feeding route, however, should remain with the patient and carers. Patients and carers can be trained to pass the NG tube and may do so nightly, allowing them to remove the tube during the day. NG tube feeding may be the preferred option in patients with oesophageal or gastric varices in whom gastrostomy placement may be contraindicated. The main disadvantages of NG tube feeding are coughing, which may displace the tube; difficulties passing the tube, particularly in those with nasal polyps; nasal irritation; and swallowing enzymes, which may be uncomfortable for some patients who have a tube *in situ*.

Gastrostomy feeding

Gastrostomy feeding is generally considered the preferential route for long term feeding. Feeding may be more comfortable, particularly during exacerbations. Tubes are often inserted endoscopically, although laparoscopic insertion may be indicated in those with previous abdominal surgery. Patients have the option of a gastrostomy tube or button device, which may be used 2–3 months after gastrostomy tube insertion.

Types of feed

There are few published data comparing the efficacy of different feed types for children with CF.

Polymeric feeds

Whole protein polymeric feeds are tolerated by most patients and are the first choice of feed in most CF centres. Patients usually tolerate a 1.5 kcal/mL (6 kJ/mL) standard paediatric feed or adult feeds depending on age or weight, e.g. Nutrini Energy Multi Fibre, Paediasure Plus Fibre, Frebini Energy Fibre, Tentrini Energy Multi Fibre, Nutrison Energy Multi Fibre, Osmolite 1.5, Fresubin Energy Fibre. There are distinct advantages in the use of these feeds: they are cheap, prescribable, have low osmolarity and are available as sterile, ready to hang packs. No difference in fat malabsorption, nitrogen absorption or weight gain has been seen when polymeric feeds, given with PERT, are compared with hydrolysed protein feeds (semi-elemental feeds) [88].

Elemental feeds

Little work has been done comparing the use of amino acid based feeds (elemental feeds) with polymeric feeds in CF. Amino acid based feeds are generally lower in fat than polymeric feeds and contain a mixture of medium and long chain fat, which in theory reduces the amount of PERT required. They are expensive, have a higher osmolarity and lower energy density than polymeric feeds, and are not the first choice of feed in many centres (Table 7.11).

High fat feeds

High fat feeds may have a theoretical advantage in patients with severe lung disease as they result in less carbon dioxide production and lower respiratory quotient. One study [89] concluded that despite the increase in carbon dioxide after being fed a high carbohydrate formula, patients who were clinically stable were able to increase their respiratory minute volume sufficiently to compensate for this. High fat feeds are not routinely used in clinical practice.

Pancreatic enzymes with feeds

Practical administration of enzymes with overnight enteral feeds varies between CF centres; however, one study showed optimum fat absorption when the enzymes were given in a divided dose, at the start of the feed and part way through the feed [90]. Patients are usually advised to take half the dose orally at the start of the feed and the other half mid feed or post feed. It is not common practice to wake patients to take their enzymes. Enzymes should be taken orally and not put down the feeding tube.

An initial dose of enzymes based on the fat content of the feed titrated against the number of enzymes required for a fat containing meal or snack is used, and adjusted based on gastrointestinal symptoms.

Enteral feeding in ventilated patients

Pancreatic enzymes are usually given orally, which is not possible in ventilated patients. The choice of feed in these circumstances is usually an amino acid based, medium chain triglyceride containing feed, e.g. Emsogen, Elemental 028 Extra, given continuously over 24 hours. The need for enzymes is reduced in these circumstances. If there are signs of malabsorption powdered enzyme preparations, mixed with water, may be administered via the feeding tube.

Vitamin, mineral and other supplementation

Exocrine pancreatic insufficiency and altered bile salt metabolism contribute to fat soluble vitamin deficiency in most patients with CF. Biochemical evidence of fat soluble vitamin deficiency has been reported in 79% of newborn screened infants at diagnosis [91] and even in screened pancreatic sufficient infants [92].

All patients should have the following plasma levels measured annually, ideally at a time of clinical stability: fat soluble vitamins A, D, E; total cholesterol; vitamin E:fasting lipid ratio; prothrombin time [50,67]. Retinol binding protein, plasma zinc levels and C-reactive protein should be measured to help in the interpretation of vitamin A levels.

All patients with PI should receive supplements of vitamins A, D and E. There is no international consensus on the need to routinely supplement with vitamin K and practice varies between countries. Plasma vitamin levels should be rechecked 3–6 months after any adjustments in dose.

In PI patients, pancreatic enzyme replacement may enhance absorption of vitamins, so it is recommended that vitamin supplements are taken at or just prior to mealtimes to coincide with enzyme administration.

Patients who are pancreatic sufficient should be monitored annually and supplementation given in response to plasma levels. A recent study of pancreatic sufficient children managed at a specialist CF centre showed that the majority required supplementation with vitamin D to achieve recommended plasma levels [93] and this highlights the need for regular monitoring.

Vitamin A

Vitamin A deficiency may be multifactorial and not just a consequence of fat malabsorption. There is an increased loss of retinol disproportionate to the degree of fat malabsorption, suggesting a possible defect in handling of retinol in the gastrointestinal tract. Low levels of retinol binding protein and zinc may also contribute.

Vitamin A deficiency may cause night blindness and also has a role in the maintenance of mucus secreting epithelial cells. Low vitamin A levels have been associated with poorer clinical status [94,95] and lower weight standard deviation scores and bone density [94].

Assessment of vitamin A status is difficult and plasma levels of retinol may not reflect body stores. Vitamin A may accumulate in the liver. The plasma level of vitamin A usually correlates with plasma retinol binding protein levels and low vitamin A levels may reflect low retinol binding protein output by the liver rather than vitamin A deficiency. Plasma retinol levels are suppressed during acute infection so levels should be checked during times of clinical stability.

Recommended dose: 4000–10 000 IU per day depending on age and plasma levels [67].

Vitamin D

The two main forms of vitamin D are ergocalciferol (vitamin D2) and colecalciferol (vitamin D3). Colecalciferol is derived from UV irradiation of 7-dehydrocholesterol in the skin and, for the majority of people in the UK, UV irradiation can provide in excess of 80% of requirements.

Vitamin D deficiency may cause osteoporosis and osteomalacia and is a risk factor in the development of low bone mineral density in CF. Assessment of plasma 25-hydroxyvitamin D gives a good indication of vitamin D status; however, seasonal variations are well recognised. A plasma level of 75 nmol/L is recommended for the general population [96] and levels between 75 and 150 nmol/L are recommended throughout the year for patients with CF [45].

Vitamin D is usually given as a combined supplement with vitamin A and it may be necessary to give additional vitamin D to maintain optimal levels. Colecalciferol has been shown to have higher effectiveness compared with ergocalciferol as a supplement [97].

> *Recommended dose*: 400–800 IU per day is usually used in children and up to 2000 IU in adolescents; however, higher doses may be required to achieve optimal year round levels.

Vitamin E

Vitamin E is an antioxidant and protects cell membranes from free radical oxidative damage. Severe vitamin E deficiency may cause neurological problems and contribute to anaemia.

Newborn screened infants have been shown to be deficient in vitamin E. Supplementation is recommended in all PI patients and in those pancreatic sufficient patients demonstrating low serum levels. Vitamin E may play a role in cognitive function and prevention of vitamin E deficiency through early nutritional intervention in screened infants has been shown to be associated with better cognitive function [98].

Serum vitamin E levels represent only a proportion of total body vitamin E and will vary according to levels of lipoprotein, so vitamin E:fasting lipid ratio should be assessed.

> *Recommended dose*: 10–200 mg per day depending on age [67].

Vitamin K

There is no international consensus on the need for routine vitamin K supplementation. A survey of practice across the UK showed that around 18% of centres routinely supplement their patients with vitamin K, with varied doses [99].

Risk factors for low vitamin K levels include CF related liver disease, frequent antibiotic therapy and short gut syndrome as a result of bowel resection [100]. There is increased focus on vitamin K and its role in bone health [101] and deficiency may be important in the development of low BMD; a lack of vitamin K results in undercarboxylated osteocalcin causing an imbalance in bone formation and breakdown. Plasma vitamin K levels are unreliable as a measure of status and undercarboxylated prothrombin (PIVKA-II) levels should be assessed. CF Trust guidance suggests that there is insufficient evidence for routine supplementation, but consideration should be given to individuals with low BMD, liver disease or prolonged prothrombin time [45].

> *Recommended dose*: in those patients who require supplementation give phytomenadione (vitamin K1) daily:
> - 300 µg/kg/day for infants
> - 5 mg for children 2–7 years of age
> - 10 mg for children >7 years of age

A summary of doses of vitamin supplements and commonly used preparations is given in Tables 11.5 and 11.6.

Water soluble vitamins

Water soluble vitamins are well absorbed and routine supplementation is not necessary.

Calcium

The degree of calcium absorption in CF is variable. Studies of children and adolescents who do not have CF have shown increased bone deposition and improved BMD when they are given calcium supplementation.

CF Trust guidance [67] suggests that calcium intake should be optimised to reduce the risk of low BMD. Intakes of 1300–1500 mg daily are recommended in children from 8 years of age. If dietary intake is poor, advice should be given to increase intake of dairy sources of calcium. Calcium supplements may be required to achieve an adequate intake in patients with a dislike of dairy foods.

Sodium

There is a lack of consensus regarding the need to routinely supplement with sodium and practices vary across the UK.

Salt supplementation in infants

Breast milk and infant formulas have relatively low sodium contents which may be insufficient

Table 11.5 Summary of vitamin supplement doses in cystic fibrosis.

Age	Vitamin A	Vitamin D	Vitamin E
<1 year	4000 IU	400 IU	10–50 mg
>1 year	4000–10 000 IU	400–800 IU	50–100 mg
Adolescents	4000–10 000 IU	400–800 IU	100–200 mg

Table 11.6 Composition of vitamin preparations used in cystic fibrosis.

Preparation (dose)	Vitamin A (IU)	Vitamin D (IU)	Vitamin E (mg)
Vitamin A and D Capsule (1 capsule)	4000	400	0
Multivitamins BPC (1 capsule)	2500	300	0
Abidec (0.6 mL)	1333	400	0
Dalivit (0.6 mL)	5000	400	0
Vitamin E (α-tocopheryl acetate) Gelcap 75 units (1 gelcap)	0	0	50
Vitamin E (α-tocopheryl acetate) Gelcap 200 units (1 gelcap)	0	0	134
Vitamin E (α-tocopheryl acetate) Gelcap 400 units (1 gelcap)	0	0	268
Calcichew D3 Forte (1 tablet)	0	400 (plus 500 mg calcium)	0
Adcal D3 Caplet (1 caplet)	0	200 (plus 300 mg calcium)	0
Calcium and ergocalciferol tablet (1 tablet)	0	400 (plus 97 mg calcium)	0
Ergocalciferol or colecalciferol solution 3000 units/mL (1 mL)	0	3000	0

to prevent sodium depletion in infants with CF. Sodium deficiency can be confirmed by analysis of urinary sodium (<10 mmol/L) and sodium supplementation can be given at a dose of 1–2 mmol/kg/day and the response monitored [67]. This should be given in divided doses to aid tolerance, and is often tolerated best when mixed with a feed. An evaluation of sodium supplementation in CF infants suggested that some require significantly more than the standard recommended dose so individual monitoring and dose adjustment is required [102].

Salt supplementation in older children

In hot weather, salt supplements are advised for all age groups. This may be given in divided doses mixed with a drink of diluted fruit drink to improve palatability and aid compliance:

- 1–7 years: 1 g sodium daily (600 mg sodium chloride = 10 mmol sodium)
- >7 years: 2–4 g sodium daily

Essential fatty acid supplementation

Essential fatty acid deficiencies particularly of linoleic acid (n-6) and docosahexanoic acid, DHA

(n-3) are seen in CF patients [103]. There is some evidence that routine supplementation with ω3 fatty acids, due to their anti-inflammatory effects, may provide some benefits particularly in terms of lung function with relatively few side effects. However, the evidence is insufficient currently to advocate routine supplementation.

Probiotics

The benefit of probiotics in CF is yet to be established. The normal balance of probiotic organisms in the gastrointestinal tract may be disturbed by illness, poor diet, infection and the use of antibiotics. There is some evidence that probiotic supplements may reduce the incidence of intestinal inflammation and severe respiratory infection in children with CF [104]; however, more research is required to establish effective doses and they are not currently used routinely in practice in the UK.

Complementary therapies

Families of children with CF may consider the use of alternative therapies to complement or replace their standard treatment. These may include the use of herbs, vitamins, minerals and changes in diet. The dietitian, medical team and pharmacist should evaluate any products being used and give advice to ensure practices are safe and do not interact adversely with medically prescribed treatments.

Appetite stimulants

Appetite stimulants are not routinely used in paediatric practice; however, they may be considered in cases of severe anorexia.

Megesterol acetate, a progesterone derivative, is reported to improve weight gain in patients with HIV and cancer, and has been observed to improve appetite in CF patients. However, side effects include adrenal suppression and glucose intolerance [105].

Cyproheptadine, an antihistamine with a secondary effect of appetite stimulation, has been shown to improve weight and height in CF patients without side effects apart from transient drowsiness [106].

Growth hormone stimulates growth and can be used as an anabolic agent. Growth hormone has been associated with increased weight, height and lean tissue mass in patients with CF following a high energy diet [107].

Pancreatic enzyme replacement therapy

Patients with PI must take pancreatic enzymes with all fat containing meals, drinks and snacks. A range of enzyme preparations is available. Enteric coated acid resistant preparations such as Creon (Abbott Healthcare), Nutrizym (Merck Serona) and Pancrease (Janssen) are more effective than the older non enteric coated powder and tablet preparations such as Pancrex V capsules or powder (Paines and Byrne). The degree of PI varies so requirements must be individualised.

Pancreatin preparations degrade over time. The dose stated per capsule is a minimum as the capsules are over-filled to compensate for this degradation. Therefore capsules with a longer shelf life will have greater potency than those near to their use by date.

On average infants and young children have a higher fat intake per kilogram body weight than older children and adults, and hence require a higher dose of pancreatin per kilogram body weight. Enzymes should be titrated according to the fat content of the meal or snack. Requirements vary from 400 IU lipase/g fat to 5000 IU lipase/g fat. Most patients require 50–100 IU lipase/g fat/kg/day [108]. In order to maintain their integrity the enzyme preparations must not be crushed or chewed and should be given at the start, midpoint and end of a meal.

Doses should be advised for each individual and adjustments made based on clinical symptoms, appearance and frequency of stools, presence of abdominal symptoms and weight gain. It is recommended that the total dose of enzyme should not exceed 10 000 IU lipase/kg body weight daily [109].

Patients and carers should be educated on recognition of symptoms and dose adjustment to achieve optimal absorption. Adjustment of enzyme dose can be a difficult area of care for parents and carers and was highlighted in the report 'Food for Thought' [16] as an area of concern for families. Time should be taken for education of families, and children as they become more independent, on their enzyme requirements and how to titrate the dose relative to the fat content of food.

Administration of enzymes

Infants should be given enzymes in a granular form, Creon Micro (Abbott Healthcare), on a spoon, mixed with a small amount of milk or fruit purée. This should be given at the start and throughout a feed if the feed takes in excess of 30 minutes to complete. Older children should be changed to a capsule preparation usually around 4–5 years of age. They should be encouraged to swallow the enzyme capsules whole as soon as possible.

As the amount of food eaten by young children can vary considerably between meals, it is recommended that the dose be split throughout the meal so that adjustments can be made according to the amount of food eaten. Pancreatin preparations available in the UK are shown in Table 11.7.

Table 11.7 Pancreatin preparations available in the UK.

Preparation	Lipase units*	Protease units*	Amylase units*	Type of preparation
Creon Micro per scoop (100 mg)	5000	200	3600	E/c granules
Creon 10 000 per capsule	10 000	600	8000	Capsules, e/c granules
Creon 25 000 per capsule	25 000	1000	18 000	Capsules, e/c pellets
Creon 40 000 per capsule	40 000	1600	25 000	Capsules, e/c granules
Nutrizym 10 per capsule	10 000	500	9000	Capsules, e/c minitablets
Nutrizym 22 per capsule	22 000	1100	19 800	Capsules, e/c minitablets
Pancrease HL per capsule	25 000	1250	22 500	Capsules, e/c minitablets
Pancrex V per capsule	8000	430	9000	Capsules, powder
Pancrex granules per gram	5000	300	4000	Granules
Pancrex V 125 per capsule	2950	160	3300	Capsules, powder
Pancrex V per tablet	1900	110	1700	E/c tablets
Pancrex V Forte per tablet	5600	330	5000	E/c tablets
Pancrex V powder per gram	25 000	1400	30 000	Powder

E/c, e/c, enteric coated. The declared enzyme content of the capsules is the minimum concentration of active ingredient.
*Enzymes expressed as international units (IU).

Adjunctive therapy to pancreatic enzymes

Pancreatic enzyme preparations can be inactivated by gastric acidity. H_2 receptor antagonists, such as ranitidine, or proton pump inhibitors, such as omeprazole, may help increase efficacy of pancreatic enzymes by reducing the volume and acid concentration of gastric secretions. Their use should be considered in patients with uncontrolled signs of malabsorption or in those requiring large doses of enzymes to control symptoms.

Practical dietary management

Infants

The introduction of newborn screening for CF has provided an opportunity to minimise the effects of CF on the infant's nutritional status early in life. However, even with the introduction of screening and early nutritional intervention, studies have shown that up to 50% of infants with CF show growth faltering by 12 months of age and require nutritional supplementation. Risk factors include meconium ileus, severe genotype and pancreatic insufficiency [110, 111].

Breast milk

Breast milk has many advantages for infants with CF:

- the lipase and amylase content may partially compensate for reduced pancreatic secretion
- its immunological properties may offer some protection against infection
- it has an optimal fatty acid profile, helping to maintain essential fatty acid status
- its nutrients are highly bio-available
- breast feeding is psychologically beneficial for the mother

In the UK 83% of mothers breast feed their infants at birth [112] and many infants at diagnosis will be breast fed. However, a large proportion of these will discontinue breast feeding over the first year of life with one study indicating that only 12% remained breast fed at the end of the first year [9]. This drop may be due to mothers' choice (mirroring the sharp reduction in breast feeding prevalence over the first year of life seen in healthy infants); for clinical reasons because of faltering growth; or due to the burden of treatment.

Early studies suggest breast fed infants can grow normally [113]; however, more recent studies have indicated a decline in nutritional status in infants who are breast fed beyond 2 months of age [114]. In clinical practice, if a mother is breast feeding her infant at diagnosis she should be encouraged to continue; however, close monitoring of the infant's nutritional status is essential and supplementary high energy feeds may be required if there is evidence of faltering growth.

Formula feeding

If the infant is bottle feeding, a whey based formula should be recommended and the infant be allowed to feed on demand.

High energy formulas

High energy formulas are useful to supplement the intake of infants whose weight gain is inadequate, whether breast or bottle fed. Three energy dense infant formulas are available in the UK: Infatrini and Similac High Energy have an energy density of 1 kcal (4 kJ) per mL; SMA High Energy has an energy density of 0.9 kcal (3.8 kJ) per mL.

Studies reviewing feeding practices of CF infants suggest that between 25% and 42% of infants with CF will require a high energy feed during the first 12 months of life [110].

Hydrolysed protein formulas

Hydrolysed protein formulas (Table 7.6) may be required following surgery for meconium ileus when there may be a secondary disaccharide intolerance, or if there is a diagnosis of cow's milk protein intolerance. There are no advantages in the routine use of protein hydrolysate feeds.

Introduction of solids

Solids should be introduced around 6 months of age, but not before 17 weeks of age, according to Department of Health guidelines [115]. Early weaning may significantly reduce the volume of breast milk or formula milk taken and should be discouraged. Parents should be encouraged to follow normal weaning guidelines and establish a good pattern of eating from early on, including the normal progression through textures and introduction of a wide range of foods, with the aim of the child being on mashed family foods by 12 months of age.

Once solids have been established in the diet, if the child shows signs of weight faltering, advice can be given to increase the energy intake from solids by:

- using full fat yoghurts, fromage frais and milk puddings as a dessert after a savoury meal
- adding grated cheese, butter or polyunsaturated or mono-unsaturated spread to savoury foods

- using full fat cow's milk or high energy formula in foods such as mashed potatoes and sauces

Pancreatic enzymes

Pancreatic enzymes should be introduced at diagnosis in infants with proven PI, as identified either by genotype or through faecal elastase measurement.

Creon Micro is the enzyme of choice for infants and should be given immediately prior to feeding, on a spoon, mixed with a small amount of milk or fruit purée. Ideally the enzyme should be given at intervals throughout the feed.

The dose should be adjusted according to symptoms, but should not exceed 10 000 units lipase/kg body weight/day. Initially 1/4 to 1/2 scoop of Creon Micro should be given per feed, and the dose adjusted as necessary in response to changes in stool frequency, stool consistency, weight gain and feed intake. Breast fed babies may require a lower dose of enzyme due to the lipase content of the milk, and should initially be started on 1/4 scoop per feed.

Pancreatic enzymes are required with any fat containing solid foods, starting with 1/4 to 1/2 scoop Creon Micro once the infant is taking more than a few spoonfuls of solids at a time, and the dose adjusted as solid intake increases.

Monitoring

The key to good outcomes for screened infants is regular monitoring and proactive management, promptly addressing any nutritional concerns. Weekly contact with families may be necessary immediately after diagnosis, to review weight gain, abdominal symptoms and feeding patterns. Once weight gain and feeding practices are established, fortnightly or monthly reviews may be sufficient.

Toddlers

Undue focus on weight gain and food intake can lead to abnormal feeding patterns and negative feeding behaviour in toddlers. Many factors precipitate food refusal, including parental anxiety, acute infections, hospitalisation, vomiting and gagging associated with GOR or coughing. Support may be needed from the psychologist to manage severe cases of food refusal, but the following guidelines may help to minimise the duration or severity of the problem.

- Encourage the family to eat together at a table so that the mealtime becomes a social occasion; a lack of structure and routine can lead to poor eating habits.
- Offer small meals and give more if the meal is finished.
- Advise parents not to force their child to eat, as the child will soon learn to control the situation and increase their negative food behaviour further.
- Initially offer a food that the child likes; then very gradually increase variety, praising good behaviour and ignoring poor eating behaviour.
- Avoid any negative focus on the child's eating behaviour, even outside of mealtimes, commenting only on good behaviour.
- If food is refused, do not offer an alternative.
- Take any uneaten food away after 20–30 minutes without comment.
- Remind parents that food preferences will change in time, so keep offering foods which have previously been rejected, although avoid foods for which the child has a very obvious strong dislike.

Pancreatic enzymes

Erratic and grazing toddler eating behaviour can make administration of the correct dose of enzyme difficult, as meals may not be finished or may take a long time to complete. Splitting the enzyme dose throughout the meal may be helpful to control this.

Many parents worry when they have given enzymes and then the food is refused, and that harm will come to their child as a result. Some may resort to giving favourite food such as chocolates or crisps if the first food is refused to minimise any potential harm. Reassurance should be given to the family that no harm will come to the child if enzymes are given and then the child refuses to eat, and that they should avoid offering alternative foods if the first food is refused; the child will soon learn to manipulate this situation.

Adolescents

Adolescence is a period of transition during which there is normally a rapid increase in height velocity and pubertal development. For many young people with CF this pubertal transition can be delayed, particularly in those with poor nutrition. Requirements for nutrients are at their highest and nutritional support in the form of overnight enteral feeding may be required to support optimal growth during this period.

During the adolescent years independence should be encouraged; however, this can lead to an increase in non-compliance with treatment as the young person learns to push the boundaries and take risks. This is a normal part of development, but can be a worrying time for parents and carers. Adolescence is also a time when there may be new challenges with the development of comorbidities such as CFRD or CFLD, and the need for increased nutritional support in the form of overnight feeding.

Denial, treatment rejection and anger are common and it is essential that the team work with the young person, avoiding a dictatorial style of clinical management, to make a treatment plan which is accepted by the young person. Psychology support may be helpful at this challenging time. Due to the increased survival, and as a result of aggressive management of CF, young people often have a complex regimen of interventions aimed at both treatment and prevention of complications.

The treatment regimen may be excessively time consuming and allow little time for normal activities outside of the school day. It is essential that the team work together to rationalise treatment and ensure that the life is manageable; compromises may sometimes need to be made.

CF related diabetes

The primary aim of treatment in CFRD is to maintain nutritional status and normoglycaemia. Individualised dietary instruction should be given by a CF specialist dietitian and the insulin treatment should be tailored to the dietary intake, rather than working the diet around the administration of insulin.

There are differences between the dietary recommendations for diabetes mellitus and those for

Table 11.8 Differences in the dietary management of diabetes mellitus and cystic fibrosis (CF) related diabetes.

	Diabetes mellitus [118]	CF related diabetes
Energy	100% EAR if BMI is 18.5–25	Individualised, but up to 120%–150% EAR depending on nutritional status
Fat	<35% total energy	40% total energy
Refined sugars	Up to 10% total energy	Allow throughout the day
Carbohydrate	45%–60% total energy	45%–50% total energy
Dietary fibre	No quantitative recommendation, but encouraged	Encouraged if well nourished, but may compromise appetite
Protein	10%–20% total energy. Not >1 g/kg body weight	200% RNI
Salt	Low intake <6 g sodium chloride daily	Increased requirement
Snacks	Scheduled meal plan including some snacks	Ad lib

EAR, estimated average requirement; BMI, body mass index; RNI, reference nutrient intake.

CFRD (Table 11.8). This apparent conflict should always be resolved in favour of the CF diet unless the patient has a BMI above the healthy range.

For diabetes mellitus, individuals are advised to follow a reduced fat, high fibre, low refined carbohydrate, low salt, controlled energy diet. In CFRD, in order to maintain adequate nutritional intake and nutritional status, there should be no restriction of refined carbohydrate or high fat foods [27,116–118]. Fibre should be given as tolerated, but care should be taken to ensure that this does not have a negative impact on appetite. Many families will be aware of the conflict between the dietary recommendations for CFRD and diabetes mellitus and all team members should be confident in their recommendation to continue with the high fat, high sugar and therefore high energy diet needed for CF.

Many CF patients have very erratic eating habits and their insulin should be tailored to this pattern. Patients should be encouraged to eat regularly,

if possible, and to aim to eat a similar amount of carbohydrate each day. Many centres recommend that refined carbohydrates are given with meals rather than eaten *ad lib* between meals; this is to reduce the glycaemic effect and to aid with the achievement of normoglycaemia. For some patients carbohydrate counting is useful, enabling them to eat to appetite and adjust insulin doses accordingly.

This should only be recommended in those patients for whom this additional advice will not be an excessive burden.

Patients using oral nutritional supplements should consider the use of polymeric supplements rather than carbohydrate only supplements. Patients receiving gastrostomy or nasogastric feeding will require long acting insulin to cover the increased carbohydrate load overnight. Advice should be given in the event that insulin is given and then the overnight feed omitted.

CF associated liver disease

The development of liver disease can further exacerbate malnutrition by increasing fat malabsorption and protein loss. Patients with CFLD have been shown to have BMI, weight and height comparable with age matched peers with CF and no liver disease, but lower arm anthropometry measurements [119]. This may be due to increased body weight as a result of hepatosplenomegaly or, in end stage liver disease, ascites. Arm anthropometry is therefore a useful measure of nutritional status in patients with CFLD.

Energy requirements may increase as a result of fat malabsorption and up to 150% requirements may be needed. The effect of fat malabsorption is likely to be more significant in end stage liver disease when medium chain triglycerides can be a helpful energy supplement, as these are readily absorbed without the use of bile salts.

Salt supplementation may need to be restricted in patients with end stage liver disease as this may precipitate the development of ascites (p. 179).

Fat soluble vitamins are required in the usual CF doses and, if the patient is not already on vitamin K, supplements should be given at a dose of up to 10 mg daily.

Patients with liver disease are more prone to developing significant anorexia, particularly those with advanced disease, and overnight supplementary feeding may be necessary to prevent worsening malnutrition. Gastrostomy feeding is contraindicated in patients with advanced disease or varices due to the risk of gastric bleeding.

Liver transplantation is considered when there is evidence of deteriorating nutritional status and lung function. BMI has been shown to be maintained up to 5 years post liver transplantation; liver transplant is considered to be an effective treatment for selected patients with CFLD [39].

Transition to adult care

The majority of children with CF will transition to adult care, there being very few mortalities during childhood. It is essential that this transition to adult care is seamless and is handled safely, sensitively and effectively. Transition to adult care is often considered a major life event for many families,

and although it is often embraced by the young person and family it can also be a time of increased anxiety. Patients should be transferred to adult care at approximately 16 years of age, but the timing should be flexible depending on the individual's health, emotional, physical, social and educational circumstances.

To be successful, transition relies on collaboration between paediatric and adult centres, effective planning and communication. There are a number of models for transition [120], but whichever model is adopted it is essential that transition is considered as a process and not a single event and that the care is gradually handed over once all parties are comfortable and ready.

Useful address

Cystic Fibrosis Trust
11 London Road, Bromley, London BR1 1BY, UK

12

Kidney Diseases

Julie Royle

Introduction

The kidneys play an essential role in the maintenance of homeostasis by excreting waste products, such as urea and uric acid, and purposely adjusting the urinary excretion of water and electrolytes (solute) to counter dietary intake and the body's endogenous production of these from metabolism. The kidneys have a major role in the secretion of hormones. This includes erythropoietin for red blood cell production, renin and angiotensin II affecting renal and systemic haemodynamics, as well as hydroxylated vitamin D affecting calcium, phosphate and bone metabolism. Other functions include peptide hormone catabolism and gluconeogenesis.

A variety of diseases can affect the kidneys leading to a sudden deterioration in renal function (acute kidney injury) or an irreversible deterioration of renal function (chronic kidney disease). Impairment of excretory, regulatory and endocrine functions is seen as kidney function deteriorates and the management of these impairments is the foundation of treatment.

Acute kidney injury

Acute kidney injury (AKI) is characterised by an abrupt and reversible decline in renal function leading to an increase in the blood concentration of urea and creatinine and the inability of the kidneys to regulate fluid and electrolyte balance effectively. An incidence of 0.8 per 100 000 total child population has been reported [1] with the highest incidence seen in the neonatal period. The incidence in children is increasing with a change in aetiology from primary renal disease to multifactorial causes [2]. In childhood, AKI may be associated with anuria (urine output <1 mL/kg/day), oliguria (urine output <0.5–1.0 mL/kg/hour), a normal urine output or high urine output. The causes of AKI in children are classified as pre-renal, intrinsic renal disease or post-renal [2] (Table 12.1).

Diarrhoea associated haemolytic uraemic syndrome (HUS) remains the commonest cause of intrinsic AKI in childhood. It leads to significant morbidity and mortality during the acute phase [3]. The most common infectious agent causing HUS is enterohaemorrhagic *Escherichia coli* (EHEC),

Table 12.1 Causes of acute renal injury in children.

Pre-renal failure	Intrinsic renal failure	Post-renal failure
Hypovolaemia (gastroenteritis, haemorrhage)	Diseases of the kidney or vessels (acute glomerulonephritis, acute tubular necrosis, haemolytic uraemic syndrome, vasculitis, hypoplasia)	Obstruction (posterior uretheral valves, calculi, tumours, trauma)
Peripheral vasodilation (sepsis, antihypertensive medications)	Myoglobinuria	
Impaired cardiac output	Intratubular obstruction (uric acid)	
Bilateral renal vessel occlusion	Iatrogenic factors (removal of solitary kidney)	
Drugs (ciclosporin, diuretics)	Tumour infiltrate	
	Nephrotoxic drugs (antimicrobials, heavy metals, insecticides, cytotoxic agents)	
	Hypoxic/ischaemic insults	

usually of the serotype 0157:H7 [3]. Foods of bovine origin including beefburgers and unpasteurised milk, as well as contact with farm animals, are major sources for human infection although EHEC has been recovered from many retail foods. HUS is classically characterised by the sudden onset of haemolytic anaemia, thrombocytopenia and the development of AKI after acute gastroenteritis, often with bloody diarrhoea.

Management of AKI

The initial management of AKI focuses on the correction of fluid balance and biochemical abnormalities including hyponatraemia, hyperkalaemia and acidosis which can be life threatening. Further injury to the kidney should be prevented through maintaining adequate blood pressure and avoiding nephrotoxic medication. Transfer to a tertiary nephrology centre is indicated in those children requiring renal replacement therapy (RRT).

Such indications for RRT include

- severe or persistent hyperkalaemia
- fluid overload with hypertension, congestive cardiac failure or pulmonary oedema
- severe uraemia
- metabolic abnormalities including acidosis, hyponatraemia or hypernatraemia, hypocalcaemia
- hyperphosphataemia
- fluid removal to allow the provision of nutrition
- removal of a dialysable drug or toxin

Choice of renal replacement therapy

The selection of RRT in acutely ill children depends upon the availability of treatment modalities and ventilatory support, the patient's requirements for fluid and solute removal and haemodynamic stability. The choice is between peritoneal dialysis (PD), continuous renal replacement therapy (CRRT) and intermittent haemodialysis (IHD). Factors determining the choice of RRT include the desired outcome of therapy and clinical condition of the child as indicated in Table 12.2 [4]. PD is the

Table 12.2 Indications for choice of renal replacement therapy in acute kidney injury.

Indication for dialysis	Clinical condition	Modality indicated
Solute removal	Stable	HD
	Unstable	CRRT, PD
Fluid removal	Stable	PD, isolated ultrafiltration on HD
	Unstable	CRRT
Solute and fluid removal	Stable/unstable	HD, PD, CRRT
Tumour lysis syndrome	Stable/unstable	HD followed by CRRT
Toxin or drug removal	Stable/unstable	CRRT, IHD for some drugs

HD, haemodialysis; CRRT, continuous renal replacement therapy; PD, peritoneal dialysis; IHD, intermittent haemodialysis.

preferred modality in children as it is well tolerated and there are no rapid fluid shifts. IHD is used when there is an urgent need for solute removal. For the critically ill child in the paediatric intensive care unit (PICU), CRRT is the favoured treatment.

Nutritional management of AKI

Children with AKI are highly catabolic. This is usually multifactorial manifesting as anorexia, the catabolic nature of the underlying disorder, increased breakdown and reduced synthesis of muscle protein, increased hepatic gluconeogenesis, nutrient losses in drainage fluids or dialysis and impaired access to food. Input from a paediatric dietitian with experience in renal disease is essential from the onset as the dietary prescription varies with clinical management and the stage of the illness [5].

Nutritional support aims to provide sufficient energy to avoid catabolism, starvation and ketoacidosis as well as to control metabolic abnormalities. The provision of nutrition is easier once dialysis is initiated since the fluid removed by ultrafiltration allows larger volumes of feed to be given. Nutritional intervention for children with AKI depends on

- clinical management: conservative versus RRT
- biochemical assessment: plasma levels of sodium, potassium, bicarbonate, urea, creatinine, albumin, glucose, calcium, magnesium and phosphate should be regularly monitored and reviewed (Tables 12.3a and 12.3b)
- cause of AKI including the involvement of other organs
- gastrointestinal functioning
- growth parameters: height (if available) and weight plotted on a growth chart [6]; weight recordings prior to the onset of AKI will help determine a more accurate estimation of dry weight
- dietary history: if the child is eating

Methods of feeding

Enteral feeding
The child with AKI may initially take oral fluids readily, driven by thirst. However, vomiting is common. Most children fail to achieve nutritional

Table 12.3   Reference ranges (Central Manchester Foundation Trust).

(a) Guidelines for normal serum values

Analyte	Age	Range
Sodium (mmol/L)	<1 month	130–145
	>1 month	135–145
Potassium (mmol/L)	<1 month	3.5–6.0
	>1 month	3.5–5.0
Bicarbonate (mmol/L)	All	20–26
Urea (mmol/L)	1 month	2.0–5.0
	1 year	2.5–6.0
	Child	2.5–6.5
	Teenager	3.0–7.5
Albumin (g/L)	<1 month	25–35
	1–6 months	28–44
	Child	30–45
Calcium (mmol/L) serum total	<2 weeks	1.9–2.8
	>2 weeks	2.2–2.7
Phosphate (mmol/L)	<1 month	1.4–2.8
	5 weeks to 1 year	1.2–2.2
	1–3 years	1.1–2.0
	4–12 years	1.0–1.8
	15 years	0.95–1.5
	Adult	0.8–1.4
PTH (pg/mL) normocalcaemic	All	10–60
Magnesium (mmol/L)	All	0.65–1.0
Ferritin (µg/L)	All	30–275
Glucose (mmol/L) fasting	<1 month	2.5–5.5
	>1 month	3–6.0

(b) Guidelines for normal serum creatinine values

Age	Serum creatinine (µmol/L)
<1 week	<100
1–2 weeks	<80
2–4 weeks	<55
1 month to 1 year	<40
1–3 years	<40
4–6 years	<46
7–9 years	10–56
10–12 years	30–60
13–15 years	40–80
16 years to adult male	40–960
16 years to adult female	26–86

Ketones interfere positively. Bilirubin interferes negatively.

targets through diet alone. As the duration of the acute illness can be prolonged, the passing of a fine bore nasogastric tube is recommended. The tube can be passed at the time of sedation or when anaesthetised for procedures including the insertion of a peritoneal dialysis catheter or arterial line [5]. This allows the provision of early nutritional support because anorexia, vomiting or food refusal can impair management and may increase parental anxiety.

A continuous 24 hour feeding regimen using an enteral feeding pump at a slow rate (10–20 mL/hour) is advantageous in the initial stages of treatment when vomiting is present. As oral intake improves, the transition from continuous to overnight feeding provides the outstanding nutritional prescription until appetite improves sufficiently to allow tube feeding to be discontinued. Those children with persistent diarrhoea may tolerate a hydrolysed protein feed (see Tables 7.6, 7.11) before considering parenteral nutrition.

Parenteral nutrition
The parenteral route is only considered when enteral nutrition is not tolerated. Standard hospital parenteral nutrition (PN) regimens are often unsuitable for the child with AKI because of their electrolyte composition and the amount of fluid they provide. An appropriate daily nutritional prescription to meet individual requirements should be agreed by the dietitian, pharmacist and medical staff. When formulating PN, nitrogen and electrolyte modified solutions, together with increased energy from carbohydrate and fat solutions where fluid allowance is limited, need to be considered. On CRRT the loss of nutrients through filtration and dialysis needs to be compensated for in the replacement fluids (see Fluid); levels need to be greater than those found in standard PN regimens. For many children PN is temporary and the enteral route is re-established as soon as gut function returns.

Nutritional considerations

There are few data on the nutritional requirements of critically ill children with AKI and on RRT. Most of the information is derived from adult data.

Energy
Little is known about the energy requirements of infants and children with AKI [7]. A minimum of the estimated average requirement (EAR) for energy [8] for healthy children of the same chronological age provides a guide (Table 12.4). These recommendations can be difficult to achieve during acute treatment; it is important to provide the maximum energy intake tolerated within the prescribed fluid allowance. The early addition of glucose polymers to water (flavoured with squash or cordial if desired) or to drinks of choice is recommended.

Table 12.4 Nutritional guidelines for the child with acute kidney injury.

	Energy* (kcal/kg body weight/day)	Protein (g/kg body weight/day)
Conservative management		
0–2 months	95–120 (400–500 kJ)	1.0–2.1
Infants/children/adolescents	EAR for chronological age	1.0
Peritoneal dialysis		
0–2 months	95–120 (400–500 kJ)	2.1–2.5†
Infants/children/adolescents	EAR for chronological age	1.0–2.5
Haemodialysis		
0–2 months	95–120 (400–500 kJ)	1.0–2.1
Infants/children/adolescents	EAR for chronological age	1.0–1.8
CRRT		
0–2 months	95–120 (400–500 kJ)	2.5–3.0
Infants/children/adolescents	EAR for chronological age	2.5

EAR, estimated average requirement [8, 9]; CRRT, continuous renal replacement therapy.
*These guidelines are rarely achieved in the acute stage when fluid is restricted.
†If dialysis is prolonged, increased protein may be required.

It is prudent to start at a concentration of 0.5 kcal (2 kJ)/mL, building up to a concentration of 1 kcal (4 kJ)/mL, or 25% carbohydrate (CHO) concentration, depending on individual tolerance. Liquid glucose polymer preparations can also be used, but require dilution with water to be tolerated by children. It is recommended to start with a 1:5 dilution of liquid glucose polymer, building up to a final 1:3 dilution. The neutral preparations can be flavoured with squash or cordial. When fluid is severely restricted, ice cubes and lollies can be prepared with these energy dense solutions and offered at frequent intervals. Energy rich CHO drinks including original bottled Lucozade Energy (17.2% CHO concentration) and Mountain Dew (13% CHO concentration) can be useful alternatives for those children who refuse to drink prescribed energy supplements.

A list of energy supplements that can be considered is given in Table 12.5. These can be successfully added to infant formulas to increase energy density:

- in infants up to 6 months of age, 0.85–1.0 kcal/mL (3.6–4 kJ/mL) is usually tolerated
- in infants from 6 to 12 months of age, 1.0–1.5 kcal/mL (4–6 kJ/mL) should be tolerated

In children over 12 months of age, or whose weight is >8 kg, a nutritionally complete paediatric feed can be considered and modified as necessary to meet individual requirements (Table 12.5). The energy density can be built up to 1.5–2.0 kcal/mL (6–8 kJ/mL). Fat emulsions can be given as a prescribed medicine during the day.

A few children develop insulin resistance and hyperglycaemia can occur. If managed on PD, this can be exacerbated by the absorption of glucose from the PD fluid together with the intake of high CHO supplements. Insulin infusions need to be considered to control blood glucose levels before the reduction of dietary CHO.

When PN is initiated, a high concentration of dextrose solution up to 25% is indicated, with lipids providing 10%–20% of non-protein energy.

Protein

In children with AKI who are being managed conservatively, protein should be limited to the reference nutrient intake (RNI) [9] level to minimise uraemic symptoms. This needs to be gradually increased as tolerated if RRT is started, with its associated increased solute removal and possible protein losses. The RNI for protein [9] is not appropriate for the child with AKI on RRT and requirements should be individually determined. The age and weight of the child, the serum biochemistry and RRT modality, when implemented, all need to be considered. Nutritional guidelines are shown in Table 12.4.

Once RRT is established, the following increments can be used as a guide to increase protein intake to the levels given in Table 12.4:

- exclude protein if the serum urea is ≥40 mmol/L
- introduce 0.5 g protein/kg if the serum urea is ≥30 mmol/L and < 40 mmol/L
- give 1 g protein/kg if the serum urea is ≥20 mmol/L and <30 mmol/L
- give the RNI for height age (infants) or chronological age (children) if the serum urea is <20 mmol/L

CRRT allows the nutritional support of highly catabolic states but contributes to nitrogen loss through the filtration of free amino acids and small peptides across haemofilters. Maxvold et al. [10] demonstrated that at similar blood and dialysate/prefiltered replacement fluid flow rates, there is an equivalent urea clearance with haemofiltration and haemofiltration with dialysis. A negative nitrogen balance occurred in children with AKI on PN containing 1.5 g/kg/day of protein and an energy intake 20%–30% above resting energy expenditure. An 11%–12% loss of dietary amino acids was found on both modalities. A significant daily accumulative glutamine loss may potentiate nitrogen imbalance. A dose adjustment of amino acid formulation may be needed to overcome negative nitrogen balance in children with AKI on CRRT. An adult study by Scheinkestel et al. [11] showed that a protein intake of 2.5 g/kg/day and meeting energy requirements increased the likelihood of achieving a positive nitrogen balance and improving survival. Nutrition therapy in AKI remains an area of many unanswered questions, especially for those managed on CRRT, and Li et al. illustrate this in their review of adult AKI studies [12]. There are few paediatric studies.

Nutritional supplements, using a nasogastric tube, are frequently used to meet protein requirements in the initial stages of treatment. For infants

Table 12.5 Nutritional supplements.

Supplement	Suggested use
Energy	
Glucose polymers	
Powder, e.g. Polycal, Super Soluble Maxijul, Vitajoule	Add to infant formula, baby juice, cow's milk, squash, fizzy drinks, tea, milk shake, ice cubes and lollies
Liquid, e.g. Polycal	Dilute with water, cordial or fizzy drinks of choice (unless fluid restricted), add to jelly
Fat emulsion e.g. Calogen, Liquigen	Add to infant formula, cow's milk, nutritionally complete supplements
Combined fat and carbohydrate e.g. Super Soluble Duocal Powder, QuickCal	Add to infant formula, cow's milk, nutritionally complete supplements
Protein	
Protein powders e.g. Protifar, Vitapro, Renapro	Add to infant formula, Liquid Duocal, modular feed components
Renal specific infant formulas	
Kindergen Powder per 100 g: 7.5 g protein, 503 kcal (2104 kJ), 93 mg phosphorus, 3 mmol potassium, 10 mmol sodium	For infants with CKD or conservatively managed AKI
20% solution (20 g powder made up to 100 mL with water): 1.5 g protein, 101 kcal (421 kJ), 18.6 mg phosphorus, 0.6 mmol potassium, 2 mmol sodium	
Renastart Powder per 100 g: 7.5 g protein, 494 kcal (2066 kJ), 92 mg phosphorus, 3 mmol potassium, 10.5 mmol sodium	
20% solution (20 g powder made up to 100 mL with water): 1.5 g protein, 99 kcal (413 kJ), 18 mg phosphorus, 0.6 mmol potassium, 2.1 mmol sodium	
Nutritionally complete feeds	
Nutrini per 100 mL: 2.8 g protein, 100 kcal (420 kJ), 50 mg phosphorus, 2.8 mmol potassium, 2.6 mmol sodium	For oral or supplementary tube feeding in children >1 year and weight >8 kg Can be combined with energy supplements
Paediasure per 100 mL: 2.8 g protein, 101 kcal (422 kJ), 53 mg phosphorus, 2.8 mmol potassium, 2.6 mmol sodium	
Nutrini Energy per 100 mL: 4.1 g protein, 150 kcal (630 kJ), 75 mg phosphorus, 4.2 mmol potassium, 3.9 mmol sodium	
Paediasure Plus per 100 mL: 4.2 g protein, 151 kcal (632 kJ), 80 mg phosphorus, 3.5 mmol potassium, 2.6 mmol sodium	
Nepro HP per 100 mL: 8.1 g protein, 180 kcal (722 kJ), 72 mg phosphorus, 2.7 mmol potassium, 3.0 mmol sodium	Consider micronutrient contribution in younger children
Low electrolyte supplements (not nutritionally complete)	
Fortijuce per 100 mL: 4 g protein, 150 kcal (640 kJ), 12 mg phosphorus, 0.2 mmol potassium, 0.4 mmol sodium	Can be diluted with water or fizzy drinks
Ensure Plus Juce per 100 mL: 4.8 g protein, 150 kcal (638 kJ), 11 mg phosphorus, 0.4 mmol potassium, 0.5 mmol sodium	
Renilon 7.5 per 100 mL: 7.5 g protein, 200 kcal (835 kJ), 3 mg phosphorus, 0.6 mmol potassium, 2.6 mmol sodium	
Vita-Bite per 25 g bar: 0.06 g protein, 137 kcal (571 kJ), <12.5 mg phosphorus, 0.63 mmol potassium, <0.1 mmol sodium	
Low protein milk substitute	
Sno-Pro per 100 mL: 0.16 g protein, 89 kcal (371 kJ), <30 mg phosphorus, <1.3 mmol potassium, <3.3 mmol sodium, <20 mg calcium	Use as a substitute for cow's milk to reduce protein and phosphate intakes
Renamil per 100 g: 4.6 g protein, 477 kcal (2003 kJ), 25 mg phosphorus, 0.2 mmol potassium, 2.6 mmol sodium	

CKD, chronic kidney disease; AKI, acute kidney injury.

standard whey based formulas (which are already low in electrolytes and phosphate) are recommended. These can be modified as required. Kindergen and Renastart, renal specific low phosphate, low potassium infant formulas (Table 12.5), can be beneficial for infants not receiving RTT or receiving intermittent haemodialysis when serum biochemistry levels are unstable. Nutritionally complete, energy dense infant formulas (Infatrini, Similac High Energy, SMA High Energy) can be useful if blood biochemistry allows when on RTT. The phosphate content of these feeds is higher than in standard infant whey based formulas so serum phosphate levels should be regularly reviewed. For the older child a number of nutritionally complete supplements are available. These can be used solely or in combinations with their protein, phosphate and potassium contents being assessed prior to use (Table 12.5). If protein hydrolysate formulas are indicated (in particular when the diarrhoeal phase is prolonged in HUS) they should be modified with respect to biochemical parameters as well as to meet individual nutritional requirements. Introduction should be gradual and delivery is usually by the nasogastric route. Once the child's appetite improves and protein intake is met through eating, energy supplemented drinks can replace nutritionally complete formulas or protein supplements.

Fluid

The volume of fluid prescribed during conservative treatment is based on insensible fluid requirements of $400\,mL/m^2$ body surface area/day or approximately $20\,mL/kg$ body weight/day, with a 12% increase for each degree Celsius above normal body temperature and a reduction if the child is ventilated. Insensible losses should be added to the previous day's urine output to give the total daily fluid allowance. On RRT, the fluid prescription is determined by monitoring the volume of fluid removed by ultrafiltration plus insensible losses. Ideally fluid removal on RRT should be flexibly managed to allow the maximum space for increased nutritional fluids. Maximal nutrient intakes using supplements should be provided within the fluid allowance and divided as evenly as possible throughout the day. A written prescription plan should be provided for the ward nurses and families.

Electrolytes and minerals

The intake of electrolytes, especially potassium, is likely to be restricted in conservative management. Serum levels and the use of RRT will dictate requirements thereafter. Any dietary restrictions should be minimised to avoid compromising nutritional intake.

Potassium rich foods including citrus fruits, fruit juices, bananas, potato crisps and chocolate are commonly brought into hospital by relatives. All carers should be advised about choosing foods with a low potassium content when serum potassium levels are elevated so that rich food sources are withdrawn (Table 12.6).

Once serum phosphate levels are above the reference ranges, the intake of phosphate rich foods should be moderated. A lower phosphate intake can partly be achieved when protein intake, particularly that of dairy products, is modified (Table 12.7). Cow's milk is generally restricted or eliminated from the diet during the acute phase because of its high protein, phosphate and potassium content. Avoidance of cow's milk also reduces the potential cow's milk protein or lactose intolerance which can follow the diarrhoeal prodrome in patients with HUS. If the milk restriction proves difficult a low protein milk substitute, such as Sno-Pro or Renamil (Table 12.5), can be advised.

Reduction in sodium intake can aid compliance when fluid intake is restricted by reducing thirst. This can be achieved by the avoidance of salted snacks and a no added salt diet (Table 12.8).

The level of the above restrictions depends on each individual child and their clinical condition. They should be frequently monitored to avoid unnecessary restrictions when their appetite is typically poor and their nutrition is easily compromised.

Micronutrients

Vitamin supplementation should be considered if dialysis treatment is prolonged. A general paediatric vitamin supplement of water soluble vitamins should be adequate for the majority of children as appetite improves. Iron supplementation may be indicated in some children during the recovery phase, particularly in those who had a poor diet history prior to the onset of AKI.

When on CRRT water soluble vitamins, especially folic acid, thiamin and vitamin C are lost.

Table 12.6 Potassium rich foods and suggested alternatives.

Potassium rich foods*	Suggested alternatives
Banana, apricots, kiwi fruit, grapes, avocado, citrus fruits, e.g. orange, grapefruit; dried fruit, e.g. raisins; tinned fruit in fruit juice; melon, plums, rhubarb, blackcurrants	Apple, pear, satsuma, blueberries, tinned fruit in syrup
Hi juice squash, fruit juices including orange, apple, tomato Instant coffee and coffee essence Malted drinks Cocoa, drinking chocolate	Squash, cordials, Lucozade, lemonade and fizzy drinks, tea
Potato crisps and potato containing snacks, nuts, peanut butter, salt substitutes, meat extract, yeast extract	Corn or rice snacks (without added potassium chloride and take account of sodium content), sweetened popcorn, jam, honey, marmalade, syrup
Jacket potatoes, chips (oven and frozen), roast potatoes	Rice (boiled or fried), spaghetti, pasta, noodles, bread, chapatti, naan, crackers
Mushrooms, spinach, tomatoes, spaghetti in tomato sauce, baked beans, pulses and hummus, tinned and packet soups	Carrots, cauliflower, swede, broccoli, cabbage
Chocolate and all foods containing it, toffee, fudge, marzipan, liquorice	Boiled sweets, jellies, mints, marshmallows
Chocolate biscuits	Biscuits: plain, sandwich, jam filled, wafer
Chocolate cake, fruit cake	Cake: plain sponge filled with cream and/or jam Jam tarts, apple pie, doughnuts, plain scones
Milk, yoghurt, evaporated and condensed milk	Low protein milk substitutes, e.g. Sno-Pro, Renamil

*Allowance will depend on individual assessment.

Requirements when on this treatment are unknown and a minimum of the RNI [9] should be given. Patients receiving CRRT also lose magnesium and calcium; this often leads to negative balances requiring additional supplementation. Zinc is also abnormally lost but serum levels do not generally fall [13, 14].

Recovery phase

As renal function improves and urine output increases, RRT is stopped. Dietary restrictions, where instigated, can gradually be relaxed. Serum electrolytes and dietary intake should be monitored closely as major losses, especially of potassium, during the diuretic phase can occur.

Prior to discharge, advice should be given on returning to a normal diet as renal function continues to improve. The opportunity to educate the child and family about the principles of a well balanced diet can also be taken if poor eating patterns were highlighted during the admission. Where appetite is slow to improve, some children may need to continue energy and vitamin supplements

for a short time, with monitoring of their progress in clinic.

Outcome of AKI

The prognosis and outcome for children with AKI depends on the underlying cause. Children with acute tubular necrosis and interstitial nephritis usually recover well. Most children with HUS make a good recovery of renal function but require long term monitoring for proteinuria, hypertension and renal impairment. Factors associated with a poor outcome include multi-organ failure and the need for RRT and these children need secondary or tertiary follow-up [1].

Chronic kidney disease

Chronic kidney disease (CKD) is characterised by an irreversible deterioration of renal function which can progressively decline to end stage renal disease [15]. It defines renal dysfunction as a continuum from mild to severe. The National Institute for Health and Care Excellence (NICE) has adopted the US National Kidney Foundation

Table 12.7 Phosphate rich foods and suggested alternatives.

Phosphate rich foods*	Suggested alternatives
Cow's milk (full cream, semi-skimmed, skimmed) Dried milk powder and other milk products	*Infants* Whey based infant formulas, e.g., Cow & Gate 1, SMA 1, Aptamil 1 for at least 1–2 years *Children* Reduced intake, consider low protein milk substitute (Table 12.5)
Large portions of meat, poultry and fish Processed meats containing phosphate additives	Reduced portion sizes
Yoghurt, fromage frais, mousse, ice cream, milk puddings including custard	Reduce intake Custard made with milk substitute
Evaporated milk, condensed milk, single cream	Double cream†
Cheese, e.g. Cheddar, Edam, processed cheese and cheese spread	Limit intake and/or encourage use of cottage cheese or full fat cream cheese
Egg yolk	Meringues
Cocoa, chocolate and chocolate containing foods, toffee, fudge	Boiled sweets, mints, dolly mixtures
Sardines, pilchards, tuna	White fish
Baked beans, pulses	Vegetables
Nuts, peanut butter, marzipan	Jam, honey, marmalade, syrup
Cola drinks and any others containing phosphoric acid	Squash, cordials, lemonade, Lucozade
Convenience and processed foods with phosphorus additives including dicalcium phosphate, disodium phosphate, monosodium phosphate, sodium tripolyphosphate, tetrasodium pyrophosphate	Foods with no phosphorus containing food additives

*Allowance will depend on individual assessment.
†Caution: vitamin A content (p. 266).

Table 12.8 Sodium rich foods and suggested alternatives.

Sodium rich foods	Suggested alternatives
Salted crisps, nuts and savoury snacks	Unsalted crisps, unsalted nuts, rice cakes, unsalted popcorn
Tinned and packet soups	Homemade soups
Pot savouries	Sweet snacks instead of savoury
Tinned foods with added salt	*Reduced salt products, e.g. reduced salt baked beans
Bacon, sausages and other processed meats and fish	Fresh meats and fish
Cheese and cheese products	Cottage cheese, ricotta and cream cheese
Stock cubes, meat and vegetable extracts	Halve the amounts used or use reduced salt varieties; add herbs and spices in their place
Pickles, sauces and chutneys	
Ready-made meals and take-away meals	Homemade meals using fresh ingredients

*Many processed/manufactured foods contain high amounts of salt and even lower salt varieties can have a high salt content.

Kidney Disease Outcome Quality Initiative (NKF KDOQI) classification of CKD into five stages (Table 12.9) [16]. This staging does not apply to children below 2 years of age where ongoing renal maturation is seen. Published UK data in 2009 reveal an incidence of CKD under the age of 16 of 7.4 per million age related population [17]; the incidence and prevalence for people of South Asian origin is greater than for the white and black population. The causes of CKD in children are different

Table 12.9 Stages of renal failure [16].

Stage	Description	GFR (mL/min/1.73 m^2)
1	Kidney damage with normal or increased GFR	>90
2	Kidney damage with mild decrease in GFR	60–89
3	Moderate decrease in GFR	30–59
4	Severe decrease in GFR	15–29
5	Kidney failure	<15 or dialysis

GFR, glomerular filtration rate.

Table 12.10 Causes of chronic kidney disease in childhood in the UK [18].

Cause	Percentage
Renal dysplasia and related conditions	28
Obstructive uropathy	20
Glomerular disease	17
Reflux nephropathy	9
Primary tubular and interstitial disorders	7
Congenital nephrotic syndrome	7
Renal vascular disorders	5
Metabolic disease	3
Polycystic disease	2
Malignant and related disorders	2

from adults and are shown in Table 12.10 [18]. Initially the poorly formed or damaged kidney adapts by increasing the filtration rate in the remaining nephrons through adaptive hyperfiltration; homeostatic mechanisms are usually maintained within reference ranges at this stage. In the longer term this leads to damage of the remaining nephrons and ultimately to end stage kidney disease.

Management of CKD

The management of children with CKD is based on a multidisciplinary team (MDT) approach within a specialist tertiary centre where the dietitian is a key team member. The aims of the team are to optimise the quality of life of the child and family whilst treating the complications of the disease and delaying or slowing the progression of renal disease, together with preparing them for RRT. The sequence of events in CKD forms the basis for management of these children irrespective of aetiology and addresses nutrition, growth, fluid

and electrolyte balance, acid–base abnormalities, renal bone disease, hypertension, slowing the progression of CKD, anaemia, cardiovascular disease, medication, education and psychosocial support.

A good knowledge of biochemical and haematological parameters is essential to identify variations from normal age specific reference ranges (Tables 12.3a and 12.3b) when formulating dietary management plans. The serum values of particular relevance include urea, creatinine, sodium, potassium, bicarbonate, albumin, calcium, phosphate, alkaline phosphatase, parathyroid hormone (PTH), glucose, cholesterol and triglycerides. Haemoglobin, ferritin and percent hypochromic cells (<10%) can be used to assess iron status in combination with serum iron and total iron binding capacity (TIBC) to calculate the percent transferrin saturation (TSAT = serum iron × 100 divided by TIBC), which should be maintained at >20%.

An assessment of the glomerular filtration rate (GFR) provides an indication of the overall level of renal function. GFR estimation by Cr51 EDTA clearance is used to predict when RRT is likely to be required. GFR should not be measured before 1 year of age as the kidney function may continue to mature during the first year of life and even beyond. GFR can be estimated using the Haycock Schwartz formula: predicted GFR = 40 × ht (cm)/serum creatinine (μmol/L).

Nutrition

The adverse effects of poor nutrition in children are manifested by their influence on the capacity to grow and develop appropriately. There is a complex interrelationship between renal dysfunction and nutrition whereby abnormalities or a decline in renal function frequently lead to changes in nutritional intake or metabolism, as well as poor nutrition complicating CKD. Malnutrition is associated with increased mortality. Early and careful nutritional therapy may improve both growth and mortality in all ages of children with CKD [19]. The aetiology of growth delay and cachexia in children with CKD is multifactorial with inadequate energy intake, uraemic toxicity, anaemia, increased inflammatory response and metabolic and endocrine abnormalities among the foremost causes. The dietitian plays an essential role in optimising the management of these causes and needs to ensure that individualised dietary prescriptions are practical and flexible to aid adherence.

Dietary and anthropometric assessment

There is no simple measure of nutritional status for children with CKD. Nutritional parameters are complicated on account of salt and water imbalances together with the inappropriateness of comparing growth to that of age matched populations. The frequency of nutritional monitoring depends on age, stage of CKD and how well the child is thriving. In order to prevent the development of malnutrition it is recommended that children with stages 3 and 4 CKD are seen 6 monthly and 1–3 monthly respectively [20]. Monthly review is recommended for children <2 years of age with stage 5 CKD and 3–4 monthly in the over 2s. A 24 hour dietary recall in clinic and an annual 3-day food diary analysis are valuable tools when estimating nutritional intakes and individual baseline requirements. Information on prescribed medications, presence or absence of nausea and vomiting, diarrhoea, constipation and energy levels can be helpful in determining the child's nutritional and medical needs. Dietary intake should be communicated to members of the MDT, where appropriate, to reinforce discussions and recommendations made with the child and family.

Height and weight plotted on growth charts are used to assess nutritional status. At each clinic visit accurate measurements of height or supine length, weight and, for children <2 years of age, head circumference should be obtained and plotted for chronological age on appropriate growth charts. Where the child is within normal percentile ranges for height (>2nd percentile), energy and micronutrient requirements can be based on recommendations for children of the same chronological age [8,9]. For the child who falls below the normal percentile ranges for height (<2nd percentile), their height age (age at which the child's height would be on the 50th percentile) should be used for comparison with recommended intakes for energy and micronutrients [8,9] and adjusted accordingly thereafter. Estimated dry weights need to be used in those children retaining fluid.

Extremes of body mass index (BMI) are associated with increased morbidity and mortality and children with CKD should avoid becoming overweight or obese. However, it is difficult to find a measure of body composition that is relevant for children with CKD. They may not have a normal body composition making a comparison with normal populations inappropriate. CKD may have a disproportionately greater effect on spinal growth and children have been shown to have a low ratio of length of trunk to limb [21]. They also have a relatively high fat mass, low lean mass and increased central adiposity [22]. BMI should not be used as a measure of fatness for children <2 years of age. It can also be misleading in adolescents with CKD due to delayed sexual maturation and linear growth which is further confounded by reduced muscle mass, reduced activity and fluid retention; if BMI is used it is suggested that it is plotted against the child's height age [23].

Mid upper arm circumference (MUAC) can be measured 6 monthly and compared to norms for age; MUAC is unlikely to be affected by oedema. Skinfold thickness may be affected by fluid retention. Reduced values for skinfold thickness have been found in children with CKD [19]. These and other measurements for determining body composition, including bioelectrical impedance, are generally used for research purposes only.

Dietary principles in CKD

Nutritional management of children with CKD requires attention to adequacy of energy intake; regulation of protein intake; fluid balance and electrolytes; regulation of calcium and phosphate intakes; adequacy of micronutrient and iron intakes.

Dietary recommendations depend upon age, stage of CKD, management and nutritional assessment. The recommended intakes of energy and protein in conservatively managed children are given in Table 12.11. Children with CKD are typically anorexic and have spontaneous energy intakes below the EAR for age. To achieve the EAR for energy, most children with CKD require energy supplements (Table 12.5). The majority of infants and many young children need to have a feed delivered by a nasogastric or gastrostomy tube to optimise nutrition [24].

Energy

The energy requirements for children with CKD are the same as those of normal children. Energy

Table 12.11 Nutritional guidelines for the child with chronic kidney disease.

Age	Energy (per kg body weight per day)		Protein (per kg body weight per day)
	(kcal)	(kJ)	(g)
Conservative management			
Infants			
Preterm	110–135	460–560	2.5–3.0
0–2 months	96–120	400–500	2.1
3–12 months	72–96	300–400	1.5–1.6
1–3 years	78–82	325–340	1.1
Children/adolescents			
4 years to puberty	Minimum of EAR for chronological age		1.0–1.1
Pubertal	(use height age if <2nd percentile for		0.9–1.0
Post-pubertal	height)		0.8–0.9
Peritoneal dialysis (APD/CAPD)			
Infants			
Preterm	110–135	460–560	3.0–4.0
0–2 months	96–120	400–500	2.4
3–12 months	72–96	300–400	1.9
1–3 years	78–82	325–340	1.4
Children/adolescents			
4 years to puberty	Minimum of EAR for chronological age		1.3
Pubertal	(use height age if <2nd percentile for		1.2
Post-pubertal	height)		1.0–1.2
Haemodialysis			
Infants			
Preterm	110–135	460–560	3.0
0–2 months	96–120	400–500	2.2
3–12 months	72–96	300–400	1.7
1–3 years	78–82	325–340	1.2
Children/adolescents			
4 years to puberty	Minimum of EAR for chronological age		1.1
Pubertal	(use height age if <2nd percentile for		1.1
Post-pubertal	height)		1.1

These guidelines are for the initiation of management and require adjustments based on individual nutritional assessment.
Protein intakes reflect the reference nutrient intake (RNI) in the UK [9] plus an increment to achieve positive nitrogen balance including any transperitoneal losses [16].
EAR, estimated average requirement [8]; APD, automated peritoneal dialysis; CAPD, continuous ambulatory peritoneal dialysis.

intakes below the EAR contribute to growth failure. The provision of adequate energy is essential to promote appropriate weight gain and growth in all children with CKD and is especially important in stages 3 and 4 to avoid the use of lean muscle mass as an energy source. The EAR for energy for either height age (if the child's height is <2nd percentile) or chronological age (if the child falls within the normal percentile range) is used as baseline guidelines (Table 12.11) [8]. Raised serum urea levels in combination with increased serum potassium levels can be suggestive of catabolism and the need to increase non-protein energy intake.

High energy, low protein foods
These include sugar, glucose, jam, marmalade, honey, syrup and should be encouraged where possible. The liberal use of polyunsaturated or mono-unsaturated oils in cooking or margarine spread on bread, toast or added to meals and vegetables can contribute significantly to the child's

energy intake. Special low protein dietary products such as bread and biscuits are rarely needed.

Energy supplements

Anorexia, nausea and vomiting are features of CKD and can be exacerbated by uraemia. These symptoms, together with an abnormal sense of taste, contribute to a reduced energy intake. Energy supplements are helpful in meeting this deficit. A number of supplements are available and enable a flexible approach (Table 12.5). Combined fat and CHO supplements or glucose polymer alone, if additional fat is not tolerated, can be successfully added to infant formulas, tube feeds and oral nutritional supplements. The concentrations of CHO and fat should be increased gradually to establish tolerance. Assuming normal gut function, the following upper limits for CHO and fat can be worked towards:

- infants <6 months: 12% CHO and 5% fat
- infants >6 months to 1 year: 15% CHO and 6% fat
- toddlers aged 1–2 years: 20% CHO and 7% fat
- older children: 32% CHO and 9% fat

Liquid glucose polymers are useful when diluted with a fizzy drink or diluted squash and the volume used will depend on the fluid allowance. Powdered glucose polymers are useful in children who drink plenty of water or squash. Each day a target amount to use should be negotiated and a personalised record chart can aid compliance.

Protein

Children, especially infants and young children, have a high requirement for protein per kilogram body weight because of the demands of growth. A recent systematic review of protein restriction for children with CKD [25] showed no significant impact on delaying progression of renal failure and there is an association with inferior growth. The correlation between dietary protein intake and proteinuria was also insignificant.

Protein intake should be optimised to allow for the maintenance of nitrogen balance and growth together with the preservation of lean body mass. In CKD, protein must provide at least 100% of the RNI for age to avoid protein becoming a limiting factor in growth [19]. The RNI for height age is advised when the child is <2nd centile for height. Insufficient protein will impact on body composition with a predominance of fat rather than lean tissue being laid down. Children achieve recommended protein intakes more easily than their energy requirements and a protein intake above 3 g protein/kg should be avoided because of the associated phosphorus load and link with cardiovascular morbidity. Where dairy proteins have been limited to restrict phosphate intake, and adequate energy intake has been ensured to promote anabolism, further protein modification is seldom needed. However, when a child's serum urea remains persistently >20 mmol/L, a gradual protein reduction based on the child's 3-day dietary record should be initiated to lower the urea level to <20 mmol/L. Protein of a high biological value should comprise 65%–70% of the total dietary protein intake.

Growth

Growth retardation is one of the major complications of childhood CKD and correlates with the age of onset. Most children do not reach their genetic height potential despite optimal management. Fall-off in growth velocity or weight can be early indicators of growth failure and potential causes must be explored. The cause of growth failure is multifactorial and includes growth hormone (GH) and insulin-like growth factor 1 (IGF-1), nutritional status, acid–base balance and bone mineralisation [26]. Cytokines are known to suppress the appetite through their action on the central nervous system. Anaemia, chronic infection, corticosteroid therapy and psychosocial factors can also play a part. The paediatric dietitian, as part of the MDT, contributes to optimising the management of these factors where appropriate.

Normal growth in childhood occurs in four phases: prenatal, infantile, childhood and pubertal. Nutrition is important in all growth phases but especially during the infantile stage when growth is at its highest and is less dependent on GH. There is a slowing of growth velocity in the childhood phase when growth is more dependent on the GH/IGF-1 axis [19]. At puberty, which is typically delayed in CKD, there is a rapid increase in growth velocity in response to sex steroids and GH; adequate nutrition is important during this anabolic phase.

The importance of satisfactory nutrition and electrolyte balance in infancy to optimise growth is well recognised [27] and is the most critical time for nutritional intervention to have an effect on catch-up growth. Supplementary feeding using the enteral route is invariably indicated in this group. There is ongoing debate as to whether older children with renal failure are able to follow their growth percentiles with the provision of adequate nutrition alone. An improvement in height standard deviation score (SDS) has been observed in a small group study [27] although other studies have not consistently shown an improvement in growth with nutritional supplements [19]. Other factors including the dysregulation of hormones and cytokines are implicated. The most recent KDOQI guidelines suggest that in older children, poor intake may be a result of inadequate growth and not the cause [28]. For children with a height or height velocity for chronological age below −2SDS, growth hormone therapy following the optimisation of nutritional management has been shown to increase height velocity and final adult height [29]. Children with CKD have an inadequate response of GH stimulating IGF-1 production despite normal or raised levels of circulating GH.

Fluid and electrolyte balance

In several causes of CKD in infancy, including obstructive uropathy and renal dysplasia, there is poor urinary concentrating capacity and sodium wasting. Sodium depletion results in contraction of the extracellular fluid volume and further impairment in renal function, as well as impairment of growth [30]. Sodium chloride supplements can be added to infant feeds or be given as a medicine. The amount should be increased until an improvement in growth is seen without the development of hypertension, peripheral oedema or hypernatraemia. Such infants typically require up to 4–6 mmol sodium/kg/day. These infants are usually polyuric and require free access to fluids in the form of supplemented feed and extra water.

In contrast, children with primary renal diseases exhibiting hypertension may benefit from a reduction in sodium intake as a no added salt diet avoiding salted snacks and encouraging fresh foods (Table 12.8).

As the GFR declines in CKD stages 4 and 5, sodium and fluid retention are commonly seen.

This can lead to volume overload and hypertension; dietary sodium and fluid restriction together with diuretics are instigated. Fluid restrictions are only instituted as urine output diminishes or oedema develops, more usually when the GFR falls below $15\,mL/min/1.73\,m^2$. Fluid prescriptions are individualised to take account of insensible losses and a typical day's urine output.

The majority of children with CKD stages 1–3 maintain potassium homeostasis. If hyperkalaemia occurs, other correctable causes including drugs such as angiotensin-converting enzyme (ACE) inhibitors, metabolic acidosis and catabolism should be excluded before initiating a potassium modified diet (Table 12.6). A haemolysed blood sample will show a falsely high serum potassium level. In stage 5 CKD, hyperkalaemia necessitates a potassium modified diet; any nutritional supplements used must be exchanged for low potassium varieties. Foods containing the preservative potassium sorbate should be minimised if hyperkalaemia persists; 100 g of food containing this additive can add an additional 1.0–2.5 mmol of potassium to the diet. Hyperkalaemia is the most dangerous of the electrolyte disturbances, affecting cardiac function.

Hypokalaemia is seen in renal tubular disorders such as cystinosis and Bartter's syndrome. Potassium supplements are usually indicated together with medication (indometacin) that reduces renal sodium, potassium and water losses [31]. Hypokalaemia can be seen in polyuric CKD as well as resulting from the use of some diuretics or with episodes of diarrhoea and vomiting.

Acid–base abnormalities

Maintenance of acid–base status is important in infants and children. Faltering growth in infancy can be associated with persistent metabolic acidosis, as can bone demineralisation and hyperkalaemia. Extracellular potassium shifts occur with metabolic acidosis as bicarbonate is lost through the kidney. Acidosis is corrected with the administration of sodium bicarbonate. Sodium bicarbonate supplements do not usually cause sodium retention until CKD stage 5 and, as such, have little effect on blood pressure control; they do not usually need to be included in an assessment of sodium intake. Dialysis will usually correct acidosis. Chronic acidosis contributes to insulin resistance and may affect growth. In older children a protein intake in excess of requirements, and hence an excess in intake of sulphur containing amino acids, can increase endogenous acid production. Protein intake should be modified in such instances.

CKD-mineral bone disorder (CKD-MBD)

The pathogenesis of CKD-MBD is complex. Children with stage 2 CKD usually have no signs of bone abnormalities but biochemical abnormalities can be evident. There is a fall in 1,25-dihydroxyvitamin D3 production; this results in an increase in PTH levels and a drop in serum calcium levels, further stimulating PTH production. Phosphate retention, as a result of reduced GFR, causes hypocalcaemia and a rise in PTH. Secondary hyperparathyroidism causes bone resorption and a further increase in serum phosphate levels when GFR is low [15]. In addition to MBD, this process can lead to calcification in other tissues including blood vessels and muscle tissue as well as phosphate acting as a uraemic toxin. Recent evidence indicates an increased prevalence of generalised vitamin D deficiency in CKD which might also contribute to CKD-MBD.

Management of CKD-MBD is a combination of limiting dietary phosphate intake and the use of oral phosphate binders. The control of phosphate levels is of fundamental importance to slow the progression of parathyroid gland morphology. Optimal control of bone and mineral homeostasis is essential for preventing debilitating skeletal complications, achieving adequate growth and preserving long term cardiovascular health. PTH levels are a sensitive marker of abnormalities in bone mineral metabolism and levels should be regularly monitored with an aim of maintaining levels within or less than twice the normal range [32].

Dietary phosphate restriction
Organic phosphorus is present in most foods. Phosphorus is naturally found in foods that are rich in protein. Bioavailability is lower from plant foods, including seeds and legumes, due to the limited gastrointestinal absorption of phytate based phosphorus. Gastrointestinal absorption of organic phosphorus is efficient at 40%–60%. Inorganic phosphorus is the main component of many preservatives and additive salts found in processed foods. This is more readily disassociated and absorption is reported as >90% [33]. These food preservatives add to the phosphorus burden of the diet and need to be factored into dietary counselling.

Phosphate restriction (Table 12.7) should start as soon as biochemical abnormalities are seen. In infants standard whey based infant formulas are used for at least 1–2 years due to their lower phosphate content. Where hyperphosphataemia persists, Kindergen or Renastart (Table 12.5), usually in combination with standard whey based infant formula, can be used to regulate serum phosphate levels. Consideration should be given to their lower calcium and potassium contents. In older children, cow's milk can be introduced in a controlled amount. Individualised targets should be given for cow's milk and cow's milk products. Where indicated, nutritional supplements with a lower phosphate content (Table 12.5) should be chosen and be included within the dietary allowance. Guidelines for phosphate intake are based on body weight as follows:

- infants <10 kg <400 mg/day
- children 10–20 kg <600 mg/day
- children 20–40 kg <800 mg/day
- children >40 kg <1000 mg/day

Care needs to be taken not to compromise protein intake whilst restricting dietary phosphate. A guide to the phosphorus content of different foods per gram of protein is given in Table 12.12. Dietary strategies should enable children and their carers to choose foods with less phosphate but to maintain an adequate protein intake. Maintenance of serum

Table 12.12 Guide to the phosphorus content of foods related to their protein content.

Type of food	Phosphorus (mg/g protein)
Poultry, meat and white fish	7–9
Pulses	12–18
Tofu	12
Shell fish, oily fish, offal	15–20
Egg	16
Hard cheese	20
Milk, yoghurt	28
Peanuts	15
Almonds	26
Walnuts	48

Table 12.13 Phosphate binders.

	Elemental calcium, mg (mmol) per tablet	Dose	Flavour	Estimate of potential binding power
Calcium carbonate binders				
Setler's Tums tablets (500 mg)	200 (5.0)	1–3 tds	Spearmint, peppermint, various fruit flavours	Approximately 39 mg phosphorus bound per 1 g calcium carbonate
Calcium carbonate (20% solution)	400 (10.0) per 5 mL	5–15 mL tds	–	
Rennie tablets Digestif/Spearmint (680 mg)	272 (6.8)	1 tds	Peppermint/ spearmint	
Remegel tablets (800 mg)	320 (8.0)	1–3 tds	Mint	
Calcichew tablets (1250 mg)	500 (12.6)	1 tds	Orange	
Adcal (1500 mg)	600 (15.0)	1 tds	Fruit flavour	
Calcium acetate binders				
Phosex tablets (1000 mg)	250 (6.25)	1–3 tds	(swallow whole)	Approximately 45 mg phosphorus bound per 1 g calcium acetate
Phosex tablets (500 mg) named patient basis	125 (3.1)	2–4 tds	(swallow whole)	
Sevelamer binders				
Sevelamer hydrochloride Renagel tablet (800 mg)	None	1–3 tds	(swallow whole)	Approximately 80 mg phosphorus bound per 1 g sevelamer
Sevelamer carbonate Renvela tablet (800 mg) or powder (2.4 g)	None	1–3 tds or 1 sachet of powder	Powder in natural or citrus flavour	

tds, three times a day.
Total intake of elemental calcium (including diet) should not be >1500 mg of calcium per day [42].

phosphate within the normal reference values for age is desirable (Table 12.3a). During conservative management and when on haemodialysis, phosphate intake will be reduced with protein modification.

Calcium intake is compromised when phosphate is restricted in the diet and may need supplementation. An average of 20%–30% of the calcium in calcium based phosphate binders is absorbed and therefore can be factored into calcium intake.

Hydroxylated vitamin D

Vitamin D is converted to the activated form 1,25-dihydroxyvitamin D3 in the healthy kidney. The decrease in activated vitamin D levels seen in CKD and the resultant hyperparathyroidism may be addressed by a reduction in phosphate intake, but usually requires supplementation with hydroxylated vitamin D3 in order to increase the absorption of calcium in the small intestine. The most common preparation used in the UK is 1α-hydroxycholecalciferol (alfacalcidol). The dose is based on serum calcium and PTH levels and is

reduced or suspended if calcium levels are above the normal range (Table 12.3a). There is current ongoing work to determine whether vitamin D supplementation, as colecalciferol, is beneficial in children with CKD.

Phosphate binders

Although dietary management can control plasma levels in early CKD stages, persistent hyperphosphataemia requires the addition of oral phosphate binding drugs to block intestinal phosphate absorption (Table 12.13). Aluminium salts, although effective phosphate binders, have been abandoned in children due to their toxicity. Calcium carbonate is the first line phosphate binder in children. Tablets should be chewed and taken preferably just before meals/snacks as a lower pH improves binding capacity. Alternatively tablets can be crushed to a fine powder or used in solution and then be added to feed bottles or overnight/daytime bolus feeds. Regular shaking is recommended as the powder can settle out. Calcium carbonate impairs the absorption of iron so should be taken separately from oral iron supplements. Approximately 20%–30% of the calcium contained in a calcium phosphate binder will be absorbed and can contribute to hypercalcaemia. Calcium acetate achieves a similar control of serum phosphate at a lower dose of elemental calcium. It is taken during meals and swallowed whole. Calcium based binders can lead to an increase of the Ca × P ion product and the development of vascular and soft tissue calcification. Soft tissue calcification has been reported in 60% of autopsies of children with renal failure [34].

To reduce positive calcium balance, non-calcium containing phosphate binders are increasingly used [35]. Sevelamer hydrochloride and sevelamer carbonate are calcium free synthetic anion exchange polymers which bind phosphate and cholesterol. Sevelamer carbonate reverses the negative effect of sevelamer hydrochloride on acid–base balance. Lanthanum carbonate has recently become available. It is also calcium free but is not currently used in children, with a lack of data on the effect on the growing skeleton.

Calcimimetic agents (cinacalcet)
Cinacalcet is a calcimimetic agent which increases the sensitivity of calcium sensing receptors to extracellular calcium ions, thereby inhibiting the release of PTH. It is gaining use in severe cases of hyperparathyroidism. Promising results have been seen in limited paediatric trials [36].

Hypertension

Hypertension is common in the late stages of CKD and is due to fluid overload and the activation of the renin-angiotensin-aldosterone system [15]. Hyperparathyroidism can also contribute. Management strategies include salt restriction (Table 12.8), exercise, carefully monitored weight loss in overweight children and strict fluid control where appropriate.

Many children readily exceed the adult daily maximum recommendation for sodium intake of 100 mmol (6 g salt) because of their penchant for salted snacks and processed foods. Dietary advice should take into account current lifestyles and the hidden salt in foods when devising targets to reduce salt intake. Advice needs to be given on interpreting food labels and giving ideas for lower salt snacks. The food industry needs to continue

Table 12.14 Recommendations on salt consumption in children.

Age range	Target daily intake of salt (g) and sodium (mmol)	
0–6 months	<1 g	<17 mmol
7–12 months	1 g	17 mmol
1–3 years	2 g	34 mmol
4–6 years	3 g	50 mmol
7–10 years	5 g	84 mmol
11–14 years	6 g	100 mmol

Target salt intakes for infants and children have been estimated as an increase in the reference nutrient intake (RNI) by a factor of 1.5 [37].

the policy of reducing the salt content of their products for the population at large. Poor compliance with salt restriction is a common observation. The Scientific Advisory Committee on Nutrition (SACN) [37] gives recommendations on salt intake for children throughout childhood which can be used as a guideline (Table 12.14).

In the absence of fluid overload, hypotensive therapy is started when the child's systolic or diastolic blood pressures are repeatedly >90th centile for age. The Dietary Approaches to Stop Hypertension (DASH) trial showed in adults that a salt reduction together with a healthy eating plan could reduce blood pressure by 11.5/5.7 mmHg in hypertensive subjects and 7.1/3.7 in normotensives [38]. It would be prudent to avoid excessive sodium intakes in this group of children.

Preservation of renal function

In most children with CKD, renal function continues to decline with the progression being greatest in infancy and puberty. Decline is also seen with progressive glomerulosclerosis, interstitial fibrosis and vascular sclerosis. Control of proteinuria and hypertension has proven to be the strongest independent predictor for progression of renal disease [39]. Proteinuria is associated with inflammatory factors in the urine which contribute to renal disease progression. ACE inhibitors have a renoprotective benefit independent of their antihypertensive effects and are prescribed in some children with proteinuria [40].

The lack of significant impact from protein restriction in children was considered earlier (p. 254). There is reluctance to recommend dietary modification in an attempt to delay the progression of chronic renal insufficiency in the early stages of CKD [41]. Similarly there is currently a lack of evidence in the paediatric literature supporting the effects of addressing hyperlipidaemia and hyperhomocysteinaemia [18].

Anaemia

The anaemia of CKD is associated with substantial morbidity, an increased risk of cardiovascular disease, reduced quality of life and reduced exercise capacity. Anaemia is seen in children when their GFR is $<60\,mL/min/1.73\,m^2$. The blood film is a normochromic, normocytic anaemia as a consequence of inadequate erythropoietin production by the damaged kidneys. The aetiology of anaemia in CKD is multifactorial with iron and folate deficiency, reduced red blood cell survival, hyperparathyroidism induced bone marrow suppression and gastrointestinal loss. Serum ferritin is used to assess iron status (Table 12.3a) and should be $>100\,\mu g/L$. Management aims are to prevent the development of iron deficiency anaemia and the maintenance of adequate iron stores. Haematology results are frequently monitored by the MDT.

Dietary assessment
Foods rich in iron, folic acid and vitamins C and B_{12} should be advised to ensure children are achieving recommended intakes for age and sex [9]. Sources of haem iron are to be recommended together with advice about non haem iron and its potential inhibition by phytates in cereal grains and legumes; polyphenols including tannin in tea, coffee and cocoa; and calcium in milk and dairy products.

Oral iron supplements
Oral iron supplements are prescribed when dietary iron intake is insufficient to maintain adequate iron stores. As the child progresses to stage 5 CKD intravenous iron therapy is used.

Iron preparations can be prescribed as liquid, tablet or capsule to aid compliance. Vitamin C enhances the absorption of non haem iron. It is important to avoid over supplementation. Oral iron is prescribed at a daily dose of 2–3 mg of elemental iron/kg body weight/day and given in two to three divided daily doses. Iron is best absorbed in the absence of medications (antacids/phosphate binders), food, infant formulas, milk or nutritional supplements. Ideally, it should be taken 1 hour before or 2 hours following a feed or meal and be taken with a micronutrient supplement where prescribed. Problems with compliance are common, particularly with the potential side effects including nausea, vomiting and constipation. The ideal prescription can be impractical and a flexible approach that is conducive to the child's feeding pattern, school and family should be advised.

Cardiovascular disease

The lifespan of children with advanced CKD remains low compared with the general paediatric population, with cardiovascular disease (CVD) accounting for the majority of deaths [42]. Cardiovascular abnormalities develop early in the course of CKD and progress as end stage is reached. Recognised risk factors in renal insufficiency include a pro-atherogenic state with left ventricular hypertrophy (LVH), hyperlipidaemia, hypoalbuminaemia, hypertension and dysregulated mineral metabolism. Hypertension and volume overload are associated with the development of LVH in children. There is consistent association between the time on dialysis and deteriorating measures of vascular function. Thickening and stiffness of the blood vessel walls have both been associated with abnormal levels of calcium, phosphorus and parathyroid hormone [42]. The lifelong nature of CKD reinforces the importance of dietetic involvement in reducing CVD risks in connection with addressing the management of fluid levels, hypertension and the regulation of the calcium-phosphorus-parathyroid hormone complex and levels of vitamin D.

Education and psychosocial support

The conservative stage of CKD management is a time for ongoing education and preparation for the child and family by all members of the renal team in preparation for stage 5 CKD management. Progressive renal failure is disruptive to a child's schooling, social life and family life. To many families, nutrition can be one of the more demanding parts of management. An understanding of the psychosocial effects of feeding such children is as important as the nutritional advice [43]. Many families travel long distances to their renal unit; regular telephone contact and visits to the home, nursery and school can be invaluable supportive measures to clinic visits. Good communication is essential with other team members to help develop practice, management strategies and share team philosophies which ultimately lead to better patient care. Adequate dietetic time is crucial to provide the close and frequent supervision which is required to monitor and maintain qualitative standards of care for each child, due to the changing needs for growth and development. Attendance on ward rounds, outpatients clinic and psychosocial team meetings are essential [43].

Medication

Several of the prescribed medications in CKD are nutrition related (including phosphate binders, oral iron, sodium supplements, vitamins) and should be periodically reviewed as part of the dietary assessment. Children and their families should be advised on the correct administration and timing of medications to ensure compliance, optimise absorption and minimise potential side effects. Ongoing discussion with education and information about each medication should be routine within each dietetic review. The practicalities of taking medications, including at school, should be identified and regimens adjusted accordingly following medical and team discussion. Adherence with medication is a significant problem, especially amongst the adolescent group.

Management of stage 5 CKD

For many children with established renal failure the treatment can be cyclical between dialysis and transplantation. The treatment of choice for all children with established renal failure is a successful renal transplant with pre-emptive transplantation occurring before dialysis is required. Transplantation provides superior long term survival and quality of life. Children are usually activated on the national waiting list for cadaveric renal transplantation at NHS Blood and Transplant when their GFR falls to approximately $10\,mL/min/1.73\,m^2$. Living donor transplantation is becoming the choice for an increasing number of families.

Pre-emptive transplantation is not always possible and is unsuitable for certain renal diseases or if the child presents in established renal failure. Dialysis is started once a patient becomes symptomatic and biochemical abnormalities and fluid overload are unresponsive to conservative management alone. Dialysis in children can be by haemodialysis (HD) or peritoneal dialysis (PD). In the UK, PD is the favoured dialysis modality for children [15].

Chronic dialysis

PD is preferable for young and small patients. It offers the advantages of being performed at home and allows regular school attendance, but gives a high level of responsibility to the child's carer. HD has the disadvantage of being a hospital based treatment which disrupts the home routine, but it can relieve the family of a great responsibility and may be used to give the carer some respite. A child will transfer to HD if there is a loss of peritoneal access or function. No comparative studies of HD and PD outcomes in children suggest that one procedure is superior to the other [44]. In the UK in 2009, of the children on dialysis 55.7% were on PD [17]. Home haemodialysis has been developed in some countries and has been introduced as a dialysis option in the UK.

The performance of PD requires a patent abdominal cavity and a functioning peritoneal membrane across which solute and fluid transport can take place. A PD catheter is inserted into the abdominal wall. PD can be performed intermittently (usually overnight) using an automated cycling machine. This automated peritoneal dialysis (APD) is the preferred option in smaller children, combining five or six overnight exchanges with a long daytime dwell of dialysate. Alternatively the child may have continuous ambulatory peritoneal dialysis (CAPD) where the child or carer carries out three to four exchanges of dialysate during the day with a long overnight dwell.

Peritoneal membrane transport capacity for solutes and ultrafiltration can be estimated using a standardised peritoneal equilibration test (PET) which is used in determining the PD prescription including dialysate dwell times. A low transporter status in the PET indicates low purification rates and potential issues in achieving creatinine clearance, but ultrafiltration is good; the number of cycles can be low over a long duration. A high solute transport rate in the PET implies good purification, but is associated with rapid glucose absorption and dissipation of the osmotic gradient needed for ultrafiltration; short dwells and increased glucose exposure are usually required to attain sufficient water removal and ultimately ultrafiltration fails [45]. These patients are classed as rapid transporters. Several new PD solutions have been introduced to improve PD therapy. Peritonitis is the single most common complication of PD and requires antibiotic therapy. Anorexia can be seen as a result of the pressure effect caused by the dialysate in the abdomen.

HD is an intermittent process lasting 4–6 hours typically three times a week; smaller children, especially anuric patients, frequently require four or more dialysis sessions a week to ensure adequate fluid removal. Small molecular weight solutes are removed from the blood by diffusion through a semipermeable membrane. Small solute clearance is typically measured by urea clearance and is dependent on the clearance characteristics of the dialyser and the blood pump flow rate [46]. The dialysis fluid composition takes into account concentrations of sodium, potassium, chloride, bicarbonate, calcium, magnesium and glucose. HD provides a greater level of small molecule mass transfer than PD. Access to the circulation is usually through a central venous catheter in younger children whilst an arterio-venous fistula is created in older children once blood vessels have developed sufficiently. Central venous catheters pose an infection risk.

Nutrition and chronic dialysis

Children treated with dialysis require a nutritional prescription dependent on their age and treatment modality. This prescription requires regular dietetic review and includes all the points highlighted in the conservative management of CKD, together with consideration of the efficiency and demands of dialysis. Evidence based clinical practice guidelines for all stages of CKD and related complications are produced by the National Kidney Foundation Kidney Disease Outcome Quality Initiative (NKF KDOQI) [47]. Nutritional guidelines for the child with stage 5 CKD based on NKF KDOQI data [16] are given in Table 12.11.

The monitoring of dialysis prescriptions (dose of dialysis, solution(s) used, ultrafiltration) and urine output should be carried out by the nephrologist, renal nurse and dietitian and is used when formulating a nutritional prescription. Dialysis dose affects growth and nutritional status in children. Dialysis adequacy can be monitored by urea kinetic modelling, in particular by calculation of Kt/V (normalised whole body urea clearance) and nPCR (normalised protein catabolic rate). Kt/V is termed as the minimally acceptable dose of dialysis and refers to the dose of dialysis below which a significant increase in morbidity and mortality would occur. The target Kt/V for patients on PD is >2.1 [45] and on HD is 1.2 [46]. Kinetic modelling software programs can be used to tailor PD prescription to the individual's characteristics and needs. In contrast to adult patients, Kt/V is difficult to define in children and scientific data demonstrating that dialysis efficacy can be predictive of morbidity and mortality are lacking [45]. Adequacy of PD in children is better expressed by the attainment of a normal fluid and electrolyte balance plus minimal phosphate and toxin build-up in a clinically asymptomatic child, with near to normal growth and psychomotor development.

Energy

The EAR for energy [8] is used as a guideline for requirements. This is corrected for height age if the child's height is <2nd percentile (Table 12.11). There is no consistent evidence that energy requirements on dialysis are different from those for normal children. Some studies suggest that HD stimulates the release of cytokines and complement which can have the direct effect of increasing resting metabolic rate [48]. However, other studies have shown a deficit of energy stores in children on HD which, when adjusted for lean body mass, gives a similar resting energy expenditure to matched healthy children [49]. Provision of 100% EAR for energy allows for catch-up growth in children <2 years of age and shows some benefit in older children. Energy intake should be increased by up to 30% daily where recurrent vomiting is an issue [19].

During PD glucose is absorbed from the dialysis fluid. Edefonti et al. reported a mean energy contribution of 9 kcal (38 kJ)/kg body weight/day [50]. Table 12.15 gives a guide to the energy from glucose absorbed from PD fluid. Energy intake for children on PD should be reduced when excess weight

Table 12.15   Glucose absorption from peritoneal dialysate (PD).

PD solution concentration	Grams of anhydrous glucose per			Osmotic effect
	1 L	1.5 L	2 L	
1.36%	13.6	20.5	27.2	Weak hypotonic solution
2.27%	22.7	34.1	45.4	Intermediate
3.86%	38.6	57.9	77.2	Strong hypertonic solution

To calculate the energy obtained from glucose absorbed from PD fluid: total the grams of glucose from all the exchanges, multiply by 4 kcal (17 kJ) per gram and then multiply by 60%–80%.

gain is seen. For those children on PD requiring additional energy intake, it is best to consider a nutritionally complete supplement (Table 12.5) in preference to a refined CHO supplement in view of the raised triglyceride levels seen in children on PD and the additional source of exogenous glucose derived from the PD fluid. These children also have increased protein requirements and benefit from complete supplements. The use of complex CHO foods such as bread, potatoes, rice and cereals should be encouraged. The replacement of glucose in PD fluid by glucose polymers (7.5% icodextrin) is beneficial in children with sodium and water overload; in addition the transperitoneal absorption rate is much lower than that of glucose [45] and so contributes much less energy. The quantity of toxic glucose degradation products is also reduced. Significantly, increased dialysis with an icodextin daytime dwell in children on overnight APD showed no effect on albumin homeostasis in the short term [51] but longer term studies are awaited. Excess weight gain is emerging as a problem in children on PD in developed countries and dietary prescriptions need to be modified accordingly.

Protein

There are limited data to demonstrate the optimal amounts of protein for children on dialysis and existing data do not include all age ranges. Protein intake must be no less than 100% RNI for children on dialysis, with an addition to compensate for the losses of protein and amino acids across the dialysing membrane. For these reasons protein intakes can be alleged to be liberal [19].

Dietary protein restriction has led to poor growth in children on HD. Druml *et al.* demonstrated a loss of 0.2 g amino acid/L filtrate in an HD session [52]. Protein intake on HD needs to be sufficient for growth, but moderated in order to minimise large variations in blood urea levels between dialysis sessions. The aim for pre-dialysis serum urea levels should be <20 mmol/L, provided the child is not catabolic. For children on HD, an added dietary protein intake of 0.1 g/kg/day should be appropriate to compensate for dialytic losses [16].

The protein requirements of children on PD are higher than when on HD to allow for the greater reported transperitoneal losses of protein and amino acids, with the greatest losses being seen in the smaller, younger child (Table 12.11). Daily peritoneal protein losses reduce from an average of 0.28 g/kg in the first year of life to <0.1 g/kg in adolescents [53]. Dietary protein sources with a high phosphate content, including cow's milk and dairy foods (Table 12.12), need to be restricted to reduce the dietary phosphorus load that is implicated in the pathogenesis of dialysis associated calcifying arteriopathy [16]. Many infants and children require complete nutritional supplements either as sip or tube feeds (Table 12.5) to meet recommended protein intakes.

Alterations to protein intake should always be made along with ensuring an adequate energy intake. Consideration of serum urea, albumin and phosphate levels are essential in tailoring an individual's protein requirements. Hypoalbuminaemia is a marker of cachexia and protein energy wasting (PEW) and has been associated with mortality in children initiating dialysis such that each 1 g/L fall in serum albumin level has been shown to relate to a 54% increase in risk of death [54]. Rapid changes in albumin levels can, however, be attributed to non-nutritional factors including PD loss of albumin, hydration status, the presence of systemic disease, liver function and a persistent nephrotic state. Supplementary tube feeding should be considered for those children who fail to consistently take sufficient nutrition by the oral route.

Protein requirements are increased in patients with proteinuria, as well as during episodes of peritonitis or other intercurrent infections. Peritonitis has a catabolic effect on the body and the permeability of the peritoneum for protein and amino acids can increase by 50%–100%. The main protein loss is albumin although other immunoglobulins are also lost. Serum albumin levels fall in these circumstances and increased intakes of nutritionally complete supplements should be prescribed and encouraged.

Amino acid containing PD solutions have been suggested to replace transperitoneal losses and to reduce glucose load. Studies have failed to show any long term nutritional benefits in children in either improved total serum protein or albumin [19]; slight increases in serum urea have been reported.

There are losses of amino acids into the dialysate during HD. There are limited and small studies on the use of intradialytic parenteral nutrition (IDPN) in children receiving HD. An early study showed no improvement in amino acid levels after supplementation; another study showed weight gain in three adolescents with organic illness after 6 weeks of starting IDPN [55]. In those patients who do not respond to enteral supplementation, IDPN could be considered in those who have been losing >10% body weight for three consecutive months [55]. The use of IDPN remains controversial and further clinical trials are needed. There are potential side effects: hyperglycaemia, cramps and long term changes to liver function.

Protein energy wasting (PEW)

In patients with CKD, especially those undergoing maintenance dialysis, PEW is the strongest risk factor for adverse outcomes and death [56]. Younger age, duration of CKD and time on dialysis together with the presence of inflammatory diseases are increased risk factors. PEW is characterised by the state of decreased body protein mass and fuel reserves. The PEW seen in CKD is a slow, progressive process. Initially, there is slightly impaired nutrient intake and absorption plus an increase in inflammatory markers in seemingly well nourished children. In the second phase, depletion of tissue levels and body stores occurs with a change in biochemical and physiological functions; these changes progress with time and marked cachexia is seen [57].

There is evidence that inflammation is an important cause of cachexia and PEW in patients with CKD. An increase in proinflammatory cytokines, tumour necrosis factor alpha and interleukin-6 are seen [58]. These act through the hypothalamus to affect appetite and metabolic rate. In turn, poor protein anabolism results in a reduction in serum albumin and pre-albumin. Levels of albumin, pre-albumin and C-reactive protein (CRP) can be used to assess the degree of inflammation or illness but should not be used as an indicator of nutritional status. Increased energy and protein alone are not enough to reverse the catabolism associated with inflammation. Body composition studies suggest that children with stage 5 CKD who were able to maintain body mass with nutritional supplements gained fat mass rather than lean body mass [22]. Adequate dialysis is essential. Current diet therapies in the early stages of investigation into the PEW of CKD are ω3 fatty acids and soya protein, used for their anti-inflammatory properties [59]. The treatment of inflammation in improving body composition and linear growth in children with CKD is likely to become a cornerstone in management.

Nutritional supplements for infants

To meet energy and protein requirements, protein powders with a lower phosphate content can be added to standard whey based infant formulas, in combination with energy supplements (Table 12.5). Alternatively, where biochemical parameters allow, infant formulas can be concentrated progressively to provide an increased balance of all nutrients or energy dense infant formulas can be used (Table 1.18). Biochemistry should be frequently monitored, particularly with respect to potassium, phosphate and urea. A combination of Kindergen or Renastart (renal specific low phosphate and potassium infant formulas) and a standard whey based infant formula is used to design a feed to correct high serum phosphate and potassium levels. For infants >12 months of age, or whose weight is greater than 8 kg, nutritionally complete supplements can be considered (Table 12.5). Combining feeds and supplements to achieve specific intakes of particular nutrients is a common practice to achieve nutritional and biochemical goals. An example is given in Table 12.16.

Nutritional supplements for children and adolescents

A nutritionally complete low phosphate supplement is frequently prescribed on the commencement of PD [60] as part of the overall nutritional and

Table 12.16 Sample feed to meet the requirements of an infant on automated peritoneal dialysis (APD).

Feed recipe	Energy (kcal (kJ))	Protein (g)	CHO (g)	Fat (g)	Na$^+$ (mmol)	K$^+$ (mmol)	PO$_4$ (mg)
An 8-month-old boy on APD: weight 8 kg; fluid allowance 800 mL; energy requirement 72 kcal (300 kJ)/kg; protein requirement 1.9 g/kg							
110 g Cow & Gate 1	534 (2232)	10.7	59.5	28.1	6.0	13.1	223
5 g Duocal	25 (104)	0.0	29.1	8.9	0.4	0.0	2
6 g Vitapro	22 (90)	4.5	0.5	0.4	0.8	1.1	19
3.4 mL 30% NaCl	0	0.0	0.0	0.0	17.0	0.0	0
+ water to 800 mL							
Total per 100 mL	73 (303)	1.9	11.1	4.7	3.0	1.8	31
Total per 800 mL	580 (2413)	15.2	89.1	37.4	24.2	14.2	244
Total per kg	73 (303)	1.9	11.1	4.7	3.0	1.8	31
The feed needs to be modified following drainage and clearance issues with the dialysis and a period off APD. His serum biochemistry shows increased levels of urea (12.3 mmol/L), K$^+$ (6.5 mmol/L), PO$_4$ (2.4 mmol/L). Fluid needs to be restricted to 500 mL per 24 hours							
112 g Renastart	553 (2300)	9.4	78.1	29.8	13.1	3.8	115
5 g Vitapro	18 (75)	3.8	0.5	0.3	0.7	0.9	16
+ water to 500 mL							
Total per 100 ml	114 (474)	2.4	14.1	5.4	2.5	0.9	24
Total per 500 mL	571 (2375)	12.2	70.5	27.0	12.5	4.3	119
Total per kg	72 (300)	1.5	8.8	3.4	1.6	0.5	15

The feed parameters need to be continually revised with ongoing biochemistry results. The calcium content of the feed is less than half the reference nutrient intake and needs to be addressed if the feed is used over a prolonged period of time.

dialysis prescription (Table 12.5). These supplements can also be required by children on HD who fail to achieve recommended intakes. Prescribed supplements should be treated as a medication; if taken orally they are best taken in divided amounts (preferably after food) during the day or as a drink before bed.

Carnitine

Carnitine is an amino acid derivative which has a key role in the regulation of fatty acid metabolism and adenosine triphosphate (ATP) formation. Altered carnitine metabolism is seen in CKD; limited protein intake, impaired carnitine synthesis, malnutrition and dialysis all contribute. A low serum free carnitine concentration can be seen in paediatric dialysis patients [61]. Carnitine supplements have been proposed as a treatment for symptoms or complications of dialysis including intradialytic arrhythmias, skeletal muscle cramps, hypertriglyceridaemia and anaemia. Further research to support the routine supplementation in children on dialysis is needed. However, in adults

there is some evidence supporting the treatment of erythropoietin-resistant anaemia with carnitine supplements [62].

Fluid and electrolytes

Fluid

Fluid allowance is prescribed for the individual depending on insensible losses, residual urine output and dialysis modality. Insensible fluid losses are calculated as 400 mL/m^2 body surface area per day or approximately 20 mL/kg body weight/day. On PD the fluid removed by ultrafiltration is also included in formulating fluid prescriptions. Fluid weight gain between HD sessions can be problematic especially if the child is anuric; the fluid allowance is based on insensible fluid losses and fluid removal between dialysis sessions. Ideally interdialytic weight gain should not exceed 5% of the child's estimated dry weight. Prolonged fluid overload in HD can cause cardiac problems, including cardiomyopathy. Accurate weighing of patients with careful interpretation of the intake and output of fluids can help with the interpretation of fluid balance.

In children and infants receiving enteral feeds, the fluid allowance needs to be negotiated with the medical staff to allow space for nutrition and to avoid over-concentration of feeds in order to meet nutritional requirements in a small volume of fluid.

Meticulous attention should be given to fluid management to avoid the cardiovascular complications of long term fluid overload. Educating children about their fluid restriction should include practical ways of reducing fluid intake, including using tablet rather than liquid medicines, and the judicious use of foods with a high water content such as jelly, gravy, sauces and yoghurt. Thirst prevention techniques, including reducing salt intake and good mouth care, should be considered. Involving younger children in devising fluid record charts can aid compliance. It is also better, psychologically, to talk about a fluid allowance rather than a fluid restriction. An example of feeding a child on HD is given in Table 12.17.

Sodium
Infants and children, especially the polyuric infant, on PD can become hyponatraemic (serum sodium <130 mmol/L) due to the sodium losses into the ultrafiltrate. To maintain sodium balance, medicinal salt supplements are prescribed if increasing dietary sodium does not correct levels. Conversely those children on PD who are hypertensive and oedematous require education regarding a no added salt diet (Table 12.8). Hypertension and excess interdialytic weight gain seen in children on HD are invariably related to salt and water overload. The importance of a sodium restricted diet needs to be reinforced to reduce both thirst and fluid intake. An intake between 1 and 3 mmol/kg body weight/day is usually acceptable.

Potassium
A child with a good urine output can cope with a more liberal potassium intake. In anuric or anephric infants and children, dietary potassium modification is invariably indicated. In adolescents on APD, or those who are having large volumes of dialysate with CAPD, a moderate intake of potassium can usually be allowed. However, advice should be targeted at preventing overindulgence of potassium rich foods and drinks; for example crisps may be taken occasionally but suitable low potassium corn snacks are preferable, squash should be drunk in preference to pure fruit juices.

Although HD is very effective at clearing potassium because of the intermittent nature of the treatment (typically three times a week), children on HD invariably require dietary potassium advice to minimise problems with hyperkalaemia (Table 12.6). Some dialysis units allow potassium treats such as crisps or chocolate whilst

Table 12.17 Sample feed to meet the requirements of a child on haemodialysis.

Feed recipe	Energy (kcal (kJ))	Protein (g)	CHO (g)	Fat (g)	Na$^+$ (mmol)	K$^+$ (mmol)	PO$_4$ (mg)
A 6-year-old girl established on haemodialysis becomes acutely unwell and requires an enteral feed. Weight 17 kg; fluid allowance 800 mL with 700 mL reserved for the feed; energy requirement 1480 kcal (6.2 MJ); protein requirement 1.1 g protein/kg. The feed should be built up gradually to ensure tolerance							
200 mL Nepro HP*	360 (1498)	16.2	41.2	19.5	6.1	5.4	144
100 ml Paediasure*	101 (420)	2.8	11.2	4.5	2.6	2.8	53
170 g Polycal powder	652 (2712)	0.0	163.2	0.0	0.4	0.2	0
80 mL Calogen	360 (1498)	0.0	0.0	40.0	0.3	0.0	0
3g Paediatric Renal Seravit + water to 700 mL	9 (37)	0.0	2.25	0.0	0.0	0.0	51
Total per 100 ml	212 (882)	2.7	31.1	9.2	1.34	1.21	36
Total per 700 mL	1483 (6170)	19.0	217.9	64.5	9.4	8.5	249
Total per kg	87 (362)	1.1	12.8	3.8	0.6	0.5	15

*Adult renal specific feeds may be useful to achieve energy and protein requirements in a restricted fluid volume, but care needs to be taken with their micronutrient profile especially if used in large quantities. Feed provides 78% of RNI for calcium and needs reviewing if feed used in the longer term.

receiving HD; these should be eaten within the first 30 minutes of HD and be given in controlled amounts so that the potassium can be cleared during the dialysis session.

Hyperkalaemia can result in fatal cardiac arrhythmias. When plasma levels are >6.5 mmol/L there is a prolongation of the PR interval and peaking of the T wave on electrocardiogram (ECG). In such instances salbutamol is prescribed to enhance cellular potassium uptake. An ion exchange resin such as calcium resonium can be used as a crisis management strategy. It can take several HD sessions following a high serum potassium level to achieve an acceptable baseline level due to the movement of potassium from the intracellular fluid.

Advice about potassium intake needs to be tailored to each individual. Intakes need to be reviewed at frequent intervals together with blood biochemistry results and dietary analysis. A photographic album of foods rich in potassium and food models can be useful educational tools. Older children need to be involved in decision making and the setting of targets when discussing serum potassium levels.

Phosphate
Phosphate restrictions continue when on dialysis (Table 12.7). In adults 800 mg of phosphate is typically removed during each HD session and 300–400 mg/day on PD. Removal figures will be lower in children due to lower flow rates and volume of dialysate used.

Micronutrients

Little is known about the essential micronutrient requirements or biochemical status of children with CKD. Individual dietary assessment is essential, taking into account intakes from diet, infant formulas and nutritionally complete supplements, the latter often being the sole source of nutrition for many younger patients. Only then can medicinal supplements be individually and safely prescribed, where indicated. The RNI [9] for healthy children of the same age and sex provides guidelines for children with CKD [63] and should be aimed for in stages 2–5 CKD, with the exception of calcium, phosphate, magnesium, sodium and potassium which may not bear any relation to recommended dietary reference values.

For children on dialysis a water soluble vitamin supplement is often prescribed as a prudent measure, although a recent study measuring serum levels of B vitamins of mainly unsupplemented children on dialysis showed normal to high levels of these in all children [64].

Adult renal studies have shown that there are potential dialysate losses of vitamins C, B_6 and folic acid [65]. Published adult recommendations for these vitamins are likely to be too high for the majority of paediatric patients. Recommended intakes based on the RNI and from the few paediatric studies available [66] would suggest daily intakes of

- vitamin C 15 mg (infants); 60 mg (children)
- vitamin B6 0.2 mg (infants); 1.5 mg (children)
- folate 60 μg (infants); 400 μg (children)

Excessive intakes of vitamin C should be avoided as elevated oxalate levels can lead to the development of vascular complications [67].

Vitamin A levels are invariably increased in the serum of children on dialysis as retinol binding protein levels increase with uraemia. Elevated levels of vitamin A in CKD have been associated with hypercalcaemia, anaemia and hyperlipidaemia [68]. An excessive intake of vitamin A should be avoided. An intake close to the RNI is a sensible practice target [69]; however, this can be difficult to achieve in practice when the vitamin A contribution from feeds and nutritional supplements is also considered.

Recent studies highlight that a high proportion of children with CKD, especially those of South Asian origin, are vitamin D deficient or insufficient. High PTH levels in children with CKD could be due to vitamin D deficiency [70] and studies are recommending early diagnosis and treatment; this is especially pertinent with the anti-inflammatory role of vitamin D.

Further research on the links between vitamin B status and homocysteine, an amino acid intermediate, with CVD may affect recommendations for children in the future [71]. Homocysteine is an intermediary of methionine metabolism which, at raised levels, is a risk factor for CVD. Hyperhomocysteinaemia is common in adult patients with chronic renal insufficiency and appears to relate to reduced clearance of plasma homocysteine. Supraphysiological folic acid treatment has been used to normalise homocysteine levels in CKD but a recent systematic review has shown that homocysteine lowering based on folic acid does not reduce cardiovascular events in people with kidney disease and should not be used as such [72].

Dietary assessments typically reveal zinc and copper intakes below recommended values. It is helpful to measure serum levels before starting supplementation as these trace elements have impaired clearance with reduced renal function.

Children more at risk of possible micronutrient deficiencies include those who are anorexic and not under the direct care of a specialist renal unit and dietitian. Children who have prolonged periods on restricted diets when conservatively managed or who have prolonged time on dialysis, complicated by peritonitis or other intercurrent infections, are also of concern. Infants and children receiving nutritional support from complete feeds, usually by the enteral tube feeding route, are less likely to require extra vitamin and minerals. Older children, with an inadequate diet and poor compliance with oral nutritional supplements, often benefit from micronutrient supplements.

Micronutrient intakes can be greater than the RNI when adult renal specific feeds are used solely or in combination for children. It needs to be borne in mind that some nutrients, including pyridoxine and magnesium, can have toxic effects at high intakes. Dietary intake should be evaluated and serum levels measured where intake far exceeds the RNI.

To aid compliance and acceptability the taste and presentation of micronutrient supplements are important factors. Ketovite tablets, providing vitamins C, E and B complex (dose 1–3 per day) are most widely prescribed. A renal specific micronutrient supplement, Dialyvit Paediatric, containing recommended dietary reference intakes for B complex vitamins plus vitamins C, E, K, copper and zinc is available [73].

Encapsulating peritoneal sclerosis (EPS)

EPS is a serious and life threatening complication of long term PD with an incidence of 1%–3% in adult CKD patients. It is rare in paediatric patients but has been reported in Japan due to the unavailability of deceased donor transplantation. EPS is characterised by partial or diffuse bowel obstruction, accompanied by sclerotic thickening of the peritoneal membrane. The clinical presentation includes abdominal pain, nausea, vomiting, weight loss, low grade fever and ultrafiltration failure [74]. Duration of PD is the largest risk factor. The treatment is surgical removal of the sclerosed peritoneum. Post surgery, parenteral nutrition is commenced for 10–14 days. The possibility of refeeding syndrome needs to be considered (p. 78). Enteral feeds are gradually reintroduced and patients can have a high degree of anxiety about recurrent abdominal symptoms.

Nutritional considerations for infants with CKD

Improved clinical experience in dialysis techniques and renal transplantation has seen increasing numbers of infants taken onto end stage management programmes. The ultimate goal is early transplantation; this is technically more complex in the very small child. Most units prefer to promote the growth of the child to a bodyweight >10 kg or length >80 cm before they are eligible for transplantation. Optimal nutrition, with or without early dialysis, is essential in the care of these infants and young children since growth is crucially nutrition dependent during the first 2 years of life. Nutrition has been one of the most important factors responsible for the improved outcomes and improved growth seen in this population [75,76]. Data on growth, without the use of growth hormone, and the dietetic contact necessary to manage and support children and their families receiving chronic PD and intensive nutrition support illustrates the essential role of paediatric renal dietitians in the management of such families [77]. The provision of adequate nutrition for growth requires frequent adjustments of nutritional prescriptions in accordance with blood biochemistry, especially in pre-school children.

Once diagnosis is established, there may be a period of conservative management to determine if renal function improves or stabilises. Supplementary enteral feeding is indicated early to achieve and maintain growth and neurodevelopmental progress. In addition, salt and water should not be restricted in the salt-wasting polyuric child [19]. Initiation of enteral feeds before height deficits were noted has been associated with superior height outcomes compared with initiation after growth had faltered [78].

For infants requiring dialysis, APD has become the preferred choice due to its capacity for fluid removal; enteral feeding programmes should be commenced before or at the initiation of dialysis using nasogastric tubes or gastrostomy devices. A gastrostomy button can be inserted at the same time as insertion of the chronic dialysis catheter in children <5 years of age and this is increasingly practised in older children when it is anticipated that there will be a struggle to meet the nutritional prescription [79, 80]. Some believe that gastrostomy tube feeding provides better growth outcomes; however, evidence for this is needed [78]. Tube feeding reduces some of the parental anxieties associated with oral feeding whilst assuring nutritional and medication prescriptions are met. It is preferable to force feeding, which can result in vomiting and/or refusal of formula or food as well as having a detrimental effect on normal oral feeding behaviour in the long term [81]. Complications of gastrostomy feeding are rare but include post-surgical peritonitis in children already on PD when the gastrostomy is formed; an open procedure reduces this risk [19].

Vomiting can be an ongoing problem for some infants; feed prescriptions should be closely monitored and altered appropriately. Some infants are sensitive to changes in their fluid balance and this should be considered in relation to vomiting. Persistent vomiting is stressful for families, particularly mothers, and close dietetic and team support is required in the long term [43]. Gastro-oesophageal reflux (GOR) and disturbances in gastrointestinal motility are common in infants with CKD [82] and investigations to detect and treat appropriately are essential. Advice about appropriate positioning of the baby when feeding should be initially advised and a thickened feed can be tried (p. 136). Gastroparesis (delayed gastric emptying) can be treated with prokinetic agents such as metoclopramide, erythromycin and domperidone. Some medications, including calcium channel blockers and calcitonin, can delay gastric emptying and should be reviewed. Persistent GOR can respond to proton pump inhibitors such as omeprazole and lansoprazole [83]. In extreme cases anti-reflux surgery may be indicated; in a review of their population of infants in stage 5 CKD Kari *et al.* found that 22% of those who received enteral nutrition to achieve nutritional adequacy required a Nissen fundoplication to manage their persistent vomiting [24]. Vomiting of a psychogenic nature can be seen in some children, particularly those living in stressful family circumstances [84]. Carers, especially those of infants, need frequent reassurance that lack of interest in food and anorexia are symptomatic of renal failure.

Weaning should be encouraged at the customary recommended age to enable the development of oral feeding experiences and the reduction of sensitisation to food. The feeding problems seen in infants and young children with CKD are multifactorial. Many of these babies commonly pass large volumes of dilute urine; this creates a thirst and preference for water rather than formula. The large number and volume of prescribed medications can contribute to refusal to take adequate formula by mouth. These babies have disordered taste perception and refuse energy dense sweetened foods in preference for salty foods. They often find difficulty in swallowing lumpy foods and fail to progress from puréed baby foods to more energy dense family foods; in extreme circumstances even puréed foods may cause choking and retching [85]. Carers need reassurance that it is typical for a child with CKD to only take small amounts of food and drink and that the early introduction of enteral feeding is recommended before growth failure is evident. Positive reinforcement with the use of dummies (pacifiers) and oral feeding whilst receiving daytime enteral bolus feeds should be encouraged to help minimise feeding issues [86].

Enteral feeding regimens that provide a balanced fat and CHO profile to meet energy requirements do not enhance the hyperlipidaemia seen in CKD [87].

Nutritional support

Prevention of growth disturbances is a major goal of nutritional therapy. The early initiation of enteral nutritional support is considered when the child's oral intake fails to meet recommended nutritional intakes and growth velocity is affected. Prolonged trials of oral supplements should be discouraged. Brief intervals of poor growth during infancy can result in significant loss of height potential. Where oral supplementation is unsuccessful, enteral tube feeding should be instigated early before significant nutritional deficits and aversive feeding interactions have developed between the child and family.

There needs to be a discussion with the family and team members as to the most appropriate feeding route for each child. Essentially, a shared team philosophy of early and sustained nutritional support is required [79]. Play preparation with the use of DVDs, photograph albums, booklets and dolls can assist in teaching, whilst some carers find it helpful to talk to other families with similar experiences.

The delivery of the feeds must be tailored to the individual child and their home circumstances. Intermittent enteral tube feeding can be given as daytime boluses or serve as a top-up if oral feeds are not completed. These bolus feeds can be given as gravity feeds or given more slowly through an enteral feeding pump. Initially, slower rates may be required for more concentrated feeds to improve tolerance [78]. A continuous overnight infusion via a pump can be beneficial in those infants with more severe GOR; however, many community healthcare professionals refuse to supervise this feeding method, especially if the child has a nasogastric tube rather than a gastrostomy device *in situ*.

Renal transplantation

Renal transplantation is the treatment of choice for children with stage 5 CKD to restore normal or near normal physiology and metabolic function without dialysis and minimal dietary restrictions. Survival of children with an allograft is superior compared with those remaining on dialysis. The donor kidney can come from a living related, living unrelated or deceased donor [26]. Pre-emptive transplantation produces improved graft survival and reduced mortality compared with dialysis followed by transplantation [15]. Children on the UK cadaveric transplant waiting list are given priority over adults and an average wait is 277 days at the time of writing [17]. Living related donor (LRD) transplantation is increasing. This has the advantages of shorter waiting times and improved graft survival. Five year paediatric allograft survival is 91% for LRD and 79% for cadaveric transplants [15]. Post transplantation medications aim to prevent graft rejection and include the calcineurin inhibitors ciclosporin and tacrolimus, mycophenolate and steroids. Minimising steroid exposure can improve linear growth and reduce metabolic disorders. Early steroid withdrawal has been shown to significantly help growth at 6 months post transplant especially in pre-pubertal children [88]; improved lipid and glucose metabolism profiles were also seen. Nutritional advice continues to be an important feature of treatment post transplant with the dietitian continuing to be involved with the ongoing management.

Initial dietary management

Immediately after transplantation, the main concerns for the recipient include the complications of rejection and infection. Feeding commences on the return of normal bowel sounds. If there are no complications, the child usually develops an appetite as renal function improves and previous dietary restrictions can be relaxed in line with biochemical results. Fluid balance is dependent on output and is assessed daily by medical staff. A high fluid intake is initially encouraged to perfuse the transplanted kidney. Serum phosphate levels typically fall below reference ranges due to the large tubular and urinary losses; dietary advice should encourage phosphate rich foods and drinks at this stage. Invariably phosphate supplements are prescribed in the early post-transplant days to match urinary losses. Serum magnesium levels can also fall and require medicinal supplementation. Those children who experience acute tubular necrosis following a renal transplant require a period of conservative management or dialysis therapy including appropriate dietary modification until adequate renal function is achieved.

In infants and children receiving enteral feeds pre transplant, concerns have been raised about a prolonged transition to exclusive oral nutrition [86]. Others have shown that long term enteral tube feeding does not preclude the transition to normal feeding and the majority of children will eat and drink after a successful renal transplant [76]. Feeding dysfunction and impaired oromotor development appear to be more evident in infants who received nasogastric feeding than in those who had gastrostomy buttons for feeding [89].

It is recommended to cease tube feeding whenever possible at the time of renal transplantation, in order to stimulate appetite as renal function is restored especially if higher doses of corticosteroids are prescribed. To do this successfully the medical staff, dietitian and team members need to provide ongoing support to families. Most children do well and resume normal eating and drinking post transplant [76, 89]. There will always be exceptions to this approach with some children requiring short periods of nutritional support, particularly in the first few weeks or months post transplantation. In such patients a planned and agreed strategy to wean off enteral tube feeding must be implemented. Common experience is that some young children take time to adapt to drinking more fluids. In such cases fluid boluses delivered via the enteral feeding tube are given short term. Severe eating difficulties present in a small number of children; these may benefit from a behaviour modification approach [90].

Although a renewed appetite is positive in the initial stages of management, excessive weight gain and obesity in the long term must be avoided. Both the child and family should be reminded of this soon after transplant. The principles of a sensible, healthy eating, well balanced diet for all the family is advised prior to discharge from hospital.

All patients on immunosuppressive therapy need to take care with food hygiene and avoid foods which carry a high risk of food poisoning organisms such as *Listeria* and *Salmonella*; this should be discussed with each child and family prior to discharge.

Hypertension can present following transplantation and antihypertensive therapy is prescribed. Early post transplantation systolic hypertension strongly and independently predicts poor long term graft survival in paediatric patients [91]. Arterial wall stiffness has been demonstrated in young adults with end stage renal disease since childhood, with hypertension being the main determinant [92]. Weight control and advice regarding salt intake, as part of the healthy eating recommendations, should be encouraged.

Dyslipidaemia is seen in some children following transplantation and requires regular assessment. An evaluation 2–3 months after transplantation and annually thereafter is recommended [71]. Studies have identified that 40% of deaths in adult renal transplant patients are attributed to CVD and they occur at a younger age than in the general population [93]. There is growing evidence that dyslipidaemia hastens the progression of renal disease itself. Disordered lipoprotein metabolism results from complex interactions among many factors including the primary disease process; use of medications such as corticosteroids; the presence of malnutrition or obesity; and diet [94]. All children with dyslipidaemia should follow the recommendations for therapeutic lifestyle changes [71]. Dietary modification should include advice favouring mono-unsaturated and poly-unsaturated fats and oils in preference to saturated fats, together with encouraging the regular consumption of ω3 fatty acids and antioxidants from fruit and vegetable intake. Moderate physical activity is recommended.

Ongoing dietary management

Children still receiving nutritional support post transplant should be regularly reviewed in the outpatient clinic. A transition period to encourage the oral route of feeding should be agreed with families. To stimulate the appetite, a reduced volume of bolus feed should be given during the day. Vitamin and/or trace mineral preparations may be required in those children whose micronutrient intakes are poor. Iron status should also be monitored. Several younger children struggle with fluid targets post transplant and require bolus top-ups with water.

Transplantation restores the conditions to promote more typical growth. However, (when used) corticosteroids as well as a low GFR in the graft kidney will both have growth suppressive effects. Steroids suppress growth mainly by interacting with the GH/IGF-1 axis, and by affecting the growth plate [95]. A nutritionally adequate balanced diet should be established to sustain normal growth whilst guarding against overnutrition.

The prevention of weight gain leading to obesity can be a difficult problem particularly for adolescents where body image is important. The patient who was anorexic prior to transplantation may not engage in discussions to modify food intake to control body weight. Adolescents who experience excess weight gain and change of body image can be susceptible to crash dieting and possible fasting to lose weight. Healthy eating and exercise should always be encouraged, including information on the health risks of alcohol and smoking. Adolescents need to be included in setting their own dietary targets.

A small number of children develop steroid induced diabetes mellitus post transplant which requires insulin therapy and appropriate dietary advice. Hyperglycaemia is also seen in a small number of children when acute rejection episodes are treated with pulses of methyl prednisolone; this effect is often transitory.

Chronic rejection of the transplanted kidney will eventually result in the child returning to dialysis with appropriate dietary intervention as for CKD.

Nephrotic syndrome

Nephrotic syndrome (NS) comprises a group of disorders characterised by heavy proteinuria (early morning urine protein:creatinine ratio > 200 mg/mmol) leading to hypoalbuminaemia (serum albumin <25 g/L) and oedema. The reduction in circulating proteins results in a fall in plasma oncotic pressure which is seen as generalised oedema. The mechanism of proteinuria in NS is a defective glomerular filtration barrier; the glomerular podocytes are seen to lose their complex morphology during active disease [96] and albumin and other proteins are lost into the urine. The salt and water retention leading to oedema is determined by this effect on the plasma albumin concentration. Dyslipidaemia is invariably present.

Nephrotic syndrome can be congenital or acquired. Congenital disease may be due to a genetic mutation or secondary to a congenital infection. Acquired disease is more common; this is typically idiopathic and is categorised according to the response to corticosteroid treatment as either steroid sensitive or steroid resistant disease. NS may also be acquired secondary to infections, pharmacological agents or neoplasia.

Idiopathic NS is the commonest glomerular disease in childhood with a reported incidence of 2 cases per 100 000 children in the UK, being four to six times more common in the UK Asian population [96]. It is more common in males (2:1) and the median age for presentation is 4 years. Minimal change nephrotic syndrome (MCNS) is the most common variant and responds well to treatment with high dose corticosteroids with 95% of children

responding within 8 weeks; these are classified as having steroid sensitive nephrotic syndrome (SSNS). Their prognosis is generally good with the likelihood of few continuing dietary problems as long term remission is usually reached before adulthood. Those children who relapse frequently and are steroid dependent usually require ongoing dietary intervention to monitor and maintain nutritional status and to prevent obesity. Growth failure, disfigurement of facial and body appearance as well as behavioural changes remain important issues in their long standing management [97].

The incidence of focal segmental glomerulosclerosis (FSGS) is increasing; this is less responsive to glucocorticoids. Those children whose proteinuria cannot be suppressed have a greater risk for progressive kidney disease [98] and require management under the direction of a paediatric nephrologist with specialist dietetic advice. Immunosuppressive drugs of various types are used to try and induce remission; these children are classed as steroid resistant.

Complications of NS can be divided into acute, relating to infections and susceptibility to thrombosis, and long term with prolonged episodes of nephrosis especially affecting growth, bones and the cardiovascular system [96]. A recent study has shown that the occurrence of growth retardation was influenced by height at diagnosis and the number of relapses; careful monitoring of growth is essential when up to 25% of these complex NS patients are seen to experience severe growth retardation during the course of their disease [97]. Reduced bone mineral density has been documented in adults who were treated with high dose corticosteroids for childhood nephrotic syndrome [98]. A recent study of 80 children with NS after short term glucocorticoid treatment has shown an inverse relationship between glucocorticoid exposure and spine areal bone mineral density and a low rate of vertebral deformities [99]. In children with long standing NS, an increase in CVD can be attributed to the use of corticosteroids, dyslipidaemia, oxidant stress, hypertension and obesity.

Dyslipidaemia results from the complex interactions between disordered lipoprotein metabolism, medications and dietary factors. The increase in hepatic lipoprotein synthesis in response to low plasma oncotic pressures plays a key role. Dyslipidaemia manifests as elevated plasma total cholesterol and triglycerides and usually corrects when the nephrosis resolves. The treatment of children with steroid resistant NS and persistent dyslipidaemia with HMG-CoA reductase inhibitors has been proposed in childhood dyslipidaemia care guidelines, but randomised studies are lacking [100].

Nutritional issues

Historically, both high and low protein diets have been advised. Studies have shown that albumin synthesis is limited by the capacity of the liver to synthesise albumin and is not increased with protein augmentation. There is no significant benefit on plasma albumin concentration or growth from a high protein intake [101, 102]. Although a decrease in albuminuria has been shown with low protein diets in animal studies [103], a low protein diet in children carries the risk of malnutrition and poor growth, especially in early childhood. High and low protein diets can be impractical, resulting in dietary imbalances and additional family anxieties.

Nutritional assessment

The dietitian should be involved following diagnosis and should obtain a detailed dietary history and chart growth parameters for both weight and height [6], including those available prior to diagnosis. These can help in both the prediction of the child's acceptable dry weight and approximate nutritional requirements. Attention to fluid balance and serum electrolytes is also important.

Nutritional management

Energy and protein
A balanced diet, adequate in both energy (EAR for children of the same chronological age) [8] and protein (RNI for chronological age) [9] is adequate for most children. Energy intake needs to be reduced if the child gains excessive weight on corticosteroid therapy. Children with severe and prolonged episodes of oedema need to be evaluated for malabsorption as the gut and surrounding tissues may also be oedematous and therefore function suboptimally. The subsequent malnutrition will require intensive nutritional support with

the possibility of supplementary feeding. Protein hydrolysate feeds may be indicated in this situation (see Table 7.11).

Sodium
Sodium intake is a major contributor to thirst and hence weight gain through fluid retention in children with NS [104]. In these oedematous cases of NS, renal sodium reabsorption in the proximal tubules is a determining factor [105]. A no added salt diet (NAS) avoiding salted snacks such as crisps, with advice about the high sodium content of manufactured foods such as tinned and packet soups, pot savouries and ready meals, is recommended (Table 12.8). Very low sodium diets and the use of specialist products are rarely necessary. A relaxed NAS diet is encouraged when the child is in remission, in line with healthy eating advice.

Fluid
Restriction of fluid is combined with a NAS diet in the initial oedematous phase. Fluid restriction is determined by the medical staff. Severe oedema may require pharmacologic intervention including loop diuretics, thiazide diuretics and, as a temporising measure, 25% albumin infusion [98]. Since diuretics can cause hypokalaemia and hyponatraemia, serum levels of potassium and sodium should be regularly monitored and responded to.

Fats
Diet is unlikely to significantly reduce the elevated lipid levels commonly seen in nephrotic patients. However, as part of the initial general healthy eating advice, the use of mono-unsaturated and poly-unsaturated margarines and oils together with a reduction of saturated fat intake should be advocated. Such advice should be given with care so as not to compromise total energy intake.

Ongoing nutritional management

For most children the introduction of steroid therapy can greatly stimulate appetite. In practice the common dietary problem is the prevention of excessive weight gain and BMI should be regularly monitored. Early anticipatory dietary advice to counsel on weight control is recommended if obesity is to be prevented. Children who are overweight at initiation of corticosteroid treatment are more likely to remain overweight after treatment for NS [106].

Children will often feel hungry whilst on corticosteroid therapy and a reduction of energy dense between meal snacks such as biscuits, crisps, sweets, chocolate and sugar containing drinks should be encouraged, together with their substitution with suitable low energy alternatives. Healthy eating advice for all the family should be reinforced and a leaflet/booklet on healthy eating can be helpful to aid compliance [107].

Nutritional support may be required in children who have prolonged anorexia or where there is evidence of malnutrition. Oral nutritional supplements or enteral feeding via a nasogastric tube should be considered (Table 12.5). An adequate calcium intake meeting the RNI [9] should be advised in children on long term corticosteroid therapy, together with the regular consumption of dietary sources of antioxidants.

Food allergy

Over the past 60 years numerous reports have suggested an association between idiopathic NS and atopic disorders. Idiopathic NS can be precipitated by allergic reactions and has been linked with food allergies and aeroallergens (pollen, dust); in addition many patients have a raised serum immunoglobulin E. Different types of dietary manipulations to remove suspected allergens have been attempted. This includes the use of elemental diets, limited exclusion diets or few foods diets (p. 314). The response to each of these diets has been inconsistent as well as the results often being confounded by the concurrent use of corticosteroids and the lack of a control group [108]. Allergies are common in children with idiopathic NS, but it is the underlying immune system in these individuals that predisposes them to both disorders.

Follow-up

It is recommended that the dietitian should see all NS patients at least once in clinic following their discharge to monitor their clinical progress and nutritional intake. Healthy eating guidelines should be reinforced to ensure that the diet is practical for all family members and not unnecessarily restrictive.

Psychosocial support

Parents are naturally anxious and concerned when they learn that their child has a chronic illness. Family friendly information about the management and treatment of NS is recommended. A parents' support group enables the sharing of experiences and can be of great benefit to parents who feel isolated.

Congenital nephrotic syndrome

Congenital nephrotic syndrome (CNS) is a rare inherited kidney disorder. Infants present at birth or within the first 3 months of life with heavy proteinuria, hypoalbuminaemia and oedema. The principal feature of CNS is the extensive leakage of plasma proteins into the urine. In the majority of cases, this is caused by mutations in genes encoding for structural or regulatory proteins of the kidney filtration barrier found in the glomerular capillary wall. About half of all nephrin gene (NPHS1) mutations are found in Finland. Other genetic types of CNS include podocin gene mutation and Wilms' tumour suppressor gene, whilst in developing countries infections are a possible aetiology [109].

In severe forms of CNS generalised oedema, a urinary protein >20 g/L and a serum albumin level <10 g/L can be detected in the newborn period. The amount of proteinuria varies with the type of CNS. Serum creatinine and urea levels are variable. In NPHS1, renal function is normal for the first months of life, whilst in the other types kidney failure can develop faster. Of note in NPHS1, the placental weight is more than 25% of the birth weight. Genetic analysis is the favoured method for the exact diagnosis of CNS and the diagnosis determines the management and genetic counselling of the family.

Management

The aims of therapy during the first months are to control oedema and possible uraemia, prevent and treat complications including infections and thromboses together with optimising nutrition to promote growth. In the majority of cases, kidney transplantation is the only curative outcome.

Heavy proteinuria of between 10 and 100 g/L leads to life threatening oedema, protein malnutrition and reduced growth. Parenteral albumin infusions are essential; these are often needed daily. Due to the protein excretion an imbalance of serum coagulation factor levels, as well as low levels of serum thyroid-binding globulin and thyroxine, are seen and need supplementing. There are marked lipid disturbances. Treatment is initially supportive with the aim of optimising nutrition and growth until the child is able to have renal replacement therapy. Unilateral or bilateral nephrectomies are performed to reduce the proteinuria and dialysis is established until kidney transplantation is possible. These patients require intensive dietetic support and intervention.

Nutritional management

The loss of proteins (90% of which is albumin with other protein losses including immunoglobulin G, transferrin and ceruloplasmin) is the main problem for infants with CNS. This leads to protein malnutrition, reduced growth and a depressed immune system. Intensive nutritional therapy is required as malnutrition increases the incidence of mortality. Energy intake should be maximised to 130 kcal (545 kJ)/kg estimated dry body weight with a protein intake of 3–4 g protein/kg. Concentrated infant formulas or proprietary energy dense infant formulas can be used to meet these requirements.

Requirements need to be adjusted according to weight gain and growth. Protein supplements can be added to the feed, with additional energy given as glucose polymers (Table 12.5). Fluid allowance should be negotiated with medical staff to allow for adequate nutrition, but is usually restricted to 100–130 mL/kg. Sodium intake is minimised and can be achieved with the use of whey based infant formulas and energy dense infant formulas.

Many infants require early enteral feeding to ensure their nutritional requirements are met, but this can be difficult to achieve on a very restricted fluid allowance, despite concentrating the feed and adding protein and energy supplements. Breast fed infants are unlikely to meet dietary requirements. Expressed breast milk can be supplemented with protein and energy supplements as illustrated in Table 12.18. Normal weaning practice is encouraged. Complete paediatric enteral feeds can be used for infants >8 kg (estimated dry weight).

Patients usually require activated vitamin D, alfacalcidol, to enhance calcium absorption. Vitamin and micronutrient intakes should meet dietary reference values [9]. Supplementary magnesium (50 mg/day) and calcium (500–1000 mg/day) are given if serum levels fall.

Some units have given rape seed oil (10–15 mL) and fish oil (2 mL) to patients with CNS to increase the P:S ratio of the diet [110], but the fatty acid

Table 12.18 Sample feed to meet the requirements of a 4-week-old girl with congenital nephrotic syndrome.

Feed recipe	Energy (kcal (kJ))	Protein (g)	CHO (g)	Fat (g)	Na$^+$ (mmol)	Calcium (mg)
A 4-week-old girl with congenital nephrotic syndrome whose mother is expressing breast milk. Weight 3.3 kg; fluid restriction 120 mL/kg = 400 mL; energy requirement = 130 kcal (545 kJ)/kg = 429 kcal (1795 kJ); protein requirement 3 g/kg						
390 mL EBM	269 (1125)	5.1	28.1	16.0	2.5	133
25 g Polycal powder	96 (402)	0	24.0	0	0.1	1.0
10 mL Calogen	45 (188)	0	0	5.0	0	0
7 g Vitapro	25 (105)	5.3	0.6	0.4	0.9	28
Total per 100 mL	109 (456)	2.6	13.2	5.4	0.9	40
Total per 400 mL	435 (1820)	10.4	52.7	21.4	3.5	162
Total per kg	132 (552)	3.2	16.0	6.5	1.1	49
The mother can no longer supply expressed breast milk (EBM). The baby is fed on a modified energy dense infant formula						
400 mL Infatrini	404 (1690)	10.4	41.2	21.6	4.4	320
10 g Polycal powder	38 (159)	0	9.6	0	0	0.4
Total per 100 mL	111 (464)	2.6	12.72	5.4	1.1	80
Total per 400 mL	442 (1849)	10.4	50.8	21.6	4.4	320
Total per kg	134 (560)	3.2	15.4	6.5	1.3	97

profile of current infant formulas and paediatric enteral feeds has made this practice largely redundant.

Renal function declines with time and dietary prescriptions need to be modified to accommodate the metabolic consequences of chronic kidney disease. Bilateral nephrectomies are performed when the infant reaches a target weight (typically 7–8 kg) which halts the protein losses in the urine and hence the nephrotic state. Dialysis is obligatory and dietary management is altered accordingly until the child receives a successful kidney transplant.

Nephrogenic diabetes insipidus

Nephrogenic diabetes insipidus (NDI) is a rare genetic disorder characterised by the kidney failing to respond to arginine vasopressin, the antidiuretic hormone (ADH). Water homeostasis is usually finely balanced by the release of vasopressin and the stimulation of thirst. Vasopressin acts in the kidneys to concentrate urine and reduce plasma osmolality. In infants with NDI there is an inability to concentrate the urine above 100 mOsm/kg H_2O; they present in the first weeks of life with polyuria, polydipsia, dehydration, hypernatraemia and growth failure. NDI can result from a genetic abnormality in any of the key components of cellular water reabsorption in the collecting duct or in the transporters involved in generating a hypertonic medulla. Most cases are caused by mutations in the X-linked AVPR2 gene and more boys than girls are affected.

The excessive fluid intake needed to excrete a normal renal solute load leads to a preference for water intake with consequent failure to thrive, exacerbated by anorexia and vomiting. Diagnosis is based on finding a low urine osmolality which is unresponsive to a water deprivation test or to ADH replacement therapy.

NDI is managed by ensuring an adequate fluid intake, decreasing the renal solute load (RSL) of the feed (which reduces the volume of urine required for its excretion) and a combination of drug treatments: a diuretic such as chlorothiazide, which has an antidiuretic effect and can reduce the polyuria by as much as 50%; and a non-steroidal anti-inflammatory drug, such as indometacin, which also reduces urinary

output [111]. Indometacin can cause gastroduodenal ulceration so should be given with a feed (or food). Ranitidine may be given to protect the stomach from mucosal injury.

Nutritional management of NDI

Infancy

A feed presenting a renal solute load of 15 mOsm/kg H_2O/kg body weight requires a fluid intake of >200 mL/kg body weight for excretion. Fluid intakes above this are hard to achieve consistently in young infants and may cause vomiting. The nutritional management of NDI is to provide sufficient fluid from a low solute feed while providing the EAR for energy [8] and the RNI for protein for height age [9]. The RSL of the feed should therefore be reduced to 15 mOsm/kg H_2O/kg body weight or less to reduce obligatory urine excretion. An estimate of the RSL of a feed can be made using the following formula:

Ion/protein	Contributory solute load (mOsm/kg H_2O)
1 mmol Na	1
1 mmol K	1
anions	$2 \times (Na + K)$
1 g protein	4

A sample feed for an infant with NDI, calculating RSL, is given in Table 12.19.

Energy supplements are routinely used to meet energy requirements as the amount of formula must be limited to control RSL. Water should be offered after each feed. Glucose polymers can be added to the water to provide extra energy without further increasing RSL. It is important to check that the feed provides the RNI for protein, vitamins and micronutrients, although this may not be achieved in the first few days after diagnosis when more dilute feeds with a lower RSL may need to be given whilst blood osmolality falls to an acceptable level.

It is particularly difficult to achieve the higher protein requirements of premature infants with NDI and it may not be possible to reduce RSL to <15 mOsm/kg H_2O/kg without compromising

Table 12.19 Sample feed for an infant with nephrogenic diabetes insipidus.

A 6-month-old boy with nephrogenic diabetes insipidus. Weight 6.8 kg. He is taking
700 mL feed with an additional 700 mL water, offered after each feed. He has
started some weaning foods. Feed volume 100 mL/kg. Water volume 100 mL/kg.
Total fluid volume 200 mL/kg

	Energy (kcal (kJ))	Protein (g)	Na$^+$ (mmol)	K$^+$ (mmol)
100g Cow & Gate 1	485 (2029)	9.7	5.4	12.2
45g Maxijul	171 (715)	0	0.4	0.1
+ water to 700 mL				
Total	656 (2745)	9.7	5.8	12.3
Per kg	96 (402)	1.4	0.9	1.8
Req/kg	96 (402)	1.6		

+ 1 g protein from weaning foods

Renal solute load of feed = Na + K + (2 × [Na + K]) + (4 × protein)
= 5.8 + 12.3 + (2 × [5.8 + 12.3]) + 4 × 9.7)
= 93.1 mOsm/kg H$_2$O
= 13.7 mOsm/kg H$_2$O/kg body weight

protein intake. The compromise may be to give a lower than ideal protein intake for a few days until the drug treatments have brought the polyuria under control.

Low sodium weaning solids should be started at the standard recommended age of around 6 months. In more extreme cases of growth failure, nasogastric or gastrostomy feeding may be necessary if insufficient nutrition is taken orally.

Childhood

Some authors suggest a sodium restriction of 1 mmol/kg/day [112] to control the craving for fluids while others consider a NAS diet to be adequate to control excessive fluid intakes [111] provided the child is on long term medication. Some support group websites that families may access suggest an unnecessary level of salt restriction. It is usual to liberalise the diet from low salt (0.6–1.0 mmol Na/kg) to NAS (1.5–2.0 mmol Na/kg) as the child enters toddlerhood. This gradual increase in dietary salt intake needs to be balanced against the craving for fluids, which can inhibit appetite for food. Salt intake may need to be reduced to a level where the child no longer desires large volumes of water. Children need to have free access to fluids day and night.

Regular dietary assessment is necessary throughout childhood to ensure that the recommended intakes for energy [8], protein and micronutrients [9] are still being met. Most children take adequate nutrition orally and feeding tends to improve with age. If weight gain is poor, an energy dense diet and energy supplements may be useful. Enteral feeding should be considered if oral intake is inadequate and growth falters.

There is little information on the long term growth of children with NDI. One retrospective study showed that the majority of children grew below the third centile of local growth standards, and that many showed an improvement of weight, height and BMI over time; those children who did not comply with treatment showed growth delay [113].

Renal stones in childhood

Renal stones, kidney stones, renal calculi, urolithiasis and nephrolithiasis are all terms used to refer to the accretion of hard, solid minerals throughout the urinary tract. The size of the stone is less important than its location and whether it obstructs or prevents urine from draining properly. Stones are uncommon in children with only 1%–3% occurring during childhood; however, the incidence is believed to be increasing. The continuing increase in childhood obesity may be contributing to the growing prevalence of childhood stone disease.

The aetiology of stones in children differs from that in adults. Young children, predominantly boys, are prone to infective stones (30% of childhood cases), although this form of calculi is falling in incidence in developed countries. 44% of stones result from a metabolic abnormality; a metabolic evaluation should be undertaken in all children with stones. Hypercalciuria is frequently seen and cystinuria and hyperoxaluria account for 5%–15% of paediatric stones. Calcium stones are found where there is hypercalciuria, hyperoxaluria and hypocitraturia. 26% of stones are idiopathic [114]. An increased rate of stone formation is seen in children born prematurely, in those with neurological problems, those on a ketogenic diet and in children with a reconstructed or augmented bladder [115]. Premature and formula fed babies have increased solute excretion, with children who were premature having a greater risk of nephrocalcinosis and nephrolithiasis [115]. Factors increasing the risk of stone formation include molecules from which stones form (including calcium, oxalate and cystine from metabolic and dietary sources); poor urine flow; urine pH; infection. Some drugs also increase the risk of stone formation: diuretics, chemotherapeutic agents, salicylates, corticosteroids and vitamins A and D [114].

Stones can develop at any age, from as early as the first 2–3 months of life. The incidence of stones is twice as high in boys as in girls. There is a greater prevalence in children <5 years mainly due to infective stones secondary to urinary tract infection; the infective organisms produce an alkaline medium which favours the precipitation of calcium phosphate and magnesium ammonium phosphate. The formation of stones requires a supersaturated urine: the greater the concentration of ions, the more likely they are to precipitate. The concentration of ions in the urine depends on the pH of the urine, the solute concentration and ionic strength. Congenital abnormalities of the urinary system can cause urinary stasis and predispose to stone formation as the solute concentration of the retained urine increases.

The main aims of treatment of renal stones are to prevent stone re-occurrence, prevent stone growth and eliminate existing stones. Treatments can be by medical therapy or surgical intervention. All children with renal stone disease should be advised to increase fluid intake, typically by 150% [114] or more. An increased fluid intake reduces the concentration of substrates in the urine together with increasing urinary flow to reduce the potential for crystallisation, stone formation or growth.

Hypercalciuria

Hypercalciuria is the most common cause of metabolic stone disease. It can be idiopathic, where children present with gross haematuria, or as a result of secondary causes through lack of renal tubular reabsorption, increased intestinal absorption or imbalance of bone formation [114]. The amount of calcium in a child's urine is age dependent with higher levels excreted by the immature nephron of the neonate; hypercalciuria needs to be assessed against reference ranges [114]. Urinary calcium excretion is influenced by many factors including diet, ethnicity, age and geography. Most children have normal serum calcium levels.

A diet history should be taken to determine fluid, sodium, calcium, animal protein, vitamin C and vitamin D intakes; all of these can contribute to an increase in urinary calcium excretion. Urinary sodium excretion correlates with calcium excretion so a diet high in sodium increases the excretion of calcium as well as high urinary pH and hence the likelihood of calcium stone formation. In the majority of children a NAS restriction (Table 12.8) to reduce calcium excretion, together with a good fluid intake (2–3 L/day) to reduce the concentration of ions in the urine is sufficient to prevent further stone formation. Restricting dietary sodium has the added benefit of promoting an increase in bone mineral density. Advice regarding fluids should preferentially encourage water rather than soft drinks which can increase the risk of calcium and uric acid stones due to their high level of sugar and phosphoric acid.

Dietary calcium restriction or the administration of sodium cellulose phosphate (which reduces calcium absorption) is not recommended for children with normocalcaemic hypercalciuria because of the potential effect on reducing bone mineralisation. However, excessive calcium intakes should be avoided with the RNI for calcium intake for chronological age [8] being advised. Excessive intakes of vitamin D and vitamin C should be avoided as these can contribute to hypercalciuria and hyperoxaluria [116]. If conservative management with diet is insufficient, thiazide diuretics are prescribed. These reduce urinary calcium by increasing calcium absorption in the proximal and distal tubule.

Oxalosis and hyperoxaluria

Oxalosis or primary hyperoxaluria is a rare autosomal recessive disorder where there is widespread deposition of calcium oxalate crystals in the kidneys, bones, heart and other organs. This occurs due to enzyme deficiencies in the liver. An increased urinary excretion of oxalate is seen. Treatment aims to keep urinary oxalate excretion <0.4 mmol/L through a high fluid intake of >2 L/day. Oral citrate can reduce calcium oxalate precipitation by making the urine more alkaline. Restriction of dietary oxalate has little influence on the disease as only 10%–15% of urinary oxalate is derived from dietary intake; 60% of urinary oxalate is produced from the endogenous metabolism of glycine, glycolate and hydroxyproline. Pyridoxine sensitivity is seen in 10%–40% of patients. In the more severe cases renal failure develops.

Secondary hyperoxaluria can be seen in patients with malabsorption syndromes including Crohn's disease or short bowel syndrome. When there is less available calcium to bind oxalate, the absorption of oxalate increases [115]. The reduction of dietary oxalate (Table 12.20) and vitamin C, which is a precursor of oxalate, can be beneficial together with ensuring an adequate calcium intake. A high animal protein intake should be avoided as this can increase the amount of oxalate absorbed and stimulate an increase in uric acid with a fall in urine pH.

Cystinuria

Cystinuria accounts for 10% of paediatric stones. It is a complex autosomal recessive disorder resulting in a defect in the transporter of L-cystine and the dibasic amino acids ornithine, arginine and lysine in the proximal tubule of the kidney [114].

A NAS diet may be beneficial in lowering cystine excretion, together with avoiding an excessive protein intake. Other dietary treatments, including a low methionine diet, are rarely used in children.

Hypercalcaemia

Hypercalcaemia results when the rate of calcium entry into the extracellular fluid is greater than the calcium excretion by the kidneys. This can be brought about by increased absorption of calcium from the intestinal tract as in Williams syndrome and idiopathic infantile hypercalcaemia; increased release of calcium from the skeleton as seen during immobilisation and malignancy; or reduced excretion of calcium from the kidney as in primary hyperparathyroidism. Infants presenting with hypercalcaemia may have feeding problems; vomiting; polydipsia and polyuria, which results in a preference for water to milk feeds. Consequently these infants often experience faltering growth.

Idiopathic infantile hypercalcaemia (IIH) is a rare disorder of unknown aetiology that presents with hypercalcaemia in the first year of life. It can also be secondary to a variety of conditions including vitamin D intoxication [117]. This hypercalcaemia resolves in the majority of children by the age of 3 years.

Williams syndrome is a genetic disorder with multisystem characteristics: dysmorphic facies ('elfin' face), CVD, developmental delay and a lack of social inhibition. Infants often have feeding

Table 12.20   Dietary sources of oxalate [121].

High oxalate content	Moderate oxalate content	Low oxalate content
Rhubarb, strawberries	Apples, apricots, oranges, peaches, pears, pineapples, plums	Banana, grapefruit, green grapes, melon
Blackberries, blueberries, raspberries and their juices	Orange juice	Apple juice
Chocolate, cocoa, tea	Coffee, cola	Lemonade, jelly
Nuts		Beef, lamb, poultry, pork, seafood Cheese, eggs, milk, yoghurt
Beetroot, beans in tomato sauce, celery, leeks, parsley, spinach, sweet potatoes	Asparagus, broccoli, carrots, tomatoes	Cabbage, cauliflower, onions, peas
		Noodles, pasta, rice and oil

difficulties and GOR is common. Raised calcium levels may persist and need ongoing monitoring [118].

In conditions such as these where there is increased intestinal calcium absorption, treatment options include a low calcium diet with a reduced vitamin D intake, corticosteroids, calcitonin and cellulose phosphate. Calcitonin inhibits osteoclastic bone resorption and enhances renal calcium excretion. Cellulose phosphate is a non-absorbable resin that binds calcium, so inhibiting intestinal absorption. Thiazide diuretics are used in cases of persisting hypercalciuria [117].

Calcium intake should be reduced so as not to exceed the RNI for age [9]. In IIH and Williams syndrome a low calcium formula with no added vitamin D, such as Locasol, can be used (<0.2 mmol calcium/100 mL when reconstituted with deionised water). The formula can be modified with energy supplements in the infant with faltering growth. The level of calcium in the local water supply should be checked as this can make a significant contribution to calcium intake in hard water areas (contributing up to 0.3 mmol calcium/100 mL). Deionised (distilled, purified) water must be used if necessary and can be prescribed under the Advisory Committee on Borderline Substances for hypercalcaemia. Other rich sources of dietary calcium, including dairy produce, need to be limited in the diet. In effect the infant and older child should follow a milk free diet with the additional advice to restrict foods fortified with vitamin D, including baby cereals, breakfast cereals and margarine. A milk free diet (Table 7.8) will provide approximately 6–7 mmol calcium/day. Low calcium diets carry a risk of iatrogenic rickets and asymptomatic hypocalcaemia [117] so children need to be monitored closely.

As serum calcium levels return to normal, sources of calcium can be gradually introduced into the diet depending on the individual child's response. This can be managed in portions of food containing approximately 3 mmol calcium, such as 100 mL cow's milk, 20 g cheese, 75 g fruit yoghurt. Vitamin supplements containing vitamin D must not be given.

From data available, less prolonged calcium restriction is safest and a normal diet should be returned to by 6–12 months in those with IIH [119]. Where there is persistent hypercalcaemia in children with Williams syndrome then continuing calcium restriction may be necessary.

Hyperuricaemia

A study has suggested that fructose induced hyperuricaemia may play a role in the metabolic syndrome [120]. This is consistent with the increased consumption in recent decades of fructose containing beverages including fruit juices and soft drinks sweetened with sugar and high fructose corn syrup. Fructose raises uric acid levels which inhibits nitric oxide bioavailability. Children with hyperuricaemia should be advised to avoid these drinks as well as avoiding foods with a high purine content (Table 12.21), moderate their intake of animal protein foods whilst increasing starchy carbohydrate and fluid intake; a plan for gradual weight loss should be instigated in those who are overweight.

Renal tubular disorders

Renal tubular disorders are a heterogeneous group of disorders affecting aspects of the functioning of the renal tubules and as such present in a variety of ways. The disorders are caused, directly or indirectly, by dysfunction of transporter proteins responsible for tubular reabsorption or secretion of various electrolytes [123]. Tubular dysfunction in childhood is rare, but when present can lead to severe electrolyte and volume disturbance. Many of these tubulopathies are salt-wasting disorders. Children with hereditary tubular dysfunction typically present in the first year of life with non-specific symptoms including poor feeding, vomiting and faltering growth. Biochemical analysis of both serum and urine are fundamental for diagnosis. The hyponatraemia, hypokalaemia, low bicarbonate and hypophosphataemia seen are consistent with generalised proximal tubular dysfunction and are known as the Fanconi syndrome.

Bartter's syndrome

Bartter's syndrome describes a number of closely related renal tubular disorders characterised by hypokalaemic metabolic alkalosis, hypochloraemia, hyper-reninaemia and hyperaldosteronism

Table 12.21 Dietary sources of purines [122].

High purine content	Moderate purine content	Low purine content
Organ meats: kidney, liver	Meat, poultry	Eggs
Game meats: duck, goose	Dried peas, beans, lentils	Nuts, peanut butter
Mackerel, sardines, mussels, scallops	Other fish and shellfish	
		All milk and milk products
	Asparagus, cauliflower, green beans, mushrooms, spinach	Most fruit and vegetables
	Wholegrain bread and cereals	Low fibre bread and cereals
	Wheat germ and bran, oatmeal	Rice, pasta
Meat extracts, yeast supplements	Meat soups, bouillon	Vegetable soups and stocks
		Cakes, biscuits
		Coffee, tea

with normal blood pressure. The underlying renal defect results in the excessive urinary loss of sodium, chloride and potassium [31].

Treatment involves the correction of dehydration and electrolyte abnormalities. Indometacin, which reduces renal salt, potassium and water losses, is prescribed along with potassium supplements. It is difficult to restore serum potassium into the normal range and most patients tolerate a potassium concentration of 2.5 mmol/L without the expected associated problems [124]. Indometacin should be given with food or milk because of the potential gastrointestinal side effects of nausea, vomiting, abdominal pain and peptic ulcer. Nutritional supplements (Table 12.5) are indicated where appetite remains poor and growth is impaired.

Cystinosis

Nephropathic cystinosis is a rare genetic storage disorder characterised by the intracellular storage of free cystine due to a defect in lysosomal cystine transport. The primary defect is in the gene CTNS which encodes for cystinosin. Cystinosin transports cystine out of lysosomes. In cystinosis the cystine becomes trapped within the lysosomes which in turn causes a malfunction of the Na-K ATPase pumps [123]. It is the most common cause of Fanconi syndrome in childhood. The accumulation of cystine crystals mainly affects the proximal tubules. Children usually present in late infancy with poor feeding, excessive thirst, delayed growth, weakness and rickets. All ethnic groups are

affected; however, the classical child is fair-haired, blue-eyed and Caucasian.

Treatment comprises rehydration and electrolyte replacement with the administration of bicarbonate, electrolyte and vitamin D supplements. Indometacin reduces the GFR and subsequent tubular losses as well as reducing often extreme polyuria. The Fanconi syndrome causes chronic renal impairment and eventually renal replacement therapy is required. A cystine depleting agent, mercaptamine (cysteamine), is given to reduce progressive glomerular damage which if untreated leads to stage 5 CKD by 10 years of age. It is now more commonly seen that dialysis or transplantation are not needed until at least the second decade of life. Renal transplantation is successful but does not correct the disorder. Cystine continues to accumulate in non-renal tissues causing multisystem dysfunction [124].

Children with cystinosis typically have very poor appetites and severely reduced growth which is disproportionate to their degree of renal dysfunction [123]. The growth failure is multifactorial with acid–base and electrolyte imbalance, poor nutrition, rickets and cystine deposition in the bones and thyroid being major factors. Oral nutritional supplements should be prescribed in the first instance; however, feeding difficulties are common with many requiring a gastrostomy. A small study demonstrated oromotor dysfunction including hypotonia, abnormal gag reflex and congested voice [125]. Hypotonia, muscle weakness, gross and fine motor dysfunction and ataxia were seen on neurology examinations. Overnight gastrostomy feeding has been shown to improve height and weight parameters [126]. The gastrostomy can also be used for the administration of medication. Gastrointestinal symptoms are common [127] and occur at a young age including GOR, pseudo-obstruction and swallowing dysfunction. In extreme cases PN has been indicated.

Long term information is needed to determine whether early oromotor problems predict the later development of progressive myopathy. Adults with cystinosis can show progressive neuromuscular dysfunction, with bulbar and upper extremity weakness.

13

Congenital Heart Disease

David Hopkins

Introduction

Congenital heart disease in infancy and childhood refers to structural abnormalities that arise in the four main chambers of the heart itself and/or the great vessels that lead to or from the heart. The type, size and combination of lesions determines the ability of the heart and lungs to respectively pump and oxygenate blood and this in turn affects the workload and utilisation of energy in these organs. Not all cardiac lesions put an infant or child at risk of faltering growth. Some lesions, however, will result in an increase in cardiorespiratory workload that affects the amount of surplus energy available for growth. In addition some patients have defects that lead to the development of congestive heart failure (CHF), which describes a set of symptoms and clinical signs where cardiac output is inadequate to meet the metabolic demands of the body.

A glossary is given, describing cardiac anomalies and corrective procedures (p. 305).

Incidence

The incidence of clinically relevant moderate to severe forms of congenital heart disease (CHD) is between 6 and 8 in every 1000 live births [1, 2] and forms the largest single group of congenital abnormalities. Eight lesions make up 80% of cases, the most common of which are ventricular septal defect, persistent ductus arteriosus, atrial septal defect and tetralogy of Fallot. Children with certain syndromes have a higher incidence of congenital heart defects, e.g. 50% of infants with Down's syndrome have cardiac defects. This percentage is even higher in children with Noonan syndrome, 80%, who present mainly with pulmonary stenosis or hypertrophic cardiomyopathy [3].

Screening and diagnosis

Some congenital cardiac anomalies are frequently detected on ultrasound at routine antenatal screening. The ability to identify these anatomical defects will depend both on the skill of the operator and the timing of the antenatal ultrasound check. Some defects are discovered during the postnatal check up within the first 24 hours of birth. For example, coarctation of the aorta (narrowing in the aortic arch) may be identified by absent femoral artery pulses and ventricular septal defect (VSD), atrial septal defect (ASD) and persistent ductus arteriosus (PDA) may initially be suspected on detection of a heart murmur. Occasionally if a lesion remains undetected the child may present acutely with cardiogenic shock and elevated blood

Clinical Paediatric Dietetics, Fourth Edition. Edited by Vanessa Shaw.
© 2015 John Wiley & Sons, Ltd. Published 2015 by John Wiley & Sons, Ltd.
Companion Website: www.wiley.com/go/shaw/paediatricdietetics

lactate levels. Alternatively a lesion may only come to light when an infant or child presents with faltering growth. A child with faltering growth whose diet history indicates a normal or above normal intake warrants a cardiac assessment as part of further clinical investigations. This is particularly so in any child who fails to gain adequate weight following optimisation of nutritional intake and the dietitian's role may be key in highlighting suspicion. Once a suspected case has been referred to a paediatric cardiac centre diagnosis is confirmed on echocardiography (ultrasound scan) or, in very rare cases, by cardiac catheterisation.

Factors associated with poor growth in congenital heart disease

Underlying physiology and energy expenditure

Energy expenditure in patients with congenital heart defects depends on both the type and severity of the lesion. Average daily total energy expenditure (TEE) in infants without cardiac defects appears to be between 60 and 70 kcal (250–290 kJ)/kg/day [4–6] and if energy intake is at the estimated average requirement (EAR) of 100–115 kcal (420–480 kJ)/kg/day then 30–55 kcal (125–230 kJ)/kg/day should be available for growth.

The most plausible explanation for why TEE should be elevated in patients with cardiac defects is the extent to which the type and severity of the lesion affects respiratory effort [6–8]. In a normal circulation blood is pumped to the lungs by the right ventricle under pressure that is about a third of that of the left ventricle. This is because the pulmonary vascular resistance of the lungs is considerably less than that of the rest of the body. Therefore a cardiac anomaly that results in a 'hole' between the left and the right sides of the circulation tends to result in a greater than normal volume of blood being pumped to the lungs. This is termed a 'left to right shunt'. If the amount of blood flow in the shunt is high, the elevated blood pressure present in the lungs is known as pulmonary hypertension [7]. This results in fluid building up in the airspaces of the lungs leading to inefficient gas exchange across the capillaries. In these cases the patient is acyanotic with adequate oxygenation of blood, but at the expense of high energy expenditure due to the increased respiratory effort. As a result patients with acyanotic lesions have a tendency to become wasted [9, 10] although length/height may also be affected if the effect is prolonged. Examples of acyanotic lesions are moderate to large VSD, PDA and atrioventricular septal defects (AVSD). If the left to right shunt is significant, congestive cardiac failure (CHF) is seen and energy expenditure is further elevated [7]. Other acyanotic lesions, however, may not cause cardiopulmonary changes that are large enough to affect energy expenditure and growth. One example is an isolated ASD where the primary repair may be carried out later in childhood with negligible effect on growth.

The presence of cyanosis appears to exert an additional independent effect resulting in stunting [11, 12]. The mechanism for this is uncertain but it has been suggested that suboptimal tissue oxygenation may be a factor [13]. Varan *et al.* [11] demonstrated that children with complex cardiac defects that cause a combination of both pulmonary hypertension and cyanosis appear to be at the greatest nutritional risk, with stunting occurring in addition to wasting.

Examples of a cyanotic and an acyanotic lesion and tetralogy of Fallot are shown in Figs 13.1, 13.2 and 13.3. Children with cardiomyopathy represent a smaller separate group of patients who tend to have high energy requirements.

The doubly labelled water technique has been used to calculate the energy expenditure of infants with a variety of cardiac lesions [6, 7, 10, 14]. Pre surgical infants without CHF have been shown to have an elevated TEE of 77–80 kcal (322–334 kJ)/kg/day, about 10% above normal [7]. Lesions with a large degree of left to right shunt, CHF and some cyanotic lesions appear to cause an even greater TEE of 87–94 kcal (364–393 kJ)/kg/day [6, 7, 14] with expenditure as high as 157 kcal (656 kJ)/kg/day in one individual case [10]. The effect of CHF in elevating metabolic rate may be quite marked even in infants as young as 1 month of age [15]. The more TEE is elevated, the less energy is available for accretion of new tissue resulting in the lower body mass index (BMI) and slower growth seen in these patients [6, 9, 11, 16, 17].

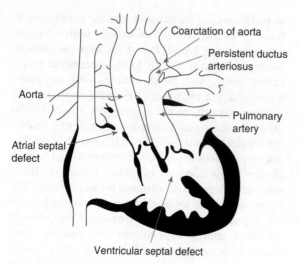

Figure 13.1 A complex cyanotic lesion.

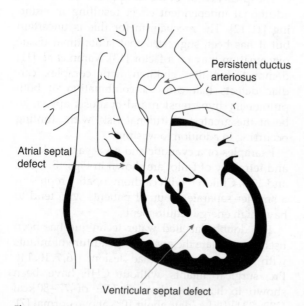

Figure 13.2 A complex acyanotic lesion.

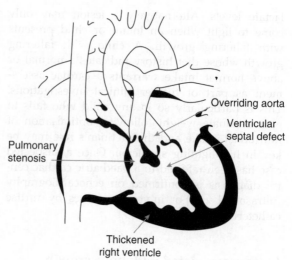

Figure 13.3 Tetralogy of Fallot.

Malnutrition itself is also known to reduce ventricular mass and cardiac output, which may exacerbate an already compromised circulation [17].

Other proposed mechanisms by which basal metabolic rate may become elevated are hypertrophy of the cardiac muscle, increases in sympathetic nerve activity, haemopoietic tissue production, episodes of pyrexia and metabolic stress [8].

Age and timing of repair

Cardiac lesions can additionally be subdivided into those that undergo primary repair in early infancy and those that require a staged repair with further operations in later infancy or childhood. Defects such as an isolated coarctation of the aorta or transposition of the great arteries (TGA), which require repair in the neonatal period, usually have limited or no effect on long term nutritional intake and should not require dietetic intervention. Infants with several or complex cardiac abnormalities, requiring staged repair with a series of operations over time, may be at higher risk of compromised growth. Growth of infants with operated TGA has been compared with those with hypoplastic left heart syndrome (HLHS) where a staged repair involving three separate operations is usually carried out over 3–4 years [18]. Those with HLHS weighed significantly less at 1 month, 6 months and 12 months of age, took twice as long to achieve a target energy intake of 100 kcal (420 kJ)/kg/day and had a far higher incidence of feeding difficulties than the TGA group (48% vs. 4%).

In a mixed group of 150 hospitalised infants, children and young adults with CHD a third were found to have wasting (<90% weight for length/height) and 64% were stunted (<90% of mean height for age) [19]. Infants were at greatest risk due to their smaller nutritional reserve with 79% wasted and 82% stunted. Older children also need to have continuing monitoring of their nutritional status as ongoing cardiac support and intervention was required in 84% of toddlers, 58% of school-age children and 38% of adolescents [19]. Nutritional deficits and secondary growth disturbances that may ultimately put children at increased surgical risk should be corrected wherever possible [20]. Both malnutrition and growth retardation are associated with more complex CHD in infancy [9, 11, 21–24] and childhood [19].

Endocrine effects

Hormone levels may also play a role in affecting the growth of children with cardiac abnormalities. Serum concentrations of insulin-like growth factor 1 (IGF-1) are reduced in children with a VSD, with lower levels correlating with increasing size of the left to right shunt and reduced BMI [25]. Hypermetabolism is thought to be the reason for this, compromising nutritional status by reducing IGF-1 synthesis, further slowing linear growth and weight gain [25].

Substrate metabolism

Lundell *et al.* [26] have looked at lipid metabolism in two groups of infants with CHD. One group had VSD; the other group had cyanotic CHD. The cyanotic group all had transposition of the great arteries and a mean oxygen saturation of 68%. Both groups were given an intravenous (IV) lipid load. Severe growth retardation in infants in both groups was correlated to higher peak levels of linoleic acid in the plasma free fatty acids after IV lipid load. The peak levels of linoleic acid in the triglyceride fraction were positively correlated to weight standard deviation score. Peak glycerol levels were higher in the most growth retarded infants, indicating faster intravascular lipolysis. They concluded that lipid metabolism is disturbed in infants with CHD with infants with cyanotic lesions having a decreased ability to oxidise fatty acids [26].

Feeding behaviour

Increased breathlessness and fatigue may cause some cardiac patients to feed repeatedly for short periods of time. However, there is uncertainty as to whether actual energy intakes of infants with cardiac lesions are affected by this type of feeding behaviour. Energy intakes between 82% and 88% of those recommended have been demonstrated in some children with CHD [10, 27] but others have demonstrated near normal energy intakes [6, 7, 14, 24, 25]. Children with cardiac defects that result in both pulmonary hypertension and cyanosis have been reported as having intakes that are significantly lower than those with pulmonary hypertension or cyanosis alone [11]. Early satiety, vomiting and anorexia, all of which may be interlinked, lead to low energy intake.

Factors affecting feeding and digestive ability

Diarrhoea

Nutritionally compromised infants are more susceptible to infections and if these are frequent the use of antibiotics may affect gut flora. Patients who develop infected postoperative sternal wounds may have antibiotic therapy that results in diarrhoea which may transiently affect absorptive capacity.

Gastro-oesophageal reflux

Infants with congenital cardiac defects have been found to have delayed gastric emptying [28] and are therefore more likely to have problems with gastro-oesophageal reflux (GOR). Positioning and feed thickeners may be used as a first line treatment if there is a suspicion of GOR (p. 136). In the intensive care setting there is often a clear correlation between deterioration in cardiac function and reduced feed tolerance, which resolves if cardiac function improves. Additional drug treatment or a resort to nasojejunal feeding may be needed to control more severe vomiting. It is therefore also worth considering other factors that may cause vomiting, e.g. cow's milk protein allergy. A trial of cow's milk free formula can be indicated if no other underlying cause is identified or the infant's vomiting becomes protracted (Table 7.6).

Pain

Pain is thought to affect both the severity and length of the catabolic response to surgery. If pain

Table 13.1   Cardiac defects and likelihood of dietetic intervention.

Low	Variable	High
Coarctation of aorta	Pulmonary atresia*	Ventricular septal defect (VSD) moderate to large
Patent ductus arteriosus (PDA) if early surgery performed	Tetralogy of Fallot*	Atrioventricular septal defect (AVSD)
Atrial septal defect (ASD)		Hypoplastic left heart*
Cor triatriatum		Truncus arteriosus*
Transposition of the great arteries (TGA)*		Aortopulmonary window
Total anomalous pulmonary venous drainage (TAPVD)*		PDA if large and if surgery is delayed
Pulmonary stenosis*		Tricuspid atresia* Ebstein's anomaly* Partial anomalous pulmonary venous drainage (PAPVD)*

*Cyanotic lesions.

is not sufficiently controlled the catabolic response following surgery might be prolonged with detrimental effects on healing [29]. In addition ongoing experience of pain might delay progression to oral feeding following surgery.

Investigations

Investigations requiring patients to be nil by mouth, such as cardiac catheterisation or computed tomography (CT) scans, will interfere with feeding regimens. Often there is limited scope to catch up with additional feeds when the patient returns to the ward and repeated investigations will compromise nutritional intake.

Faltering growth in CHD is therefore multifactorial, but from the available evidence it appears that the major factor is that of elevated energy expenditure affecting the surplus of energy that should be available for growth. An understanding of the primary cardiac anatomy helps to identify those patients who are at risk. Table 13.1 categorises the various cardiac lesions in terms of potential nutritional risk. Although most patients have improved growth postoperatively, some continue to exhibit growth failure even after haemodynamic correction [16].

Nutritional management

If sufficient energy is provided appropriate weight gain and linear growth can be achieved [30–32].

Yahav et al. [30] found a good correlation between energy intake and weight gain, but in the most severely nutritionally depleted infants a consistent weight gain was observed only when energy intake exceeded 170 kcal (710 kJ)/kg/day. Barton et al. recommended intakes of 150 kcal (630 kJ)/kg/day in order to achieve adequate growth [10]. Nevertheless the studies measuring TEE seem to indicate that an intake of approximately 30 kcal (125 kJ)/kg/day above the EAR for energy should be sufficient to compensate for the elevated energy expenditure and achieve adequate growth in most infants [6,7,14,33]. A reasonable starting point with an infant who has faltering growth would be 120–130 kcal (500–545 kJ)/kg/day, with further increase in energy intake should adequate weight gain not be achieved.

The use of growth charts is essential to plot weight and length measurements so that energy requirements can be assessed. Whilst some may require increased energy intakes to ensure adequate growth, others may be at risk of disproportionate weight gain if they continue to be given even normal energy intakes. The author's experience is that energy intakes as low as 70 kcal (230 kJ)/kg/day are necessary to prevent excessive weight gain in some stable long term ventilated infants with cardiac defects. In these cases it is important to ensure protein, vitamin and mineral requirements are met with appropriate supplementation. Vitamin and mineral intakes of young children with CHD have been shown to be lower than those of the normal population but, with the exception of vitamin D, they still appear to meet the reference nutrient intake (RNI) [27].

Types of feed

Breast feeding or expressed breast milk, as with most infants, is the feed of choice for infants with CHD. The mechanism of breast feeding may cause less cardiorespiratory stress resulting in lower oxygen desaturation episodes [34] and has even been attempted within 1 week of heart transplant [35]. If there is ongoing fluid restriction (less than 100 mL/kg/day) beyond the first week following surgery or inadequate weight gain, fortification of the breast milk is necessary. This may be done by using one of the commercially available breast milk fortifiers for the premature infant or by adding 2%–5% infant formula powder (see Table 1.14). Addition of a commercial fortifier has been shown to have a negligible effect on delaying gastric emptying [36]. If glucose polymer is used alone to fortify breast milk or is used in combination with a fat supplement, care should be taken to ensure that the protein:energy ratio of the feed is not compromised as it may lead to a disproportionate accretion of fat at the expense of lean tissue.

If breast milk is not available or is insufficient, a suitable infant formula should be provided. Infants with CHD who have elevated energy requirements may be offered a formula with a higher energy and nutrient density:

- Infatrini 100 kcal (420 kJ)/100 mL 2.6 g protein/100 mL
- Similac High Energy 100 kcal (420 kJ)/100 mL 2.6 g protein/100 mL
- SMA High Energy 91 kcal (380 kJ)/100 mL 2.0 g protein/100 mL

Table 13.2 shows a comparison of the energy and protein obtained from standard infant formula and nutrient dense infant formula fed at increasing volumes, illustrating how nutritional requirements for growth may be met.

A high to very high energy feed may be needed to achieve adequate weight gain and appropriate catch-up growth in some infants with CHD. If there are doubts regarding an infant's tolerance of commercial nutrient dense formulas then standard infant formula may be used initially, gradually increasing the concentration to 15%–17% to provide 72–90 kcal (300–375 kJ)/100 mL depending on the brand, before progressing to the nutrient dense formula. The strength and volume of feed can be increased as shown in Table 13.3.

If weight gain is unsatisfactory on 1 kcal (4 kJ)/mL feed fed at 150 mL/kg, and it is not possible to increase the volume of feed, then a further gradual increase in energy density of the feed should be undertaken with the addition of glucose polymer or Duocal (fat and carbohydrate) in 1% daily increments up to a maximum of 4% until weight gain is achieved. At this level of fortification a reasonable protein:energy ratio of 9% is maintained. The final feed provides an energy density of 1.2 kcal (5 kJ)/mL. Alternatively if the protein:energy ratio needs to be better preserved then addition of infant formula powder in 1% increments up to 4% may be considered, achieving a protein:energy ratio of approximately 10%. As these infants are often at risk of GOR [28] a fine balance has to be made between giving a feed of sufficient energy density to achieve adequate growth whilst limiting vomiting, malabsorption or, if feeding via nasogastric tube, occurrence of large gastric aspirates.

The patient in the paediatric intensive care unit

Energy expenditure

Following cardiac surgery the majority of patients are sedated, paralysed and mechanically ventilated whilst in the paediatric intensive care unit (PICU). Unfortunately predictive energy expenditure equations have been found to be inadequate in calculating nutritional requirements for these patients [37, 38]. One study using indirect calorimetry in infants and young children in the PICU found an average energy expenditure of 68 kcal (284 kJ)/kg/day [37]. Cyanosis did not appear to have any effect on postoperative metabolic rate [37] but those patients who underwent cardiopulmonary bypass appear to have had higher postoperative energy expenditure (74 kcal (309 kJ)/kg/day) than those who did not (58 kcal (242 kJ)/kg/day). Avitzur et al. [39] found lower levels of postoperative energy expenditure, but

Table 13.2 Comparison of standard infant formula and nutrient dense infant formula.

A 3-month-old infant with a congenital cardiac defect resulting in faltering growth,
weight 3.9 kg (<0.4th percentile)
Feed volumes 100, 120 and 150 mL/kg

		Energy		Protein
		(kcal)	(kJ)	(g)
Feeding 100 mL/kg				
Total fluid intake 360 mL				
Feeding 45 mL × 3 hourly × 8 feeds				
(a) 360 mL standard infant formula		245	1025	5
	per kg =	70	293	1.4
(b) 360 mL of 1 kcal/mL formula		360	1505	9.4
	per kg =	100	418	2.7
DRV	per kg =	100 (EAR)*	420	2.1 (RNI)†
Initial aim	per kg =	120+	500+	3+
Feeding 120 mL/kg				
Total fluid intake 440 mL				
Feeding 55 mL × 3 hourly × 8 feeds				
(a) 440 mL standard infant formula		299	1250	6.6
	per kg =	85	355	1.9
(b) 440 mL of 1 kcal/mL formula		440	1840	11.4
	per kg =	125	525	3.3
DRV	per kg =	100	420	2.1
Initial aim	per kg =	120+	500+	3+
Feeding 150 mL/kg				
Total fluid intake 520 mL				
Feeding 65 mL × 3 hourly × 8 feeds				
(a) 520 mL standard infant formula		341	1425	7.8
	per kg =	97	405	2.2
(b) 520 mL of 1 kcal/mL formula		520	2175	13.5
	per kg =	150	620	3.9
DRV	per kg =	100	420	2.1
Aim if growth falters	per kg =	140+	590+	3.5+

DRV, dietary reference value.
*Estimated average requirement (dietary reference values).
†Reference nutrient intake (dietary reference values).

Table 13.3 Increasing feed strength and fluid volume using a staged approach.

	Fluid mL/kg		Feed kcal (kJ)/100 mL	Energy kcal/kg	kJ/kg
Day 1	100 mL	15% standard infant formula	72–78 (300–325)	72–78	300–325
Day 2	120 mL	SMA High Energy	91 (380)	109	455
Day 3	120 mL	Infatrini or Similac High Energy	100 (420)	120	50
Day 4	140 mL	Infatrini or Similac High Energy	100 (420)	140	585
Day 5	150 mL	Infatrini or Similac High Energy	100 (420)	150	630

again no difference between acyanotic and cyanotic patients, 62 kcal (259 kJ) vs. 59 kcal (247 kJ)/kg/day. Infants with HLHS in the immediate 3 days following their first complex Norwood stage 1 operation have been shown to have even lower energy expenditure, 39–43 kcal (163–180 kJ)/kg/day [40], although energy intakes failed to meet even these requirements.

Energy requirements during the first few postoperative days therefore appear to be close to or even below normal. However, once the patient comes off the ventilator, changes in metabolic rate will depend on any residual lesion that affects cardiopulmonary function.

Fluid restrictions

There is a need to limit the amount of fluid in the circulatory system postoperatively as cardiopulmonary bypass causes oedema of all the body's tissues which compromises organ function. Keeping the lungs relatively dry also helps to wean the patient off the ventilator. As a result there is often a limited fluid volume for feeding in the first day or so after operation. In small infants with a large number of IV drug infusions, e.g. 5–6 mL/hour, there is usually limited space for meaningful volumes of feed until at least an 80% fluid allowance is reached and intensive dietetic intervention may not be feasible (see example below). As energy intake is limited during this period, blood sugar monitoring is required with correction being made if they are found to be low. The permitted amount of fluid in the days immediately following surgery varies between units, but inevitably results in insufficient volume to achieve adequate nutrition. However, fluid restrictions are usually temporary and there is opportunity to improve intake as the feed volumes increase.

Fluid allowances on cardiac intensive care units are often expressed in terms of a percentage and are calculated cumulatively as follows:

- 4 mL/kg/hour for the first 10 kg in weight
- 2 mL/kg/hour for the second 10 kg in weight
- 1 mL/kg/hour for every kilogram above 20 kg

These volumes provide a patient with a '100%' fluid allowance. This may not, however, equate to normal fluid requirements, particularly for an infant or small child, and nutrition can easily be compromised.

Worked example: Infant weighing 3.5 kg
100% fluid allowance provides 4 mL/kg/hour
= 4 × 3.5 × 24 = 336 mL/day
Total fluid allowance: 96 mL/kg/day compared with a usual fluid requirement of 150 mL/kg/day. In the unlikely event that all of this fluid allowance was available for feeds a standard infant formula would provide on average 65 kcal (270 kJ)/kg/day

Worked example: Child weighing 30 kg
100% fluid allowance provides
For the first 10 kg: 4 mL/kg = 4 × 10 = 40 mL/hour
For the second 10 kg: 2 mL/kg = 2 × 10
= 20 mL/hour
For the third 10 kg: 1 mL/kg = 1 × 10 = 10 mL/hour
Total fluid allowance: 70 mL/hour

If the child has a 50% fluid restriction then he/she will receive only 50% of the calculated volume, i.e. 35 mL/hour. Fluids used to flush intravascular arterial and venous pressure monitoring lines and intravenous drugs are then usually deducted, leaving the remaining hourly fluid volume for feeds

Table 13.4 illustrates how fluid allowances might be increased following surgery depending on whether the patient has undergone cardiopulmonary bypass or not. Volumes of intravenous drug infusions are included in the total fluid allowance leaving limited room for feed in the days immediately after surgery.

Infants and children without cardiac defects are known to be at risk of developing malnutrition following admission to the PICU, with those admitted from wards and other hospitals being at greatest risk [41], and aggressive nutritional

Table 13.4 Fluid allowance during admission to the paediatric intensive care unit after cardiac surgery.

Day post surgery	Cardiopulmonary bypass	Non cardiopulmonary bypass
1	50%	80%
2	60%	90%–100%
3	70%	120%
4	80%	Free fluids
5	90%	
6	100%	
7	120%–135%	
8	150%	

therapy may improve some biochemical markers of nutritional status (p. 72). Should the clinical condition and/or fluid balance of the patient result in fluid restrictions continuing beyond the expected time frame steps should be taken to ensure nutritional requirements are met. Less than a third of children undergoing cardiac surgery have been shown to achieve their estimated energy requirement whilst on the intensive care ward and have significant falls in weight during their stay [42].

Following discharge from the PICU the fluid allowance of patients is often increased and provides an opportunity to improve feed intake. Infants provided with an 80 kcal (334 kJ)/100 mL feed on day 1 of discharge from the PICU, increasing to 100 kcal (420 kJ)/100 mL feed on day 3, have demonstrated significant improvements in weight gain at discharge compared with controls [43]. Increases in the energy density of feeds may be well tolerated by some but may also result in vomiting necessitating use of anti-reflux treatments.

Methods of feed administration

The majority of patients admitted to the PICU are fed via nasogastric tube for the first few days following cardiac surgery. However, once discharged to the ward most should have transitioned or be in a position to transition to oral feeds. On discharge from hospital the majority of cardiac infants should be taking feeds orally, but some may fail to complete feeds and others may require ongoing tube feeds. This may be due to fatigue brought on by the effort of sucking, anorexia or early satiety. Factors that have been shown to have a detrimental effect on oral feeding capability are vocal chord injury, long postoperative ventilation and poor weight at surgery [44].

If an infant is regularly failing to complete feeds one of the following strategies should be employed:

- offer smaller more frequent feeds orally
- complete feeds via nasogastric tube
- give small frequent bolus feeds via nasogastric tube
- top up small frequent daytime feeds with continuous feeds overnight via an enteral feeding pump

- give feeds continuously over 20–22 hours via an enteral pump, allowing the gut to rest for a short period and gastric pH to return to normal

Feeding an infant or young child overnight via a nasogastric tube, whether in hospital or at home, requires a risk assessment. There have been a number of studies looking at the efficacy of methods of feed administration in infants with CHD. Children with complex congenital heart lesions who fail to achieve adequate weight gain with oral fortified feeds have been shown to have greater energy intakes and weight gain using the same feeds given as continuous nasogastric infusions [20]. It has been suggested that continuous feeding causes a smaller rise in basal metabolic rate and heart rate than occurs after bolus feeds [45]. Feeding 1 kcal (4 kJ)/mL formulas orally; or as oral daytime feeds plus 12 hours overnight continuous nasogastric feeding; or as 24 hours continuous nasogastric feeds has been compared in a group of infants with CHD and CHF [46]. During the 5 months of the study only the group of infants receiving 24 hours continuous nasogastric feeds achieved target intakes in excess of 140 kcal (585 kJ)/kg/day. However, others have demonstrated improvements in energy intake and body weight with nutritional counselling alone [31].

Improved standard deviation scores (SDS) for weight has been demonstrated in 37 patients with cardiac defects who had undergone percutaneous gastrostomy placement [47]. Comparison with nasogastric fed controls is difficult, however, due to differences in starting SDS for weight. Patients who require long term tube feeding may benefit from a gastrostomy as it may present less of an impediment to the development of oral feeding skills. The timing of weaning off gastrostomy feeds to allow for the development of independent feeding skills should be addressed for each individual child.

Other nutritional issues

Sodium supplementation of infant feeds

Some infants with CHD fail to gain weight on an energy intake in excess of 140 kcal (585 kJ)/kg. The use of diuretics makes electrolyte depletion a possibility. If this is suspected a 24 hour urine sodium balance should be done to establish urinary sodium losses and sodium supplementation should be considered. An infant feeding 150 mL/kg of a standard infant formula receives 1.0–1.3 mmol Na+/kg, depending on the formula, compared with the RNI for sodium for an infant aged 0–3 months of 1.5 mmol Na+/kg. Infants feeding 150 mL/kg of one of the commercially available higher energy formulas will receive between 1.4 and 1.65 mmol Na/kg.

Anticoagulation and the vitamin K content of feeds

Children undergoing Blalock–Taussig (BT) and Glenn shunts, total cavo-pulmonary connection (TCPC or Fontan operation), pulmonary artery reconstruction and some operations requiring tissue homografts are given either aspirin or warfarin postoperatively for anticoagulation. Vitamin K has an antagonistic effect on some of the anticoagulation drugs and may be given in some instances to counter excessive anticoagulation, the dose being 300 µg/kg/day. While most cardiac infants tolerate whole protein feeds there may occasionally be a need to use a hydrolysed protein formula (Table 7.6), some of which have high vitamin K content, e.g. Pregestimil. An infant weighing 5 kg feeding 150 mL/kg/day of such a formula may receive an additional 60 µg of vitamin K per day. If a patient is anticoagulated the international normalised ratio (INR) should be monitored in the days following the introduction of such formula.

Outcome of patients with specific cardiac lesions

Advances in surgical expertise in recent years has meant that increasing numbers of infants with severe cardiac lesions are surviving and being discharged into the community. The nutritional status of infants and children with CHD depends on both the type of lesion and the number of operations that they require. The more complex the lesion and the greater the number of planned operations, the greater the nutritional risk to the patient. The following two lesions, however, present a relatively low nutritional risk in spite of their complexity and for two separate reasons.

Transposition of the great arteries (TGA)

With TGA the two main arteries exit from alternate ventricles from those they would normally use. The aorta exits from the right ventricle rather than the left and the pulmonary artery exits from the left ventricle. The patient is able to survive because blood can mix through a patent foramen ovale (PFO) and a PDA. The patient is almost always given prostaglandin to try to keep the PDA open. In about 25% of patients the PFO is enlarged, using a cardiac catheter in a procedure called a balloon atrial septostomy, and this allows for better mixing of blood. The patient is then allowed to recover before an operation is carried out at about 1 week of age in which the arteries are switched over to their correct position; the hole between the atria is repaired and the PDA is closed. Unlike most infants with congenital heart defects, those with TGA tend to have normal birth weights [12,16] although the reason for this is uncertain. As they undergo the repair of this complex defect within the first few weeks of life they are able to be discharged, feeding normally, usually with no need for dietetic intervention.

Tetralogy of Fallot

There are four separate aspects to this complex cyanotic defect: a ventricular septal defect; an overriding aorta in which the aorta straddles the two ventricles; obstruction of pulmonary blood flow from the right ventricle (sub pulmonary stenosis) and right ventricular hypertrophy (Fig. 13.3). A ventricular septal defect on its own will usually cause a left to right shunt with excessive blood flow to the lungs and the patient being at risk of developing pulmonary hypertension and associated faltering growth. However, with tetralogy of Fallot the right ventricular outflow tract obstruction protects them from excessive lung blood flow. Due to the obstruction the workload of right ventricle is increased resulting in it becoming hypertrophied but this does not appear to affect growth. Rarely, if the patient is very blue (cyanosed) a Blalock–Taussig (BT) shunt operation is initially performed (p. 305) early in life to try to normalise pulmonary blood flow.

Once stabilised or after recovery from the shunt operation the infant is able to be discharged home after a short inpatient stay and most cases achieve adequate weight gain. However, those who have undergone a BT shunt may be at risk of developing a degree of excessive pulmonary blood flow thereby increasing respiratory effort, which may require nutritional support. At about 4–6 months of age when the infant has had a chance to grow the reparative operation is carried out with the VSD being closed, the outflow obstruction repaired and (if necessary) the BT shunt being taken down. On discharge they usually require no further nutritional support.

Hypoplastic left heart syndrome

In contrast to the above two conditions, patients who have undergone the first stage of repair (the Norwood operation) for HLHS constitute a group that is at particular nutritional risk. Almost a third of patients with HLHS have been shown not to meet normal energy requirements during their hospital stay with almost 60% not regaining their birth weight by discharge following their first operation [48]. Introducing standardised management protocols, including home surveillance programmes, has been shown to improve intraoperative survival rates and poor weight gain is used as one of the indicators for earlier surgical intervention [49, 50]. Within this group of patients, a gastrostomy has been linked to improved survival independently of weight gain [50]. It may be that improved survival is linked to reduced use of nasogastric tubes with these being a route for hospital acquired infection.

Complications of congenital heart disease affecting nutritional status

Chylothorax

Normal transport of chyle

After digestion in the intestinal lumen dietary fats are absorbed into the mucosal cells as glycerol and fatty acids. Long chain fatty acids of 12 or more carbon atoms are re-esterified to triglycerides and pass into the thoracic lymph duct as chyle. Sixty to seventy per cent of absorbed dietary fat passes through the lymphatic system at a concentration of between 5 and 30 g/L. Flow increases markedly after ingestion of a high fat meal with lesser but

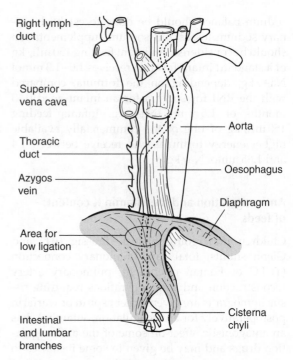

Figure 13.4   Anatomy of the thoracic duct, (Source: Merrigan *et al.* [57].)

definite increases after mixed meals of protein, carbohydrate and fat [51]. The principal function of the thoracic lymph duct is to transport chyle to where it enters the venous system near the junction of the left internal jugular and subclavian veins [52] and these vessels then drain into the superior vena cava. Figure 13.4 shows the anatomy of the thoracic lymph duct.

Chylothorax is caused by a fistula between the thoracic lymph duct and the pleural cavity resulting in the accumulation of chyle in the pleural cavity itself. Chyle contains lymphocytes, immunoglobulin, enzymes, triglycerides, cholesterol and fat soluble vitamins the loss of which, if unchecked, would invariably lead to serious metabolic deficit.

Fistulas

There are three types of fistula.

- *Traumatic fistula*: the thoracic duct drains into the vessels close to where some cardiac surgical procedures are carried out. As the thoracic duct is difficult to see there is an increased risk of disruption and damage to the duct during surgery, resulting in a traumatic fistula.

- *Obstructive fistula*: these result from increased pressure in the thoracic lymph duct itself which causes its walls to become leaky. This may be secondary to increased venous pressure due to sluggish blood flow or clots in the veins distal to where the thoracic duct empties. Patients with right-sided obstructive cardiac lesions require venous to pulmonary artery shunt operations to achieve longer term oxygenation. Theoretically procedures that affect venous return on the right side of the heart are more likely to result in obstructive chylothorax. The Glenn and TCPC shunt operations are two examples where the venous return is plumbed directly into the pulmonary vasculature to try to achieve adequate oxygenation. Under these circumstances the blood flow in the lungs is increased resulting in 'back pressure' into the pulmonary arteries and the newly connected systemic veins. As a result the lymph does not drain well into the veins and the lymphatic vessels themselves become engorged and leaky, with chyle passing into the thoracic cavity. However, it appears that the increased risk of developing chylothorax only occurs with the larger TCPC shunt [53]. An exacerbating factor may be the development of either a chest infection or a postoperative pleural effusion and chylothorax may occur some days after operation. A list of cardiac defects that may require these operations is shown in Table 13.5.
- *Congenital fistula*: some children may develop congenital chylothorax [54], with children having Noonan syndrome being at higher risk.

Diagnosis

As chyle contains fat from the intestinal lacteal system it has a characteristically milky appearance that often raises suspicion when it appears in post surgical pleural chest drains. A chest drain sample with a triglyceride content of >1.1 mmol/L, a total cell count >1000/μL with a predominance of lymphocytes or the presence of chylomicrons has been used to confirm diagnosis [53, 55] although others use a combination of these [56]. As the concentration of triglycerides in chyle is higher than that of plasma this has also been used to differentiate chylous pleural effusions from those of other origin [57].

Table 13.5 Conditions requiring Glenn and/or total cavo-pulmonary connection (TCPC) shunt operations (see p. 305 for definitions).

Heart defect	Operation
Ebstein's anomaly	TCPC*
Pulmonary atresia with/without intact ventricular septum	Glenn shunt and TCPC
Tricuspid atresia	TCPC
Single ventricle physiology	Glenn shunt and TCPC
Hypoplastic left heart	Norwood stage 2 and 3[†]

*TCPC is one of a number of surgical options in Ebstein's anomaly.
[†]The second stage of the Norwood procedure may be similar to a Glenn shunt or TCPC and the third stage may be a TCPC operation.

Incidence and duration

The incidence of chylothorax is between 1.34% and 9.2% following cardiac surgery for CHD [53, 55, 58]. Low body weight, longer cardiopulmonary bypass time and secondary chest closures are all associated with increased risk of developing chylothorax [58]. A higher incidence of chylothorax has been noted in patients undergoing repair of tetralogy of Fallot, the TCPC procedure and heart transplantation [53].

A median duration of 9–15 days is expected before chest drain output ceases [53, 58] although up to a quarter of cases have continued outputs beyond 30 days [53]. The amount of chylous drainage varies between 2 and 40 mL/kg in most cases [55, 58, 59] with high outputs >100 mL/kg/day being indicative of dietary treatment being unsuccessful [58].

Treatment options

Chylothorax can be treated conservatively using a minimal long chain triglyceride (LCT) diet [53, 55, 58, 60] or total parenteral nutrition (TPN) [55]. However, it has been proposed that some suspected cases of chylothorax may be self-limiting with a median resolution time of 1 week following presentation [56].

The aim of the minimal LCT diet is to reduce the lymph flow and so allow the fistula to heal. Dietary fat is mainly composed of LCT. Normally medium chain triglycerides (MCT), with 6–10 carbon atoms in the fatty acid chain, do not constitute more than a

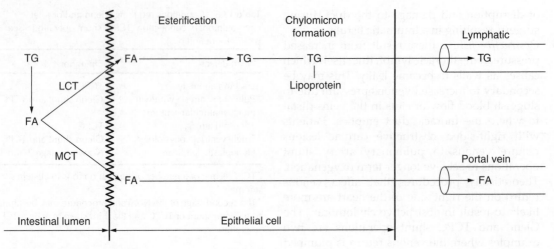

Figure 13.5 Scheme of the pathways of absorption of long chain triglyceride (LCT) and medium chain triglyceride (MCT). FA, fatty acid; TG, triglyceride.

minor proportion of dietary fats. However, as they are absorbed directly into the portal vein as 'free fatty acids' bound to albumin (Fig. 13.5) they constitute a useful additional source of energy in a diet that may otherwise be low in energy. Restriction of free water intake during the treatment period may have a beneficial effect on outcome.

There have been individual case reports of the hormone somatostatin or an analogue octreotide, both of which have antisecretory and antidiarrhoeal properties, being used in isolation or as an adjunct to a minimal LCT diet or PN to treat refractory chylothorax. A dose of 1–4 μg/kg/hour is recommended [61,62] although benefit has been noted on smaller doses [63]. Despite some promising case reports [61–64] results appear to be inconsistent [55]. Surgical ligation of the thoracic lymph duct is usually reserved for patients who do not respond to 3–4 weeks of dietary and medical treatment [55,65].

Prognosis

The conservative dietary approach has a success rate of between 70% and 80% [53,58,60]. A useful algorithm for the management of chylothorax has been produced by Cormack *et al.* [60] and is shown in Fig. 13.6. However, development of chylothorax has been shown to almost triple the duration of hospital stay [53].

Dietary treatment of chylothorax

A general guide has been to give not more than 1 g LCT per year of life up to a maximum of 4–5 g LCT/day. The origin of this practice is *Diets for Sick Children*, 4th edition, 1987, Dorothy Francis. However, the evidence base for this is poor and the guidance is often breached, particularly in older infants and younger children where 1–2 g LCT/day is very difficult to manage.

Minimal fat feeds for the infant with chylothorax

- Monogen
- MCT Pepdite
- Minimal LCT modular feed based on Pepdite Module 767

Monogen

Monogen is a whey protein based infant formula with low LCT content. The fat sources are fractionated coconut oil and walnut oil. Monogen was previously thought to contain 0.21 g of LCT per 100 mL formula at standard dilution (17.5%). However, recent analysis by the manufacturer has revealed that the amount of LCT is closer to 0.38 g/100 mL (Table 13.6).

If the infant has previously been tolerating normal or concentrated feeds prior to the development of chylothorax, it should be possible to introduce Monogen at full strength despite the relatively high carbohydrate content (12%). If the baby has

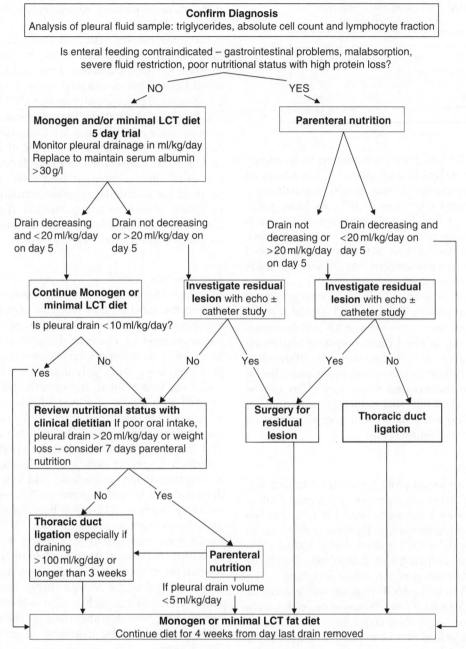

Figure 13.6 Chylothorax algorithm.

had limited enteral nutrition then, as a precaution, Monogen may be introduced at half strength, i.e. 9% dilution in the first 12–24 hours. Standard dilution provides 74 kcal (310 kJ)/100 mL. In cases of severe fluid restriction it has previously been advocated to gradually increase the concentration of the feed in order to meet requirements. In view of the current higher LCT content of the feed, it might be prudent to increase energy density using either glucose polymer (in 1% increments) or MCT

Table 13.6 Nutritional content of standard Monogen per 100 mL.

Energy	74 kcal/310 kJ
Protein equivalent	2.2 g
Carbohydrate	12 g
Fat	1.9 g
MCT	1.52 g
LCT	0.38 g

emulsion (in 1%–2% increments) up to an energy density of 90 kcal (375 kJ)/100 mL. This allows an increase in energy density whilst maintaining a protein:energy ratio close to 10%. As Monogen is a complete infant formula supplementation with essential fatty acids (EFA) should not be needed. However, falls in EFA status have been noted following commencement on Monogen feeds (personal communication).

In order to achieve adequate energy intake to facilitate growth the total LCT intake may be greater than the 1 g per year of life recommendation. As long as chest drain output is unaffected then a higher LCT intake should be allowed to continue. If chest drains are not *in situ* then clinical signs such as increased respiratory effort can be used to monitor tolerance to increasing amounts of LCT. A chest x-ray may confirm re-accumulation of chyle in the pleural cavity.

MCT Pepdite
If whole cow's milk protein is contraindicated, e.g. where the infant has a proven cow's milk protein allergy, Monogen cannot be used. MCT Pepdite has been used on some units (personal communication) but it has a higher LCT content: 0.68 g/100 mL (25% of total fat) compared with 0.38 g/100 mL (20% of total fat) in Monogen. An infant weighing 3.5 kg feeding 150 mL/kg MCT Pepdite will receive in excess of 3.5 g LCT/day. In some cases this may provide too much long chain fat and a minimal LCT modular feed may be required to reduce chyle flow adequately.

Minimal LCT modular feed
A modular feed can be designed using Pepdite Module 767 as a minimal fat protein source. It is free of cow's milk protein. To produce a nutritionally adequate infant feed it is necessary to add carbohydrate, a suitable fat source, electrolytes,

minerals and vitamins. An example of this feed is shown in Table 13.7.

Once the full strength feed is tolerated, weight gain should be reviewed. It may be necessary to increase the energy density of the feed to facilitate weight gain. This should be done by the incremental addition of glucose polymer and MCT emulsion, e.g. Liquigen. A total of 12% carbohydrate as glucose polymer and 4% fat as MCT emulsion should be tolerated. If sufficient quantities of a vitamin and mineral preparation, e.g. Paediatric Seravit, are added to the modular feed there should be no need for additional supplementation with the exception of sodium and potassium. If the infant consistently takes <150 mL/kg then the need for supplementation should be assessed.

Essential fatty acids
EFA in phospholipids are important for maintaining the function and integrity of cellular and subcellular membranes. They also participate in the regulation of cholesterol metabolism, being involved in its transport, breakdown and ultimate excretion. Long chain polyunsaturated fatty acids (LCP) are important in the growth and development of term infants and their addition to the diet in appropriate quantities is safe [66]. A deficiency state arising from an inadequate intake of linoleic acid has been demonstrated in children [67]. Although a specific deficiency state arising from inadequate dietary α-linolenic acid has not been demonstrated in healthy humans, it is regarded as a dietary essential [67]. It has been recommended that the neonate requires at least 1% of energy intake from linoleic acid (C18:2) and at least 0.2% of energy from α-linolenic acid (C18:3) [68]. On re-analysis it appears that Monogen has slightly over the required percentage energy from linoleic acid whilst having slightly less α-linolenic acid. Table 13.8 gives a comparison of EFA content of feeds used in the treatment of infants with chylothorax.

EFA supplementation of feeds
If EFA need to be added to a feed this may be done using walnut oil; the fatty acid content provides linoleic and α-linolenic acids in an acceptable quantity and ratio. Walnut oil contains 55 g linoleic and 12 g α-linolenic acids per 100 mL (Table 19.4). The

Table 13.7 A modular feed for treating chylothorax.

A 3-month-old infant develops a chylothorax post cardiac surgery. Whole cow's milk protein is contraindicated

Weight 4 kg, fluid volume 150 mL/kg

	Na+ (mmol)	K+ (mmol)	Energy (kcal/kJ)	CHO (g)	Protein (g)	MCT (g)
16 g Pepdite Module 767			55/230		13.8	
60 g glucose polymer	0.5	neg	232/970	58		
24 mL Liquigen	0.3		108/450			11.8
17 g Paediatric Seravit	0.15		51/215	12.8		
5 mL KCl (2 mmol/mL)		10				
4 mL NaCl (1 mmol/mL)	4					
+ water to 600 mL						
Totals	4.9	10	446/1865	70.8	13.8	11.8
per 100 mL	0.8	1.6	74/311	11.8	2.3	2
per kg	1.2	2.5	111/466		3.4	

Day 1	Day 2	Day 3
4 g Pepdite Module 767	8 g Peptide Module 767	12 g Pepdite Module 767
15 g glucose polymer	30 g glucose polymer	45 g glucose polymer
6 mL Liquigen	12 mL Liquigen	24 mL Liquigen
6 g Paediatric Seravit	12 g Paediatric Seravit	17 g Paediatric Seravit

Aims in constructing feed: 3+ g protein per kg; 74 kcal (310 kJ) per 100 mL; 12% carbohydrate concentration.
The feed concentration should be gradually increased daily as shown to achieve the full strength.

Table 13.8 Percentage energy derived from linoleic and α-linolenic acids in minimal LCT feeds.

	Energy from C18:2 (%)	Energy from C18:3 (%)
Monogen	1.1	0.17
MCT Pepdite	5.1	0.75
Minimal LCT modular feed	0	0

addition of 0.15 mL of walnut oil to 100 mL of the minimal LCT Pepdite Module 767 based feed will provide EFA (and at the same time contribute a minimum amount of LCT) to a minimum of 1% energy from linoleic acid and 0.2% energy from α-linolenic acid. As the energy content of the feed is increased it will be necessary to increase the EFA supplementation proportionately.

Minimal LCT weaning diet
The following foods contain minimal LCT and can be introduced as weaning solids:

- puréed vegetables, e.g. potato, carrots, swede, green beans
- puréed fruit, e.g. pears, apples, banana, peaches
- puréed boiled rice mixed with minimal fat milk
- baby rice reconstituted with minimal fat milk
- tins and jars of baby foods containing less than 0.2 g LCT per 100 g may be included in the diet (mainly the fruit based tins and jars). Other commercial baby foods may contain too much LCT and need to be avoided

Even when solids are introduced into the diet of the infant, a minimal LCT formula will continue to form a major part of the nutritional intake providing energy, protein, vitamins and minerals and is an essential part of the diet until at least 1 year of age. A sample day's menu for the toddler on a minimal LCT diet is given in Table 13.9.

A minimal fat milk may replace the minimal LCT formula from 1 year if nutritional intake is not compromised by doing so. This minimal fat milk can be flavoured with Nesquik powder, fruit Crusha syrups or low fat chocolate flavour topping. It can also be used on breakfast cereals, to make custard or in cereal puddings. The quantities of the ingredients may be varied to taste if needed, to provide 70–90 kcal (230–375 kJ)/100 mL. Extra energy can be added to the diet by increasing the

Table 13.9   Sample day's menu for a toddler on a minimal LCT diet.

Minimal fat milk (MFM)	
60 g skimmed milk powder	Provides 500 kcal (2090 kJ)
35 mL Liquigen	22 g protein
30 g glucose polymer	0.8 g LCT
8 g Paediatric Seravit	
+ water to 600 mL	
Use throughout the day for drinks and mixed with appropriate foods	

Breakfast	10 g Rice Krispies + 60 mL MFM
	Glass MFM (100 mL)
Mid morning	Glass MFM (100 mL)
	2 MCT biscuits
Lunch	80 g baked beans + 50 g MCT chips
	50 g very low fat fromage frais
	Glass fruit squash + glucose polymer
Mid afternoon	Glass MFM (100 mL)
	Meringue or Rice Krispie cake
Supper	40 g white fish steak fried in MCT oil
	Fat free mashed potatoes plus 2 teaspoons Liquigen
	40 g carrots
	50 g very low fat ice cream
	Jelly
Bedtime	Glass MFM (100 mL)

Total LCT intake for the day 2 g

concentration of glucose polymer in the milk or by using a 10%–15% solution of glucose polymer to make up fruit squash. Increased energy intake can be achieved by the addition of Liquigen to suitable foods such as mashed potatoes or other root vegetables.

Feeding the older child and adolescent with chylothorax

Keeping the LCT intake to a minimum necessitates the exclusion of many foods including animal and vegetable fats such as butter, lard, margarine and vegetable oils. It also makes it necessary to strictly limit or exclude protein foods that also have a high fat content such as meat, fatty fish, full fat milk, cheese and eggs. All cakes, pastry and biscuits

made with LCT fats must also be avoided. An important part of the diet is skimmed milk fortified with carbohydrate and MCT as a source of energy, protein, minerals and vitamins.

MCT can be used in the diet in the form of MCT oil or MCT emulsion. MCT oil allows fried foods to be included, such as fried fish, chips and crisps. Both MCT oil and MCT emulsion can be used in baking, cakes, biscuits, pastry; all these foods are valuable sources of energy and can greatly enhance the palatability of the diet to the patient. The final diet may contain 40–70 g MCT, depending on the age and energy requirement of the patient. This should be gradually introduced over a period of 7–10 days in order to avoid abdominal discomfort. Table 13.10 lists foods containing minimal LCT, which can be used freely in the diet.

The weights and fat contents of foods which can be used to construct a day's meals containing minimal fat for the child or adolescent with chylothorax are given in Table 13.11. A review of some suitable low fat foods indicates that there may be up to a threefold variation in fat content of some meat and fish products depending on the brand. To make the diet more manageable the family can be taught to calculate minimal LCT exchanges as follows:

$$0.2 \text{ g fat exchange}$$
$$= \frac{0.2}{\text{grams of fat/100 g of food}} \times 100 \text{ g}$$
$$0.5 \text{ g fat exchange}$$
$$= \frac{0.5}{\text{grams of fat/100 g of food}} \times 100 \text{ g}$$

Table 13.10   Free foods for minimal LCT diet.

All fruits fresh, tinned or frozen (except olives and avocado pear)
All vegetables, fresh, tinned or frozen
Sugar, honey, golden syrup, treacle, jam, marmalade
Jelly and jellied sweets such as Jelly Tots, Jelly Babies, wine gums or fruit pastilles
Boiled sweets, mints (not butter mints)
Fruit sorbets, water ices, ice lollies
Meringue, egg white, Rite-Diet egg replacer
Spices and essences
Salt, pepper, vinegar, herbs, tomato ketchup, most chutney, Marmite, Oxo, Bovril
Fruit juices, fruit squashes, Crusha fruit flavouring syrups, Nesquik fruit flavouring powder, chocolate flavour topping, bottled fruit sauces
Fizzy drinks, lemonade, cola, Lucozade

Table 13.11   LCT content of foods suitable for use in minimal LCT diet.

Food	LCT (per 100 g)	Average portion size (g)	LCT per portion (g)
Breakfast cereals			
Branflakes	2.0	35	0.7
Cornflakes	0.9	25	0.2
Frosties	0.6	20	0.1
Sugar Puffs	1.6	25	0.4
Special K	1.0	20	0.2
Cocopops	2.0	20	0.4
Just Right	2.5	40	1.0
Rice Krispies	1.0	25	0.25
Ricicles	0.7	20	0.1
Weetabix	1.9	37.5 (2 biscuits)	0.7
Puffed Wheat	2.5	15	0.4
Frosted Shreddies	1.4	35	0.5
Weetaflakes	1.6	30	0.5
Bread			
White, large thin slice	1.6	35	0.4
Granary	1.7	35	0.6
Matzos	1.0	20	0.2
Crumpets (toasted)	1.0	45 (1 crumpet)	0.45
Dairy foods			
Reduced fat cottage cheese	1.4	50	0.7
Very low fat fromage frais	0.1	100	0.1
Condensed milk, skimmed sweetened	0.2-1.0	50	0.1 - 0.5
Very low fat yoghurt (Muller Light)	0.1	200	0.2
Very low fat ice cream	0.4	50	0.2
Fish			
White cod fillet, raw	0.1-0.7	100	0.7
White cod steak, raw	0.6	100	0.6
Grilled white haddock fillet	0.6	100	0.6
Steamed whiting	0.9	100	0.9
Steamed smoked haddock	0.9	100	0.9
Fish finger	7.2	25 (1 fish finger)	1.8
Tuna	0.2-0.6	100	0.2 - 0.6
Shell fish			
Prawns (peeled)	0.5-1.7	80	0.4-1.4
Crabsticks	0.1	50	neg
Crab (canned)	0.9	50	0.4
Crab (white meat only)	0.1	100	0.1
Shrimps (canned)	1.2	50	0.6
Cockles (boiled)	0.3-3	50	0.1-1.5
Mussels	2-3	50	1.0-1.5
Meat, poultry and alternatives			
Roast turkey, light meat	1.4	70	1.0
Roast chicken, light meat	4.0	25	1.0
Roast lamb, lean	8.0	25	2.0
Roast beef, lean only topside	4.0	45	1.8
Silverside, lean only	4.9	40	2.0
Thin sliced packet beef cooked with added water	2.6	30	0.8
Ham	2.3-7.0	40	1.2 - 2.8
Quorn mince	2.0	50	1.0
Legumes, pasta, rice			
Baked beans in tomato sauce	0.5	200	1.0
Tinned spaghetti in tomato sauce	0.1	200	0.2
White rice (boiled)	0.3	150	0.4
White pasta (boiled)	0.8	130	1.0

A sample day's meal for a 14-year-old boy with chylothorax is shown in Table 13.12 and Table 13.13 gives a nutritional analysis of the diet.

Vitamin and mineral supplementation
Since a wide range of foods must either be excluded from the diet or taken in reduced quantities, it is essential to check the vitamin and mineral content of the diet, giving supplements if needed.

Table 13.12 Sample day's meals for a 14-year-old boy with chylothorax. Aim 4–5 g LCT per day.

Daily milk allowance	
Fortified skimmed milk (FSM)	*20% glucose polymer solution*
100 g skimmed milk powder 100 g glucose polymer 50 mL Liquigen + water to 1000 mL	40 g glucose polymer + water to 200 mL

1000 mL FSM provides 950 kcal (3970 kJ), 36 g protein, 1.3 g LCT

Breakfast	25 g cornflakes + FSM 120 mL orange juice and glucose polymer Apple
Mid morning	Glass of FSM + meringue + 2 MCT biscuits
Lunch	70 g roast turkey (light meat only) 150 g mashed potatoes + 15 mL Liquigen 60 g carrots 120 g tinned fruit + 120 mL custard made with FSM Glass fruit squash made with glucose polymer solution
Mid afternoon	250 mL FSM + 1 sachet strawberry Build Up + banana + 2 MCT biscuits
Supper	200 g baked beans + 100 g MCT chips Apple pie made with MCT pastry + 100 g very low fat fromage frais
Bedtime	Glass of FSM

Table 13.13 Nutritional analysis of minimal LCT diet for a 14-year-old boy showing comparison with dietary reference values.

			DRV
Energy	(kcal)	2700 (11.3 MJ)	2200 (9.2 MJ)
Protein	(g)	87	42
LCT	(g)	5	
Na	(mmol)	100	70
K	(mmol)	130	80
Ca	(mmol)	42	25
Fe	(μmol)	330	200
Vitamin D	(μg)	13	10*
Vitamin A	(REμg)	1200	600
Vitamin C	(mg)	165	35

DRV, dietary reference values; RE, retinol equivalent.
*At risk individuals with little sunlight exposure.

Length of treatment period

The traditional length of treatment on a minimal LCT diet is 4–6 weeks, but the evidence base for this is limited. Cormack *et al.* [60] have suggested a return to normal diet 4 weeks after removal of a pleural drain that has not resulted in recurrence of chylothorax, while others suggest 2–4 weeks continued treatment following chest drain removal [52]. A more recent study has indicated that breast feeding/normal diet could be reintroduced within a week following 10 days of diet which resulted in successful resolution of symptoms [58]. However, the specific details are limited, with the dietary treatment described as 'long chain fatty acid free' with the addition of only 1%–2% MCT. For infants, the risk of limiting the supply of EFA during what is probably a critical point in brain and retinal development should be balanced against the possibility of achieving faster resolution of chylothorax.

Following reintroduction of a normal diet clinical signs usually confirm whether chylothorax has recurred or not, but a chest x-ray may help in clarifying diagnosis.

If an older child with chylothorax requires tube feeding 'juice' style oral nutritional supplements, e.g. Ensure Plus Juce, Fortijuce, Fresubin Jucy or Paediasure Plus Juce, may be used as the feed base as they do not contain any fat. These feeds require supplementation with some electrolytes and EFA from walnut oil to make them nutritionally complete (Table 13.14). They may be diluted if

Table 13.14 Supplementation of 'juice' style oral nutritional supplements to make them nutritionally complete for a 9-year-old boy.

Oral nutritional supplement	Supplementation required
Ensure Plus Juce	Sodium, potassium, calcium*, magnesium*, phosphorus, fluoride, vitamin D[†]
Fortijuce	Sodium, potassium, calcium*, magnesium, phosphorus
Fresubin Jucy	Sodium, potassium, magnesium, phosphorus
Paediasure Plus Juce	Sodium, potassium, calcium*, magnesium*, folate, fluoride, vitamin D[†]

Calculations are based on these supplements being used to provide the estimated average requirement (EAR) for energy.

Fresubin Jucy provides 2–4 times as much vitamin K as the other supplements when used to meet the EAR for energy, but the amount per kilogram body weight should not affect clotting.

All of the above require an essential fatty acid supplement.

*Relatively small amounts of additional mineral required to meet reference nutrient intake (RNI).

[†]Vitamin D intake relatively low, although no RNI is set for this age.

necessary should a 1.25–1.5 kcal (5–6 kJ)/mL feed not be tolerated.

Necrotising enterocolitis

The overall incidence of necrotising enterocolitis (NEC) in infants with congenital heart defects is approximately 10 times that found in term infants without such defects. A review of cases of NEC in a large cohort of term and preterm infants with CHD (n = 643) demonstrated an incidence of 21 cases (3.3%); seven had a gestational age <36 weeks; six term infants had developed an episode of poor systemic perfusion or shock [69]. Of the eight remaining term infants who developed NEC all had lesions which put them at risk of low blood flow in the systemic circulation. Hypoplastic left heart and truncus arteriosus/aortopulmonary window were identified as defects that increased the risk of the infant developing NEC [69].

In addition, lesions requiring high doses of prostaglandin (>0.05 µg/kg/min), to keep the ductus arteriosus open to ensure adequate blood flow to the lungs, may also place the patient at increased risk of NEC. The use of prostaglandin introduces a theoretical risk of blood being 'stolen' from the systemic circulation to the lungs, resulting in reduced mesenteric blood flow and perfusion of the associated gut tissue. Disturbed mesenteric artery blood flow in infants with such systemic to

pulmonary circulatory shunts has been demonstrated [70]. However, in a separate smaller study involving neonates with HLHS none developed NEC despite proven reduced mesenteric artery blood flow [71].

Cases of NEC have also been reported in patients with cyanotic lesions, TGA and pulmonary atresia following cardiac catheterisation [72]. The aetiology of NEC in this group of patients remains unclear; possibly hypoxia, resulting in splanchnic vasoconstriction along with catecholamine release due to the stress of cardiac catheterisation, might result in reduced blood flow to the gut. As a precaution it is suggested that feeds might be introduced more cautiously in these patients following catheterisation.

Coarctation of the aorta has not been identified as a predisposing factor for NEC despite the reduced systemic blood flow which theoretically could reduce mesenteric blood flow artery and intestinal tissue perfusion. These infants may be admitted with a history of taking feeds at near normal volumes with no signs of intolerance. However, if they are admitted in clinical shock with an acidotic picture, then feeds might be withheld temporarily until the infant is more clinically stable.

It is common practice for infants with HLHS to have feeds withheld in the first few days after birth before the first staged repair (Norwood Stage 1 or Sano procedure) with PN providing preoperative nutritional support. However, del Castillo *et al.*

reported that up to one-third of their patients are fed preoperatively with no apparent increase in NEC although details on quantities and type of feed are lacking [73].

Postoperative feeding protocols and algorithms provide guidance on the introduction of feeds to try to reduce the incidence of NEC in patients with HLHS [73, 74]. Introduction of feeds at around 7 days postoperatively using either breast milk or a hydrolysed protein feed, with a slower increase in volumes, achieving full feeds after a further 7 days has been proposed [73]. Braudis et al. have suggested that an adequate cardiac output is required with low requirement for ionotropes and good peripheral perfusion before considering commencing enteral feeds [74]. However, once initiated they propose a fairly rapid increase in feeds, initially at 1 mL/kg/hour but then increasing by 2 mL/kg/hour every 4 hours until target volumes are met, and report no incidence of NEC. Breast milk with its known benefits in preventing NEC in premature infants [75] should remain the feed of choice in cardiac infants at high risk of NEC [73].

Protein losing enteropathy

Children with a cardiac anatomy that gives them a single functional ventricle undergo a series of operations in which the venous return is eventually plumbed directly into the arteries of the lungs (TCPC procedure) which has the benefit of improving oxygenation and reducing the load on the ventricle. Protein losing enteropathy occurs in CHF [76] and there is a growing body of evidence that it occurs in 10%–25% of patients who have undergone a TCPC procedure [77, 78]. This may resolve as cardiac function improves following surgery or heart transplant [79]. Localised lesions have been treated by partial bowel resection [77]. There is limited evidence for the dietary treatment of protein losing enteropathy, but a useful starting point would be to follow that for intestinal lymphangiectasia (p. 125). The diet should provide 5–10 g fat per day and be high in protein using MCT to improve energy intake.

Hepatic dysfunction

The TCPC operation is known to cause 'back pressure' on the liver, predisposing patients to hepatic dysfunction. Some go on to develop moderate to severe liver disease [80]. Prothrombin time becomes progressively deranged from the time of operation and it has been proposed that this, along with the ability to eliminate galactose, is used as a test of liver dysfunction in this population [80]. Dietary treatment will depend on the degree of liver failure and its progression.

Vocal cord palsy and feeding difficulties

Vocal cord palsy (VCP) is a well documented complication of certain neonatal cardiac procedures [44, 81–83]. Any surgery close to the aortic arch (where the left recurrent laryngeal nerve branches off the vagus nerve), along with the pulmonary arteries, carries an increased risk. In particular, surgery to ligate a PDA has an increased probability of development of VCP due to nerve damage. Smaller infants undergoing ligation of PDA seem to be particularly at risk with up to two-thirds of extremely low birth weight infants developing VCP after surgery [83]. These infants needed long term tube feeding, longer ventilatory support and had longer hospital stays compared with age matched controls. Patients with VCP have abnormal swallowing patterns and are less able to protect their airways resulting in greater chance of aspiration [84]. Up to 63% of infants with VCP in one series required long term gastrostomy feeding to meet their nutritional requirements [82].

Case studies to illustrate the nutritional management of CHD

Case study 1

Baby boy, antenatal diagnosis made on ultrasound scan at 33^{+2} weeks' gestation, working diagnosis of double outlet right ventricle (DORV) with a VSD, interrupted aortic arch and coarctation of aorta.

Born at 38^{+3} weeks gestation, Caesarean section for breech presentation.

Birth weight 2.91 kg (>9th percentile), head circumference 34.4 cm (50th percentile).

Day 1: Echocardiogram confirms diagnosis of DORV and aortic arch is found to be hypoplastic (small) rather than interrupted (closed off). Also has a subaortic VSD.

Day 2: Intravenous fluids stopped and encouraged to feed orally with a fluid allowance of 80 mL/kg.

Day 3: Fluid allowance increased to 100 mL/kg. Good oxygen saturations of 98% whilst in air. Feeding a combination of expressed breast milk (EBM) and normal infant formula via nasogastric tube.

Day 4: Fluid allowance increased to 135 mL/kg.

At 1 week of age: Undergoes first cardiac operation. Repair of hypoplastic aortic arch and excision of coarctation tissue with an end-to-end anastomosis of aortic tissue. Has an uneventful PICU stay; fluid allowance gradually increased to 150 mL/kg. (Table 13.15 illustrates how fluid allowance, feed type and volume and resultant energy intake changed over the postoperative course.)

Post op day 5: Tachycardia with mild recession of sternum noted. Weight 2.61 kg, having been 2.81 kg the previous day. Referred to dietitian: breast milk fortifier added to EBM (½ strength initially, 1 sachet per 100 mL). Fluid allowance increased to 165 mL/kg.

Post op day 6: Commenced on 'test dose' of Captopril to try to reduce afterload on heart. Fluid allowance further increased to 185 mL/kg and concentration of breast milk fortifier increased to full strength, 1 sachet per 50 mL.

Post op day 7: 2% glucose polymer added to fortified breast milk.

Post op day 11 onwards: Changed to 2 hourly feeds due to increased respiratory rate and some vomiting. Continued on fortified feed with 2 hourly regimen for a further 3 weeks. Overall weight gain during this time 940 g (~310 g/week). Subsequent weight gain slowed to 40 g in the following week.

Aiming for closure of VSD when he weighs 4.5 kg: Glucose polymer in feed changed to Duocal to improve energy intake. Feed administration changed to 50 mL × 2 hourly bolus feeds during the day and 25 mL/hour continuous feeds overnight to maximise feed tolerance, providing 145 kcal (605 kJ) and 3.5 g protein/kg/day.

Surgery to close VSD 9 weeks after initial operation to repair coarctation of the aorta: Weight 4.385 kg. Total weight gain 1775 g (average weight gain per week 197 g). By postoperative day 7 oral feeds had begun to be re-established, with 20–25 mL taken at each feed having initially used a syringe to introduce small amounts of feed (5 mL) by mouth. A change to a slow flow teat with support of the patient's jaw during feeds was found to reduce/stop gagging with bottle feeds. He had also successfully latched onto the breast. Speech and language therapist advised to allow him to feed before every nasogastric feed was due if he was awake and alert, but not for extended periods due to uncoordinated suck and risk of tiring.

Table 13.15 Postoperative changes in fluid allowance and modifications to feed.

Postop day	Working weight (kg)	Feed type	Total fluid allowance (mL/kg)	IV infusions (mL/hour)	Feed regimen	Energy intake (kcal/kg)	Protein intake (g/kg)
1	2.91	EBM	80	5	13 mL × 3 hourly × 4	12 (50 kJ)	0.2
2		EBM	100	3.5	24 mL × 3 hourly × 8	45 (190 kJ)	0.85
3		EBM	120	1	40 mL × 3 hourly × 8	76 (320 kJ)	1.4
5	2.81	EBM	150	0	53 mL × 3 hourly × 8	103 (430 kJ)	2.0
6	2.61 (working weight 2.81 kg)	EBM + ½ strength BMF	165	0	58 mL × 3 hourly × 8	136 (570 kJ)	3.4
7	2.60	EBM + BMF + 2% glucose polymer	185	0	60 mL × 3 hourly × 8	151 (630 kJ)	3.6
11	2.69	As day 7	180	0	40 mL × 2 hourly × 12	151 (630 kJ)	3.6

EBM, expressed breast milk; BMF, breast milk fortifier; IV, intravenous.

Discharge to local hospital 10 days after closure of VSD: Fortified EBM taken orally with nasogastric top-up feeds to complete target volumes.

Case study 2

Baby boy, tricuspid atresia, hypoplastic right ventricle, moderate size VSD of 4.5 mm and ASD. Born at 38+5 weeks' gestation. Birth weight 3.00 kg (9th–25th percentile), head circumference 33.4 cm (9th–25th percentile).

Previous medical history: Admitted to Special Care Baby Unit postnatally for observation. Nasogastric tube removed on day 4 of life. Mum was advised on checking for worsening cyanosis. Oxygen saturations were 90% when he was self-ventilating in air. Good blood flow across the atrial and ventricular septal defects so a Blalock–Taussig not necessary. Transferred to his local hospital on day 5 and subsequently discharged home. Discharge weight 2.84 kg.

Admitted to PICU at 11½ weeks of age: Following Glenn shunt operation along with an atrial septectomy. VSD had become small enough not to require an operation to close it. Weight 4.36 kg (0.4th percentile), length 55.5 cm (2nd percentile).

Post op day 2: Chylothorax suspected due to the milky colour of chest drain output. Sample sent to laboratory to check for triglycerides. Triglyceride content of 1.8 mmol/L confirms chylothorax.

Usual intake was a standard infant formula, 90–120 mL every 2–2½ hours during the day, total 750 mL, 117 kcal (490 kJ)/kg. Minimal LCT formula Monogen started at full strength, fluid allowance 80 mL/kg, feeding regimen 44 mL × 3 hourly × 8 nasogastric bolus feeds providing 59 kcal (248 kJ)/kg, 1.8 g protein/kg, total of 1.3 g LCT/day.

Post op day 4: Fluid allowance is increased to 120 mL/kg. Concentration of Monogen increased from usual 17.5% to 19% increasing energy content from 73.5 kcal (309 kJ)/100 mL to 80 kcal (335 kJ)/100 mL. A feeding regimen of 65 mL × 3 hourly feeds provides 95 kcal (399 kJ)/kg, 2.8 g protein/kg, total of 2.1 g LCT/day.

Post op day 6: Nasogastric tube is removed following, allowed to feed on demand. Weight 4.8 kg but thought to be retaining some fluid. Concentration of Monogen remains at 19%. He is taking 75–100 mL × 7 feeds a day, total 630 mL,

~130 mL/kg. Based on his current weight this provides 105 kcal (440 kJ)/kg, 3.1 g protein/kg, total of 2.6 g LCT/day.

Post op day 8: Clinically much better and is considered well enough to be discharged home.

Post op 5 weeks: Seen in outpatient clinic. Weight 5.8 kg (9th percentile). Clinically well and changed back to a normal infant formula.

Case study 3

6½-year-old girl with a diagnosis at birth of double inlet left ventricle, VSD, ASD and persisting ductus arteriosus. Birth weight 3.4 kg (50th percentile).

Previous medical history: Ligation of PDA and pulmonary artery band at 1 month of age. Weight at operation 3.48 kg (9th percentile). At 19 months of age developed signs of exertion and cyanosis on playing. Readmitted for a Glenn shunt with the superior vena cava anastomosed to the right pulmonary artery. Weight 9.9 kg (25th–50th percentile). At 5 years 6 months of age referred for cardiac catheter to assess blood flow before her final operation.

At 5 years and 10 months of age final TCPC operation: On admission weight 17.0 kg (9th percentile), height 111 cm (25th percentile).

Post op day 7: Weight 16.2 kg (>2nd percentile) and looks thin. Intake assessed. Breakfast: 1½ slices of toast with butter. Lunch: small ham sandwich, ½ packet crisps, jelly. Dinner: half portion of spaghetti bolognese, few spoons of ice cream. Snacks: 1 packet Quavers, ½ banana. Offered high energy milk shakes and powdered high energy high fat supplements to mix with full fat milk. Discharged postop day 16, weight 16.7 kg (<9th percentile).

Post op day 55: Readmitted having developed a chylothorax. Chest drain output started to become opaque and a triglyceride content of 3 mmol/L confirms chylothorax. Weight 16.5 kg (2nd–9th percentile).

Dietary management of chylothorax: 5 g LCT fat total. 4.5 g LCT fat from food (5 × 0.5 g fat exchanges and 10 × 0.2 g fat exchanges) with 0.5 g LCT fat from 500 mL skimmed milk. Skimmed milk fortified with 5% glucose polymer and 4% MCT emulsion (Liquigen), providing 76 kcal (320 kJ) and 3.3 g protein per 100 mL, 380 kcal (1600 kJ) per day. Build Up added to improve the protein, vitamin and mineral content of the special skimmed milk. 10 g Paediatric Seravit added to further improve vitamin and mineral intake.

Intake while on ward (MCT oil used in cooking):

Protein foods: turkey mince, turkey cottage pie, plain roast chicken, wafer thin ham, baked beans, plain roast beef
Staple foods: plain pasta, mashed potato
Vegetables: peas, carrots, sweet corn
Low fat sauces: low fat bolognese sauce, low fat sweet and sour sauce
Dessert items: plain fruit, tinned fruit, jelly, sorbet
Snacks: breakfast cereal with special skimmed milk, toast with jam
Drinks: Build Up strawberry milk shake, squash with 20% glucose polymer, lemonade mixed with 'juice' style supplement

Review 1 week after discharge: weight 16.6 kg (2nd–9th percentile).

Review 5 weeks after discharge: weight 17.2 kg (9th percentile). Advised to revert to a normal diet.

Review aged 6 years 3 months: weight 17.8 kg (9th percentile), height 113 cm (<25th percentile).

Future research and unanswered questions

At present there is uncertainty as to whether the level of LCT in currently used feeds (0.38 g/100 mL) is low enough to treat chylothorax satisfactorily and treatment failures may be due to this amount of LCT.

A number of studies have now identified energy requirements of patients on intensive care who have undergone specific operations. Further evaluation of postoperative energy requirements in specific patient groups may enable better targeting of nutritional support.

The issue of whether patients with hypoplastic left heart should be fed preoperatively or not and with what type of infant milk has not been resolved. In view of the potentially devastating effects of development of NEC, in conjunction with the cardiac defect, this may be an issue that proves difficult to resolve.

Glossary

Aortopulmonary window: A hole, or 'window', is present between the aorta and the pulmonary artery. This results in higher pulmonary blood pressure with more blood than usual going to the lungs and less to the systemic circulation.

Atrial septal defect (ASD): A hole between the right and left atria. There is malformation of the septum between the two chambers. The defect may have anomalous pulmonary drainage associated with it, in which some of the venous return from the lungs enters the right atrium rather than the left.

Blalock–Taussig (BT) shunt: A procedure in which the subclavian artery is connected to the pulmonary artery in order to provide adequate blood flow to the lungs. Used when the defect results in no direct connection between the right ventricle and the pulmonary circulation, e.g. pulmonary atresia. A modified version of this procedure is to use a Gore-Tex graft between the subclavian and pulmonary arteries (modified BT shunt).

Coarctation of the aorta: A narrowing of the aortic arch near to where the ductus arteriosus connects in the foetal circulation. One of the signs is reduced or absent femoral pulses. Surgical repair is either with an end-to-end anastomosis, with the narrowed section being cut out, or by using a flap of subclavian artery.

Cor triatriatum: A membrane divides the inside of the left atrium interfering with blood flow into the left ventricle.

DiGeorge syndrome (22Q11 microdeletion): Cardiac defects that affect the pulmonary artery and aorta are associated with this syndrome. Parathyroid hormone is absent and infants often need calcium supplementation postoperatively. The thymus is also affected resulting in poor immune function and the need for irradiated blood products to be given if transfusion is required.

Double outlet right ventricle (DORV): Both aorta and pulmonary arteries exit from the right ventricle. A VSD is present allowing blood to exit from the left ventricle.

Ductus arteriosus: This is a connecting vessel between the pulmonary artery and the aorta. Its function is to allow blood to bypass the lungs in the foetal circulation. If it remains open once the infant is born it is known as a 'patent ductus arteriosus'. This causes excess blood flow to the lungs.

Ebstein's anomaly: A deformed tricuspid valve, with missing leaflets, arises lower than normal from the wall of the right ventricle. This results in a small functional right ventricle with the pulmonary artery exiting from above the tricuspid valve. Poor pulmonary blood flow results.

Glenn shunt: A procedure in which the superior vena cava is disconnected from where it enters the right atrium and is attached to the right pulmonary artery. The venous return from the upper part of the body therefore flows directly into the pulmonary arteries. This is used as a means of oxygenating blood when there is a non-functioning right ventricle usually due to stenosis of the pulmonary valve or atresia of either the tricuspid valve or pulmonary artery.

Hypoplastic left heart syndrome (HLHS): Due to embryological defects the size of the left ventricle is severely reduced. The aortic and mitral valves are also defective or absent and the aorta is reduced in size.

Interrupted aortic arch: The aorta exits from the left ventricle but fails to continue round to form the usual arch. The descending part of the aortic arch remains connected to the pulmonary circulation via the ductus arteriosus.

Partial anomalous pulmonary venous drainage (PAPVD): As for TAPVD but fewer pulmonary veins are misdirected.

Patent ductus arteriosus (PDA): The hole that exists between the pulmonary artery and aorta in foetal circulation persists postnatally. Some cardiac lesions require this hole to remain open in order to get blood to the lungs and so be compatible with life. Prostaglandin E1 is used to keep the duct patent.

Patent/persisting foramen ovale (PFO): The hole between the two atria that is normally present in the foetal circulation persists postnatally.

Pulmonary atresia: The outflow from the pulmonary artery is completely restricted either at the site of the pulmonary valve or the artery itself. A VSD may or may not be present and this will affect the surgical course.

Pulmonary stenosis: The valve of the pulmonary artery is not formed correctly resulting in reduced blood flow to the lungs. There are three types with areas of tissue above or below the valve or the valve itself being affected.

Shunt: The redirection of blood flow from one area of the circulation to another via a 'short circuit'. This may be due to a physiological defect as in the movement of blood from the left to right ventricle across a VSD or due to an operation

such as a BT shunt in which blood is redirected from the systemic to pulmonary circulation (see Blalock–Taussig shunt above).

Tetralogy of Fallot (Fig. 15.3): There are four aspects to this defect: a ventricular septal defect, pulmonary stenosis, right ventricular hypertrophy and an overriding aorta in which the aorta straddles the two ventricles.

Total anomalous pulmonary venous drainage (TAPVD): The four pulmonary veins usually return blood to the left atrium. In TAPVD all of these veins empty into a variety of other locations: the superior vena cava, the inferior vena cava, the hepatic vein, hepatic portal vein or the right atrium.

Total cavo-pulmonary connection (TCPC): An operation in which the inferior vena cava is connected directly to the right pulmonary artery. This operation follows on from a Glenn shunt (see above) and occurs when a child is older. These operations are used where there are right-sided obstructive cardiac lesions resulting in deoxygenated blood flowing from the body directly into the pulmonary circulation without going through the right side of the heart.

Transposition of the great arteries (TGA): The aorta exits from the right ventricle and the pulmonary artery exits from the left ventricle. Blood is able to mix due to a patent foramen ovale and patent ductus arteriosus. Initially the PFO is enlarged, using a cardiac catheter in a procedure called a balloon atrial septostomy, to allow for better mixing of blood. Surgical repair in which the arteries are cut and switched over is carried out at about 2 weeks of age.

Tricuspid atresia: The tricuspid valve between the right atrium and right ventricle fails to from. A PFO or ASD along with a VSD ensures that this lesion is compatible with life.

Truncus arteriosus: A single large vessel exits from above the two ventricles due to the pulmonary artery and the aorta failing to divide in the embryo. There is only one single valve to this large vessel, having 3 to 6 leaflets. A VSD is also present just beneath where the vessel leaves the heart. Truncus arteriosus is classified into four types depending on where the right and left pulmonary arteries arise.

Ventricular septal defect (VSD): A hole between the two ventricles. There are various types. The most common is a perimembranous defect in which the hole is located at the 'top' of the ventricle near to where blood exits. Muscular VSDs are located near the 'bottom' or apex of the ventricle.

Acknowledgements

Dr Alison Hayes, Consultant Paediatric Cardiologist, for Figs 13.1–13.3 and for checking medical details in the text. Mr Andrew Parry, Consultant Paediatric Cardiac Surgeon for checking medical and surgical details. Ms Camille Jankowski for provision of additional references on chylothorax. Mrs Rachel Meskel, Mrs Sonal Patel, Mrs Philippa Wright and the Paediatric Cardiac/PICU Dietitians Interest Group for contributing to debate and discussion on a range of dietetic treatments in cardiac surgery. Mrs Sheila Hopkins for proof reading.

Further reading

Congenital heart disease

Krauss A, Auld A Metabolic rate of neonates with congenital heart disease. *Arch Dis Child*, 1975, **50** 539–41.

McDonnell N *The Paediatric Cardiac Surgical Patient*, 3rd edn. University of Brisbane, 2003. Copies available by e-mail mcdonnem@ozemail.com.au.

Mitchell I, Davies P, Day J *et al.* Energy expenditure in congenital heart disease before and after cardiac surgery. *J Thorac Cardiovasc Surg*, 1994, **107** 374–80.

Chylothorax

Hopkins RL, Akingbola OA, Frieberg EM Chylothorax: key references. *Ann Thorac Surg*, 1998, **66** 1845–6.

Gracey M, Burke V, Anderson CM Medium chain triglycerides in paediatric practice. *Arch Dis Child*, 1970, **45** 445–52.

Ramos W, Faintuch J Nutritional management of thoracic duct fistula. A comparative study of parenteral verus enteral nutrition. *J Parenter Enteral Nutr*, 1986, **10** 519–21.

Bond SJ, Guzzetta PC, Snyder ML *et al.* Management of paediatric postoperative chylothorax. *Ann Thorac Surg*, 1993, **56** 469–72.

Kosloke AM, Martin LW, Schubert WK Management of chylothorax in children and medium chain triglyceride feedings. *J Ped Surg*, 1974, **9** 365–71.

14

Food Hypersensitivity

Rosan Meyer and Carina Venter

Introduction

Many symptoms are correctly or incorrectly attributed to food hypersensitivity and as a result can lead to confusion when it comes to diagnosis and management. In an effort to improve diagnosis, treatment and general understanding of allergic reactions the Nomenclature Review Committee of the World Allergy Organization issued a report proposing revised nomenclature [1]. This report states that any reaction to food that causes objectively reproducible symptoms or signs, even when the food is eaten unknowingly (blind), should be described as food hypersensitivity. If immunological mechanisms can be demonstrated then the reaction can be described as a food allergy. If immunoglobulin E (IgE) is involved in the reaction then the term IgE mediated food allergy should be used and the term non-IgE mediated food allergic reactions used for immune mediated reactions that are not mediated by IgE. All other reactions should be described as non-allergic food hypersensitivity, as there is no immunological mechanism involved (Fig. 14.1).

Important factors concerning food hypersensitivity reactions

- A food hypersensitivity reaction is known as a food allergy where the immune system is involved. These reactions may involve immunoglobulin IgE or may involve other immune mechanisms (non-IgE mediated food allergy) (Fig. 14.1, A and B).
- Some food hypersensitivity occurs as a result of enzyme deficiency such as lactase deficiency or disorders of amino acid or intermediary metabolism, e.g. phenylketonuria. These reactions are non-allergic hypersensitivities, are well documented and are discussed elsewhere in this book (Fig. 14.1, C).
- Some foods may cause unpleasant symptoms, e.g. caffeine in coffee and cola; vasoactive amines in cheese and wine; phenylethylamine in chocolate. These effects are pharmacological and are non-allergic (Fig. 14.1, D).
- Some food induced reactions are non-immune mediated and of unknown origin. These may include a variety of gastrointestinal symptoms related to different foods, e.g. abdominal cramping with garlic or wheat fibre (Fig. 14.1, E).

Over recent years a significant amount of research has been undertaken in this area. This chapter can only provide an introduction to food hypersensitivity and further reading is recommended (see References and Further reading). Dietetic principles have been concentrated on, but it is essential to understand some of the immunological mechanisms involved to ensure dietetic management is optimal.

Clinical Paediatric Dietetics, Fourth Edition. Edited by Vanessa Shaw.
© 2015 John Wiley & Sons, Ltd. Published 2015 by John Wiley & Sons, Ltd.
Companion Website: www.wiley.com/go/shaw/paediatricdietetics

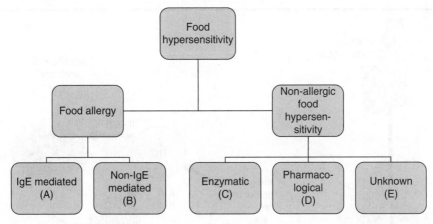

Figure 14.1   Classification of food hypersensitivity (adapted from Johansson *et al.* [1]).

IgE mediated allergy

IgE is an immunoglobulin normally present at very low levels in the plasma of non-allergic individuals, but levels are raised in patients suffering from allergic conditions such as asthma, atopic dermatitis, allergic rhinitis and anaphylaxis. When atopic individuals are exposed to a food protein (antigen) via the skin, gastrointestinal tract or lung mucosa, the antigen is taken up and transported to local lymph nodes by specialist processing cells called antigen presenting cells. These cells break down and present the antigen to T and B cells within specific areas of the lymph node. The type of T cell involved in this encounter is important in determining whether IgE [as opposed to other antibody isotypes (IgA or IgG)] is produced. T-helper 2 cells play an important role in determining IgE production by B cells. These surround the antigen and present the antigen to T-helper 2 cells. This stimulates B cells to produce IgE specific antibodies, which then bind to mast cells or basophils via high affinity receptors. This cascade of immune reactions then leads to the symptoms associated with an immediate food allergy (Fig. 14.2). A variety of cytokines are released which may induce the IgE mediated late response. Neutrophils and eosinophils invade the site of response and infiltrated cells are activated. These then release a variety of mediators including platelet activating factor, peroxidase, eosinophil major basic protein and eosinophil cationic protein leading to a second phase allergic response that is often more severe than the initial response. In the subsequent 24–48 hours, lymphocytes and monocytes infiltrate the area and establish a more chronic inflammatory picture [2].

Clinical manifestation of IgE mediated food allergy

Symptoms generally appear within 0–2 hours after a small amount of food has been consumed. Immediate symptoms may affect the gut, the skin and/or the lungs and common symptoms are summarised in Table 14.1 [3].

Symptoms of upper airway obstruction (laryngeal oedema), lower airway obstruction (bronchoconstriction), hypotension, cardiac arrhythmias and even heart failure constitute the most severe and sometimes life-threatening reactions. This is known as anaphylactic shock and first symptoms may include sneezing and a tingling sensation on the lips, tongue and throat followed by pallor and feeling unwell, fearful, warm and light-headed. The presentation of anaphylaxis is varied but the major causes of death are obstruction to the upper airway or shock, hypotension and cardiac arrhythmia [4–6]. The results of double blind placebo controlled food challenges (DBPCFC) from several studies in the USA and UK have shown that the most common foods to provoke immediate reactions are peanuts, tree nuts, milk, egg, soy and wheat, fish and shellfish. Seeds (e.g. sesame) may also cause this type of reaction.

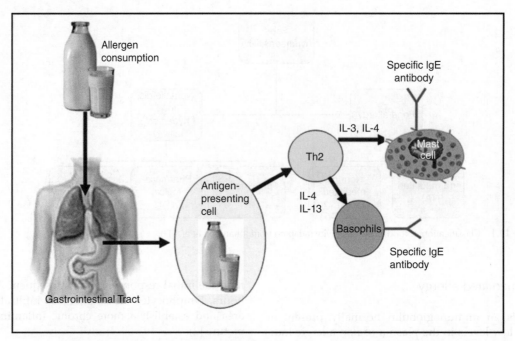

Figure 14.2 Immunological basis for food allergy.

Table 14.1 Symptoms of food allergy modified from Sackeyfio et al. [24] with permission from NICE [10].

	IgE mediated Immediate onset	Non-IgE mediated Delayed onset
Gastrointestinal	Angioedema of the lips, tongue and palate	Reflux
	Oral pruritis	Abdominal pain, bloating
	Nausea	Vomiting
	Colicky abdominal pain	Gastro-oesophageal reflux
	Vomiting	Loose frequent stools
	Diarrhoea	Blood and/or mucus stool
		Infantile colitis
		Food refusal/aversion
		Constipation
		Perianal redness
		Pallor and tiredness
		Faltering growth and one or more of the gastrointestinal symptoms above (with or without serious atopic eczema)
Cutaneous	Acute urticaria	Pruritis
	Acute angioedema	Atopic eczema
	Erythema	Erythema
	Pruritis	
Respiratory	Upper respiratory tract symptoms (nasal itching, sneezing, rhinorrhoea)	Asthma
	Lower respiratory tract symptoms (cough, chest tightness, wheezing or shortness of breath)	
Systemic	Anaphylaxis	

Non-IgE mediated food allergy

These reactions are immune mediated delayed hypersensitivity reactions with symptoms appearing more than 2–48 hours after antigen exposure. Although the mechanism of this reaction is not yet fully understood, it is thought that it involves sensitised T cells reacting with the antigen to produce cytokines, which mobilise non-sensitised cells to fight the antigen. This causes inflammation, tissue damage and the formation of epitheloid and giant cells [7].

Clinical manifestation of non-IgE mediated food allergy

These reactions to foods may develop slowly after hours or days and the exposure dose evoking a reaction varies from small to larger amounts [8, 9]. As with immediate symptoms, adverse reactions can affect the skin, gastrointestinal tract or lungs. Symptoms include chronic diarrhoea, vomiting which in severe persistent cases may lead to hypovolaemic shock, diarrhoea abdominal pain, faltering growth, infantile colic, constipation, eczema and asthma [10]. Gastrointestinal symptoms are further discussed in Chapter 7.

Mixed IgE and non-IgE food allergy

It is now recognised that patients can present with a mixed picture including both the immediate type IgE mediated and the delayed type non-IgE mediated reactions. An example of this overlap is atopic dermatitis and eosinophilic oesophagitis [11, 12]. The same child may show signs of both IgE mediated allergy, e.g. to egg, and non-IgE mediated allergy, e.g. to milk [13].

Symptoms often associated with both IgE and non-IgE mediated food allergy

It is important to recognise additional features that are often present in children with food allergies and these may have implications in the nutritional management. These include faltering growth; vitamin D, calcium and iron deficiency; aversive feeding; pallor and tiredness [14, 15].

Non-allergic food hypersensitivity

The most well known non-allergic food hypersensitivity is lactose intolerance (p. 124). Symptoms arise due to the osmotic effects of lactose and fermentation thereof by intestinal bacteria. This may cause excessive flatus, explosive diarrhoea, perianal excoriation, abdominal distension and pain [16]. The overlap in symptoms with non-IgE mediated gastrointestinal food allergies often causes confusion with the diagnosis, but is distinctly different due to the absence of an immunological mechanism.

More controversial problems which may be related to non-allergic food hypersensitivity are migraine, rheumatoid arthritis, migraine with epilepsy, enuresis, autism and attention deficit hyperactivity disorder (ADHD). Dietary manipulation (elimination and challenge) is the mainstay for diagnosis and treatment of these conditions [2]. It is important to consider nutritional adequacy when such a diet is implemented (p. 320).

Diagnosis of food hypersensitivity

IgE mediated allergy

Skin prick tests

The skin prick test (SPT) indicates the presence of allergen specific IgE. It can be performed in a medical setting equipped to deal with anaphylaxis and yields an immediate result, which is very useful for clinicians and parents. Drops of food extract, positive (histamine) control and negative (saline) control are applied using lancets. In general, food allergens eliciting a wheal size at least 3 mm larger than those induced by the negative control are considered positive. Venter *et al.* provide more specific information on 'cut-off points' for SPT results [17]. It is important to note that the positive predictive accuracy of SPTs is less than 50% compared with results from DBPCFC. Negative predictive accuracy is 95% [18, 19]. This means that negative SPT responses are a worthwhile means of excluding IgE mediated allergies, but positive SPT responses only indicate an atopic individual with a tendency to react to this food. Exclusion diets should not be based on these results alone.

Specific IgE test

Specific IgE is an *in vitro* assay for identifying food specific IgE antibodies from serum. It is more expensive than SPT and the results are not available to the clinician immediately, possibly delaying diagnosis. This test may be preferred when patients have dermatographism, severe skin disease or a limited surface area for testing (e.g. in severe atopic dermatitis); when patients have difficulty discontinuing antihistamines; or when patients have exquisite sensitivity to certain foods [18]. Interpretation of results is as difficult as with SPTs. For more information on the interpretation of specific IgE see Venter *et al*. [17]. However, SPTs and specific IgE tests provide useful contributory information towards a diagnosis when added to the clinical history and are interpreted by clinicians with appropriate competencies [18, 19].

Intradermal test

A report of the British Society for Allergy and Environmental Medicine with the British Society for Nutritional Medicine [20] and the recent USA guidelines [21] do not recommend the use of intradermal tests. Unacceptably high false positive rates as well as safety concerns, such as systemic reactions (including fatal anaphylactic responses), are associated with this allergy skin test [22].

Other diagnostic tests

To date there are no additional diagnostic procedures to those described above which can be recommended as useful tests in the diagnosis of IgE and non-IgE mediated food allergy. IgG testing has received a significant amount of attention in the lay press for assisting in the 'diagnosis' of non-IgE mediated reactions. The European Association for Allergy and Clinical Immunology [23], the American Academy for Allergy Asthma and Immunology and the UK National Institute for Health and Care Excellence (NICE) [24] advise against the use of this 'test' for diagnosing any type of food allergy due to lack of research and the concern that misinterpretation may lead to nutritionally incomplete diets. Other tests that have also been shown to be of no benefit in the diagnosis of food hypersensitivity include vega testing, hair analysis, cytotoxic test, kinesiology, iridology, electrodermal testing and sublingual provocative food testing [25].

Non-IgE mediated allergy

There are currently no validated *in vitro* or *in vivo* tests which can identify foods responsible for non-IgE mediated food allergies [26]. It has been suggested that atopy patch testing could be used to aid the diagnosis of non-IgE mediated food allergy; however, this has not been confirmed by studies. It may be that combining SPT with patch testing can improve the diagnosis, but there is insufficient data for the routine use of this test in non-IgE mediated allergy [21, 24, 27, 28]. Currently, the symptomatic improvement on an allergen exclusion diet, followed by a return of symptoms on allergen reintroduction or a food challenge remains the gold standard for diagnosing this food allergic condition [21, 29].

Non-allergic food hypersensitivity

As for food allergy, there is no proven test for the diagnosis of non-allergic food hypersensitivity. Advertised diagnostic methods such as applied kinesiology, hair tests or electrodermal tests were evaluated in a Consumer Association report [30, 31]. The verdict was that known allergies in individuals were not picked up, the services exaggerated the number of allergies and this could result in unnecessarily restricted and inadequate diets. The report suggests that people should not waste their money on these tests. Vega testing has also been assessed in a double blind study and was shown to be unable to accurately diagnose food hypersensitivity of any mechanism [32].

Elimination diets for diagnosis of IgE and non-IgE mediated food allergies

Sometimes clinical history and diagnostic tests give a strong indication as to the food(s) causing symptoms. In this case, advice on dietary exclusion is given to manage the symptoms and reintroduction of these foods into the diet will not occur until there is an indication that the allergy may have been outgrown. However, in some cases (particularly for non-IgE mediated food allergy and non-allergic food hypersensitivity) it may not be clear if particular foods are involved. It may therefore be necessary to first devise a 'diagnostic' elimination diet. Before this is embarked upon it is essential to consider whether the child/parent is sufficiently motivated and able to adhere to the diet. The length of time required on an elimination diet to confirm/refute a food allergy is poorly researched and may vary from 2 to 6 weeks. In the absence of any clear, well researched guidance, a decision on the period of elimination should be made for the individual and the following factors should be taken into account:

- type of suspected food allergy (IgE mediated symptoms tend to resolve faster than non-IgE mediated symptoms)
- frequency of symptoms
- degree of restriction of diet (i.e. one food versus many foods)
- nutritional status of the child

Any improvement of symptoms has to be followed by reintroduction or a challenge with the offending foods, resulting in reproducible deterioration and then recovery on re-elimination in order to confirm the presence of a food allergy. The NICE guidelines recommend that challenges for IgE mediated allergy should be performed in a clinical setting, and food challenges (food reintroduction) for delayed symptoms can be performed at home [10].

Phase 1: diagnostic elimination diet

Taking a full diet history is mandatory before embarking on an elimination diet; this may indicate provoking foods. The accuracy of the diet history needs to be taken into account, as it is not uncommon for parents to be mistaken as to which foods affect their child and problems with staple foods eaten several times a day, such as milk and wheat, often go unnoticed [2]. Keeping a food symptom diary before starting a diet may provide a baseline but seldom adds any useful information about suspect foods which has not been revealed by diet history. The initial diet may exclude one food (e.g. cow's milk) or a number of foods (e.g. cow's milk, soya and eggs). The choice of diet is a matter of clinical judgement taking into account age, severity and type of symptoms and whether other elimination diets have already been tried [2]. There are three levels of dietary restriction: an empirical diet, a few foods diet or an elemental diet (Fig. 14.3).

Empirical diet

An empirical diet is used where food hypersensitivity is suspected and causative agents are not known. One or several of the most commonly provoking foods are avoided. Cow's milk, hen's egg, wheat, soy, peanut, tree nut, sesame and kiwi are responsible for the majority of IgE mediated food induced allergic reactions in young children [2]. Fin fish, shellfish, tree nuts and peanut are more common food allergens in older children [2]. In children with atopic dermatitis (mixed IgE and non-IgE mediated) the offending foods are similar to those in IgE mediated allergies; however,

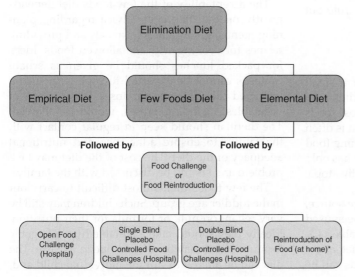

Figure 14.3 Using elimination diets and food challenges/reintroduction to aid diagnosis.
* Only if there is no risk of an immediate severe reaction.

studies of common allergens in delayed reactions yield anecdotal results. The most common foods in a paediatric population with non-IgE mediated gastrointestinal food allergies, according to Meyer *et al.*, were milk, soy, egg and wheat [33]. It is not unusual for paediatric gastroenterologists to suggest a diet free from milk and soy (most cases) and egg and wheat in the more severe cases (Tables 7.8, 7.9, 7.10).

Many parents report allergic type symptoms related to fruit and occasionally to vegetables. It is important to elicit the type of reaction and also the time of year these occur. Pollen allergy syndrome (otherwise known as oral allergy syndrome) in older children may need to be ruled out [2]. In infants and young children citrus and tomato are often blamed for exacerbation of atopic dermatitis. Flare up of eczema may occur around the mouth/face due to the pH of the fruit and its histamine content, but specific research supporting this is absent. Fruit and vegetables contribute important micronutrients to the diet; it is therefore important not to eliminate these foods from a diagnostic exclusion diet without ensuring dietary adequacy. Practical advice is to cover the area around the mouth with petroleum jelly (e.g. Vaseline) prior to eating these fruits and vegetables.

Problems can occur with empirical diets when excluded foods are inadvertently replaced by others which can cause adverse reactions, e.g. a child on a milk free diet may drink soy milk or orange juice instead and it is possible to be equally reactive to these foods. Failure to respond to an empirical diet does not always therefore rule out the possibility of food hypersensitivity.

Few foods diet

A few foods diet is a diet consisting of a small number of hypoallergenic foods. This diet may be useful if there is a perception that most foods cause an allergic type reaction. Although it is often suggested as a dietetic option for establishing food induced hypersensitivity reactions, its use has only been extensively studied in patients with atopic eczema [34–36].

Diets using one meat, one carbohydrate source, one fruit and one type of vegetable have been used [37]. Examples of such diets are given in Table 14.2. If no improvement occurs with the first diet, a second diet containing a different set of foods can be

Table 14.2 Two examples of few foods diets.

A	B
Turkey	Lamb
Cabbage, sprouts, broccoli, cauliflower	Carrots, parsnips
Potato, potato flour	Rice, rice flour
Banana	Pear
Soya oil	Sunflower oil
Calcium and vitamins (Table 14.3)	Calcium and vitamins (Table 14.3)
Tap water	Tap water
Hypoallergenic formula (<2 years)	Hypoallergenic formula (<2 years)

Possible additions: milk free margarine, sugar for baking. Possible variations: bottled water; rabbit instead of above meats; peaches and apricots, melon, pineapple instead of above fruits.

used. Nutritional adequacy should be monitored carefully [2, 38, 39]. In extreme circumstances more rarely eaten foods such as rabbit, venison and sweet potatoes could be included [38]. As these diets are nutritionally demanding, it is suggested that they should not be followed for more than 4 weeks.

Since the above diets are extremely rigorous, less restricted diets have been used to improve adherence (Table 14.3) [38]. It is much more difficult to find a completely different set of foods for a second attempt if the first is not helpful. However, it is possible to monitor progress closely and adjust or further restrict the diet during the third or fourth week in an attempt to achieve eventual success.

The acceptability of the few foods diet depends greatly on the dietitian's advice regarding planning menus, giving ideas for meals and providing recipes for cooking with the allowed foods. Ideas for packed lunches should be given as school canteens cannot be expected to cope with such a restricted diet. For vegetarians a larger range of vegetables, including pulses, would be allowed. The dietitian should keep in regular contact with the family to ensure adherence and nutritional adequacy of the diet. The cost of the diet may be a problem and should be discussed with the family.

The few foods diet is most difficult to carry out in the toddler age group. Such children may still be very reliant on milk or formula for their nutrition. Ideally they should take a suitable hypoallergenic formula, but it may be refused due to its taste. The diet can be altered to suit the individual child and,

Table 14.3 Less restricted few foods diet.

This diet should be used for no more than 4 weeks. Children under 2 years require a nutritionally adequate substitute for milk

Choose two foods from each food group

Meat	Lamb, rabbit, turkey, pork
Starchy food	Rice, potato, sweet potato
Vegetables	Broccoli, cauliflower, cabbage, sprouts (brassicas)
	Carrots, parsnips, celery
	Cucumber, marrow, courgettes, melon
	Leeks, onions, asparagus
Fruit	Pears, bananas, peaches and apricots, pineapple
Also included	Sunflower oil, whey free margarine
	Plain potato crisps
	Small amount of sugar for baking
	Tap or bottled water
	Juice and jam from allowed fruits
	Salt, pepper and herbs in cooking

A calcium (350–500 mg/day) and vitamin supplement is advisable for children who are not consuming a hypoallergenic formula: calcium gluconate effervescent 1 g × 3 daily; or calcium lactate 300 mg × 6 daily; or Sandocal 400 g × 1 tablet daily; or Calcium Sandoz liquid 15 mL daily; Dalivit/Abidec 0.6 mL daily

in some circumstances, can be made less restricted by including a larger range of meats, fruits and vegetables.

Few foods diets are usually carried out in the home environment. It is important that the child's lifestyle is not altered; otherwise changes in symptoms could be attributed to factors other than change in diet. Regular medication should not be changed before or during the diet trial for the same reason. Children on regular medication such as anticonvulsants should remain on these but be switched to a colour/preservative free version if possible. Attention should be paid to non-food items which may be consumed by small children such as toothpaste (a white toothpaste should be used), chalks and play dough [38].

Elemental diet

Hypoallergenic or elemental diets based on amino acids (e.g. Elemental 028 Extra, Neocate Advance for children or Neocate LCP, Nutramigen AA for infants) can occasionally be justified where there has been no response to a restricted diet, but this treatment should be very much a last resort as suitable products are very unpalatable and tube feeding may be necessary to achieve adequate nutrition. This will involve a hospital admission. Suitable products are listed in Tables 7.7 and 7.11. These feeds have been used mainly for

children with severe atopic dermatitis and for severe gastrointestinal food allergies [29, 36, 38].

Phase 2: food challenges and reintroduction foods

Following improvement on the diagnostic diet, the dietitian will need to perform either a food challenge in hospital, in particular for IgE mediated symptoms, or a reintroduction plan/prolonged food challenge at home for the delayed type reactions.

Food challenges

History taking
Prior to considering any food challenge it is important to gather all the history relevant to performing the challenge safely. Taking a history will provide important information on

- the age of the patient to determine how difficult it may be to perform the food challenge and to help in identifying the possible food causing the symptoms
- the type of food or foods causing reported symptoms, e.g. raw egg versus cooked egg
- the age of onset of symptoms as well as the frequency and reproducibility of the reaction

- the time of onset of symptoms in relation to food consumption; the clinical manifestation and duration of the symptoms
- the quantity of food causing symptoms in order to prevent false negative food challenges
- a thorough description of the most recent reaction is also very important in designing challenges; the details of the most recent reaction may be more helpful than those of more distant reactions
- sometimes more than one food or factor is needed to elicit a positive challenge outcome (e.g. a combination of foods eaten together, exercise induced anaphylaxis or with concomitant drug intake)
- a list of foods that are well tolerated and that could be used as a placebo or vehicle to mask the challenge food [40]

Challenges can be performed as either open food challenges (OFC), single blind placebo controlled food challenges (SBPCFC) or DBPCFC (Fig. 14.3) [40].

Open food challenges
During OFC both the clinician and patient (or parent) is informed of the food being administered and these challenges should be sufficient to either confirm or refute most reported food hypersensitivity. However, many children are very reluctant to eat a food which they do not remember having eaten before or which they have previously been told to avoid. Indeed it is not uncommon for children who have had previous severe reactions to foods to exhibit some degree of food avoidance. It is therefore often advisable to provide the challenge in a 'single blind' form (culprit food mixed with another food acceptable to the child) simply to ensure that the child consumes it [41, 42].

OFC are mainly used in the clinical setting and are useful for the diagnosis of objective symptoms [42]. Although factors such as starting dose, dose increment and final dose may not be that critical, it is essential that the patient has consumed an adequate amount of food during the challenge to make a diagnosis accurate [43, 44].

Single blind placebo controlled food challenges
During the SBPCFC, both active and placebo challenges are given. The health professionals involved know which food is active and which is placebo,

but the patient does not. Sufficient masking of the challenge food is very important. SBPCFC are particularly useful when performing food challenges in children who do not want to ingest a specific food.

Double blind placebo controlled food challenge
The gold standard for confirming or refuting food allergy is the DBPCFC [40, 45], although in practice open challenges are more common. One of the strengths of the DBPCFC is that neither the patient nor the investigator knows when the active or the placebo challenge is performed. It therefore rules out reporting bias from the clinician and any psychological effect from the patient.

The DBPCFC is mainly used for research purposes and can be time consuming and difficult to manage. It needs to be used only in clinical practice where there is a possibility that any observed reaction could be caused by anxiety or in diagnosing subjective symptoms such as abdominal pain, nausea [40, 42, 44].

Considerations when performing food challenges

Elimination period
Prior to a food challenge, the identified food should be excluded from the diet as discussed above.

Challenge dose
Guidance on performing food challenges (OFC and DBPCFC) such as the dosages given and foods used is discussed in the PRACTALL consensus guidance [45]. The PRACTALL recommendations suggest the following doses for food challenges [45]: 4.334 g of protein divided into 3 mg, 10 mg, 30 mg, 100 mg, 300 mg, 1000 mg and 3000 mg doses. In terms of amount of food given this equates to

- *Milk*: 12.428 g of skimmed milk powder (8.3 mg; 27.8 mg; 83.3 mg; 277.8 mg; 833.3 mg; 2777.8 mg; 8333.3 mg)
- *Soya*: 134.6 mL of soya milk (0.1 mL; 0.3 mL; 0.9 mL; 3.0 mL; 9.1 mL; 30.3 mL; 90.9 mL)
- *Egg*: 9.45 g of egg powder (6.4 mg; 21.3 mg; 63.8 mg; 212.8 mg; 638.3 mg; 2127.7 mg; 6383.0 mg); 34.711 g of egg (23.4 mg; 78.1 mg; 234.4 mg; 781.3 mg; 2343.8 mg; 7812.5 mg; 23 437.5 mg)

- *Wheat*: 5.5538 g of gluten powder (3.8 mg; 12.5 mg; 37.5 mg; 125 mg; 375 mg; 1250 mg; 3750 mg)
- *Peanut*: 8.886 g of peanut flour (6 mg; 20 mg; 60 mg; 200 mg; 600 mg; 2000 mg; 6 000 mg); 18.5126 g of peanut butter (12.5 mg; 41.7 mg; 125 mg;   416.7 mg;   1250 mg;   4166.7 mg; 12 500 mg)

This amount of food, however, should still be followed up with an age appropriate portion of the food at the end of a negative challenge [45]. The interval between doses can be anything between 15 and 60 minutes but the timing between each dose should be dependent on the patient's history and sufficient to allow symptoms to develop.

There are currently no specific recommendations regarding the dose or design to be used when performing food challenges to diagnose delayed symptoms, e.g. atopic dermatitis or constipation, apart from that the amount normally known to cause a reaction should be used, or a normal portion of the food [44]. This raises practical issues where the patient is a very vague historian. Another difficult issue is that some reactions only occur when the causative food is eaten in sufficient doses on consecutive days and this must be planned for when designing the food challenge. The advantage of these challenges is that the reactions are not life threatening so the whole challenge can be completed at home.

Challenge duration
For immediate symptoms, if no reaction has occurred after all doses have been consumed the child can go home (after 1–2 hours) with instructions to incorporate that food gradually into the diet. A longer challenge period (1–4 weeks) is recommended when looking for delayed reactions [45–48].

Challenge food used
Dried, cooked or raw food, as indicated by the history, should be used in order to mimic the history as close as possible [49, 50].

Challenge location
It is recommended to perform a food challenge in hospital if there is a history of immediate reactions and/or if the patient is sensitised to the offending food. If there is the slightest concern that the child may experience an immediate or IgE mediated reaction the challenge should be performed under professional supervision in experienced hospital units; all other challenges can be performed at home [42, 44, 45].

Considerations when performing double blind placebo controlled food challenges

Time between active and placebo challenges
When dealing with immediate symptoms at least 2 hours, but ideally 3–4 hours, should be allowed between the active and placebo challenge. In practice, it is very difficult to perform two challenges in a child in one day. In the case of delayed symptoms 1 week between the active and placebo challenge should be allowed [40, 43, 51]. The patient's history will play a major role in the final decision.

Masking of the challenge food
The challenge food should be blinded (masked) in terms of smell, flavour and texture. Ideally, the active and placebo challenges should be identical regarding taste, appearance, smell, viscosity, texture, structure and volume; blindness should also be assessed by standard tests [44, 52]. Although this is paramount in performing food challenges for research purposes, it may not be necessary when performing DBPCFC for a clinical diagnosis or when doing DBPCFC in young children.

There are a number of factors that should be taken into account when choosing a challenge vehicle or placebo:

- the fat content of the vehicle can influence the challenge outcome [53]
- the vehicle must also allow for enough challenge food to be used [44]
- cooking, canning, roasting can have different effects on the allergenicity of different foods [54–56, 57–60]. The food challenge should always conclude with consumption of a normal portion of the food, prepared according to the history to eliminate this issue [57, 58]

A variety of foods can be used for blinding. It is often helpful to use foods that are readily accepted by children such as ice cream, yoghurt, milkshake, milky puddings, fruit purée, mashed potatoes, soup, chocolate pudding, fruit juice, cocoa/carob, peppermint [49, 50]. Many commercial products such as cakes, biscuits or pastas that are free of egg, milk and wheat can be used as placebo. Finding a suitable and acceptable vehicle/placebo is particularly difficult if children suffer from multiple food hypersensitivity [50].

Capsules are not recommended to be used in DBPCFC as the challenge food bypasses the mouth. The early oral symptoms seen in some food allergic individuals will not occur which could warn against later serious reactions when the challenge food hits the gut. Also the symptoms of oral allergy syndrome will be missed in older children (p. 331).

Interpretation of food challenges

The final and most important part of the challenge is the interpretation of the symptoms during the challenge [53, 59]. This is not always easy as there are some confounding effects, such as disease patterns for eczema and chronic urticaria. Presence of aero-allergens, particularly during the hay fever season, may also affect the challenge outcome [60, 61].

The outcome of the food challenge should be documented on either a food challenge chart (hospital challenge) or a food and symptom diary (home challenge). Any symptoms at home should be verified by the study clinician if possible [2]. The final outcome of the food challenge should be decided by the supervising doctor and dietitian involved, based on the history of the child and the symptoms experienced. There are no clear guidelines regarding the point at which a challenge should be considered positive, but some advice is summarised in the PRACTALL guidance [45]. This is based on clinical expertise rather than substantiated by evidence. In addition, Koplin et al. [62] have published guidelines on performing OFC in children suspected of IgE mediated food allergies. Food challenge involved gradually increasing doses on day 1 in the hospital and continued ingestion of the maximum day 1 dose (1 teaspoon of peanut butter or tahini paste or 1 whole raw egg white) on day 2 through to day 7. The HealthNuts standardised cessation criteria for a positive OFC result were any of the following signs occurring within 2 hours of ingestion [62]:

- three or more concurrent non contact urticaria persisting for at least 5 minutes

- perioral or periorbital angioedema
- vomiting (excluding gag reflex)
- evidence of circulatory or respiratory compromise (anaphylaxis, e.g. persistent cough, wheeze, change in voice, stridor, difficulty breathing and collapse)

The food challenge result was also considered positive if any of the above reactions occurred within 2 hours of ingestion of the food on days 2 to 7 of the challenge at home.

Reintroduction of foods

In the case of suspected non-IgE mediated symptoms or non-allergic food hypersensitivity an elimination diet can be followed by the reintroduction of offending foods: to confirm the food related reaction; to expand the variety of foods consumed in the case of a few foods and elemental diet. The reintroduction of foods is often a very difficult step, especially if significant symptom relief has been experienced. Very little guidance exists on the reintroduction of foods following a few foods diet or elemental diet and practice varies between allergy centres, depending on

- the type of food allergy and symptoms
- the most likely offending foods (which are introduced at the end)
- the nutritional status of the child and nutritional adequacy of the existing diet
- the foods the child misses most

Foods should be reintroduced singly in order to try and identify trigger foods. Each new food may be tried in a small test quantity, then given in normal amounts every day for a week and then incorporated into the diet as desired. A guide to reintroduction of foods is given in Table 14.4.

After food challenge or food reintroduction, the food should continue to be consumed if there is no reaction, or avoided (maintenance diet) if there is a reaction to the food. Despite the clear need for food introduction or challenge, some parents/carers may refuse to give a particular food if the child has improved a great deal when it has been eliminated. The dietitian will have to accept this and continue to provide support to the family – the offending food should be introduced at a later stage.

There is no published literature regarding food reintroduction at home apart from a recent

Table 14.4 Open reintroduction of foods.

Each food should be given in normal quantities daily for 4–7 days before being allowed freely in the diet. Smaller doses on the first day of introduction may be recommended initially [17]. The order of reintroduction depends on the child's preference and on which foods were avoided initially

Oats	Porridge oats, Scottish oatcakes, homemade flapjacks (if sugar is already allowed)
Corn	Sweetcorn, homemade popcorn, cornflour, maize flour, cornflakes if malt is tolerated
Meats	Try meats (including offal) singly e.g. chicken, beef, pork
Wheat	Wholemeal or unbleached white flour for baking, egg free pasta, Shredded Wheat, Puffed Wheat, Weetabix
Yeast	Pitta bread; ordinary bread (this usually also contains soya)
Rye	Worth trying if wheat is not tolerated; pure rye crispbread; pumpernickel
Cow's milk	Fresh cow's milk, cream, butter, plain yoghurt, milk containing foods with tolerated ingredients, e.g. rice pudding. Try cheese separately later
Cow's milk substitute	If cow's milk is not tolerated try substitutes one by one Infant soya formula (if >6 months) or infant hydrolysate formula Sheep milk, goat milk for >1 year olds (boiled or pasteurised). Supermarket liquid soya milk (>2 year olds), supermarket rice milk (>4 1/2 year olds) with additional calcium
Egg	Use one whole fresh egg per day for test period. It may be preferred to begin with small amounts of egg in baking
Fish	Fresh or frozen (not smoked, battered etc.), e.g. cod, herring. If one type is not tolerated others may be. Try shellfish separately later
Tomatoes	Fresh tomatoes, canned and puréed tomatoes, ketchup
Peas/beans	These include peas, green beans, kidney beans, lentils, baked beans in tomato sauce if tomato is tolerated
Orange	Pure orange juice, oranges, satsumas. If oranges are tolerated all citrus fruit probably is too
Sugar	Use ordinary sugar on cereal, in drinks and baking. Some parents comment that small amounts are tolerated whereas larger amounts are not
Chocolate	Try only if sugar is tolerated. If diet is milk free, use milk free chocolate Cocoa powder in drinks and cooking
Carob	Carob confectionery can be tried if chocolate is not tolerated. Check other ingredients – it may contain milk or soya
Tea/coffee	Add milk if this is already in the diet
Peanuts	Plain or salted peanuts (not for <4 year olds) Peanut butter
Other nuts	Try singly or mixed
Malt	Malt/malt flavouring is present in most breakfast cereals. Try Rice Krispies if rice is tolerated
Nitrite/nitrate	Corned beef if beef is tolerated, ham and bacon if pork is tolerated
Sodium benzoate	Supermarket lemonade provided other ingredients are tolerated
Sodium glutamate	Stock cubes, gravy mixes, flavoured crisps, provided the other ingredients are tolerated
Sodium metabisulphite	Some squashes, sausages provided the other ingredients are tolerated, dried fruit
Vitamins Minerals	These may be given if needed to enhance nutritional adequacy and introduced singly to test tolerance

Other foods, e.g. fruit and vegetables, can be introduced gradually as desired. Manufactured foods such as ice cream, biscuits can be introduced taking into account known sensitivities. Many additives, e.g. colours, flavours, will be introduced as mixtures in manufactured foods such as sweets and canned/bottled drinks. For children with multiple cereal intolerances, flours such as buckwheat, soya, gram (chickpea), wheat starch may be tried. Some of the special dietary products for gluten free and low protein diets may be suitable but other ingredients must be checked (they may not be prescribed for food hypersensitivity)

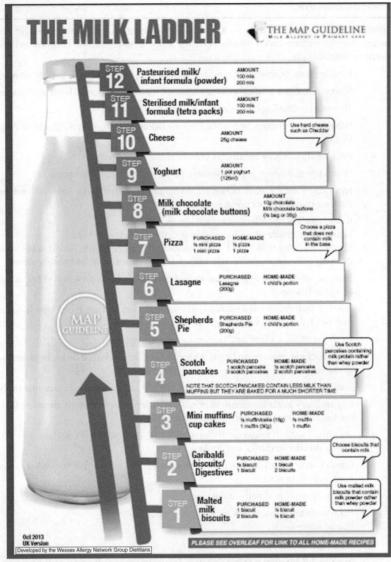

Figure 14.4   Milk ladder for reintroduction of cow's milk at home [63].

publication by Venter *et al.* [63] regarding the gradual reintroduction of cow's milk after a period of avoidance (Fig. 14.4).

Phase 3: maintenance diet

The maintenance diet is achieved when the introduction of all foods has been attempted and the child is having the widest possible variety of foods.

The maintenance diet for the child with diagnosed food allergies must be nutritionally adequate.

Nutritional requirements and dietary management

Currently, the only treatment for any food hypersensitivity is dietary avoidance of the causative allergen. Although symptom improvement is significant with such diets, the nutritional impact must be taken into account.

Nutritional requirements

Although it is well known that faltering growth is common in this population and that there is a higher risk of nutritional deficiencies in children with food allergies [29, 64–67], there is very little research on their requirements. Many factors specific to the allergic child may impact on nutritional requirements, as highlighted in Table 14.5. In the absence of specific guidelines the prudent approach would be to ensure that the allergic child achieves at least the normal requirements for a child of that age (p. 11) and that any deficiencies are corrected.

Dietary Management

The principles of dietary avoidance in children with food hypersensitivity are as follows:

- which foods need to be avoided
- suitable alternatives to these foods
- practical advice for living on a restricted diet

Which foods need to be avoided

Information on foods which may contain 'hidden' allergens, and where these allergens may be found in non-food items, is the mainstay of any advice about dietary avoidance. The EC labelling laws that came into effect in November 2005 have been helpful [68]. In the past food labels did not have to state the presence of an ingredient if it made up less than 25% of the final product. Individuals may have unknowingly eaten a forbidden food, with subsequent adverse reactions. However, the new labelling laws require the presence of 14 potential food allergens, in any quantity, to be declared on the label. These foods are celery, cereals containing gluten (wheat, barley, rye and oats), crustaceans, molluscs, eggs, fish, milk, mustard, tree nuts, peanuts, lupin, sesame seeds, soybeans and sulphites (at levels above 10 mg per kg or litre). Foods that are not pre-packed do not come under this legislation so it is important to ensure patients and their families are aware of this. If a child has a life threatening reaction to a food it is often the safest option to advise that only pre-packaged foods are bought so that the label can be checked. However, dietitians should be aware that EU labelling laws will change in December 2014 and will stipulate that non pre-packed foods will also require written

Table 14.5 Factors that may impact on nutritional requirements.

Factors	Explanation	Possible nutritional deficiencies				
		Energy	Protein	Vitamins	Minerals	Trace elements
Elimination diet	Many foods contribute significantly to the child's diet (e.g. cow's milk)	x	x	x	x	x
Severe eczema	Increased itching and possible skin healing may increase energy/protein requirements	x	x			
Poor sleeping pattern	Disrupted sleep may increase energy requirements	x	x			
Enteropathy/colitis	Diarrhoea and possible malabsorption of nutrients may lead to deficiencies	x	x	x	x	x
Vomiting	Excessive losses	x	x	x	x	x
Irritability/pain	Reduces food intake	x	x	x	x	x
Aversive feeding	Leads to reduced intake	x	x	x	x	x
Medication	Some medications used for treatment have side effects that may impact on nutritional requirements (e.g. corticosteroids)				x	x

allergen advice. In the UK some flexibility has been allowed for verbal allergen advice to be given. However, if this advice is given verbally, it should be consistent and verifiable on challenge, i.e. available in a written format such as on recipes or takeaway menus (see Useful Addresses).

Labels stating 'may contain traces' or 'made in a factory with' or any version of text used for precautionary labelling have caused significant confusion [69]. Although the UK Food Standards Agency brought out guidance in 2006 to improve food labelling for people suffering from food allergies, in particular addressing the issue of 'may contain', this guidance is not compulsory [70]. According to this document: 'advisory labelling on possible cross-contamination with allergens should be justifiable only on the basis of a risk assessment applied to a responsibly managed operation. Warning labels should only be used where there is a demonstrable and significant risk of allergen cross-contamination, and they should not be used as a substitute for Good Manufacturing Practices' [70].

Parents should take this warning seriously and the dietitian should discuss this issue with them. The dietitian also needs to address contamination issues. This is particularly relevant when buying loose foods from bakeries and delicatessens and eating out of the home [71]. Obviously, where reactions only occur to large doses of food allergen it is important to stress that there is no need to worry about contamination issues and 'may contain' labelling.

Some food manufacturers and some supermarkets produce 'free from' lists for their products. These are very useful in managing food avoidance diets and parents/carers should be encouraged to use these to identify products that can be included in the diet.

It is important for parents/carers to be able to identify the sources of allergens in composite foods and to recognise the terminology that may be used for each allergen (Table 14.6). The dietitian needs to take into account the nutrients that the offending foods contribute to the diet, so that these can be replaced with suitable alternatives.

Suitable alternatives

It is important for dietitians to familiarise themselves with suitable alternatives for foods that must be avoided. Advice should be given on available products (e.g. peanut free confectionery, milk substitutes, egg free cakes, wheat free pasta) and where to find them. Products and ingredients change constantly. It is therefore essential that dietitians dealing with food allergy constantly update themselves with new products and review existing products. This task can be made easier by joining a specialist support group where this information is shared (see Useful addresses). Dietitians should also be aware of suitable website and phone applications that can help families with the availability of suitable foods.

Food allergies, in particular cow's milk allergy, most commonly occur during the first year of life [29], when breast milk or infant formula are the sole or main source of nutrition. The young child is particularly vulnerable to nutritional deficiencies and growth failure [65, 66] so it is important that dietitians can advise parents on suitable alternatives.

Human milk

Breast milk should be encouraged for all infants. Occasionally infants exhibit allergic symptoms whilst being exclusively breast fed. It is known that allergens from the mother's diet can appear in breast milk [72] and breast fed infants with multiple food allergies have been described [73]. The mother should be encouraged to avoid all suspected food (p. 313) which appears to upset the infant when she eats it [73]. If symptoms cannot be controlled by maternal allergen avoidance, as a last resort the mother may need to stop breast feeding. Isolauri et al. [74] and Hill et al. [75] have found this to be the case in infants with severe atopic dermatitis and impaired growth. Breast feeding mothers on exclusion diets should be reviewed by a dietitian to check the adequacy of their diets as they may need supplements, especially of calcium and vitamin D [76].

Hypoallergenic formulas suitable for children with cow's milk protein allergy

There are currently two definitions widely used in the EU to define products suitable for management of cow's milk protein allergy (CMPA). The first such definition for labelling infant formulas with reduced allergenicity is arbitrarily based on a content of <1% immunoreactive protein of total nitrogen, which translates into the majority of

Table 14.6 Common allergens, their sources and nutrient contribution (adapted from [118]).

Allergen	Sources	Terminology	Macronutrient and micronutrient
Milk	Butter and most fat spreads, cheese, cow's milk, sheep and goat milk, evaporated and condensed milk, cream, ghee, yoghurt, ice creams, custard, dairy desserts and manufactured foods using milk or butter in their ingredients	Casein, caseinates, curd, lactoglobulin, lactose, milk solids, whey, buttermilk, milk sugar, whey sugar, whey syrup sweetener	Protein, energy, vitamin A, vitamin D, riboflavin, pantothenic acid, vitamin B_{12}, calcium, phosphorus
Egg	Egg white and yolk, cakes, biscuits, speciality breads, mayonnaise	Albumin, dried egg, egg powder, egg protein, frozen egg, globulin, lecithin (E322), livetin, ovalbumin, ovomucin, ovovitellin, vitellin, pasteurised egg	Protein, vitamins A, D, E and B_{12}, riboflavin, pantothenic acid, biotin, selenium, iodine, folate
Soy	Soya sauce, soya products, meat substitutes, breads, vegetarian and vegan foods, processed meat	Soya beans, soya flour, soya protein, soya gum, soya starch, texturised (or hydrolysed) vegetable protein, soya flavouring, soya lecithin (E322)	Protein, fibre, thiamin, riboflavin, pyridoxine, folate, calcium, phosphorus, magnesium, iron, zinc
Wheat	Bread, breakfast cereals, pasta, cakes, biscuits, crackers, cold cooked meat, pies, batter, flour, semolina, couscous, bottled sauces and gravies	Bran, cereal filler, farina, starch, wheat, durum wheat, spelt, kamut, wheat bran, wheat gluten, wheat starch, wheat germ oil, hydrolysed wheat protein, triticale, bulgar wheat	Energy, thiamin, riboflavin, niacin, iron, folate (if fortified)
Nuts	Peanuts/tree nuts, nut oil, nut flour, nut butter, some sprouts, confectionery, frozen desserts, Asian dishes, nut snacks, trail mix, some rice crackers, some cereal bars, some cookies, some brownies, nut toppings on ice cream, vegetarian and vegan foods, satay sauce, some breakfast cereals, some liquors and sauces	Arachis oil and hypogeaia (peanut), prunus (almond), juglans (walnut), corylus (hazelnut), peanut protein, groundnut, earth nut, monkey nut	Protein, vitamin E, niacin, magnesium, manganese, chromium. Some nuts may contain a significant amount of essential fatty acids
Fish	All types of white and fatty fish, anchovy (Worcester sauce), aspic, caviar, surimi, Caesar salad, Gentleman's Relish, kedgeree, caponata, fish sauce, paella, bouillabaisse, gumbo		Protein, iodine Fish bones: calcium, phosphate Fatty fish: omega-3 fatty acids, vitamin A and vitamin D

peptides being <1.5 kDa [77]. However, there is no evidence that this threshold would prevent a clinical reaction. There has therefore been a drive by official bodies for hypoallergenic formulas to be tested in clinical trial, using another criterion that stipulates that a formula suitable for management of CMPA should be tolerated by at least 90% of children with a CMPA with a 95% confidence interval [77]. Only extensively hydrolysed formulas

(eHF) and amino acid formulas fall within either of these definitions and dietitians should be aware that partial hydrolysates are not suitable for the treatment of CMPA [77–79]. Although the majority of peptides will be <1.5 kDa in all eHF, as per the first definition, not every feed has gone through a clinical trial testing its tolerance according to the latter definition. However, many eHF have been used with success without these clinical trials and some contain similar peptide lengths to feeds that have gone through clinical trials. It is therefore up to the clinical judgement of the dietitian to choose the correct eHF suitable for the allergic child based on the type of protein, the extent of hydrolysis and also the available research.

Extensively hydrolysed infant formulas

An eHF is often the choice for an infant with immediate or delayed adverse reactions to cow's milk (Table 14.7). Casein hydrolysates have been successfully used for over 60 years; whey hydrolysates were introduced in the 1990s and hydrolysates of pork and soya are also available but rarely used for CMPA [29, 79] (Table 7.6). There is some variation in the degree of hydrolysis in these formulas, casein products being the most highly hydrolysed with >90% of the peptides being smaller than 1.5 kDa.

Much of the literature on the use of these formulas relates to IgE mediated allergy. As far as cow's milk associated gastrointestinal allergies are concerned, both extensively hydrolysed casein and whey formulas have been shown to be satisfactory. However, the incidence of intolerance to eHF is higher (29.7%) in children with delayed type food allergy compared with the immediate type (IgE mediated) cow's milk allergy (around 10%) [12, 33, 75]. Therefore some infants (>10%) may react to hydrolysed formulas. Anaphylactic reactions have been described with both casein and whey hydrolysates [80–83]. Also, late onset adverse reactions to eHF have been reported by Hill and Hosking [8]. However, the majority of cow's milk allergic infants will tolerate any of the eHF. A detailed discussion on cow's milk allergy and the formulas available in the UK is given by Du Toit *et al.* [29].

Amino acid based formulas and amino acid based nutritional supplements

Amino acid formulas (AAF) (Table 14.7) consist of pure synthetic amino acids and have been shown to be tolerated by infants and children with both IgE and non-IgE mediated food hypersensitivity [81, 83]. They are particularly useful for those infants who fail to tolerate an eHF and may be useful in some allergic infants as first line treatment. Hill *et al.* [75] found that children with non-IgE mediated food induced gastro-enterocolitis, proctitis syndromes with faltering growth, severe atopic

eczema, or with symptoms during exclusive breast feeding may benefit from an AAF. As AAF are significantly more expensive than eHF, it is important that the most suitable choice of hypoallergenic formula is made. Choice of formula is guided by

- the type of allergic disorder
- the severity of symptoms
- growth status
- the previous tolerance of breast milk

Infants who have previously tolerated breast milk will also tolerate an eHF. This is related to the residual β-lactoglobulin (0.84–14.5μg/L) detected in eHF made from cow's milk, which is similar to breast milk. If an infant has a history of anaphylactic reactions or eosinophilic oesophagitis, first line choice should be an AAF [84, 87]. There is some evidence that improved longitudinal growth has been seen with an AAF so it may therefore also be useful in infants who have severe faltering growth [63, 75, 80].

The choice of formula remains a challenge for dietitians where the clinical need and the cost of the formula have to be weighed up. A number of key publications have made some suggestions regarding formula choice, which are summarised in Table 14.8. This guidance, however, does not replace the clinical expertise of the dietitian. The problem dietitians face is that there are very few randomised controlled trial studies that have performed direct comparisons between two different formulas, the studies are relative poor quality, numbers are small and clinical profiles of the infants included are poorly described.

Table 14.8 summarises the current available international guidelines on the use of hypoallergenic formulas in the diagnosis and management of CMPA if breast milk is not available. Current research indicates that the majority of children with CMPA will improve on an eHF. The guidelines therefore suggest the use of an AAF, as a first option, only for more severe presentations of CMPA such as a history of anaphylaxis, Heiner syndrome, eosinophilic eosophagitis and severe gastrointestinal and/or skin presentations, usually in association with faltering growth. In addition AAF is useful for infants presenting with symptoms whilst exclusively breast fed who fail to respond to a maternal elimination diet where a hypoallergenic formula is required. Some question

Table 14.7 Hypoallergenic formulas suitable for the management of food allergy [29, 79].

Formula	Protein source	Tested for hypoallergenicity*	Molecular weight of proteins (Da)‡	Osmolality (mOsm/kgH$_2$O)	Additional information
Nutramigen Lipil 1 and 2	eHF casein	Yes [84]	60.4% <500 35% 500–1000 4.1% 1000–2000 0.2% 2000–3000	280 and 340	Clinically insignificant lactose content. Nutramigen Lipil 2 is suitable from 6 months of age. With LCP
Pregestimil Lipil	eHF casein	No†, but same peptide mixture as Nutramigen Lipil 1 and 2	60.4% <500 35% 500–1000 4.1% 1000–2000 0.2% 2000–3000	280	Contains 55% MCT. Clinically insignificant lactose content. For allergy and/or fat malabsorption/ maldigestion. With LCP
Similac Alimentum	eHF casein	Yes [82]	73 % < 500 20 % 500–1000 6 % 1000–2000 1% 2000–3000	374	Clinically lactose free. Contains 33% MCT With LCP.
Pepti-Junior	eHF whey	No, but similar peptide mixture to Pepti 1 and 2	39.3% < 500 27.2% 500–1000 22.1% 1000–2000 8.1% 2000–3000	210	Contains 50% MCT. Clinically insignificant lactose content. For allergy and/or malabsorption/ maldigestion.
Pepti 1 and 2	eHf whey	Yes [85]	50.5% < 500 27.3% 500–1000 Further peptide size not available in comparable categories	280 and 290	Contains prebiotics. Pepti 1 contains 41% lactose § and Pepti 2 36% lactose. Pepti 2 is suitable from 6 months of age.
Althera	eHF whey	Yes [86]	92% < 500 7.3% 500–1000 0.7% 1000–2000 0.02% 2000–3000	335	Contains 53% lactose §.
Pepdite	eHF pork collagen and soya	No	Peptide size not available in comparable categories	237	Suitable for children <1 year of age. Not suitable for patients requiring Halal or Kosher diet. Rarely used for CMPA.
MCT Pepdite	eHF pork collagen and soya	No	Peptide size not available in comparable categories	290	Suitable for children <1 year of age. Contains 75% MCT. Not suitable for patients requiring Halal or Kosher diet. Rarely used for CMPA, mainly used for malabsorption.
Pepdite 1+	eHF pork collagen and soya	No	Peptide size not available in comparable categories	460 for 91 kcal/100 ml 580 at 100 kcal/100 ml	Suitable for children >1 year of age. Not suitable for patients requiring Halal or Kosher diet. Rarely used for CMPA.

Table 14.7 (continued)

Formula	Protein source	Tested for hypoallergenicity*	Molecular weight of proteins (Da)‡	Osmolality (mOsm/kgH₂O)	Additional information
MCT Pepdite1+	eHF pork collagen and soya	No	Peptide size not available in comparable categories	460 for 91 kcal/100 ml 580 at 100 kcal/100 ml	Suitable for children >1 year of age. Contains 75% MCT. Not suitable for patients requiring Halal or Kosher diet. Rarely used for CMPA. Mainly used for malabsorption.
Infatrini Peptisorb	eHF whey	No	47.3% < 500 23.2% 500–1000 21.1% 1000–2000 8.4% 2000–3000	360	Energy dense eHF. Suitable for children with malabsorption and other gastrointestinal disorders requiring an eHF.
Neocate LCP	AAF	Yes [83]	100% Amino Acids	360	Truly hypoallergenic, no CMP β-lactoglobulin. Lactose free. With LCP
Nutramigen AA	AAF	Yes	100% Amino Acids	348	Truly hypoallergenic, no CMP β-lactoglobulin. Lactose free. With LCP
Alfamino	AAF	Data not available at the time of publishing as product just available on the UK market	100% Amino Acids	360	Truly hypoallergenic, no CMP β-lactoglobulin. Lactose free. With LCP
Neocate Active	AAF	No, but same amino acid mix as Neocate LCP	100% Amino acid	510	Suitable for children >1 year of age.
Neocate Advance	AAF	No†, but same amino acid mix as Neocate LCP	100% Amino acids	610	Suitable for children >1 year of age.
Nutrini Peptisorb	eHF whey	No	47.3% < 500 23.2% 500–1000 21.1% 1000–2000 8.4% 2000–3000	345	Energy dense eHF suitable for children >1 year of age.

*Tolerated by 90% of children with CMPA with a 95% confidence interval (CI)

†Studies have been performed using this formula in CMPA, however these were not set out to establish hypoallergenicity, as per definition of "tolerance of 90% of children at a 95% CI".

‡Dalton sizes may differ slightly depending on measurement method as well as batch of product

§Lactose free from cow's milk protein

LCP long chain polyunsaturated fatty acids

MCT medium chain triglycerides

CMP cow's milk protein

Table 14.8 Choosing the most appropriate formula for infants and children with cow's milk protein allergy [63].

Clinical presentation	DRACMA first choice [87]	ESPGHAN first choice [88]	USA first choice [21, 119, 120]	Australian Consensus Panel first choice [121, 121]
Anaphylaxis	AAF	AAF	No recommendation	AAF
Acute urticaria or angioedema	eHF	No specific mention, but eHF in general as first line treatment for CMPA apart from specific indications for AAF	No recommendation	eHF if <6 months SF if >6 months
Atopic eczema/ dermatitis	eHF	No specific mention, but eHF in general as first line treatment	No recommendation	eHF if <6 months SF if >6 months eHF if >6 months if also presenting with faltering growth
Immediate gastrointestinal allergy	eHF	No specific mention, but eHF in general as first line treatment	No recommendation	eHF if <6 months SF if >6 months eHF if >6 months if also presenting with faltering growth
Allergic eosinophilic oesophagitis	AAF	AAF (as well as for other eosinophilic disorders of the gut)	AAF/hypoallergenic formula (NIAID)	AAF
Gastroesophageal reflux disease	eHF	No specific mention but eHF in general as first line treatment	No recommendation	eHF if <6 months SF if >6 months eHF if >6 months if also presenting with faltering growth
Cow's milk protein-induced enteropathy	eHF	AAF (severe enteropathy complicated by faltering growth and hypoproteinaemia)	eHF/AAF	eHF if <6 months SF if >6 months eHF if >6 if also presenting with faltering growth
Food protein-induced enterocolitis syndrome (FPIES)	eHF	AAF	Hypoallergenic formula (NIAID) eHF/AAF	eHF
Cow's milk protein induced gastroenteritis and proctocolitis	eHF	No specific mention, but eHF in general as first line treatment		Gastroenteritis: eHF if <6 months SF if >6 months eHF if >6 months if also presenting with faltering growth Proctitis: eHF
Severe irritability (colic)	eHF	No specific mention, but eHF in general as first line treatment	Hypoallergenic formula	eHF if <6 months SF if >6 months

AAF, amino acid formula; eHF, extensively hydrolysed formula; SF, soy formula; CMPA, cow's milk protein allergy; NIAID, National Institute of Allergy and Infectious Diseases.

the use of hypoallergenic formulas containing lactose in children with CMPA. The European Society for Paediatric Gastroenterology, Hepatology and Nutrition (ESPGHAN) advises that adverse reactions to lactose in children with CMPA are not reported and states that complete avoidance of lactose may not be needed in the majority of cases [88]. It may be important, however, to consider not using these formulas in children who have an enteropathy with severe diarrhoea where there is secondary lactose intolerance [63].

The introduction of complementary foods can often be very challenging, particularly in infants with multiple food allergies and faltering growth. Neocate Spoon is an amino acid based food supplement (with vitamins C and D, calcium and iron) which can be given in addition to breast milk or a hypoallergenic formula to support the introduction of complementary foods. It can be mixed with sweet or savoury foods. This product is not nutritionally complete and must never be given as a sole source of nutrition.

Formulas based on whole soy protein isolate
Infant formulas based on whole soy protein isolate have been available without prescription for many years. In the past, soy based formulas were used widely as an alternative to cow's milk formula in those infants with CMPA. However, in 2004 the UK Chief Medical Officer advised against the use of soy formula in infants under the age of 6 months unless there is a specific medical indication due to their high phytoestrogen content [89]. The Committee on Toxicity of Chemicals in Food, Consumer Products and the Environment is reviewing more recent research in this area.

The prevalence of concomitant soy allergy in infants with CMPA differs between IgE and non-IgE mediated disease. Klemola *et al.* and Zeiger *et al.* found that 10% and 14%, respectively, of infants with IgE mediated CMPA have concomitant soy allergy, whereas associated soy allergy in non-IgE mediated CMPA is much higher (up to 50%), especially in enterocolitis and enteropathy syndromes [90–92]. These data may vary between countries, however.

The use of soya formula in the diagnosis and management of CMPA is a highly debated topic, with clear differences between different countries and professional bodies (Table 14.8). Soya formula

can be given for the treatment of CMPA in infants over the age of 6 months if it has been proved that they do not have soy allergy and they have failed to take other hypoallergenic formulas due to the taste preferences of the child or if there are strong parental preferences (e.g. vegan diet). Soya containing products such as soya desserts enhance the variety in a cow's milk free diet and can be given from 6 months of age [92].

Sheep and goat milk
Sheep and goat milk are not suitable for infants with CMPA as their nutritional composition is unsuitable for infant feeding, there is sometimes concern about microbial content and their proteins can be as sensitising as cow's milk protein. Dean *et al.* have shown that there is strong cross-reactivity *in vitro* between allergens in all mammalian milks (except human milk) [93]. An infant formula based on goat milk is not suitable for the treatment of CMPA.

Practical advice
It is important to provide families with practical advice on how to manage their child's food allergy. This starts with some practical hints on how to introduce the hypoallergenic formula.

• The formula should be offered when the infant is hungry and thirsty
• It may sometimes be easier if the first bottles are not given by the main carer
• Mixing hypoallergenic formula with weaning foods may help the child to get used to the taste of the formula
• If the child is able to hold a bottle (usually over 6 months of age) then a baby beaker with free flow may also be useful
• Vanilla essence may be helpful to improve the taste, but take care as if too much is added it may make the formula more bitter
• Flavourings should be avoided but, if all else fails, a milk and soy free milk shake powder or syrup can be added

Parents also need information on the availability of products to suit their child's exclusion (avoidance) diet. Although children with wheat allergy are not eligible for prescription gluten free foods, some general practitioners will prescribe items like bread and pasta if requested. It is very helpful for parents to have lists of gluten and wheat starch free foods which are also egg, milk and soya free if necessary. They may choose to buy these items as many are not prescribable. It is also useful to tell parents about wheat free items readily available in supermarkets, e.g. puffed rice cakes, Thai rice noodles. Most food manufacturers and supermarkets have a customer helpline and these telephone numbers can be given to parents so they can get information themselves.

Parents find recipes very useful. Some examples are cakes without egg, biscuits and cakes without wheat, and gravy and sauces without wheat. A general discussion about menu planning is helpful. Advice may include ideas for weaning foods and packed lunches. Other carers may need to be contacted, e.g. school caterers. Parents also appreciate tips on how to get a child to take a new food. For example, wheat free products are often better accepted initially if given with other flavours, e.g. jam on bread, sauce on pasta. A carer other than the main carer is often able to persuade the child to take the new food. It is also important to discuss the management of food allergies at nursery, school and when the family travels abroad.

Dietary supplements

Whenever a food is removed from the diet there is the likelihood that the diet will no longer meet nutritional requirements (Table 14.6); the more foods that are eliminated the greater the risk of a deficiency. Infants who consume less than 500–700 mL, depending on the hypoallergenic formula used, and all infants more than 6 months of age who are fully breast fed will require a multivitamin preparation containing, in particular, vitamins A and D [29]. In addition, a calcium supplement will be required in children with CMPA who do not consume sufficient formula or calcium containing foods. Family doctors are generally happy to prescribe supplements but sometimes an over-the-counter supplement may be more readily accepted, especially in older children. Vitamins and minerals must be free from the offending allergens. Vitamin and mineral supplements are often forgotten in infants less than 6 months; if dietary consumption is suboptimal and maternal dietary intake has not been good during pregnancy and lactation then vitamins and minerals should be given without any hesitation.

A case study to illustrate the management of a child with food allergy is given in Table 14.9.

Monitoring

It is essential that children following an exclusion diet are followed up regularly. Children's diets vary enormously as they get older and nutritional requirements also change. In addition, there may be advances in knowledge that may affect treatment strategies and it is also important to ensure that as the child gets older they themselves understand their diet.

The key aspect of monitoring childhood food allergies is establishing when the child has outgrown their allergies. Food challenges or reintroduction of food at home form an important part of this process.

The dietary management of food hypersensitivity consists primarily of educating patients and their families so they can avoid the causative food whilst still meeting all nutritional requirements. No dietary manipulation is easy so it is the role of the dietitian to give information not only on how to avoid the causative food but also on how to make the resultant diet as palatable as possible. Before any advice is given it is essential to consider how strict the diet needs to be. It is not necessary for a family to strive for complete avoidance of an allergen if reactions only occur when relatively large doses of the food are taken. On the other hand, when life threatening reactions occur when exposed to tiny doses advice on complete avoidance is essential.

Natural progression

Food allergy is most commonly acquired during the first year of life with a peak incidence between 2.2% and 5.5% during the first year of life in the UK [94]. The prevalence falls to 2.3% in teenagers and then plateaus at 1%–2% through adulthood. These figures may be higher in tertiary centres [95]. The majority of reactions to foods in infants and young children are milk, egg, nuts, soy, fish and wheat [2]; however, in adulthood the most common food allergens include hazelnut, apple, peach and shrimp [96]. Although the tendency to develop allergies clearly has a genetic component (Table 14.10), it is strongly influenced by

Table 14.9   Case study: management of food allergy.

Presentation
A 3-month-old baby girl presented with chronic diarrhoea and mild-to-moderate eczema across her body and face. Weight = 25th centile.

Formula fed from birth. Her family history: mother has asthma and father has hayfever. Born at full term, normal delivery. Maternal history of eczema, asthma and hay fever, but no paternal history of allergy.

This infant was seen by a paediatrician, an allergy nurse and a paediatric allergy dietitian, who provided advice regarding skin care and changed her formula to an eHF, in line with current guidelines [78, 84]. Skin prick tests (SPT) were not conducted at this stage, based on her current symptoms, which suggested a non-IgE mediated allergy. Written and verbal advice on low allergen weaning foods (i.e. milk, egg, soy, nut, wheat and fish free) was provided, as her mother wanted to start weaning when her baby reached age 4–5 months.

Follow-up
Returned to the allergy clinic at age 6 months; her diarrhoea had resolved and her eczema had cleared, with only the occasional flare. On examination, she was found to be well and thriving, with a normal physical examination. Weight = 25th centile.

Full blood count, clotting profile and liver function were all within the normal range.

Because she was weaning, SPT were performed to determine which foods could be safely introduced.

Skin prick tests: results at ages 6 months and 12 months

Test	Wheal size at 6 months (mm)*	Wheal size at 12 months (mm)*
Milk	3	1
Egg	2	1
Wheat	0	0
Soya	0	0
Peanut	0	0
Positive control	3	4
Negative control	0	0

* SPT are considered positive if the wheal is ≥3 mm larger than the negative control; for further information see [2].

The SPT for milk was positive, which suggested that hypersensitivity to cow's milk may have played a role in her eczema flares in the past. Together with her improved symptoms since switching to eHF, this allowed a diagnosis of cow's milk protein allergy (CMPA) to be made. A second, smaller wheal suggested a potential allergy to egg. In consultation with the paediatrician and dietitian, the baby's mother was advised to use milk and egg free weaning foods and given recipes and website addresses. It was also recommended that all other foods could be introduced one at a time, with the precautionary exclusion of soya, because infants with non-IgE mediated CMPA are commonly sensitised to soy [92]. In addition, the baby's formula was changed to a follow-on eHF, which contains more calcium and is therefore suited to babies >6 months of age.

At age 9 months
Weight = 50th centile

Thriving. Eczema was under control and the diarrhoea had not returned. She was feeding a follow-on eHF and solid foods, excluding milk, egg and soy. An oral challenge with one boiled egg was performed in hospital, with a negative result. Therefore it was recommended that she should be given a well cooked scrambled egg at home the next morning, returning to the children's ward if symptoms reappeared.

At age 12 months
Weight = 50th centile

Thriving. Eating a varied diet and consuming 355–415 mL eHF per day with additional supplement of vitamins A and D. SPT showed negative results for cow's milk and soya, so oral challenges with these foods were given. The soya challenge, conducted over a period of a week at home, was negative. However, the cow's milk challenge, which was conducted in hospital, resulted in an immediate flare of her eczema, with diarrhoea the following morning. It was recommended that soya yoghurts and puddings could be introduced to increase variety in her diet, but she should continue to avoid all milk products.

Table 14.9 *(continued)*

2 years
SPT for milk produced a 2 mm wheal. On analysing this toddler's diet, her nutritional intake was found to be adequate. As a result, it was recommended that the milk free diet was continued and calcium enriched soy milk could be introduced.

Four months later, the girl accidentally drank a cup of milk at nursery, without an adverse reaction. Consequently, oral challenge was given in hospital, which continued at home for a week. As she showed no allergic symptoms, the mother was advised that milk products could be gradually reintroduced. Subsequently, she occasionally experienced eczematous symptoms, which were treated with emollients, antihistamines and a little hydrocortisone.

3 years
SPTs were negative for all allergens tested and she was tolerating all foods.

eHF, extensively hydrolysed formula.

Table 14.10 Risk of a child developing allergies [2].

Family members with food allergy	Percentage risks
Both parents with identical allergies	72%
Both parents with non-identical allergies	43%
One parent with allergy	20%
Neither parent allergic	12%
One sibling with allergy	32%

environment and lifestyle factors. These include air pollution, environmental tobacco smoke exposure, maternal and infant nutrition, environmental allergen exposure, family size, infections and hygiene [97].

It has long been established that most children grow out of these allergies [1], in particular milk and egg allergy. However, recent studies performed in tertiary centres have shown that some of these allergies are more persistent and children outgrow them later than previously thought. Approximately half of egg allergic children will be tolerant by the age of 3 years and 66% by 5 years of age [98]. For milk, about 80%–90% of children may become tolerant based on population based studies [95, 99]. It is commonly thought that peanut allergy does not resolve although Skolnick *et al.* [100] have shown that it may be outgrown in 21.5% of patients. Tree nut, fish and shellfish allergies tend to develop in older children and are unlikely to be outgrown.

Although many children grow out of their initial food allergies, it is evident that allergic disorders change and progress from eczema and food allergy in early childhood to asthma and rhinitis related to pollen allergy in later childhood. This phenomenon is referred to as the 'allergic march' [101].

Oral allergy syndrome (pollen allergy syndrome)

Some older children report symptoms of itching or unpleasant sensation in the oral mucosa after eating some types of fruit. This is termed oral allergy syndrome. These reactions are due to cross-reactivity, usually with pollens such as birch and grass, but occasionally latex. Such cross-reactivity does not always indicate that avoidance of all these foods is necessary, with clinical history being indicative of the requirement to avoid certain foods. These mucosal reactions are normally to raw fruit so advice regarding cooking the food or trying tinned varieties can often result in the child being able to eat the fruit. This advice is important in helping the child maintain their fruit intake. Oral allergy syndrome is more fully described elsewhere [102].

Transition to adult care

Although many children will outgrow their allergies, some will continue to have their allergies into adulthood and some may develop new food hypersensitivities. The transitional stage, starting during teenage years, is the time when children will have to take responsibility for their own management. A recent study by Monks *et al.* [103] found that the majority of teenagers reported eating foods labelled 'may contain' an allergen as they perceive that the foods are actually very unlikely to contain an allergen. Many of the teenagers only carried their self-injectable adrenaline (required for anaphylactic patients who accidentally consume an offending allergen) when they thought they were particularly at risk of a reaction; some did not know how to treat themselves if a reaction should occur. A recent systematic review looking into strategies that improve transition between paediatric and adult care in children with chronic illness found four broad categories that improved transition: patient directed intervention (educational programmes, skills training); staff intervention (named transition coordinators); joint clinics run by paediatric and adult physicians; and changes to service delivery (separate young adult clinics, out of hours phone support, enhanced follow-up). All these interventions have been shown to improve care [104].

Problems with dietary management in food hypersensitivity

Food hypersensitivity remains a controversial area of medicine and it is important to avoid giving inappropriate emphasis to dietary treatment. However, people who feel that diet plays a role in their child's illness should have the opportunity to discuss in an unbiased fashion the possibilities of dietary treatment and, where appropriate, have the opportunity to trial an exclusion diet. A lack of sympathetic approach may lead to self-imposed diets (likely to be inadequate) or self-referral to an unqualified practitioner. Whatever the prejudices of the professionals involved, the question of diet must be discussed as the child may be on an inadequate and inappropriate diet. Although some children may be on unhelpful diets, others benefit dramatically from the correct exclusion diet. The role of the dietitian is to assist in maintaining helpful diets and to broaden the diet as much as possible. It is equally important to encourage people to abandon exclusion diets where they confer no benefit. An open-minded approach is necessary. Occasionally parents will not take advice and in exceptional cases the dietary restrictions imposed by the parent on the child may be regarded as a form of child abuse [105, 106].

Controversial elimination diets

Migraine and epilepsy

Cheese, chocolate and red wine sometimes provoke migraine, allegedly owing to the presence of a pharmacologically active ingredient, tyramine. Children with severe migraine who have failed to benefit from avoidance of cheese and chocolate have been shown to respond to a few foods diet and the most common provoking foods on food reintroduction were those which are implicated in food hypersensitivity in general [107, 108]. When migraine attacks are less than one per week it is difficult to use a diet approach. If symptoms are infrequent, 3 weeks of a few foods diet would not be long enough to assess change in rate of attacks and the reintroduction phase would be very muddled. However, for children with severe frequent migraine who have not responded to medication, a diet trial is a worthwhile procedure.

Sometimes children with severe migraine have other symptoms and epilepsy may be one of these. A minority of children with epilepsy who also have migraine respond to dietary elimination whereas children with epilepsy alone do not [109]. As with migraine, the diet approach cannot be tried unless seizures are frequent. A trial of diet for such children who have not responded to conventional treatment is worth considering.

Attention deficit hyperactivity disorder (ADHD)

The question of diet and ADHD is very controversial. In 1975 Feingold, an American allergist, claimed that hyperactive children would benefit from avoiding foods containing salicylates together with artificial flavours and colours. Later, food preservatives were also excluded. The results of studies aimed at testing Feingold's hypothesis indicated that only a few hyperactive children responded to the elimination of food additives from their diets. Problems with methodology and interpretation of these studies have been discussed by Taylor [110]. Five studies have looked at the relationship between food (not just additives) and behaviour [111]. More recently, McCann et al. [112] performed a double blind randomised controlled study using two additive mixtures and found that artificial colours or a sodium benzoate preservative (or both) in the diet resulted in increased hyperactivity in 3-year-old and 8–9-year-old children in the general population. At the time of publishing this study, the exact mechanism of worsening ADHD through food additives was not known. Since then, the same group has discussed how food additives can exacerbate ADHD symptoms and cause non-IgE dependent histamine release from circulating basophils. The fact that some children reacted worse than others was found to be related to specific genes influencing the action of histamine, which may explain the inconsistency between previous studies [113].

From a practical dietetic point of view, food colourings and sodium benzoate are found in processed foods, often with high sugar and salt content. Parents of a child with ADHD should in the first instance be advised to ensure a healthy balanced dietary intake. For children with severe ADHD whose parents wish to explore the dietary approach (free from colourings and sodium benzoate) they should be given the opportunity to do so with the support of a dietitian; otherwise they will be tempted to experiment with the diet unsupervised, which may lead to nutritional deficiencies.

Other treatments such as behaviour modification or stimulant medication may be more effective than dietary management although some children may end up on a combination of these treatments.

Future research needs and unanswered questions

Prevention of food allergies

See Chapter 31 for details of prevention strategies for food allergy.

Probiotics

A probiotic is defined as 'an oral supplement or a food product that contains a sufficient number of viable microorganisms to alter the microflora of the host and has the potential for beneficial health effects' [114]. Two Cochrane reviews assessed the use of probiotics for treatment and management of allergies. Both found that there was insufficient evidence to suggest that probiotics were effective for the prevention of allergic disease and treatment of atopic dermatitis. Although there was a reduction in clinical eczema, this effect was not consistent between studies [115]. Inconsistencies were most probably due to the difference in probiotic strains and research methodologies. Further research is required prior to recommending routine supplementation of probiotics in allergic children [116].

Prebiotics

There are some data to suggest that prebiotics may play a role in the prevention of allergic diseases when added to a hypoallergenic feed in high risk infants [116, 117]. Further information on allergy prevention is covered in Chapter 31.

Acknowledgements

We would like to acknowledge Kate Grimshaw, who wrote this chapter for the third edition. We have used much of her original text.

Further reading and useful links

Skypala I, Venter C *Food Hypersensitivity*. Oxford: Wiley-Blackwell, 2009.

Venter C, Arshad SH Epidemiology of food allergy. *Pediatr Clin North Am*, 2011, **58** 327–49.

Venter C, Meyer R Session 1: Allergic disease: the challenges of managing food hypersensitivity. *Proc Nutr Soc*, 2010, **69** 11–24.

Sampson HA Update on food allergy. *J Allergy Clin Immunol*, 2004, **113** 805–19.

Sicherer SH Food allergy. *Lancet*, 2002, **360** 701–10.

Joneja JV *Dietary Management of Food Allergies and Intolerances. A Comprehensive Guide*, 2nd edn. Vancouver: JA Hall, 1998.

Leung DYM, Sampson HA, Geha RS, Szefler SJ (eds) *Pediatric Allergy. Principles and Practice*. St Louis, MO: Mosby, 2003.

Holgate S, Church MK, *Lichtenstein LM* Allergy, 2nd edn. London: Mosby, 2002.

Sicherer SH Food allergy: when and how to perform oral food challenges. *Pediatr Allergy Immunol*, 1999, **10** 226–34.

Committee on Toxicity of Chemicals in Food, Consumer Products and the Environment (COT) Adverse Reactions to Food and Food Ingredients, Department of Health, London, 2000.

Roberts G Food allergy – getting more out of your skin prick tests. Editorial. *Clin Exper Allergy*, 2000, **30** 1495–8.

British Dietetic Association Food Allergy and Intolerance Specialist Group

www.bda.uk.com (non members)
www.members.bda.uk.com/groups/faisg/index

Anaphylaxis Campaign

PO Box 275, Farnborough, Hampshire, GU14 6SX
Tel. 01252 373793
www.anaphylaxis.org.uk

Allergy UK

3 White Oak Square, Swanley, Kent, BR5 7AG
Tel. 01322 619898
www.allergyuk.org

European Association for Allergy and Clinical Immunology

www.eaaci.net

INDANA – International Network for Diet and Nutrition in Allergy

www.indana-allergynetwork.org

Food Allergy Network

www.foodallergy.org

American Academy of Allergy Asthma and Immunology

www.aaaai.org

Food Standards Agency of the UK

food.gov.uk/policy-advice/allergyintol/label/

15 Immunodeficiency Syndromes, HIV and AIDS

Natalie Yerlett, Julie Lanigan and Lisa Cooke

Immunodeficiency Syndromes

Natalie Yerlett

Introduction

In an environment abundant with microorganisms, the immune system acts to protect the body from their potential harm. The human immune system has two functionalities, different, but both complementing each other to enhance effectiveness.

'*Innate*' *immunity* is the body's first line defence, immediately having phagocytic cells ready to engulf and digest microorganisms. This response does not rely upon previous exposure to the antigen and does not produce antigen specific antibodies. Due to this, innate immunity is crucial to survival in early life. Innate immune responses are important in containing an infection and include complement cascade reactions and phagocytic cytokine release to induce inflammation. Innate immunity is non-specific and does not confer lifelong immunity to a repeat infection. These first line responses are triggered whilst awaiting the second line adaptive immune response [1].

'*Adaptive*' *immunity* is the more specific, tailored second line defence system. This enables the body to recognise and remember specific pathogens and subsequently mount a stronger immune response on each further exposure. Central to this is the production of an array of immune cells: B cells, T cells and natural killer (NK) cells, some of which produce specific antibodies to a particular antigen [1]. Adaptive immunity is paramount after infancy.

There are four main types of pathogens that should illicit an immune response:

- fungi, e.g. *Aspergillus fumigatus*
- parasites, e.g. *Leishmania donovani*
- bacteria (extracellular or intracellular), e.g. *Streptococcus pneumonia*
- viruses, e.g. influenza, cytomegalovirus

Defects or failures in any part of the complex immune system may lead to immune-pathological reactions and disease, often as a result of not being able to mount an immune response against an antigen, thus allowing it to successfully infiltrate and cause harm. Disorders of the immune system can be:

- primary genetic mutations where elements of the immune cell nomenclature can be missing altogether
- secondary to immune suppression therapy

These can be differentiated into disorders of B cell maturation and/or their ability to produce antibodies; T cell defects; combined T cell/B cell defects; disorders of phagocytes; complement deficiencies [1, 2].

Common immunodeficiency syndromes are listed in Table 15.1 together with their possible dietetic considerations.

B and T cells

B cells

B cells are derived from haematopoietic stem cells in the bone marrow and remain there during maturation. B cells make up a 'humoral' immune response and their main function is to produce antibodies (immunoglobulins), namely IgA, IgD, IgG, IgM and IgE [1]. Therefore, B cells help to protect against extracellular pathogens, e.g. bacteria. There are two types of B cells:

- B_1 cells – are polyspecific with low affinity for many antigens
- B_2 cells – are constantly renewed in the bone marrow

B_2 cells then progress through a further maturation process, which results in more specific B cell subsets [1]. These include:

- plasma B cells (effector B cells) – already exposed to antigens, subsequently producing and secreting antibodies
- memory B cells – made from activated B cells specific to a previous antigen; they are secreted quickly on encounter with the same antigen for the second time
- marginal zone B cells – resident in the spleen
- follicular B cells – resident in lymphoid tissues

Table 15.1   Summary of some immunodeficiency syndromes and possible dietetic considerations.

Immunodeficiency	Possible dietetic considerations
B cell defects	
IgA deficiency	Malabsorption, coeliac disease [4], gastrointestinal infection
IgG subclass deficiency	Malabsorption, possible food allergy/colitis [9, 10]
Common variable immunodeficiency	Abdominal pain, diarrhoea [28]
T cell defects	
Autoimmune enteropathy	Protracted diarrhoea of infancy, severe faltering growth, often failure of normal nutritional interventions [12, 13], hypoallergenic diet may be required
Class II MHC deficiency	Chronic diarrhoea, severe infections
Wiskott–Aldrich syndrome	Malabsorption, bloody diarrhoea [1]
T and B lymphocyte defects	
SCID	Diarrhoea, malabsorption, vomiting, GORD, infectious diarrhoea, faltering growth, increased nutritional requirements [20], hydrolysed protein formulas often required
Autosomal recessive	Increased nutritional requirements
X-linked ADA, PNP deficiency, Omenn syndrome	Skin losses, possible fluid/electrolyte imbalance
Phagocyte defects	
Chronic granulomatous disease	Diarrhoea, protein-losing enteropathy, pancolitis, frequent infections, intolerance of high feed volume, increased nutritional requirements requiring early use of nutrient dense enteral feeds [1, 19]
Leucocyte adhesion deficiency	Mucosal infection and inflammation [19]

MHC major histocompatability complex; SCID, severe combined immune deficiency; GORD, gastro-oesophageal reflux disease; ADA, adenosine deaminase; PNP, purine nucleoside phosphorylase.

B cell defects

B cell defects can range in type and severity. They may encompass:

- absent B cells – severe reduction in all antibodies such as XLA [1, 2]
- low B cell count but deficient B cell subclass, resulting in a variable degree deficiency such as low IgA/IgG
- normal B cell count but with light chain deficiency/isotype – selective IgA deficiency

Selective IgA deficiency

IgA deficiency is the most common of the primary immune deficiency diseases. Patients may have a deficiency or a total absence of IgA, but usually have normal levels of the other immunoglobulins. Patients may be asymptomatic with 'silent IgA deficiency' or may require immunoglobulin treatment. IgA acts to protect mucosal surfaces; deficiency therefore leads to recurrent or chronic infections such as sinusitis, pneumonia, bronchitis and gastrointestinal infections.

The incidence of IgA deficiency in the general population is 1 in 700 people of European origin [3]. The prevalence of coeliac disease is up to 30% higher in patients with IgA deficiency compared with the general population [4], and this IgA deficiency persists when following a gluten free diet despite the return of a normal mucosa [5]. IgA antibodies against both tissue transglutaminase (tTG) and endomysial antibodies (EMA) are relied upon for serum screening of coeliac disease; therefore patients with IgA deficiency will not have a reliable tTG/EMA serum level and should have IgG tTG and EMA testing when available [6]. IgA plays a vital role in mucosal integrity; therefore it is also associated with the onset of food allergy [7].

IgG and IgG subclass deficiency

Children may have deficiencies in one or more of the IgG subclass (IgG1–4). Clinical presentation depends on the severity and combination of the deficiency, with some individuals being asymptomatic. Most commonly, children may present with recurrent infections [8]. It has been shown previously that patients with IgG deficiency may present with food allergy or food allergic colitis [9]; however, the literature in this area is limited.

Food allergy testing involving IgG is not recommended [10]. The dietetic management of food allergy is described in Chapters 7 and 14.

T cells

T cells develop from haemopoietic stem cells in bone marrow which then migrate to the thymus. Here, they undergo maturation, differentiation into T cell types and finally undergo positive/negative selection to ensure that the resulting T cells will not over- or under-recognise host 'self' antigens. T cells illicit a 'cell mediated', intracellular immune response; therefore they can help to fight off intracellular pathogens such as viruses. There are three main categories of T cells [1]:

- naïve T cells
- memory T cells
- effector T cells

T cell defects

T cell defects range in type and severity, for example:

- complete insufficiency of T cell/T cell function, with/without concurrent B cell defect such as severe combined immune deficiency (SCID), including Omenn syndrome and major histocompatibility complex (MHC) Class II deficiency
- partial or complete insufficiency of T cell function such as DiGeorge syndrome (often associated with absent thymus) or Wiskott–Aldridge syndrome
- T cell dysregulation, i.e. autoimmune enteropathy

Autoimmune enteropathy

A primary immune dysregulation can result in immune mediated damage to the intestinal mucosa, commonly presenting with protracted diarrhoea of infancy and malabsorption [11]. The disease may be caused by immune dysfunction of varying natures, including activation of mucosal T cells causing persistent damage to the gut mucosa [12] or by auto-antibodies present on the gut mucosa [11]. Severe inflammation, villous atrophy with crypt hyperplasia and increased mitosis may be seen histologically. These changes in the small intestinal mucosa may resemble those found in coeliac disease [13]. Such infants present with severe faltering growth and may be unresponsive to normal enteral nutritional interventions [14]. Intense nutritional management is crucial as poor nutritional status can worsen mucosal integrity. In such cases immunosuppression is often required to control the disease. In patients with life threatening autoimmune enteropathy resulting from a primary autoimmune dysregulation, and in most cases where the disease has proved unresponsive to conventional immunosuppressive therapy, a bone marrow transplant can be a successful treatment [15, 16]. It is now possible to identify such primary genetic defects of gut mucosal integrity in early infancy and treat with stem cell transplant [17].

Current nutritional management of patients undergoing gastroenterological stem cell transplantation is similar to that of post graft versus host disease (GvHD) (p. 340). Post-transplant, patients are usually maintained on a milk, egg, wheat and soya free diet for up to 2 years. Extreme caution should be applied when challenging with new feeds or foods.

Defects in phagocytes

Phagocytic cells, including macrophages, neutrophils and monocytes, are important in host defence against pyogenic bacteria and other intracellular organisms. These cells leave the bone marrow and migrate to peripheral tissues, particularly at sites of infection or inflammation. Phagocytes ingest pathogens and degrade them; therefore phagocyte defects can lead to severe infection and as a result may be fatal [1]. Some patients may present with gastrointestinal complications similar to those of inflammatory bowel disease [18]. The clinical presentations of some phagocyte defects are

- chronic granulomatous disease (CGD) where phagocytes cannot produce superoxide radical so cannot degrade pathogens after ingestion
- deficiencies in any stage of the migration, adherence or transmigration of leucocytes where the finding and destruction of pathogens at the site of an infection is prevented

Children with CGD present with frequent infections, such as pneumonia, which are difficult to

cure. These frequent infections increase nutritional requirements and decrease the appetite for food and tolerance of adequate volumes of oral feeds. It is therefore often necessary to initiate enteral feeding as soon as an acute episode begins to prevent excessive weight loss. Energy dense feeds are often tolerated. Diarrhoea is usually common due to intensive antibiotic therapy. Patients may be treated with stem cell transplantation.

Combined immunodeficiencies

Wiskott–Aldrich syndrome

Wiskott–Aldrich syndrome (WAS) is an X-linked immunodeficiency syndrome causing small platelet size. These platelets are mopped up by the spleen with a resultant thrombocytopenia. Immunoglobulin concentrations, T cells and antibody production are also affected [1]. Patients have numerous chronic infections due to reduced immunity, early infantile eczema and they often bleed easily, including bloody diarrhoea. This bleeding results in anaemia which needs to be corrected with iron supplements. Some children may benefit from amino acid based formulas (p. 114).

Severe combined immune deficiency

Infants with combined immune deficiency, including SCID, have a gene mutation characterised by deficiencies of one or more of the three main lymphocyte subsets (T, B and NK cells). The condition is fatal if untreated. Infants may present at birth or after 3 months of age once maternal immunoglobulin protection has worn off. Infants often present with recurrent severe infections which may be bacterial, fungal or viral. These infections often persist despite treatment [1, 2].

Dietetic management of infants with SCID

Infants diagnosed with SCID often face a nutritional challenge. They may suffer from diarrhoea, malabsorption, vomiting, gastro-oesophageal reflux [19], respiratory infections and/or faltering growth despite a seemingly adequate oral intake. Barron et al. have shown that some of their population of infants with SCID have increased nutritional requirements as a result of hypermetabolism [20]; 100% of the infants presenting with diarrhoea, independent of pneumonia, were at risk of hypermetabolism and subsequent faltering growth. Infants with a diagnosis made between 3 and 12 months of age were at greatest risk.

The use of an energy dense formula, e.g. 0.9 kcal (3.8 kJ)/mL or 1 kcal (4 kJ)/mL, given orally and/or via a nasogastric tube can be indicated, if tolerated. A nasojejunal tube can be considered in infants with ongoing gastro-oesophageal reflux or delayed gastric emptying that is preventing the establishment of oral or nasogastric feeding.

Infants with adenosine deaminase (ADA) deficient SCID often display faltering growth. Once a diagnosis has been made, polyethylene glycol–adenosine deaminase (PEG-ADA) enzyme replacement can be given which may temporarily restore some immune function, thus improving nutritional status.

Parenteral hydration and nutrition may be necessary where an infant requires stabilisation pre or post diagnosis. Some infants with very high requirements may require parenteral nutrition (PN) alongside enteral and/or oral feeds. It may not be possible to meet full requirements with PN alone. Sodium status (urinary and serum) can be a useful tool to ensure adequate sodium levels for growth [21]. In practice, a urinary sodium level <20 mmol/L may indicate poor sodium status (despite normal serum sodium), and sodium supplements may be necessary or the sodium content of PN increased in increments of 1 mmol/kg/day. Urinary sodium levels should then be monitored weekly or biweekly until a level >20 mmol/L is maintained. There is limited evidence for this practice, but clinically this can be effective, especially for infants with chronic diarrhoea who may have high sodium losses. Where full PN is given (except at times of complete gut rest) trophic feeds should be given to help maintain the integrity of the gut mucosa.

Reintroduction of feeds following period of gut rest

At all times reintroduction of enteral feeds should be considered a priority and started as soon as the infant is medically stable. Oral rehydration solution may be given first; if this is tolerated then a suitable formula feed can be introduced.

Reintroduction of feeds should be done slowly, often in 1 mL increments as tolerated. Continuous feeding over 20–24 hours is recommended to begin with. Extensively hydrolysed protein formulas (p. 113) or amino acid based formulas (p. 114) are likely to be better tolerated than a whole protein formula. These formulas have higher osmolality than standard formulas; therefore it may be beneficial to start with half standard concentration, building up concentration gradually at 1%–2% at a time. Once standard concentration is achieved and tolerated, it is often necessary to increase the concentration further to achieve higher energy and nutrient density. This should be done with caution, increasing by 1% at a time, usually not exceeding a concentration of 1 kcal/mL (4 kJ/mL). It is often possible to offer the infant a proportion of their feed (however small) orally. This will help to promote oromotor skills, avoid oral sensitisation and can also be a valuable input to the infant's care by the parent(s).

In older children or infants of weaning age, food can be introduced as early as tolerated. Initially, the diet may be milk, egg, wheat and soya free. This is usually necessary following bone marrow transplant for autoimmune enteropathy and in patients who have developed GvHD post transplant. In addition, foods may be kept 'bland', with introduction of one new food at a time. Once immune function has stabilised following transplant, and in the absence of gastrointestinal symptoms, restricted foods can be added in one by one.

Treatment for SCID

Treatment for SCID is primarily haematopoietic stem cell transplantation (HSCT), or more recently by *ex vivo* gene therapy. Gene therapy may be useful when a well matched donor is not available for HSCT. Stem cells are extracted from the patient, a working copy of the gene is then inserted by retrovirus carrier and the cells are then returned to the patient. Both gene therapy and HSCT are potentially curative and have been proved successful in many patients [22].

Nutritional status may be compromised if chemotherapy such as Melphalan is given for conditioning prior to gene therapy treatment. Dietetic management is similar to that outlined for HSCT (p. 341).

Haematopoietic stem cell transplantation

In this treatment donor haematopoietic stem cells, usually derived from bone marrow, umbilical cord blood or peripheral blood stem cells, are transplanted into the patient. HSCT remains a risky procedure; however, for patients with SCID or autoimmune enteropathy HSCT can be an effective cure. Transplantation of SCID patients from a matched sibling donor has 90% 3 year survival rate, with mismatched transplants having a 65% success rate [23]. Regardless of diagnosis prior to transplant, maintaining nutritional status pre, peri and post transplant is essential and significantly affects clinical outcome [16, 24]. Energy requirements can be estimated and Schofield equations for predicting resting energy expenditure in children pre transplant have been shown to be suitable [16].

Children receiving an allogeneic haematopoietic stem cell transplant are given myeloablative immunosuppressive conditioning drugs for about 10 days prior to transplant depending on the individual protocol planned for each child. During this time, gut rest is often initiated and PN started, if not already being given.

Reduced intensive conditioning transplant can be used in some SCID patients. This is used where possible due to fewer side effects compared with standard HSCT. This type of transplant may be used where there is a good, matched sibling donor.

When children have coexisting organ damage myeloablative conditioning therapy has been associated with increased treatment toxicity and morbidity. Low intensity conditioning regimens have been shown to be as effective in promoting engraftment and donor immune reconstitution, with minimal toxicity and improved survival.

Infection remains life threatening to children having HSCT and all patients are treated in a reverse isolation unit with high efficiency particulate air filter. Meals may be provided by a designated ward or diet kitchen, or main hospital menus may be adapted following 'clean' precautions to reduce the risk of infection from food borne microorganisms (p. 30). Oral and enteral feeds may be pasteurised as an additional precaution. Some centres may allow commercial bottled water to be taken orally; however, common practice is to only allow water that has been boiled, whether tap or bottled water. Pharmacy grade sterile water can be used, but is often unpalatable. Food restrictions

usually continue for 3–6 months post transplant or longer if diagnosed with GvHD.

Complications following HSCT leading to impaired nutritional status

Mucositis

Mucositis is inflammation and/or ulceration of the mucous membranes. This may be present throughout the digestive tract but is most commonly in the mouth making eating or passing a nasogastric tube painful. It is often treated with gut rest.

Graft versus host disease

Graft versus host disease (GvHD) may be present in the mucosa, liver, lungs or skin. GvHD of the gut results in profuse watery diarrhoea, exacerbated by feed/food with a concurrent rapid decline in nutritional status [25]. GvHD is treated with gut rest and/or steroids in severe cases; therefore PN is often needed during this time.

Continuous, low volume amino acid based formula can be initiated once stool frequency has decreased. In severe cases it may be necessary to start with half strength feeds to reduce osmotic load. In some patients, feeds are not tolerated and instead a simple 'few foods' diet, e.g. plain chicken with potato or rice, may be gradually reintroduced. Some patients tolerate feed or food better than others, with no known explanation. Oral diet often starts as milk, egg, wheat and soya free, with the later introductions of these foods sequentially once the child is medically stable.

Venous occlusion disease

Venous occlusion disease (VOD) is a condition where the tiny blood veins in the liver become blocked as a result of chemotherapy. Whilst PN has been the preferred method of nutritional support post transplant, especially during times of gut rest, enteral feeding can be used successfully [26]. Almost all patients will require PN for a period of time if they develop severe gut problems.

If VOD is suspected, fluid restriction is indicated and lipid free PN may be necessary. The evidence base for this practice is lacking. Some patients are at higher risk of VOD than others, depending upon their conditioning regimen. It is important to monitor the situation and restart lipids as soon as possible. Lipid free PN is unlikely to meet energy requirements, particularly as resting energy expenditure may be increased [16]. Supplementation with walnut oil (p. 601) to meet essential fatty acid requirements should be considered early on, particularly if lipid free PN is used for prolonged periods, or if the patient is a young infant.

Dietetic management of HSCT

A suggested protocol is to pass a nasogastric tube prior to the start of conditioning, i.e. day 5 HSCT (day 0 is when the stem cell infusion is given), before mucositis may develop. Passing a nasogastric tube when the patient already has severe mucositis may be very traumatic.

Dietetic management of HSCT is similar to that described for SCID patients. Hydrolysed protein formulas are usually better tolerated post transplant than whole protein formulas. Patients may initially require a continuous feeding regimen, building up to an overnight feed, daytime boluses and oral diet. A normal 'clean' diet, including cow's milk protein, is usually tolerated and can be encouraged. Oral intake is often slow to recover to achieve full nutritional requirements, so some children may require enteral feeds for several months after discharge from hospital.

Regular follow-up and monitoring post transplant is crucial. Advice is needed regarding weaning off enteral feeds where appropriate and reintroducing any restricted foods to normalise intake; this will also decrease parental anxiety.

HIV and AIDS

Julie Lanigan and Lisa Cooke

Introduction

Human immunodeficiency virus (HIV) is a retrovirus that attacks the human immune system. Acquired immunodeficiency syndrome (AIDS) is a disease complex occurring as a result of HIV induced cell mediated immune deficiency which may cause life threatening opportunistic infections, tumours and other conditions. More than 30 million people are infected worldwide, including 3.4 million children under 15 years [27]. The majority of cases are from sub-Saharan Africa which accounts for about 70% of all infections.

The main source of HIV infection in young children is mother to child transmission. The virus may be transmitted during pregnancy, labour and delivery, or by breast feeding. Improved antenatal testing, perinatal antiretroviral therapy for both infant and mother, planned vaginal or elective caesarean birth and safe infant formula feeding have dramatically reduced mother to child transmission to less than 1% in the UK [28]. Avoidance of all breast feeding by HIV infected women is recommended in the UK to prevent transmission of HIV by this route [29].

Most children seen in the UK are of sub-Saharan African origin. Many of these present with undiagnosed HIV infection whilst others have received inappropriate treatment. Understanding the natural history of HIV and its progression in untreated children is central to their nutritional assessment and management. This chapter focuses mainly on the nutritional care of children in the UK but also includes a global perspective.

UK incidence and prevalence

National surveillance of paediatric HIV was established in 1986 and is carried out by the National Study of HIV in Pregnancy and Childhood (NSHPC) based at the Institute of Child Health, London [30]. In total 2355 children under the age of 16 diagnosed with HIV in the UK had been reported to the NSHPC by March 2011. To date only about 15% of these have died and monitoring is carried out by the Collaborative HIV Paediatric Study (CHIPS). CHIPS was set up in 2000 to monitor clinical, laboratory and treatment information on infected children living in the UK and Ireland

and is a collaboration between the Clinical Trials Unit of the Medical Research Council, the paediatric centres looking after infected children and the NSHPC [31].

Perinatal HIV transmission

To minimise the risk of perinatal transmission all pregnant women should be recommended an HIV test at the time of antenatal booking. Antiretroviral therapy (ART) can be started at an appropriate time, depending on gestation at diagnosis, previous obstetric history and other relevant considerations. All infected women should continue taking ART during labour; in most cases this will be their usual oral regimen. Following uncomplicated deliveries the infant is given single drug prophylaxis, but where problems arise during delivery which increase the risk of transmission the paediatric team may decide that triple therapy is required. Guidelines for treatment during pregnancy, labour and delivery and postnatal management of the mother and infant can be found on the website of the Children's HIV Association (CHIVA) [28].

Breast feeding

Breast feeding is a route of HIV transmission from mother to child and this poses a dilemma not least because of its importance in child development both biologically and emotionally. In the UK, to prevent the transmission of HIV infection during the postpartum period, the joint British and Children's HIV Associations (BHIVA/CHIVA) recommend the complete avoidance of breast feeding for infants born to HIV infected mothers, regardless of maternal disease status, viral load or treatment. The World Health Organization (WHO) infant feeding guidelines recommend formula feeding only when certain conditions are met [32]. These include availability of safe clean water, affordability of infant formula and hygienic conditions for feed preparation. In less developed settings mothers known to be HIV infected (and whose infants are HIV uninfected or of unknown HIV status) should exclusively breast feed their infants for the first 6 months of life, introducing appropriate complementary foods thereafter, and continue breast feeding for the first 12 months of life.

Breast feeding should then only stop once a nutritionally adequate and safe diet without breast milk can be provided. Once the decision to breast feed has been made, however, adherence to exclusive breast feeding is recommended to help minimise the risk of transmission. There are many factors which influence the risk of transmission through breast feeding. High viral load, reduced CD4 count, breast pathology (e.g. mastitis), presence of infection and prolonged duration of breast feeding (>6 months) are all strongly related to increased transmission risk. Other related factors include non exclusive breast feeding during the first 6 months of life, maternal vitamin deficiencies (B, C and E) and infant oral lesions [29]. Safer breast feeding can be achieved by encouraging

- exclusive breast feeding up to 6 months of age
- good lactation management
- abstaining from breast feeding during mastitis
- prompt treatment of oral thrush

For mothers choosing to breast feed it is important that exclusivity is maintained to maximise the protective effect of breast feeding on the gut mucosa, thereby minimising the risk of viral transmission from breast milk. Abrupt cessation of breast feeding is no longer advisable because of negative effects for the mother and infant. When mothers known to be HIV infected decide to stop breast feeding, infants should be provided with safe and adequate replacement feeds to enable normal growth and development.

Diagnosis

The most widely available test worldwide (HIV-ELISA) detects antibodies to HIV rather than the virus itself. All babies born to infected women will have passively acquired antibodies to HIV which may persist, on average, to 10 months of age and in some cases up to 18 months. It is therefore not possible to reliably diagnose infants on the basis of antibody presence until beyond this age. There is a highly sensitive and specific test available in the UK that can detect the presence of viral DNA, HIV DNA polymerase chain reaction (PCR); this can be used as a diagnostic test in infants. Infection can be diagnosed in the majority of non breast feeding infants by 1 month of age using this method. Testing should be carried out before the child is

48 hours old, repeated at 1–2 months and again at 3–6 months. Diagnoses in children over the age of 18 months can be reliably made on the presence of HIV antibody.

Antiretroviral therapy should be started in all infants irrespective of clinical or immunological stage as soon as the diagnosis of infection is confirmed. Treatment in children is based on a paediatric clinical and immunological staging system for HIV infection (Tables 15.2, 15.3). Guidelines for HIV testing in children can be found on the CHIVA website [33].

Disease progression

In children the course of disease has a more rapid progression to AIDS than in adults. Under the age of 5 years children have higher viral loads and are susceptible to more frequent recurrent bacterial infections than is usual in childhood. Their immature immune system makes them more vulnerable to the opportunistic infections characteristic of HIV infection that take an aggressive course and can be life threatening.

Diseases such as pneumocystis carinii pneumonia (PCP) and cytomegalovirus (CMV) are common in children with PCP being the leading AIDS defining illness and cause of death in HIV infected infants. Lymphocytic interstitial pneumonitis, a lung disease rarely seen in adults, also occurs frequently in HIV infected children.

Paediatric HIV disease often presents as growth faltering, diagnosed by a downward crossing of growth percentiles, and may be accompanied by frequent recurrent infections. In infants neurodevelopment and motor skills, such as crawling and walking, may be delayed. There have been considerable advances in treatment of HIV infection in infants and children in the last 10 years following the introduction of highly active antiretroviral therapy (HAART). Growth faltering in HIV positive children is now rarely seen in the UK in those who attend clinic for regular monitoring. However, children recently arrived from HIV endemic areas may present with untreated HIV infection that is frequently accompanied by growth faltering.

A small subset of human immunodeficiency virus type 1 (HIV-1) infected individuals who are therapy naive – referred to as long term non progressors – maintain a favourable course and

may be asymptomatic for many years [36]. Such children do not require ART. It is important to preserve treatment options for all children to minimise the risk of resistance. Therefore, beyond infancy, HAART is usually delayed until clinical symptoms develop or there is evidence of declining immune function. A broad spectrum antibiotic cotrimoxazole (Septrin) should be prescribed to all infected infants under the age of 1 year and to those at high risk of transmission. It is also used in HIV infected children of all ages who show signs of declining immune function. Adherence to treatment regimens is extremely important both to ensure maintenance of therapeutic levels and to prevent development of drug resistance.

A multidisciplinary approach to care planning is essential involving close liaison with doctors, nurses, occupational therapists, physiotherapists, psychologists and social workers. Where possible, links with the community team should also be made. Families with HIV need access to high quality medical care. A strategy to develop clinical networks for paediatric HIV treatment and care is currently under development [35] with the paediatric sub-group of the London HIV Consortium aiming to establish clinical networks which employ lead clinicians who should develop common protocols and shared care guidelines, in collaboration with CHIVA.

Social problems

Many HIV infected children in the UK are born to mothers from high prevalence countries, particularly sub-Saharan Africa; a very small number may have contracted HIV from mothers using intravenous drugs. Associated poor/temporary housing facilities, isolation, physical and mental health of other family members may contribute to poor nutrition. Confidentiality and fears of disclosing the diagnosis of HIV can hinder liaison with appropriate health and social support providers. HIV is a disease with a great degree of social stigma attached and appropriate disclosure is an essential part of successful management. For many families the fear of friends and neighbours being made aware of the diagnosis can be greater than the fear of the disease itself and may lead to a loss of compliance with medication, diet and even with accessing treatment. For children this can be

Table 15.2   Centers for Disease Control (CDC) classification for paediatric HIV infection.

Clinical category	Symptom severity	Type of symptoms
N	No symptoms	Children who have no symptoms considered to be the result of HIV infection or only one of the symptoms listed in category A
A	Mildly symptomatic: children with 2 or more symptoms in category A, but none of the symptoms in category B or C	Lymphadenopathy; hepatomegaly; splenomegaly; dermatitis; parotitis; recurrent upper respiratory tract infection, sinusitis or otitis media
B	Moderately symptomatic: children have symptoms in category B	Anaemia, neutropenia or thrombocytopenia; single serious bacterial infection (e.g. pneumonia, bacteraemia); candidiasis, oropharyngeal (thrush); cardiomyopathy; cytomegalovirus infection; diarrhoea (recurrent or chronic); hepatitis; herpes stomatitis, recurrent; lymphoid interstitial pneumonia; nephropathy; persistent fever >1 month; varicella zoster (persistent or complicated primary chickenpox or shingles)
C	Severely symptomatic: examples of conditions in clinical category C together with any condition listed in the 1987 surveillance case definition for AIDS, with the exception of lymphoid interstitial pneumonia. See link for more details [61]	**1** Serious bacterial infections, multiple or recurrent **2** Opportunistic infections Candidiasis (oesophageal, pulmonary); cytomegalovirus disease with onset of symptoms at age >1 month; cryptosporidiosis with diarrhoea persisting 1 month; *Mycobacterium tuberculosis*, disseminated or extrapulmonary; *M. avium* complex or *M. kansasii*, disseminated; *Pneumocystis carinii* pneumonia (PCP); progressive multifocal leukoencephalopathy; toxoplasmosis of the brain with onset at age >1 month **3** Severe failure to thrive/wasting syndrome Crossing at least two percentile lines on growth chart (e.g. 90th to 50th, or 50th to 10th) or <3rd percentile and continuing to deviate downwards from it over a 3 month period, or >10% loss of body weight in older child *plus* **(a)** chronic diarrhoea >30 days OR **(b)** documented intermittent or constant fever >30 days **4** HIV encephalopathy At least one of the following progressive findings for at least 2 months in the absence of a concurrent illness other than HIV infection that could explain the findings: **(a)** failure to attain or loss of developmental milestones or loss of intellectual ability, verified by standard developmental scale or neuropsychological tests **(b)** impaired brain growth or acquired microcephaly demonstrated by head circumference measurements or by brain atrophy demonstrated by computerised tomography or magnetic resonance imaging (serial imaging for children <2 years of age) **(c)** acquired symmetric motor deficit manifested by two or more of the following: paresis, pathologic reflexes, ataxia or gait disturbance **5** Malignancy

Source: Adapted from MMWR, 1994 [64].

Table 15.3 Revised human immunodeficiency virus paediatric classification system: immune categories based on age-specific CD4+ T cell count and percentage, 1994.

Immune category	<12 months		1–5 year		6–12 year	
	No./mm^3	(%)	No./mm^3	(%)	No./mm^3	(%)
Category 1: No suppression	≥1500	(≥25%)	≥1000	(≥25%)	≥500	(≥25%)
Category 2: Moderate suppression	750–1499	(15%–24%)	500–999	(15%–24%)	200–499	(15%–24%)
Category 3: Severe suppression	<750	(<15%)	<500	(<15%)	<200	(<15%)

Source: Adapted from MMWR, 1994 [64].

particularly distressing. In many cases parents are unwilling to disclose the diagnosis and it is essential that the professional involved in the family's care is informed of the disclosure status within the family unit before attempting to give advice.

Nutritional considerations

HIV affects nutrition in many ways and a combination of increased energy expenditure, malabsorption and altered macronutrient metabolism can lead to negative energy balance and weight loss. Although studies among apparently healthy children infected with HIV show no difference in resting metabolic rate (RMR), studies among children suffering opportunistic infections show they have raised energy expenditure [36]. Children infected with HIV may have increased energy requirements of around 10%, and whilst recovering from illness this may increase by 50%–100%, above established requirements of healthy uninfected children [37].

Providing optimal nutrition to children with HIV is critical for two reasons: it provides the greatest opportunity for normal growth and development; and it supports the optimal functioning of the immune system [38].

When planning nutritional advice for HIV infected children several related aspects also need to be considered such as disease state, growth and development, social factors and geographical location, e.g. children living in developing countries may be undernourished whereas in the UK excess nutrition is more common. Side effects of treatment regimens and their interactions with foods should be taken into consideration. Details of antiretroviral drugs and food interactions can be found on the Paediatric European Network for Treatment

of AIDS website [39] and are summarised in Table 15.4.

Nutritional requirements

Energy

Increased RMR is an important contributor to energy imbalance in HIV infected patients [40]. Energy requirements of children with HIV are best estimated to meet 100% of the estimated average requirement for age, with adjustments made for mobility, infection, weight loss and malabsorption. When assessing requirements these should be based on the child's actual size (or height age) rather than expected weight/length for age, i.e. the age that corresponds to the child's height falling on the 50th percentile. This provides a better estimate for achievable food intake.

Protein

HIV infection is associated with a loss of lean body mass and it is well established that this depletion has adverse effects on morbidity and mortality [41]. Loss of body protein is the result of decreased dietary intake, malabsorption and metabolic change. During energy restriction fat stores are depleted first but, in HIV infection, several studies have shown that there is a preferential loss of body protein [42]. Evidence suggests that the metabolic mechanisms underlying changes in body composition that occur during HIV infection differ from those present during chronic food restriction and other diseases associated with rapid weight loss. Protein requirements for HIV infected children are not yet established, and although these have been estimated to be 150%–200% of the recommended daily allowance [43] there is insufficient

Table 15.4   Highly active antiretroviral therapy (HAART): food restrictions, drug interactions and side effects.

Drug	Food interactions	More common side effects	Drug interactions	More severe/rare side effects
Nucleoside reverse transcriptase inhibitors (NRTI)				
Lamivudine (3TC, Epivir), liquid, tablets	None – pre-dose meal may reduce nausea	Nausea or vomiting, abdominal pain, diarrhoea or constipation, headache, fatigue	None known	Pancreatitis MT
Zidovudine (ZDV, AZT, Retrovir), liquid, capsules	None	Nausea, vomiting, headache, muscular pain, sleep disturbance	Not to be prescribed with Stavudine	MT Liver toxicity Myopathy Myositis
Stavudine (D4T, Zerit), liquid, capsules	None – pre-dose meal may reduce nausea	Peripheral neuropathy, headache, nausea or vomiting, diarrhoea or constipation	Not to be prescribed with AZT	LDS MT Raised liver enzymes
Abacavir (ABC, Ziagen), liquid, tablets	None – pre-dose meal may reduce nausea			Hypersensitvity (fever, fatigue, nausea, vomiting, diarrhoea and abdominal pain or respiratory symptoms) Raised LFT Raised CPK Lymphopenia MT
Didanosine (ddI, Videx), liquid, capsules	Taken at least 1 hour before or 2 hours after food	Diarrhoea, nausea, stomach cramps, vomiting, rash	Food H_2 antagonists	Peripheral neuropathy Electrolyte disturbances Retinal depigmentation Hyperuricaemia Raised liver enzymes
Non-nucleoside reverse transcriptase inhibitors (NNRTI)				
Efavirenz (Sustiva), liquid, capsules, tablets	None	Skin rash, CNS disturbance (insomnia, nightmares, agitation)		Continuing CNS disturbance Liver toxicity
Nevirapine (Viramune), liquid, tablets	None	Skin rash, possibly life threatening (fever, nausea, headache)		Hepatitis, possibly life threatening (liver damage/failure)
Emtricitabine Emtriva), liquid, capsules	None	Headache Nausea Raised creatine kinase	Not known	Not known
Tenofovir (Viread), tablets	None	GI disturbance, renal disturbance (hypophosphataemia, increased serum creatinine, glyosuria, proteinuria, calciuria, phosphaturia)	Lactic acidosis, hepatomegaly and steatosis seen with use of nucleoside analogues	Based on animal studies, at high doses there is a risk of osteomalacia (none reported in children)
Protease inhibitors (PI)				
Amprenavir (APV, Agenerase), liquid, capsules	None – pre-dose meal may reduce nausea	Diarrhoea, vomiting, rash, perioral paresthesia (unusual feelings around the mouth)	None known	LDS DM Rash (possible sign of life threatening syndrome, Stevens–Johnson) Haemolytic anaemia

Table 15.4 (continued)

Drug	Food interactions	More common side effects	Drug interactions	More severe/rare side effects
Nelfinavir (NFV, Viracept), tablets, powder	With or after food (helps absorption and reduces nausea)	Diarrhoea (can be controlled with loperamide), nausea	In adults – not to be recommended in conjunction with rifampicin	Persistent diarrhoea Abdominal pain LDS Hyperglycaemia, ketoacidosis and DM
Ritonavir (RTV, Norvir), liquid, capsules	Best with food (reduces GI side effects and increases absorption) Bitter tasting – can be disguised with strong tasting foods or fluids, e.g. blackcurrant cordial, peanut butter	Headache, nausea or vomiting, diarrhoea, tingling/numbness in mouth, tiredness	Ritonavir and ddl should be taken 2 hours apart from each other	LDS Renal disturbance DM Dyslipidaemia
Atazanavir (Reyataz), capsules	Take with food to increase absorption	Raised unconjugated bilirubin, headaches, fever, dizziness, nausea, vomiting, diarrhoea, sleep disturbances	Take at least 1 hour before or after antacid or ddl	LDS Hyperglycaemia DM Pancreatitis Ketoacidosis Hepatitis
Indinavir (IDV, Crixivan), capsules	1 hour pre or 2 hours post food (except when taken with RTV) Ensure well hydrated If given with ddl take 1 hour apart and on an empty stomach	Nausea, GI pain, headache, taste changes, dizziness, hyperbilirubinaemia	NVP or EFV often decrease IDV levels	LDS Hyperglycaemia Ketoacidosis DM
Lopinavir + Ritonavir (LPV/r, Kaletra), capsules, liquid	Take with food to maximise absorption Bitter tasting liquid – can be disguised with strong tasting foods or fluids, e.g. blackcurrant cordial, peanut butter	Mild to moderate diarrhoea, nausea, vomiting, GI disturbance	ddl 1 hour before or 2 hours after Increase dose if given with NNRTI or previous PI exposure	Dyslipidaemia LDS Pancreatitis Hyperglycaemia Ketoacidosis DM Hepatitis
Saquinavir (SQV, Invirase, Fortovase), tablets	Take within 2 hours after a meal Do not take with grapefruit juice (interacts with cytochrome P450 to increase PI concentration)	Diarrhoea, nausea, rash, fatigue, headache, peripheral neuropathy, numbness, dizziness		LDS Photosensitivity (use UV protection) Hyperglycaemia Ketoacidosis DM
Fusion inhibitors (FI)				
Enfuvirtide (T20, Fuzeon), powder	Administered by injection	Not known	Not known	Not known

CNS, central nervous system; CPK, creatine phosphokinase; DM, diabetes mellitus; GI, gastrointestinal; LDS, lipodystrophy syndrome; LFT, liver function tests; MT, mitochondrial toxicity; PI, protease inhibitors; UV, ultraviolet light.
Source: Adapted from PENTA guidelines, 2009 [39].

evidence to suggest that additional protein can prevent loss of stores during the acute phase of infection. Moreover, clinical status may deteriorate if overfeeding occurs during sepsis [44]. Overall, existing evidence suggests that protein intake should be increased by about 10% to maintain body stores during the chronic asymptomatic phase of infection. During opportunistic infections requirements for both energy and protein are likely to increase to about 30%–50% above usual requirements but it is unlikely that an unwell child will be capable of achieving an intake above an additional 10%, which should therefore be advised. Once the acute infection is resolved, further increases can be encouraged to help achieve nutritional recovery.

Vitamins and minerals

Vitamin and mineral requirements are not known for certain. To date, with the exception of vitamin A supplementation in developing countries, no randomised controlled trials have investigated the effects of micronutrient supplementation in children and these should therefore be given with caution [45]. Evidence suggests that regular megadose vitamin A supplementation may reduce diarrhoeal disease and mortality and all cause morbidity and mortality in children under 5 years [46, 47]. Supplements of individual nutrients are not prescribed unless there are concerns that the reference nutrient intake (RNI) is not being met. Following dietary assessment, if requirements cannot be met by dietary intake alone, multivitamin/mineral supplementation may be advisable to achieve 100% RNI.

Complications associated with HIV infection

Frequent bacterial infections can lead to complications such as fever, more severe secondary infections and protracted diarrhoea with dehydration which may result in nutritional problems and hospital admissions. HIV infected children often suffer from candidiasis, a yeast infection that can cause severe nappy rash in infants and infections in the mouth and throat in children of all ages, making eating difficult. HIV related enteropathies are common, leading to food intolerance and malabsorption. Any one of these complications may lead to reduced appetite and dietary intake thereby compromising growth and development in childhood.

Growth faltering

Maintaining adequate growth of HIV infected children is a priority. Growth is an important predictor of morbidity and mortality and impairment is associated with increased gastrointestinal and respiratory infections [48, 49]. Energy intake is the main determinant of energy balance [41] and in HIV infected children reduced intake leads to growth failure [36].

Periods of decreased dietary intake associated with frequent episodes of infections are commonly reported by parents of children who lose weight between clinic visits. In combination with optimal nutrition, HAART may reverse growth failure and where HAART is available and access to food is not compromised chronic growth failure is not common. However, when growth faltering is diagnosed the contributory factors are often complex and interventions difficult to manage. Children who display suboptimal growth may not meet diagnostic criteria for initiation of HAART. In the absence of treatment the role of the dietitian is central to support growth, development and nutritional status.

Growth assessment

Growth assessment is essential for effective management. It is important to consider the child's genetic and environmental history, e.g. a child who presents with low height and/or weight for age may be genetically predetermined to be smaller than average and assessment of mid-parental height and weight can help to clarify this. Using the UK-WHO growth charts it is possible to calculate the mid-parental centile and identify a growth percentile range that reflects normal growth for a child based on their genetic potential (p. 6). In many cases an infected child may not reach their genetic potential due to early growth faltering as a result of disease, malnutrition or a combination of the two. In all cases a realistic growth target should be set with the aim of maintaining growth along the centiles that have been accepted as appropriate for the individual child.

Downward centile crossing of two major centile lines (one centile space) is indicative of growth faltering and in general height and weight should not deviate by more than two centile spaces. Low height for age (stunting) is commonly reported and linear (length/height) catch-up growth cannot usually be achieved by nutritional intervention beyond the age of 2 years as the child's growth trajectory has become established. In clinical practice growth charts are essential and can be used to reassure parents that their child is growing healthily. Upward centile crossing of weight should be closely monitored as this may indicate the onset of obesity. Measurements of body composition (e.g. skinfold thickness and waist, hip and limb circumferences) allow monitoring of adiposity and should be part of a child's routine assessment.

Gastrointestinal complications

Some children arrive in the UK with undiagnosed HIV infection and are therefore untreated. They may present with food intolerance, malabsorption, constipation and diarrhoea, all features of HIV infection. These are often transitory and can result either from HIV related enteropathies in undiagnosed children or as side effects of treatment following diagnosis. Protein hydrolysate and/or amino acid based feeds may be required in the short term while the infection is stabilised and the treatment regimen is adjusted (Tables 7.7, 7.11). Lactose intolerance is particularly prevalent in this group who are largely of sub-Saharan African origin (a region where this condition is more common). Carbohydrate malabsorption occurs often in HIV infected children, even in those who are free from gastrointestinal infections, and can be severe among immune compromised children [50]. Specific advice for food intolerance should be provided together with supporting information regarding how to obtain and prepare appropriate foods.

When nutritional needs cannot be met orally, supplementary tube feeding may be used as an adjunct to the normal diet; if long term nutritional support is predicted, gastrostomy feeding may be considered. Enteral feeding is an unusual step to take in the UK as food is more plentiful and affordable and oral nutritional supplements are available free on prescription.

Dyslipidaemia and the lipodystrophy syndrome

The HIV associated lipodystrophy syndrome (HIV-LDS) is characterised by redistribution of adipose tissue which can manifest as a marked loss of subcutaneous fat in the periphery (lipoatrophy) and/or increases in intra-abdominal fat (lipohypertrophy). Changes in body fat may be accompanied by features of the metabolic syndrome including insulin resistance, impaired glucose tolerance and dyslipidaemia.

Diagnosis of HIV-LDS is difficult in the absence of widely accepted objective diagnostic criteria but it is nevertheless an important consideration in the treatment of HIV infected children who are already known to be at increased risk of cardiovascular disease [51].

Dyslipidaemia is seen in association with HIV infection in children regardless of treatment and is thought to arise in part secondarily to fat redistribution but also as a result of drug toxicity [52]. The classical changes observed in the lipid profile are elevated serum total cholesterol (TC), low density lipoprotein cholesterol (LDL-C), triglycerides and reduced high density lipoprotein cholesterol [27–30].

Studies investigating the relationship between HAART and the lipid profile in children have reported hypercholesterolaemia (HC), defined by the American Heart Association as TC concentration >95th percentile for age and gender (≥5.2 mmol/L), in 13%–47% of treated children [53, 54]. Raised plasma TC has been reported in children treated with non nucleoside reverse transcriptase inhibitors (NNRTI) but the greatest effects have been seen in association with protease inhibitors (PI). Synergistic effects have been reported for PI in combination with NNRTI [55].

The obvious concern of these findings is the implication that HAART and particularly PI treatments may increase the risk of cardiovascular disease in adult life. Assessment of endothelial dysfunction, an accepted risk factor for development of atherosclerosis, through measurement of brachial artery flow mediated dilatation found that children receiving therapy had reduced vascular function compared with those not receiving treatment; children on a PI inclusive regimen were worst affected [51].

Rare complications

Mitochondrial toxicity (MT) may result from therapy with certain classes of ART drugs (Table 15.4) and is implicated in a wide range of toxicities including neurological disease in infants, peripheral neuropathy and hepatic stenosis. Lactic acidosis is a rare but serious side effect of MT and is potentially fatal; however this has rarely been reported in children. There have been increasing reports of osteonecrosis and abnormalities of bone mineral metabolism in patients receiving HAART [56, 57].

Nutritional assessment

At baseline all children should receive a nutritional assessment including

- weight
- length/height
- head circumference (infants and children <2 years)
- waist, hip and mid upper arm circumferences. Longitudinal measurements (6 monthly) will allow monitoring of changes in body composition
- detailed diet history, with special attention to food intolerance, feeding difficulties, use of supplements
- medication history, with special attention to drug interactions, vitamin and mineral supplements, alternative therapies
- biochemical assessment, with special attention to cholesterol/triglycerides and vitamin D

This assessment should be repeated annually; a form has been designed for dietitians working in paediatric HIV in the UK to use and can be downloaded from the CHIVA website [58]. Some measurements should be carried out more frequently, e.g. to monitor effects of HAART when commencing treatment or changing regimen. Plasma lipid concentrations should be measured about 3 months after commencement of therapy

and after a change has been made. Biochemical monitoring is a routine aspect of HIV care and where possible dietetic surveillance should be used to help identify children at risk of metabolic abnormalities. The lipid profile should be assessed following each routine clinic appointment and monitored at annual dietetic assessment. Children with raised TC or LDL-C or triglycerides on two consecutive occasions should be referred for lipid management. Initially this should be managed conservatively through diet and lifestyle intervention but in children aged >8 years protracted cases may be considered for pharmaceutical intervention.

Height and weight should be measured at each clinic visit (ideally 3 monthly) and plotted on UK-WHO growth charts [59]. Downward or upward crossing of centiles indicates the need for nutritional assessment and possible dietetic intervention.

Dietary treatment for children

Based on disease severity children fall into two broad categories: asymptomatic and symptomatic. However, children will cross categories throughout the course of treatment, e.g. a child once referred for growth faltering may present at a later stage in treatment with overweight/obesity and/or lipid abnormalities. There is a wide range of symptoms and disease severity within the symptomatic category of children and careful assessment is needed for accurate dietetic diagnosis. The aims of advice and treatment are to

- provide optimal nutrition
- support regeneration of the immune system
- maintain growth, development and activity
- help adherence to medication
- preserve lean body mass
- prevent overweight and obesity
- encourage cardioprotective diet
- encourage healthy eating
- provide advice on food safety and hygiene

For most children a balanced diet should provide all essential nutrients (with the exception of vitamin D). In the UK it is recommended that all children <5 years are given supplements of vitamins A, C and D (p. 731). Serum vitamin D levels are frequently low in HIV infected children and supplementation above UK recommendations may be necessary. Guidelines for vitamin D supplementation are currently under development. In symptomatic children additional dietary advice may be needed to alleviate disease symptoms and redress deficiencies.

A full diet history will give the best estimate of the quality of the diet and its nutritional adequacy. This method poses the least burden on families who are often having difficulties managing the disease and their lives. Particular attention should be paid to traditional diet and ways of cooking. Many families are refugees or immigrants and may be living in temporary accommodation with limited cooking facilities. Furthermore, knowledge of foods available in the UK may be poor and the dietitian will need to glean information relating to eating practices in the country of origin and translate to advice appropriate to the UK. Families need to be equipped with the knowledge and skills necessary to provide a balanced diet that is affordable, culturally acceptable and palatable. Showing knowledge and understanding of traditional foods and eating practices is central to the successful transmission of dietary advice for the specific population it is aimed at. Careful questioning should collect the following information:

- in infants and young children, intake of milk and solids
- weaning practices, including timing and usual foods
- quantity and variety of sources of protein, carbohydrate, fat, vitamins and minerals
- textures managed, e.g. puréed, soft, hard foods
- meal pattern and time taken to eat main meals
- type and timing of snacks and drinks
- amount of food eaten outside the home, e.g. at nursery or school
- feeding problems
- cooking facilities and equipment
- financial status

Some children, in particular those newly diagnosed, present with feeding problems which may affect their nutritional intake. Many of these require referral to and discussion with other members of the multidisciplinary team after which appropriate dietetic interventions can be implemented. Social workers should be included and are invaluable in assessing the need for and accessing financial and practical aid. Some common problems and suggested dietary interventions are given in Table 15.5.

Delays in growth and development may occur and the infant/child's developmental age rather than the actual age should be used when assessing the most appropriate food textures, feeding position and utensils.

Advice should be food based wherever possible; if an increased energy and nutrient intake is required the usual diet should be fortified in the first instance. Convenient high energy snacks can be recommended in the short term but it should be stressed that these foods are for the treatment of an acute infection or period of growth failure and that in the long term healthy eating should be encouraged. If further short term nutritional support is required then age appropriate oral nutritional supplements may be considered (Table 11.3).

Diet and HIV related dyslipidaemia

There are currently no evidence based dietary guidelines specific to prevention or treatment of HIV related dyslipidaemia. In their absence the most appropriate dietary advice for children with a normal lipid profile is to follow healthy eating guidelines. Most national guidelines are similar to the recommendations of the American Academy of Pediatrics [60] which advises the gradual adoption between the ages of 2 and 5 years of a diet containing around 30% energy from fat and consumption of adequate energy to support growth and development. The recommended diet for children with abnormal lipid profile is similar to that recommended for the population, but saturated fat should be restricted to 7% of total energy and dietary cholesterol to 200 mg/day. Data from randomised clinical trials in children as young as 7 months of age have demonstrated that these dietary recommendations are safe and do not interfere with normal growth, development and sexual maturation [61, 62].

The amount of saturated fat is generally too high in the modern diet and can be reduced by keeping foods that are highly processed, especially those based on animal fats, to about a third of fat intake. Replacing saturated fats with polyunsaturated fats, e.g. omega-3 (found in fish, green leafy plants, seeds and nuts) and omega-9 fatty acids (found in olive oil) should be encouraged. These fats have been shown to have beneficial effects on the lipid profile.

Table 15.5 Dietary interventions in paediatric HIV.

Problem	Assessment	Referral/discussion	Intervention
Delayed weaning	Diet history Milk and solids intake Meal pattern Sleep and activity pattern		Assess and advise on appropriate milk intake for age, e.g. excessive milk intake and timing of feeds may reduce appetite for other foods
	Medical history Oral health Gastrointestinal problems	Refer to medical team if problems are reported, e.g. sore mouth, reflux diarrhoea, constipation	Consider medical conditions and advise appropriately Food intolerance – may need hydrolysed protein/amino acid based feed Diarrhoea – avoid spicy and fried foods; fibrous foods, e.g. wholegrain cereals and salad vegetables; caffeinated drinks, e.g. tea, coffee and cola Foods high in lactose may also affect some people, i.e. foods containing milk Bland foods, e.g. potatoes, white plain boiled rice, bread and pasta should be advised Assess fluid loss and intake Constipation – increase fibre and fluid if appropriate
	Social history Financial status Cultural beliefs Isolation	Refer to social work team if there are financial or social barriers to weaning	Provide weaning advice adapted to cultural needs Direct to support groups and aid sources, e.g. Food Chain
Neuro-developmental delay	Diet history Feeding techniques Meal pattern Behaviour	Refer to speech and language therapist	Modify food consistency Encourage finger foods Encourage daily routine Consider supplementary tube feeding/gastrostomy
Eating difficulties: swallowing and/or chewing; inflamed/sore mouth	Diet history Meal pattern Feeding techniques	Refer to speech and language therapist	Modify food consistency Advise on meal pattern
	Medical history Oral health	Dental problems Side effects of medicines	Soft, non acidic foods Avoid spicy foods and drinks Use straw to bypass lesions Suck ice lollies
Growth faltering	Diet history Appetite changes Meal pattern Timing of snacks and drinks Fluid intake Eating away from the home	Refer to medical team to identify/eliminate organic cause	Encourage energy and nutrient dense meals with small nutrient dense snacks in between Space drinks and snacks away from meals Discourage excessive fluid intake
	Disease progression Effects of medicines Social/cultural influences Behavioural problems	Refer to psychosocial team	Encourage energy dense foods: full fat milk, cheese, fats (include PUFA and MUFA and moderate SFA, use of omega-3), sauces, sugar/honey, jam Use age appropriate supplements if unable to meet requirements through usual diet and where child is severely immunodeficient and/or symptomatic and losing weight

MUFA, mono-unsaturated fatty acids; PUFA, polyunsaturated fatty acids; SFA, saturated fatty acids.

There may also be benefits from eating foods rich in soluble fibre. Examples of these include oats, legumes (pulses: lentils, peas and beans), fruits and vegetables. In addition to this children should be advised to reduce consumption of sugar and high sugar foods such as fruit juice, fizzy drinks and confectionery.

Obesity prevention and treatment

HIV and obesity are concurrent epidemics and dietary advice given for the management of dyslipidaemia in HIV is also relevant to obesity. In the UK, guidance for prevention, management and treatment of childhood obesity has recently been issued from the National Institute for Health and Care Excellence (NICE) [63]: include advice on achieving a healthy diet; address lifestyle risk factors within the family and social settings; incorporate strategies for behavioural change. Importantly, interventions must include at least one other family member. The guidance also recommends that nurseries, schools and childcare facilities should minimise sedentary activities and provide regular opportunities for active play and structured physical activity.

Useful links

Immune Deficiency Foundation

idf@primaryimmune.org

Bubble Foundation UK

www.bubblefoundation.org.uk

Children's HIV Association (CHIVA)

http://www.bhiva.org/chiva/index.html

Avert

http://www.avert.org/

Nam

http://www.aidsmap.com/

Children with AIDS Charity (CWAC)

http://www.cwac.org/

The Food Chain

http://www.foodchain.org.uk/

16

Ketogenic Diets

Georgiana Fitzsimmons and Marian Sewell

Introduction

The ketogenic diet is very high in fat, very low in carbohydrate with sufficient protein to allow for growth. The diet was first used to treat epilepsy in the 1920s [1]. Following observations that fasting decreased seizure frequency, the diet was designed to induce a similar metabolic response. Use of the diet decreased when new antiepileptic drugs were introduced in the 1950s. It has more recently regained popularity internationally due to concerns about side effects of medications and is considered when medications fail to control seizures. Current guidelines from the UK National Institute for Health and Care Excellence (NICE) for childhood epilepsy recommend considering the ketogenic diet to treat children with medication resistant epilepsy [2].

Approximately 60 000 children in the UK have epilepsy [3] and first line treatment is antiepileptic medication; however, in approximately 25% seizures cannot be controlled this way. After a first medication fails, there is only a 15% chance the second will be effective and only a 20% chance it will stop the seizure activity [4]. The ketogenic diet provides an alternative treatment option.

Ketogenic diets in other disorders

The diet is the treatment of choice for children with glucose transporter 1 (Glut 1) deficiency syndrome [5]. In this disorder an inherited protein defect causes disruption of glucose transport from the blood vessels into the brain. The diet is considered first line treatment because neurological symptoms, including seizures, are regarded as consequences of the energy deficit of the brain. The high fat ketogenic diet produces ketone bodies which the brain uses as an alternative energy source to glucose. Treatment with diet is currently recommended in Glut 1 patients at least until puberty.

Ketogenic diets may also be used as a treatment for pyruvate dehydrogenase (PDH) deficiency [6] and there is also increasing interest in the efficacy of the diet for children presenting with fever induced refractory epilepsy of childhood syndrome (FIRES) [7].

How the ketogenic diet works

The precise mechanism(s) of how the diet works to reduce seizures in epilepsy remains unknown, but

Clinical Paediatric Dietetics, Fourth Edition. Edited by Vanessa Shaw.
© 2015 John Wiley & Sons, Ltd. Published 2015 by John Wiley & Sons, Ltd.
Companion Website: www.wiley.com/go/shaw/paediatricdietetics

there are numerous studies investigating this. It may be due to the direct action of the ketone bodies producing an anticonvulsant effect, or to metabolic changes associated with ketosis. Hypotheses of anticonvulsant effects include:

- *Changes to energy metabolism in the brain.* Failure to meet brain energy needs may contribute to the initiation and spread of epileptic activity; the ketogenic diet increases brain energy reserves by bypassing less efficient glycolysis pathways and maximising tricarboxylic acid cycle function. This may influence seizure activity by increased production of inhibitory neurotransmitters, improved ability to buffer the extracellular milieu, or altering the resting membrane potential [8].
- *Alteration of brain amino acid handling.* Utilisation of ketone bodies as a brain substrate alters the metabolism of glutamate, an important excitatory neurotransmitter. Reduced transamination of glutamate to aspartate increases glutamate availability for synthesis of the main inhibitory brain neurotransmitter, gamma amino butyric acid (GABA), both directly and via glutamine production [9].
- *Role of neuropeptides and norepinephrine.* Anticonvulsant neuropeptides, galanin and neuropeptide Y, are regulated by energy states and may mediate action of the ketogenic diet [10], with increased levels being released in the brain [11]. Norepinephrine, an inhibitory neurotransmitter, may also contribute to the anticonvulsant mechanism of the diet [12].
- *Calorie restriction.* Calorie (energy) restriction may underlie the anticonvulsant mechanism of the diet; this alone has been shown to reduce seizure susceptibility in mice [13]. Calorie intake is not restricted to less than normal requirements when using the ketogenic diet as it is important to optimise the child's growth.

Figure 16.1 shows how the brain metabolises energy.

Types of ketogenic diet

Until recently there have been two types of ketogenic diet: the classical and the medium chain triglyceride (MCT) diet. Two further diets have been developed: the modified ketogenic diet (MKD) and the low glycaemic index treatment (LGIT). All types of diet are high in fat and restricted in carbohydrate.

Classical diet

The classical diet is based on a ratio of grams of fat (long chain triglycerides) to grams of carbohydrate and protein [fat:(carbohydrate + protein)]. A 4:1 ratio equates to 90% calories from fat with the remaining 10% from protein and carbohydrate (Fig. 16.2).

MCT diet

A modification of this diet was introduced in the 1970s using MCT as an alternative fat source [14]. MCT yields more ketones per calorie of energy than long chain triglycerides (LCT); MCT is absorbed more efficiently and carried directly to the liver in the portal blood. This increased ketogenic potential means less total fat is needed in this diet and thus allows inclusion of more carbohydrate and protein. The traditional MCT diet has approximately 75% of calories from fat, 45%–55% calories from MCT and 21%–25% from LCT (Fig. 16.2). MCT oil or Liquigen, a 50% MCT emulsion in water, can be used as the source of MCT.

Modified ketogenic diet (MKD) or modified Atkins diet

This is a modification of the Atkins diet and recent studies show similar results in efficacy to the classical and MCT diets in both children [15, 16] and adults [17]. At the authors' centre this diet is referred to as the modified ketogenic diet; in the USA it is known as the modified Atkins diet. This diet allows a free intake of protein; it is very low in carbohydrate and requires a liberal fat intake (approximately 75% of daily calories). It is frequently used in older children and adolescents who may not cope with the dietary restrictions of the classical or MCT diets.

Low glycaemic index treatment (LGIT)

The LGIT is designed to limit increases in post prandial blood glucose levels by restricting the quantity

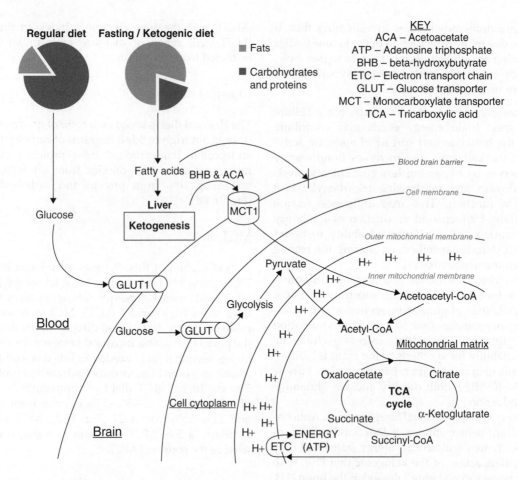

KEY
ACA – Acetoacetate
ATP – Adenosine triphosphate
BHB – beta-hydroxybutyrate
ETC – Electron transport chain
GLUT – Glucose transporter
MCT – Monocarboxylate transporter
TCA – Tricarboxylic acid

In the fasting state fatty acids cannot provide energy for the brain but ketone bodies produced in the liver enter the brain via MCT1 transporter providing energy during prolonged fasting.
The ketogenic diet replicates this metabolic state to give an alternative fuel source to the brain and the ketones possibly exert an anticonvulsive effect.

Figure 16.1   Energy metabolism in the brain.

of carbohydrate to 10% total calories and using only carbohydrate with low glycaemic index (GI) of <50; 60% of calories come from fat and 30% from protein [18, 19].

Efficacy of the ketogenic diet

Seizure reduction

Many studies have reported efficacy of the ketogenic diet. Freeman *et al.* [20] found approximately 30% of 150 children achieved 90% seizure reduction and 50% achieved 50% reduction. In a systematic review of 11 studies in 2000, Lefevre and Aronson [21] concluded there was sufficient evidence to determine that the diet is efficacious in children with refractory epilepsy although they were concerned about the lack of randomised controlled studies. A Cochrane review of the diet also noted this [22]. A recent randomised controlled trial showed success in treating children with epilepsy with no difference in efficacy between classical and MCT diets [23, 24].

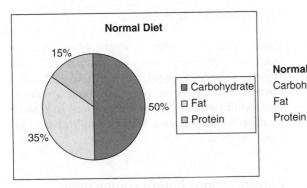

Normal diet

Normal diet	
Carbohydrate	50%
Fat	35%
Protein	15%

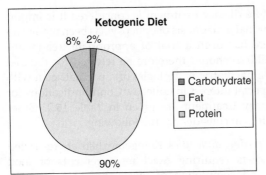

Classical ketogenic diet

Classical ketogenic diet	
Carbohydrate	2%
Fat	90%
Protein	8%

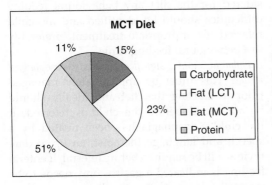

MCT diet

MCT diet	
Carbohydrate	15%
LCT fat	23%
MCT fat	51%
Protein	11%

Figure 16.2 Percentages of macronutrients in normal diet, classical ketogenic diet and MCT diet.

Seizure types

The diet has traditionally been reported to be most successful in treating patients with myoclonic-astatic seizures, or the mixed seizures seen in Lennox–Gastaut syndrome, although Freeman *et al.* [20] found no significant difference in seizure control between different types of seizure or epilepsy syndrome. The diet is increasingly used as a treatment for infants with infantile spasms [25–27].

Other benefits

Whilst few studies have systematically reviewed the improvements in development and behaviour reported by parents, one study noted significant improvements in development quotient, attention and social functioning whilst on the diet [28]. Although only some children become free of seizures, a larger proportion show a reduction in seizure frequency. Fewer seizures and side effects caused by antiepileptic medications may lead to children being more alert and able to make better developmental progress.

Successful ketogenic diet therapy may result in cost benefits as it may be possible to reduce antiepileptic medications for some children on the diet and some may be able to discontinue medications altogether [29]. Improved seizure control on the diet could potentially also reduce hospital admissions, emergency department attendances and GP visits with both cost benefits and improved quality of life for families [30].

Patients with epileptic seizures often have sleep abnormalities. Hallbook *et al.* found the diet increased rapid eye movement sleep which contributed to improvement in quality of life [31].

Some children have sustained reduction in seizures following discontinuation of the dietary treatment. A study by Martinez *et al.* in children who were free of seizures on the ketogenic diet showed the risk of seizure recurrence after discontinuation of the diet was slightly lower than after stopping anticonvulsants, and similar to that following surgery [32].

Possible side effects of the ketogenic diet

Many of the side effects of the diet can be resolved with dietary modifications as shown in Table 16.1.

Raised lipid levels

Raised serum cholesterol and triglyceride levels are common [37, 38]; this may be less of a problem on the MCT diet [39]. There is no evidence from case reports that the diet causes any adverse effects on cardiovascular function later in adulthood [40].

Delayed growth

Many children on the diet show a reduction in growth velocity [41–44]. Weight gain may be slower than before commencement of diet, particularly during the first 6 months, and the weight centile may drop gradually [45]. Weight and height should therefore be monitored and dietary prescriptions reviewed regularly.

Other reported side effects

These include cardiac complications due to selenium deficiency [46], pancreatitis [47] and hypoproteinaemia [48]. Haematological disturbances have been reported, both impaired neutrophil function [49] and alterations in platelet function with increased tendency to bruising and bleeding [50].

Considerations before commencing the diet

Before dietary treatment is considered it is important that a diagnosis of epilepsy has been made and there has been a trial of appropriate treatments. Children should therefore be referred for the diet by a paediatric neurologist or a paediatrician with a special interest in epilepsy. Contraindications for dietary treatment are given in Table 16.2. Other factors to consider are the following.

- *Feeding difficulties.* Ketogenic diets are restricted diets requiring exact measurements of food and completion of meals. Before being considered for the diet any behavioural feeding difficulties should be identified and the child referred for appropriate treatment, preferably to a behavioural feeding clinic.
- *Dysphagia and significant gastro-oesophageal reflux.* This must be appropriately managed prior to starting the diet and ideally should be addressed before the child is referred. If the child's dysphagia has been treated by a speech and language therapist, an up to date review will be required before referral. If enteral feeding is indicated a gastrostomy needs to be inserted prior to starting the diet.
- *Dietary restrictions and food allergy.* Although not a contraindication, multiple food allergies may make a ketogenic diet impractical; each child's case should be assessed individually by the dietitian.
- *Medical history.* Children with renal stones or hyperlipidaemia and those taking diuretics or medications which increase the risk of acidosis may be unsuitable for dietary treatment and should be assessed by a paediatric neurologist.

Table 16.1   Possible side effects of the ketogenic diet.

Side effects	Contributing factors	Possible dietary manipulations
Constipation	Limited fibre intake	Increase intake of low carbohydrate, high fibre vegetables Add fibre supplement, e.g. Resource Optifibre
	Insufficient fluid intake	Increase fluid intake Add sugar free laxative, e.g. Movicol Paediatric
Excess ketones	Incorrect administration of diet by family/carers	Check how diet is administered Treat with fruit juice (see Managing illness, p. 377)
	Fat intake too high	Reduce LCT/MCT (see Troubleshooting, p. 376)
Nausea, vomiting, diarrhoea	Incorrect administration of fat intake	Check how diet is administered
	Can occur on initiation of diet or if unwell	Introduce fat more slowly
Food refusal	Excess ketones	See Managing illness
	Calorie prescription overestimated	Adjust calories (see Troubleshooting)
	Dislike of meal choices	Offer alternative menu ideas Consider change of diet type
	Excess ketones	See Troubleshooting
	Underlying food behavioural problems	Offer alternative meal ideas, involve parent support groups to assist with menu planning Consider referral to specialist feeding team
Elevated blood lipids	High fat diet	Check blood lipid profile regularly Repeat fasting lipid profile if initial test non fasting Exchange saturated fats for mono-unsaturated fats and polyunsaturated fats
Exacerbation of reflux	High fat diet resulting in delayed gastric emptying	Smaller more frequent feeding Add/optimise anti-reflux medication Referral to specialist gastrointestinal team for further investigation
Renal stones	Occur in 3%–6% of patients [33, 34] Causes may include: (1) Dehydration	Optimise fluids Renal ultrasound is required prior to ketogenic therapy
	(2) Some antiepileptic medications, Topirimate, Zonisamide, Acetozalomide, can increase risk of renal stones [35]	Monthly urine dip stick test for protein recommended for all patients – if three consecutive positive tests will need renal ultrasound
Metabolic acidosis	Excess ketones Increased risk due to decreased blood pH if on Topiramate, Zonisamide or Acetozalomide	See Troubleshooting Medication may need adjusting – discuss with neurologist
Bone demineralisation and increased risk of fractures	Inadequate calcium, vitamin D supplementation [36] Chronic acidosis Previous use of steroids Non compliance with vitamin/mineral supplements	Supplement with sufficient calcium and vitamin D (see Monitoring the diet, p. 374) Consider alternative vitamin/mineral preparations
	Immobility Possible effect of antiepileptic medications, e.g. sodium valproate	Bone density scan Discuss with neurologist

Table 16.2 Contraindications for dietary treatment.

Definite contraindications [51]	Possible contraindications
Fatty acid oxidation defects	Concomitant steroid use will limit ketosis
Organic acidurias	
Pyruvate carboxylase deficiency	
Familial hyperlipidaemia	
Hypoglycaemia under investigation	
Ketoneogenesis/ketolysis defects	
Diabetes mellitus	
Severe gastro-oesophageal reflux	
Severe liver disease	
Non compliance of patient/carers	

Practical management of the ketogenic diet

Energy intake is expressed as calorie intake throughout this section on dietary management.

Implementation of the ketogenic diet can be difficult and success depends on core staff: a dietitian trained in the use of the ketogenic diet; a paediatric neurologist or a paediatrician with a special interest in epilepsy and experience of the diet; a specialist nurse. This multidisciplinary team (MDT) must be able to advise and assist families when they encounter problems either caused or exacerbated by the diet. Community support and easy hospital access must be available at all times. The support of a dietetic assistant, pharmacist and clinical biochemist may also be helpful for the core team.

Implementing and supporting a child on the ketogenic diet requires sufficient dietetic time. The authors' centre advises one whole time equivalent (WTE) dietitian for a caseload of 20 children (based on an audit of the time taken to establish children on the MCT or classical diet). However, with additional input from 0.3WTE dietetic assistant the dietitian to patient ratio can be increased to 1:24.

Hospital or home initiation

The diet can be initiated in an outpatient setting, but only if the dietitian can be in telephone contact with the family regularly to provide support; this needs to be daily for the first few weeks. Once established on the diet families require ongoing support to monitor and make dietary adjustments (p. 374).

Some centres prefer a hospital admission to start the diet. Infants should start the diet in hospital as they require particularly close monitoring.

Commitment from the family

The success of the diet requires the family and carers to be committed and willing to comply with the dietary regimen and monitoring. Families are required to monitor and record the child's weight, test and record twice daily urine or blood ketones, keep a seizure diary, communicate frequently with the dietitian and attend regular clinic appointments. The extent of the dietary restrictions and the need to weigh all food accurately must be stressed from the outset.

Preparing for the diet

Medical investigations and screening tests may be required before starting the diet, at the discretion of the paediatric neurologist. Any potential side effects should be discussed with the family at the initial screening visit (Table 16.1).

Laboratory tests and urinalysis

Urine organic acids and a blood spot carnitine test should be completed before the diet is initiated to screen for metabolic disorders that would contraindicate its use (see Table 16.2). These may have already been done to help determine a diagnosis. As these tests take time to be analysed they should be completed early in the assessment period.

Establishing the goals of dietary treatment

Realistic expectations should be discussed with the patient and family. Treatment goals should be agreed and documented before the diet is started and be reviewed at follow-up appointments to help decide if continuing treatment is indicated.

Dietetic assessment

A 3–4 day food diary is essential to assess suitability for ketogenic dietary treatment and give an indication of the child's food preferences and eating patterns (Table 16.3). This is used to help decide which diet is most suitable for the child and forms a basis for meal plans.

Pre diet meal manipulation

Some children may benefit from a reduction in sources of concentrated carbohydrate (CHO) and the introduction of high fat foods such as cream and mayonnaise, if not already part of the usual diet. Caution is required as introducing too much

Table 16.3 Factors to consider in the pre ketogenic diet dietetic assessment.

3–4 day food record diary to assess current dietary intake, eating patterns and nutritional status
Food preferences and restrictions
Behavioural issues with food
Food allergies or intolerances
Swallowing difficulties
Developmental feeding skills, food textures, thickened fluids
Fluid intake and types

Anthropometric measurements and recent growth trends

- Weight
- Height (for measuring children for whom height/length is not possible see page 5)
- Head circumference (<2 years old)
- Plot on centile charts to establish recent growth trends

Level of mobility and activity; immobile children may need fewer calories than active children
Vitamin and mineral supplements

Bowel habits

- Frequency
- Foods, medications or nutritional products used to treat constipation

Others involved in the child's care

- Family members, respite carers, nursery, school
- Health professionals: local team, school nurse, speech and language therapist

Seizures may influence energy requirements

- Type
- Frequency

Medications

- Formulations and carbohydrate content
- Side effects

Baseline bloods and urinalysis completed (p. 374)

fat before starting the ketogenic diet could cause excessive weight gain. Samples of Ketocal (p. 363) Betaquik or Liquigen can be given to try depending on the type of diet proposed.

Ketogenic meals appear much smaller than normal meals due to so many of the calories being provided by high fat foods. Sample menus illustrate what a typical ketogenic meal looks like and helps families understand all that is involved in meal preparation, e.g. accurate weighing and incorporating fat.

Pre diet manipulations should be supervised by a dietitian as excessive CHO restrictions could lead to hypoglycaemia, hyperketosis, weight loss or other detrimental effects. It may not be advisable to restrict CHO intake pre diet for children with Glut 1 deficiency.

Deciding which ketogenic diet to use

The 3–4 day food diary will form the basis for the type of diet chosen, but the child's and family's preference should be taken into account as well as palatability and ease of use. It is possible to change from one diet to another if the initial diet is unsuitable. The advantages and disadvantages of each type of diet are shown in Table 16.4.

Duration of dietary treatment

In most cases there is a 3 month trial period. Progress is then reviewed at an MDT clinic appointment and it is decided with the family if continuing treatment is appropriate. If the diet is of no benefit it should be discontinued. Some reasons for discontinuing the diet are

- child and family finding the diet too difficult and do not wish to continue
- diet is not effective in controlling seizures or not achieving goals set at baseline
- side effects outweigh benefits of the diet, e.g. poor growth
- non compliance

If the diet continues then 6 monthly reviews are necessary. In the authors' a trial off diet is suggested at 2 years to determine the ongoing efficacy of the treatment.

Initiating ketogenic diets

Calculating the diet

The diet prescription needs to be adjusted over time depending on the child's weight, level of ketosis,

Table 16.4   Advantages and disadvantages of different diet types.

Diet type	Advantages	Disadvantages
Classical	Uses 'normal' foods More experience in use of classical diet and more widely used EKM can be used to calculate meal plans Suitable for tube feeds (Ketocal p. 370)	Meals appear small because of the high fat content Very restricted CHO and protein
MCT	Less total fat allows more protein and CHO so meals may appear more 'normal' May be suited to those with limited food choices, high intakes of carbohydrate or the more selective eater	Possible gastrointestinal side effects or laxative effect MCT required with every meal/snack
MKD	Free protein, calories No weighing of foods, household measures used May help families or teenagers engage with a ketogenic diet who might otherwise find it too difficult	Generous fat intake still required (75% of calories) Very restricted CHO (10–20 g/day) May make dietetic management difficult as no control on calories May require more parent/carer input in designing meals
LGIT	Food not weighed, uses simple exchanges Currently limited experience in the UK	Limited CHO (10% total calories) Generous fat intake still required (60% of calories)

EKM, electronic ketogenic manager; CHO, carbohydrate; MCT, medium chain triglyceride; MKD, modified ketogenic diet; LGIT, low glycaemic index treatment.

seizure control and activity. For example if seizure activity decreases, mobility may increase and with it energy requirements (p. 376). Although fasting has been traditionally used to initiate the diet this has now been shown to be unnecessary [52, 53].

Calorie requirements

Calorie intake is carefully controlled on the ketogenic diet as excess or limited calories may compromise ketosis and seizure control. All calculations for the diet are expressed in (kilo) calories as the unit of energy and daily intake is based on the estimated average requirement (EAR) for energy as advised by the UK Department of Health [54]; however, requirements should be individualised.

Protein requirements

Protein requirements are based on safe levels for growth [55]. At the authors' centre the classical diet includes the protein content of vegetables in the daily allowance so it is important to give a minimum of 1.0–1.2 g protein/kg/day. This may need to be higher for younger children to ensure optimal growth [56].

Diet prescription for the classical diet

The calculation is based on

- calorie requirements
- protein requirements
- ratio of fat : (protein + CHO), e.g. 4:1 = 4 g fat : 1 g (protein + CHO)

Proportions of fat for different classical diet ratios are given in Table 16.5. A worked example of the classical 4:1 diet is given in Table 16.6 and an example meal prescription is given in Table 16.7.

An alternative method for calculating the diet is outlined in Kossoff *et al.*'s book *The Ketogenic Diet* [57].

On the classical diet, each meal and snack must be in the correct ketogenic ratio. The actual amounts may need to be rationalised so that the diet prescription can be translated into food, but the quantity of protein should not be reduced in

Table 16.5 Proportions of fat for different classical diet ratios.

Ratio	Approximate percentage of calories from fat (remainder from protein and CHO)
4:1	90
3.5:1	89
3:1	87
2.5:1	85
2:1	82
1.5:1	77
1:1	69

CHO, carbohydrate.

order to do this. The amounts of food per meal can be given as food choices calculated using UK food composition tables [58]. A sample menu is given in Table 16.8. Some centres have devised their own systems of food choices; these are not standardised, but are individual to each centre. Alternatively, a computer calculation tool Electronic Ketogenic Manager (EKM) is available to calculate and plan meals.

Electronic ketogenic manager (EKM)

EKM (MicroMan2000 Ltd) can be used with the classical diet to reduce time spent calculating meal plans. It is available as a free download for dietitians at www.edm2000.com. Parents can also use this tool but only if working in conjunction with a dietitian who provides target figures for meal calculations (confirmation from the medical/dietetic team is needed before download for parents is authorised). An example of a classical diet menu recipe worked out using EKM is shown in Table 16.9.

Meal replacements

In the event of a child being unwell with cough/cold/sore throat and not wanting to complete their usual meals, a drink can be given as a meal replacement to ensure that the child does not lose weight. Ketocal LQ is a nutritionally complete liquid preparation in a 4:1 ratio, designed to be taken orally. The calories for each prescribed meal/snack are matched by the calories in the Ketocal LQ (Table 16.10). The ratio should be kept the same as the child's usual prescription so glucose polymer

Table 16.6 Worked example for classical 4:1 diet.

A 22-month-old boy with late onset infantile spasms
Weight 12.45 kg (75th centile) Height 86.3 cm (50th centile)
Food diary analysis 1100 kcal/day
Weight centile > height centile therefore plan = 1000 kcal/day

Calculation
4:1 ratio = 90% kcal from fat

$90/100 \times 1000 = 900$ kcal
900 kcal/9 kcal per gram fat = 100 g fat

Remainder for protein and CHO

1000 kcal – 900 kcal = 100 kcal for protein and CHO
(100 kcal/4 kcal per g protein or CHO)
= 25 g protein and CHO

Safe level protein [55] = 0.97 g/kg
Aim: 1.2 g/kg = 15 g protein (60 kcal)
CHO = 25 g – 15 g = 10 g (40 kcal)

Daily prescription
1000 kcal/day
100 g fat
15 g protein
10 g CHO
Use the family's food diary to estimate calorie distribution for meals and snacks
Work out grams of nutrients per meal/snack
Divide kcal required for meal/total kcal per day
e.g. for a 300 kcal meal: 300/1000 × 15 g protein per day = 4.5 g protein/meal
300/1000 × 10 g CHO per day = 3 g CHO/meal
300/1000 × 100 g fat per day = 30 g fat/meal

CHO, carbohydrate.

Table 16.7 Example meal prescription for classical 4:1 diet: 1000 kcal diet, 3 meals and 1 snack.

Meal/snack	Amount of fat, protein, CHO
100 kcal snack	10 g fat 1.5 g protein 1 g CHO
200 kcal breakfast	20 g fat 3 g protein 2 g CHO
350 kcal lunch and supper	35 g fat 5.25 g protein 3.5 g CHO

CHO, carbohydrate.

can be added to the Ketocal LQ to achieve the required ratio. Alternatively Ketocal 4:1 powder (p. 370) (also nutritionally complete in a 4:1 ratio at the standard 20% concentration) or Ketocal 3:1 powder can be used and glucose polymer added to lower the ratio as required.

Initiating the classical diet

It is unusual to start the diet with a 4:1 ratio; this should only be done in hospital with caution. Most UK centres recommend starting at home with a 2:1 ratio and building up to 3:1 or 4:1 ratio over a period of days or weeks depending on the child's tolerance and level of seizure control at each step. Diet ratios can be increased more gradually for those who have problems tolerating the amount of fat, e.g. 2:1 to 2.5:1 to 3:1 etc. If a child has good seizure control on a low ratio it may not be necessary to increase to a 4:1 ratio.

Diet prescription for the MCT diet

The calculation is based on

- calorie requirements
- 45%–55% calories from MCT
- 10% calories from protein
- 15%–17% calories from CHO
- remaining calories from LCT

Table 16.8 Sample menu for classical 4:1 diet.

Meal	Prescription	Menu
Breakfast: Scrambled egg with bacon	20 g fat 3 g protein 2 g CHO	11 g raw whole egg, 5 g raw lean back bacon, 47 g raw tomato, 12 g butter, 18 g double cream
Lunch: Salmon and coleslaw	35 g fat 5.25 g protein 3.5 g CHO	17 g smoked salmon, 37 g mayonnaise, 5 g olive oil, 25 g raw cabbage, 25 g raw carrot
Snack: Cream and yoghurt	10 g fat 1.5 g protein 1 g CHO	17 g full fat Greek yoghurt, 17 g double cream
Dinner: Chicken with mushroom sauce	35 g fat 5.25 g protein 3.5 g CHO	14 g chicken, 20 g carrot, 35 g mushroom, 66 g double cream, 3 g olive oil

CHO, carbohydrate.

Table 16.9 Electronic ketogenic manager screen.

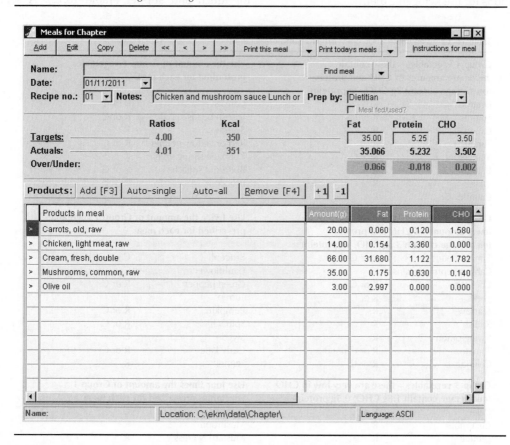

Table 16.10   Meal replacement drink for classical 4:1 diet.

Calories in meal 4:1 ratio		Amount of Ketocal LQ (100 mL Ketocal LQ = 148 kcal)
Lunch and supper	350 kcal	237 mL Ketocal LQ (1 × tetrapak)
Breakfast	200 kcal	135 mL Ketocal LQ
Snack	100 kcal	68 mL Ketocal LQ

Table 16.11   Choices for calculating MCT meals.

Choice	Average macronutrient content (g) per choice	kcal per choice
Protein	6 g protein and 3 g fat	51
Fat	5 g fat	45
CHO	10 g CHO 1.5 g protein	46
MCT oil	per 100 g = 100 g MCT	8.3 per g MCT
Liquigen	per 100 g = 50 g MCT	8.3 per g MCT

MCT, medium chain triglyceride; CHO, carbohydrate.

The calorie content of MCT is controversial. Original studies used 8.3 kcal/g [14, 23, 59, 60], although more recent literature suggests that this value may be nearer 7 kcal/g or lower [61]. European labelling law [62] requires a value for MCT that is in line with that of LCT, i.e. 9 kcal/g. This may be amended in the near future, but until this issue is resolved a figure of 8.3 kcal/g is recommended for calculations for the ketogenic diet.

The MCT ketogenic diet is planned to allow for greater flexibility and to give more CHO in the diet. The authors' centre uses an exchange system or 'choices' for protein, fat and CHO using the values listed in Table 16.11.

A weighed allowance of vegetables is given for lunch and supper (Table 16.12). A separate

Table 16.12   Vegetable allowance for MCT and classical diets.

Group 1 vegetables – these contain moderate amounts of CHO and protein (on average contain 7g CHO, 2g protein)		Use the amount of Group 1 vegetables prescribed for each meal	
Beetroot	R	Carrots	R or C
Sprouts	R or C	French beans	R or C
Onion	R	Swede	R
Turnip	R	Red or yellow pepper	R or C
Mangetout	R or C	Cabbage/spring greens	R
Beansprouts	R	Butternut squash	R or C
Okra	R or C	Broccoli	R
Cauliflower	R		
Group 2 vegetables – these contain lower amounts of CHO and protein (on average contain 3.5g CHO, 1g protein)		**Use twice the amount of Group 1 vegetables prescribed for each meal**	
Runner beans	R or C	Broccoli	C
Cabbage/spring greens	C	Cauliflower	C
Courgette	R or C	Green pepper	R or C
Leeks	R or C	Turnip	C
Marrow	R	Pumpkin	R or C
Radish	R	Spinach	R or C
Spring onion	R	Swede	C
Tomato	R or canned	Curly kale	R or C
Celeriac	R or C	Fennel	R
Group 3 vegetables – these are very low in CHO (on average contain 1.8g CHO, 0.5g protein)		**Use four times the amount of Group 1 vegetables prescribed for each meal**	
Celery	R or C	Marrow	C
Cucumber	R	Mushroom	R
Lettuce	R	Mustard & cress	R
Fennel	C		

CHO carbohydrate; R, raw; C, cooked.

list of CHO, protein and fat choices from foods is also given (Tables 16.13–16.15). Values have been calculated using *McCance and Widdowson's The Composition of Foods* [58].

A worked example for the MCT diet is given in Table 16.16. A sample meal prescription is given in Table 16.17 and a sample menu in Table 16.18.

MCT diet meal replacement milkshake

If a child is not completing their full meals a replacement milkshake can be given (Table 16.19). This milkshake is not nutritionally complete and should only be used for 2–3 days. It may not be tolerated if the child has diarrhoea and vomiting (p. 377). The calories for each meal/snack are replaced by using the milkshake. For convenience, one of the two specially designed ketogenic diet products, Ketocal (4:1 or 3:1 powder) or Ketocal

Table 16.13   10 g carbohydrate choices for MCT diet; each provides an average of 1.5 g protein.

Rice and pasta
12 g rice (dry weight)
13 g pasta or noodles (dry weight)

Breads and crackers
24 g wholemeal bread
22 g white bread
19 g scones or teacakes
15 g cream crackers

Breakfast cereals
14 g Branflakes
11 g Cornflakes
11 g Rice Krispies
13 g Weetabix
17 g porridge oats (dry weight)

Vegetables
58 g potato without skin (raw or boiled weight)
39 g roast potato
38 g sweetcorn, canned and drained

Fruits
150 g raspberries, strawberries or blackberries
100 g apple, orange, pear, peach or plum (no stones)
65 g grapes
43 g banana (without skin)

Other
13 g flour (white, wholemeal, plain, self-raising)
100 g semi-skimmed milk = $\frac{1}{2}$ CHO choice + $\frac{1}{2}$ protein choice

Table 16.14   6 g protein choices for MCT diet; fat adjusted – each provides an average of 3 g fat.

Fish
22 g tuna, tinned in oil
30 g white fish with an extra 3 g oil or 4 g butter, margarine, mayonnaise
30 g smoked mackerel
25 g sardines, tinned in oil

Meat
26 g raw beef
20 g roast beef
30 g raw lamb
21 g roast lamb
28 g raw pork with an extra 2 g oil or 3 g butter, margarine or mayonnaise
19 g roast pork with an extra 2 g oil or 3 g butter, margarine or mayonnaise
30 g raw mince (beef, lamb or pork)
27 g raw chicken meat with an extra 3 g oil or 4 g butter, margarine or mayonnaise
20 g roast chicken breast with an extra 2 g oil or 3 g butter, margarine or mayonnaise
33 g ham with an extra 2 g oil or 3 g butter, margarine or mayonnaise

Cheese
24 g Cheddar (count as 1 fat choice)

Other
1 small egg (approximately 50 g)
43 g Quorn
100 g semi-skimmed milk = $\frac{1}{2}$ protein choice + $\frac{1}{2}$ CHO choice

Table 16.15   5 g fat choices for MCT diet.

1 portion = 1 × fat choice
6 g butter
5 g oil
6 g mayonnaise
10 g double cream

LQ could also be used p. 363. Liquigen does not need to be added as these products are designed in a 3:1 or 4:1 fat to protein + CHO ratio and so will continue to encourage ketosis.

Initiating the MCT diet

MCT can cause symptoms of gastrointestinal discomfort: abdominal cramps, diarrhoea, nausea,

Table 16.16 Worked example for MCT diet.

A 8¹/₂-year-old girl in main stream school with teaching support
Weight 31.3 kg (75th centile) Height 130.6 cm (50th centile)
Food diary analysis 1900 kcal. A mixed diet, three meals a day, after school snack, takes a packed lunch to school and eats foods of normal texture. Enjoys pasta, potatoes and bread

Calculation
50% total kcal from MCT fat
Weight centile > height centile, therefore plan = 1800 kcal/day

50% kcal from MCT = 50/100 × 1800 kcal = 900 kcal
                 900 kcal/8.3 kcal/g MCT = 108 g MCT
                 (or 216 mL/216 g Liquigen per day)

10% kcal from protein = 10/100 × 1800 kcal = 180 kcal
                 180 kcal/4 kcal/g protein = 45 g protein
                 45 g protein ÷ 6 g protein/choice = 7.5 protein choices * (382 kcal)

Allow for 3 g fat per protein choice
                 7.5 protein choices × 3 g fat per protein choice
                 = 22.5 g fat (202 kcal)
                 (202 kcal + 180 kcal = 382 kcal)
                 This will be deducted from the final LCT allowance

15% kcal from CHO = 15/100 × 1800 kcal = 270 kcal
                 270 kcal/4 kcal/g CHO = 67.5 g CHO
                 67.5 g CHO ÷ 10 g CHO/choice = 6.5 CHO choices * (260 kcal)

Allow for 1.5 g protein per CHO choice
                 6.5 CHO choices × 1.5 g = 9.75 g protein (39 kcal)
                 39 kcal + 260 kcal = 299 kcal

Allow 40 g group 1 vegetables twice a day (allow 0.9 g CHO + protein/10 g group 1 vegetables) = 28 kcal

Subtotal kcal

MCT 109 g (216 g Liquigen)	896
7.5 protein choices (51 kcal/protein choice)	383
6.5 CHO choices (46 kcal/CHO choice)	299
40 g group 1 vegetables × 2	28
	1606 kcal

Remainder of kcal to come from LCT fat
                 1800 kcal − 1605 kcal = 195 kcal = 21.6 g LCT fat
                 1 fat choice = 5 g LCT fat = 21 g fat ÷ 5 g = 4 fat choices * (180 kcal)
Total kcal   180 kcal + 1606 kcal = 1786 kcal

CHO, carbohydrate; MCT, medium chain triglyceride.
*Round to the nearest ¹/₂ choice.

Table 16.17 Example meal prescription for MCT diet: 1793 kcal diet, 3 meals and 1 snack.

Total 1793 kcal	Divided as MCT = 109 g (905 kcal)	6 1/2 CHO choices* (299 kcal) 7 1/2 protein choices* (382 kcal) 4 fat choices* (180 kcal)	Plus vegetable allowance
Breakfast (470 kcal) 56 g Liquigen 1 fat choice 2 CHO choices 2 protein choices	Lunch (578 kcal) 72 g Liquigen 1 fat choice 2 CHO choices 2 1/2 protein choices 40 g group 1 vegetables*	Supper (600 kcal) 72 g Liquigen 1 1/2 fat choices 2 CHO choices 2 1/2 protein choices 40 g group 1 vegetables*	Snack (145 kcal) 18 g Liquigen 1/2 fat choice 1/2 CHO choice 1/2 protein choice

CHO, carbohydrate; MCT, medium chain triglyceride.
*See Tables 16.12–16.15.

Table 16.18 Sample menu for MCT diet, for meal prescription in Table 16.17.

Meal	MCT/Liquigen	Choices	Food	Weight
Breakfast	56 g Liquigen or 28 g MCT oil	2 protein	Scrambled egg	100 g
		2 CHO	Bread fried in MCT oil	48 g
		1 fat	Double cream to mix with egg	10 g
Lunch	72 g Liquigen or 36 g MCT oil Use 72 g Liquigen to mix with diet lemonade to make a drink	2 1/2 protein	Ham (1 1/2 protein) Cheddar cheese (1 protein)	49 g 24 g
		2 CHO 1 fat	Bread Mayonnaise Butter	48 g 3 g 3 g
		40 g group 1 vegetables*	Cucumber, celery Fresh tomato	40 g of each 40 g
Snack	18 g Liquigen or 9 g MCT oil	1/2 protein 1/2 CHO 1/2 fat	Cheddar cheese Banana Double cream	24 g 21 g 5 g
Supper	72 g Liquigen or 36 g MCT oil	2 1/2 protein	Chicken raw (use 8 g olive oil to cook)	67 g
		2 CHO 1 1/2 fat	Rice (uncooked weight) Double cream	24 g 15 g
	Serve sugar free jelly made with rest of MCT allowance, i.e. 62 g Liquigen	40 g group 1 vegetables*	Mushrooms Carrots Use 5 g MCT to cook	40 g 30 g

CHO, carbohydrate; MCT, medium chain triglyceride.
*See Table 16.12.

vomiting; however, if it is introduced slowly over 7–10 days these problems can be prevented. Calorie intake will be reduced while building up the amount of MCT in the diet so there needs to be an individualised plan to compensate for this by giving extra choices of protein, CHO and fat or 1–2 extra snacks for the first few days. MCT can be given as MCT oil or as Liquigen. MCT should be included in all meals and snacks. A snack containing MCT given as late as possible

Table 16.19 Sample meal replacement for MCT diet, provides 575 kcal.

Ingredients (extra water can be added to dilute)	CHO choices 2	Protein choices 2½	Fat choices 1
300 mL semi-skimmed milk	1½	1½	
10 g double cream			1
6 g Protifar		1	
5 g sugar*	½		
72 g Liquigen			
or use 388 mL Ketocal			
LQ (100 mL = 148 kcal)			

*Sugar is not usually given as a CHO choice but can be used for convenience for a meal replacement drink.

before bed may help maintain the best possible ketosis overnight.

Diet prescription for the modified ketogenic diet (MKD)

Currently there is no consensus among UK centres on how the MKD is administered. There are differences in the amount of CHO prescribed per day; how to give adequate fat; whether or not to measure protein. The daily CHO allowance ranges from 10 to 30 g. It may be reduced to optimise seizure control. Kossoff *et al.* looked at the ideal level of CHO when starting a child on a modified Atkins diet, whether 10 g or 20 g per day produced a more significant seizure reduction. Kossoff proposes that 10 g initially may be ideal, with an increase to 20 g per day after 3 months to improve tolerance of diet [63].

The authors' current practice is

- establish calorie requirements
- limit CHO initially to 20 g/day
- fat to provide 75% total energy
- a simple system for fat and CHO choices, spread evenly throughout the day, based on household measures
  - ∘ 10 g fat per choice
  - ∘ 5 g CHO per choice
- guidance on protein portions

In practice as protein is not limited it is unlikely that minimum requirements will not be met. Household measures are used rather than accurate weighing of foods as energy intake is not strictly controlled. The CHO intake of the child's diet is reduced and the fat intake increased gradually over 1–2 weeks until the diet prescription is achieved.

A worked example for the MKD is given in Table 16.20 and a sample menu is given in Table 16.21. Fat and CHO (including vegetables) choices are given in Table 16.22.

Enteral feeding

Ketocal

Ketocal is a specially designed nutritionally complete formula. It is available in either a 3:1 or 4:1 powder preparation, which can be used for tube feeding. It can be prescribed by the family doctor (general practitioner, GP) in the UK on the dietitian's advice and is currently only available direct from the company to the family home, not via pharmacies. The ratio of the feed can be altered by adding CHO or protein modules, by adding calculated quantities of the child's usual formula (pre ketogenic diet), or can be calculated in the same way as an oral classical diet. The administration of the feed can be similar to the child's usual regimen. Feeds are introduced slowly starting at a low classical ketogenic ratio of 1:1 or 2:1 and then gradually increased in a similar way to the oral classical diet. If a more gradual introduction is required then half ratio increments could be considered. Calorie content should be kept the same throughout the introductory period or during any increase in ratio. Macronutrient and micronutrient levels should be checked and vitamin and mineral supplements given as required (p. 372). These should not be added to the feed as they may cause the feed to

Table 16.20   Worked example for modified ketogenic diet.

A 14-year-old boy referred for a ketogenic diet would like to be independent as far as possible with preparation of his meals and is keen not to appear too different to his peers

Weight = 47.2 kg (25th centile); height = 164 cm (25th centile)

Food record diary 2000 kcal

As both height and weight on 25th centile give approximately 2000 kcal per day

Plan: 75% total kcal from fat (1.5:1 ratio approximately)

$$75/100 \times 2000 = 1500 \, kcal$$
$$1500 \, kcal/9 \, kcal/g \, fat$$
$$= 166 \, g \, fat \, (round \, to \, nearest \, ^1\!/_2 \, choice)$$
$$= 17 \times 10 \, g \, fat \, choices \, (1530 \, kcal)$$

Allow 15 g CHO (+ allow 5 g CHO from vegetables) = 20 g CHO per day

$$20 \, g \, CHO \times 4 \, kcal/g \, CHO$$
$$= 80 \, kcal$$
$$= 4 \times 5 \, g \, CHO \, choices$$

Total kcal from fat and CHO   = 1610 kcal

The remainder of kcal to be provided by protein: 3 average servings of protein rich foods per day

Diet plan: 17 fat choices and 3 CHO choices per day
Distribute vegetable portions over the day with meals and/or snacks (Table 16.21)

Table 16.21   Sample menu for modified ketogenic diet.

Diet plan: 17 fat choices*, 4 CHO choices*
In addition: up to 2 small servings (small cereal bowl) of salad vegetables per day

	Food	*Number of choices*
Breakfast	Scrambled egg with bacon or cheese	
4 fat choices	6 tsp butter	3 fat choices (to mix into egg)
	3 tsp oil OR 3 tsp double cream	1 fat choice (to cook bacon or add cream to egg if not having bacon)
1 CHO choice	$^1\!/_2$ slice bread OR 5 strawberries	1 CHO choice
Lunch	Smoked salmon	
	1 small cereal bowl of salad vegetables	
5 fat choices	9 tsp mayonnaise	3 fat choices
	40 mL Calogen as drink	2 fat choices
1 CHO choice	$^1\!/_2$ slice bread OR $^1\!/_2$ kiwifruit	1 CHO choice
Snack	Ham or chicken with cheese	
3 fat choices	9 tsp mayonnaise	3 fat choices
1 CHO choice	$^1\!/_2$ apple	1 CHO choice
Supper	Chicken for stir fry	
	Chicken	
	1 small cereal bowl of salad vegetables	
1 CHO choice	Bean sprouts	2 tbsp $^1\!/_2$ CHO choice
	Cabbage – shredded	1 tbsp $^1\!/_2$ CHO choice
5 fat choices	9 tsp olive oil	3 fat choices (use to cook chicken and vegetables)
	6 tsp double cream	2 fat choices (freeze the cream with sweetener to make 'ice cream' dessert)

tsp, teaspoon (5 mL); Tbsp, tablespoon (15 mL).
*See Table 16.22.

Table 16.22 Carbohydrate and fat choices for modified ketogenic diet.

CHO choice	Quantity
Fruit	
Apple	$^1/_2$ apple
Kiwifruit	$^1/_2$ kiwifruit
Orange	$^1/_2$ orange
Pear	$^1/_2$ small pear
Strawberries	5 strawberries
Starchy foods	
Bread	$^1/_2$ thin slice
Mashed potato	$^1/_2$ tablespoon
Vegetables	
Cabbage boiled or raw	2 tablespoons
Bean sprouts raw	4 tablespoons
Courgette raw or cooked	2 medium
Onion chopped	2 tablespoons
Carrots raw	2 medium
French beans cooked	4 tablespoons
Tomato	1 medium

Fat choices	
Butter	2 teaspoon
Margarine/oil	3 teaspoons
Double cream	3 teaspoons
Calogen	20 mL

1 carbohydrate choice is equivalent to 5 g CHO.
1 fat choice is equivalent to 10 g fat.

separate out. A worked example of an enteral feed is given in Table 16.23.

Modular feeds

Ketocal is based on cow's milk protein and is therefore unsuitable for a child with cow's milk protein allergy. If possible a milk challenge is advisable prior to starting the diet to determine if the child is still allergic to milk. If so, a modular ketogenic feed will be necessary. A worked example of a 3:1 ketogenic feed is given in Table 16.24.

Managing the ketogenic diet

Fluid

Fluid restriction is no longer thought to be necessary [52, 64]. Children should be encouraged to take adequate fluids to meet normal requirements.

Vitamin and mineral supplements

The diet requires full vitamin and mineral supplementation and preparations must be CHO free. Phlexy-Vits or Frutivits are suitable; the dose must be calculated for the individual to meet requirements (p. 21). Forceval Adult (1 capsule alternate days) is suitable for older children (7–10 years) who are able to swallow capsules. A calcium supplement may also be required, e.g. Sandocal. This may not be necessary with the MCT diet if an adequate intake of dairy products is consumed. The intake of all vitamins and minerals should be closely monitored to ensure nutritional adequacy.

Vitamin D

It is not uncommon for children starting the diet, or during treatment with the diet, to have low levels of 25-hydroxyvitamin D. Levels should be checked at baseline and 6 monthly thereafter. At the authors' centre normal ranges for 25-hydroxyvitamin D are considered to be >80 nmol/L for this patient group (personal communication); low levels are supplemented with 1000 IU (25 µg) vitamin D daily . The vitamin D content of the diet and any vitamin and mineral supplements are taken into account and the dose of vitamin D titrated accordingly.

Other supplements and medications

Potassium citrate

Some UK centres routinely give prophylactic medication to alkalise the urine to reduce the risk of renal stones forming (p. 277) [65].

Carnitine

Serum carnitine levels (both free and total) should be checked at baseline and then regularly monitored. Carnitine is involved in transport of LCT into mitochondria for oxidation and requirements may increase when following a high fat diet. If deficiency is found, a supplement of 50–100 mg/kg/day should be given [66], starting with 10 mg/kg to ensure tolerance. Although most children do not require supplementation [67] those most at risk of deficiency are in the younger age groups and those on sodium valproate medication.

Table 16.23   Worked example of a ketogenic tube feed.

A 14-month-old girl in status epilepticus is on multiple medications to try to control seizures. Seizure activity affects her swallowing. A nasogastric tube is *in situ*.

Current feeds: 800 mL standard infant follow-on milk, 160 mL bolus feeds given 5 times per day = 540 kcal (68 kcal/100 mL) plus 150 mL water

Total fluids 950 mL/day

Weight 9.3 kg (25th centile); she is gaining weight appropriately

Calculation

Ketocal **4:1 ratio** provides 146 kcal/100 mL at 20% concentration; 160 g made up to 800 mL with cooled boiled water = 1186 kcal

75 g Ketocal (9.4% dilution)	= 548 kcal	11.44 g protein	2.25 g CHO	54.8 g fat
per 100 mL	= 68 kcal	1.43 g protein	0.3 g CHO	6.8 g fat
		= 1.24 g protein/kg		

Start with 2:1 ratio and gradually increase to 3:1 and then 4:1 as tolerated and dependent on ketosis and seizure control
To lower the ratio add the girl's usual formula to Ketocal

2:1 ratio made up to 800 mL with cooled boiled water = 546 kcal

61 g Ketocal (7.6% dilution)	= 445 kcal	9.3 g protein	1.83 g CHO	44.5 g fat
19 g follow-on formula	= 101 kcal	2.28 g protein	10.8 g CHO	5.32 g fat
per 100 mL	= 68 kcal	1.45 g protein	1.6 g CHO	6.2 g fat
		= 1.26 g protein/kg		

3:1 ratio made up to 800 mL with cooled boiled water = 548 kcal

70 g Ketocal (8.8% dilution)	= 511 kcal	10.68 g protein	2.10 g CHO	51.1 g fat
6 g follow-on formula	= 32 kcal	0.72 g protein	3.42 g CHO	1.68 g fat
per 100 mL	= 68 kcal	1.42 g protein	0.7 g CHO	6.6 g fat
		= 1.24 g protein/kg		

CHO, carbohydrate.

Table 16.24   Worked example of a modular 3:1 ratio ketogenic feed.

7-year-old boy, weight 16.4 kg. Usual feed is 600 mL Neocate Advance, providing 618 kcal and 0.98 g protein/kg

Product	Energy (kcal)	Protein (g)	CHO (g)	Fat (g)	Na (mmol)	K (mmol)
140 g Calogen	630	0	0	70	0.42	0
23 g Complete Amino Acid Mix (code 0124)	75	18.86	0	0	0	0
4 g Phlexy-vits	0.12	0.01	0.02	0	0.22	0.02
16 g KCl oral solution (2 mmol/mL)	0	0	0	0	0	32
35 g NaCl oral solution (1 mmol/mL)	0	0	0	0	35	0
4 g Maxijul	15.2	0	3.8	0	0.03	0
Plus water to 700 mL						
per 100 mL	103	2.7	0.5	10.0	5.10	4.57

CHO, carbohydrate. Feed 600 mL of this recipe.

Minimising the carbohydrate content of medications

All medications should be as low in CHO as possible as extra CHO can affect ketosis and seizure control may be compromised. Sugar derivatives ending in 'ose' or 'ol' are usually converted to glucose in the body (cellulose is an exception and is acceptable). Sugar free medications often contain sorbitol which contributes some CHO to the diet and this needs to be considered if used. Syrups, elixirs and chewable tablets should be avoided as these generally contain more CHO than other presentations. Pharmacists can advise on the lowest CHO preparations of medications.

Adding interest to the diet

To help incorporate the high fat content of the diet a range of recipe ideas have been developed. Examples can be found on helpful UK and US parents' support groups websites (see Useful resources). These can be adapted for the individual child's diet prescription. MCT oil can be used for frying and roasting (beware its low smoke point). Liquigen can be used

- for making sugar free jelly, ice lollies, 'ice cream' dessert
- as an ingredient of 'quiche', scrambled eggs, mashed potato, sauces and soups
- as a drink to have with a meal (diluted with water with added flavouring such as sugar free squash or diet fizzy drink)
- for mixing with an allowance of semi-skimmed milk (full fat milk may be too thick)
- as a 'shot' of medicine

Ideas for using the fat and cream in the classical ketogenic diet:

- add butter, margarine or oil to vegetables or to the meal before eating, or use in cooking
- serve cream with allowed fruit and/or sugar free jelly or freeze to make 'ice cream' – add flavourings or sweetener
- add water to cream and use as 'milk'
- dilute 1 part cream to 1 part diet fizzy drink/ sparkling water as a drink
- oil hides well in 'ice cream', fruit purée
- mix mayonnaise with cream or oil or mix into cooked chopped meats or fish, or use as a salad dressing

Free foods

Water can be taken freely and up to 1000 mL of low CHO squash (CHO content <0.3 g/100 mL undiluted drink). The volume is limited as squash contains some CHO. Diet fizzy drinks are suitable. Sweeteners free of CHO, such as saccharin, are suitable. But powdered sweeteners should be checked as they may contain maltodextrin. A pinch of spices and a few drops of flavour essences can be used to flavor foods.

Monitoring the diet

Children should have blood and urine samples taken at baseline and throughout the course of this treatment. Full details of recommended laboratory tests and frequency are shown in Table 16.25 and other factors to consider at clinic reviews are suggested in Table 16.26. Although each centre has its own protocol for monitoring, national guidelines are similar. Frequency of monitoring at the discretion of the paediatric neurologist. Once established on the diet children should be reviewed in a MDT clinic at 3 and 6 months and then 6 monthly thereafter.

Daily monitoring provides essential information for any necessary dietary manipulations.

Seizures

Keeping a seizure diary, recording the frequency and type of seizures before and during the diet is essential to assess the benefits of the diet.

Ketones

Ketones can be measured in either urine or blood and should be measured twice a day, in the morning before breakfast and before bed. Once the diet is established and stabilised ketone testing may be done less frequently. Testing gives an indication of compliance with the diet and checks that ketone levels are not too high. Some children may have good seizure control with lower ketone levels. It is important to focus on seizure control rather than achieving certain ketone levels. Ketones are typically lower in the morning reflecting the overnight fast. It is important to note that levels can be affected by a number of factors other than the diet itself (p. 376).

Table 16.25   Suggested baseline and ongoing monitoring laboratory investigations.

	Baseline	At 3 months	At 6 months and 6 monthly thereafter
Blood investigations			
Plasma amino acids	√		
Full blood count	√	√	√
Renal profile includes	√	√	√
sodium			
potassium			
urea			
creatinine			
bicarbonate			
albumin			
Liver function tests	√	√	√
Calcium and phosphate	√	√	√
Magnesium	√	√	√
Glucose	√	√	√
Lipid profile*	√	√	√
Total cholesterol			
Triglycerides			
Vitamins			
A, E	√	√	√
D (plasma 25-hydroxyvitamin D)	√		√
Vitamin B_{12}	√		√
Folate	√		√
Copper	√		√
Vitamin C	√		√
Ferritin	√		√
Trace elements	√	√	√
Zinc			
Selenium			
Blood ketones and free fatty acids (beta-hydroxybutyrate and non-esterified fatty acids)	√	√	√
Plasma lactate	√		
Free and acylcarnitine profile (blood spot on Guthrie card)	√	√	√
Urine investigations			
Check for haematuria monthly at home/GP (using dipstick)			
Urine organic acids	√		
Calcium:creatinine	√	√	√
Urine urate	√	√	√

*If the sample is *not* a fasting sample and values are elevated, repeat test on a fasting sample.

- *Urine ketones* A dipstick is used to test for acetoacetate. Aim: 4–16 mmol/L.
- *Blood ketones* Blood ketone monitors are available; these test β-hydroxybutyrate. This method may be easier and more accurate than urinary ketone testing but depends if the child accepts having their finger pricked twice daily. Aim: minimum 2 mmol/L, although seizure control has been shown to be optimal when blood β-hydroxybutyrate levels are 4 mmol/L or above [68].
- *Hyperketosis or acidosis* Blood ketone levels >5 mmol/L, or urine ketones >16 mmol/L, should be monitored carefully to assess for hyperketosis or acidosis.

Weight and height checks

Weekly or fortnightly checks are used to assess if energy intake is appropriate. Height should be measured at the start of the diet and monitored at each outpatient appointment if possible.

Table 16.26 Considerations at clinic reviews.

Investigation	Review
Progress on diet	Achieving goals set at diet initiation?
Growth monitoring	Height
	Weight
	Head circumference (<2 years)
	Plot on centiles
Laboratory screening	See table 16.25
Nutritional assessment by dietitian to ensure diet remains nutritionally adequate	Food record diaries repeated as indicated
Seizure record diary	Daily diary recording pre diet and ongoing
Ketone record (blood or urine)	Daily diary recording pre diet and ongoing
Medications	Current antiepileptic drugs Possible to wean medications?
Education and behaviour	
Decision to proceed/wean diet	Review all of the above

Troubleshooting

Short term complications during diet initiation

These can include dehydration, drowsiness, hypoglycaemia, nausea, vomiting and diarrhoea [60]. Symptoms usually resolve after a few days, but it is important to initiate the diet slowly in order to minimise early side effects. This is especially important in children taking Topiramate due to increased risk of acidosis and excess ketosis.

Hypoglycaemia

Hypoglycaemia occasionally occurs on the diet and some centres recommend blood sugar levels are checked during the first few weeks of diet initiation and at clinic review. It is not unusual for children on the diet to have blood glucose levels in the range of 2.5–4 mmol/L (normal range 3.5–5.5 mmol/L); this is not a problem unless symptoms develop. Infants may be more prone to low blood glucose levels and should be monitored at diet initiation and until they are established on the diet and levels are stable.

Symptoms of low blood sugar include sweating, pallor, dizziness, becoming cold and clammy, jittery, confused or aggressive. Symptomatic hypoglycaemia, or blood glucose levels of ≤2.5 mmol/L, should be treated immediately by giving a drink containing CHO, e.g. 15–30 mL fruit juice. A doctor should be contacted; ongoing monitoring of blood sugars is necessary and further treatment may be needed.

Excess ketosis

The signs of hyperketosis are rapid, panting breathing; increased heart rate; facial flushing; irritability; vomiting; unexpected lethargy. This should be treated as for hypoglycaemia. If symptoms do not improve after 15–20 minutes, treatment should be repeated and a doctor contacted. It will be necessary to alter the diet ratio if excessive ketone levels persist.

Possible causes of low ketones

This may be due to

- extra CHO given (in food or medication)
- excess energy given in diet prescription
- the child developing an intercurrent illness
- after exercise (consider giving an extra ketogenic snack before or after exercise)
- starting steroid medication

Commonly asked questions

Table 16.27 gives some questions commonly asked by parents.

Check list for changes in ketone levels or seizure control

A change in ketone levels or seizure control should prompt these questions:

- Are ketones and seizures being tested and monitored correctly and regularly?
- Do all carers understand the diet (e.g. respite carers, school, grandparents)?
- Is extra food being taken/given?
- Is the child completing all the fat in the meals? (any measured fat used for cooking must be eaten and the plate well scraped of fat)
- Is the child unwell?
- Has a new medication been added that contains extra carbohydrate?
- Is weight gain appropriate? (insufficient/ excessive weight gain: ↑/↓ energy by 50–100 kcal/day)

- Do carers have the correct composition of any food/recipe changes?
- Are all foods being measured accurately using scales?
- Are vegetable/fruit choices being used correctly?
- Is the child drinking carbohydrate containing fluids? (check the type and quantity taken; if these contain some carbohydrate swap to a lower CHO version or limit the the quantity taken.)

To achieve better seizure control the ratio (for the classical diet) or percentage energy from MCT and/or carbohydrate (for the MCT diet) may need increasing or decreasing. If the amount of MCT is increased, the corresponding amount of LCT fat can be reduced to keep the same total percentage energy from fat in the diet. For the MKD, carbohydrate may need to be reduced.

Managing illness while on the diet

Ketone levels often drop just before a child becomes unwell and develops any symptoms of an intercurrent illness. This may be caused by a combination of factors, such as the infection itself and decreased physical activity. Although ideally ketosis should be maintained during an intercurrent illness, the priority is to treat the illness.

Close liaison between the ketogenic MDT and the investigating local hospital or GP may be necessary during times of illness, surgery or other hospital admissions. Clinical guidelines for health professionals for managing illness, nil by mouth status and surgical procedures are available [37, 69]. The child's local paediatrician and GP should be advised when the diet is started and provided

Table 16.27 Commonly asked questions on the ketogenic diet.

Question	Answer
How quickly will a response to the diet be seen?	Each child responds to the diet differently and it depends on the time taken to establish the diet. It may take several weeks before an improvement is seen
Is it normal for my child to be so tired?	When children start the diet they may feel sleepy and be more lethargic; this usually improves with time
Should the diet be adjusted if my child steals extra food?	No, but ketone levels may drop as a result. Continue the diet as normal at the next meal. If the child continues to take extra food the diet prescription may need to be adjusted to provide more calories so that extra food is not sought

with a copy of guidelines for managing illness in children on KD. Parents should also have a copy in a handheld patient file in case of an emergency admission to a hospital not familiar with the diet.

Illness may cause loss of appetite. Offering smaller more frequent meals containing less fat may be helpful. If the child is unable to tolerate full fat meals, it may be necessary to reduce the fat in the diet until recovery. Half the prescribed amount of cream, butter, oil and/or mayonnaise (or MCT if on the MCT diet) should be given at each meal and slowly increased to normal as tolerated. If the child is unable to complete their meals, having the food mixed together will ensure that what is eaten is in the correct proportion of fat to protein and CHO. This will help maintain some level of ketosis.

Sugar free drinks should be offered regularly to prevent dehydration.

If a child has diarrhoea, and/or is vomiting, oral rehydration solutions may be used, e.g. Dioralyte. These do not usually cause a significant loss of ketones; additional fluid should be given for each vomit or loose bowel motion.

If fluids are not tolerated orally (or through the tube if on enteral feeds) intravenous (IV) fluids may be required to prevent dehydration. Saline is recommended to limit disruption to ketosis. Dextrose infusions should be avoided unless there are concerns about symptomatic hypoglycaemia, or if IV fluids are needed for a significant length of time [69].

Additional calories in the form of extra meals or snacks may be necessary for a few days after an illness, e.g. if the child has been unwell and missed meals for 3 days, then one extra meal can be given for three consecutive days until the child is better and tolerating their full diet.

If the child has a febrile illness the diet can be continued as long as the child tolerates the food and is happy to eat. If not, a meal replacement drink can be offered. For example, if half a meal is eaten, then half a meal replacement drink.

If a child is on tube feeds these may need to be stopped when there is vomiting or diarrhoea. Some children may still tolerate smaller more frequent feeds, or continuous feeds. If feeds need to be stopped, water can be given to ensure adequate fluid intake. If symptoms continue for longer than 24 hours then an oral rehydration solution may be required. If the child is not able to tolerate enteral

fluids they should be seen by a doctor as IV fluids and additional treatment may be required.

Since ketogenic feeds are high in fat, when reintroducing feeds, half strength should be given for 24–48 hours, then gradually built up to full strength, as tolerated, over a few days.

Some children have an increase in seizures during times of illness. Families should be encouraged to contact their medical team if this occurs.

Pain relief medications

Low CHO pain relief medications can be used on the diet, e.g. sugar free Paracetamol, Medinol and Paracetamol suppositories.

Ketone and glucose monitoring during illness

Ketones

During illness it is important that families continue to check ketone levels twice a day (or more frequently if indicated) to establish if there has been a change in the usual level of ketosis, to make sure ketones are not too high and to check that the child is not ketoacidotic. Signs of ketoacidosis may include excessive fatigue or lethargy; nausea; vomiting; very strong fruity smell on breath; rapid panting breathing; increased heart rate (see troubleshooting section).

Blood glucose

Blood glucose levels may need to be checked regularly if there are concerns the child has symptomatic hypoglycaemia. This is particularly important in babies and children <2 years old. Blood glucose checks should follow any time of fast, e.g. on waking in the morning or if meals have been missed or not completed because of illness. For the treatment of symptomatic hyperketosis and low blood sugars (see troubleshooting section).

Discontinuing the diet

There are few formal studies to give guidance on how or when to safely withdraw the diet [70, 71]. The time taken to wean off the ketogenic diet varies for each child. The longer they have been on the diet, and the more successfully it has controlled seizures, the more gradual should be the change back to a normal diet. Weaning is done in a step-wise progression. When weaning the diet it is best to avoid making adjustments when the child is unwell, or if they are having more frequent seizures. An individualised weaning plan is required.

Seizures should be monitored throughout the weaning period. If at any time the seizures increase during weaning the diet is kept at the same level for a time or the child reverts to the previous step of the wean until seizures settle again. However, the usual pattern of seizure activity needs to be taken into account and any changes should be discussed with the neurologist.

The time taken to wean may be influenced by parental anxiety about the return of seizures and hence their resistance to weaning. Extra support may be required for these families. Advice may need to be given about normal healthy eating, particularly when children have been on the diet for 2 years or more. In most cases vitamin and mineral supplementation can be stopped once on a normal diet. The reintroduction of refined carbohydrate should only take place gradually once the child is established on an otherwise normal diet without ill effects.

If the diet is completely discontinued successfully but seizures recur some time later, parents may wish to return to using the diet again, or opt for medication. For the majority of cases this will be effective [71].

Weaning the classical diet

At the authors' centre the classical diet is weaned by gradually reducing the diet ratio stepwise from 4:1 to 3:1, to 2:1, to 1:1 usually over a period of weeks depending on seizure activity. Recommendations from the Johns Hopkins Hospital suggest that if the classical diet has been successful in treating seizures the ratio is reduced from 4:1 to 3:1 for 6 months and then to 2:1 for another 6 months, followed by a gradual normalisation of the diet [71].

Weaning the MCT diet

Discontinuing the MCT diet should follow a step-wise, gradual process with the amount of MCT slowly reduced. This can be achieved by reducing MCT in the diet by 5 g per meal daily, or in the same way that it was introduced into the diet. Gradually more protein and carbohydrate choices should be added to the diet while keeping the calorie content the same.

Weaning the MKD

Every 4–7 days the fat choices should be reduced by a half or one choice and the number of starchy carbohydrate choices increased by one until a normal diet is achieved.

Weaning the low GI diet

Information regarding weaning the LGIT diet can be found in *Dietary Treatment of Epilepsy. Practical Implementation of Ketogenic Therapy*, Oxford: Wiley Blackwell, 2012.

Transition to adult care

There is little data on the use of the ketogenic diet in adults. The 2012 NICE guidelines for childhood epilepsy [2] suggest that a randomised controlled trial of ketogenic diet in adult patients with drug?resistant epilepsy should be conducted to help determine the efficacy of the diet in adults. Currently there are few adult services where older children on the ketogenic diet can be transitioned to. At the time of writing few dietitians looking after adults have the resources or support from a neurologist to support the continuation of the diet. Currently teenagers are slowly weaned off the ketogenic diet before they go to adult services.

Future research

- Ongoing research into the exact mechanisms of the diet
- Establishing the genetic basis of why some children respond to diet and others do not
- Further research to determine the efficacy of the newer treatments: MKD and low GI diets
- Further research to determine the most appropriate method for discontinuing the diet

- Ongoing research studying the diet for adults and conditions other than epilepsy, where there is a possible neuroprotective role such as Alzheimer's disease, Parkinson's disease, migraines, cancer/brain tumours, autism and diabetes

Useful resources for dietitians

KetoPAG (Ketogenic Diet Professional Advisory Group)

KetoPAG is a group of dietitians, doctors and nurses who are involved with the use of the ketogenic diet in the UK. The group provides a useful support structure for dietitians involved with these diets and has an email forum for health professionals. Dietitians can request to be included by contacting the authors.

Dietary Treatment of Epilepsy

Practical Implementation of Ketogenic Therapy, 1st edn. Oxford: Wiley Blackwell, 2012.

Parent support groups
Specific to the ketogenic diet
Matthew's Friends (UK)
www.matthewsfriends.org

The Daisy Garland Charity (UK)
www.thedaisygarland.org.uk

The Charlie Foundation (US)
www.charliefoundation.org

The Carson Harris Foundation (US)
www.carsonharrisfoundation.org

About epilepsy
The National Society for Epilepsy
www.epilepsynse.org.uk
Tel: 01494 601300

Young Epilepsy
www.youngepilepsy.org.uk
Tel: 01342 832243

Epilepsy Action
www.epilepsy.org.uk
Tel: 01132 108800

USA Epilepsy Website
www.epilepsy.com

17 Disorders of Amino Acid Metabolism, Organic Acidaemias and Urea Cycle Disorders

Marjorie Dixon, Anita MacDonald, Fiona White and Jacky Stafford

Introduction to Inherited Metabolic Disorders

Fiona White

Metabolism

Metabolism describes the chemical processes which occur in the body's cells to produce energy and other substances needed for normal body functioning. It comprises two elements: anabolism and catabolism. Anabolism is the formation and storage of complex compounds needed for growth, tissue repair and energy storage from simpler molecules. Catabolism is the breakdown of large complex molecules to provide energy for cellular activity and smaller compounds, e.g. amino acids, needed for anabolic reactions or for elimination from the body. Commonly the term metabolism defines the breakdown of food and how its components (carbohydrates, fats and proteins) are transformed into energy via a sequence of chemical reactions (metabolic pathways) which are controlled by large numbers of different enzymes.

Enzymes themselves are proteins. These biochemical reactions frequently involve cofactors, often vitamins, which help the specific enzyme function, e.g. vitamin B_6 is the cofactor for the enzyme cystathionine β synthase which converts the amino acid homocysteine into cystathionine. Figure 17.1 illustrates the metabolic processes involved in the overall metabolism of carbohydrates, fats and protein including the catabolic processes to produce energy and urea (the product of the detoxification of the nitrogen moiety of amino acids) and anabolic processes to form tissue protein and energy stores, glycogen and lipids.

Carbohydrate metabolism

Cellular carbohydrate (CHO) metabolism involves both catabolic (glycolysis, glycogenolysis) and

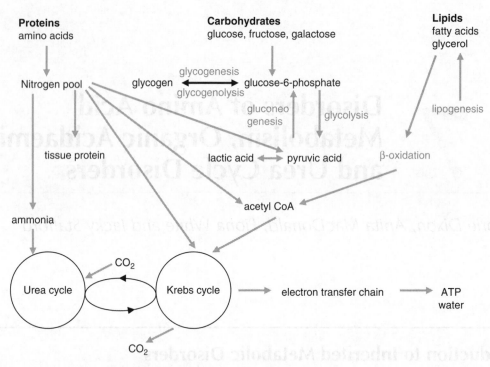

Figure 17.1   Summary of metabolism of carbohydrates, fats and proteins.

anabolic processes (glycogenesis, gluconeogenesis). Carbohydrates, as monosaccharides (glucose, fructose, galactose), are absorbed in the intestine and then transported to the liver where excess glucose, galactose and fructose are converted to glucose-6-phosphate (G-6-PO$_4$). Depending upon energy needs G-6-PO$_4$ undergoes either catabolism to form energy or anabolism to form glycogen, the storage form of glucose, in liver and muscles. To produce energy G-6-PO$_4$ (derived from monosaccharides from dietary CHO or produced from glycogen degradation by glycogenolysis) is converted by a series of enzyme reactions in the glycolytic pathway to form pyruvate or lactic acid, then to acetyl-CoA, which is also produced from fatty acid oxidation and degradation of the carbon skeleton of glucogenic amino acids (Table 17.1). Acetyl-CoA enters the Krebs cycle, also known as the citric acid or tricarboxylic (TCA) cycle, within the mitochondria. Within the Krebs cycle acetyl-CoA, combined with oxaloacetate, undergoes cycles involving eight enzymes, in which reducing equivalents are produced which then enter the electron transfer chain for the production of energy as adenosine triphosphate (ATP). When

Table 17.1   Classification of amino acids.

Glucogenic only	Ketogenic only	Ketogenic and glucogenic
Alanine	Leucine	Isoleucine
Arginine	Lysine	Phenylalanine
Asparagine		Threonine
Aspartate		Tyrosine
Cystine		Tryptophan
Glutamate		
Glutamine		
Glycine		
Histidine		
Methionine		
Proline		
Serine		
Valine		

cells do not require G-6-PO$_4$ for energy production it undergoes glycogenesis to be stored as glycogen until required to restore blood glucose levels. G-6-PO$_4$ can also be produced via pyruvate from protein catabolism of glucogenic amino acids (Table 17.1) or breakdown of glycerol from lipids (gluconeogenesis).

Fat metabolism

Dietary fat is present mainly as long chain triglycerides, comprising a glycerol backbone and fatty acids. Dietary fats, and lipids produced endogenously from acetyl-CoA, are initially hydrolysed by lipases into glycerol and free fatty acids. Glycerol is then oxidised to acetyl-CoA via pyruvate. Lipid transport is a complex process and is discussed in Chapter 19. Fatty acids enter the mitochondria via the carnitine transport cycle (medium chain fatty acids enter independently of carnitine) into the β-oxidation spiral in which fatty acids, via a series of enzymes, produce acetyl-CoA and electron carriers. Acetyl-CoA can enter the Krebs cycle or form ketone bodies in the liver. Electron carriers ($FADH_2$ and NAD) enter the electron transfer chain to produce ATP. Acetyl-CoA in excess of requirements for energy production via the Krebs cycle is converted via lipogenesis to stored lipids in adipocytes.

Protein metabolism

Dietary protein is broken down into 20 individual amino acids for absorption. Of these nine are essential or indispensible (histidine, isoleucine, leucine, lysine, methionine, phenylalanine, threonine, tryptophan, valine) as they cannot be synthesised by the body. The other 11 (alanine, arginine, asparagine, aspartic acid, cystine, glutamic acid, glutamine, glycine, proline, serine, tyrosine) are classified as non essential amino acids (NEAA), or dispensable, as they can be produced from the breakdown of essential amino acids (EAA). A few of the NEAA become conditionally essential in certain disorders or at times of stress. These include arginine, cystine, glutamine, glycine, proline and tyrosine and in such circumstances must be provided in the diet.

Amino acids enter the body's nitrogen pool (Fig. 17.2) and are used to form tissue protein for growth and body tissue repair, or are catabolised by two processes. The amine group (nitrogen moiety) undergoes transamination, in which it is transferred to a keto acid producing a keto acid and an amino acid, and then deamination to produce ammonia which is detoxified via the urea cycle to produce urea, which is then excreted in urine. The carbon skeletons of amino acids (organic acids) are glucogenic, ketogenic or both (Table 17.1).

Glucogenic amino acids degrade

- directly to Krebs cycle intermediates
- via acetyl-CoA or acetoacetyl-CoA to oxaloacetate which is either used in the Krebs cycle or can be converted to phosphoenolpyruvate and used to produce G-6-PO$_4$ via gluconeogenesis
- to pyruvate which can either be used to produce G-6-PO$_4$ via gluconeogenesis or converted irreversibly to acetyl-CoA by the pyruvate

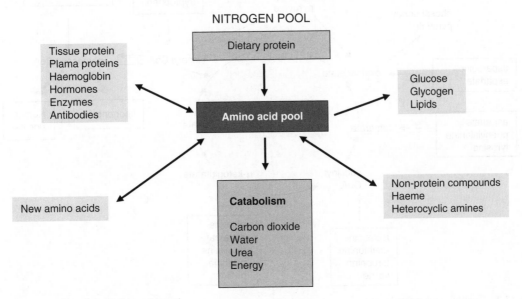

Figure 17.2 Function of the amino acid pool.

dehydrogenase (PDH) complex. Acetyl-CoA can then enter the Krebs cycle

Ketogenic amino acids degrade to acetoacetate or acetyl-CoA and are used in fatty acid synthesis or ketone body production (Fig. 17.3).

Control and regulation of metabolism

To maintain homeostasis within cells metabolic pathways have to be finely balanced (Fig. 17.4). This is achieved by either

- flux through pathways, increasing or decreasing by intracellular self-regulation of reactions (feedback) by responding to concentrations of substrates or products, e.g. a decreased concentration of an essential product causes enzyme activity in the metabolic pathway to increase and produce more product from the substrate
- responding to signals from other cells, involving hormones and growth factors

Influence of hormone regulation

Hormones are released according to the metabolic status including whether in the fed or starved state and stress. Their regulation of metabolic pathways play a crucial role by

- altering the availability of substrates, e.g. sympathetic response during exercise increasing the mobilisation of fatty acids, insulin being released in response to high blood glucose levels and glucagon being released when glucose levels are low
- influencing enzyme activity, e.g. epinephrine, a fight and flight hormone, increases phosphofructokinase (PFK) activity, an important enzyme in glycolysis. In addition glucocorticoids and thyroid hormones also affect energy metabolism

Table 17.2 summarises the action of hormones on metabolic pathways.

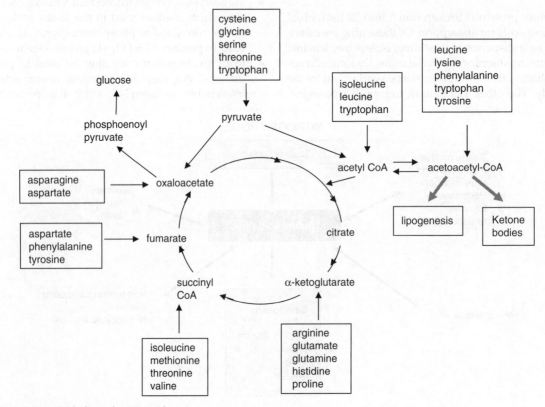

Figure 17.3 Catabolism of amino acids.

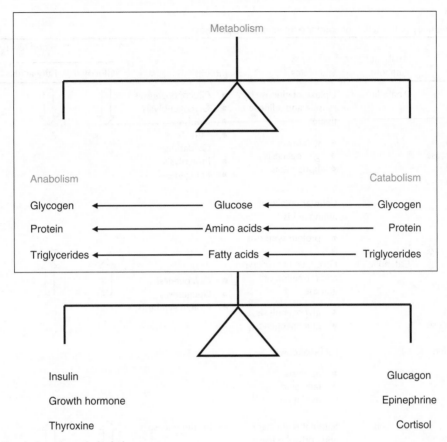

Figure 17.4   Regulation of metabolic balance.

Inherited metabolic disorders

Inherited metabolic disorders (IMD) are genetically inherited biochemical disorders of specific enzymes or proteins causing a block in a normal metabolic process of protein, CHO or fat metabolism. As a result there is an abnormality in the normal metabolic process and accumulation of intermediary metabolites which cannot be further metabolised. This concept of IMD was originally conceived by Garrod [1] in 1902 and in 1908 he went on to describe such disorders including alkaptonuria, albinism, pentosuria and cystinuria [2] which are all inherited in an autosomal recessive trait. IMD can be categorised in a number of ways. Based on their pathophysiology they can be considered in three distinct groups.

1 **Disorders of intermediary metabolism leading to intoxication**
   These include disorders in which the enzyme deficiency leads to accumulation of intermediary metabolites proximal to the block (B) and the formation of alternative products (D) producing acute or chronic toxic effects which result in disease manifestations and may also lead to deficiencies of products downstream of the block (C).

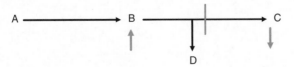

Table 17.2   Summary of the action of hormones on metabolic pathways.

Hormone	Anabolic/ catabolic	Stimulates	Inhibits	Blood levels		
				Glucose	Fatty acids	Amino acids
Insulin released in response to • increased blood glucose • increased blood amino acids	Anabolic	Uptake of glucose by muscle and adipose tissue • glycolysis • glycogenesis • lipogenesis Cellular uptake of amino acids • protein synthesis	• Gluconeogenesis • Glycogenolysis • Lipolysis • Fatty Acid Oxidation • Proteolysis • Ketogenesis	↓	↓	↓
Glucagon released in response to • decreased blood glucose • decreased blood amino acids	Catabolic	Glycogen breakdown and formation of glucose • glycogenolysis • gluconeogenesis Fat breakdown • lipolysis • fatty acid oxidation	• Glycogenesis • Lipogenesis • Protein synthesis	↑	↑	↔
Epinephrine released during exercise and stress (stimulation of sympathetic nervous system)	Catabolic	Stimulates glucagon and cortisol release Glycogen breakdown and formation of glucose • glycogenolysis • gluconeogenesis Fat breakdown • Lipolysis	• Insulin release	↑	↑	↔
Cortisol Released due to physiological and emotional stress Supports effects of decreased insulin and increased glucagon secretion	Catabolic	Decreased glucose, fatty acid and amino acid uptake by all tissues except brain • gluconeogenesis • lipolysis		↑	↑	↑

Table 17.2   *(continued)*

Hormone	Anabolic/ catabolic	Stimulates	Inhibits	Blood levels		
				Glucose	Fatty acids	Amino acids
Growth hormone Released in response to • hypoglycaemia • increased plasma amino acid levels • increased metabolism associated with growth, exercise	Anabolic	Muscle protein synthesis Mobilisation of free fatty acids • lipolysis Reduced cellular glucose uptake • gluconeogenesis	Glucose uptake by muscles (glucose sparing)	⇧	⇧	⇩
Thyroxine Slow response to metabolic changes Increases sensitivity to epinephrine, glucagon and growth hormone Increases basal metabolic rate	Catabolic	Increases ATP production • glycolysis • glycogenolysis • lipolysis • fatty acid oxidation		indirectly ⇩		

Examples of such disorders include the amino acidopathies (phenylketonuria, maple syrup urine disease, homocystinuria, tyrosinaemias); organic acidaemias; urea cycle disorders; disorders of sugar intolerance (galactosaemia, hereditary fructose intolerance); metal intoxication disorders (Menkes disease, Wilson disease) and porphyrias. These disorders all have a symptom free period after birth and then present with acute (either in the neonatal period or a later onset) or chronic signs of 'intoxication'. Acute symptoms can be triggered by dietary intake, catabolism, fever, intercurrent illness. Chronic, progressive presentations include developmental delay, failure to thrive, cardiomyopathy, hepatomegaly, lens dislocation.

2 **Disorders of intermediary metabolism involving energy metabolism**
These include disorders in which the enzyme deficiency results in lack of energy production or energy utilisation within organs including liver, muscle, brain, myocardium. These disorders can be subdivided into defects of mitochondrial or cytoplasmic energy:
  ○ mitochondrial energy disorders include disorders of fatty acid oxidation, ketone body defects, congenital lactic acidaemias, respiratory chain disorders
  ○ cytoplasmic energy disorders include disorders of glycolysis, glycogen metabolism, gluconeogenesis, glucose transport and hyperinsulinism and disorders of creatine metabolism
Symptoms may include hypoglycaemia, lactic acidosis, hepatomegaly, cardiomyopathy, myopathy, hypertonia, failure to thrive, sudden infant death.

3 **Disorders involving complex large molecules**
These are disorders in which complex molecules are incompletely catabolised and accumulate in organelles resulting in varied symptoms including progressive loss of function of affected body systems, organomegaly

and dysmorphic features. They include disorders of lipoprotein and cholesterol metabolism, lysosomal storage disorders, peroxisomal disorders, disorders of glycosylation, disorders of sterol synthesis and disorders of purine and pyrimidine metabolism.

Management

A significant number of IMD are treatable, often by therapeutic dietary intervention. The main forms of nutritional therapy in IMD are:

1 *substrate reduction* in which the metabolite which accumulates, due to the enzyme deficiency, is restricted (if it is an essential nutrient) or as far as possible removed from the diet. Such a treatment strategy is employed in managing

   ○ disorders of amino acid metabolism
   ○ disorders of galactose and fructose metabolism
   ○ lipoprotein disorders
   ○ disorders of fatty acid oxidation
   ○ some peroxisomal disorders, e.g. Refsum's disease

2 *provision of products normally produced downstream of the block* and which, as a result of the block, are conditionally essential to prevent deficiency

   ○ tyrosine supplementation in phenylketonuria
   ○ arginine in urea cycle disorders
   ○ maintaining normoglycaemia by regular feeding and/or CHO supplements in
      • glycogen storage disorders
      • disorders of fatty acid oxidation
   ○ cholesterol in Smith–Lemli–Opitz syndrome
   ○ mannose in CDG 1b (phosphomannose isomerase deficiency)

3 *stimulation of residual enzyme activity* by use of pharmacological doses of cofactors, often vitamins

   ○ vitamin B_{12} in methylmalonic acidaemia
   ○ pyridoxine (vitamin B_6) in homocystinuria
   ○ riboflavin (vitamin B_2) in multiple acyl-CoA dehydrogenase deficiency

   ○ sapropterin in some forms of biopterin responsive phenylketonuria

4 *providing alternative substrates*

   ○ use of glucose and medium chain triglycerides in long chain fat oxidation disorders
   ○ use of the ketogenic diet in Glut 1 deficiency syndrome to produce ketones as an alternative energy source to glucose by the brain

In many IMD the promotion of anabolism and avoidance of catabolism is vital to prevent metabolic decompensation occurring. Where acute metabolic decompensation occurs with the risk of further irreversible damage, particularly neurological, the use of emergency dietary regimens is imperative. Detailed discussion of dietary treatment approaches are given in the relevant sections of this and the following chapters.

Patients with IMD are invariably complex to treat and it is important they are managed by an experienced metabolic team including doctors, specialist dietitians, clinical nurse specialists, biochemists, pharmacists and psychologists in a metabolic centre. Local professionals and hospital teams also form an integral part of the care for metabolic patients.

Newborn screening

Early detection is important to ensure a good outcome in many IMD, starting treatment before significant or any damage is done. Newborn screening (NBS) aims to detect affected infants before symptoms occur to allow early implementation of treatment. Phenylketonuria was the first IMD to be part of NBS (from the end of the 1960s); screening has been expanded to include a variety of other disorders, depending on local health policy. Further information is given in disorder specific sections.

Inheritance

The concept of IMD being due to a block in a metabolic process, with the accumulation of intermediary metabolites leading to disease, was introduced by Garrod [1, 2]. In 1911 Johannsen [3] introduced the theory that genes were responsible for inheritance and in 1941 Beadle and Tatum [4]

hypothesised the one gene, one enzyme theory. The molecular disease concept in which gene mutations alter protein structure by changing a single amino acid within the protein was introduced by Pauling *et al.* [5] and Ingram [6] with their work on sickle cell anaemia.

The structure of DNA was described by Watson and Crick in 1953. DNA contains information as a code made up of four different chemical bases. The sequence of bases provides information for building and maintaining body structures. DNA sequences are made up of exons and introns. Exons are coding sequences which contain information to encode for a protein. Introns, which occur between exons, do not code for proteins. The process of a gene expressing for a protein involves two significant steps, transcription and translation. Transcription, within the cell nucleus, involves the transfer of information in the DNA to messenger RNA (mRNA). mRNA carries this information out of the nucleus into the cytoplasm for translation where ribosomes read the sequence of mRNA bases. Three base (codon) sequences code for specific amino acids (AA). Transfer RNA (tRNA) then assembles the protein by sequentially adding AA until a stop codon (a three base sequence which does not code for an AA) is reached [7].

Genetic disorders arise due to mutations (change) in the DNA sequence. An error in the coding sequence of a gene can result in no protein or an abnormal protein or enzyme being produced. Many mutations are benign (silent) whereas others lead to variable severity of defect. Mutation types include point mutations, missense mutations, nonsense mutations, deletions, insertions, inversions, duplication, frameshift mutations (Table 17.3). Further information can be obtained at www.genetichealth.com and www.ghr.nlm.nih.gov/handbook/mutationsanddisorders/possiblemutations.

Gene mutations result in a genotype which predicts residual enzyme activity. Single genes do not function independently but interact with other genes and the individual's environment resulting in the disease phenotype. There is not always an exact genotype–phenotype correlation.

Patterns of inheritance

Autosomal recessive (AR) inheritance

In AR inheritance faulty (mutated) copies of the gene have to be inherited for the disease to be expressed (Fig. 17.5). Parents are obligate

Table 17.3 Types of mutations.

Mutation type	Change in amino acid (AA) code	Effect
Point	Single base pair change	Benign unless causes change in AA code
Missense	Single base pair change	Substitution of one AA for another in the protein chain. Can have serious consequences
Nonsense	Single base pair change or premature termination of AA code (stop codon)	Signals cell to stop building a protein, thus producing a shortened protein which may function improperly or not at all
Insertion	Adds a piece of DNA which changes number of DNA bases	Protein product produced may not function correctly
Deletion	Removes piece of DNA	Function of resulting protein may be altered
Duplication	Piece of DNA abnormally copied once or multiple times	Resulting protein function may be altered from normal
Frameshift	Loss or addition of one or more DNA bases causing change in grouping of the triplet base pair coding for AA. Deletions, insertions and duplications can also result in frameshift mutations	Usually results in non functioning protein
Splice site mutations	Introns (bulk of the DNA within a gene which is not translated) not spliced from mRNA	Incorrect protein is produced

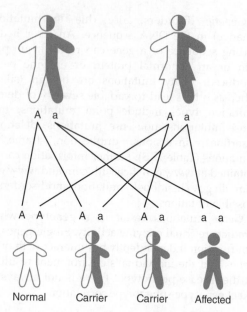

Figure 17.5   Autosomal recessive inheritance (http://www
.geneticseducation.nhs.uk).

heterozygotes (carriers) but do not have the disease. They may carry the same or a different gene
fault (mutation). Affected offspring are either
homozygous with two copies of the same gene
fault (mutation) or compound heterozygotes with
two different gene faults (mutations). There is a
25% (one in four) risk of having an affected child
with each pregnancy. Unaffected children have a
66% (two out of three) chance of being a carrier.
Many IMD are inherited in this way including
phenylketonuria (PKU), maple syrup urine disease
(MSUD), galactosaemia, glycogen storage disease
(GSD) Ia, medium chain acyl CoA dehydrogenase
deficiency (MCADD).

When individuals affected with an AR disorder have children they will all inherit the faulty
(mutated) copy of the gene. The risk of their
children actually having the same AR disorder
depends upon whether their partner is affected
with the same AR disorder or carries a faulty
(mutated) copy of the same gene. Children of parents who both have the same AR disorder will all
inherit the disorder. The risk of offspring inheriting
the disorder when one parent has an AR disorder
depends upon the carrier frequency rate for the
disorder. For example PKU has a carrier frequency
of approximately 1 in 50 which gives a 1 in 100 (1%)

chance of any child of a parent with PKU inheriting
the condition.

Autosomal dominant (AD) inheritance

AD inheritance only requires one copy of a faulty
(mutated) gene to inherit the disorder; this can be
inherited from either parent (Fig. 17.6). There is a
50% risk of occurrence with each pregnancy. Unaffected offspring will have two normal copies of the
gene. Dominant mutations can occur sporadically
(*de novo*) with both parents having no mutations.
This is often seen in Glut 1 deficiency syndrome.
Occasionally an AD disorder can occur as the result
of a germ line mutation; parents usually have a
normal phenotype but one of the parents has a
mutation occur in some of his/her sperm/eggs.
AD conditions can occur in a homozygous state in
which case they can be very severe or lethal. Familial hypercholesterolaemia (FH) is an autosomal
dominant disorder; heterozygotes are symptomatic
but homozygotes are more severe, often dying
from fatal myocardial infarction in early adult life.
Individuals with heterozygous AD disorders (only
one copy of the faulty gene) have a 50% chance of
passing on the faulty gene. All children to individuals with homozygous AD disorders will inherit
the disorder.

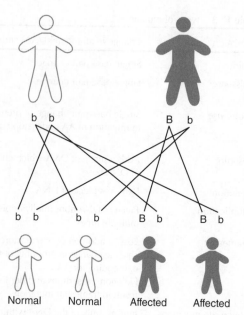

Figure 17.6   Autosomal dominant inheritance (http://www
.geneticseducation.nhs.uk).

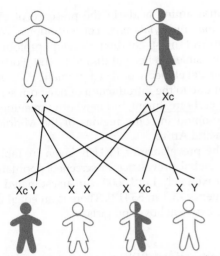

Affected son Normal daughter Carrier daughter Normal son

Figure 17.7   X-linked inheritance (http://www.genetics education.nhs.uk).

X-linked inheritance

Mutations occur in genes on the X chromosome (Fig. 17.7). X-linked recessive single gene defects affect males as they only have one X chromosome and if the gene fault/mutation is passed on from a carrier mother then they are affected. Females carry the gene fault/mutation on one of their two X chromosomes. Depending upon the degree of X inactivation (how many of the mutant X chromosomes are active) females can be symptomatic to a greater or lesser extent, e.g. in ornithine transcarbomylase (OTC) deficiency some carrier females present with hyperammonaemia. Males with X-linked disorders will pass on the faulty gene to all of their daughters; sons are unaffected. Examples of X-linked IMD include adreoleukodystrophy, OTC deficiency, X-linked GSD type IX.

Mitochondrial inheritance

Mitochondria contain their own DNA, which originates in the egg and encodes for enzymes involved in electron transport and energy metabolism. Some mitochondrial encoded polypeptides join with nuclear originated protein to form a complete enzyme. Thus mitochondrial disorders can be inherited in maternal, recessive, X-linked or dominant fashion dependent upon the defective polypeptide.

Cells contain multiple mitochondria and therefore many alleles for one gene. When some alleles are mutated the cells contain a mixture of normal and mutated alleles, known as heteroplasmy. Depending on the number of mutated mitochondria in the cell or tissue, diseases with the same mutation can be expressed differently. Examples of mitochondrial inherited IMD include Leigh syndrome, Pearson syndrome, mitochondrial encephalomyopathy lactic acidosis and stroke like episodes (MELAS).

Summary

There are over 500 different IMD currently identified. A significant number are treatable, often by therapeutic dietary intervention as the sole treatment, or in combination with pharmacological agents. These are discussed further in the following sections.

Amino Acid Disorders

Anita MacDonald and Fiona White

In this section the following amino acid disorders are considered: phenylketonuria (PKU) and tetrahydrobiopterin (BH4) deficiencies, maple syrup urine disease (MSUD), homocystinuria (HCU) and tyrosinaemia. For each condition, the prevalence, biochemistry, genetics, pathophysiology, diagnosis, outcome and non dietetic treatment is described separately. All these amino acid conditions share the same principles of dietary management. Therefore, the dietary management for all conditions is considered in one section, with any specific feature for each condition being individually discussed.

The following definitions are used throughout this chapter:

- substrate/precursor amino acid: an amino acid that cannot be catabolised due to an enzyme defect in a metabolic pathway, e.g. phenylalanine in phenylketonuria; methionine in homocystinuria.
- L-amino acid: an amino acid, with the exception of glycine, that can be found in two stereoisomeric forms (L and D forms). Only L-amino acids are used by cells. D-amino acids are not naturally found in proteins but are important in the structure of bacteria.
- protein equivalent: the amount of protein provided by an L-amino acid supplement. Total protein equivalent refers to protein sourced from an L-amino acid supplement and natural protein from the diet.
- tandem mass spectrometry (MS/MS): the analysis technology commonly used in newborn screening. It consists of a specialised instrument that detects molecules by measuring their weight or mass electronically and results are displayed (graphically) in the form of a mass spectrum.

Phenylketonuria

PKU is an autosomal recessive inborn error of amino acid metabolism, caused by a deficiency of the hepatic enzyme phenylalanine hydroxylase (PAH) (phenylalanine 4-mono-oxygenase, EC 1.14.16.1), which catalyses the hydroxylation of phenylalanine to tyrosine, the rate limiting step in phenylalanine catabolism. The enzyme deficiency leads to increased phenylketones (hence phenylketonuria); accumulation of phenylalanine resulting in hyperphenylalaninaemia; low tyrosine concentrations; lower dopamine, norepinephrine and serotonin production [8].

This high level of brain phenylalanine is possibly the chief cause of neurotoxicity [9]. It is thought to interfere with cerebral protein synthesis [10], increases myelin turnover [8] and inhibits neurotransmitter synthesis [11], the latter caused by impaired uptake of non phenylalanine large

neutral amino acids in the presence of elevated plasma phenylalanine concentrations. Without treatment most children develop profound and irreversible intellectual disability [12]. Fortunately in the developed world symptomatic PKU is rarely seen due to the introduction of newborn screening and early treatment, but newborn screening is still uncommon in some regions of the Middle East, Asia and Africa.

The prevalence of PKU is given in Table 17.4. The global prevalence in screened populations is approximately 1 in 12 000 with an estimated carrier frequency of 1 in 55 [13]. There is an equal gender ratio between boys and girls.

Classification of PKU

There is a broad continuum of phenotypes in PKU ranging from severe to milder forms. The need for diet therapy and the amount of dietary phenylalanine tolerated gives an indication of severity [24]. PKU is generally classified by the severity of hyperphenylalaninaemia at diagnosis.

- Classical or severe PKU is usually characterised by blood phenylalanine concentrations

Table 17.4 Prevalence of PKU.

Population	Prevalence
Turkish [14]	1 in 4000
Irish [15]	1 in 6200
Eastern Europe [15]	1 in 3000 to 1 in 33 000
Arabic population [16]	Up to 1 in 6000 although variable between Arab countries
China [17, 18]	1 in 10 000 to 1 in 17 000
Western Europe [15]	1 in 7000 to 1 in 33 000
West Midlands (UK) [19]	1 in 12 600 northwest Europeans 1 in 14 500 Pakistani population
Southern Europe [15]	1 in 4000 to 1 in 36 000
Poland [15]	1 in 8000
Russia [15]	1 in 8000
USA [20]	1 in 15 000
Finnish [21]	1 in 100 000
African [22]	1 in 100 000
Japanese [23]	1 in 70 000

Countries use different upper 'cut-off' phenylalanine concentrations to diagnose PKU.

>1200 μmol/L, with a phenylalanine toler-
ance no greater than 250 mg/day to maintain plasma phenylalanine concentrations
<360 μmol/L [25].
- Moderate PKU is classified with diagnostic phenylalanine concentrations of 600–
1200 μmol/L. Most patients with moderate/
severe PKU tolerate between 200 and 700 mg/
day phenylalanine whilst maintaining plasma
phenylalanine concentrations <360 μmol/L.
- Patients with persistent hyperphenylalaninaemia, or mild PKU, present with plasma
phenylalanine concentrations between 120 and
600 μmol/L on a normal diet. If phenylalanine
concentrations are maintained within these
limits without treatment, there is little evidence
to suggest patients are at risk of intellectual,
neurological or neuropsychological impairment [26]. Some centres, however, advocate
treatment when phenylalanine concentrations
are >360 μmol/L [25, 27, 28].

Tetrahydrobiopterin deficiencies

About 1%–2% of hyperphenylalaninaemia is
caused by mutations in genes coding for enzymes
involved in tetrahydrobiopterin (BH4) cofactor
biosynthesis or regeneration [29], affecting phenylalanine homeostasis and catecholamine and
serotonin biosynthesis [30]. The BH4 deficiencies are treated with neurotransmitters with or
without BH4 supplementation (Table 17.5). A low
phenylalanine diet may be prescribed for hyperphenylalaninaemia. Without treatment [except
pterin-4-α-carbinolamine dehydratase (PCD) defi-
ciency] the disorders are generally characterised
by progressive developmental delay, irritability,
motor dysfunction, impaired muscle tone, movement disorders and seizures [13, 31]. Symptoms
may be subtle only in the newborn period [13].

Biochemistry

Phenylalanine hydroxylase catalyses the hydroxylation of phenylalanine to tyrosine in the presence
of the cofactor BH4 and several enzymes that serve
to regenerate BH4, e.g. dihydropteridine reductase
and pterin-4-α-carbinolamine [32] (Fig. 17.8).

Normally hydroxylation of phenylalanine
contributes up to 50% of the tyrosine that is incorporated into tissue protein [33]. In PKU there is
an inability to convert phenylalanine into tyrosine.
Subsequently low to normal or reduced concentrations of tyrosine are common in untreated patients.

Table 17.5 Tetrahydrobiopterin deficiencies with raised phenylalanine concentrations: treatment and use of low phenylalanine diet [31].

Condition	Mean (range) plasma phenylalanine (μmol/L) before onset of treatment	Treatment	Use of low phenylalanine (phe) diet
GTP cyclohydrolase deficiency (GTPCH deficiency)	533 (55–2930)	L-dopa/carbidopa, 5-hydroxytryptophan, BH4	≤5% given low phe diet
6-pyruvoyl-tetrahydropterin synthase deficiency (PTPS deficiency)	Severe: 829 (121–2251) Mild: 1111 (41–3805)	L-dopa/carbidopa, 5-hydroxytryptophan, BH4	15% given low phe diet
Dihydropteridine reductase deficiency (DHPR deficiency)	717 (22–3207)	L-dopa/carbidopa, 5-hydroxytryptophan, folinic acid	Many given low phe diet*
Pterin-4-alpha-carbinolamine dehydratase deficiency (PCD deficiency)	533 (183–1850)	Transient and benign without neurotransmitter deficiency or neurological symptoms	May be treated with BH4/low phe diet

*In DHPR deficiency BH4 supplementation may lead to an increased risk of central nervous system folate deficiency [13].

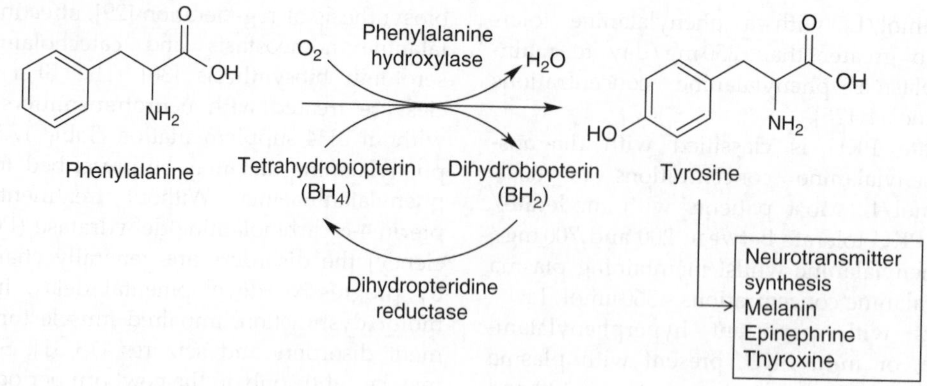

Figure 17.8   Hydroxylation of phenylalanine.

In addition the phenylalanine:tyrosine ratio, normally around 1:1, is significantly increased. Tyrosine is essential for the synthesis of the catecholamine neurotransmitters such as dopamine and norepinephrine.

Genetics

PKU is caused by mutations in the gene encoding the phenylalanine hydroxylase enzyme (PAH). The gene is on the long arm of chromosome 12 in the band region of q22-q24.1 [34]. There are more than 800 disorder causing mutations in the PAH gene [35, 36]. Different mutations affect the activity of PAH dissimilarly ranging from little or no effect to complete suppression of the activity of the enzyme [24]. There is a good correlation between genotype and phenotype [37]. Consequently genotypes with more severe mutations will result in a moderate to classical phenotype with higher untreated blood phenylalanine concentrations. Mild mutations in PAH will result in a phenotypically less severe form of PKU. In those cases where a patient is heterozygous for two mutations of PAH (i.e. each copy of the gene has a different mutation) the milder mutation will predominate. Spain has an especially high prevalence of mild PKU [25].

There are a small number of patients with so called severe PKU mutations who have escaped intellectual disability despite high blood phenylalanine concentrations and poor dietary control. These patients appear to have near normal brain phenylalanine concentrations despite high blood phenylalanine levels [38].

Diagnosis

In the UK PKU is detected on routine neonatal screening by collecting blood spots from the heel onto filter paper between days 5 and 8 of life, which are then analysed by tandem mass spectrometry (MS/MS) [39] (see www.newbornscreening-bloodspot.org.uk for screening guidelines for PKU in the UK). Infants with a phenylalanine level >240 µmol/L should be referred to a designated PKU team and assessed within 24 hours of a positive screening result. A repeat blood sample to recheck phenylalanine and tyrosine measurements, together with blood for dihydropteridine reductase and blood samples for pterins (neopterin and biopterin) to diagnose tetrahydrobiopterin deficiencies, should be taken. A low phenylalanine diet should be commenced immediately providing blood phenylalanine concentrations are ≥400 µmol/L (although some centres commence treatment when blood phenylalanine concentrations are ≥600 µmol/L [27]). It is a UK standard that all infants have commenced dietary treatment by 14 days of age [39].

It is good practice to test any new sibling of a proband case with PKU at 48–72 hours and then repeat at the usual newborn screening time (days 5–8). In the UK DNA analysis is used mainly for prenatal testing only or to detect carrier status of an 'at risk relative' [38].

Treatment guidelines

Diet is the basis of treatment for patients with PKU with blood phenylalanine concentrations consistently ≥400 µmol/L. It consists of a limited and controlled amount of natural protein derived from food sources to provide essential phenylalanine requirements, with the majority of nutrient requirements being met by a phenylalanine free source of L-amino acids, usually supplemented with added micronutrients (a protein substitute). The overall aim of treatment should be to 'achieve an optimal cognitive and psychological development and well being of the child' [40]. Published guidelines have been unanimous in their requirement for neonatal screening and strict blood phenylalanine control in the first 10 years of life [20, 41–43], but there has been little agreement about the upper blood phenylalanine threshold to commence treatment, phenylalanine target concentrations for adolescents and adults, the need for long term treatment, frequency of blood phenylalanine monitoring and use of alternative treatments such as large neutral amino acids (LNAA) and sapropterin. Currently a group of health professionals, working with the European Society for PKU (ESPKU), are developing PKU guidelines which, it is hoped, will be adopted throughout Europe and beyond. Recommended blood phenylalanine concentrations are given in Table 17.6.

Recent meta-analysis of blood phenylalanine concentrations and intelligence quotient (IQ) [44] support the approach that treatment should be continued in adulthood. Furthermore, recent meta-analysis of data from reaction times studies suggested that upper phenylalanine concentrations should be 320 µmol/L for children aged 7–13 years; 570 µmol/L for adolescents aged 14–18 years [45].

Outcomes in early diet treated PKU

Neurocognitive and neuropsychological

If untreated, PKU leads to global intellectual disability [46], significant delays in developmental milestones, hyperactive behaviour with autistic features, seizures, eczema, musty body odour and light pigmentation (eyes, hair and skin). If treatment is started within the first 3 weeks of life, irreversible intellectual disability is prevented. Most early treated children who have commenced diet by 4 weeks of age fall within the broad normal range of general ability, attain expected educational standards and lead independent lives as adults [25]. Outcome, however, is dependent on the quality of blood phenylalanine control [47] and children may have subtle defects in IQ, attention, processing speed, fine motor skills and perception and visual-spatial abilities [48]. Executive function (working memory, planning, organisation and inhibitory control) may be impaired [49, 50] (Table 17.7). Sustained attention and reaction time is reduced [51]. In adolescents meta-analysis indicates that any relaxation of blood phenylalanine concentrations >600 µmol/L is associated with slower processing speed [45]. Psychological and psychiatric disturbances may develop including anxiety related disorders (phobias/panic attacks), low

Table 17.6 Recommended blood phenylalanine concentrations throughout life.

| Age | Target blood phenylalanine concentrations (µmol/L) | | | |
	UK [43]	Germany [42]	USA [20]	France [40]
0 months to 6 years	120–360* At school age (4–5 years) upper phenylalanine level is increased to 480 µmol/L	40–240	120–360	120–300
7–9 years	120–480	40–240	120–360	120–300
10–12 years	120–700	40–900	120–360	<900
13–15 years	120–700	40–900	120–600	<900
16–18 years	120–700	40–1200	120–900	<900
>18 years	120–700	40–1200	120–900	<1500

Normal physiological plasma phenylalanine concentration in infants, children and adolescents is approximately 60 µmol/L [8].

Table 17.7   Neurocognitive and neuropsychological outcome reported in PKU.

Suboptimal neurocognitive/neuropsychological outcome	Authors
Effect on IQ A meta-analysis of 40 studies indicated that during the critical periods (0–12 years of age) every increase of 100 µmol/L of phenylalanine over target was associated with a 1.3–3.1 point reduction in IQ. Similar significant correlations were observed between lifetime IQ and mean lifetime phenylalanine level for early treated patients where each 100 µmol/L increase in phenylalanine predicated a 1.9–4.1 reduction in IQ	[47]
A meta-analysis examining neuropsychological and intellectual presentations in continuously treated adolescents and adults (113 patients with PKU compared with 107 controls) found a substantially lower average IQ than the control group. They also differed from control adults on processing speed, attention, inhibition and motor control	[54]
A regression model of the relationship between IQ, lifetime blood phenylalanine concentrations and blood phenylalanine variability from 46 children aged 2–15 years showed that IQ decreased by 4.3 points for every 1 point increase in standard deviation (SD) of blood phenylalanine	[55]
Tremor, deficits in fine motor abilities: hand–wrist steadiness, finger–hand dexterity and hand–wrist speed	[56]
Deficits in motor speed and motor control	[57–59]
Deficits in working memory	[60, 61]
Reduced reaction times	[51, 62]
Deficits in sustained attention	[63]
Information processing slower and less efficient in children and adults with PKU	[45, 58, 62, 64–66]
Children and adolescents with PKU showed lower performance in several executive functioning skills including initiation of problem solving, concept formation and reasoning	[49, 50, 66, 67]
Autism, attention deficit hyperactivity	[68]
Psychiatric emotional and behavioural characteristics in children Attention problems, school problems, less achievement motivation, decreased social competence, decreased autonomy and low self-esteem	[67, 69]
Psychiatric emotional and behavioural characteristics in teenagers/adults Depressed mood, generalised anxiety, phobias, decreased positive emotions, low self-esteem, social maturity deficits, social isolation or withdrawal, delayed autonomy, lower rate of forming normal adult relationships	[52, 63, 67, 69–73]

level depression, attention deficit/hyperactivity, low mood and agoraphobia [52]. Associations between the quality of blood phenylalanine control and behaviour problems, sustained attention and lower IQ are well documented [52, 53].

Quality of life

Health related quality of life in PKU is generally comparable to a healthy population [63, 73–75]. In a group of 172 adults with PKU 76% were in full-time employment, 23% had obtained university degrees and 67% remained single [76]. In a further study more adults with PKU lived with their parents with fewer having children compared with controls [73]. Increasing non adherence in adolescents is associated with better quality of life [77] although parents worry more about school performance when their child's blood phenylalanine concentration results are poor [78]. In direct contrast returning to a low phenylalanine diet in adults is associated with improved quality of life [79, 80].

Growth and nutrition

Growth

There are few differences in growth [81, 82] and body composition [83] between children with PKU and the general population. In the 1990s there were studies describing low length for age in infants and young children [84–86], but height for age improved with time [85].

Overweight

Early studies indicated that PKU children may have a higher prevalence of overweight [87–89]. Although the rate of overweight [81, 90, 91] and percentage of body fat is high in older girls, particularly over the age of 11 years, many researchers have demonstrated it is comparable to the general population [92–94]. Factors associated with overweight in PKU include relaxation of strict diet therapy, a high carbohydrate intake and low activity levels [93].

Bone health

Low bone mineral density (BMD) in children [95] and osteopenia in adults has been reported [96, 97]. There is some suggestion of increased spontaneous osteoclastogenesis [98], consistent with increased bone resorption markers, in affected patients [96, 98]. It is unclear if the deficits in bone mineralisation relate to the disorder or its treatment. Possible reasons for poor BMD include amino acid imbalances; inadequate intake of natural protein, calcium, phosphorus, magnesium [99], vitamin D [96] or n-3 polyunsaturated fatty acids [100]; low calcium/protein ratios; poor dietary adherence with micronutrient supplemented L-amino acids [101, 102]; low plasma magnesium, zinc and copper concentrations [99]; elevated plasma phenylalanine concentrations [103]; lack of weight bearing exercise [95].

Vitamin B$_{12}$ deficiency

Vitamin B$_{12}$ deficiency is mainly reported in adolescents or adult patients who have either relaxed their diets and are less adherent with phenylalanine free L-amino acid supplements; or stopped treatment but are not eating a normal protein intake particularly animal protein which is the major source of vitamin B$_{12}$ [104–107]. Symptoms such as spastic paraparesis, tremor and slurred speech are associated with deficiency, but patients may be unaware of the early manifestations of vitamin B$_{12}$ deficiency as they appear insidiously [105].

Minerals and trace minerals

In the early years of PKU treatment biochemical selenium deficiency was common [108–110]. Selenium is now added to the majority of phenylalanine free L-amino acid supplements, thereby improving selenium status [111]. Low plasma zinc concentrations are still described [112–114], despite generous zinc supplementation in phenylalanine free L-amino acid supplements. Iron deficiency anaemia [115, 116], low haemoglobin [117] and ferritin [117, 118] concentrations are documented in children on diet therapy.

Antioxidants

Altered antioxidant capacity is observed in PKU both in human and animal models [119, 120] and markers of lipid, protein and DNA damage have been reported. Although this may be associated with an increased free radical generation, it may also be due to depletion of the antioxidant micronutrients [121] or a combination of both [122].

Other treatment options

A number of new treatment options, either as an adjunct therapy to a low phenylalanine diet or to replace diet, are available or in development.

Large neutral amino acids

Large neutral amino acids (LNAA) – histidine, isoleucine, methionine, phenylalanine, threonine, tryptophan, tyrosine, valine – are carried into the brain via the L-type amino acid carrier. They compete for the carrier and their rate of entry into the brain depends upon plasma concentrations. High concentrations of plasma phenylalanine will reduce the entry of the other LNAA into the brain and result in higher brain phenylalanine levels. In PKU, giving large amounts of phenylalanine free LNAA competes with phenylalanine and may reduce its influx into the brain [123, 124]. It may increase both brain neurotransmitter concentrations and brain essential amino acid concentrations [125]. It is suggested that LNAA may have a secondary effect by decreasing blood phenylalanine concentration and inhibiting phenylalanine entry into the circulation [126]. Transport of LNAA across membranes (from gut to blood and from blood to brain) is facilitated by the transporter proteins, which selectively bind to the LNAA. Clinical studies are summarised in Table 17.8.

The use of phenylalanine free LNAA supplements may be considered in older patients with PKU unable to adhere to diet therapy. They have not been tested in children under the age of 11 years and are not advocated in pregnancy. This treatment is not used widely, there are limited LNAA supplements available and no preparation is on ACBS prescription in the UK. There is little advantage in using LNAA in patients who are adherent to their diet therapy.

Glycomacropeptide

Glycomacropeptide (GMP) is a low phenylalanine protein source used as an alternative to L-amino acids in the treatment of PKU. GMP constitutes 15%–20% of the protein found in whey. Pure GMP contains 47% (weight/weight) of indispensible amino acids. It contains no aromatic amino acids including phenylalanine, tyrosine, tryptophan, histidine, arginine and cysteine. It is also low in methionine and leucine but contains elevated amounts of threonine and isoleucine. To ensure GMP is low in phenylalanine it undergoes special processing through chromatography, ultrafiltration/diafiltration and lyophilisation to reduce phenylalanine content to <2 mg/g of GMP [133]. Commercially adapted GMP protein substitutes that are currently available are high in isoleucine and threonine (compared with phenylalanine free L-amino acids) and have required supplementation with some L-amino acids including tyrosine, tryptophan, histidine and leucine [134].

There is some evidence that GMP, when given to PKU mice, competitively inhibits phenylalanine transport into the brain and PKU mice show comparable growth and reduced concentrations of plasma and brain phenylalanine compared with a conventional amino acid source [135]. The concentrations of isoleucine and threonine in plasma showed a significant two- to three-fold increase in the GMP fed mice. Human research is very limited and there is very little long term outcome data,

Table 17.8   Studies examining large neutral amino acids (LNAA) in PKU.

Study detail	Authors
• Mice with PKU (with features of classical PKU) were given 0.5 g/kg and 1 g/kg LNAA over 48 hours and compared with control and sham fed mice. Blood phenylalanine was reduced in the LNAA treated mice by an average of 15% (0.5 g/kg) and 50% (1 g/kg) in 48 hours. The control and sham fed mice maintained high blood phenylalanine levels	[127]
• Treatment of six PKU patients (aged 20–34 years) on a normal/very relaxed diet with phenylalanine free LNAA tablets (0.4 g/kg body weight) enriched in tyrosine and tryptophan, increased blood concentration of tyrosine and tryptophan to normal levels. Furthermore, the brain phenylalanine concentrations showed a significant reduction over a 6 month period. No adverse symptoms were reported. All six subjects reported increased energy and improvement of demeanour	[128]
• In 19 patients with severe intellectual disability due to untreated PKU, a prospective double blinded placebo controlled crossover 6 month trial examined the effects of LNAA tablets. They experienced improved concentration and the development of a meaningful smile. They were more aware of external stimuli and had less self-injury	[129]
• LNAA were given at 0.5 g/kg/day (eight subjects) and 1 g/kg (three subjects) for 1 week. The patients were not on strict diet therapy but eight were taking some L-amino acid supplement. Blood phenylalanine decreased by 50%	[130]
• In a short randomised crossover trial, LNAA were given at 0.5 g/kg/day (20 subjects, aged 11–32 years). Blood phenylalanine decreased by a mean of 39% from baseline on LNAA	[131]
• In a randomised double blind four phase controlled trial, 16 subjects with PKU (aged 11–45 years) were given (1) LNAA + usual L-amino acids; (2) usual L-amino acids; (3) LNAA only; (4) no LNAA or L-amino acids. Plasma phenylalanine decreased with LNAA when patients were not taking their phenylalanine free L-amino acids. There was no correlation between plasma and brain phenylalanine when plasma phenylalanine was <1200 μmol/L	[132]

no information about nutritional status or any information outlining GMP's safety in children <11 years of age. Short term data, however, in older patients suggest fasting phenylalanine concentrations were significantly lower with the GMP compared with an L-amino acid supplement. Blood urea nitrogen was also significantly lower with GMP [136]. There is some suggestion that it lowers postprandial concentrations of the appetite stimulating hormone ghrelin and may help promote satiety [137]. Low phenylalanine GMP products that can be used to replace phenylalanine free L-amino acid supplements are obtainable in the USA; they are not available in the UK on ACBS prescription.

Biopterin-responsive phenylalanine hydroxylase deficiency

Sapropterin dihydrochloride is the biologically active synthetic form of tetrahydrobiopterin (BH4), the naturally occurring essential cofactor for the enzyme PAH [138]. Some mutant PAH enzymes show enhanced activity in the presence of pharmacological doses of sapropterin [139], so it is effective in a subset of patients mainly with mild or moderate phenotypes of PKU [140]. Sapropterin has been demonstrated to lower blood phenylalanine concentrations [141] and improve phenylalanine tolerance [142, 143]. It is an oral medication given as an adjunctive therapy with a 'relaxed' low phenylalanine diet, or it may replace diet therapy depending on the individual response to the drug [144]. Approximately 20%–40% of patients achieve ≥30% reduction in blood phenylalanine concentration with a BH4 loading test, with a dose of 20 mg/kg [140, 145]. The dose of sapropterin is titrated to individual patient requirements (5–20 mg/kg) [146]. Long term data describing blood phenylalanine control, neuropsychological outcome and nutritional status are limited. There is evidence to suggest that even with sapropterin patients still require careful long term monitoring to prevent loss of dietary control associated with poor dietary adherence, excessive natural protein intake and catabolism associated with infections [147].

Phenylalanine ammonia lyase enzyme substitution therapy

Phenylalanine ammonia lyase (PAL; EC 4.3.1.5) is an enzyme that degrades phenylalanine into trans-cinnamic acid and ammonia [148]. It does not require a cofactor. Although its administration lowered blood and brain phenylalanine concentrations in mice [149], its repetitive and extended exposure induced an immune response [150]. This has led to the development of a pegylated phenylalanine ammonia lyase (PEG PAL) to aid the suppression of immune recognition with repeated PAL injections [151].

The use of PEG PAL is being investigated in humans. The drug Phenylase™ (PAL) (Biomarin Pharma) is given by subcutaneous injections to patients >16 years with PKU. In Phase 2 clinical trials it has been administered to 25 subjects for 1 year and it lowered blood phenylalanine on average by 68% compared with pretreatment levels, with all 25 patients maintaining blood phenylalanine concentrations <600 μmol/L. The main principal adverse reaction reported is hypersensitivity type reactions (injection site reactions, disseminated skin reactions or joint pain). This occurs during the initial dosing of the drug [152]. In theory tyrosine supplementation should still be required [148].

Genome targeted gene therapy

Liver directed gene therapy, by using recombinant adenoassociated virus (AAV) vectors, has corrected hyperphenylalaninaemia to normal in PAH deficient mouse models. AAV vectors produce minimal immune response and give longer lasting effects compared with the initial vectors used in gene therapy [153]. This does not, however, lead to permanent correction of liver PAH deficiency. Skeletal muscle has also been successfully used as an alternative target for gene therapy in PAH deficient mouse models [154].

Pharmacological chaperones

There is progress in identifying alternative pharmacological chaperones to BH4 that will enhance the thermal stability and activity of PAH [155, 156].

Maple syrup urine disease

Maple syrup urine disease (MSUD) is a neurotoxic, autosomal recessive disorder of branched chain amino acid (leucine, isoleucine and valine) catabolism. The first step in the catabolism of branched chain amino acids (BCAA) is their transamination to form the branched chain keto acids (BCKA): 2-oxoisocaproic acid (leucine), 2-oxo-3-methylvaleric acid (isoleucine) and 2-oxoisovaleric acid (valine) [157] (Fig. 17.9).

In MSUD, there is a deficiency of the multienzyme α-ketoacid dehydrogenase (BCKAD; EC.1.2.4.4.) complex, which is required for the second shared step in the degradation of BCKA. BCKAD is composed of three enzymes: a 2-oxodecarboxylase (E1) that requires thiamin as a cofactor, dihydrolipoyl acyltransferase (E2) and dihydrolipoyl dehydrogenase (E3).

Deficiency of BCKAD causes accumulation of high concentrations of leucine, valine, isoleucine and alloisoleucine as well as their corresponding BCKA in plasma and cerebrospinal fluid. Neurological sequelae are present in most patients. Although increased plasma concentrations of leucine and/or its keto acid 2-oxoisocaproic acid are considered the main neurotoxins [158] the mechanisms underlying the brain damage are not well established. Brain injury in MSUD is also

associated with demyelination [159,160], neurotransmitter disturbances, induction of oxidative stress [161], apoptosis and energy deficit [162]. The neurotoxicity of leucine may be associated with its ability to inhibit transport of other LNAA across the blood–brain barrier (BBB), reducing the brain supply of amino acids such as tryptophan, tyrosine, phenylalanine, valine and threonine [163,164]. There appears little apparent toxicity associated with increased plasma concentrations of isoleucine or valine [158].

Prevalence

MSUD has an estimated frequency of approximately 1 in 116 000 [165]. In the Mennonite populations of Pennsylvania, Kentucky, Indiana and Wisconsin, USA, it occurs in approximately 1 in 176 newborns [158]. The frequency is also high in the Ashkenzi Jewish population and in countries where consanguineous marriage is common [160].

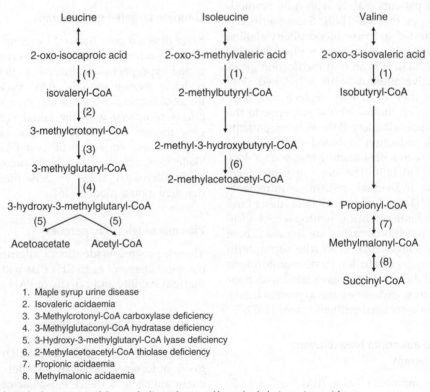

1. Maple syrup urine disease
2. Isovaleric acidaemia
3. 3-Methylcrotonyl-CoA carboxylase deficiency
4. 3-Methylglutaconyl-CoA hydratase deficiency
5. 3-Hydroxy-3-methylglutaryl-CoA lyase deficiency
6. 2-Methylacetoacetyl-CoA thiolase deficiency
7. Propionic acidaemia
8. Methylmalonic acidaemia

Figure 17.9 Selected inborn errors of the catabolic pathways of branched chain amino acids.

Classification

MSUD is a genetically and phenotypically hetero-geneous disorder of variable clinical severity from a severe classical form to a milder variant. Five clinical and biochemical phenotypes are known (Table 17.9).

Biochemistry in classical MSUD

The following are seen:

- ↑ 2-ketoacids in plasma, urine and cerebrospinal fluid
- ↑ accumulation of BCAA. On presentation, plasma leucine levels are commonly in the range 1000–5000 μmol/L (normal reference range 65–220 μmol/L)
- L-alloisoleucine (>5 μmol/L), formed from the tautomerisation of isoleucine, is present in plasma
- presence of ketonuria without treatment, poor metabolic control or catabolic stress
- elevated molar ratio of leucine to other amino acids such as alanine, glutamine and tyrosine [163, 170].

Genetics

MSUD is an inherited autosomal recessive condition. Over 100 causal mutations [23] in four genes that encode for the BCKAD complex [BCK-DHA (E1α), BCKDHB (E1β), DBT (E2), DLT (E3)] give rise to the various phenotypes. The chromosomal location of E1α is on chromosome 19q 13.1-13.2 [171].

Diagnosis

Elevated plasma leucine, L-alloisoleucine and isoleucine (combined) in MSUD can be detected by MS/MS in extended newborn screening programmes (In England, MSUD newborn screening was approved May, 2014. www.screening.nhs.uk). Newborn screening should reduce diagnostic time and thereby lessen exposure to very high leucine concentrations. In the UK pilot project [165], however, as screening is between days 5–8 of life, infants may be symptomatic by the time positive screening results are available. Without newborn screening, infants with a classical presentation of MSUD are commonly encephalopathic by the time the diagnosis is suspected. Early diagnosis is hampered by the lack of routinely detectable metabolic abnormalities (such as hyperammonaemia, hypoglycaemia or metabolic acidosis) as well as the striking similarity of the initial presentation to neonatal meningitis [172]. The presence of L-alloisoleucine is a diagnostic marker for MSUD [173].

Treatment guidelines

Dietary restriction of BCAA (leucine, valine and isoleucine) whilst avoiding their deficiency, maintaining growth and nutritional status and avoiding catabolism is the mainstay of therapy. The aim is to maintain plasma BCAA concentrations within a target treatment range that is not associated with neurotoxicity. Meticulous treatment, using an emergency regimen (p. 502) for any catabolic stress (infection, surgery, trauma) that may lead to metabolic decompensation, is essential. There is little outcome based evidence to set guidelines for target treatment concentrations of BCAA. However, best possible intellectual performance is associated with leucine not exceeding normal concentrations of 200 μmol/L [164] and as a consequence some recommend maintaining 2–3 hour postprandial leucine concentrations close to normal concentrations (80–200 μmol/L) [157, 160]. Others suggest that in order to meet leucine requirements for protein synthesis and avoid protein deficiency, leucine concentrations could be maintained up to 1.5 times the upper range (100–300 μmol/L) [163]. The UK expanded newborn screening group suggest maintaining an upper leucine concentration of 400 μmol/L [165] (Table 17.10)

It is recommended that valine and isoleucine concentrations are maintained between 200 and 400 μmol/L. This is to avoid deficiency so that they do not become rate limiting for protein synthesis and to overcome BBB transport competition with leucine [170]. Valine supplementation may be particularly important because it has a low affinity for the BBB LAT1 transporter and it is especially vulnerable to competitive inhibition by leucine [163].

Table 17.9 Clinical phenotypes of MSUD [163, 166–168].

Type and BCKAD (% of normal activity)	Age of onset	Clinical signs and symptoms	Biochemistry	Dietary treatment

Classic (0%–2%)	Neonatal presentation	• Poor feeding
		• Sweet, malty caramel like smell
		• Episodic vomiting
		• Irritability
		• Hypoglycaemia
		• Lethargy
		• Encephalopathy
		• Cerebral oedema
		• Seizures
		Delay in diagnosis may result in neurological damage or death
		Long term problems include
		  ◦ attention deficits
		  ◦ impulsivity
		  ◦ hyperactivity
			↑ plasma BCAA
			↑ plasma allo-isoleucine
			↑ 2-ketoacids in urine
			Ketonuria
				Low BCAA diet
				Leucine tolerance is low
				Requires emergency regimen during illness, fasting, infection or surgery

Intermediate (3%–30%)	Presents at any age	• Faltering growth • Hypotonia • Feeding problems • Progressive developmental delay • Seizures • Ketoacidosis • Vulnerable to acute and chronic neurological sequelae as in classic form	Similar to classic phenotype but quantitatively less severe	Low BCAA diet [167] Requires emergency regimen during illness, fasting, infection or surgery
Intermittent (5%–20%)	Infancy to adults	• Episodic ataxia/acute behaviour change and ketoacidosis (often with intercurrent illness or increased protein intake)	Normal BCAA and urine organic acid profile when well Abnormal BCAA and urine organic acid profile when unwell	Generally tolerate normal/moderate restriction of leucine intake when well [163] Requires emergency regimen during illness, fasting, infection or surgery [167]
Thiamin responsive (a cofactor for BCKD complex) (2%–40%)	Late onset	• Similar to intermediate phenotype	Leucine tolerance and biochemical profiles improve with thiamin therapy	Requires dietary restriction [169] but less severe than classic MSUD Responds to thiamin therapy Acts on E2 subunit Requires emergency regimen during illness, fasting, infection or surgery [167]
Dihydrolipoamide dehydrogenase deficiency (E3 deficiency) (8%–20%)	During infancy	• Severe hypotonia • Developmental delay • Microcephaly • Spasticity • Ketoacidosis • Reduced ATP synthesis • Leigh's disease	↑ blood lactate ↑ pyruvate ↑ plasma alanine, glutamate, glutamine and BCAA ↑ BCKA and α-ketoglutarate in urine	Low BCAA diet tried but thought not to be helpful

BCKAD, α-ketoacid dehydrogenase; BCAA, branched chain amino acids.

Table 17.10 Suggested guidelines for blood branched chain amino acid concentrations in MSUD.

Amino acid (μmol/L)	Hoffman *et al.* 2006 [164]	Strauss *et al.* 2009 [163]	UK Expanded Newborn Screening 2012 [165]	GMDI Consensus Guidelines 2013 [169]	Normal reference range
Leucine	≤200 (lower level not stated)	100–300	200–400	≤ 5 years of age: 50–200 >5 years of age: 50–300	65–220
Valine	Not stated	200–400	200–400	200–400	90–300
Isoleucine	Not stated	200–400	200–400	200–400	26–100

GMDI, Genetic Metabolic Dietitians International.

Other treatment options

Thiamin
Pharmacological doses of thiamin may improve BCAA tolerance in patients with a thiamin responsive phenotype. Leucine restriction is still advocated with thiamin supplementation [169].

Liver transplantation
Orthotopic liver transplantation is an effective therapy for classic MSUD, associated with an increase in BCKD activity to at least the level seen in the very mild MSUD variant. Alloisoleucine may still remain elevated [158]. Patients should no longer require diet therapy and the risk of metabolic decompensation is removed [160]. Successful domino transplantation has also been reported [174].

Outcome

Without early and effective treatment children develop severe and permanent brain damage, including spasticity, and may die within the first few months of life. With early diagnosis and assiduous dietary management the outcome is improving. Average intellectual performance, however, is clearly below that of normal subjects [175] although some will attend normal schools and have normal IQ scores. The intellectual outcome is related to length of time after birth that plasma leucine concentration is >1000 μmol/L and is dependent on the quality of long term metabolic control [164]. In addition some children may have inattention and hyperactivity disorder and older patients may show generalised anxiety, panic or depression resulting in poor educational

and social achievement [164]. Although there are reports of college graduates with MSUD [158], low educational achievement, high unemployment and low autonomy (still living with their parents) have been reported in adults [176]. Children with milder forms of MSUD tend to have better outcomes [176] but all patients are vulnerable to rapid deterioration associated with catabolic stress.

Some patients present with pancreatitis during treatment for acute intercurrent illness/leucine intoxication [163].

Nutritional outcome

A number of nutritional deficiencies have been reported on low BCAA diets including deficiency of valine, isoleucine [177–180], n-3 fatty acids [170], erythrocyte glutathione peroxidase and selenium [161]. Low BMD was reported in 90% of adolescents with MSUD [163].

Homocystinuria

Classical homocystinuria (HCU) (OMIM 236200) is an autosomal recessive disorder of methionine catabolism. It is due to deficiency of the enzyme cystathionine β-synthase (CBS) (EC 4.2.1.22) located on the long arm of chromosome 21. Methionine is initially converted into the amino acid homocysteine by a series of enzyme dependent steps (Fig. 17.10). Homocysteine, which is not a constituent of protein and thus not required for protein synthesis, is then normally either degraded through the trans-sulfuration pathway or recycled back to methionine by the remethylation pathway [181]. The trans-sulfuration pathway converts homocysteine via cystathionine, with the addition of a

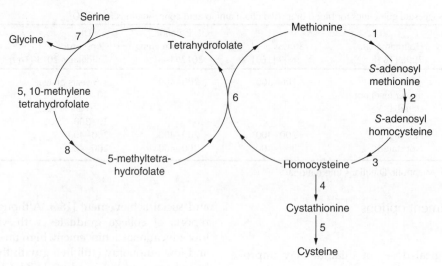

Figure 17.10   Metabolic pathways of homocysteine metabolism.

serine group, to cysteine. There are two remethylation pathways of homocysteine to methionine:
(i) involves methionine synthase, vitamin B_{12} and
folic acid and (ii) involves betaine-homocysteine
methyltransferase and occurs in certain tissues,
e.g. liver, kidney [182]. The first step in the
trans-sulfuration of homocysteine requires CBS
and pyridoxal-5-phosphate (vitamin B_6) as a cofactor. A deficiency of CBS results in increased plasma
concentrations of methionine, homocysteine and
other sulphur containing metabolites (mixed
disulphides) and low levels of plasma cysteine,
cystathionine and serine. In addition homocystine
is present in large amounts in the urine (hence

the condition being termed homocystinuria).
Two main phenotypes of HCU exist: pyridoxine
responsive HCU, which is the milder phenotype;
and pyridoxine non responsive HCU.

There are several other inherited metabolic disorders associated with methionine or homocysteine
metabolism (Table 17.11). These involve either the
trans-sulfuration pathway, by which methionine
is catabolised, or the remethylation pathway by
which homocysteine is normally recycled back to
methionine [181]. A number of the remethylation
defects are inherited disorders of the cofactor vitamins (B_{12}, folic acid) involved in the metabolic
pathways of homocysteine metabolism (Fig. 17.10).

Table 17.11   Other disorders of methionine and homocysteine metabolism.

Disorder	Biochemistry	Treatment
Methionine S-adenosyltransferase (MAT) deficiency	Increased methionine	Generally not required
5,10-methylenetetrahydrofolate reductase (MTHFR) deficiency	Low-normal methionine Increased homocysteine	Betaine Folic acid, B_{12}
Methionine synthase deficiency	Low-normal methionine Increased homocysteine	B_6, B_{12}, folic acid Possibly betaine and methionine
Cobalamin (B_{12}) defects – CblC	Increased homocysteine Low-normal methionine Methylmalonic acidaemia	B_{12} Betaine Possibly methionine

The management of the remethylation disorders is based on cofactor vitamin, betaine and methionine supplementation [181]. These will not be further described.

Genetics

Classical HCU was first described in 1962 [183, 184]. It is caused by mutations in the gene encoding for the cystathionine β-synthase (CBS) enzyme (EC 4.2.1.22) [185] found on the long arm of chromosome 21 [185] and is expressed mainly in the liver and kidneys [181]. HCU is inherited as an autosomal recessive trait. At least 160 mutations have been identified, with the majority being private (i.e. only occurring within that family) [186]. The worldwide incidence of HCU is approximately 1 in 344 000 [187], but there are large population differences, being highest in ethnic populations where there is a high level of consanguinity. In the Republic of Ireland the incidence is at least 1 in 65 000 [188]. The incidence may be underestimated due to the infrequency of newborn screening for the disorder. DNA screening studies of newborn infants in a number of countries have shown that the overall incidence may be as high as 1 in 20 000 [189]. The highest reported incidence is in Qatar where there is a high carrier frequency (1% population) of a common mutation, with an incidence of 1 in 1800 [190].

Biochemistry

In healthy normal subjects plasma homocysteine is present in several forms [191]:

- 10%–20% is present as free, non protein bound homocysteine (fHcy) comprising homocysteine (reduced form <2%), homocystine (disulphide of homocysteine) and mixed disulphide (homocysteine-cysteine)
- the largest proportion, 80%–90%, is present as protein (albumin) bound homocysteine

Plasma total homocysteine (tHcy) concentration is the sum of all the different forms. In plasma from normal subjects free homocysteine (fHcy) is usually undetectable and tHcy is 5–15 μmol/L [192]. fHcy only becomes detectable when tHcy exceeds 60 μmol/L [193]. At diagnosis plasma tHcy in HCU

patients will be significantly increased with levels often >200 μmol/L. In addition plasma methionine levels are elevated and cysteine levels are low.

Pathophysiology

Individuals who have HCU are clinically normal at birth. CBS deficiency results in accumulation of methionine, homocysteine and their S-adenosyl derivatives and deficiency of cystathionine and cysteine. Without early diagnosis and treatment there is a progressive onset of the multisystem clinical features of HCU, in extreme cases appearing early in childhood [194], thought to be caused by the accumulation of homocysteine [194, 195]. The major clinical features involve

- the ocular system – lens dislocation, iridodenesis, myopia, glaucoma
- skeletal system – osteoporosis, scoliosis, elongation and thinning of the long bones, marfanoid appearance
- vascular system – thromboembolisms, malar flush
- central nervous system – developmental delay, learning difficulties, electroencephalogram changes, epilepsy, psychiatric disturbance

Other clinical features include pancreatitis [196] and spontaneous pneumothorax [197, 198].

The ocular symptoms may be a result of abnormal formation of zonular fibres which are composed of glycoprotein normally containing high concentrations of cysteine [199]. Thromboembolisms are probably the result of homocysteine induced platelet abnormalities [194]. Excess homocysteine may cause abnormal collagen crosslinking, resulting in development of osteoporosis and abnormalities of skin, joints and skeleton [194]. Unfortunately genetically modified animal models have so far not added to knowledge of the pathophysiology; the CBS knockout mouse has a rapidly lethal phenotype [200] and other genetically modified mouse models have phenotypes very different to human phenotypes [194].

Diagnosis

HCU is diagnosed from analysis of quantitative amino acid in plasma which has been immediately processed showing raised methionine, fHcy and tHcy, and low plasma cysteine and cystathionine. HCU may be diagnosed from screening in the neonatal period. Historically, few centres have specifically screened for the disorder, although over recent years it has been added around the world as newborn screening (NBS) has expanded. NBS is only likely to identify pyridoxine non responsive HCU as plasma homocysteine levels are unlikely to be sufficiently elevated in pyridoxine responsive HCU at the time of NBS. Consequently a significant proportion will only be diagnosed following the onset of clinical symptoms.

In the UK screening for HCU is currently not a routine part of NBS. In England six centres are undertaking an expanded NBS pilot between July 2012 and March 2014 [165] of which pyridoxine unresponsive HCU is one of a panel of five disorders being additionally screened for. Initial screening is on measurement of methionine in dried blood spots measured by tandem MS/MS. If methionine is ≥50 μmol/L then tHcy is measured; if ≥15 μmol/L this is considered a positive screen and the infant is referred for diagnostic tests of plasma amino acids, including methionine and tHcy, and vitamin B_{12} levels. Screening, diagnostic and clinical management guidelines can be accessed from the website [165].

Treatment

Treatment is aimed at reducing homocysteine levels and will depend upon factors such as whether pyridoxine responsive or non responsive and age of diagnosis. All newly diagnosed patients should initially have a 7 day trial with a pharmacological dose of pyridoxine (vitamin B_6): 50 mg twice daily in those diagnosed on NBS [165] and 100–200 mg three times daily in older children [201], together with 5 mg folic acid to assess for pyridoxine responsiveness.

Pyridoxine responsive HCU

The enzyme CBS requires pyridoxal-5-phosphate, formed from pyridoxine (vitamin B_6), as its cofactor. A significant number of CBS deficient individuals show clinical and biochemical response to pharmacological doses of pyridoxine, up to

500 mg/day [202]. Pyridoxine supplementation should be kept to the minimum effective dose as doses >1000 mg/day have been associated with peripheral neuropathy [194]. The defect in pyridoxine responsive cases is still caused by mutations within the CBS protein and is not due to either deficient pyridoxine status or a disorder of pyridoxine metabolism. Pyridoxine, in this situation, is acting to increase residual CBS activity.

Worldwide up to 50% of cases of CBS deficiency HCU are pyridoxine responsive showing a decrease in plasma methionine and almost complete elimination of homocysteine from plasma (free homocysteine <5 μmol/L) and urine [188, 203]. There are population differences with a much smaller percentage showing pyridoxine responsiveness in certain populations, e.g. Britain and Ireland. In CBS deficiency folic acid requirements are probably increased due to an increased flux through the remethylation pathway [204]. It is therefore essential to also give folic acid, 5 mg daily, and to ensure that plasma vitamin B_{12} levels (required for folate metabolism) are adequate. In those individuals with pyridoxine responsive HCU treatment with pyridoxine and folic acid can prevent further deterioration in symptoms except for advanced eye disease [202].

Pyridoxine non responsive HCU

In this group plasma homocysteine levels do not fall following pharmacological doses of pyridoxine. Treatment strategies aim at reducing homocysteine levels by

- decreasing the intake of the substrate methionine by use of a methionine or protein restricted diet to reduce plasma methionine and thereby homocysteine levels
- giving an additional pharmacological dose of folic acid, 5 mg daily, to ensure adequate supply of folate for the remethylation pathway
- utilising alternative pathways to remove homocysteine by giving betaine (a methyl donor) which remethylates homocysteine back to methionine and so reduces plasma homocysteine levels. If betaine is used plasma methionine levels will usually be elevated

The decision on which treatment option to use varies between metabolic centres possibly depending upon factors including age and mode of diagnosis, i.e. screened or clinically presenting, and previous treatment experiences. Those diagnosed on NBS are more likely to be solely diet treated, at least in the early years, than those clinically presenting at a later age.

Dietary management of HCU

The principles of dietary management, in common with other amino acid disorders, are based on decreasing the load on the affected pathway and supplementing deficient products beyond the metabolic block. Early dietary treatments were described in 1966 in Manchester [205] and later in Vancouver [206]. The primary aims of dietary treatment are to correct abnormal biochemistry (reduce plasma methionine levels to within or slightly above the normal age related reference range unless on betaine therapy), decrease plasma homocysteine levels and increase plasma cysteine levels to within the normal range (Table 17.12). Further details of dietary management are given see page 416.

Betaine therapy

Betaine is a methyl donor, derived from choline, and promotes the remethylation reaction of homocysteine to methionine via the enzyme betaine-homocysteine methyltransferase (Fig. 17.11). Use of betaine in HCU, at a maximum dose of 150 mg/kg/day (6–9 g/day maximum in adults) in two to three divided doses [194, 207], results in a decrease in plasma homocysteine levels and will normally result in plasma methionine levels being significantly increased, although this is not universal [208, 209]. Pharmacokinetic studies demonstrated that doses of betaine above 200 mg/kg/day in two to three divided doses were of no additional value in decreasing tHcy levels [207].

Oral betaine can be useful in improving biochemical control in circumstances where dietary

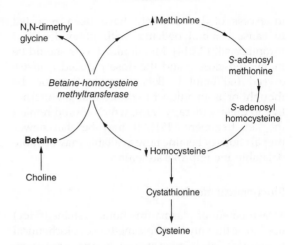

Figure 17.11 Methyl group donation by betaine.

adherence is poor, e.g. adolescents, adults and those late diagnosed. However, adherence with betaine is not always good, with fHcy levels in 13 patients in one study not being significantly altered with betaine (mean 35 µmol/L pre treatment and 33 µmol/L on treatment), and it is unlikely to replace dietary therapy [202], although a recent European survey [210] identified significant individuals treated with betaine alone. In the 'human only' HCU mouse betaine efficacy in reducing homocysteine decreased significantly over time [211] which may add to the need to combine with dietary therapy.

The reduced long term effect of betaine at lowering homocysteine levels may in part be due to oxidative stress impairment of the function of betaine-homocysteine methyltransferase [212], which could be prevented by the concurrent administration of taurine, an antioxidant, in the HCU mouse. Taurine given with betaine may potentially improve the therapeutic effects of long term betaine use [212]. The significantly raised plasma methionine levels, which occur with betaine use, do not appear to affect the pathophysiology of the disease [202]. Very high levels of plasma methionine,

Table 17.12 Biochemical monitoring in HCU.

	Plasma methionine	Plasma cysteine	Plasma fHcy	Plasma tHcy
B_6 responsive	Normal range	Normal range	<10 µmol/L	<50 µmol/L
B_6 non responsive, diet alone	Normal range	Normal range	<10 µmol/L	<100 µmol/L
B_6 non responsive + betaine	<1000µmol/L	Normal range	<10 µmol/L	<100 µmol/L

in excess of 1000 µmol/L, have been reported to cause cerebral oedema, without evidence of thrombosis [213, 214]. Methionine levels should be monitored closely and the dose reduced if levels exceed 1000 µmol/L. Betaine might therefore be thought of as an adjunct to rather than an alternative to dietary therapy [213], which should remain the key treatment [181]. It may be that newer preparations of betaine now available may be more palatable and improve adherence.

Biochemical monitoring

Measurement of plasma free homocysteine (fHcy) used to be the only available method of biochemical monitoring of homocysteine. Routine measurement of plasma total homocysteine (tHcy) has only become available over the last decade [215] and is increasingly used. Levels of fHcy <10 µmol/L indicate good biochemical control [202]. Data on acceptable tHcy levels in HCU are still limited and as yet data on lifelong tHcy and clinical outcome are not available. In the normal population tHcy levels are 5–15 µmol/L [192] and fHcy is only detectable when tHcy ≥60 µmol/L [193]. To achieve tHcy <60 µmol/L fHcy would need to be undetectable. It is known, however, that achieving lifelong fHcy <10–11 µmol/L reduces the probability of complications developing [188, 202].

The UK expanded NBS project recommendations [165] are given in Table 17.12, with an aim of tHcy <100 µmol/L. Lower levels are more achievable in pyridoxine responsive patients, with around 10% responding fully with normalisation of fasting plasma tHcy, methionine and cystine [187]. Until more data are available on tHcy levels and clinical outcome both plasma fHcy and tHcy should ideally be monitored.

Regular monitoring of plasma methionine, cysteine, fHcy and tHcy should be undertaken [165]:

- weekly from start of treatment until levels are stable for 4 consecutive weeks, then
- fortnightly to 1 year of age
- monthly to 2 years of age
- thereafter 3 monthly

Monitoring of homocysteine is technically challenging to ensure results are accurate. No dried blood spot method for monitoring is currently in routine use; thus samples must be taken at a hospital. Liquid blood samples have to be deproteinised within 10 minutes to preserve fHcy; otherwise it will be bound to plasma proteins and lead to underestimation. For accurate tHcy measurement samples also have to be rapidly dealt with to separate blood cells from the sample [201].

In addition to monitoring plasma homocysteine, methionine and cysteine levels, vitamin B_{12} and folate status should be assessed as low levels of these could cause inadequate response to treatment due to their intimate roles in homocysteine metabolism.

Manipulation of the diet

Methionine intake

- if fHcy/tHcy are towards lower target ranges then an increase in methionine/protein intake, by 10–20 mg methionine or 0.5–1 g protein per day, should be advised
- if fHcy/tHcy are higher than target ranges then a decrease in methionine/protein intake, by 10–20 mg methionine or 0.5–1 g protein per day, should be advised

Factors such as illness, growth rate and dietary adherence should be taken into account. (Tables 17.33 (high blood concentrations) and 17.34 (low blood concentrations) give guidance on interpretation of substrate blood amino acid results.)

Cysteine

Cysteine becomes a conditionally indispensable amino acid in HCU (Table 17.15). Monitoring plasma cysteine is problematic; it has been shown that fHcy concentrations increase significantly when total cysteine (tCys) concentrations are <170 µmol/L [216]. If tCys levels are <170 µmol/L supplementation should be considered as it may be beneficial in reducing fHcy.

Clinical outcome

Good long term biochemical control in HCU can prevent the onset of complications in early diagnosed individuals and can curtail further progression, but not reversal, of the disorder in late diagnosed cases, apart from the eye disease [202]. Published outcome data from follow-up of patients treated over many years show that lifelong median fHcy <11 μmol/L significantly reduces the probability of developing complications [188] and levels of fHcy <10 μmol/L indicate good biochemical control [202]. Normal IQ has been reported [202, 217] in pyridoxine unresponsive HCU with good treatment adherence since diagnosis in the neonatal period. In a review of 46 patients treated at the National Centre, Dublin, over a 38 year period [218], 65% were diagnosed from NBS (77% of whom had good/moderate control). The cmplication rate was 2% for those diagnosed on NBS and under good control, 17% for those diagnosed on NBS but with poor control and 45% for those not identified on NBS. Tertiary education was achieved by 84% of those diagnosed on NBS compared with 43% who were clinically presenting cases. Ectopia lentis is likely to develop where fHcy >12.3 μmol/L. Cognitive outcome in children is related to exposure to homocysteine and is best where cumulative exposure up to age 4 years is <100 μmol/L.

Vascular events have been shown to be the commonest cause of death in HCU with the risk of a vascular event at 25% below 16 years of age and at 50% by age 30 years in undiagnosed or poorly controlled HCU [219]. If factor V Leiden mutation, another risk factor for thrombotic events, is also present in addition to HCU this further increases the risk [220]. The actual frequency of factor V Leiden in the HCU population is unknown, with reports of 64% in 11 patients from seven families with a high rate of consanguinity [220] and 20% in 15 non consanguineous patients [221]. Cardiovascular risk is greater in pyridoxine non responsive HCU [203]. Adverse vascular changes are thought to be caused by effects of increased circulating homocysteine levels on endothelial smooth muscle cells; fHcy is more relevant to endothelial cell function and its interactions with circulating blood [222].

Maternal HCU

Pregnancy in women with pyridoxine responsive HCU, provided they are on treatment, appears to carry no significant risk to either the woman or offspring [194]. In pyridoxine non responsive HCU, however, pregnancy appears to be associated with a higher incidence of spontaneous abortion. There is little evidence of other adverse effects on the foetus [203]. Betaine appears to be safe during pregnancy with infrequent reports of abnormalities being observed in offspring [202, 203]. Both pregnancy and homocystinuria are risk factors for thromboembolism. Increased levels of homocysteine in the first few weeks postpartum have been reported which can be alleviated by anticoagulation therapy [223, 224]. Management of pregnancy in women with HCU includes good metabolic control and the use of anticoagulant therapy during the later stages of pregnancy and first 6 weeks postpartum to safeguard the mother's health.

Tyrosinaemia

Tyrosine, an amino acid found in dietary protein and also endogenously synthesised from the hydroxylation of phenylalanine, is used for protein synthesis as well as being a precursor for a number of important body chemicals including dopamine, epinephrine, norepinephrine, melanin and thyroxine. Tyrosine is catabolised by a series of enzyme dependent reactions to fumaric acid and acetoacetate (Fig. 17.12). There are three inherited disorders of tyrosine metabolism: hereditary tyrosinaemia types I, II and III. In addition to these, raised tyrosine levels may be found in neonates, particularly preterm infants, on NBS. This is most commonly transient tyrosinaemia of the newborn probably due to immaturity of the enzyme 4-hydroxyphenylpyruvate dioxygenase (Fig. 17.12) [225]. This may respond to vitamin C supplementation to induce enzyme activity, with rapid normalisation of tyrosine levels. Another rare cause of raised tyrosine levels is in infants fed unmodified goat's milk which has a high protein content and can give rise to suspicion of tyrosinaemia type I, with raised tyrosine and a metabolic acidosis [226].

Tyrosinaemia type I

Hereditary tyrosinaemia type I (HTI) (OMIN 276700) is an autosomal recessive disorder of tyrosine catabolism. HTI is caused by reduced activity of the enzyme fumarylacetoacetate hydrolyase (FAH, EC 3.7.1.2) which catalyses the final step of tyrosine degradation (Fig. 17.12). The metabolic block results in accumulation of fumarylacetoacetate (FAA) and maleylacetoacetate (MAA), with FAA being further metabolised to

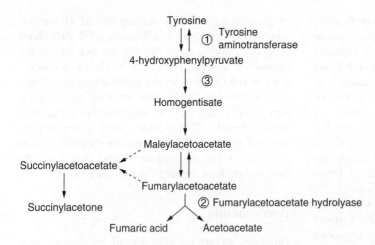

Figure 17.12   Pathways of tyrosine degradation. 1 Tyrosinaemia type II. 2 Tyrosinaemia type I. 3 4-Hydroxyphenyl-pyruvate dioxygenase (site of action of 2-(2-nitro-4-trifluoromethylbenzoyl)-1,3-cyclohexanedione, NTBC).

produce succinylacetone (SA). These metabolites are considered toxic. HTI can present at different ages with varying degrees of severity. Most affected infants will present clinically unless born in a region where NBS for HTI is performed, had early testing due to an affected sibling or had been identified on NBS with abnormal amino acid levels. NBS allows identification and institution of treatment prior to the onset of symptoms [227]. Currently HTI is not included in the NBS panel of inherited metabolic diseases in the UK.

Genetics

HTI is caused by mutations encoding for FAH. The gene is located on chromosome 15 with over 40 mutations having been identified [228]. Certain FAH mutations occur more frequently in particular areas or ethnic groups including French-Canadian (over 90% alleles are the same mutation), Mediterranean countries, Finns, Turks and Pakistanis. There is no clear genotype–phenotype correlation [229]. The worldwide incidence of HTI is approximately 1 in 100 000, being more common in certain areas, e.g. in Quebec, Canada, where it is around 1 in 1846 [230]. In Birmingham, UK, the higher incidence of 1 in 20 791 is associated with South Asian ethnicity and consanguinity [231].

Biochemistry

Normal plasma concentrations of tyrosine are around 30–120 µmol/L. Plasma tyrosine levels in

HTI are usually only moderately elevated, around two to four times the upper end of the range, as the defect occurs later in the tyrosine degradative pathway rather than in the early steps. This makes the measurement of tyrosine unhelpful as a marker for screening for HTI. FAA, MAA and SA are found in significantly increased concentrations in both plasma and urine. The presence of SA is pathognomonic for HTI. SA inhibits δ-aminolevulinic acid (δ-ALA) dehydratase resulting in accumulation of δ-ALA, which is excreted in high concentrations in urine.

Clinical features and pathophysiology

The metabolites FAA, MAA and SA are thought to be responsible for the clinical features of progressive liver failure with increased risk for hepatocellular carcinoma (HCC), renal tubular dysfunction with hypophosphataemic rickets and δ-ALA for a porphyria like syndrome [232, 233]. FAA, MAA and SA bind to sulphydryl groups and this may result in tissue injury [234]. Other manifestations include cardiomyopathy and pancreatic cell hypertrophy which can cause hyperinsulinism [234]. Plasma methionine concentration can also be markedly increased, due to secondary inhibition of S-adenosylmethionine synthetase [232], and this may affect normal liver function [235].

HTI can present clinically at any age from the neonatal period until adulthood. It can manifest with a variety of clinical symptoms and severity and is usually classified according to age of onset of symptoms, broadly correlating with severity of disease [227, 236]:

- acute – the most common form presents before 6 months of age with acute liver failure, the most severe before 2 months
- sub acute – presents between 6 months and 1 year of age with progressive liver failure, hepatosplenomegaly, coagulopathy, faltering growth and rickets
- chronic – presents over 1 year of age with chronic liver or renal disease and rickets or with porphyria like episodes; some may also have cardiomyopathy

Diagnosis

The main diagnostic metabolite for HTI is SA measured in plasma, dried blood spot or urine. Plasma quantitative amino acids, showing raised tyrosine ± methionine, are found in any severe liver disease and are not specific for HTI. Alpha-fetoprotein (AFP) levels are normally markedly raised, even in those identified on NBS, but again this is not specific [227]. Infants rarely present with clinical symptoms in the first few days, although biochemical abnormalities may be present soon after birth, including raised SA and AFP levels.

Treatment

The treatment of HTI has been revolutionised since the use of nitisinone (2-(2-nitro-4-trifluoromethyl-benzoyl)-1,3-cyclohexanedione, NTBC, Orphadin®) was described in 1992 [237]. Prior to the discovery of nitisinone, HTI was treated with a low tyrosine, low phenylalanine diet to minimise formation of toxic metabolites. A reduced methionine intake was also used initially. Dietary treatment was shown to improve renal tubular dysfunction and growth. Liver function (in particular prothrombin time) sometimes improved a little but dietary management could not completely prevent the production of toxic metabolites (including SA) or the development of HCC. Some patients developed progressive liver failure or lethal porphyric crises. Liver transplantation was the only really effective treatment for HTI.

Nitisinone works by inhibition of the enzyme 4-hydroxyphenylpyruvate dioxygenase, blocking the tyrosine degradation pathway at this point, the defect in tyrosinaemia type III (HTIII) (Fig. 17.12). This prevents the formation of the hepatotoxic and nephrotoxic compounds and SA (which probably plays an important role in neurotoxicity) but instead leads to an increase in plasma tyrosine. Nitisinone treatment leads to rapid improvement in hepatic and renal function and prevents neurological dysfunction in most patients [238]. In those who have started nitisinone treatment early in life, the risk of early development of HCC is markedly reduced. For patients who start nitisinone treatment late, there remains a considerable risk for liver malignancy [239]. Nitisinone is now established as a very effective alternative to liver transplantation.

Treatment with nitisinone must be continued without interruption otherwise serious complications, including acute liver failure, neurological crisis or malignant liver changes, may occur [227]. The usual dose of nitisinone is 1 mg/kg/day in two divided doses; however, it has been demonstrated that a single daily dose can maintain adequate plasma NTBC levels [240]. There have been compliance issues with taking nitisinone regularly [241] so once daily dosing may be beneficial in improving adherence and thus metabolic control.

Although nitisinone is highly affective in suppressing the production of SA and related toxic metabolites it does lead to a further increase in plasma tyrosine. Studies on healthy volunteers showed that following a single dose of nitisinone plasma tyrosine concentrations increased from around 100 μmol/L at baseline to approximately 1100 μmol/L [242]. In tyrosinaemia type II (HTII) high plasma tyrosine concentrations are the probable cause of the oculocutaneous manifestations and may also be associated with the mental retardation reported in some patients [232]. To reduce the risks with high plasma tyrosine concentrations, patients with HTI on nitisinone are treated with a low tyrosine/low phenylalanine diet (in practice a low protein diet with tyrosine and phenylalanine free L-amino acid supplements) to maintain blood tyrosine levels within the target treatment range. The target treatment range for tyrosine was 200–500 μmol/L as reported in much of the literature, but the upper limit in the main UK centres is now more commonly 400 μmol/L in view of concerns regarding intellectual outcome. A target range of 200–400 μmol/L is given as a guide in the recent published international recommendations on management of HTI [227].

If HTI is suspected because of liver disease, then once appropriate investigations (including plasma amino acids, urine organic acids, investigations for galactosaemia and, if age appropriate, tests for hereditary fructose intolerance) are undertaken nitisinone should be started. A low tyrosine, low phenylalanine diet should also be commenced pending confirmatory results. It is not normally necessary to restrict methionine as plasma levels will normalise as liver function improves. Whilst waiting for diagnostic results galactose and fructose should be withheld from the diet until galactosaemia and hereditary fructose intolerance have been excluded [227].

Dietary management in HTI treated with nitisinone

The principles of dietary management, in common with other amino acid disorders, are based on decreasing the load on the affected pathway and supplementing deficient products beyond the metabolic block. The primary aims of dietary treatment are to correct abnormal biochemistry, maintain blood tyrosine levels within 200–400 μmo/L, and maintain blood phenylalanine in the normal range.

The intake of natural protein is reduced, thereby limiting tyrosine and phenylalanine intakes, and is altered according to plasma tyrosine concentrations. The amount of natural protein tolerated varies between patients. It has been reported to decrease from a peak of 1.8–2.4 g protein/kg/day at 4–5 months to around 1 g protein/kg/day in late infancy (with mean plasma tyrosine levels ranging from 322 to 497 μmol/L) [243]. This high peak of protein intake may be related to catch-up growth following diagnosis. Thereafter, once the patient has stabilised, the total protein intake usually varies little, irrespective of age, except during growth spurts. This scenario is also observed in the author's (FW) cohort of HTI patients where natural protein allowance changes little with increasing age, even in the most adherent patients. Average

natural protein intake per kilogram decreases with age in this cohort, average intakes being at 1–4 years age 0.6 g/kg/day (median 8 g/day), at 5–10 years 0.4 g/kg/day (median 8 g/day) and ≥11 years 0.2 g/kg/day (median 14 g/day, the majority in this age group always having an intake around this). There is intra-individual variation in natural protein tolerance, as is seen in all disorders of amino acid metabolism, with intakes varying between 7 and 16 g/day. One centre has reported that daily natural protein intake increased with age in 6/11 patients [244]; however, median intakes were not dissimilar to the author's patient group. Further details of dietary management are given on p. 416.

Biochemical monitoring and dietary manipulation

Recent management recommendations suggest maintaining blood tyrosine levels between 200 and 400 μmol/L [227] and blood phenylalanine concentration within the normal reference range. High tyrosine concentrations are risk factors for neurotoxicity and corneal opacities [245]. Eye complications are said to be rare with tyrosine concentrations <800 μmol/L [227]. A study of 11 patients treated with nitisinone reported no ophthalmic side effects despite some patients in the group having consistently elevated concentrations of tyrosine. They suggest that corneal problems may only arise if plasma tyrosine approaches a much higher concentration of 2000 μmol/L [246]. Regular monitoring of blood or plasma tyrosine and phenylalanine concentrations should be undertaken. Generally dried blood spots are taken at home and sent in to the laboratory for analysis:

- weekly in infants because growth is rapid, or in newly diagnosed patients until stable
- every 1–2 weeks in 1–4 year olds
- monthly thereafter or more frequently if levels are unstable

Blood tyrosine concentration is used to determine natural protein intake (Table 17.13). Factors such as illness, growth rate and dietary adherence should be taken into account when assessing and interpreting blood monitoring results. (Tables 17.33 (high blood concentrations) and 17.34 (low blood

Table 17.13 Manipulation of diet with blood tyrosine levels.

Blood tyrosine level	Protein intake
>400–700 µmol/L	Decrease by 1–2 g protein
<200 µmol/L	Increase by 1 g of protein

Table 17.14 One and 2 year survival probability after the onset of symptoms prior to 1992 [236].

Age of onset of symptoms	Survival rates	
	1 year	2 years
Very early onset <2 months	38%	29%
Early onset 2–6 months	74%	74%
Late onset >6 months	96%	96%

concentrations) give guidance on interpretation of substrate blood amino acid results.)

Once there is stability on diet following diagnosis it would be usual to have a minimum of two results outwith the target range before making dietary changes.

The plasma amino acid profile is also used to check that all other essential amino acids do not fall below the normal reference range, in particular phenylalanine. Low plasma phenylalanine concentrations have been observed in patients with HTI on restricted tyrosine/phenylalanine intakes [247, 248]. If plasma phenylalanine concentrations remain low they may become rate limiting for protein synthesis and plasma tyrosine levels will remain high. In addition low plasma phenylalanine levels are known, in PKU, to be associated with decreased IQ and this has also been observed in HTI where the lowest IQ was seen in those who had phenylalanine levels <40 µmol/L in the first 2 years of treatment [249]. It is therefore important to monitor phenylalanine levels, noting that there is diurnal variation [227] and if blood phenylalanine levels are consistently below the lower reference range a phenylalanine supplement is given usually starting with 50 mg/day. In practice supplementing around 10 mg phenylalanine/kg/day normalises plasma phenylalanine level when plasma concentrations are low [250] but care needs to be taken to ensure that supplementation does not increase tyrosine levels [227]. Ideally the phenylalanine supplement should be given as a divided dose along with the L-amino acid supplement.

Monitoring of NTBC levels, SA and AFP levels should all be done regularly at clinic reviews. Methods for determining NTBC levels in dried blood spots have been developed which enable easier monitoring.

Clinical outcome

Prior to nitisinone treatment survival rates were clearly related to age of onset of symptoms with death from liver failure, neurological crisis or HCC usually by 10 years of age [236] (Table 17.14).

Nitisinone is now the mainstay of treatment for HTI with over 600 patients worldwide having treatment [225]. A small proportion, fewer than 10%, of patients presenting acutely with liver failure do not respond. Jaundice and worsening coagulopathy progress and mortality is high without an urgent liver transplant if there is no improvement within 7 days [225]. Treatment with nitisinone and a low tyrosine/phenylalanine diet have resulted in an over 90% survival rate with normal growth, improved liver function, prevention of cirrhosis and correction of the renal tubular dysfunction [251] and absence of porphyria like crisis [241].

Despite nitisinone treatment, there remain some unresolved long term outcome issues including concerns regarding neurological outcome [241, 249, 252], optimal dosage of nitisinone, evaluation for HCC risk and pregnancy [253]. Outcome studies on 46 French [241], 10 Belgian [249] and seven German (over 3 years of age) [252] patients treated with nitisinone and diet show high incidence of educational difficulties and cognitive impairment in up to 35% of the French cases of school age [241] and in five of the seven German cases [252]. Performance skills were found to be affected more than verbal abilities [225]. The cause of the cognitive deficits is unclear but may be the result of high tyrosine levels due to poor adherence with the dietary treatment. The French study reported 36% patients had tyrosine levels >500 µmol/L [241] and in the Belgian study only 3/10 patients achieved tyrosine <500 µmol/L [249]. Chronic high tyrosine levels are associated with cognitive difficulties in HTII and some cases of HTIII [241, 249]. Tyrosine is a precursor for the neurotransmitters dopamine and norepinephrine. High tyrosine levels may alter the synthesis of these [249] and rat studies have shown association between dopamine activity and impaired performance [254]. Some patients have low plasma phenylalanine concentrations [247, 249]. There is a known association in PKU between low phenylalanine levels and low IQ [249] where patients with the lowest IQ had mean phenylalanine <40 μmol/L in the first 2 years of treatment. Phenylalanine and tyrosine are both neutral amino acids and they compete for entry at the BBB; thus high tyrosine levels with low phenylalanine concentrations will limit the amount of phenylalanine transported into the brain, potentially being rate limiting for brain protein synthesis. The ratio of Tyr:Phe should indicate phenylalanine availability in the brain in HTI [249] as the Phe:Tyr ratio informs of tyrosine availability in PKU [255]. It may be that the previous upper target for tyrosine was too high at 500 μmol/L and that the treatment range should be 200–400 μmol/L [241].

Pregnancy

Safety of nitisinone treatment in pregnancy and the effects of high tyrosine levels are not yet fully understood; however, babies have been born to three women with HTI on nitisinone who were normal at birth and on early follow-up [227]. There have been two published reports of pregnancies in two women with HTI, one in which the baby was unaffected with HTI [256] and the second in which the baby also had HTI [257]. In both cases the infants were normal at birth, both had raised tyrosine levels (higher than the maternal levels due to positive gradient across the placenta) and nitisinone was detectable in neonatal blood at birth with levels comparable to simultaneous levels in the mothers. Tyrosine levels normalised within 4 weeks in the unaffected child but increased in the affected child. Both infants were reported to have normal development. These reports suggest that to date there have been no detrimental effects of foetal exposure to nitisinone, high tyrosine or low phenylalanine levels. In fact in the case where both mother and baby had HTI, exposure to nitisinone had suppressed the disease in the foetus [257].

Tyrosinaemia type II: Richner–Hanhart syndrome

Tyrosinaemia type II (HTII) (OMIN 276600) is an autosomal recessive disorder of tyrosine catabolism

caused by deficiency of hepatic tyrosine aminotransferase (TAT, EC 2.6.1.5) which catalyses the first step of the tyrosine degradation pathway (Fig. 17.12). The metabolic block results in accumulation of tyrosine with plasma tyrosine concentrations usually >1200 μmol/L (normal reference range 30–120 μmol/L) at presentation. These high concentrations of tyrosine result in tyrosine crystals depositing within cells which cause inflammation and lead to some of the clinical features which may affect the eyes, skin and mental development. Unless diagnosed on NBS the disorder will normally present in the first few months of life.

Genetics

HTII is caused by mutations encoding for the enzyme tyrosine aminotransferase (TAT, EC 2.6.1.5). The gene is located on chromosome 16. Seventeen mutations have been described [258]. Most cases of HTII have not been confirmed by enzyme or mutation analysis; therefore some cases may actually be HTIII not HTII [225]. HTII occurs in fewer than 1 in 250 000 individuals [259].

Biochemistry and diagnosis

TAT deficiency causes plasma tyrosine levels to be grossly elevated, usually >1200 μmol/L at diagnosis with tyrosine levels also increased in cerebrospinal fluid. If the tyrosine concentration is less markedly increased HTIII should be considered. There is gross elevation of the phenolic acids 4-hydroxyphenyl -pyruvate, -lactate and -acetate in the urine, probably due to direct deamination of tyrosine by the kidneys or tyrosine catabolism by mitochondrial aminotransferase to 4-hydroxyphenylpyruvate. N-acetyltyrosine and 4-tyramine are also increased [225].

Clinical features and pathophysiology

HTII affects the eyes and skin (oculocutaneous tyrosinaemia) and central nervous system with the main clinical features being [225]

- ocular lesions – occur in around 75% cases; corneal damage is due to tyrosine crystals disrupting corneal epithelial cell function and leading to an inflammatory response

- skin lesions – occur in around 80% of cases and affect pressure areas, most commonly the palms and soles; this is possibly caused by excessive intracellular tyrosine causing structural abnormalities of the epidermal keratinisation [260]
- neurological complications – occur in around 60% cases; some develop normally while others have varying degrees of developmental delay including seizures, self-mutilation and behavioural difficulties [261]

Treatment

HTII is treated with a tyrosine/phenylalanine restricted diet and tyrosine/phenylalanine free L-amino acid supplements to reduce high plasma tyrosine concentrations. The principles of dietary management used for HTI can be applied to HTII. Methionine restriction is not necessary. With dietary treatment, the skin and eye problems usually improve rapidly. Skin and eye symptoms do not generally occur if tyrosine concentrations are <800 µmol/L [225]; however, to minimise the risk of high tyrosine levels contributing to developmental delay lower plasma tyrosine levels are recommended [262], aiming at 200–500 µmol/L [225].

Biochemical monitoring and dietary manipulation

The recommendations for HTI for tyrosine and phenylalanine monitoring can be used.

Pregnancy

Case reports on the outcome of maternal tyrosinaemia are variable: maternal hypertyrosinaemia may have caused foetal neurological abnormalities, e.g. microcephaly, seizures, developmental delay; other untreated pregnancies had normal foetal outcomes [261,263]. There has been one case report of pregnancy treated with diet where tyrosine levels were maintained in the range 100–200 µmolL with a normal foetal and maternal outcome [264].

Tyrosinaemia type III

Tyrosinaemia type III (HTIII) (OMIN 276710) is an autosomal recessive disorder of tyrosine metabolism. HTIII is due to reduced activity of 4-hydroxyphenylpyruvate dioxygenase (4-HPPD) (EC1.13.11.27) which is expressed in the liver and kidney and catalyses the second step in the tyrosine degradation pathway (the step that is inhibited by nitisinone in the treatment of HTI) (Table 17.12). The metabolic block results in elevated plasma tyrosine and increased excretion of its phenolic derivatives in urine [225]. Some cases are identified through NBS because of elevated tyrosine levels.

Genetics

HTIII is caused by mutations in the enzyme 4-HPPD gene located on chromosome 12. Five mutations have been described [225] but without specific genotype–phenotype correlation. It is a very rare disorder with only 13 cases described in the literature to date. In some enzymatically diagnosed cases no mutations have been identified [265,266].

Biochemistry and diagnosis

At presentation plasma tyrosine levels are usually in the range 300–1000 µmol/L with accompanying increased excretion of 4-hydroxyphenyl -pyruvat, -lactate and -acetate. Diagnosis is possible by enzyme analysis of liver or kidney biopsy or mutation analysis [225].

Clinical features

If not identified on NBS the presenting clinical features are neurological symptoms including developmental delay, ataxia, microcephaly, seizures and increased reflexes [225,265]. Liver and renal function are normal and there are no reports of the oculocutaneous features seen in HTII [265].

Treatment and outcome

HTIII is treated with a tyrosine/phenylalanine restricted diet with tyrosine/phenylalanine free L-amino acid supplements to reduce high plasma tyrosine concentrations, aiming to maintain plasma tyrosine levels between 200 and 500 μmol/L. The principles of dietary management used for HTI can be applied. There are reports that after infancy many patients with HTIII are able to maintain tyrosine levels within the target treatment range without the need for dietary treatment [267]. This has also been observed in the author's (FW) unit. Intellectual impairment is the commonest long term complication reported in 75% of cases [265, 268].

General principles of low amino acid diets

Dietary treatment is essential for the amino acid disorders PKU, MSUD, HCU and HTI, II and III. They all share the same principles of dietary management with the aim of correcting abnormal biochemistry by

- decreasing the substrate amino acid(s) load on the affected pathway
- supplementation of any deficient amino acids beyond the metabolic block

Diet may be the sole therapy or used in combination with other treatments, e.g. sapropterin in PKU, betaine in homocystinuria, nitisinone in HTI. Although straightforward in principle diet therapy is highly restrictive, complex for patients and carers and requires careful ongoing management and monitoring by an experienced specialist metabolic/paediatric dietitian.

There are nine important goals of dietary management for amino acid disorders.

1 To restrict foods high in natural protein to prevent excess accumulation of the 'substrate' amino acid(s). Foods such as meat, fish, eggs, cheese, nuts and seeds are not permitted unless it is a very mild phenotype of the disorder.

2 To limit the amount of natural protein to maintain 'substrate' blood amino acids within the target treatment range. The types of natural food sources allocated for substrate amino acids are usually from cereal, potato and potato products, some vegetables and milk products. They are given in the form of an exchange system, whereby one food can be exchanged or substituted for another of equivalent natural protein (or specific amino acid) content.

3 Provision of L-amino acids that are free of 'substrate' amino acids to meet at least safe levels of protein/nitrogen requirements.

4 Provision of indispensible/conditionally indispensible amino acids that may become deficient as a result of the enzyme block or dietary treatment (e.g. tyrosine in PKU, phenylalanine in HTI, II and III, cystine in HCU) (Table 17.15).

5 To maintain a normal (but not excessive) energy intake by encouraging foods naturally low in protein and specially manufactured low protein foods such as bread and pasta. Children with neurological disability are likely to have lower energy requirements.

6 Provision of all vitamins, minerals, essential fatty acids and long chain polyunsaturated fatty acids (LCPUFA) to meet dietary reference values/requirements. These can be provided by the L-amino acid supplements (Appendix I) or given as separate products.

7 To achieve healthy growth, normal body composition and optimal nutritional status.

8 To prevent catabolism and metabolic decompensation during illness or trauma. This is particularly important with MSUD.

9 Provision of a diet that is palatable, varied and 'easy' to maintain.

Protein requirements in amino acid disorders

Proteins provide an essential structural and functional role and amino acids serve as the building blocks of all vital organs, muscle (including heart muscle), hormones and biological fluids such as blood. As the human body is incapable of maintaining reserves of protein, a constant supply of good quality protein is needed to maintain growth and other physiological functions [269]. The body is in a dynamic state; its proteins and other nitrogenous compounds are being degraded and resynthesised continuously. This process is not completely efficient, and as some amino acids are lost by oxidative catabolism there is a requirement for dietary nitrogen and nutritionally essential amino acids [270]. The magnitude of daily protein synthesis in adults is three to four times greater than the intake of protein (5- to 6-fold greater in growing children) [271].

Table 17.15   Indispensible/conditionally indispensible amino acids 'at risk' of deficiency.

Amino acid disorder	Substrate amino acid	Indispensible/conditionally indispensible amino acids 'at risk' of deficiency	Supplementation of indispensible/conditionally indispensible amino acids
Phenylketonuria	Phenylalanine	Tyrosine Maintain within normal age related reference range	Daily requirement usually added to phenylalanine free L-amino acids
Maple syrup urine disease	Leucine, valine and isoleucine	Valine, isoleucine (intake may be lower than requirements on a leucine restriction so may require extra supplementation) Maintain within target treatment range as deficiency may be rate limiting for protein synthesis	Titrate valine/isoleucine supplements according to blood target treatment range of valine/isoleucine During illness add valine/isoleucine supplements routinely to natural protein free emergency feeds, supplemented with BCAA free amino acid supplements
Homocystinuria	Methionine	Cystine Maintain within normal age related reference range	Added to methionine free L-amino acids Additional supplementation may be necessary
Tyrosinaemia type I, II and III	Tyrosine	Phenylalanine Maintain within normal age related reference range	Titrate phenylalanine supplements according to normal reference blood targets for phenylalanine

BCAA, branched chain amino acids.

Anabolism, including protein synthesis, increases in tissues following the ingestion of foods. In particular, amino acids are used to support anabolism throughout the day, but especially following meal ingestion (foods containing carbohydrate, fat and protein). The form and nature of dietary proteins may influence amino acid utilisation within the body. L-amino acids do not require digestion and are directly available for absorption by the small intestine [272]. This leads to rapid absorption [273, 274] and this may cause a transient imbalance among amino acids in the systemic circulation. In particular they cause plasma amino acids to rise more quickly, and to higher concentrations, but also to fall more quickly than following ingestion of whole protein such as casein [274]. In addition nitrogen retention and weight gain following ingestion of L-amino acids is less efficacious than with casein rich protein suggesting a less efficient transfer of amino acids into tissue and plasma proteins [273, 275]. There is also a suggestion of increased oxidation when amino acid supplements are taken in large single doses [276].

Amino acid requirements in healthy infants and children

For healthy infants up to 6 months of age, the amino acid content of breast milk is recognised as the best estimate of amino acid requirements. The average essential amino acid content of mixed human milk proteins is given in Fig. 17.13. However, in amino acid disorders *ad lib* breast milk intake without supplementation with suitable L-amino acids would be in excess of their tolerance.

The FAO/WHO/UNU [277] report on *Protein and Amino Acid Requirements in Human Nutrition* used a factorial calculation approach to estimate the amino acid requirements of children (Table 17.16). These were based on the rates of growth, protein deposition for children of different age groups, the

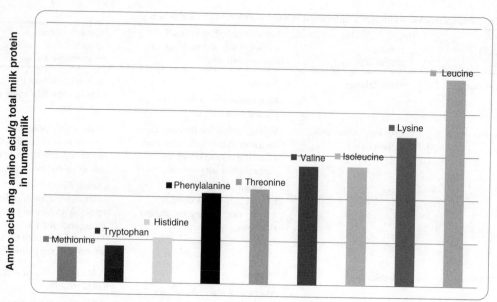

Figure 17.13   Amino acid composition of mixed human milk proteins [277].

Table 17.16   Amino acid requirements of healthy children determined using the factorial approach [277].

Age (years)	Essential amino acid requirements (mg/kg/day)								
	His	Ile	Leu	Lys	SAA	AAA	Thr	Trp	Val
0.5	22	36	73	64	31	59	34	9.5	49
1–2	15	27	54	45	22	40	23	6.4	36
3–10	12	23	44	35	18	30	18	4.8	29
11–14	12	22	44	35	18	30	18	4.8	29
15–18	11	21	42	33	16	28	17	4.5	28

For school aged children the estimated requirement for branch chain amino acids (leucine, valine, isoleucine combined) using the factorial approach is 96 mg/kg/day and by the IAAO technique is 147 mg/kg/day [280].

amino acid composition of whole body protein, as well as the efficiency of dietary protein utilisation [278]. Amino acid requirements have more recently been determined using a stable isotopic technique, the indicator amino acid oxidation method (IAAO) [279].

Total protein requirement in amino acid disorders

In patients with amino acid disorders who require severe restriction of natural protein intake, the provision of a suitable precursor free L-amino acid supplement is essential to both prevent protein deficiency and optimise metabolic control. In the majority of patients it is likely that precursor free amino acids will supply >75% of the total protein intake [281]. The optimal protein intake, accounting for inefficiency of precursor free amino acids, is not agreed. Some allow an inefficiency factor for L-amino acid sources of 1.2 [282]. Long term intake of precursor free L-amino acids has been linked to proteinuria and decreased glomerular filtration rate (GFR) in PKU [277], although this has not been studied in a controlled way.

In the UK a higher protein intake than FAO/WHO/UNU [277] safe levels of protein intake is recommended in children with PKU to compensate for the inefficiency of L-amino acids and is supported by studies investigating metabolic control on differing dosages of free L-amino acids [283, 284].

Table 17.17 Guidelines for total protein requirements for amino acid disorders (protein equivalent from protein substitute and natural protein/amino acid exchanges).

Age (years)	Total protein (g/kg body weight/day)
0–2	3.0
3–10	2.0
11–14	1.5
>14	1.0 (maximum 80 g/day)

This will also help minimise any disturbance of flux of amino acid across the BBB [285]. Recommended daily total protein intakes per kilogram body weight are given in Table 17.17. In the absence of disorder specific research this guidance for protein intake is used for other amino acid disorders.

L-amino acid supplements

Nutritional composition of L-amino acid supplements

The composition of L-amino acid supplements was originally based on the amino acid profile of breast milk [286]. Appendix I gives the nutritional composition of L-amino acid supplements available for amino acid disorders in the UK. There are two main groups of L-amino acid supplements: age group targeted L-amino acids with added nutrients; L-amino acids only.

Age group targeted L-amino acid supplements with added nutrients

All infant L-amino acid formulas contain a macronutrient and micronutrient profile similar to normal infant formula but have a higher protein equivalent content of approximately 2 g/100 mL of formula. They usually contain LCPUFA and some contain novel nutrients such as prebiotics.

L-amino acid supplements designed for older infants and young children usually contain added carbohydrate ± fat and LCPUFA. There has been a tendency to reduce the amount of added carbohydrate in products designed for school children and teenagers as adequate energy can be provided by food. This is not usually associated with loss of metabolic control [287–289]. Some of these products contain minimal quantities of sodium and

potassium as it is assumed they will be provided by the diet.

The addition of vitamins and minerals to age targeted L-amino acid supplements is advantageous as it prevents the need for separate fortification. It is intended that the amount of vitamins, minerals (except sodium and potassium) and trace elements added to each product meets the dietary requirements of children and teenagers when an average dose is prescribed. If an L-amino acid supplement is being prescribed outside the intended age range, or if only a small dose of L-amino acid is prescribed (e.g. when sapropterin/betaine is prescribed with relaxed intake of natural protein in PKU or HCU), the vitamin and mineral intakes (from diet and L-amino acid supplement) need to be carefully assessed to ensure an adequate intake is provided.

L-amino acid supplements only

L-amino acid powders only usually provide a protein equivalent of approximately 80 g/100 g of product and do not contain any macronutrient or micronutrient fortification. They are used less commonly in daily dietary management but can be very useful in emergency regimens for MSUD (p. 453) and glutaric aciduria type 1 (p. 486). They can be given via an enteral tube to deliver the required dosage of L-amino acids in relatively small volumes. L-amino acid tablets are available for PKU.

Presentation of L-amino acid supplements

For children >12 months of age L-amino acid supplements are mainly presented as flavoured/unflavoured powders (cans, premeasured sachets) and ready to drink liquids (pouches, bottles, tetrapaks). Powders are designed to be given either as a gel or drink. One flavourless preparation has been designed to mix with food (Add-ins). Additionally in PKU a low volume semisolid weaning product, capsules and tablets are available (Appendix I). Suitable infant amino acid formulas are discussed in the section on Feeding and management of newly diagnosed infants (p. 433).

Adherence with L-amino acid supplements

Adherence is a major issue [290, 291] mainly associated with the bitter taste of the supplements. Failure to take the prescribed amount is coupled with poor metabolic control [292, 293]. However, the improved range, taste, volume, presentation and availability (through home delivery) of existing preparations for PKU has improved long term adherence, particularly in teenagers taking liquid L-amino acid supplements [288, 294]. Study evaluations have proven UK ACBS prescribable L-amino acids to be safe and efficacious. Even though the range of suitable products has expanded, the number, range of flavours and presentations of L-amino acid supplements for amino acid disorders other than PKU is still limited.

Timing of L-amino acid intake

It is best to give L-amino acids in small frequent doses, three to four times spread evenly throughout the day rather than once or twice daily only [295]. Infrequent administration of large doses increases nitrogen excretion as well as amino acid oxidative utilisation so this practice is not advocated [296]. Theoretically it is advantageous that L-amino acid supplements are given with some of the natural protein allowance. Carbohydrate added to the L-amino acids may reduce leucine oxidation and increase net protein synthesis [297].

Administration of L-amino acid supplements

L-amino acid supplements can be taken as a drink, paste/gel via a spoon or as tablets. It is not usually advocated that they are added to food as this will spoil the taste of the food and it cannot be guaranteed that all the food will be eaten. However, one flavourless L-amino acid supplement (Add-ins) has been developed specifically to mix with food for patients ≥4 years. The following should be considered when administering L-amino acids.

- They are hyperosmolar, ranging from 600 to 2700 mOsm/kg H_2O (manufacturers' data), depending on their dilution with water. If they are given in a small volume of water or as a paste they may cause abdominal pain, diarrhoea or constipation. An additional drink of water should always be given with L-amino acid supplements if they are diluted with less water than recommended.
- When powders are prepared in a drink format, the tyrosine is hydrophobic and so tends to form an insoluble layer. Children often refer to

this as the 'froth' and either have it skimmed from the drink surface or leave it in the bottom of the cup. In PKU, it is important to explain the importance of tyrosine to ensure all of the preparation is consumed.
- They can be given as a paste/gel. A small amount of water (usually 1–1.5 mL water per 1 g of powder) is added to each dose to make a spoonable paste or gel. Spoonable paste/gel is a successful way of administering L-amino acids and it needs to be introduced in this format early in a child's life (preferably from 6 months of age). One to two teaspoons prior to solids is a useful way to accustom a young child to the taste in the weaning period. Their contribution to mineral and vitamin intake should be considered. Artificial flavours should not be added to unflavoured L-amino acid supplements before the age of 1 year.
- Ideally paste/gel supplements should be prepared immediately prior to use and receive minimal handling as excessive mixing may release sulphur containing amino acids.
- Giving liquid L-amino acids from pouches helps disguise their colour and smell.

Useful strategies for parents and other carers to encourage L-amino acid intake in their children are given in Table 17.18.

Provision of conditionally indispensible/essential amino acids

Tyrosine supplementation in PKU

Tyrosine becomes an indispensible amino acid because it is not supplied endogenously via phenylalanine hydroxylation or only to a limited degree. It is therefore essential to supplement it in the diet. L-tyrosine is important for the biosynthesis of the brain neurotransmitters (epinephrine, norepinephrine and dopamine), thyroxin and melanin skin pigments. The PKU MRC Working Group [43] suggested that L-amino acid supplements supply 100–120 mg/kg/day of tyrosine which is five times the amount recommended for non PKU school children [298]. Tyrosine is added to all ACBS prescribable L-amino acid supplements (9%–11% of the amino acids). Provided adequate L-amino acid supplement is given to meet protein requirements, it will supply the daily tyrosine requirement

Table 17.18 Strategies for encouraging L-amino acid supplement intake in children.

Strategies
• Caregivers should be patient, calm and encouraging whilst maintaining a persistent and determined approach
• Establish a routine for L-amino acid supplement: always give at the same time each day
• Continue to offer L-amino acid supplement even when a child refuses or is unwell. Giving a child a 'day off' from L-amino acid supplements will adversely affect their metabolic control and give the wrong message. Stopping an L-amino acid supplement, even for 24 hours, may create difficulties with its reintroduction, particularly in young children
• If taken with meals, offer L-amino acid first to ensure it is taken
• Ensure they understand from an early age that their L-amino acid supplement is just as important as any medicine
• If more than one person administers the L-amino acid supplements ensure that all caregivers involved apply the same strategies in the same way
• It is good practice to ensure that no L-amino acid supplement is left behind in containers or pouches
• An adult should always supervise the intake of L-amino acid supplements at home, nursery or school

making additional supplementation unnecessary in infants and children.

Diurnal variations in blood tyrosine concentrations are wide. Fasting tyrosine concentrations may be low but then peak immediately following L-amino acid supplement intake [299]. Therefore, in PKU, tyrosine supplementation produces marked but unsustainable increases in plasma tyrosine concentrations.

Cystine supplementation in HCU

Cystine is a conditionally indispensable amino acid because of the metabolic block preventing cysteine being produced from cystathionine. Although all the methioine-free L-amino acid supplements contain added cystine (30–50 mg/g protein equivalent) plasma cysteine concentrations are commonly low.

Cysteine and homocysteine-cysteine is present in plasma in three different forms: free cysteine, bound to homocysteine forming a mixed disulphide, or bound to protein. With increased concentrations of plasma homocysteine, the amount of cysteine present as the mixed disulphide homocysteine-cysteine increases and cysteine and protein bound cysteine decrease [300]. When monitoring diet treated patients, total plasma cysteine (free and bound) should ideally be assessed but it is difficult to measure. As biochemical control improves with decreasing homocysteine concentrations, cysteine levels increase.

If total cysteine concentrations are very low, a cystine supplement of 1–2 g/day can be administered. Cystine has a poor solubility, so care is required to ensure it does not precipitate out of solution when added to water.

Phenylalanine supplementation in HTI, II and III

Low plasma phenylalanine concentrations have been observed in HTI patients on restricted tyrosine/phenylalanine intakes [247, 248]. If plasma phenylalanine concentrations remain low, they may become rate limiting for protein synthesis and plasma tyrosine levels will remain high. It is important to monitor phenylalanine concentrations and to supplement with additional phenylalanine if consistently low. In practice, it should be noted that there is significant diurnal variation between morning and afternoon phenylalanine concentrations (a morning phenylalanine may be within target concentration but afternoon concentration low) and so interpretation is challenging [248]. Plasma phenylalanine should always be measured at the same time of day [227]. A starting dose of 50 mg/day of phenylalanine is given for fasting phenylalanine consistently (≥2 consecutive concentrations) below normal laboratory reference range, but additional phenylalanine may increase tyrosine concentrations and any supplementation should be carefully monitored.

Valine and isoleucine supplementation in MSUD

Although there is inability to catabolise leucine, valine and isoleucine it is leucine that is reported to be particularly toxic. For simplicity the natural protein allocation in the diet is measured in leucine food exchanges rather than a complex system involving all three amino acids. The valine and isoleucine content (approximately 4%–7%) of protein in food, however, is lower than its leucine content (approximately 10% of protein) (Table 17.19). Therefore, the amount of valine and isoleucine consumed from leucine exchanges may not meet requirements and consequently lead to low blood levels of valine and/or isoleucine. Deficiency of these will become rate limiting for protein synthesis making supplementation necessary. The need for valine and isoleucine supplementation is individual. In older infants and children a suggested starting dose of 50–100 mg/day of valine and or isoleucine should be given if isoleucine and or valine are below target treatment range and the dose is then titrated according to plasma valine and isoleucine concentrations. In addition, when plasma leucine concentrations are high and those of valine and or isoleucine low, a rapid fall of leucine can only be achieved by combining a reduced leucine intake with a temporary increased supplement of valine and isoleucine [160]. (Dosage with emergency feeds is given on p. 449 and in newly diagnosed infants on p. 436.)

Administration of conditionally indispensible/ essential amino acid supplements

Individual amino acid supplements are available as powders either as L-amino acids only or in a sachet format with added carbohydrate (Table 17.20). Quantities and strengths of amino acid in sachets vary. Amino acids can be administered in three even doses throughout the day, best added to the total daily dose of the usual L-amino

acid supplement providing it is fully consumed and the product is well mixed. It is difficult to add individual amino acids to 'ready to drink' pouches of L-amino acid supplements so they may best be added to milk replacements (e.g. Sno-Pro or Prozero) or food such as fruit purée. For both breast and bottle fed infants, they can be added to at least three bottles of L-amino acid infant formula but care should be taken to ensure it is consumed. The carbohydrate contribution should be calculated if single amino acids in sachets (supplemented with carbohydrate) are added to infant feeds or emergency feeds in MSUD, as this can be significant when generous doses are given.

Substrate amino acid requirement/tolerance supplied by natural food sources

The amount of tolerated amino acids from natural food sources, in the different amino acid disorders, will vary depending on the severity of the patient's phenotype, age and adjunct drug therapy. Other factors affecting substrate amino acid tolerance are listed in Table 17.21.

Natural protein/amino acid tolerance is defined as the amount of disorder specific substrate amino acid that maintains the blood amino acid within a target treatment range. The amount of natural protein/amino acid from infant formula or food should be systematically titrated until the substrate amino acid(s) are stable within the target treatment range. With the exception of very mild presentations for each condition, amino acid tolerance is likely to be less than the minimum amount recommended for healthy infants and children. In healthy children

Table 17.19 Percentage of selected essential amino acids found in milk products, cereals, vegetables and fruits.

	Per cent of protein contributed by each amino acid from cereals, milk products	Per cent of protein contributed by each amino acid from vegetables	Per cent of protein contributed by each amino acid from fruits
Phenylalanine	5%	3%–4%*	3%
Tyrosine	5%	3%–4%*	3%
Leucine	10%–11%	3%–6%*	5%
Valine	6%–7%	4%–5%*	3%–4%
Isoleucine	4%–6%	3%–5%*	3%–4%
Methionine	2%–3%	1%*	1%

*Spinach is an exception and contains a higher proportion of each amino acid and needs to be measured as part of each exchange system [301].

Table 17.20 Individual amino acid supplements available in the UK.

		Tyrosinaemia	PKU	PKU	MSUD	MSUD	MSUD	MSUD	HCU	HCU
Product		Phenylalanine 50	L-Tyrosine	Tyrosine 1000	L-Valine	Valine 50	L-Isoleucine	Isoleucine 50	L-Cystine	Cystine 500
Company		Vitaflo	Nutricia	Vitaflo	Nutricia	Vitaflo	Nutricia	Vitaflo	Nutricia	Vitaflo
Amount of L-amino acid	g/100 g	1.25	100	25	100	1.25	100	1.25	100	12.5
Amino acid per sachet	mg/sachet	50	N/A	1000	N/A	50	N/A	50	N/A	500
Weight of tub	g	N/A	100	N/A	100	N/A	100	N/A	100	N/A
Weight of sachet	g	4	N/A	4	N/A	4	N/A	4	N/A	4
Energy	kcal/100 g	384	360	370	338	384	345	384	370	370
Energy	kcal/sachet	15	N/A	15	N/A	15	N/A	15	N/A	15
Energy	kJ/100 g	1607	1532	1548	1438	1607	1467	1607	1573	1548
Energy	kJ/sachet	63	N/A	63	N/A	63	N/A	63	N/A	63
CHO	g/100 g	95	0	72.5	0	95	0	95	0	82.5
CHO	g/sachet	3.8	N/A	2.9	N/A	3.8	N/A	3.8	N/A	3.3
Protein equivalent	g/100 g	1	90.1	20	84.6	1	86.3	1	92.5	10

Table 17.21 Factors affecting substrate amino acid tolerance for each disorder.

- Residual enzyme activity in the disorder
- Net protein catabolism
- Non protein:energy ratio
- Growth rate
- Age
- Gender
- Dietary adherence
- Dosage of substrate free L-amino acids
- Drug treatment in PKU/HCU/HTI
- Target treatment substrate blood amino acid concentrations

substrate amino acid(s) requirements are highest in early infancy with, after the age of 1 year, a slow and steady decline in tolerance per kilogram body weight (Table 17.22). This is in parallel with decreasing growth rate and protein requirements.

Indispensible amino acid deficiency

For all the disorders it is important to avoid amino acid deficiency, excess or imbalance (Table 17.23). Infants and young children are particularly at risk of deficiency due to higher requirements, increased requirements post recovery from illness/trauma,

or due to food refusal during the toddler years. Deficiencies can result in inadequate weight gain, faltering growth and poor wound healing. In MSUD low plasma concentrations of isoleucine and valine occur [177] and decreased isoleucine concentrations are associated with an acrodermatitis enteropathica like syndrome. Isoleucine is an essential amino acid for normal growth and differentiation of keratinocytes and its depletion has been reported to cause growth arrest in keratinocyte cultures [304]. In addition, failure to provide adequate isoleucine and valine for protein synthesis during acute metabolic decompensation slows the rate at which blood leucine decreases.

Prescription of substrate amino acids (natural protein)

A prescribed amount of each substrate amino acid (natural protein) is allocated, mainly determined by target treatment blood amino acid concentrations. Systems for allocating substrate amino acids vary throughout Europe [308]. In the UK the amino acid is allocated in the form of a daily food exchange system, with different exchange systems for the four disorders (Table 17.24). Each patient is allocated a total daily amount of substrate amino

Table 17.22 Tolerance of individual substrate amino acids.

Age	PKU Phenylalanine	MSUD Leucine	Valine	Isoleucine	HTI mg/kg/day Tyrosine	HCU mg/kg/day Methionine
	mg/kg/day					
0–6 months	25–60*	80–110[†] 100–110[‡]	Give supplements until plasma concentrations are between 200 and 400 µmol/L		140–50[§]	15–60[¶]
7–12 months	25–40*	40–50[‡]			40–50[§]	12–43[¶]
	mg/day					
1–10 years	200–700*	400–600[‡]	Give supplements until plasma concentrations are between 200 and 400 µmol/L		150–500[§]	Median 230**
11–16 years	220–1000*	400–600[‡] 500–700[†]			250–800[§]	

This may not take into consideration the small, additional quantities consumed from low protein free foods, and fruits and vegetables allowed without measurement/calculation in the diet.

*MacDonald A. Unpublished clinical data: maintaining plasma phenylalanine 110–360 µmol/L in 1–10 years; and 110–700 µmol/L in 11–16 years.

[†]de Baulny et al. [160]: maintaining leucine concentrations 80–200 µmol/L.

[‡]Dixon [302]: maintaining leucine concentrations 200–400 µmol/L.

[§]Daly A. Unpublished clinical data: maintaining plasma tyrosine 200–400 µmol/L.

[¶] van Calcar [303]: maintaining total homocysteine <50 µmol/L.

**White [300]: maintaining free homocysteine <10 µmol/L.

Table 17.23 Signs and symptoms of amino acid deficiency [170, 304–307].

Amino acid deficiency	Signs and symptoms of deficiency
Phenylalanine	Amino aciduria, anorexia, listlessness, alopecia, osteopenia, perineal rash, poor growth, death
Phenylalanine/tyrosine	Amino aciduria, anorexia, listlessness, hypotonia, poor growth
Leucine	↓ appetite, apathy, irritability, ↓ weight, infections, ↑ plasma isoleucine and valine
Isoleucine	Weight loss, acrodermatitis enteropathica-like rash
Valine	Poor appetite, drowsiness, excess irritability, crying in infants, weight loss and ↓ albumin
Methionine	Poor weight gain
Inadequate protein intake	Inadequate weight gain, decreased muscle mass, osteopenia, hair loss, low prealbumin and ↓ tolerance to substrate amino acids

Table 17.24 Examples of amino acid/protein exchange systems for amino acid disorders.

Amino acid disorder	Exchange system	Approximate protein equivalent	Examples of number of exchanges for different amounts of daily amino acid allocated
PKU	50 mg phenylalanine	1 g	200 mg phe daily 4 × 50 mg exchanges = 4 g protein 300 mg phe daily 6 × 50 mg exchanges = 6 g protein
MSUD	50 mg leucine	0.5 g	400 mg leucine daily 8 × 50 mg exchanges = 4 g protein 500 mg leucine daily 10 × 50 mg exchanges = 5 g protein
Homocystinuria	20 mg methionine	1 g	100 mg methionine daily 5 × 20 mg exchanges = 5 g protein 200 mg methionine daily 10 × 20 mg exchanges = 10 g protein
Tyrosinaemia	1 g protein	1 g	4 g natural protein daily = 4 × 1 g protein exchanges 8 g natural protein daily = 8 × 1 g protein exchanges

phe, phenylalanine.
If the amino acid analysis is available then this figure is used to estimate the weight of food for each exchange. When amino acid analysis is unavailable it is acceptable to estimate amino acid content from protein analysis (e.g. 1 g protein yielding 50 mg phe, 100 mg leucine, 20 mg methionine). This applies to most foods but fruit and vegetables generally contain lower concentrations of some of the essential amino acids.

acid and then the number of exchanges to make up this daily allowance is calculated. One food can be exchanged or substituted for another of equivalent substrate amino acid content. The allowance is divided evenly over the day and given with the L-amino acid supplement (Table 17.25). No more than 50% of the natural protein allowance should be given at any one meal.

Change in substrate amino acid tolerance throughout life

Although amino acid requirements decrease per kilogram body weight throughout childhood there are no reports of longitudinal tolerance in any of the amino acid disorders. It is possible that some patients consume a higher intake of substrate amino acids than prescribed or reported because, if blood amino acids are within the target treatment ranges, dietary intake of substrate amino acids may not be estimated with accuracy. From the age of 2 years, in each amino acid disorder, if there is stability of control with low variability of blood substrate concentrations [313] the amino acid tolerance should be re-examined from time to time, but particularly at the times of rapid growth. Some adults with PKU have been reported to tolerate more natural protein than their paediatric

Table 17.25   Guide to using natural protein exchange foods.

1   Exchange foods are generally sourced from low biological protein foods like potatoes, peas, sweetcorn, rice, pasta and breakfast cereals. Yoghurt or milk is a useful protein source in older infants and toddlers when appetite may be poor. The percentage of amino acids found in milk products, cereals, vegetables and fruit is given in Table 17.19

2   It is preferable to weigh foods with digital scales rather than using household measurements which are not accurate [309]. It has been shown that in PKU, however, with increasing age of the child some parents [310] and teenagers [311] stop weighing exchange foods and estimate instead without loss of metabolic control

3   Ideally exchanges should be spread evenly throughout the day so that a load of dietary substrate amino acid is not given at any one time. In PKU, it has been shown that plasma phenylalanine concentrations increase above baseline by 10%–18% when 50% of the total daily phenylalanine allowance is given at one time and by 8%–26% when 75% of the daily allowance is given at one time [312]

4   It is useful to teach parents and patients to calculate 1 g protein exchanges directly from food packages and 'pocket size protein calculators' are helpful

5   Theoretically any foods can be eaten as exchanges but high protein foods can only be accommodated in tiny amounts. Many young children do not understand exchange systems and have difficulty in understanding why they cannot eat more of these foods. It may be unfair to accustom their taste to high protein foods and if they became used to eating ordinary bread, biscuits or chocolate for their exchange foods any equivalent low protein special foods may be less acceptable

clinics had prescribed [314, 315]. Any challenge with additional substrate amino acids should be conducted carefully, introducing small measured quantities (equivalent to 0.5–1 g/day natural protein) systematically.

Lists of basic food and drink exchange weights for the different amino acid disorders are given in Tables 17.26 and 17.27.

Fruits and vegetables counted as part of the exchange system

This varies for each amino acid disorder. In MSUD and HCU any fruits and vegetable containing >1 g protein/100 g food are counted as part of the exchange system. In PKU, most fruits and vegetables only yield 30–40 mg phenylalanine/g protein [318]. There is evidence that all fruits and vegetables with a phenylalanine content ≤75 mg/100 g food do not elevate plasma phenylalanine concentrations [319]. In addition, vegetables containing phenylalanine between 76 and 99 mg/100 g food do not increase plasma phenylalanine concentrations when eaten in small portions [319]. The NSPKU [316] permits one serving per day (by definition 'a handful') of any fruit and vegetable containing 76–99 mg phenylalanine/100 g food. Use of similar 'free fruits and vegetables' by other countries has not been shown to adversely affect blood phenylalanine control in PKU [320, 321].

Energy requirements and low protein food sources

For all amino acid disorders, it is important that age related average energy requirements are met for optimal dietary protein utilisation. Although it is aimed to give a percentage distribution of carbohydrate and fat similar to recommendations for a healthy population, only 20%–25% of energy is provided from fat [322, 323] due to a low intake of higher fat/protein containing foods.

It has long been established that utilisation of dietary protein is influenced by energy intake [324–326]. Protein synthesis and catabolism are energy dependent and thus are sensitive to dietary energy deprivation. Insulin is secreted in response to carbohydrate (and protein) promoting cellular uptake and use of amino acids. Energy and/or glucose depletion will result in amino acid (especially branched chain) breakdown (gluconeogenesis) to meet minimal glucose requirement, which can ultimately lead to a loss of metabolic control.

There are some foods which are naturally very low in protein so can be eaten in normal portion sizes in the diet without measurement (Tables 17.28–17.30).

Essential fatty acids and LCPUFA

A strict low amino acid diet is devoid of natural dietary sources of n-3 LCPUFA such as eggs,

Table 17.26 Basic exchanges for PKU, HT I, II, III and HCU.

Food	PKU [316, 317] 50 mg phe exchanges	Tyrosinaemia [300, 317] 1 g protein exchanges	HCU [300, 301, 317] 20 mg methionine exchanges
Milk			
SMA First infant formula	85 mL	75 mL	75 mL
Cow & Gate First infant formula	90 mL	75 mL	65 mL
Aptamil First infant formula	90 mL	75 mL	65 mL
Cow's milk	30 mL	30 mL	20 mL
Single cream*	30 mL	30 mL	30 mL
Double cream*	60 mL	60 mL	45 mL
Yoghurt (natural/flavoured)	20 g	20 g	20 g
Custard	30 g	30 g	20 g
Cereals			
Rice – raw	15 g	15 g	15 g
Rice – boiled	45 g	45 g	40 g
Vegetables			
Asparagus, boiled	1 'handful' per day[†]	1 'handful' per day[†]	1 'handful' per day
Baked beans (canned)	20 g	20 g	35 g
Broad beans, boiled	20 g	12 g	75 g
Broccoli, boiled	1 'handful' per day[†]	1 'handful' per day[†]	45 g
Brussels sprouts, boiled	1 'handful' per day[†]	1 'handful' per day[†]	75 g
Cauliflower, boiled	1 'handful' per day[†]	1 'handful' per' day[†]	65 g
Lentils, raw	5 g	5 g	10 g
Lentils, boiled	12 g	12 g	30 g
Mushrooms (fresh)	unrestricted[§]	unrestricted[§]	35 g
Peas, fresh, frozen, tinned, petit pois, boiled	25 g	15 g	35 g
Spinach, boiled	25 g	45 g	20 g
Spring greens, boiled	35 g	55 g	100 g
Sweetcorn (canned)	35 g	35 g	25 g
Yams, boiled	1 'handful' per day[†]	1 'handful' per day[†]	85 g
Potato			
Main crop, boiled, jacket, flesh only (average value)	80 g	50 g	70 g
Roast	55 g	35 g	45 g
Chips	45 g	25 g	35 g
Fruit (edible portion)			
Avocado	1 'handful' per' day[†]	1 'handful' per' day[†]	30 g
Dried fruits, e.g. raisins, currants, sultanas	1 'handful' per' day[†]	1 'handful' per' day[†]	75 g[‡]

phe, phenylalanine.

*There are a many different dairy creams available with variable fat content, therefore protein content. Always check protein content on the individual product nutritional analysis label.

[†]The National Society for PKU (NSPKU) permits one serving (by definition a 'handful') of one portion daily of any fruit and vegetable containing 76–100 mg phenylalanine/100 g. By limiting to one portion per day the natural protein from these sources is controlled. The same rule has been applied to tyrosinaemia. The individual weights of the amount of fruit and vegetable that yield 1 g protein are given in Table 17.55.

[‡]This is an average amount for dried fruits.

[§]The non protein nitrogen is high in mushrooms.

Table 17.27   50 mg leucine exchanges for MSUD.

Food	Weight (g)	Protein (g)*	Leucine (mg)[†]	Isoleucine (mg)[†]	Valine (mg)[†]
Milk					
SMA First infant formula[‡]	35 mL	0.5	47	26	27
Cow & Gate First infant formula[‡]	35 mL	0.5	54	31	33
Cow's milk	15 mL	0.5	50	27	36
Single cream	20 mL	0.5	48	26	36
Double cream	35 mL	0.6	52	30	38
Yoghurt (natural/flavoured)	10	0.4	57	31	34
Custard	15 mL	0.4	57	31	42
Ice cream (non dairy)	15	0.5	53	28	36
Cereals					
Rice – raw	10	0.7	56	26	39
Rice – boiled	25	0.6	47	22	32
Vegetables					
Asparagus boiled as served	65	2.2	49		
Baked beans (canned)	15	0.8	51		
Broccoli, boiled	45	1.4	51		
Brussels sprouts, boiled	35	1.0	53		
Cauliflower, boiled	40	1.2	53		
Mushrooms (fresh)	50	0.9	53		
Okra (fried in oil)	35	1.5	52		
Peas, boiled	15	1.0	45		
Petit pois, boiled	15	0.8	51		
Spinach, boiled	20	0.4	54		
Spring greens, boiled	25	0.5	51		
Sweetcorn (canned)	15	0.4	50		
Yams, boiled	45	0.8	49		
Potato[§]					
Boiled, jacket	60	1.3	55		
Roast	45	1.3	53		
Chips	35	1.3	46		
Fruit (edible portion)					
Avocado	45	0.9	52		
Bananas	55	0.7	53		
Kiwi fruit	90	1.0	51		
Dried fruits[¶]	60	1.4	56		

Figures for the weight of food are rounded to the nearest 5 g, although many families use electronic scales which are accurate to between 1 and 2 g.
Table adapted from [302],
*[317],
[†][301] and Leatherhead Food RA, Randalls Road, Leatherhead, Surrey, UK, 1994, for fruits and vegetables; no data available for isoleucine or valine.
[‡]Manufacturers' data for infant formulas.
[§]Potato – the leucine content of potato varies between old, new and different varieties; an average figure has been used.
[¶] Dried fruits – the leucine content of different dried fruits is similar, so an average figure has been used.

meat, milk or fish. The diet is low in fat [323], α-linolenic acid, arachidonic acid and devoid of any sources of eicosapentaenoic acid (EPA) and docosahexaenoic acid (DHA) [327]. Evidence suggests that children with PKU and adults with MSUD have reduced concentrations of DHA in plasma and membrane phospholipids compared with controls [322, 328–331]. Controlled trials with

Table 17.28 Foods that can be allowed without measurement in amino acid disorders.

Food group	Examples of suitable foods
Fruits and vegetables	Fruits and vegetables that can be given without measurement are given in Tables 17.29 and 17.30. Fruit crisps, e.g. apple and pineapple
Fats	Butter, margarine, ghee, lard, dripping, vegetable oils
Starches	Cassava flour, arrowroot, cornflour, custard powder, potato starch, sago, tapioca, tapioca starch
Sugars	Sugar, glucose, jam, honey, marmalade, golden syrup, maple syrup, treacle, sweets containing <0.3 g protein/100 g
Miscellaneous	Vegetarian jelly, agar-agar, salt, pepper, herbs, spices, vinegar; tomato and brown sauce; baking powder, bicarbonate of soda, cream of tartar; food essences and colouring; gravy mixes containing <0.3 g protein/100 mL; cook in sauces containing <1.0 g protein/100 g
Drinks	Water, squash, lemonade, cola drinks, fruit juice; black tea, fruit tea, green tea, coffee: tonic water, soda water, mineral water. Rice milk drink is very low in protein but is unsuitable for children under 5 years of age All drinks given to children with PKU have to be free of aspartame*
Pickles	All clear pickles in vinegar, e.g. pickled onions, gherkins, red cabbage
Low protein special foods	A selection of low protein breads, flour mixes, pizza bases, pasta, biscuits, egg replacers and milk replacements are available. Some vegan, protein free cheeses (e.g. Violife/Veganic) based on vegetable oil and plant starches may be purchased
	Other low protein specialist products contain some natural protein/amino acids, e.g. modified soya based cheeses, low protein snack pots, burger mixes, milk replacements, but can be incorporated into the diet as part of the natural protein exchange system. Many have been approved for ACBS prescription. A suitable list of low protein special foods is available from the NSPKU website (www.nspku.org). Any special food containing ≥0.5 g/100 g of protein should be calculated into the natural protein allowance
Energy supplements	If appetite is poor and energy intake is low, in order to maintain metabolic control it may be necessary to add energy supplements such as glucose polymer, fat emulsions or combined energy/fat supplements. In children with MSUD with neurological impairment, nasogastric/gastrostomy feeding may be necessary to ensure adequate energy, L-amino acid supplements and nutrient intake

*Aspartame (E951) is an artificial sweetener derived from a dipeptide composed of phenylalanine and the methyl ester of aspartic acid. It is added to squashes, fizzy drinks, chewing gums, sweets, desserts, tabletop sweeteners and some savoury snacks, e.g. flavoured crisps. It should be avoided in PKU. Other artificial sweeteners such as sucralose, saccharin or Acesulphame K are suitable.

DHA ± arachidonic acid supplements [332, 333] have led to improvement in LCPUFA status. It is important that consideration is given to supplementation with EPA and DHA if these are not already added to the precursor free L-amino acid supplement. Many L-amino acids have added DHA ± EPA (Appendix I). Alternatively separate DHA ± EPA supplements can be administered. The optimal dosage of DHA/EPA in children is not established but between 200 and 500 mg daily are provided by L-amino acid supplements for children aged between 2 and 16 years.

Micronutrients

There have been few reports describing vitamin and mineral intake from natural foods and precursor free L-amino acid supplements in amino acid disorders. The optimal intake of micronutrients on a low amino acid diet is unknown and may differ from the normal population since the majority of micronutrients are chemically derived. No tailored micronutrient dietary reference values have been established for amino acid disorders. As a consequence, normal population dietary

Table 17.29 Fruits and vegetables allowed without measurement in PKU and HT I, II, III.

Fruit

Fresh, frozen or tinned in syrup (≤75 mg phenylalanine or tyrosine/100 g)

Apple	Jack fruit	Pomegranate
Apricots	Kiwi fruit	Prickly pear
Bananas	Kumquats	Prunes
Bilberries	Lemon	Quince
Blackberries	Limes	Raisins
Blackcurrants	Loganberries	Raspberries
Clementines	Lychees	Redcurrants
Cherries	Mandarins	Rhubarb
Cranberries	Mango	Satsumas
Currants, dried	Melon	Sharon fruit
Damsons	Medlars	Star fruit
Dragon fruit	Mulberries	Strawberries
Figs – not dried	Nectarines	Tamarillo
Figs – green, raw	Olives	Tangerines
Gooseberries	Oranges	Water melon
Grapefruit	Pawpaw	Mixed peel
Grapes	Peaches (not dried)	Angelica
Greengages	Pineapple	Glace cherries
Guava	Plums	Ginger

Vegetables

Fresh, frozen or tinned vegetables (≤75 mg phenylalanine or tyrosine/100 g)

Artichoke	Fennel	Parsley and all herbs
Aubergine	Garlic	Parsnips
Baby sweetcorn	Gherkins	Pak choi
Beans – French, green	Gourd	Parsnip
Beetroot	Karela	Peppers
Cabbage	Kohl rabi	Pumpkin
Carrots	Lady's finger (okra)	Radish
Capers	Leeks	Squash – acorn, butternut
Cassava	Lettuce	Swede
Celeriac	Mangetout	Sweet potato
Celery	Marrow	Tomatoes
Chicory	Mooli	Tomato purée
Courgette	Mustard and cress	Turnip
Cucumber	Onions	Watercress
Endive	Spring onion	Water chestnuts

All fruits and vegetables containing phenylalanine content 76–99 mg/100 g: *allow 'one handful' per day of any one of these fruits or vegetables in PKU and HT I, II, III*
Asparagus, avocado, beansprouts, broccoli, brussel sprouts, cauliflower, plantain/yam

Table 17.30 Fruits and vegetables allowed without measurement in MSUD and HCU.

Fruit

Fresh, frozen or tinned in syrup (<15 mg methionine and/or <1 g protein/100 g or <30 mg leucine/100 g)

Apple	Guava	Pawpaw*
Apricots	Kiwi fruit	Pears
Blackberries*	Lemon	Pineapple
Blackcurrants*	Limes*	Plums
Clementines	Lychees*	Pomegranate
Cherries	Mandarins	Raspberries
Cranberries	Mango*	Rhubarb
Damsons	Melon	Satsumas
Fruit salad	Mulberries*	Strawberries
Figs – green, raw	Nectarines (for HCU see below)†	Tangerines
Gooseberries*	Olives	Water melon
Grapefruit	Oranges	
Grapes	Passionfruit	

Vegetables

Fresh, frozen or tinned (<20 mg methionine and/or <1 g protein/100 g or <100 mg leucine/100 g)

Artichoke‡	Endive‡	Parsley‡
Aubergine	Fennel‡	Parsnips§
Beans – French, green§	Garlic‡	Peppers
Beansprouts+	Gherkins‡	Plantain§
Beetroot	Gourd#	Pumpkin
Cabbage§	Fennel	Radish
Carrots	Leeks*	Swede
Celery	Lettuce§	Sweet potato
Chicory	Marrow‡	Tomatoes
Courgette*	Mustard and cress	Tomato purée
Cucumber	Onions	Turnip
	Spring onion	Watercress‡

From [301, 317] and Leatherhead Food RA, Randalls Road, Leatherhead, Surrey, UK, 1994.
*No leucine data are available for these fruits and vegetables. They are included on the free list because they contain <1 g protein/100 g or are consumed in small amounts infrequently.
†Nectarines contain 36 mg methionine/100 g. Allow up to 1 nectarine daily only.
‡No leucine data are available for these vegetables but they are consumed in small quantities.
§These vegetables contain 50–100 mg leucine/100 g and so it is better to use them in small quantities in the diet.

reference values for micronutrients are used as a guideline.

Vitamins and minerals are added to most L-amino acid supplements so, providing an adequate dose is prescribed, there should be no need

Table 17.31 Prescribable micronutrient supplements (UK).

Product	Company	Daily dosage	Age	Comments
Fruitivits	Vitaflo	6 g sachet	3–10 years	Orange flavoured powdered vitamin, trace element and mineral mix, contains minimal amount of carbohydrate, sodium and potassium. Mix with water
Paediatric Seravit	SHS	Suggested daily dose: Age 0–6 months 14 g Age 7–12 months 17 g Age 1–7 years 17–25 g Age 7–14 years 25–35 g	0–14 years	Powdered vitamin, trace element and mineral mixture containing only trace amounts of sodium and potassium on a carbohydrate base; designed for infants and children; unflavoured and pineapple flavour. Mix with water or suitable fruit juice
Phlexy-Vits	SHS/Nutricia	7 g sachet or 5 tablets	>11 years	Unflavoured comprehensive vitamin and mineral supplement; does not contain sodium and potassium; available in powder and tablets. Powder can be mixed with water or fruit juice; better to consume immediately after mixing
Forceval soluble Junior	Alliance	Suggested daily dose: 2 daily if no vitamins and minerals added to L-amino acid supplement	≥5 years	Effervescent tablet. Contains all vitamins and minerals but contains no calcium, phosphorus and sodium, inositol and choline and only a small amount of potassium and magnesium. Dissolve in 125–200 mL water
Forceval soluble and Forceval capsules	Alliance	Suggested daily dose: 1 capsule/tablet daily if there are no vitamins and minerals added to L-amino acid supplement	≥12 years	Capsule or effervescent tablet. Contains all vitamins and minerals except vitamin K, inositol and choline but contains no sodium and only a small amount of potassium, calcium, phosphorus and magnesium. Dissolve tablet in 125–200 mL water

In order to improve micronutrient availability, it is better to administer all vitamin and mineral supplements in 2–3 equal doses throughout the day. Nutritional content is given in Table 1.23.

for additional supplementation. Data suggest that micronutrient adherence is better when they are added to L-amino acid supplements [296] than when taken as a separate supplement [334]. However, if a non supplemented L-amino acid is given, a comprehensive vitamin and mineral supplement is essential. Suitable prescribable supplements are given in Table 17.31.

Nutritional and biochemical monitoring

Regular monitoring of growth along with measures of protein and overall nutritional status is indicated (Table 17.32).

Monitoring the diet by serial measurements of substrate blood amino acid levels

In all amino acid disorders serial monitoring of substrate amino acid levels is essential to assess metabolic control. In infancy and early childhood it is good practice to measure blood levels weekly, with guidelines for PKU [43] suggesting that blood levels should be measured once every 2 weeks in children aged 5–10 years and monthly in teenagers, although this will be influenced by the stability of metabolic control and severity of the condition.

In HCU, regular blood sample monitoring is challenging as blood samples for total homocysteine require centrifugation within 1 hour of

Table 17.32 Monitoring of nutritional status and suggested frequency.

Assessment	Frequency
Diet history	Each clinic visit
Growth (weight, length/height, BMI)	Each clinic visit
Waist circumference from the age of 5 years	
Clinical examination, e.g. skin, hair	Each clinic visit/hospital admission in MSUD
Quantitative plasma amino acids (3–4 hour fasting)	Annual
Albumin, prealbumin [335]	Annual
25-hydroxyvitamin D	Annual
DEXA scan	Baseline DEXA scan at 11 years and repeat every 5 years, in the absence of osteopenia or osteoporosis
FBC, plasma zinc, selenium, ferritin, folic acid, vitamin B_{12}	Annual
Essential fatty acids	Annual

DEXA, dual-energy x-ray absorptiometry; FBC, full blood count.

collection [336] so blood samples are usually taken at a local hospital.

In PKU, MSUD and HT I, II and III parents should be taught by a specialist nurse how to collect heel or thumb prick blood samples at home. In PKU and HTI dried blood spots are usually collected. In MSUD parents may be taught how to collect either dried blood spots or samples of liquid blood. Different acceptable BCAA reference ranges may be used for dried blood spots versus plasma samples. Blood samples are posted to the hospital and analysed usually by MS/MS for PKU and tyrosinaemia and by amino acid analyser or MS/MS for MSUD. The dietitian should promptly inform the parents/patients of substrate amino acid blood results, discuss their interpretation and give instruction about any necessary dietary change.

Blood amino acid concentrations should be taken at a standard time each day preferably before the first dose of L-amino acid supplement in the morning when blood amino acid concentrations are at their highest after an overnight fast [248, 337, 338]. In PKU, for example, blood phenylalanine concentrations may vary by 150 µmol/L over 24 hours [337].

Interpreting blood 'substrate' amino acid results

Guidelines on interpreting blood substrate amino acids are given in Tables 17.33 and 17.34.

Dietary management in later diagnosed cases

Homocystinuria

Individuals diagnosed late after the onset of clinical symptoms, or as a result of investigation following a sibling being diagnosed with HCU, are commenced on treatment. Management will depend upon the individual's circumstances and may be by dietary methionine/protein restriction alone, dietary restriction with betaine or betaine alone. In the author's unit (FW) a diet restricting methionine intake to 200 mg/day is initiated, together with an age appropriate methionine free amino acid substitute (Appendix I) to make up the total protein requirement for age. If, from diet history, the normal dietary protein intake prior to diagnosis has been exceptionally high, a larger methionine allowance may be given. Subsequent methionine allowance is adjusted according to plasma methionine and homocysteine levels so as to achieve acceptable control (Table 17.12). Dietary adherence in this group can in some cases be difficult to achieve because they are used to a normal unrestricted diet. Most will have learning difficulties and so understanding the need for such a radical change in diet can be difficult to achieve. Individuals may cheat with high protein foods, take additional methionine exchanges, or refuse the methionine free protein substitute. These problems need to be addressed. A positive family attitude and support from the multidisciplinary team, including clinical psychologist, are important if dietary treatment is to succeed.

In some late diagnosed individuals in whom all attempts to give the methionine free protein substitutes have failed a modified low protein diet, using the minimum safe level of protein intake [277] to minimise protein catabolism and poor growth, is used in conjunction with oral betaine therapy. More recently management with betaine alone has been used in one late presenting case. A recent European survey [210] of dietary practices in 181

Table 17.33   Interpretation of substrate blood amino acid results: high concentrations.

Cause of high substrate amino acid concentrations	Action
Fever/infection/trauma (see emergency illness management for specific guidance for all amino acid conditions, p. 449)	1 Increase energy intake 2 Ensure intake of L-amino acid supplements 3 In MSUD, reduce leucine intake but administer BCAA free amino acids with valine/isoleucine supplements* 4 Identify and treat souce of infection as clinically indicated 5 Antipyretics as clinically indicated
Excess natural protein intake	1 Check understanding/calculation of exchanges, dietary adherence and hidden sources of natural protein 2 Check that any special products used are low protein and not gluten free by mistake
Inadequate intake of precursor free L-amino acid supplements	1 Check adherence (at home, nursery, school) 2 Timing of amino acid supplements administration (should be spread out evenly over 24 hours) 3 Check adequate home supplies of L-amino acid supplements 4 Recalculate L-amino acid requirements and adjust the dosage appropriately
Incorrect precursor free L-amino acid supplements	Check type of L-amino acid supplement. Occasionally the wrong L-amino acid supplement may accidentally be prescribed or delivered
Over prescription of phenylalanine in tyrosinaemia	High tyrosine concentrations may be due to excess phenylalanine supplementation. A reduction of phenylalanine supplements should be considered if tyrosine concentrations consistently >400 µmol/L
No obvious reason	1 If substrate blood levels are consistently high, consider a reduction in natural protein/substrate amino acid by approximately 0.5–1 g/day protein or exchange equivalent. Total daily natural protein should not be decreased below 3 g/day (or amino acid exchange equivalent) 2 It is good practice to recheck blood amino acids before reduction in natural protein

patients showed wide variety in treatment with 62% on measured methionine/protein restriction (of whom 92% also had betaine), 34% on betaine alone and 3% on unmeasured, moderate protein restriction and betaine. The use of diet alone decreased with age with the converse for use of betaine only.

Tyrosinaemia type I

Individuals diagnosed late after the onset of clinical symptoms, or as a result of investigation following a sibling being diagnosed with HTI, are commenced on dietary treatment and nitisinone. Initially natural protein intake is decreased to 0.5–1 g/kg body weight/day and an age appropriate tyrosine/phenylalanine free L-amino acid supplement introduced (Appendix I) to maintain age appropriate total protein intake/kg/day (Table 17.17). Natural protein intake is then adjusted according to plasma tyrosine results to maintain within target reference ranges (p. 412).

Feeding and management of newly diagnosed infants

Infants with PKU

Although practices differ internationally [27], in the UK infants with blood phenylalanine concentrations consistently >400 µmol/L are treated for

Table 17.34   Interpretation of substrate blood amino acid results: low concentrations.

Cause of low substrate amino acid concentrations	Action
Inadequate intake of natural protein	1 Ensure all prescribed intake of natural protein is eaten 2 Check understanding of exchange system
Anabolic phase following an intercurrent infection	1 Ensure all prescribed intake of natural protein is eaten and energy intake is adequate 2 Repeat blood substrate amino acid concentration and, if still low, consider an increase of natural protein by approximately 0.5–1 g protein or equivalent exchanges but monitor blood substrate amino acid levels carefully
Rapid growth spurt such as puberty	1 Increase natural protein by 0.5–1 g protein or equivalent exchanges if blood substrate amino acid levels below target range 2 Increase by a further 1 g protein or equivalent exchanges for every 3 consecutive blood levels below target range. Monitor substrate blood levels carefully during any increase in natural protein/exchanges
Excess intake of L-amino acid supplement or overnight consumption of L-amino acids (particularly by infant/young child or with tube feeding)	Infants may take suitable L-amino acid infant formula overnight, which may lower morning blood concentrations. Consider reducing amount of overnight L-amino acid supplements if appropriate
No obvious reason or explanation	1 Consider an increase of natural protein by approximately 0.5–1 g protein or equivalent exchanges 2 Monitor substrate blood levels carefully during any increase in natural protein/exchanges 3 It is good practice to recheck blood amino acid concentrations before any increase in natural protein

It is better to consider trends in blood results before increasing/decreasing natural protein intake. It is advisable to adjust substrate amino acids/natural protein intake after more than one blood amino acid result is available unless blood concentrations are very low or very high.

PKU. The initial treatment will depend upon the diagnostic phenylalanine concentration.

- *Phenylalanine concentration >1000 μmol/L:* The phenylalanine source (breast milk or infant formula) is temporarily stopped and replaced by a phenylalanine free infant formula given at a minimum volume of 150 mL/kg/day. This is to achieve a rapid fall in plasma phenylalanine concentrations; a decrease of between 300 and 600 μmol/L per day is expected. Breast milk or 50 mg/kg/day phenylalanine from standard infant formula is introduced when phenylalanine concentrations are approaching 1000 μmol/L or below. This should be given with a phenylalanine free infant formula. Although breast feeding is stopped for a minimal time, mothers should be encouraged

to regularly express breast milk at this time. Mothers require a breast feeding pump and support from a midwife.

- *Phenylalanine concentrations 600–1000 μmol/L:* It is not necessary to stop the phenylalanine source. Either breast feeds or 50 mg/kg/day phenylalanine from standard infant formula is given with a phenylalanine free infant formula.
- *Phenylalanine concentrations 400–600 μmol/L:* Phenylalanine concentrations should be monitored weekly to ensure concentrations are consistently >400 μmol/L before dietary treatment is started. Minimal restriction of phenylalanine may be all that is necessary but depends on the individual baby. Dietary restriction of phenylalanine should always be given

in combination with a phenylalanine free infant formula.

Breast feeding

Breast feeding, together with a phenylalanine free infant formula, is associated with long term satisfactory blood phenylalanine control and growth. Breast milk has several advantages in PKU:

- it is low in phenylalanine (46 mg/100 mL compared with approximately 60 mg/100 mL in whey based infant formula)
- it contains LCPUFA
- it is convenient and reduces the number of bottles which need to be given and helps establish good mother–infant bonding
- it gives the mother some control over the feeding process

Breast feeding is based on the principle of giving a measured volume of a phenylalanine free infant formula before each feed, so inhibiting the baby's appetite and hence suckling, thus reducing the amount of breast milk taken and therefore phenylalanine intake. Babies can still feed on demand, varying the quantity of feeds from day to day provided the phenylalanine free infant formula is always given first. Blood phenylalanine concentrations are used to determine the volume of phenylalanine free infant formula to be given. The volume at each feed will vary according to plasma phenylalanine concentrations, age of diagnosis and frequency of breast feeds, varying from 30–50 mL phenylalanine free infant formula at each feed. Most breast fed babies will take 6 to 8 feeds of phenylalanine free infant formula daily. Once blood phenylalanine concentrations are stabilised within target treatment ranges, if phenylalanine concentrations increase >360 μmol/L the phenylalanine free infant formula is increased by 10 mL per feed; the amount of breast milk decreases accordingly. If

phenylalanine concentrations are <120 μmol/L the phenylalanine free infant formula is decreased by 10 mL per feed, with breast milk being increased by similar quantities. Local practices vary.

Initially blood phenylalanine concentrations should be checked twice weekly until they have stabilised to enable trends in blood phenylalanine concentrations to be established; it also helps provide reassurance to the mother that the baby is taking sufficient breast milk, particularly if she is worried the baby is slow to recommence suckling. Local practices vary and some centres prefer to do weekly checks from diagnosis. The baby should be weighed weekly for the first 6–8 weeks. Breast feeding can continue as long as mother and baby desire and the baby should continue to be weighed weekly.

Bottle feeding

Once phenylalanine concentrations are <1000 μmol/L, 50 mg/kg/day of phenylalanine from standard infant formula should be introduced (Table 17.35). The total daily amount of calculated infant formula is divided between 6–7 feeds. Traditionally it is recommended that the standard infant formula is given first to ensure the entire phenylalanine source is given, followed by the phenylalanine free infant formula which can be fed to appetite, with guidance on an acceptable minimal volume to provide the ideal amount of precursor free amino acids. Alternatively the calculated volume of normal infant formula and phenylalanine free infant formula can be mixed together but it is essential then that the full volume is consumed. A disadvantage of mixing the source of phenylalanine (standard infant formula) with phenylalanine free infant formula is that the infant will not easily adapt to the taste of the L-amino acid infant formula. Therefore when phenylalanine from food exchanges is introduced, and the quantity of normal infant formula is reduced, the

Table 17.35 Amino acid content of whey dominant infant formulas.

Formula	Protein g/100 mL	Phenylalanine	Tyrosine	Leucine	Valine	Isoleucine	Methionine
		mg/100 mL					
Cow & Gate First	1.3 g	53	52	135	70	65	30
Aptamil First	1.3 g	53	52	135	70	65	30
SMA First	1.3 g	60	69	134	78	74	27

phenylalanine free infant formula may be less acceptable and may be refused.

Ensuring that a minimal volume of phenylalanine free infant formula is consumed is just as important as ensuring that all the phenylalanine source is taken (some infants may require phenylalanine free infant formula first to ensure a minimal volume is consumed). The total volume provided by the two formulas should equate to a feed volume of 150–200 mL/kg/day. The phenylalanine free infant formula and the source of phenylalanine (standard infant formula) should be given at the same feed to deliver the correct balance of all essential amino acids.

The quantity of standard infant formula is adjusted by 25–50 mg phenylalanine/day according to blood phenylalanine concentrations. If plasma phenylalanine concentrations are <120 µmol/L the standard infant formula is increased. If the plasma phenylalanine is >360 µmol/L, the daily dietary phenylalanine is decreased by 25–50 mg providing the infant is well and drinking adequate quantities of phenylalanine free infant formula.

An example feeding plan is given in Tables 17.36 and 17.37. There is a case study on p. 455.

Infants with MSUD

The classic unscreened MSUD infant is likely to present within the first 10 days of life with a history of poor feeding, vomiting and irritability, with encephalopathy and will require intensive care management. Plasma leucine concentrations

Table 17.36 Example of a daily feeding plan for a 4 kg infant with PKU on infant formula.

Aim: to provide 50 mg phenylalanine/kg/day and 3 g total protein/kg/day

- Total fluid intake 200 mL/kg/day (= 800 mL daily)
- 90 mL Cow & Gate First = 50 mg phenylalanine
- Total number of feeds = 6

Phenylalanine requirement 50 mg/kg/day = 4 × 50 mg = 200 mg phenylalanine/day

- Daily formula intake from Cow & Gate First = 4 × 90 mL = 360 mL daily

L-amino acid supplement

- Total fluid requirement = 800 mL
- Fluid from Cow & Gate First = 360 mL
- Deficit = 440 mL (800 – 360 mL)

Feed deficit made up with phenylalanine free L-amino acid infant formula, e.g. PKU Anamix Infant/PKU Start = 440 mL/day

Feeding plan

First feed: 60 mL × 6 feeds of Cow & Gate First
Second feed: 75 mL × 6 feeds of PKU Anamix Infant/PKU Start (more can be given if the infant is hungry)
However, in this calculation, a 'generous' intake is already provided and a differing day to day volume of phenylalanine free L-amino acid infant formula may lead to a more uneven blood phenylalanine profile

will be greatly elevated (>1000 µmol/L up to 3000 µmol/L or more) and emergency treatment requires rapid leucine reduction to target treatment levels [157]. The stimulation of a high rate of protein synthesis and elimination of catabolism is essential to aid removal of leucine from the plasma pool.

Table 17.37 Nutritional analysis of daily feeding plan for a 4 kg infant with PKU on infant formula.

Aim: to provide 50 mg phenylalanine/kg/day and total protein equivalent 3 g/kg/day

	Energy		Protein equivalent	Phenylalanine intake	Carbohydrate	Fat	Fluid
	kcal	kJ	g	mg/day	g	g	mL
360 mL Cow & Gate 1 (41 g dry weight)	238	990	4.7	191	26.6	12.2	360
450 mL PKU Anamix Infant (68 g dry weight)	311	1292	9	0	33.3	15.8	450
Total	549	2282	13.7	191	59.9	28	810
Intake per kg	137	571	3.4	48	15	7	202

Treatment of the infant with MSUD includes:

- Immediate removal of toxic metabolites by continuous venovenous extra corporeal therapies (CECRT) including haemodialysis and haemofiltration. This is very effective at rapidly reducing plasma leucine concentrations [339]. It has been shown to reduce leucine to almost 1000 μmol/L or lower within 24 hours irrespective of initial leucine concentration in neonates [340]. Newborn screening by MS/MS, however, may lead to earlier treatment and prevent the need for CECRT [341] with dietary treatment alone normalising leucine levels within 2–3 days [160]. It has been suggested that the rate of decrease of blood leucine concentrations should exceed 750 μmol/L per 24 hours [168].
- Enteral feeding should be commenced as early as possible. Provision of a BCAA free infant formula, e.g. MSUD Anamix Infant, will stimulate protein synthesis. 150 mL/kg/day of BCAA free infant formula (providing 2 g/100 mL protein equivalent) will provide 3 g/kg/day BCAA free protein equivalent. If fluid is restricted, it may be necessary to supplement BCAA free infant formula with additional concentrated BCAA free amino acid mixes only (MSUD Aid 111 or MSUD Amino 5) (see Appendix I) to enable provision of 3 g/kg/day BCAA free protein equivalent. A feeding plan is give in Table 17.38.

- A high energy intake, usually administered by a continuous tube feed, is also necessary to promote anabolism. An energy intake supplying 120–140 kcal (500–585 kJ)/kg/day is advocated [157]. Glucose polymer is usually added to BCAA free infant formula to provide a total of 10 g carbohydrate (CHO)/100 mL and 79 kcal (330 kJ)/100 mL. Fat emulsion (e.g. Calogen) can also be added if necessary. If enteral feeds are not well tolerated, it may be necessary to supplement with intravenous fat emulsion (e.g. Intralipid at 2 g/kg/day) and intravenous 10% dextrose with additional electrolytes [165]. Any hyperglycaemia requires insulin administration.
- Plasma leucine will not decrease if isoleucine and/or valine are deficient (as they become rate limiting for protein synthesis) and it has been suggested that 60–90 mg/kg/day (varying between 200 and 400 mg/day) of isoleucine and valine should be given [157, 160] to support maximal rates of protein synthesis. There is little toxicity associated with increased plasma concentrations of isoleucine and valine [341] but levels are likely to fall quickly with haemodialysis/haemofiltration. Sachets of valine (50 mg/sachet) and isoleucine (50 mg/sachet) supplements in a CHO base (3.8 g/CHO per sachet) may be used. The energy sources from these supplements contribute to the overall energy intake and should be considered in any dietary calculations.

Table 17.38   Example of daily feeding plan for 8-day-old 3 kg infant with MSUD.

Newly diagnosed by newborn screening with leucine concentration of 1200 μmol/L

Ingredients	Amount	Energy kcal (kJ)/day	Protein equivalent g/day	CHO g/day	Fat g/day	Leucine mg/day	Valine mg/day	Isoleucine mg/day
MSUD Anamix Infant	450 mL	311 (1300)	9	33.3	15.8	0	0	0
Valine 50 sachets	16 g	60 (250)	0.2	15.2	0	0	200	0
Isoleucine 50 sachets	16 g	60 (250)	0.2	15.2	0	0	0	200
Total daily intake		431 (1800)	9.4	63.7	15.8	0	200	200
Intake kg/day		144 (600)	3.1			0		
Per 100 mL		96 (400)	2.1 g	14 g	3.5 g	0	44 mg	44 mg

Administration: 19 mL/hour over 24 hours via nasogastric feeding tube.
Total carbohydrate concentration of feed is high due to the carbohydrate content of the valine/isoleucine 50 sachets. However, valine/isoleucine supplied by the supplementary sachets will decrease as natural protein is introduced from breast milk or standard infant formula (according to tolerance/titrated according to blood leucine concentrations). This will decrease the overall carbohydrate concentration of the feed.

- As the infant clinically improves, oral feeding can usually be re-established. Leucine is introduced in the form of standard infant formula/expressed breast milk when plasma leucine is <800 µmol/L. Although young infants with MSUD are likely to tolerate between 300–400 mg/day of leucine [160], it may be prudent to start with 100 mg/day (70 mL infant formula) of leucine (divided equally throughout the daily feeds) and increase and titrate intake according to blood concentrations, aiming to maintain plasma leucine at 200–400 µmol/L. However, if the plasma leucine is <400 µmol/L, then 200 mg is advised to prevent very low levels of leucine occurring [165].
- As leucine intake from infant formula increases, this natural protein will also provide a source of isoleucine and valine and so these individual supplements should be reduced and adjusted to maintain them within target treatment reference ranges. It is important to maintain a total protein intake of 3 g/kg/day from standard infant formula and BCAA free infant formula. Once oral feeding is established, similarly to PKU, the BCAA free infant formula should be administered in a separate infant feeding bottle. Plasma BCAA should be monitored frequently, preferably daily in the early stages

of management. Feeding plans are given in Tables 17.39 and 17.40.
- An infant with MSUD can be breast fed, although reports are very limited [342, 343]. During the initial stabilisation period, BCAA free L-amino acid infant formula (with valine and isoleucine supplements) is given until leucine levels are <800 µmol/L, with the mother expressing breast milk. It may be better to give expressed breast milk (by tube) during initial stabilisation of leucine concentrations to within target treatment range. The baby can then be breast fed on demand, but always with a measured quantity of BCAA free L-amino acid infant formula before breast feeds, with the volume of the latter being titrated according to BCAA amino acid concentrations. The process should be very similar to PKU.

Infants with HCU

Infants with HCU who fail to respond to a pharmacological dose of pyridoxine are commenced on dietary therapy. The dietary management guidelines pathway developed for the expanded newborn screening project is given in Fig. 17.14.

Formula fed infants

Initially all natural protein (methionine) intake is stopped and the infant is fed entirely on

Table 17.39 Example of daily feeding plan for 18-day-old 3.3 kg infant with MSUD.

Feeding 150 mL/kg/day, tolerating 80 mg/kg/day leucine (264 mg/day) and 200 mg/day of valine and isoleucine

	Energy		Protein equivalent	Carbohydrate	Fat	Leucine	Isoleucine	Valine
	kcal	kJ	g	g	g	mg	mg	mg
200 mL Cow & Gate First (27 g dry weight)	132	554	2.6	14.8	6.8	270	130	140
300 mL MSUD Anamix Infant (45 g dry weight)	207	869	6	22.2	10.2	0	0	0
MSUD Aid 111, 4 g dry weight	16	67	3	0	0	0	0	0
Valine 50 sachets, 4 g dry weight	15	63	0.04	3.8	0	0	0	50
Isoleucine 50 sachets, 6 g dry weight	22	95	0.04	5.7	0	0	75	0
Total	392	1648	11.7	46.5	17	270	205	190
Per 100 mL	78	330	2.3	9.3	3.2			
Intake per kg	119	499	3.5	14	5.2	81	62	58

Valine/isoleucine supplementation is titrated according to blood valine/isoleucine concentrations.

Table 17.40 Example of daily feeding plan for 2-month-old 4.5 kg infant with MSUD.

Feeding 165 mL/kg/day to provide 400 mg leucine (8 leucine exchanges) and 200 mg/day of valine and isoleucine

Feeding plan

First feed: 50 mL × 6 feeds of Cow & Gate First

Second feed: 75 mL × 6 feeds of MSUD Anamix Infant

	Energy		Protein equivalent	Carbohydrate	Fat	Leucine	Isoleucine	Valine
	kcal	kJ	g	g	g	mg	mg	mg
300 mL Cow & Gate 1 (41 g dry weight)	197	827	4	21.7	10.5	406	193	209
450 mL MSUD Anamix Infant (68 g dry weight)	311	1291	9	33.3	15.8	0	0	0
Total	508	2032	13	55	26.3	406	193	209
Per 100 mL	68	271	1.7	7.3	3.5			
Intake per kg	120	504	3.1	13.1	6.3	97	46	50

Valine/isoleucine supplementation is titrated according to blood valine/isoleucine concentrations. One exchange of leucine is equivalent to 50 mg.

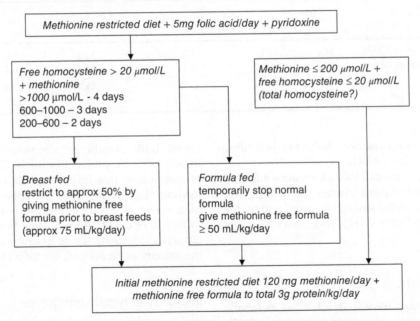

Figure 17.14 Homocystinuria (pyridoxine unresponsive) dietary management pathway [165].

a methionine free infant formula, e.g. HCU Anamix Infant, aiming to give approximately 3 g methionine free protein equivalent/kg body weight/day and normal energy requirements for age. (Other methionine free formulas are available outside the UK: www.abbottnutrition.com, www.meadjohnson.com, www.milupametabolics .com.)

Subsequently a measured amount of natural protein, initially to provide 120 mg methionine/day, from normal infant formula is reintroduced after a period of time, depending on initial biochemistry (Fig. 17.4). The normal infant formula is divided equally between several feeds (5–6 times daily) and is offered first followed by HCU Anamix Infant to appetite after each normal feed and at additional

Table 17.41 Example of a daily feeding plan for a 4 kg infant with homocystinuria.

Aim: 120 mg methionine/day and 3 g total protein/kg

- Total fluid intake 180 mL/kg/day (= 720 mL daily)
- 66 mL Cow & Gate First = 20 mg methionine
- Total number of feeds = 6 daily

Methionine requirement: 120 mg/day = 6 × 66 mL Cow & Gate First = 400 mL Cow & Gate First daily

L-amino acid supplement

- Total fluid requirement = 720 mL
- Fluid from Cow & Gate First = 400 mL
- Deficit = 320 mL (720 – 300 mL)

Therefore feed deficit made up with methionine-free L-amino acid infant formula, e.g. HCU Anamix Infant = 320 mL/day

Feeding plan

5 feeds per day of

> 80 mL × 6 feeds of Cow & Gate First followed by
> 65 mL HCU Anamix Infant (more can be given if hungry)
> Additional feeds of HCU Anamix Infant can be given if hungry

	Energy		Protein equivalent	Carbohydrate	Fat	Fluid
	kcal	kJ	g	g	g	mL
400 mL Cow & Gate First	264	1100	5.2	29.6	13.6	400
325 mL HCU Anamix Infant	241	933	6.5	24.1	11.4	325
Total	505	2033	11.7	53.7	25.0	725
Intake per kg	127	508	2.93	13.4	6.25	181

feeds as the infant demands. An example feeding plan is given in Table 17.41.

The quantity of normal infant formula is adjusted according to subsequent plasma methionine and homocysteine levels, aiming to keep within the desirable limits (Table 17.12). There is a case study on p. 455.

Breast fed infants

A survey of breast feeding in inherited metabolic disorders reported five cases with HCU [342]. As yet, however, there has been no published practical experience of breast feeding early diagnosed infants (newborn or at risk screening) with classical HCU. In theory it should be possible for such an infant to be breast fed using the principles employed in the management of PKU. Guidelines developed as part of the expanded newborn screening project in England [165] are that if initial plasma fHcy is >20 μmol/L with methionine >200 μmol/L

breast milk should be decreased by approximately 50% by giving the infant 75 mL/kg/day of methionine free infant formula prior to breast feeding (Fig. 17.14). The prescribed quantity of methionine free infant formula would then be increased or decreased according to blood methionine/homocysteine levels in order to manipulate the amount of breast milk the infant takes.

Infants with tyrosinaemia type I

Breast fed infants

Infants with HTI can be successfully breast fed whilst maintaining satisfactory biochemical control [344] using the principles employed in the management of PKU whereby a measured amount of tyrosine/phenylalanine free infant formula, e.g. Tyr Anamix Infant, to provide 1 g amino acids/kg/day is given prior to 5–6 breast feeds per day and the infant breast fed to appetite after these feeds and at any additional feeds. Tyrosine levels are monitored regularly and if tyrosine is >400 µmol/L the volume of Tyr Anamix Infant is increased to suppress breast milk intake; if tyrosine is <200 µmol/L the volume of Tyr Anamix Infant is decreased to stimulate appetite for breast milk. (Other tyrosine/phenylalanine free formulas are available outside the UK: www.abbottnutrition.com, www.meadjohnson.com, www.milupametabolics.com.)

Formula fed infants

In formula fed infants, initial management will depend upon plasma tyrosine levels. If the initial plasma tyrosine level is not >500 µmol/L then initially natural protein intake will be decreased to 1 g/kg/day, divided into 5–6 feeds, and a tyrosine and phenylalanine free infant formula offered to appetite after each feed and at additional feeds as the infant demands, aiming to give a total of 3 g protein equivalent/kg body weight/day and at least normal energy requirements for age depending on current weight.

If initial plasma tyrosine levels are >500 µmol/L, which may be the case particularly if nitisinone has been commenced prior to dietary treatment, all natural protein (tyrosine and phenylalanine) intake is stopped and the infant is fed entirely on a tyrosine and phenylalanine free infant formula aiming to give approximately 3 g tyrosine and phenylalanine free protein equivalent/kg body weight/day and at least normal energy requirements for age depending on current weight. Subsequently, as plasma tyrosine levels fall, a measured amount of natural protein, initially to provide 1 g protein/kg/day as normal infant formula, is reintroduced. An example feeding plan is given in Table 17.42. The quantity of normal infant formula is adjusted according to subsequent plasma tyrosine levels, aiming to keep within the desirable limits.

Table 17.42   Example of a daily feeding plan for a 4 kg infant with tyrosinaemia type I.

Aim: 1 g natural protein/kg/day and 3 g total protein/kg

- Total fluid intake 180 mL/kg/day (= 720 mL daily)
- 75 mL SMA First = 1 g protein
- Total number of feeds = 6 daily

Protein requirement: 1 g/kg/day = 4 × 1 g = 4 g protein/day = 4 × 75 mL SMA First = 300 mL SMA First daily

L-amino acid supplement

- Total fluid requirement = 720 mL
- Fluid from SMA First = 300 mL
- Deficit = 420 mL (720 – 300 mL)

Therefore feed deficit made up with tyrosine and phenylalanine free L-amino acid infant formula, e.g. Tyr Anamix Infant = 420 mL/day

Feeding plan

6 feeds per day of

> 50 mL × 6 feeds of SMA First followed by
> 70 mL Tyr Anamix Infant (more can be given if hungry)
> Additional feeds of Tyr Anamix Infant can be given if hungry

	Energy		Protein equivalent	Carbohydrate	Fat	Fluid
	kcal	kJ	g	g	g	mL
300 mL SMA First	198	825	4	22.2	10.2	300
420 mL TYR Anamix Infant	311	1206	8.4	31.1	14.7	420
Total	509	2031	12.4	53.3	24.9	720
Intake per kg	127	508	3.1	13.3	6.2	180

Introduction of solids

The principles of weaning onto solid foods are the same for all amino acid disorders. Solids should be introduced around 17–26 weeks of age [345]. Introducing solids before the recommended age of around 6 months for the general population may be beneficial as the neophobic response to food is less persistent, possibly leading to better acceptance of foods naturally low in protein.

- Start with 1–2 teaspoons of low protein natural foods that can be allowed without restriction such as homemade purée fruits and vegetables (Tables 17.29 and 17.30), e.g. apple, pear, carrot, butternut squash and sweet potato. Encourage parents to introduce a wide variety of homemade weaning foods in the early weaning process.
- Low protein weaning foods are usually offered after the breast or formula feeds so as not to inhibit appetite for the natural protein source and suitable L-amino acid infant formula. The intake of infant L-amino acid formula should be carefully monitored to ensure the amount is adequate.
- Many low protein weaning foods have a low energy density so higher energy weaning foods should be encouraged: homemade low protein rusks or Aminex low protein rusks, mixed with cooled boiled water to a smooth paste; low protein Promin Hot Breakfast cereal; low protein Promin pasta meal added to savoury foods; and custard made with diluted protein free liquid milk replacements, e.g. Prozero, Sno Pro. Weaning foods are gradually increased to three times daily.
- Once the infant is taking 8–12 teaspoons at a time, natural protein/amino acid exchange foods are given instead of the equivalent quantity of infant formula or a breast feed. (One breast feed in combination with L-amino acid infant formula is likely to provide approximately 1–1.5 g natural protein, but this amount is determined by the number of breast feeds consumed in 24 hours and the amount of L-amino acid infant formula.) Introduce 1 g natural protein (or equivalent amino acid exchange food) at a time, gradually replacing all breast or formula feeds with equivalent natural protein/amino acid source from solid food. Foods such as purée potato, peas, yoghurt, ordinary rusks, baby rice or vegetable based weaning foods in jars or tins are useful natural protein exchange foods. Moderate protein containing powdered cheese or white sauce mixes (when made up to 100 mL with water providing approximately 1 g natural protein) can be introduced as part of the natural protein exchange allowance from the age of 6 months.

- Gradually introduce more texture and lumpier food from 6–8 months. Introduce breakfast cereals, e.g. wheat biscuits or oat based cereal and mashed potato for natural protein exchanges.
- Finger foods can be given from 7 months of age: fingers of low protein toast; soft fruits such as bananas, strawberries and peaches; soft vegetable sticks; fingers of low protein cheese (as natural protein exchange); homemade low protein bread sticks; low protein rusks and biscuits. The infant protein substitute or a protein free milk replacement can be given from a feeder beaker at 7 months of age.
- From 9 months introduce low protein pasta dishes; sandwiches made with low protein bread; chopped low protein burgers or sausages; finger exchange foods such as pieces of boiled potato, potato products, e.g. mini-waffles, potato shapes and rice cakes. An example meal plan for a 9-month-old baby with PKU is given in Table 17.43.

Introduction of second stage L-amino acid supplement

As solids are introduced, the infant may be unable to drink adequate L-amino acid infant formula, so from the age of 5–6 months will struggle to meet total protein requirements of 3 g/kg/day. At this stage, it becomes necessary to introduce a more concentrated protein substitute (second stage L-amino acid supplement). This is gradually introduced and systematically increased to meet protein equivalent requirements unmet by natural protein and L-amino acid infant formula. This can be in the form of an L-amino acid supplement only, e.g. PK Aid 4, MSUD Aid 111 (Appendix I) or an unflavoured vitamin and mineral containing L-amino acid mixture in a spoonable or gel presentation, e.g. MSUD Gel, Tyr Gel, HCU Gel, PKU Gel,

Table 17.43 Sample menu for infant aged 9 months with classical PKU.

Weight 8.4 kg   Food exchanges 4 × 50 mg

On waking: 190 mL phenylalanine free infant formula, e.g. PKU Anamix Infant/PKU Start

Breakfast
10 g PKU Anamix First Spoon/PKU Gel as a paste
1 × 50 mg phenylalanine exchange
10 g Weetabix (1 exchange) plus Prozero/Sno-Pro
Low protein toast and butter/margarine
120 mL phenylalanine free infant formula, e.g. PKU Anamix Infant/PKU Start

Midday
10 g PKU Anamix First Spoon/PKU Gel as a paste
2 × 50 mg phenylalanine exchanges
80 g mashed potato (1 exchange)
Chopped, soft free vegetables
Homemade free vegetable sauce
20 g yoghurt (check protein value of food brand)
(1 exchange)
Banana or soft fruit
Fruit juice or diluted liquid Prozero

Evening meal
10 g PKU Anamix First Spoon/PKU Gel as a paste
1 × 50 mg phenylalanine exchange
50–60 g tinned spaghetti (check protein value of food brand) (1 exchange)
Low protein toast
Low protein custard and fruit
Fruit juice or diluted liquid Prozero

Bedtime
190 mL PKU Anamix Infant/PKU Start

Expected daily protein equivalent intake (g) (Table 17.17)
500 mL PKU Anamix Infant/PKU Start = 10.8 g protein equivalent
30 g (3 × 10 g) PKU Anamix First Spoon/PKU Gel = 12 g protein equivalent
4 × 50 mg phenylalanine exchanges = 4 g natural protein

Total = 26.8 g/day or 3.2 g/kg/day protein equivalent

PKU Anamix First Spoon. These can be mixed with a small quantity of water (1 g powder to 1 mL or 1.5 mL water depending on product) and given as a paste before meals.

Generally with L-amino acid gel/spoonable supplements, 5 g of product will provide approximately 2 g protein equivalent. A plan for introducing these products is given in Table 17.44. The entire L-amino infant formula should not normally be replaced with the second stage L-amino acid supplement until infants are at least 1 year old as infants still require some L-amino acid infant formula to ensure adequate energy intake. The L-amino acid infant formula can be stopped at 1 year; if it is continued it is usually as a social drink perhaps given in the morning or evening.

These products are hyperosmolar and should be given with extra fluid. They should be cautiously introduced and their effect on stool frequency and consistency closely monitored as infants may develop diarrhoea or constipation. Additional trace minerals and vitamins may be needed with unsupplemented L-amino acid mixtures if the volume of L-amino acid infant formula is <500 mL daily and the diet does not provide adequate amounts. Figure 17.15 gives a suggested weaning process.

Toddlers

As with normal healthy children feeding problems are common in young children with amino acid disorders [346, 347]. MacDonald *et al.* [346] reported that 47% of mothers of young children with PKU perceived their children to have at least three feeding difficulties. Principal problems were slowness to feed, a poor appetite, a dislike of sweet foods and a limited variety of foods consumed. Parents also perceived their children to have more gastrointestinal symptoms such as diarrhoea or constipation.

Feeding problems

The reasons for feeding difficulties are multifaceted; some are a consequence of the treatment and issues surrounding the disorder; others have similar causes to the general population.

- The CHO containing L-amino supplements contribute approximately 20% of the energy intake. Caregivers rarely comprehend this and may misperceive their children as eating inadequate energy if their appetite is less good than other children without amino acid disorders.
- L-amino acid supplements should be administered during illness. However, with illnesses such as coughs, colds, vomiting and diarrhoea they may cause nausea, gagging, vomiting and abdominal pain. Children are likely to refuse L-amino acid supplements if associated with discomfort and pain.

Table 17.44 Plan for introducing spoonable L-amino acid supplements in infants from the age of 5–6 months.

A boy aged 5–12 months with PKU on 4 g natural protein (200 mg phenylalanine) daily and 3 g/kg/day protein equivalent (Table 17.17)

Age of infant Weight of infant	5 months 7 kg	6 months 8 kg	8 months 9 kg	12 months 10 kg
			Protein equivalent (g/day)	
4 g/day natural protein from 4 × 50 mg phenylalanine exchanges	4	4	4	4
PKU Anamix Infant/PKU Start daily	12 (from 600 mL amino acid infant formula)	12 (from 600 mL amino acid infant formula)	12 (from 600 mL amino acid infant formula)	8 (from 400 mL amino acid infant formula)
PKU Anamix First Spoon/PKU gel	5 (from approximately 12 g of either product)	8 (from approximately 20 g of either product)	11 (from approximately 28 g of either product)	18 (from approximately 45 g of either product)
Total protein equivalent	21	24	27	30
Protein equivalent intake kg/body weight/day	3	3	3	3

If the infant takes less L-amino acid infant formula then the amount of spoonable protein substitute (PKU Gel/PKU Anamix First Spoon) should increase.

- Psychological factors in the mother including maternal depression, depressive symptoms, anxiety and poor general health [348] may contribute to feeding difficulties (these are not just seen in mothers of children with a disorder). It is unclear if maternal depression and anxiety may be the cause or result of a feeding problem. The impact of an amino acid diagnosis may heighten maternal depression and anxiety, potentially exacerbating some of the feeding difficulties.
- Caregivers who eat unhealthily, have an irregular meal plan, or who are inexperienced at parenting may be more likely to have toddlers with feeding difficulties. Additionally, if there is family dysfunction (associated with arguments and confrontation) it may lead to inappropriate mealtime conditions. Any mother with a child with feeding problems may be more insensitive, less flexible, accepting and affectionate; they may be apt to use physical punishment, tend to force feed, have difficulty receiving signals from their children and have poor social communication in both feeding and play [348].
- Many young children both with or without amino acid disorders appear food neophobic [346, 349] and commonly reject new and novel foods in favour of familiar ones. This may be as a result of lack of exposure to a wide variety of foods in the weaning period, fear of eating unsuitable foods, or unpleasant associations with trying new L-amino acid supplements or other dietary products. Generally, children who present with feeding problems as young as 6 months appear to persist with these for some time.
- Some of the strategies used by caregivers to improve feeding may have the reverse effect. Strategies such as distracting, coaxing, toys, reprimanding and allowing breaks from eating have been shown to worsen behaviour in over two-thirds of children. In addition, over control and the use of rewards have a negative effect [350].

Strategies to overcome feeding problems

As for all childhood feeding problems, early behavioural intervention can play an important role in normalising feeding behaviours and mealtime interactions, which in turn promote independence and other self-help skills in the child. Any approach to overcoming feeding problems should not only consider the day-to-day practical solutions but

Early infancy breast milk/standard infant formula started + suitable L-amino acid infant formula

From 17 weeks small amounts of natural low protein foods added to develop taste preference, e.g. puree vegetables and fruits

From 20 weeks to 12 months breast milk/standard infant formula gradually replaced with natural protein exchange foods

Low protein cereals and puree fruit and vegetables added to introduce new textures (calculate natural protein exchanges as necessary)

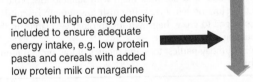

From 7 months
Self feeding encouraged with pieces of apple, cooked carrot, low protein toast

From around age 6 months no more than 600 mL/day L-amino acid infant formula (provides 12 g protein equivalent/day). Additional L-amino acid requirements to be met by second stage L-amino acid supplements, e.g. paste/gel fed from a spoon

Foods with high energy density included to ensure adequate energy intake, e.g. low protein pasta and cereals with added low protein milk or margarine

By 12 months breast milk or standard infant formula should be mainly replaced with natural protein sources from foods and suitable L-amino acid spoonable paste/gel should be the main source of L-amino acid supplement

Figure 17.15   Suggested weaning process in amino acid disorders (adapted from [345]).

also tackle any psychological causes. Many of the approaches advised in healthy children should be applied to children with amino acid disorders and the caregiver's attitudes and behaviour are central in improving feeding behaviour (Table 17.45).

Eating in nurseries or other childcare centres

It is increasingly common for young children to spend part of their day in nurseries, other childcare centres or with child minders. Nursery teachers and other childcare workers should understand the basic principles of the diet, foods permitted and forbidden, necessity for L-amino acid supplement and natural protein exchanges. Ideally they should receive one-to-one verbal explanation from the dietitian or a specialist IMD nurse and they should, at least, receive written information about the diet. Parents should be encouraged to supply suitable drinks, low protein milk replacements (e.g. Sno-Pro, Prozero), fruit or low protein biscuits

Table 17.45   Strategies to improve feeding problems in children with amino acid disorders.

Strategies

- Give caregivers guidance on child feeding development, normal expected feeding behaviour, the importance of hunger and satiety cues
- Caregivers should eat with children so positive role modelling can occur and also to promote social interaction [347, 351]. Eating together, with at least one suitable low protein shared dish, lets children watch caregivers try new foods and helps with communication of hunger and satiety, as well as enjoyment of specific foods. Caregivers need to understand the impact of negative role modelling, particularly if they are negative about the low protein diet, refuse to eat or share low protein foods and eat alternative foods without, at least, a suitable and equivalent alternative for the child with an amino acid disorder
- Establish consistent and predictable mealtime routines, with mealtime determined by the caregiver and not the child [347, 349]. By developing mealtime routines, caregivers help children learn to anticipate when they will eat. Children should not graze throughout the day, so that they develop an expectation and an appetite around mealtime; the intake of sweetened drinks or low protein milk should be controlled and children should not be fed when they are tired. Caregivers need to be firm, clear and consistent and expect acceptable behaviour at mealtimes, e.g. always sit down to eat. They should be encouraged to enlist the help of the extended family but ensure there is one coherent message to the child
- Caregivers should control both the type of food that is offered and the mealtime atmosphere. Their job is to ensure that children are offered a suitable, healthy and a varied low protein diet. Offering a child too many food choices is confusing and may cause conflict and toddler tantrums
- Caregivers should be provided with easy to follow information regarding appropriate portion sizes for children and be given guidance on expected weight gain
- Caregivers should allocate adequate time for the meal. When mealtimes are too brief (<10 minutes) children may not have enough time to eat, particularly when they are acquiring self-feeding skills and may eat slowly. Contrastingly sitting for >20–30 minutes is often difficult and mealtimes may become aversive
- In any child, increasing familiarity with the taste of a food increases the likelihood of acceptance [352, 353]. Caregivers can 'pair' the new food with a preferred food and present the new food repeatedly until it is no longer novel
- Administer L-amino acid supplements in three equal doses, following the same consistent routine, at the same time each day. The child should always be seated and distractions minimised
- Caregivers should encourage their children to play at 'cooking' with their foods as early as possible, e.g. they can put icing (made from icing sugar and water) onto low protein biscuits and decorate them with suitable low protein sweets. Alternatively, they can help to choose the toppings for their low protein pizza, or crush low protein biscuits to use as a biscuit base for a dessert. Young children may be encouraged to grow their own low protein vegetables in the family garden. All of this helps to create an interest in food and eating
- Suggest to caregivers that they invite friends to low protein birthday parties, teas and picnics. If low protein food is eaten and enjoyed by peers it will make the diet more acceptable

for snacks, a small tin of suitable sweets for treats and a packed lunch. Parents should liaise closely with the nursery about cookery sessions or parties so alternative, suitable low protein food can be provided.

Example meal plans for 4-year-old children are given in Tables 17.46 and 17.47. Suitable low protein recipe books and cards are available from all the specialist low protein manufacturers (contact details are given on p. 525).

School children

By the time children start school they spend increasingly more time away from their parents.

Primary school teachers need basic information about the amino acid disorder and any day-to-day practical implications of the special diet. Ideally a medical care plan, that all school staff adhere to, should be developed for each child to try and avoid the negative school experiences that have been reported, particularly in MSUD [354].

Most parents give their children a packed lunch as the majority of school dinner systems are only able to offer a limited choice of foods and are not usually able to prepare special dishes from low protein flour mixes. A typical lunch box usually consists of low protein sandwiches (filled with low protein cheese, salad, fruit spread or jam); salad vegetables; low protein pasta; fresh fruit; small packets of dried fruit; low protein biscuits;

Table 17.46   Menu plan for a 4-year-old girl with PKU.

Weight 16 kg

5 × 50 mg phenylalanine exchanges and phenylalanine free L-amino acid supplement to provide 2.5 g/protein/kg (Table 17.17)

Total protein equivalent requirement = 40 g (5 g from natural protein/phenylalanine exchanges and 35 g from L-amino acid supplement, e.g. 90 g PKU Anamix First Spoon or PKU Gel)

Breakfast
Phe free L-amino acid supplement (¹/₃ of daily dose), e.g. 30 g PKU Anamix First Spoon or PKU Gel
1 × 50 mg phenylalanine exchange
10 g Weetabix (1 exchange) + protein free milk replacement
Low protein toast + grilled mushrooms
Fruit juice (aspartame free)

Midday
Phe free L-amino acid supplement (¹/₃ of daily dose), e.g. 30 g PKU Anamix First Spoon or PKU Gel
1 × 50 mg phenylalanine exchange
Low protein bread + butter or margarine
25 g 'Cheezly' low protein cheese (1 exchange)
1 apple
Fruit juice (aspartame free)

Mid-afternoon
1 × 50 mg phenylalanine exchange
1 cereal bar (1 exchange)

Evening meal
Phe free L-amino acid supplement (¹/₃ of daily dose), e.g. 30 g PKU Anamix First Spoon or PKU Gel
2 × 50 mg phenylalanine exchange
80 g jacket potato (1 exchange)
20 g baked beans (1 exchange)
Salad vegetables or homemade coleslaw
Low protein fruit crumble + low protein custard
Fruit juice (aspartame free)

Bedtime
Protein free milk replacement, e.g. Prozero, Sno-Pro

Phe, phenylalanine.

Table 17.47   Sample menu plan for a 4-year-old girl with MSUD.

Weight 14 kg

8 × 50 mg leucine exchanges and branch chain free L-amino acids supplement to provide 2.5 g protein/kg (Table 17.17)

Total protein equivalent requirement = 35 g (4 g from natural protein/8 × 50 mg leucine exchanges and 30 g from L-amino acid supplement, e.g. 105 g MSUD Anamix Junior or 3 × 87 mL red MSUD Cooler 10)

Breakfast
Branch chain amino acid free L-amino acid supplement (¹/₃ of daily dose), e.g. 35 g MSUD Anamix Junior or 1 × 87 mL red MSUD Cooler 10
2 × 50 mg leucine exchange
10 g Weetabix (2 exchanges) + protein free milk replacement
Low protein toast + grilled mushrooms
Fruit juice

Midday
Branch chain amino acid free L-amino acid supplement (¹/₃ of daily dose), e.g. 35 g MSUD Anamix Junior or 1 × 87 mL red MSUD Cooler 10
3 × 50 mg leucine exchange
Low protein pasta salad wth 15 g sweetcorn (1 exchange)
Celery or cherry tomatoes
20 g yoghurt (2 exchanges) mixed with purée fruit

Mid-afternoon
1 pear or grapes

Evening meal
Branch chain amino acid free L-amino acid supplement (¹/₃ of daily dose), e.g. 35 g MSUD Anamix Junior or 1 × 87 mL red MSUD Cooler 10
3 × 50 mg leucine exchange
Vegetable curry made with free vegetables
Low protein nan bread
75 g boiled rice (3 exchanges)
Salad vegetables
Low protein jelly (thickened with pectin or carrageenan)
Fruit juice

Bedtime
Protein free milk replacement, e.g. Prozero, Sno-Pro

fruit juice; crisps or a cereal bar for natural protein exchanges. The packed lunch need not look different from their peers' packed lunches.

Ideally, the L-amino acid supplement should be given three times daily, including at school. Teachers can be helpful in supporting a young child take this at school and to ensure that a good routine is maintained. However, care should be taken with older children taking L-amino acid supplements at

school as it may single them out as being different and inadvertently lead to bullying. In addition, some children complain of halitosis post L-amino acid supplement administration which may cause issues. For older school age children, it may be better to administer L-amino acids with breakfast, immediately after school and at bedtime, provided some of the daily natural protein is given with each dose (Table 17.48).

School children spend time eating away from home, e.g. at friends' homes, parties, after school activities, breakfast clubs and sleepovers. It is important that a low natural protein diet does not restrict social activities. Children have to be trusted to eat the right foods and it is helpful if they have a good knowledge of their diet, particularly exchange foods, their portion sizes and foods they can eat without restriction. They also need to have a supply of appetising low protein foods. This will help adherence with dietary management.

By the time a child is attending school it is important they have some knowledge about their condition. They need ongoing education about the foods they can eat, exchange foods, why they take the L-amino acid supplements and the need for blood tests. The hospital IMD team may do one-to-one teaching or run group teaching sessions. Parents also need to take responsibility in ensuring their child becomes gradually more involved in their own treatment to aid future independence.

Teenagers

Many teenagers who have closely adhered to their diet as children will still continue to maintain good control in their adolescent years. However, some teenagers regard their condition as a burden and poor dietary adherence with deteriorating blood amino acid control are persistent issues in older patients [355–357]. This is even more of an issue in MSUD where there is risk of acute decompensation [358]. Teenagers may feel discriminated against when other people either amplify or minimise the importance of their medical condition and dietary needs. They may consider it embarrassing to be seen as different in the eyes of others [359]. Some, who have only been diagnosed in childhood and so started dietary treatment late (e.g. in non screened HCU patients), may especially struggle with their dietary management in teenage years. Also, in amino acid disorders, behaviour problems such as aggression and episodic depressions add to healthcare professionals' difficulties in being able to convince teenagers that diet therapy is essential [360, 361].

Lack of adherence with vitamins and minerals or micronutrient supplemented L-amino acids

Table 17.48 Menu plan for an 8-year-old boy with HCU.

Weight 27 kg

10×20 mg methionine exchanges and methionine free L-amino acid supplement to provide 2 g protein equivalent/kg (Table 17.17)

Total protein equivalent requirement = 54 g (10 g from natural protein/methionine exchanges and 44 g from L-amino acid supplement, e.g. 3 × HCU Cooler 15 or 2.5 HCU Lophlex LQ)

Breakfast
Methionine free L-amino acid supplement, e.g. 1 × HCU Cooler 15 (130 mL) or 1 HCU Lophlex LQ (125 mL)
3×20 mg methionine exchange
105 g baked beans (3 exchanges)
Low protein toast
Fruit juice

Mid-morning
Fruit
Water

Midday
3×20 mg methionine exchange
Low protein pasta salad + 25 g boiled sweetcorn (1 exchange)
Chopped peppers or tomato or cucumber
Low protein bread and margarine
1 cereal bar (2 exchanges)
1 pear
Fruit juice or water

Mid-afternoon
Methionine free L-amino acid supplement, e.g. 1 × HCU Cooler 15 (130 mL) or ½ HCU Lophlex LQ (62.5 mL)
1×20 mg methionine exchange
1 packet crisps (1 exchange)

Evening meal
2×20 mg methionine exchange
Low protein pizza
Free salad vegetables
Low protein garlic bread (with garlic butter)
60 g ice cream (2 exchanges)
Fruit juice or water

Bedtime
Methionine free L-amino acid supplement, e.g. 1 × HCU Cooler 15 (130 mL) or 1 HCU Lophlex LQ (125 mL)
1×20 mg methionine exchange 10 g cornflakes
Protein free milk replacement, e.g. Prozero, Sno-Pro

compromises nutrient intake in teenage years. In PKU, low vitamin B_{12} concentrations have been reported in older teenagers associated with failure to take prescribed supplements [362]. Powdered L-amino acid supplements have to be prepared which requires effort, causes inconvenience, embarrassment and there is a general unwillingness to consume these in the presence of others. However, liquid ready-to-use L-amino acid supplements are popular and long term studies indicate they improve adherence, metabolic control and nutritional status in teenagers [294]. Monitoring of overall nutrient intake is particularly important during this vulnerable time and regular contact and communication with teenagers is essential.

Transition from paediatric to adult services

As children mature, they are expected to take more responsibility for their diet therapy. In the UK paediatric IMD centres transfer their patients to specialist adult services. Although the transition between paediatric and adult services involves a change of health professional care, it also involves a change in management from being parent/caregiver directed to patient controlled.

If the transition process is successful, patients should have acquired self-efficacy skills, accepted more responsibility for their own care, be able to make their own decisions and feel informed and in control of their health. If the process is unsuccessful or poorly managed it could lead to loss of patient cooperation, poor dietary adherence, hostility toward the new healthcare team and failure to attend hospital appointments [363]. However, in PKU with careful planning, close liaison between paediatric and adult teams and patient and caregiver involvement, the majority of patients are able to make a successful transition to adult care [364].

Although many patients are keen to take on more responsibility for their own management, in others it causes anxiety and in all amino acid disorders there may be a degree of cognitive dysfunction, poor executive skills and psychiatric problems which mean that some care support from others is necessary. Caregivers may find transition unsettling and stressful, particularly if they feel excluded from care decisions or that treatment messages are conflicting and inconsistent between teams and individuals within teams. Caregivers commonly have a close, trusted and long term relationship with their paediatric team, they worry about their teenager's capacity to responsibly manage their own health and may feel adult providers do not want their involvement [365]. However, the commitment, support and assurances that caregivers give to their teenager during the transition process are central to its success and the patient's acceptance of their new adult care team [366].

Table 17.49 shows the process for transition for teenagers requiring low amino acid diets.

Teaching

Patient education lies at the core of managing restricted amino acid diets successfully and is fundamental to bringing about a change in eating behaviour and family lifestyle. Education should foster life long self-care that will ensure optimal metabolic control and social outcomes. Educational strategies are given in Table 17.50. The NSPKU produce a helpful teaching skills guide 'Let's learn about PKU', designed to aid dietitians and nurse specialists.

Management of illness

PKU, HCU, HTI, II and III

In PKU, HCU and HTI, II and III a formal emergency regimen (ER) is not normally necessary during illness as acute metabolic decompensation does not occur. However, in order to prevent an excessive rise in blood substrate amino acid concentrations, it is prudent to encourage L-amino acid supplements and high CHO drinks during illness. High tyrosine concentrations have been reported to cause eye lesions in tyrosinaemia type II during illness [262]. Factors to consider in the management of illness are given in Table 17.51.

MSUD

During intercurrent infections, surgery and injury plasma BCAA concentrations may rise rapidly, particularly leucine due to inadequate energy intake [374] and the direct catabolic effect of the infection [178]. This may cause rapid neurological deterioration, with neurotoxic levels of leucine and BCKA

Table 17.49   Transition process for patients requiring low amino acid diets.

Written healthcare transition plan

- Individualised clear plan with detailed information about the adult centre
- Jointly written with teenagers, caregivers and health professionals
- Include treatment goals, timetable for transfer and ensure there is consistent approach between all health professionals
- Provide a mutual understanding of the transition process
- Ideally a key worker should be appointed for each patient who has training, skills and experience to support a family through transition

Supplementary notes

- Include information about target treatment substrate amino acid ranges, frequency of home blood monitoring, educational needs and skills training required by the patient
- Identify any deficits in training or care needs prior to and at the time of transition to help with smooth transfer of care
- Review the transition plan at each clinic visit

Knowledge and skills for independent living

- Dietary knowledge (protein exchanges, function of L-amino acid supplements, suitable low protein foods, meal planning and food preparation, ordering of dietary products on prescription, stock checking, travel/holidays, eating away from the home)
- In MSUD, recognition of signs of intercurrent illness, knowledge and understanding of emergency management and knowing when to seek hospital admission is paramount
- Good understanding of their condition, treatment, consequences of non adherence, desirable metabolic control and their individualised monitoring plan

- Education should begin in the early treatment years with both caregivers and paediatric health professionals working in partnership
- Dedicated time should be allocated for education
- Use education systems that are acceptable to teenagers, e.g. 'diet apps', Twitter updates, 'You Tube' clips
- Teenagers must understand about the preparation and administration of suitable emergency feeds

Home blood taking/blood results

- Learn how to take home blood samples competently, order blood equipment and return samples according to agreed schedules
- Encourage teenagers to receive their own blood results and discuss results directly with health professionals

- Results can be sent by text, telephone or computer websites (provided permitted by hospital IT privacy policies)

Lifestyle issues

- Consider: overweight, body image, healthy lifestyle, exercise, extreme sports, smoking and its cessation, alcohol, recreational drugs, pre pregnancy planning and contraception, genetics

- Education about potential long term health issues such as osteoporosis, vitamin B_{12} deficiency should be explored

Psychological and social support

- Peer support, effective strategies to cope with bullying, feelings of social isolation should be explored
- Consider provision of 'role model' peer support, peer support groups, suitable and monitored 'Facebook' or internet chat lines
- Information and support regarding changes in financial allowances, grants and prescription charges
- Consider 'supported' summer camps for adolescents and adults to share and discuss issues that concern them

- A psychologist may be able to advise IMD teams on the best way to support patients
- Listen to the concerns of each adolescent and focus on them as individuals to build their trust

Table 17.49   *(continued)*

Supporting the caregivers

- Involve parents/caregivers at all stages, give information and listen to their concerns; they will need time to develop trust in the adult IMD team
- Give information about the philosophy of transition so they can prepare for 'letting go'
- Identify any differences in the care practice between adult and paediatric units so these can be openly discussed
- Ensure at every stage of transition (particularly following last clinic visit at paediatric unit and first visit at adult unit) that the patient knows who is leading their care and is responsible for follow-up

- Caregivers have a key role in supporting self-care which remains steadfast when health professionals may move 'in and out' of young people's care; they should not be excluded once their children reach the adult unit
- If there is unclear care team–patient responsibility it may lead to lack of follow-up and poor patient engagement with potential for the patient choosing to opt out of care systems

Transfer timing

- Consider other changes and events in a patient's life: exams, school leaving, starting university and relationships; consider developmental readiness

- Although the transition process should begin by secondary school age, there is no right time or age for the subsequent transfer to take place; some flexibility may be required

Preparing for adult service

- Teenagers should be seen in clinic without parents/caregivers but parents still need the opportunity to discuss any concerns they may have
- Early introduction of adult team and attendance of adult team at paediatric transition clinics from the age of 14 years
- Pre transfer visit to the hospital may be helpful with at least one return visit made to the paediatric clinic to discuss concerns
- Ensure a member of the paediatric team attends the first few clinic visits at the adult hospital to ensure continuity of care and a familiar face

- It is important that teenagers are prepared for transferring to an adult clinic and are able to speak for themselves within a clinic setting
- They should receive written information with a photograph of each of their adult team members, their role explained and contact numbers; this could be placed on a hospital website
- They need to know how to seek help in an emergency, how to make appointments and obtain supplies of equipment, dietary products and medication

Patient involvement and communication

- Organise focus groups/advisory groups of teenagers/adult patients who have gone through the transition process to seek their opinions on the process
- Arrange meetings with other patients who have gone through the transition process
- Regular audit and review of the service is important

[363, 364, 366–372].

being reached within hours [160]. Patients may present with symptoms such ataxia, irritability, vomiting, lethargy, seizures [160, 375] so any acute metabolic decompensation is seen as a medical emergency [376]. It is essential to start emergency feeds (Table 17.52) at the first sign of illness:

- aim to provide the child's usual intake of branch chain free amino acids and at least the normal energy requirement for age [169, 374]

- if this is difficult to achieve because oral intake is poor, tube feeding should commence without delay
- the usual leucine intake should be stopped or substantially decreased
- valine and isoleucine supplements should be added to the BCAA free L-amino acid supplement
- as a starting point valine and isoleucine should replace the amount provided by the natural

Table 17.50 Educational strategies to help with teaching.

- One-to-one demonstration of practical aspects of diet and blood taking is essential. 'Virtual' or direct supermarket tours discussing suitability of foods favoured by patients are useful
- Issue picture books of all foods allowed so that parents, children, siblings and extended family can easily identify free foods. Develop step-by-step picture books for administering L-amino acid supplements, preparing recipes and blood sample taking
- Teach parents and children how to interpret food labels so they can fully utilise all free foods on the market
- Offer low protein cookery workshops, demonstrations and cookery help lines for parents, children and the wider family
- Issue families, schools and nurseries with low protein recipe books, recipe cards and cookery DVDs, website addresses for recipes
- Group practical sessions encourage self-management and develop social support networks. Provide hands-on activities. Children may plan meals, shop for food, measure ingredients and prepare meals and snacks. Keep all activities highly interactive, creative and fun
- A home support worker with personal experience of amino acid disorders and working one-to-one with families can help others build confidence, improve cooking skills, diet knowledge and overall parenting skills [373]
- Encourage parents and patients to support each other. They may swap recipe ideas, cooking tips and practical issues
- Health professionals should guide patients to reliable and accurate internet information. Giving information on the 'top 10' most reliable and informative websites is a useful tool. The internet is a major source of information for families with PKU, particularly using the ESPKU, NSPKU and USA websites (addresses and website details are on p. 524)

Table 17.51 Factors to consider in the management of illness in amino acid disorders.

	Advice	PKU	HCU	HTI, II, III
L-amino acid supplement	Maintenance of L-amino acid supplement intake to support protein synthesis It may be better for this to be given in smaller, frequent doses throughout the day	√	√	√
High CHO intake	Encourage frequent high CHO drinks, e.g. Lucozade, Ribena (not sugar free) or glucose polymer solution	√	√	√
Natural protein intake	There is no need to formally omit natural protein. Catabolism will probably increase blood substrate amino acid concentrations more than natural protein. However, in practice, a reduced appetite leads to a lower natural protein intake	No change	No change	No change. In HTI if plasma tyrosine is high (>1000 µmol/L) it may be necessary to temporarily reduce natural protein intake and maximise energy intake
Medications	All treatment specific medication should be continued during illness Medications should be free of aspartame in PKU	Continue sapropterin if prescribed	Continue betaine and other medicines if prescribed	Continue nitisinone and any other prescribed medicines
Treat precipitating factors	For example, antipyretics for fever; antibiotics (aspartame free in PKU) for infections	√	√	√

In PKU, blood phenylalanine concentrations are likely to rise quickly during illness. For the immediate and short term treatment of infections (until a suitable aspartame free medication is sourced) it may be better to use aspartame containing medications rather than leave a child without treatment.

Table 17.52   Emergency feeding management in MSUD.

Diet	Essential	Daily dose
BCAA free amino acid supplements to support protein synthesis	Yes	0–3 years: 3 g/kg protein equivalent 4–5 years: 2.5 g/kg protein equivalent 6–10 years: 2 g/kg protein equivalent 11–14 years: 1.5 g/kg protein equivalent 15–16 years: 60 g protein equivalent
Valine and isoleucine intake	Yes	Give at least 150 mg of each during illness to avoid them becoming deficient and rate limiting for protein synthesis
Glucose polymer intake	Yes	CHO concentration and volume as per standard emergency regimen for age (p. 502)
Fat source	If tolerated	A high energy intake is required to promote anabolism. If fat is tolerated, add 3–5 g per 100 mL (in the form of 50% fat emulsion) enteral feed
Natural protein intake (leucine exchanges)	Stop or reduce by at least 50% (depending on severity of illness)	
Fluid	Maintain fluid requirements for age	Fluid requirements as per standard emergency regimen for age (p. 502)
Administration	Give orally or via a tube continuously over 24 hours	Tube feeding should be used without delay if oral intake is compromised. BCAA parenteral amino acids (with valine and isoleucine) should be considered with gastrointestinal dysfunction
Monitoring	Monitor BCAA concentrations to determine metabolic control/reintroduction of leucine Urine ketones	Daily during acute illness
Treat precipitating factors	For example, antipyretics for fever; antibiotics for infections	Daily during acute illness

protein allowance and in addition to the usual valine and isoleucine supplements, but this may vary from child to child

- valine and isoleucine supplements are necessary to promote protein synthesis which is the major route of removal of leucine from the plasma pool; if branch chain free amino acids are not given, other amino acids will become rate limiting for protein synthesis and leucine levels will remain high
- plasma BCAA must be monitored daily during illness and the valine and isoleucine content of emergency feeds titrated accordingly
- glucose polymer is added to the BCAA free supplement to the same concentration as recommended for standard emergency feeds to provide energy requirements; addition of fat emulsion should be considered if tolerated (some BCAA free supplements contain fat and CHO, see Appendix I).

With timely introduction of the ER with mild or moderate illnesses, most patients can be safely managed at home [163]. It is essential to maintain close contact with parents/caregivers during illness management (at least every 4 hours in daytime hours) to assess if prescribed emergency feed is being achieved, any feed intolerance and progression of clinical symptoms.

Urine ketone monitoring

Ketonuria is a physiological result of catabolism in late infancy, childhood and even adolescence. In MSUD, daily home monitoring using standard test strips for ketonuria is useful in illness [163] and it is a surrogate marker for metabolic instability, but should be used in combination (and not replace) plasma BCAA monitoring. A positive result indicates catabolism and supports the immediate analysis of plasma BCAA concentrations. Usually the result is expressed as negative or positive with a grade of 1 to 4. Testing should be performed according to manufacturer's instructions on fresh uncontaminated urine. Urine test reagents deteriorate with exposure to air (so should be kept in a tightly sealed container) or if used after expiry date. The use of old or incorrectly stored test reagents may lead to false negative results. Some centres outside the UK advocate home urine testing with the DNPH (2,4-dinitrophenylhydrazine) test which is a more sensitive marker for metabolic instability in MSUD than ketone testing. This is a more complicated test for parents to administer and requires the storage of potentially harmful chemicals. For this reason this form of monitoring is not widely practised in the UK.

Intravenous therapy

If emergency feeds are not tolerated and the patient is vomiting, has diarrhoea or very high temperature then intravenous (IV) fluids (at least 10% dextrose) are given. Some patients may require higher concentrations of dextrose, insulin and Intralipid to promote anabolism [157, 377]. Accompanying enteral BCAA free amino acid supplements, e.g. MSUD Aid 111 or MSUD Amino 5, providing up to a maximum concentration of 8 g/100 mL protein equivalent [378] together with valine and isoleucine supplements administered via a continuous tube feed are essential. These BCAA free amino acid supplements without additional nutrients may be best tolerated, but if they are unavailable it is necessary to use BCAA free amino acids with added nutrients. If vomiting is persistent or a patient requires a prolonged period with no gastric feeding, consideration should be given to nasojejunal feeding as, in the UK, there are no BCAA free parenteral amino acid solutions available. However, in France, such a solution has been successfully developed and used to treat acute decompensation in adult patients with MSUD [376].

Careful monitoring of hydration, electrolytes and neurological status is necessary to prevent cerebral oedema [169, 377].

Acute illness resulting in elevated plasma leucine is usually well managed without the need for CECRT (e.g. haemodialysis or haemofiltration). However, if the plasma leucine is >1000 μmol/L CECRT should be considered [339]. The GMDI [169] also suggest CECRT with the following indications: gastrointestinal intolerance, comatose state or deteriorating neurological condition despite appropriate nutritional therapy [169, 339, 340, 379]. Different dialysis modalities are associated with varying rates of leucine clearance [380] but the choice of dialysis is influenced by the treatment centre's experience. If clinically safe, aggressive enteral nutritional support including energy, fluid and BCAA free amino acid supplements with valine and isoleucine supplements should be given in combination with dialysis [163, 169].

In variant forms of MSUD, an ER and attentive care is required during catabolic stress, e.g. illness, trauma and surgery [169]. In thiamin responsive individuals, thiamin supplementation should be maintained.

Introduction of natural protein post illness

Many studies suggest reintroduction of leucine when it reaches the upper treatment target range [163, 381]. Others recommend graded reintroduction over 3–4 days when leucine concentrations are <800 μmol/L (Table 17.53) (www.expandedscreening.org). Isoleucine and valine supplements need to be adjusted according to intake provided by leucine exchanges and plasma concentrations.

Table 17.53 Introducing dietary leucine post illness.

Leucine concentrations (μmol/L)	Amount of dietary leucine to introduce
Leucine <800	25% usual leucine intake
Leucine >400<600	50% usual leucine intake
Leucine <400	75% usual intake
Repeat leucine <400	Usual leucine intake

Case studies

Case study of a newborn screened infant with PKU on breast feeds

A healthy breast fed term infant was screened for PKU on day 5 of life. She had a positive screening result with a blood phenylalanine level of 1200 µmol/L. The result was reported to the PKU team on day 9 of life. On the same day, the family were contacted by a specialist nurse (from the PKU centre) and general practitioner (GP) to explain the likely implications of this initial screening result and the parents were given the 'PKU is suspected' leaflet. A repeat blood spot was taken to confirm the diagnosis of PKU by the specialist nurse and returned to the PKU centre immediately so the result would be available for the hospital consultation with the family. Also on the same day, the parents and baby attended the PKU centre and were seen by IMD paediatrician, dietitian and nurse. The repeat blood phenylalanine concentration was 1710 µmol/L. A blood sample for pterins was also taken to exclude tetrahydrobiopterin deficiencies (this was negative). The infant weighed 3.2 kg, was well and breast fed on demand. There were no issues with feeding.

Breast feeding was stopped for 24 hours only. The infant was started on a phenylalanine free L-amino acid infant formula which was given on demand and the mother kept a daily record of all formula taken (the amounts and times) to estimate total feed intake. The mother was advised to express breast milk at least six times in 24 hours and her local midwife was contacted to provide support. Supplies of the specialist formula were organised (with parental consent) through a home delivery company who liaised with the GP.

The infant drank 60–90 mL of the phenylalanine free L-amino acid infant formula every 2–3 hours. Twenty-four hours after the commencement of this formula, the blood phenylalanine had rapidly lowered to 1210 µmol/L. At this stage, breast feeding was recommenced and 50 mL of phenylalanine free L-amino acid infant formula was introduced prior to each breast feed. Within 48 hours the blood phenylalanine reduced to 210 µmol/L and the specialist formula was then lowered to 40 mL prior to each breast feed. The mother was worried the baby was taking too little breast milk but with encouragement and reassurance she was happy to continue breast feeding in combination with the specialist formula. The baby was weighed weekly for the first 6 weeks and gained weight satisfactorily. The blood spot phenylalanine concentrations were measured twice weekly and within 2 weeks the parents had both learnt how to take blood samples. The dietitian reported results to the parents on the same day of availability.

In the first 10 weeks of life there was little variability in the blood phenylalanine concentrations and almost all were between 120 and 360 µmol/L. Gradually, phenylalanine concentrations increased to >300 µmol/L. The baby was only taking six breast feeds in 24 hours and was feeding for a longer duration at each feed. The phenylalanine free L-amino acid infant formula was increased to 50 mL and then 60 mL before each breast feed until almost all phenylalanine concentrations were maintained well within the target treatment range. The infant was weaned at 22 weeks; at 26 weeks the number of breast feeds was further decreased with phenylalanine from food (50 mg phenylalanine exchanges) replacing breast feeds at breakfast, midday and evening meal. The mother continued to give two to three breast feeds daily until the baby was 10 months old.

Case study of a newborn infant with HCU

Prior to expanded newborn screening project and before regular use of tHcy monitoring.

A female infant had a positive newborn screening test with a methionine level of 221 µmol/L. She was seen in the metabolic clinic the following day and blood samples taken for plasma quantitative amino acids. These showed methionine 681 µmol/lL, fHcy 34 µmol/L and cysteine 12 µmol/L. These results were consistent with classical homocystinuria and the baby was commenced on a 7 day trial of pyridoxine and folic acid to test for pyridoxine responsiveness. After 7 days repeat plasma quantitative amino acids were methionine 956 µmol/L, FHcy 59 µmol/L and cysteine 17 µmol/L. This showed she had the pyridoxine non responsive form and dietary treatment was instituted.

She was bottle fed on Cow & Gate First, taking 120–180 mL 4 hourly. Initially methionine intake was stopped and the baby fed solely on a methionine free formula, HCU Anamix Infant. She continued on a reduced dose of pyridoxine 20 mg per day and folic acid 1 mg per day. After 48 hours she was restarted on 120 mg methionine as 330 mL Cow & Gate First, divided into six feeds of 55 mL. At six feeds each day she was given 55 mL Cow & Gate First, followed by HCU Anamix Infant to appetite afterwards. If more than six feeds per day were demanded she was given additional feeds of HCU Anamix Infant alone. Methionine and fHcy levels were monitored weekly initially and then fortnightly, with the following results and dietary changes over her initial 6 months:

Week	Methionine µmol/L	fHcy µmol/L	Change in methionine intake
0 – start of diet	956	59	Zero for 48 hours, then 120 mg
1	54	18	Decreased to 80 mg
2	Not detected (ND)	ND	Increased to 120 mg
3	7	1	Only taken 110 mg/day, increased to 120 mg
4	6	1	Increased to 140 mg
5	13	ND	Increased to 150 mg
7	98	27	No change
8	48	13	No change
10	59	20	Teething, no change
12	48	17	No change
14	39	10	No change
16	39	11	No change, teething
22	54	2	No change

Low protein weaning advice was given and solids introduced from 21 weeks of age. Initially free fruits, vegetables, commercial weaning foods containing <0.5 g protein/100 g and low protein rusk were used. As solids were taken well the second stage of weaning was started around 26 weeks of age with the introduction of 20 mg methionine exchanges. Initially one exchange was introduced to replace 20 mg methionine as Cow & Gate First (55 mL), with further exchanges added in and the Cow & Gate First reduced. As weaning progressed and her appetite increased additional low protein products including bread, pasta, biscuits were introduced. By 1 year of age she was on 140 mg methionine per day, all taken as solids, using a combination of 20 mg methionine and 1 g protein exchanges together with a range of low protein foods. A second stage L-methionine free amino acid supplement, HCU Gel, 2½ sachets per day, was introduced at a year of age, giving a total protein intake of 3 g/kg/day.

Organic Acidaemias and Urea Cycle Disorders

Marjorie Dixon

Dietary management – general principles of low protein diets

Introduction

A low protein diet is an essential part of the management of organic acidaemias (OAA), e.g. methylmalonic acidaemia (MMA), propionic acidaemia (PA), isovaleric acidaemia (IVA), glutaric aciduria type 1 (GA1); and the urea cycle disorders (UCD). These disorders arise due to enzyme defects in the catabolic pathways of certain amino acids (in the case of OAA) and of waste nitrogen excretion

(in the case of UCD). The aim of the low protein diet is to limit the substrate load (amino acids in OAA and nitrogen in UCD) on the 'blocked' metabolic pathway, to reduce the production of toxic metabolites which can cause overwhelming neurological sequelae. As such, these are classified as 'intoxication' type disorders of intermediary metabolism (p. 385).

This section describes the provision of a low protein diet and acute management, common to these disorders. Dietary treatment is generally combined with pharmacological treatment to reduce the substrate load on the pathway (e.g. nitrogen scavengers in UCD); or to increase excretion of toxic interme-diates (e.g. carnitine and glycine to excrete isova-leric acid in IVA); or to replace a deficient product (e.g. arginine in UCD). Medical aspects and disor-der specific dietary treatments are described under each separate condition. Patients with an OAA or UCD are invariably complex to treat and it is essen-tial they are managed at specialist metabolic cen-tres. Local professionals and hospital teams should also form an integral part of their care package.

Protein requirements

Proteins are involved in nearly all cell functions. They are essential for growth and repair of body tissue; different proteins work as antibodies, enzymes, hormones and neurotransmitters and in the formation of haemoglobin. A constant dietary supply is needed as the body does not maintain reserves of protein.

Low protein diets must provide at least the minimum amount of protein, nitrogen and indis-pensable amino acids to meet the body's require-ments. 'Safe level of protein intake' (Table 17.54) and requirements for indispensable amino acid intake have been set by FAO/WHO/UNU Expert Committees since 1957, most recently in 2007 [277]. Protein intakes (g/kg/day) decrease with age throughout childhood. It is important to be aware that safe levels of protein intake have been cal-culated as the mean requirement +2 standard deviations (SD), so as to meet or exceed the requirements of most individuals. However, for some, a protein intake below the safe intake may be adequate for growth, particularly if protein is mainly from high biological value (HBV) sources. More recent advances in determining protein and amino acids requirements in humans is by Indicator Amino Acid Oxidation, a stable isotope method [382]. Using this technique mean and safe protein intake in children aged 6–10 years is reported to be 1.3 and 1.55 g/kg/day which is much higher than current FAO recommenda-tions; there is an urgent need for reassessment of these [382]. Further information is provided about the background to protein requirements in the section on amino acid disorders (p. 416).

Ideally the protein source in low protein diets should be mainly from HBV protein, but this is not

Table 17.54 Safe level of protein intake for infants, children and adolescents.

Age	Safe level (g protein/kg/day)
For infants < 6 months of age (months)	
1	1.77
2	1.5
3	1.36
4	1.24
6	1.14
For weaned infants (sexes combined) (years)	
0.5	1.31
1	1.14
1.5	1.03
2	0.97
3	0.9
4	0.86
5	0.85
6	0.89
7	0.91
8–9	0.92
10	0.91
Girls	
11	0.9
12	0.89
13	0.88
14	0.87
15	0.85
16	0.84
17	0.83
18	0.82
Boys	
11	0.91
12–13	0.90
14	0.89
15	0.88
16	0.87
17	0.86
18	0.85

Adapted from [277].

necessarily common practice because a greater vari-ety of foods and a higher energy intake per gram of protein can be provided from low biological value (LBV) protein foods. Children on low protein diets who frequently consume a limited range of LBV protein foods may be at risk of one or more indispensable amino acids becoming rate limiting for protein synthesis, e.g. lysine in predominantly cereal based diets. It is therefore important that a variety of LBV protein foods (potato, cereals, rice, pasta, pulses, vegetables) are eaten to ensure an adequate intake of all indispensable amino acids. If the protein prescription is generous enough, more HBV proteins should be included to improve the protein quality of the diet. A new method of calculating protein quality was published by the FAO in 2013 [383]. However, without more up to date and extensive amino acids analysis of foods, this is difficult and time consuming to calculate. There are no publications describing an optimal ratio of HBV to LBV foods in low protein diets for these disorders. The majority of patients in the UK consume some HBV foods as part of their daily protein allowance in urea cycle disorders [384].

Protein tolerance will vary depending on residual enzyme activity of the specific disorder, growth rate, age and sex. During early infancy growth is at a maximum so protein requirements per kilogram body weight are greatest at this time. If the child has had a period of slow growth, protein intake may need to be temporarily increased during the following period of catch-up growth. Even in the normal population protein requirements for catch-up growth are not well defined [277]. Protein requirements may also be temporarily increased if a child has had repeated intercurrent infections or episodes of metabolic decompensation associated with poor enteral intake and inadequate protein intakes, e.g. children with MMA and gastrointestinal complications can have frequent episodes of vomiting and reflux, intolerance of enteral feeds and requirement of hospital admission for intravenous (IV) 10% glucose. Protein and amino acids deficiencies can cause severe cutaneous lesions in these disorders. Tabanlıoğlu *et al.* have proposed a term acrodermatitis dysmetabolica to describe this deficiency state seen in children with metabolic disorders [304]. Clinical and biochemical monitoring are essential to help prevent such deficiencies and to guide protein prescription in these disorders (p. 463).

Provision of a low protein diet

Protein

In OAA and UCD a daily protein allowance is prescribed. Protein intake (g/kg/day) will decrease with age but the total intake will increase (Table 17.54). For infants, protein is provided by breast milk or infant formula and in older children by food (unless they are tube fed). Protein intake from LBV protein foods can be measured by an exchange system, i.e. one exchange equals the amount of food which provides 1 g of protein. This allows greater variety in the diet as foods can be substituted for each other and still provide a similar protein content. Protein can be provided by basic foods such as potato, rice, pasta, pulses, vegetables. Table 17.55 provides a list of 1 g protein exchange weights for these and some infant formulas. Protein can also be provided by manufactured foods such as bread, pitta, chapatti, breakfast cereals, biscuits, cake, potato based foods, vegetable fingers. Most manufactured foods have nutritional labels where protein content is expressed as grams of protein/100 g food; it is often also expressed as grams of protein per portion. Parents should be taught how to interpret the food label and calculate exchanges. For manufactured foods one exchange (1 g protein) is calculated as follows:

- 100 ÷ (g protein per 100 g of food)
- if more than 1 g protein is desired this is multiplied by that number of exchanges, e.g. cornflakes = 7 g protein per 100 g
- 100 ÷ 7 = 14 g cornflakes = 1 g protein
- if 2 g of protein is desired then 14 g × 2 = 28 g cornflakes

Ideally the protein intake should be evenly distributed between main meals with some for snacks, to avoid giving a protein load at any one meal. Protein food exchanges should be weighed, at least initially. Digital scales which weigh in 1 or 2 g increments are recommended. If parents are unable to cope with the concept of protein exchanges or weighing, then a set menu with handy measures for foods is used.

The energy provided by exchange foods has a wide variation, e.g. an exchange of baked beans provides 20 kcal (85 kJ) and crisps 110 kcal (460 kJ). It may be helpful, particularly if the child has a poor appetite, to give parents advice on choosing protein exchanges which are more energy dense and provide >60 kcal (250 kJ) per exchange.

If HBV protein foods are included in the diet 3 or 6 g protein exchanges can be used (i.e. one exchange is the amount of food which provides 3 or 6 g protein). Table 17.56 provides a list of 6 g protein exchange weights for higher protein foods. This can also be useful for older children or those

Table 17.55   Basic list of 1 g protein exchange foods for low protein diets.

	Food	Weight (g) = 1 exchange = 1 g protein
Infant formula	SMA First	75
	Cow & Gate First	75
	Aptamil First	75
Milk and dairy	Cow's milk	30 mL
	Single cream	30 mL
	Double cream	60 mL
	Yoghurt*	25
	Fromage frais*	20
	Ice cream*	30
	Milk chocolate*	15
	Plain chocolate*	20
	Cream/processed cheese e.g.	
	Philadelphia*	10
	Boursin*	15
	Dairylea*	10
Potatoes and starchy vegetables†	Potato, old (boiled)	55
	Potato, new (boiled)	70
	Jacket potato (flesh only)	45
	Jacket potato (flesh and skin)	25
	Chips (fresh, frozen)	25
	Roast potato	35
	Crisps	15
	Sweet potato	90
	Plantain	125
	Yam	60
Pulses†	Baked beans*	20
	Beans aduki, broad, butter, haricot, black-eye, mung, red and white kidney	12
	Chick peas	12
	Lentils	12
	Peas	15
Vegetables†	Asparagus	30
	Beansprouts	35
	Brussels sprouts	35
	Broccoli tops	30
	Cauliflower	30
	Gourd/karela	65
	Mangetout	30
	Okra	40
	Spinach	45
	Spring greens	55
	Sweetcorn	35

(continued overleaf)

Table 17.55　(continued)

	Food	Weight (g) = 1 exchange = 1 g protein
Fruit	Avocado	55
	Banana	85
	Dried fruit – varies depending on fruit, check individually	
	Currants, raisins, sultanas	45
	Peaches	30
	Pears	65
Cereals	Cornflakes*	10
	Rice Krispies*	15
	Sugar Puffs*	20
	Weetabix*	10
	Oatmeal	10
	Rice	
	raw	15
	boiled	45
	Macaroni (white) (boiled)	35
	Spaghetti (white) (boiled)	30
	Semolina (raw)	10
	Flour (white)	10
	Flour (wholemeal)	8
Breads	White, wholemeal, brown*	12
	Rolls (soft, crusty)*	10
	Chapatti*	15
	Nan*	15
	Pitta*	10

Food Standards Agency *McCance and Widdowson's the Composition of Foods*, 6th summary edn. Cambridge: Royal Society of Chemistry, 2002.
*For manufactured foods the weight for one exchange will be more accurate if calculated from the nutritional label on the food. The figures given can be used as a guide.
†The weight of one exchange is for cooked (boiled) weight (except for baked beans).

with milder disorders who are on a more generous protein allowance.

L-amino acid supplements

Precursor free amino acid supplements (i.e. free of the amino acids which cannot be metabolised) are used in the treatment of some OAA and will be discussed under the specific disorders as their role and use varies between disorders. Similarly, the use of essential amino acid supplements will be reviewed in the UCD section. Administration of amino acid supplements is discussed on p. 420.

Energy

Low protein diets may not provide sufficient energy because the intake of many foods is restricted. This must be avoided as an inadequate energy intake causes poor growth and metabolic instability with endogenous protein catabolism resulting in increased production of toxic metabolites, e.g. ammonia in UCD. The aim is to provide around normal energy requirement for age and sex. However, this is not appropriate for all patients as children with physical disability are likely to have lower energy requirements due to reduced mobility, such as children with MMA who have

Table 17.56 Basic list of 6g protein exchange foods for low protein diets.

Food	Weight (g) = 1 exchange = 6 g protein
Eggs (medium)	1 egg
Meat, trimmed of all fat, e.g. beef, pork, lamb, chicken	20
Processed meats, e.g. sausage, burger, salami, ham vary greatly – calculate from nutritional label on the food	
Fish	
White fish, e.g. cod, haddock, plaice	30
Oily fish, e.g. salmon, mackerel, sardines	30
Shellfish, e.g. prawns, crab	30
Scampi in breadcrumbs	65
Fish fingers – check nutritional label on the food	2 fish fingers
Cheese	
Cheddar, Edam, Gouda	25
Feta	40
Cottage cheese	45
Nuts	
Peanuts	25
Peanut butter	25
Cashew	30
Chestnuts	50

Food Standards Agency *McCance and Widdowson's the Composition of Foods*, 6th summary edn. Cambridge: Royal Society of Chemistry, 2002.

had a metabolic stroke; others may have increased energy requirements, such as children with GA1 with severe dystonia. Energy requirements need to be adjusted for the individual's needs considering metabolic stability, rate of weight gain and activity.

Dietary energy can be provided by both the protein exchanges and the following groups of foods which are allowed without restriction in the diet:

- foods naturally low in or free of protein: sugar, fats and a few commercial foods (Table 17.28)
- fruits and vegetables with <1.0 g protein/100 g (Table 17.57)
- specially manufactured low protein foods, e.g. bread, pasta, biscuits (Table 17.28)
- energy supplements: glucose polymer, fat emulsions or combined fat and glucose polymer supplements

Manufactured low protein foods are not always popular, although low protein milk replacements, e.g. Prozero, Loprofin Drink, are useful and can be well accepted. Some children obtain sufficient energy from normal foods and prefer to eat these. In contrast others with a poor appetite, inability to suck or swallow due to neurological disability, or vomiting, reflux and retching depend on energy supplements as their main energy source, which are invariably part of a modular tube feed. If energy supplements are given it is important to maintain a healthy balance between fat and CHO energy.

Vitamins, minerals and trace elements

Mineral deficiencies, particularly associated with low protein diets, have been reported in patients with OAA and UCD [385–388]. Vitamin and mineral supplements are almost always essential as their intake will be severely limited. An adequate intake of vitamins A and C and folic acid can be provided by fruits and vegetables, if eaten in amounts recommended for healthy children. Iron, zinc, copper, calcium, vitamin B_{12} and D are most likely to be deficient in low protein diets based mainly on LBV protein foods. Some patients are at greater risk of vitamin D deficiency such as those who are less mobile or children of Asian origin because of their dark skin. Together, the diet and vitamin and mineral supplement should provide at least the reference nutrient intakes (RNI) for vitamins and minerals [389], except for children with MMA who have chronic kidney disease (CKD) (p. 473).

The amount of supplement required varies depending on the child's diet and must be assessed for the individual. The supplement is best given as a divided dose to enhance absorption. Table 17.31 provides a list of ACBS prescribable micronutrient supplements. These vary in format (powders, capsules, effervescent tablets). Paediatric Seravit provides a comprehensive vitamin and mineral supplement (except for sodium, potassium and chloride). It can be added to infant formula or modular tube feeds, taking into account what the feed already provides, or mixed into a strong flavoured drink to mask its unpleasant flavour. Fruitivits is a comprehensive vitamin and mineral supplement which can be used from age 3 years and is palatable. Alternatively for older children Forceval Soluble Junior (suitable from age 6 years)

Table 17.57   Low protein fruits and vegetables allowed freely in the diet.

Fruit and vegetables with a low protein content

Fruit – fresh, frozen or tinned (fruit only weight) <1 g protein/100 g

Not dried fruits

Apple	Jack fruit	Pomegranate
Apricots	Kiwi fruit	Pear
Bananas	Kumquats	Prunes
Bilberries	Lemon	Quince
Blackberries	Limes	Raisins
Blackcurrants	Loganberries	Raspberries
Clementines	Lychees	Redcurrants
Cherries	Mandarins	Rhubarb
Cranberries	Mango	Sharon fruit
Damsons	Melon	Star fruit
Dragon fruit	Medlars	Strawberries
Figs – not dried	Mulberries	Tamarillo
Figs – green, raw	Nectarines	Tangerines
Gooseberries	Olives	Water melon
Grapefruit	Oranges	Mixed peel
Grapes	Pawpaw	
Greengages	Peaches	
Guava	Pineapple	
	Plums	

Vegetables

Fresh, frozen or tinned (vegetable weight only) <1 g protein/100 g

Artichoke	Fennel	Parsley
Aubergine	Garlic	Parsnip
Beans – French,	Gherkins	Peppers
green	Herbs	Pumpkin
Beetroot	Leeks	Radish
Cabbage	Lettuce	Squash – acorn,
Carrots	Marrow	butternut
Capers	Mustard and	Swede
Cassava	cress	Tomatoes
Celeriac	Onions	Tomato purée
Celery	Spring onion	Turnip
Chicory		Watercress
Courgette		
Cucumber		

Food Standards Agency *McCance and Widdowson's the Composition of Foods*, 6th summary edn. Cambridge: Royal Society of Chemistry, 2002.

or Forceval Soluble or Capsules (suitable from age 12 years) can be given. Forceval Soluble Junior does not contain calcium, phosphorus or sodium, inositol and choline and only small amounts of magnesium. A separate calcium supplement must be given. Forceval Soluble and Capsules differ in composition from Soluble Junior; they contain no sodium or vitamin K and only a small amount of calcium, phosphorus and potassium. An additional calcium supplement is needed. Phlexy-Vits (powder or tablets) is a comprehensive vitamin and mineral supplement suitable from age 11 years. The powder is generally taken mixed with a strong flavoured drink. If commercial vitamin and mineral supplements available from supermarkets and pharmacies are used, it is essential their composition is checked as this varies greatly between brands and invariably will not provide an adequate intake of all necessary micronutrients.

Essential fatty acids

Children on low protein diets may be at risk of inadequate intakes of essential fatty acids (EFA) and their longer chain derivatives docosohexaenoic acid (DHA) and arachidonic acid (AA). Sanjurno *et al.* reported a long chain polyunsaturated acid (LCPUFA) deficiency, specifically DHA in patients with UCD and MMA, and recommended supplementation [390]. Vlaardingerbroek *et al.* reported low plasma and red cell DHA concentrations in patients with UCD and branched chain organic acidurias [391]. The actual synthesis of LCPUFA in clinically stable patients with PA is reported not to be affected [392]. It is therefore important that low protein diets and modular feeds are assessed for EFA content and consideration should also be given to intakes of LCPUFA. In the UK at least 1% of total energy intake from linoleic acid and 0.2% from α-linolenic acid is recommended for normal infants [389]. The FAO/WHO 2008 [393] recommends an adequate daily intake for children >6 months to be 3%–4% linoleic acid and 0.4%–0.6% α-linolenic of daily energy intake, and DHA for infants to be based on amounts in breast milk and for children 100–150 mg for 2–4 years, 150–200 mg for 4–6 years, 200–300 mg for 6–10 years. Red cell and plasma fatty profiles should be measured if there are concerns about possible deficiency. DHA is added to some of the disorder specific precursor free amino acid supplements used in treatment of OAA such as the Infant Anamix and Cooler ranges.

Monitoring

Nutritional aspects of low protein diets

Protein and mineral deficiencies have been reported in patients with IMD on restricted protein intakes [304, 385–388, 394]. This type of diet, comprising mainly LBV proteins, is often used in children with OAA and UCD; therefore protein and amino acid intakes need to be carefully monitored. This should be done at all clinic appointments: clinical examination (skin and hair, looking specifically for signs of protein deficiency such as skin rashes), anthropometric measurements, biochemical assessment (quantitative amino acids, albumin and electrolytes) and dietary assessment (checking all nutrients). Periodic assessment of the following is also important: plasma status of vitamins, minerals and trace elements (Table 1.6); bone mineral density scans; plasma and red cell status of EFA and LCPUFA.

Growth and diet in infants

The nutritional intake of infants needs to be monitored frequently as they grow rapidly during the first few months and year of life. Newly diagnosed neonates and young infants should be weighed weekly to two weekly at local baby clinics; this can usually be decreased to monthly intervals by 1 year of age. Parents should initially be contacted every 1–2 weeks to review weight gain and assess feed intake; thereafter the frequency can be based on progress. Adjustments to low protein feeds are then made based on weight gain (to give the safe level of protein intake, provided the child is metabolically stable) and guidance given on the feeding pattern, including frequency of feeding. This regular contact can also identify at an early stage any feeding problems. Faltering growth does occur in some of these disorders; therefore regular monitoring is essential.

Emergency regimen

Frequent use of emergency regimens (ER) for management of intercurrent illnesses or vomiting and retching (a common finding in some patients with MMA) may result in protein deficiency due to interruption of daily protein supply. It is important to monitor frequency of use of the ER at clinic reviews, counting the number of days zero or reduced protein is given. Additional protein may be needed temporarily, if the ER is often necessary.

Initial dietary treatment of the critically unwell, newly diagnosed patient

Patients with intoxication type disorders generally present following a symptom free period, which can be acute or chronic. Neonates and young infants may present with a history of poor feeding, lethargy, hypotonia with relentless deterioration and progression to coma. Older children or even adults may present acutely at the time of an intercurrent infection or other catabolic event. The newly diagnosed patient may be very sick with metabolic encephalopathy, in intensive care with a severe metabolic acidosis and/or hyperammonaemia requiring ventilation and extracorporeal procedures and drug management to remove toxic compounds. Reversal of catabolism is essential to prevent further production of toxic metabolites and to help stabilise the patient.

Management

The principles of dietetic treatment to promote anabolism are similar for both OAA and UCD.

- Stop all protein sources temporarily (to reduce the production of toxic metabolites from endogenous sources).
- Give a protein free, high energy intake to promote anabolism: IV fluids comprising 10% glucose (or higher via a central line), electrolytes, ± Intralipid, combined with or progressing to continuous nasogastric feeds of 10%–20% glucose polymer (depending on age) ± fat emulsion; infants can be given a protein free feed such as Energivit, as tolerated. Some patients progress directly to introduction of protein (below) and may not have a period of protein free feeds. Fluid restrictions in the ventilated child can make an adequate enteral energy intake difficult; a higher energy intake

can often be achieved from parenteral nutrition (PN) via a central line and may be preferable during the initial stabilisation period. Assess for the individual.

- Reintroduce protein within 24–36 hours once the acute metabolic derangement, including the acidosis, has been corrected and the plasma ammonia is less than or around 100 µmol/L (normal <40 µmol/L). Protein is usually commenced with 0.5 g protein/kg body weight/day and increased to the final 'safe' level of protein intake (Table 17.54) within a few days (typically 2–3 days). An age appropriate feed is used: for infants either infant formula or expressed breast milk; for older children a paediatric enteral feed. If enteral feeds are not tolerated PN is given. A standard parenteral amino acid solution such as Vaminolact can be used but should only provide the desired amount of protein (amino acids g/kg/day). For example, to provide 2.2 g amino acids/kg for a 3.5 kg infant, Vaminolact provides 65.3 g amino acids/1000 mL; therefore 120 mL provides 7.8 g amino acids = 2.2 g/kg, administered as 5 mL/hour for 24 hours. This is given with IV glucose, lipid and vitamin and mineral solutions to provide the total energy and nutrient requirements.

- As the child stabilises the IV fluids or PN is gradually decreased and enteral feeds (with the same protein and energy content) increased concurrently, so tolerance can be assessed and an adequate energy intake and the desired protein prescription constantly provided.

- Additional electrolytes (sodium and potassium) may need to be added to the feed to provide normal requirements for age, taking into account any contribution of these from IV fluids and medicines such as sodium bicarbonate (to treat acidosis) and sodium benzoate (to treat hyperammonaemia). Blood electrolytes should also guide intake.

- For infants, if the mother wishes to breast feed she should be encouraged to express several times a day to maintain a good supply of breast milk until the baby becomes more metabolically stable; then breast feeding can be reintroduced. This changeover from nasogastric (NG) to breast feeding (BF) may take a few days in a baby who is still not fully alert post extubation and has been encephalopathic.

Initially a combination of some BF and NG feeds may be best with progression towards BF as the infant's oral feeding improves. Careful monitoring is necessary to ensure the infant receives an adequate intake during this period. Expressed breast milk (EBM) can be used to provide the protein requirement until BF is fully established. Protein free feeds may need to be given in combination with BF while metabolic stability is being established, and even long term in some patients.

- For older children, a low protein diet may be needed or a low protein tube feed (short or long term) for those with a severe neurological insult. When starting a low protein diet, taking a diet history is important as some children may already self-select a low protein diet and/or have specific eating habits and food choices. This is seen typically, but not exclusively, in those with UCD. This information is useful to plan the low protein diet and to help the family cope. It may be possible to continue with a self-selected low protein diet and just ensure adequate protein free energy, vitamins and minerals are given.

- Once the child transitions from acute to chronic management, refer to provision of low protein diets (p. 458). Practical aspects of feeding and ongoing dietary treatment are described below.

- Prior to discharge the parents need to be fully educated and given clear written instructions about the dietary treatment and emergency management of illness (discussed in detail under specific disorders) and a list of contact information for the metabolic team. Liaison with local healthcare professionals, such as health visitors and the local hospital team, is also an essential part of the care package.

Examples of a nutritionally complete low protein infant feed, older child's diet and tube feed are provided in Tables 17.58, 17.59, 17.60 respectively.

Infant feeding

Breast feeding

Breast milk or a whey based infant formula should provide the main protein source for infants. Breast milk has many immunological and nutritional

Table 17.58 Low protein feed for 3-month-old male infant

Weight 5 kg, to provide 1.36 g protein/kg

	Energy (kcal)	(kJ)	CHO (g)	Protein (g)	Fat (g)	Sodium (mmol)	Potassium (mmol)
540 mL (68 g powder) SMA First	362	1520	39	7	19	3.8	9.2
40 g Maxijul*	152	638	38	–	–	0.4	<0.2
5 g Paediatric Seravit†	13	57	3.3	–	–	–	–
Plus water to 750 mL							
Totals	527	2423	80	7.0	19	4.2‡	9.4‡
per 100 mL	70	294	10.7	0.9	2.5	0.6	1.2
per kg	105	485	–	1.4	–	0.9	1.9
DRV per kg 0–3 months§	115–100	480–420				1.5	3.4
Safe protein intake¶				1.36			

*Instead of glucose polymer a combined fat and CHO supplement could be used, e.g. Duocal.
†Vitamins and minerals are added so that the combined intake from infant formula and supplement provides the same amount as if all vitamins and minerals were provided from full strength infant formula (with no protein restriction) and/or meets normal requirements for age.
‡Additional sodium and potassium will be necessary. Note that some medicines provide electrolytes and this needs to be taken into account when calculating intake.
§Dietary reference values [389].
¶FAO/WHO/UNU safe level of protein intake (Table 17.54).

benefits. In the normal population breast fed babies produce significantly less propionic acid compared with bottle fed babies [395], so theoretically infants with disorders of propionate metabolism (MMA, PA) who are breast fed may have the additional benefit of reduced gut propionate production. There are, however, few published reports of babies with these disorders being breast fed [396–398]. Demand breast feeding can be successful in UCD and OAA provided there is regular monitoring of growth and metabolic status. During the initial stabilisation period at diagnosis when no protein is given the mother needs to express breast milk to maintain a supply and the infant is given a protein free feed. Once stabilised either EBM or breast feeding is gradually reintroduced. If demand BF provides too much protein intakes can be reduced by supplementary bottle feeding of either a protein free, or precursor amino acid free, infant formula before some or all breast feeds. Choices are discussed in more detail in the disorder specific sections. Examples of suitable specialised infant formulas include

- protein free, otherwise nutritionally complete, feed containing CHO, fat, vitamins and minerals suitable for UCD and OAA, e.g. Energivit

- disorder specific infant formula free from precursor amino acids for OAA, e.g. MMA/PA Anamix Infant, GA1 Anamix infant
- modular protein free feed suitable for UCD and OAA (Table 17.61)

Similar products are available for all of these outside the UK (www.abbottnutrition.com, www.meadjohnson.com, www.milupametabolics.com).

The volume of specialised infant formula to give before breast feeds can be calculated: (daily fluid requirements) – (volume of breast milk to provide prescribed amount of protein) = volume of specialised infant formula required.

For example, for a 4 kg infant, age 1 month:
total daily fluid requirements = 170 mL/kg/day; safe level of protein intake = 1.77 g/kg/day (Table 17.54) = 7 g protein/day
daily fluid requirements = 680 mL – 540 mL breast milk (1.3 g protein/100 mL = 7 g protein)
= 140 mL total specialised infant formula given as 35 mL before four breast feeds

Bottle feeding

If a whey based infant formula is used, the amount is adjusted to provide at least the safe level of

Table 17.59 Low protein diet for 6-year-old girl.

Weight 18 kg, to provide safe protein intake of 0.89 g protein/kg (16 g protein)

	Protein (g) (using 1 g protein exchanges)
Breakfast	
20 g Cornflakes and sugar	2
Protein free milk*	
Potato waffle	1
Mid morning	
Biscuit, crisps, cake	2
Packed lunch	
2 thin slices bread	4
Butter or margarine	
Lettuce, tomato, cucumber and mayonnaise	
40 g fromage frais	2
Portion fresh fruit	
Evening meal	
135 g savoury fried rice (chopped onion, garlic, tomato, green beans)	3
35 g sweetcorn	1
30 g ice cream	1
Tinned fruit in syrup	
Bed time	
Protein free milkshake*	

Energy supplements: a daily dose of glucose polymer and/or fat emulsion may be necessary if insufficient energy is provided by the diet

Low protein special foods: can provide extra energy and variety in the diet as necessary (Table 17.28)

Vitamin and mineral supplement: e.g. 1 sachet of Fruitivits or 25 g Paediatric Seravit is recommended for this age, but a lower dose may provide an adequate intake depending on vitamins and minerals provided by the diet

*Protein free milk alternatives, e.g. ProZero, Sno-Pro, Loprofin Drink.

protein intake for age (Table 17.54) or more if clinically indicated. Additional fluid, energy, vitamins and minerals are added, aiming to make a nutritionally adequate feed which gives around the RNI [389] for all vitamins and minerals and is comparable to a normal full strength infant formula. It is important to ensure the intake of sodium and potassium is adequate. Table 17.58 provides an example of a modular low protein feed suitable for infants. Alternatively, a combination of infant formula and a protein free formula such as Energivit is given: the infant formula provides the prescribed safe level of protein intake for age and Energivit provides the additional energy, fluid, vitamins and minerals. This is much easier for parents than making a multi-ingredient modular feed. In newborn screened infants with GA1, the total protein allowance is always provided by a combination of natural protein and precursor free amino acids (p. 481). Some centres may provide the prescribed protein allowance from a combination of natural protein and precursor free amino acids in MMA, PA, IVA, or natural protein and essential amino acids in UCD.

Weaning

Weaning is started at the usual time of around 6 months (26 weeks) of age. Normal weaning practices are followed: solids are introduced at one meal then two and three times per day and the infant progresses from smooth purées to lumpier foods and finger foods during the first year. The first solids given are protein free such as fruit or low protein vegetable purées (Table 17.57); or very low protein rusk or cereal (Table 17.28) which are available on ACBS prescription; or commercial baby foods containing <0.5 g protein/100 g (predominantly fruit purées) so that if they are refused the total protein intake is not affected. Once these are accepted protein containing solids are introduced from either commercial baby foods or homemade foods such as potato, vegetables or cereals. It is best to have a flexible approach as to when the protein food should be given; some infants may take this best before (if not too hungry) or between feeds. One gram of protein from infant formula is replaced by 1 g of protein from solids. This is less easy to regulate in the breast fed infant as the protein intake is not known. Therefore an aim for total protein intake (usually the safe level of protein intake) is set; each breast feed will then equate to an amount of protein, e.g. one feed = 2 g protein, and as the protein exchanges from solids are introduced the number of breast feeds is reduced to compensate.

It is important to ensure that an adequate energy intake is provided by exchanges and free foods, otherwise breast feeds will not be reduced sufficiently. The energy content of protein exchanges

Table 17.60   Low protein tube feed for a 4-year-old girl.

Weight 15 kg

	Energy		CHO	Protein	Fat	Sodium	Potassium
	(kcal)	(kJ)	(g)	(g)	(g)	(mmol)	(mmol)
550 mL Paediasure	556	2335	60.5	15.4	27.5	14.3	15.4
170 g Maxijul	646	2713	161.5	–	–	1.5	0.2
60 mL Calogen	270	1134	–	–	30.0	0.2	–
5 g Paediatric Seravit	24	102	6.0	–	–	–	–
100 mL Normasol						15.4	
8 mL KCl solution (2 mmol/mL)							16.0
Plus water to 1200 mL							
Totals	1496	6283	228	15.4	57.5	31.4	31.6
Per 100 mL	125	524	19	1.3	4.8	2.6	2.6
Per kg	100	420		1.0		2.1	2.1
DRV 4–6 years*	1460	6120		1.1			
Safe level of protein intake†				0.86			

Electrolytes, vitamins and minerals need to be individually determined taking into account any additional intake from food or medicines.
*Dietary reference values [389].
†FAO/WHO/UNU safe level of protein intake (Table 17.54).

Table 17.61   Protein free modular feed.

	Energy		CHO	Protein	Fat	Sodium	Potassium
	(kcal)	(kJ)	(g)	(g)	(g)	(mmol)	(mmol)
55 g Maxijul	209	888	52	–	–	0.5	0.1
40 mL Calogen	180	756	–	–	20	0.1	–
10 g Paediatric Seravit *	30	126	7.5	–	–	0.1	0.1
25 mL Normasol						3.9	
5 mL KCl solution (2 mmol/mL)							10.0
Plus water to 600 mL							
Totals	419	1770	61	–	20	4.6	10.2
Per 100 mL	70	295	10.2	–	3.3	0.8	1.7

*The dose of Paediatric Seravit is adjusted according to normal recommendations [389] taking into account the amount provided by infant formula (i.e. the protein source).

can be increased by adding butter or margarine to savoury foods and sugar to desserts. In both the bottle and breast fed infant this process of introduction of solids is continued throughout the first year of life or so and is dictated by what the infant can manage, until all the protein is provided by solid food. Ideally the protein exchanges should be evenly distributed between main meals. During this changeover period it is important to ensure that vitamin and mineral intakes are adequate. The vitamin and mineral supplement is increased or introduced (more likely in the breast fed infant) with the progressive change to solids, as these foods are a poorer source of micronutrients than infant formula and breast milk. Some patients never progress onto solids or take very small amounts because of feeding difficulties. This is discussed in more detail in disorder specific sections. If precursor free amino acids form part of the diet, progression to a product suitable for older infants or children is appropriate.

Diet in childhood

Throughout childhood protein intake is increased to provide around the safe level of protein intake (Table 17.54) for age or more if clinically indicated. This is given in conjunction with an adequate energy, vitamin and mineral intake for age as described above. It is important to ensure the child consumes a variety of LBV protein foods (Table 17.55). HBV foods can also provide some of the protein in the diet (Table 17.56) including thin sliced meats (ham, chicken or turkey), tuna in oil, cheeses (processed cheese triangles, cream cheese), hot dog sausages, fish fingers, eggs, fromage frais and yoghurt (choosing the highest energy varieties), custard style desserts. Some children may not achieve an adequate energy intake from the diet; this can be increased as necessary by

- frying foods, adding butter, margarine, vegetable oil, mayonnaise or double cream (1 g protein and 270 kcal (1.1 MJ) per 60 mL) to savoury foods such as pasta, rice or potato
- adding sugar, glucose polymer or double cream to desserts
- high CHO drinks (>10% concentration) or adding glucose polymer to drinks to a final concentration of 15%–25% CHO, depending on age
- low protein crisps, e.g. cassava snacks, prawn crackers, corn curls
- very low protein milks, e.g. Prozero, Sno-Pro, can be used to make milkshakes and desserts and can be poured onto breakfast cereals

If the child does not consume all the daily protein allowance as food, it should be replaced with fluids; cow's milk with added glucose polymer to 15%–20% CHO is often the simplest way to do this. Table 17.59 provides an example of a low protein diet.

If the infant does not progress onto solids then a change from infant formula to a paediatric enteral feed during early childhood is indicated to provide the base of low protein feed. This may be an oral or tube feed, or combination of both.

Feeding problems and tube feeding

Some children with UCD [384, 399] and OAA [400, 401] have extensive feeding difficulties and tube feeding is necessary to maintain metabolic stability and promote normal growth (particularly difficult to achieve in patients with MMA and PA). Feeding issues may be due to neurological impairment, poor appetite, slow feeding and food refusal, vomiting, retching, gastro-oesophageal reflux (GOR). Some of these problems can be present from diagnosis or be acquired, particularly during episodes of metabolic decompensation. Poor appetite, limited food variety and lengthy mealtimes have been reported as the main feeding problems identified by carers of children with OAA and UCD [399]. This pilot study also identified inadequate attention to the social aspects of eating as a key issue, with most children regularly eating alone. Involvement of a speech and language therapist and psychologist at an early stage may help manage some feeding and behavioural problems. Strategies to help prevent and manage feeding problems are given in Table 17.45.

If tube feeding is necessary a low protein modular feed is designed to meet the specific therapeutic dietary needs of the child's disorder. A measured volume of a standard paediatric feed is used to provide the prescribed protein intake, with other ingredients added to meet normal energy and nutrient requirements: glucose polymer, fat emulsions, vitamins, minerals and electrolytes. It is important to ensure adequate fluids and fibre are given. Some children have increased fluid requirements including those with GA1 who have increased muscular tone or with MMA and CKD. The additional fluid is given as water, either between feeds or extra water with tube feed flushes, depending on tolerance. An example of a low protein feed is shown in Table 17.60. Gastrostomy feeding is recommended in preference to NG feeding for children who require long term tube feeding; a Nissen fundoplication may be performed in some patients with severe vomiting and GOR.

Evans *et al.* stress the importance of adequate training in safety aspects of home enteral feeding and regular training updates for carers as incorrect practices may increase a child's risk of metabolic decompensation [402].

Disorders of Propionate Metabolism

The disorders of propionate metabolism, methylmalonic acidaemia (MMA) and propionic acidaemia (PA) share common biochemical and clinical features due to accumulation of propionyl-CoA and other metabolites. Both disorders can be classified into

- early onset form: patients present in the neonatal period or early infancy with a severe metabolic acidosis (although not always) [403] and hyperammonaemia with poor feeding, vomiting, lethargy, hypotonia and dehydration which can progress to coma and death if untreated
- late onset form: patients may present later in infancy or childhood with less severe symptoms including failure to thrive and developmental delay, acute metabolic decompensation and acidosis; a movement disorder may also develop [404, 405]

Biochemistry and genetics

These defects occur in the final steps of the catabolic pathways of the four essential amino acids isoleucine, valine, threonine and methionine. Cholesterol side chain, thymine and uracil metabolism are also affected but are of lesser significance (Fig. 17.16). MMA and PA are autosomal recessive inherited disorders.

- PA results from mutations in the PCCA or PCCB genes encoding the α- and β-subunits respectively of propionyl-CoA carboxylase, a biotin dependent enzyme which catalyses the conversion of propionyl-CoA to methylmalonyl-CoA. Defects cause high plasma and urinary propionic acid levels and excretion of multiple organic compounds, including methylcitrate, 3-hydroxypropionate and propionylcarnitine [405].

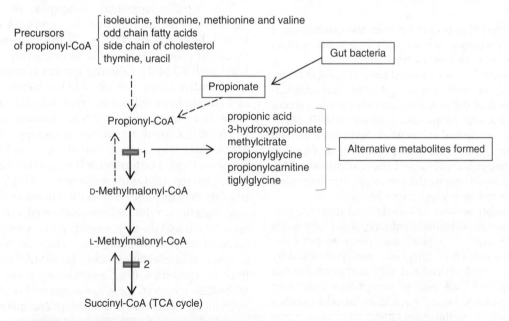

1 **Propionic acidaemia due to deficiency of propionyl-CoA carboxylase, a biotin dependent enzyme**
2 **Methylmalonic acidaemia due to deficiency of Methylmalonyl-CoA mutase, an adenosylcobalamin dependent reaction**

Figure 17.16 Disorders of propionate metabolism.

- MMA results from mutations in the MUT locus encoding the methylmalonyl-CoA mutase-apoenzyme causing reduced (mut−) or absent (mut°) activity; or by the genes required for provision of its cofactor 5-deoxyadenosylcobalamin, classified as cobalamin (cbl) A, B or D-variant 2. The conversion of methylmalonyl-CoA to succinyl-CoA (for entry into the Krebs cycle) is impaired, so methylmalonyl-CoA accumulates with greatly increased amounts of methylmalonic acid in plasma and urine. Also the compounds found in propionic acidaemia accumulate (as above) [405].
- Accumulation of propionyl-CoA is also considered a possible cause of the hypoglycaemia, hyperlactataemia, hyperammonaemia and hyperglycinaemia seen in both disorders.

Sources of propionate

It is important to appreciate that propionate (in the form of propionyl-CoA) is formed from three main sources, not just from amino acid catabolism. Estimates of the contributions of these sources are as follows.

- Around 50% is derived from the catabolism of the precursor amino acids isoleucine, valine, threonine and methionine [406].
- Around 25% is produced from anaerobic bacterial fermentation in the gut [406]. Oral administration of the antibiotic metronidazole reduces gut bacteria propionate production [407]. However, its clinical efficacy has never been proven in randomised controlled trials. Administration of metronidazole varies between centres and the benefits of one method compared with another have not been properly validated.
- Probably around 25% is derived from the oxidation of odd-numbered long chain fatty acids (C15 and C17) [408] and other metabolites. These odd-chain fatty acids are synthesised by the normal pathway of fatty acid synthesis but propionyl-CoA acts as the primer instead of acetyl-CoA; hence the additional odd number of carbons in the chain [409].

Outcome and complications

The outcome of these disorders can vary widely. Survival rates have improved in the last decade but early deaths still occur [401, 410, 411]. Early onset is associated with poorer outcome. In MMA, outcome is best predicted by vitamin B_{12} responsiveness, enzymatic subgroup, age at onset and birth decade. Mut° and cblB patients have the poorest outcome, then mut− and cblA. B_{12} responsive patients have a much better long term outcome, although they remain at risk of metabolic decompensation and long term complications such as CKD [410, 411]. The mechanisms of toxicity are complex and not well understood; a detailed review of the current concepts of the pathophysiology is given by Kölker et al. [412]. Multiple body systems can be affected in both disorders and recognised complications include acute injury of the basal ganglia (known as metabolic stroke) causing mental and motor retardation and movement disorders; cardiomyopathy [413], long QT syndrome (in PA) [414], pancreatitis [415], optic nerve atrophy [416], immune dysfunction, recurrent infections and pancytopenia, and CKD (in MMA) [417, 418]. These complications may arise during episodes of metabolic decompensation and/or are due to a more chronic deterioration of organ function [411].

The IQ/developmental outcomes in both disorders range from normal to significant intellectual disability [401, 411]. In PA the frequency of metabolic crises is reported to be negatively correlated with IQ [401]. Faltering growth is common; the causative factors are likely to be multifactorial and remain to be fully elucidated [401, 411]. Early onset and progressive growth retardation is seen in PA [401]. Growth retardation is also reported in MMA (404); CKD may be one of the contributing factors as this is a feature of CKD per se [419]. Failure to thrive is reported as more common in MMA mut° patients than the other enzymatic subgroups [410]. Although the survival rate has improved, outcome on conventional therapy remains poor. Alternative forms of therapy are being used. There are reports of liver transplantation and, in MMA, kidney, liver or combined liver and kidney transplants [420–422]; however, these are associated with significant risk at the time of transplant and metabolic complications may still arise post transplant such as metabolic stroke [423]. Protein restriction may still be necessary post transplant. MMA children with a kidney transplant need to remain on a low protein diet. In PA, low protein diet is reported to be both discontinued and liberalised [422, 424].

Treatment guidelines

Recommendations for the chronic management and health supervision of individuals with PA and acute management of PA have been published following a PA consensus conference in the USA, 2011 [425,426]. The therapeutic interventions are predominantly based on expert opinion. The European registry and network for Intoxication Type Metabolic Diseases (E-IMD) (www.E-IMD.org) are working on management guidelines for MMA and PA.

Dietary management

The main aim of dietary treatment is to reduce production of the toxic organic acids propionic or methylmalonic acid by

- restriction of precursor amino acids (isoleucine, valine, threonine and methionine) using a restricted protein diet
- avoidance of fasting to limit lipolysis and thus the oxidation of odd-chain fatty acids
- provision of an adequate energy intake to limit catabolism

The precursor amino acids (isoleucine, valine, threonine and methionine) do not accumulate in plasma in these disorders so it is not possible to use the measurement of their plasma levels to determine the intake of natural protein. Treatment is to restrict dietary protein intake to around the safe level for age (Table 17.54) with caution; too low a protein intake can have serious effects, such as poor growth, skin rashes, hair loss, vomiting and metabolic decompensation [304,385,386]. Dietary protein is increased according to age, weight, clinical condition and quantitative plasma amino acid concentrations. However, it can be difficult to achieve a balance between provision of sufficient protein for growth and avoiding an excess of protein which may precipitate illness. Practical aspects of provision of low protein diets and feeds have been discussed (p. 456).

Precursor free amino acids

Some centres provide part of the protein intake as supplements of L-amino acids (free from precursor amino acids) to further reduce the intake of precursor amino acids in an effort to improve metabolic stability, or improve the quality of the low protein diet. This appears to be a more common practice in some central European metabolic centres [401,411,427] and the USA [428]. Prescription of precursor free amino acids is highly variable providing up to 40%–50% of total protein intake [401,427,428]. However, the clinical value of these supplements remains controversial and no long term controlled studies have been published. Metabolic balance can be achieved without them; they are unpalatable and can be difficult to administer to children unless they are tube fed. One study of two patients with MMA showed that, although there was increased nitrogen retention when the low protein diet was supplemented with precursor free amino acids, there was no improvement in growth or decrease in methylmalonate excretion [429]. Touati et al. in a retrospective review of 137 patients with either MMA or PA concluded that amino acid mixture supplementation did not seem to have an important role in the long term nutritional and developmental outcome [400]. Yanicelli et al. have reported improved growth and nutrition status in a short term study of children using a precursor free amino acid feed; however, energy intakes also increased in those patients whose growth in height improved [430].

Precursor free amino acid supplements are available as infant formula, e.g. MMA/PA Anamix Infant, or drink mixes, gels or pure amino acids which are designed for different ages, e.g. XMTVI Maxamaid >1 year, XMTVI Maxamum >8 years; MMA/PA gel from 6 months; MMA/PA Cooler and Express 15, both from 3 years. All of these products contain added energy (CHO ± fat) and vitamins and minerals. For details of presentation, composition, age suitability and preparation refer to the manufacturers' websites: www.nutricia.co.uk, www.vitaflo.co.uk. Similar products are available outside the UK (www.abbottnutrition.com, www.meadjohnson.com, www.milupametabolics.com).

There are no evidence based guidelines for the amounts of precursor free amino acids to give, although it is suggested they may contribute up to half of the daily protein prescription [428]. If used, they should provide only part of the total protein intake and be based on growth and biochemical parameters including protein status such as plasma amino acids and albumin. Dietary intakes of isoleucine, valine, threonine, methionine should also be calculated to avoid deficiency states.

Avoidance of fasting

It is recommended that long fasts are avoided to limit the production of propionyl-CoA from the oxidation of odd-numbered long chain fats [408]. Mobilisation of fatty acids can be suppressed by regular three to four hourly daytime feeding and overnight tube feeding. Currently, overnight tube feeding is not used universally although many do receive this because of feeding problems. In one MMA patient, uncooked cornstarch was used to minimise lipolysis at night during pregnancy [431].

Energy requirements

Resting energy expenditure (REE) has been measured in children with disorders of propionate metabolism and is reported to be decreased in some patients when they are well [432]; however, others have described no difference between predicted and reported REE [433]. Standard predictive equations of REE may not be a good guide to energy requirements in children with MMA as they can have an altered body composition (increased fat mass, reduced fat free mass) and decreased renal function, which are both known to affect REEnobreak [434].

Medical management – pharmacotherapy

Patients are treated with some or all of these medicines:

- L-carnitine – this conjugates with propionic acid to form propionylcarnitine and increases its excretion in urine. The standard dose of 100 mg/kg/day is routinely given to all patients. A lower carnitine dose may be given in MMA patients who have deteriorating kidney function and have high plasma concentrations of propionylcarnitine.
- Metronidazole – is an antibiotic given to suppress gut production of propionate. It is usually given intermittently.

- B_{12} – is the cofactor for methylmalonyl-CoA mutase and some patients with MMA show a good response to pharmacological doses. B_{12} is given routinely to MMA-B_{12} responsive patients.
- Sodium bicarbonate – is given to correct any acidosis in MMA.
- N-carbamylglutamate – is used by some centres for treatment of severe episodes of hyperammonaemia in PA.
- Additional medicines are given to treat specific complications such as CKD in MMA.

MMA B_{12} responsive patients

In responsive patients, vitamin B_{12} is given as an intramuscular injection or rarely as an oral supplement. The dose frequency is individualised. Some urine methylmalonic acid is still produced; concentrations vary between patients and may typically range from 200 to 900 μmol/mmol creatinine (normal 0–30 μmol/mmol creatinine) which is significantly less than non responsive patients where concentrations can be >20 000 μmol/mmol creatinine. Plasma methylmalonate is also much lower, typically <0.2 μmol/L (normal 0–0.28 μmol/L) in B_{12} responsive compared with non responsive patients. Concentrations of methylmalonate increase with loss of kidney function. Dietary treatment of a low protein diet and emergency regimen is the same as for B_{12} non responsive patients, although a more generous protein allowance may be possible.

Complications of methylmalonic acidaemia and propionic acidaemia

Metabolic decompensations

Repeated hospital admissions for episodes of metabolic decompensation (some with acidosis and/or hyperammonaemia) are seen in some patients with MMA [435] and PA [401]; this may be related to intercurrent illness or a feature of the disorder itself. Intensive care treatment may be necessary. These episodes are treated in a similar manner to intercurrent illness initially with a protein free, high energy intake from either IV glucose or oral/enteral glucose polymer emergency regimen, to minimise catabolism (p. 502).

MMA and chronic kidney disease

Impaired renal function is a common complication in non B_{12} responsive MMA, manifesting initially with a defect of urinary concentrating and acidification ability due to renal tubular dysfunction [436]. Glomerular failure can develop at an early age with progression to chronic, then end stage renal failure (ESRF) during childhood or adolescence [411, 418, 435]. Deterioration of kidney function is likely to be multifactorial with methylmalonic acid itself considered nephrotoxic [437]. Development of CKD correlates with urinary MMA excretion, manifesting earlier in those with highest mean MMA concentrations [410] and in those with mut° [411]. Kidney function can deteriorate markedly during episodes of dehydration which can be caused by gastrointestinal (GI) complications such as vomiting and reflux, inadequate fluid intake, repeated illness and metabolic decompensations. At the author's centre the glomerular filtration rate is measured by the IOHEXOL method, 1–2 yearly from age 2 years in MMA patients. The management of MMA and CKD (undertaken jointly with nephrologists) can be particularly challenging and involves ongoing modification of nutrient intakes, fluids and medicines based on biochemical monitoring results and clinical symptoms.

Dietary manipulations

- The low protein diet used for MMA is also appropriate dietary treatment for CKD.
- Increased fluid requirements are needed to prevent dehydration. The amount given is determined by kidney losses, blood pressure, blood urea and electrolytes.
- Phosphate, calcium and vitamin D. Renal bone disease is complex and begins even in the milder stages of CKD, seen biochemically as a rise in parathyroid hormone (PTH). Renal bone disease is managed by a combination of medicines and diet:
  - vitamin D analogues, e.g. 1α-hydroxycholecalciferol (alfacalcidol) to increase calcium absorption from the gut.
  - if plasma phosphate is increased dietary phosphate is restricted, although intakes may already be low because patients are on tube feeds or do not eat high phosphate foods because of protein restriction. Phosphate binders are given to lower plasma phosphate, either calcium based (e.g. calcium carbonate) or a calcium free binder if there is hypercalcaemia (e.g. sevelamer hydrochloride).
  - dietary calcium should provide at least the lower RNI [389]. Around 20%–30% of calcium from calcium based phosphate binders is reported to be absorbed and contributes to daily intake.
- Electrolytes
  - supplements of sodium bicarbonate are often needed both to replace sodium losses and reduce acidosis.
  - if blood pressure is raised, dietary sodium intake may need to be reduced.
  - hyperkalaemia is not usually a problem until the end stages of kidney disease when potassium intake may need to be reduced.
- Vitamin A can accumulate in serum in CKD and this may be linked to hypercalcaemia [438]. Because of this a practice guideline in the UK has been that vitamin A intake in CKD (non MMA) should be less than twice the RNI; however, recent work suggests that even this amount may be too high [439]. In MMA vitamin A intake should be assessed, particularly the contribution from vitamin and mineral supplements and any precursor free amino acid supplements. A vitamin A intake of around the RNI seems sensible, but this may need to be reduced if plasma concentrations are increased.
- Anaemia is a chronic complication of CKD and is treated with iron supplements and injections of erythropoiesis stimulating agents: erythropoietin β or darbepoetin α. It is important to ensure adequate iron is provided from the low protein diet (most likely to be provided from a combination of feeds and vitamin and mineral supplements).

Chapter 12 provides a more detailed account of dietary treatment in CKD, but it is important to be aware that protein recommendations for CKD given in Chapter 12 are not appropriate for the CKD found in children with MMA, where protein restriction is an essential part of management. Haemodialysis or peritoneal dialysis can cause symptomatic and biochemical improvement in ESRF, with fewer episodes of metabolic decompensation [417, 440–442]. On dialysis the dietary restrictions remain necessary and are modified according to biochemical results; protein intake may be slightly increased compared with intake pre dialysis. Some patients may go straight to kidney transplant without a period of dialysis. Parenteral nutrition is given initially post renal transplant, providing the child's usual protein intake and an increased energy intake (compared with normal), returning to usual enteral feeds depending on clinical progress (personal communication). A low protein diet remains necessary post renal transplant.

Gastrointestinal and feeding problems

Gastro-oesophageal reflux, recurrent vomiting and retching are common in MMA B_{12} non responsive patients and often necessitate hospital admission [400]. In the author's cohort, 7/14 patients had GI symptoms; all were treated with anti-reflux medicines and additionally a continuous overnight feed with slow daytime bolus feeds given via an enteral feeding pump was beneficial [443]. A hydrolysed protein feed helped some with GI symptoms, including diarrhoea.

Constipation is a problem observed in some patients with PA. Maintenance of gut motility to prevent constipation is important as it may reduce propionate production. In a small study of four children, Senokot (vegetable laxative) was reported to be biochemically beneficial and to reduce transit time [444]. Use of laxatives has been recommended in treatment guidelines for PA [425]. Movicol is the laxative of choice at the author's centre. Adequate fluids and feeds containing fibre (in tube fed patients) may also help prevent constipation.

Feeding problems and tube feeding

Anorexia and feeding problems of varying degrees are almost invariably present in children with more severe disorders [400, 401]. Feeding problems can be present at diagnosis and may not improve with treatment. Food and fluid refusal can be acquired during the course of the disease and is frequently associated with repeated intercurrent infections. The causative factors of feeding problems are unclear, but increased plasma propionate is a possibility. Many children have a poor appetite for solid foods. Some will only eat a few selected foods in very small amounts, occasionally changing the type of foods that they will eat. Some are difficult feeders; parents complain of children being slow, fussy, retching or self-inducing vomiting with foods. Children with MMA have a preference for salty foods, e.g. crisps, tomato ketchup, chips and salt, and may do this to compensate for increased urinary losses of sodium.

Achieving optimal growth in MMA and PA can be difficult. Enteral feeding via gastrostomy (particularly if there is vomiting) or NG tube is essential to provide an adequate dietary intake, to prevent metabolic decompensation and to help the parents cope with a child who is difficult to feed. In the author's 12/14 patients with B_{12} non responsive MMA had feeding problems, 11/14 needed long term tube feeding; feeding problems were much less common in MMA B_{12} responsive patients and only 1/12 was tube fed [443]. In a European cohort gastrostomy feeding was necessary in 27/55 patients with PA to ensure growth and metabolic stability [401]. Early insertion of a gastrostomy in infants and young children has been recommended [425]. A percutaneous endoscopic gastrostomy tube with a jejunal extension tube (PEG-J tube) can also be helpful in the management of episodes of vomiting and pancreatitis.

Pancreatitis

Pancreatitis is a recognised complication of both MMA and PA and may be either a single acute episode or recurrent acute episodes [401, 411, 415]. In some cases it is associated with an intercurrent illness. The pathophysiology of pancreatitis is not clear. The child's usual dietary restrictions should continue irrespective of the feeding intervention used to treat pancreatitis. A period of PN may be necessary; alternatively NG/gastrostomy/jejunal feeds may be possible. Chapter 9 provides for further details about the dietetic management of pancreatitis.

Initial dietary treatment of the newly diagnosed patient

The newly diagnosed patient may be very sick and in intensive care with a severe metabolic acidosis (with increased anion gap), ketonuria and hyperammonaemia requiring ventilation and dialysis (to remove ammonia and toxic compounds). Reversal of catabolism is a crucial part of the management to help stabilise the child (p. 463).

Clinical and biochemical monitoring in MMA and PA

Monitoring of the nutritional aspects of a low protein diet has been discussed earlier (p. 463). Routine biochemical monitoring is shown in Table 17.62.

Emergency regimens for management of intercurrent illness and episodes of metabolic decompensation

During intercurrent infections patients are at risk of developing metabolic acidosis and encephalopathy. Development of new neurological signs, including metabolic stroke, are reported following episodes of acute metabolic decompensation [401, 446]. In MMA there is the added risk of dehydration and

deterioration of kidney function. To help prevent metabolic decompensation the standard emergency regimen (ER) (p. 502) is given and the child's usual medicines are continued (such as carnitine, metronidazole, sodium bicarbonate). A high energy intake from glucose polymer is given either orally at frequent 2 hourly intervals or more typically via a tube as a continuous 24 hour feed. This will reduce protein catabolism and lipolysis and hence production of toxic metabolites. If this is not tolerated or the full volume cannot be administered at home the child should be admitted to hospital without delay, because of risk of metabolic acidosis, for treatment with IV fluids (10% glucose and saline) and medicines. The British Inherited Metabolic Disease Group (BIMDG) (www.bimdg.org) provide emergency protocols for IV management. The usual protein intake is stopped for the minimum time possible to prevent protein deficiency which

Table 17.62 Routine biochemical monitoring in methylmalonic acidaemia and propionic acidaemia.

Bloods	Comments
Quantitative plasma amino acids	Glycine is usually increased
	Alanine is generally increased if lactate is increased
	If precursor amino acids or indispensable amino acids are low, consider increasing natural protein
Plasma acylcarnitines	Propionyl carnitine is increased
	Higher concentrations are seen in MMA as kidney disease progresses
	Other acylcarnitines can also be increased, e.g. free acetyl
Plasma methylmalonate (MMA only)	Increases to higher concentrations as kidney function deteriorates in MMA
Urea, creatinine and electrolytes	Urea is often low on a restricted protein diet
	Urea and creatinine increase as kidney function deteriorates in MMA
Full blood count	May have neutropenia, particularly during illness
Blood gas, bicarbonate	Possible metabolic acidosis
Ammonia	May be raised
Lactate	May be raised
Urate	May be raised, treated with allopurinol
Glutathione (GSH), glutathione disulfide (GSSG) oxidised and reduced	Not routinely measured in all centres. It is a measure of oxidative stress [445]. Concentrations can be low
MMA only – urine monitoring	
Urine MMA/creatinine μmol/mmol	Much lower concentrations in B_{12} responsive MMA
Urine methylcitrate/creatinine μmol/mmol	Much lower concentrations in B_{12} responsive MMA
MMA only – to monitor kidney function	
PTH, vitamin D, calcium, phosphate, alkaline phosphatase	To monitor renal bone disease
Ferritin, Hb, TIBC,TSAT	To monitor iron status and anaemia of chronic kidney disease
Vitamin A	Can be raised
Lipids – triglycerides and cholesterol	Can be raised
Glomerular filtration rate	1–2 yearly from age 2 years, less frequently may be appropriate in B_{12} responsive MMA

could greatly exacerbate the effects of illness. Protein is normally reintroduced early (within 24–48 hours) and over a period of 1–2 days depending on the clinical condition of the child. Obviously, a more rapid reintroduction of protein is beneficial. Practical advice on protein reintroduction is given on p. 464. Continuation of an adequate energy intake is important throughout this period.

Inadequate nutrition in these disorders leads to catabolism, making the metabolic disturbance worse. If a child is unable to be re-established on their normal diet and protein intake within a few days, or is experiencing repeated intercurrent infections with inadequate protein intake, then an early resort to PN becomes essential. PN can reverse the catabolic spiral and improve the metabolic state. If PN is indicated a normal amino acid solution can be used, but the daily volume is limited to provide only the child's usual protein intake (more may be needed in a malnourished patient); IV glucose and lipid are given to provide the energy intake. Placement of a portacath may be considered in any child who has frequent episodes of illness and if their IV access is difficult. However, this needs to be carefully considered because of the risk of line infection precipitating metabolic decompensation [425].

Methylmalonic acidaemia – additional recommendations

In MMA a generous fluid intake needs to be given to prevent dehydration and deterioration of kidney function. The ER should provide at least the child's usual maintenance fluid intake and more (this needs to be assessed on an individual basis taking into account the child's kidney function); 24 hour continuous tube feeds are suggested to administer the full fluid intake. The usual dose of sodium bicarbonate may need to be increased. The BIMDG emergency protocols suggest for IV fluids that maintenance fluids are given with 20% added.

Isovaleric acidaemia

Biochemistry and genetics

Isovaleric acidaemia (IVA) is caused by a deficiency of the enzyme isovaleryl-CoA dehydrogenase, which catalyses the third step of leucine catabolism: the conversion of isovaleryl-CoA to 3-methylcrotonyl-CoA (Fig. 17.9). Isovaleryl-CoA, isovaleric acid, isovaleryl (C5) carnitine and other metabolites accumulate. During remission the majority of isovaleryl-CoA is conjugated to isovalerylglycine which is not toxic and is excreted in large amounts in urine. Isovaleryl-CoA is also conjugated to carnitine to form isovalerylcarnitine which is also excreted in the urine. However, during acute episodes the natural capacity of this detoxification pathway is exceeded and isovaleryl-CoA is deacylated to produce large amounts of toxic isovaleric acid which may cause an overwhelming illness [447]. The actual mechanism of toxicity is not understood. IVA is an autosomal recessive inherited disorder. Mutations in the IVD gene are highly heterogeneous and no genotype–phenotype correlation has been identified [447], except in those diagnosed on newborn screening with the c.932C>T mutation, who have a much milder phenotype [448].

Classification

Clinical cases of IVA can be classified into two groups [449]:

- acute neonatal form: neonates present within the first week of life [450], commonly with poor feeding, vomiting, metabolic acidosis, hyperammonaemia (in some) and lethargy progressing to coma. Their subsequent course follows the chronic intermittent course. A characteristic smell of 'sweaty feet' may occur when the child is unwell.
- chronic form: children may present with more chronic, non-specific symptoms of failure to thrive and/or developmental delay or mental retardation. There is a wide spectrum of presentation with chronic forms.

Expanded newborn screening

A number of countries worldwide undertake expanded newborn screening for IVA, using tandem mass spectrometry, and this has identified a common milder phenotype (c.932C>T mutation) for which less dietary modification is required. A normal diet can be given (protein restriction is not necessary) but an ER for management of illness is recommended [448]. IVA is one of the disorders being evaluated in the pilot project of expanded newborn screening (since July 2012) in parts of England. Screening is by measurement of C5 acyl-carnitines in dried blood spots using tandem mass spectrometry. More information on screening, diagnostic and clinical management protocols can be found at www.expandedscreening.org.

Outcome and complications

The outcome of IVA is variable ranging from normal neurocognitive outcome/psychomotor development to, less commonly, severe mental retardation [450]. A recent review of 155 cases reports that neonatal presentation is associated with a high mortality, but those who survive the acute episode have a better neurocognitive outcome than patients with a late diagnosis [450]. Expanded newborn screening may improve the mortality of neonatal onset, provided screening is done early enough, as those with neonatal onset will present within the first week. IVA is not considered to be a progressive disorder. There are no reported major long term complications. Acute pancreatitis has been reported pre diagnosis in three cases [449], post diagnosis in one child aged 3.5 years with neonatal onset form [451] and one other child [450], but the author is aware of several other unpublished cases in the UK.

Treatment guidelines

Currently there are no published consensus treatment guidelines for IVA.

Dietary management

The main aim of dietary treatment is to minimise the formation of isovaleric acid by

- limiting the dietary intake of leucine (by means of a restricted protein diet)
- provision of an adequate energy intake to prevent catabolism and promote normal growth and development
- provision of an ER to limit catabolism during intercurrent illness

Leucine does not accumulate in plasma so it is not possible to use measurement of this to determine protein intake.

Usually a modest protein restriction (around 2 g/kg in infants and young children decreasing to between 1.5 and 1 g/kg in older patients, although some have higher intakes and remain metabolically stable) combined with an adequate energy intake is sufficient to help limit the production of isovaleric acid in the well child. Infants can be successfully exclusively breast fed [398] or given a leucine free feed before breast feeds to limit protein intake [452]. The author has experience of four partially breast fed infants: two received standard formula top-up feeds and two had protein free feeds before breast feeds. Four other breast fed infants (two sibling screens) all had leucine free formula (20 mL × 5 feeds) given pre breast feeds (personal communication). There are reports of giving leucine free amino acids in combination with a low protein diet, although no specific details of intake were provided [450]. However, in the author's experience use of leucine free amino acids is generally not warranted in the long term diet.

Some patients are not on a 'counted' protein intake and remain stable on a self-selected low protein diet (often those who present later) or just avoid high protein foods, which can be the case in older patients who are on a more relaxed diet [453]. Although many patients are not on very low protein diets it is still important to ensure that an adequate intake of all vitamins and minerals is provided as there is a risk of deficiency of some micronutrients. Practical management of low protein diets and feeds has been given (p. 456). Most children with IVA have a reasonable appetite and grow normally but major feeding problems can occur in some and tube feeding may be necessary [450, 454]. A review of the feeding habits of 29 children with IVA from three UK metabolic centres identified eight children with poor appetite (six of whom were tube fed) and two with 'bizarre' feeding habits.

If a child develops pancreatitis the usual dietary restrictions should continue irrespective of the feeding intervention used to treat the pancreatitis. A period of PN may be necessary; alternatively jejunal or NG/gastrostomy feeds may be possible. Chapter 9 provides for further details about the dietetic management of pancreatitis.

Medical management – pharmacotherapy

Two main medicines, L-glycine and L-carnitine, are used in the management of IVA. Patients are treated with either or both of these medicines. Both conjugate with isovaleric acid producing non toxic conjugates (isovalerylglycine, isovalerylcarnitine) which are excreted in urine; hence isovaleric acid levels are reduced [455–457]. These medicines are particularly important during periods of metabolic decompensation. The need for both medicines in a stable child is controversial [458, 459] and prescribed doses vary [450]. Medicines should be individually prescribed as response can vary [460].

Prescribed doses are [461]

- L-glycine (150–300 mg/kg/day)
- L-carnitine (50–100 mg/kg/day)

Initial dietary treatment of the newly diagnosed patient

The newly diagnosed infant with IVA may be very sick with hyperammonaemia and metabolic acidosis and in intensive care. Reversal of catabolism is a crucial part of the management to help stabilise the child (p. 463). The initial management aims to promote anabolism, to reduce production of isovaleric acid and to increase its excretion by giving IV glycine and carnitine.

Clinical and biochemical monitoring

There is no established laboratory marker for monitoring this disorder and therapeutic control. Plasma levels of leucine are not elevated in IVA. Plasma amino acids and carnitine should be monitored at routine clinic reviews. Patients treated with glycine generally have increased plasma glycine levels. Isovalerylcarnitine concentrations are increased. Monitoring of the nutritional aspects of a low protein diet has been discussed (p. 463).

Dietary management during illness – emergency regimen

During intercurrent infections protein catabolism greatly increases production of isovaleric acid and patients are at risk of metabolic decompensation. To help prevent this, the standard ER (p. 502) of frequent 2 hourly drinks/feeds of glucose polymer is given day and night. It is essential that glycine and carnitine continue to be given with the doses increased temporarily as necessary. If the ER is not tolerated or the full volume cannot be given at home, then the child is admitted to hospital for IV fluids (10% dextrose and saline 0.45%) and medicines. Only carnitine can be given intravenously; there is no IV glycine preparation. The BIMDG provide emergency protocols for IV management.

Protein intake is stopped temporarily (24–48 hours) and reintroduced over 1–2 days depending on the clinical condition of the child; a more rapid reintroduction is best. Practical advice on protein reintroduction is given on p. 464. Continuation of an adequate energy intake is important throughout this period. Episodes of metabolic decompensation appear to be less frequent with age [454]. Grünert *et al.* reported no episodes beyond age 9 years in 21 patients [450] although the author is aware of episodes in older children in UK metabolic centres.

Glutaric aciduria type 1

Glutaric aciduria type 1 (GA1) is a neurometabolic disorder, first described in 1975 [462]. It is caused by deficiency of the enzyme glutaryl-CoA dehydrogenase (GCDH) in the catabolic pathway of the amino acids L-lysine, L-hydroxylysine and L-tryptophan and catalyses the dehydrogenation of glutaryl-CoA to glutaconyl-CoA and its decarboxylation to crotonyl-CoA (Fig. 17.17). Biochemically there is accumulation of the metabolites glutaric acid, 3-hydroxyglutaric acid, glutaryl-CoA, glutaconic acid (to a lesser extent) and glutaryl carnitine in body fluids (urine, plasma and cerebrospinal fluid) and tissues [463]. Patients can have either low or high urinary excretion of metabolites, termed low or high excretors; irrespectively they both remain at the same risk of striatal damage. GA1 is an autosomal recessive disorder due to mutations in the GCDH gene, with more than 200 mutations identified [464]. Worldwide the incidence is reported as 1 in 100 000 although there is a much higher incidence in some specific communities: up to 1 in 300 in Irish travellers [465], the Amish community in Pennsylvania [466] and the Canadian Oji-Cree

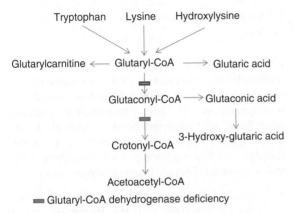

Tryptophan   Lysine   Hydroxylysine

Glutarylcarnitine ⟵ Glutaryl-CoA ⟶ Glutaric acid

Glutaconyl-CoA ⟶ Glutaconic acid

Crotonyl-CoA   3-Hydroxy-glutaric acid

Acetoacetyl-CoA

▬ Glutaryl-CoA dehydrogenase deficiency

Figure 17.17 Glutaric aciduria type 1 – catabolic pathway of lysine, hydroxylysine and tryptophan.

Indians [467]. There is no genotype/clinical phenotype correlation although there is some correlation with biochemical phenotype; those with residual GCDH activity have a low urinary metabolite excretion whilst those with high excretion have no residual GCDH activity; this does not, however, predict severity [468].

Expanded newborn screening

A number of countries worldwide undertake expanded newborn screening for GA1, using tandem mass spectrometry. Early detection by screening and pre symptomatic initiation of treatment can greatly improve the outcome, preventing the neurological handicap which develops with the clinical presentation and onset of neurological crises [469]. GA1 is one of the disorders being evaluated in the pilot project of expanded newborn screening (since July 2012) in parts of England. Screening is by measurement of glutaryl carnitine in dried blood spots using tandem mass spectrometry. More information on screening, diagnostic and clinical management protocols can be found at www.expandedscreening.org.

Clinical presentation and outcome

Typically babies with GA1 usually appear normal in the first months of life, although many will have macrocephaly. The majority of children present before 2 years of age with a median age of 9 months [470] following an intercurrent illness such as a respiratory or GI illness which precipitates to an acute encephalopathic crisis. Characteristically this causes irreversible striatal damage and a complex movement disorder. Severely affected patients are consequently left with a severe dystonic-dyskinetic disorder that is similar to cerebral palsy and ranges from extreme hypotonia to choreoathetosis to rigidity and spasticity [471]. There is loss of mobility (partial), swallowing difficulties and dysarthria. Intellectual function is generally preserved initially. Morbidity and mortality is high in patients who have had a crisis. A minority of patients have a more insidious onset or later onset neurological disease with no obvious encephalopathic episode preceding the development of the movement disorder.

Some cases of GA1 never present clinically, despite never having being treated, and may only be diagnosed on sibling screening following presentation of the index case [472, 473]. Patients appear to be at greatest risk of striatal injury during a finite period of brain development, between birth and 6 years. The neuropathogenesis of GA1 is not fully delineated; a recent overview is given by Jafari *et al.* [468]. Intraneuronal accumulation of high concentrations of glutaric acid (GA) and 3-hydroxyglutaric acid (3-OH-GA) formed by *de novo* synthesis in the central nervous system during catabolic episodes is considered to be the most important factor in precipitating neuronal damage, probably via several mechanisms: excitotoxic cell damage, impairment of energy metabolism and oxidative stress [468]. As the transport capacity for GA and 3-OH-GA across the blood–brain barrier (BBB) is low they accumulate in very high concentrations during catabolic episodes (10- to 1000-fold higher than in plasma) and are 'trapped' in the brain [474]. Studies in GCDH deficient mice provide evidence that lowering lysine intake, L-arginine (or homoarginine) supplementation and an increased glucose intake reduces the concentration of GA and 3-OH-GA in brain; carnitine supplementation increases formation of non toxic glutarylcarnitine but does not alter GA and 3-OH-GA [475, 476].

For those diagnosed on expanded newborn screening the outcome is much more positive. The onset of striatal damage and neurological symptoms can be prevented in most patients provided there is good adherence to treatment, particularly during illness [477], although cerebral changes can still be seen on neuroimaging [478] and some may still have fine motor and speech deficits [479].

Treatment guidelines

Treatment guidelines for GA1 were first published in 2007 [480] and revised in 2011 [481]. These provide comprehensive information on pathogenesis, screening and diagnosis, treatment strategies (including dietary management, Table 17.63), monitoring and outcome. Treatment involves a low lysine diet, carnitine supplementation and crucially an ER for treatment of intercurrent illnesses to prevent striatal injury and onset of a complex movement disorder. Heringer et al. [477] report that patients diagnosed on newborn screening who adhered to the treatment guidelines, particularly emergency management, and had follow-up in a metabolic centre, had a better outcome than those who did not adhere, developing motor disorder and encephalopathic crises much less frequently. Patients with delayed start of emergency treatment during acute intercurrent illness had the worst outcome, with onset of movement disorder. Emergency treatment is probably the most important aspect of treatment.

Dietary management of pre symptomatic patients

Lowering cerebral lysine influx and lysine oxidation limits production and accumulation of neurotoxic GA and 3-OH-GA and is considered neuroprotective in pre symptomatic patients who have not experienced a neurological crisis [477, 481]. Dietary management is the same for high and low excretor patients and those with insidious onset. Dietary intervention involves

- restriction of protein intake or more specifically lysine and tryptophan, the precursor amino acids
- provision of an adequate energy intake to limit catabolism, specifically lysine oxidation
- strategies to limit uptake of lysine across the BBB by competitive inhibition
- prompt implementation of an ER during intercurrent illness

The precursor amino acids lysine and tryptophan do not accumulate in plasma. It is therefore not possible to use plasma measurement of these to determine their dietary intake. For practical reasons provision of a low lysine diet varies; either a low lysine or a low protein diet is used.

Table 17.63 Maintenance dietary treatment for glutaric aciduria type 1, adapted from [480,481].

Treatment	Age				
	0-6 months	7-12 months	1-3 years	4-6 years	>6 years
Low lysine diet					Avoid excessive intake of natural protein (with a low lysine content), according 'to safe levels'.
Lysine (natural protein source) – mg/kg/day*	100	90	80-60	60-50	
Tryptophan – mg/kg/day*	20	17	17-13	13	
Amino acid supplement – g/kg/day	1.3-0.8	1.0-0.8	0.8	0.8	
Protein (natural) g/kg/day† [480]	1.4-1.3	1.5-1.3	1.4-1.3	1.3-1.1	
Protein (total) – g/kg/day† [480]	2.7-2.1	2.5-2.1	2.2-2.1	2.1-1.9	

*Lysine and Tryptophan recommendations are based on the 1st European Workshop on GA1 (Heidelberg 1993) and international dietary recommendations available at that time. A lysine free amino acid supplement needs to be administered in addition to the lysine (natural protein) intake. If the diet is not supplemented, natural protein intake should provide the 'safe levels of protein intake' or more, if necessary, to ensure adequate daily lysine intake.
†Recommendations were given for protein and total protein intake in the 2007 guideline only. The lysine/protein ratio of protein foods varies considerably. Thus the natural protein intake can be very variable dependent on food choice.

Low lysine diet

As lysine is more abundant than tryptophan in natural protein, 2%–9% versus 0.6%–2%, the diet is based on lysine rather than tryptophan intake. The guideline treatment recommendations for lysine and tryptophan intake (mg/kg/day) are based on clinical practice (from Germany) and published safe intakes at that time for the normal population (Table 17.63) [480, 481]. More recent publications (WHO/FAO/UNU 2007 [277]) set safe intakes for lysine lower, e.g. 45 mg/kg/day for 1–3 year olds, compared with 80–60 mg/kg/day in the guideline. Use of the WHO/FAO/UNU 2007 values has not been reported in clinical practice and it is therefore not known if further restriction of lysine would have any therapeutic advantage. It should also be borne in mind that a good outcome can be achieved with the current guideline recommendations. Limiting lysine intake in accordance with the guideline recommendations (Table 17.63) reduces the intake of natural protein to below normal growth requirements and a supplement of lysine free, tryptophan reduced amino acids becomes essential to prevent a deficiency state and to promote normal growth.

Recommendations for intakes of amino acid supplements are given in Table 17.63: 1.3 g/kg/day in early infancy decreasing to 0.8 g/kg/day by 1 year of age. A potential benefit of giving amino acid supplements is that they provide a good source of arginine. Lysine and arginine share the same cerebrovascular cationic transport system (y+ system), and arginine competes with lysine for uptake at the BBB and inner mitochondrial membrane. Supplementation of arginine has been shown to lower cerebral concentrations of GA and 3-OH-GA by reducing uptake of lysine through competitive inhibition in GA1 patients (using calculated cerebral amino acid influx studies) [482] and in studies of GCDH deficient mice on low lysine diet supplemented with arginine [475, 476]. Strauss et al. [482] used a dietary lysine/arginine ratio of arginine intake 1.5 to 2 times lysine intake.

Lysine free, tryptophan low amino acid supplements are available as infant formula, e.g. GA1 Anamix Infant, or powdered drink and gel mixes, which are designed for different ages, e.g. XLYS LOW TRY Maxamaid >1 year and XLYS LOW TRY Maxamum >8 years; GA gel from 6 months;

GA Express15 >3 years. These products all contain added energy ($CHO \pm fat$) and vitamins and minerals. The tryptophan content of amino acid supplements available in the UK is 4–6 mg/g of amino acids and arginine 69–78 mg/g of amino acids. XLYS TRY Glutaridon and GA amino5 are pure amino acid supplements. XLYS TRY Glutaridon differs in amino acid composition from the other products, being tryptophan free. If tryptophan free amino acid supplements are used it is essential the diet provides the requirement for tryptophan as deficiency can induce neurological dysfunction [483]. The WHO/FAO/UNU 2007 requirements [277] for tryptophan are: at 1 month 29 mg/kg/day, 6 months 16 mg/kg/day, 1–2 years 6.4 mg/kg/day and 3–10 years 4.8 mg/kg/day; these are mostly lower than the guideline [480]. For details of presentation, composition, age suitability and preparation refer to the manufacturers' websites: www.nutricia.co.uk, www.vitaflo.co.uk. Similar products are available outside the UK (www.abbottnutrition.com, www.meadjohnson.com, www.milupametabolics.com).

Low protein diet

The analysis of lysine content of foods in the UK is very limited and old [301]. It is therefore not possible to accurately and safely provide a low lysine diet, except in early infancy when the lysine and tryptophan content of infant formula is known. Instead, as weaning progresses, the diet is based on the safe level of protein intake (Table 17.54); a lysine free, low tryptophan amino acid supplement is given too. This type of diet is successfully used in the UK [484] and elsewhere in the world. A more generous protein intake of 2–2.5 g protein/kg has been given in seven patients without consequent neurological sequelae [485]. Despite these differences in provision of the diet, all patients have an aggressive emergency management plan for intercurrent illness as this is known to prevent neurological crisis.

The lysine content of different foods varies significantly, e.g. in cereal and cereal based foods there is 20–40 mg lysine/g of protein whereas milk, meat and fish products contain 70–90 mg lysine/g of protein [486]. For the same total protein intake a diet consisting mainly of cereal foods will therefore be much lower in lysine content than a diet based on milk and meat. Indeed, the lysine intake could easily be inadequate if using predominantly cereal foods to provide the safe level of protein intake and needs to be considered when planning the diet. Recommendations for natural and total protein intake (natural protein and amino acid supplement) in g/kg/day are given in the 2007 guideline [480] but not in the revised 2011 guideline [481] because the natural protein intake can be very variable depending on types of food consumed to provide lysine. A combination of cereal, vegetable and milk based foods is best to ensure an adequate lysine intake. If the diet is predominantly cereal based a higher protein intake than the safe level of protein intake will be necessary to provide sufficient lysine. Even if the diet is based on safe level of protein intake lysine free, low tryptophan amino acid supplements are given according to, or at least in similar amounts to, the guideline recommendations. Biochemical and haematological nutritional status is better in patients on lysine free, low tryptophan supplements with added vitamins and minerals [484].

Infants

On receipt of a positive newborn screening result, treatment (diet and carnitine) should be commenced promptly even before confirmation of diagnosis by enzyme and/or mutation analysis. Infants can be breast and/or bottle fed. The guideline recommends lysine intake is reduced to 100 mg/kg/day and 1.3–0.8 g protein/kg/day be provided from a lysine free amino acid supplement for age 0–6 months (Table 17.63). Lysine intake from either breast feeds or infant formula is restricted by giving supplementary lysine free, low tryptophan infant formula, e.g. GA1 Anamix Infant formula.

Breast fed infant

Breast milk provides around 68 mg lysine/g of protein or 89 mg lysine/100 mL [277]. Demand breast feeding of 150–200 mL/kg/day would provide 133–178 mg/kg/day of lysine. To limit lysine intake from breast milk the lysine free, low tryptophan infant formula is given before breast feeds. Providing 1 g/kg/day of protein equivalent from the formula will limit breast milk intake to around the desired intake of 100 mg lysine/kg/day. The total volume of infant formula is divided and distributed evenly before five to six breast feeds.

Example of a breast feeding regimen for an infant, weight 4 kg, age 3 weeks

Aim: limit lysine to 100 mg/kg/day (400 mg lysine) from natural protein and provide 1.3–0.8 g protein equivalent/kg/day from lysine free, low tryptophan infant formula
Total fluids = 170 mL/kg = 680 mL/day
Aim: 4 g protein equivalent = 1 g/kg/day
    = 200 mL GA1 Anamix Infant
Give: 40 mL × 5, before five breast feeds; additional breast feeds can be given on demand
Estimated intake of breast milk = 480 mL
    (680 mL – 200 mL)
Provides 427 mg lysine = 107 mg lysine/kg/day

Bottle feeding infant

Normal infant formula provides around 88 mg lysine/g of protein or 114 mg lysine/100 mL. Demand feeding of infant formula at 150–200 mL/kg would provide 171–228 mg/kg/day of lysine. The volume of infant formula is limited to restrict lysine to around 100 mg/kg/day (which equates to 1.1 g protein/kg) and divided between six to eight feeds, depending on feeding frequency. Lysine free, low tryptophan formula, e.g. GA1 Anamix Infant, is then fed to appetite after the normal infant formula, aiming to provide 1.3–0.8 g/kg/day of protein equivalent, but more can be given.

Example of a bottle feeding regimen for an infant, weight 5 kg, age 2 months

Aim: limit lysine to 100 mg/kg/day (500 mg lysine) from natural protein and provide 1.3–0.8 g protein equivalent/kg/day from lysine free, low tryptophan infant formula
Total fluids = 160 mL/kg = 800 mL/day
Normal infant formula of 440 mL = 501 mg lysine
    = 100 mg/kg/day
GA1 Anamix Infant (800 mL – 440 mL) = 360 mL
    = 7.2 g protein equivalent = 1.4 g/kg
Feeds = 100 mL × 3 hourly × 8 feeds
First feed 55 mL normal infant formula followed by second feed 45 mL GA1 Anamix Infant to appetite (more is given if the infant is hungry)

A nutritional analysis for the daily feed plan is given in Table 17.64.

Table 17.64 Nutritional analysis of daily feed plan for infant with glutaric aciduria type 1.

Age 2 months, weight 5 kg

	Energy		Protein	Protein equivalent	Lysine	Tryptophan	Fluid
	kcal	kJ	g	g	mg/day	mg/day	mL/kg
440 mL Cow & Gate First (60 g powder)	290	1210	5.7	–	501	91	88
360 mL GA1 Anamix Infant (54 g powder)	248	1033		7.2	–	36	72
Totals	538	2243	5.7	7.2	501	127	
Intake/kg/day	107	448	1.1	1.4	100	25	160
Aim/kg/day	100–95*	420–400		1.3 g/kg/day†	100†	20‡ 29§	150–170

*[389].
†[481].
‡[480].
§[277].

Weaning

Only the practical aspects of a low protein diet based on a safe level of protein intake (Table 17.54) will be described. Details for implementing a low lysine diet using lysine exchanges are available in Kölker *et al.*'s paper ([481], Supplementary Table 8) or a resource booklet (in German only) can be downloaded from http://www.awmf.org/uploads/tx_szleitlinien/027-018p_S3_Glutarazidurie_Typ_I_2011-05.pdf.

Weaning is started at the usual time of around 6 months (26 weeks) of age and proceeds in a similar method to low protein and amino acid diets, described in more detail on p. 416. Normal weaning practices are followed: solids are introduced at one meal then two and three times per day and the infant progresses from smooth purées to lumpier foods and finger foods during the first year. An overview of weaning stages:

- Introduce free weaning foods, e.g. fruits, vegetables, low protein manufactured foods (Tables 17.28 and 17.57).
- Start second stage lysine free, low tryptophan amino acid supplement, e.g. GA Gel. Practical aspects of introducing more concentrated amino acid supplements are given on p. 421. Less supplement is given compared with the amino acids disorders. One teaspoon of GA Gel is introduced from around 6 months at one

meal. The quantity is then gradually increased and given at two then three meals before solids. As this is increased, less GA1 Anamix is given but ensuring adequate energy, vitamins and minerals are provided by the diet and lysine free, low tryptophan supplement. GA1 Anamix infant feeds may continue to be given on waking and before bed until around 1 year of age. The guideline recommends 1.0–0.8 g protein equivalent/kg/day from the supplement for infants aged 7–12 months (Table 17.63).

For a 10 kg child, aged 1 year, one sachet of GA Gel provides 10 g protein equivalent = 1 g/kg and 67 mg tryptophan (= 6.7 mg/kg/day) which does not provide the guideline amount of 17 mg/kg/day [480] but does provide the more recent recommendation of 6.4 mg/kg/day [277]. The diet will provide more tryptophan.

- Introduce 1 g protein exchanges to provide at least the safe level of protein intake for age from a variety of foods (Table 17.54). More protein will be needed to ensure adequate lysine intake if the diet is mainly cereal based, rather than from a combination of different foods. Protein from infant formula or breast milk is replaced by food, gradually introducing 1 g exchanges of natural protein at a time using purée potato, lentils, yoghurt, vegetables or commercial weaning foods (dried or wet varieties in jars, pouches, packets) such as ordinary rusks, baby cereals or vegetable based savoury foods or milk based desserts.

• Introduce other manufactured low protein foods as necessary, e.g. low protein rusk or cereal, to provide extra energy and variety (Table 17.28).

Some vitamins and minerals will be provided by the lysine free, low tryptophan supplement (if enriched with vitamins and minerals). It is important to assess intake and if the child eats only a limited range of protein foods, supplement the diet as necessary.

Children

During early childhood the diet is provided by a combination of a low protein diet based around the safe level of protein intake and the lysine free, low tryptophan supplement, providing around 0.8 g/kg/day of protein equivalent (Table 17.63). The supplement alone should provide the tryptophan requirement for 1–2 year olds of 6.4 mg/kg/day [480]. As striatal damage occurs only during a finite period of brain development, the low lysine diet can be relaxed beyond 6 years of age [481]. The guideline recommends avoidance of an excessive intake of natural protein and to use natural protein with a low lysine content according to safe levels of protein intake. No specific guidance is given on continued use of amino acid supplements. Current practice varies, with some centres continuing the supplement whilst others change to a more relaxed controlled protein intake without using amino acid supplements.

Dietary management of symptomatic patients

Dietary treatment in symptomatic patients is reported to be of no or limited neurological benefit [470, 487, 488]. It is known that protein restriction cannot reverse neurological damage which has already occurred and dietary protein restriction alone is not sufficient to prevent brain injury [487–489]. The rationale for a restricted lysine or protein diet in symptomatic patients is unclear but for some it may be helpful in prevention of progressive neurological deterioration [471, 489] and is used in some centres.

Feeding problems

Feeding problems are common in the group of patients with neurological disease and include chewing and swallowing difficulties due to dyskinesia and GOR and vomiting due to truncal hypotonia. The extent of these feeding problems is related to the severity of the neurological disease, with acute onset being much worse than insidious onset. Dietary advice needs to be tailored to the individual child's needs: use of thickened fluids, energy dense foods of the correct consistency and energy supplements may be required to achieve an adequate nutrient and fluid intake. Tube feeding is often essential to maintain an adequate energy intake and to achieve satisfactory growth. Nissen fundoplication (and insertion of gastrostomy) may be necessary in some patients for treatment of GOR and vomiting. Assessing energy requirements in this group of patients can be difficult; the worst patients cannot walk so should need less energy, but energy expenditure is reported to often be increased due to high muscle tone and dystonic movements and to disturbances in temperature control [471], thus emphasising the need for adjusting the diet to the requirements of the individual. Additional fluids may be required in patients who have disturbances in temperature control with excessive sweating. An example of a low protein/lysine tube feed for a symptomatic patient is given in Table 17.65.

Medical management – pharmacotherapy

In addition to diet, carnitine supplementation (100 mg/kg/day) is given to facilitate production of non toxic glutarylcarnitine from glutaryl-CoA and to avoid secondary carnitine deficiency as a consequence of its increased formation. A higher dose of carnitine may be needed if free carnitine levels are low. During illness the dose of carnitine is doubled to 200 mg/kg/day. Management of the movement disorder is complex and beyond the scope of this publication; recommendations are made in the guideline [480, 481].

Nutritional and biochemical monitoring

The nutritional monitoring of low protein diets has been discussed on p. 463. Severe protein and

Table 17.65 Low protein/lysine gastrostomy feed for a symptomatic girl with glutaric aciduria type 1.

Age 4 years, weight 13 kg

	Energy		Protein g	Protein equivalent g	Lysine mg/day	Tryptophan mg/day	CHO g	Fat g	Sodium mmol	Potassium mmol	Fluid mL
	kcal	kJ									
450 mL Paediasure Fibre	454	1899	12.6	–	945	180	50.4	22.4	12	12.7	450
55 g XLYS LOW TRY Maxamaid	170	721	–	13.7	–	88	28	<0.5	13.8	11.8	
80 mL Calogen	360	1480	–	–	–	–	–	40	0.3	tr	
130 g Maxijul	494	2099	–	–	–	–	124	–	tr	tr	
Add water to 1200 mL											1200
Totals	1478	6199					202.4	62.4	26.1	24.5	1200
per 100 mL	123	517					16.9	5.2			
Intake/kg/day			1.0	1.0	73						
Aim/kg/day	1460*	6120*	0.86†	0.8‡	60–50‡	13‡			30*	28*	1200

Additional electrolytes may be necessary. Adequate vitamins and minerals are provided from the combination of Paediasure Fibre and XLYS LOW TRY Maxamaid. A fibre containing feed is used to help maintain normal bowel function.

*[389].
†[277].
‡[481].

mineral deficiencies have been reported in GA1 patients on low protein diets [394, 490]. Biochemical monitoring of maintenance treatment is difficult as there is no reliable biochemical marker. Urine GA, 3-OH-GA and plasma glutarylcarnitine do not correlate with outcome [480]. The guideline gives recommendations for routine biochemical monitoring and frequency (from 1 to 6 monthly in children <6 years of age): quantitative plasma amino acids (in particular lysine and tryptophan) to assess nutritional status; carnitine to check depletion and adherence; full blood count; liver function tests; albumin and bone chemistry. The aim is to maintain plasma lysine in the normal reference range [480], although in practice lysine can be in the lower normal reference range [491]. It is the author's practice to maintain plasma lysine in the lower normal reference range. If plasma lysine is lower than this the diet is reviewed as an increase in natural protein or change in type of food, i.e. more milk based foods if the diet is high in cereal content, may be necessary. Growth needs to be regularly monitored particularly in dystonic patients as weight gain can be significantly reduced [491].

Dietary management of illness

Prompt and aggressive treatment of intercurrent illness by implementation of a high energy ER is critical to prevent neurological damage in pre symptomatic patients and further injury in symptomatic patients [477, 481]. Delayed treatment can have serious consequences with irreversible striatal damage and a complex movement disorder. Strategies to help prevent this need to be in place and include written treatment protocols for home and local hospital, adequate education and training of parents/carers [481]. With increasing age, and in particular from 6 years of age, the risk of acute neurological insult appears to be reduced; however, use of an ER remains an important part of management.

The main aim of the ER is to reduce production and accumulation of neurotoxic GA and 3-OH-GA by

- provision of a high energy intake, at least normal requirements for age to prevent catabolism; 120% of daily energy requirement is recommended by some centres [481]

- omitting or temporarily reducing (by 50%) natural protein intake
- provision of lysine free, low tryptophan amino acids
- increased carnitine supplementation to 200 mg/kg/day (can also be given IV)

The general principles of implementation, administration of the ER and reintroduction of usual diet are the same as the standard ER. It is particularly important to implement the ER for any episode of vomiting, diarrhoea (even if no fever) or high temperature. For very minor illnesses, a change to ER may not always be necessary and continuation of the usual diet is appropriate. It is essential this provides the normal energy intake (extra energy supplements may be needed) and the usual amount of lysine free, low tryptophan amino acids.

Composition of the ER:

- natural protein: stop temporarily for 24 hours to a maximum of 48 hours.
- lysine free, low tryptophan amino acids: give 1 g/kg/day protein equivalent in children aged <6 years. Pure lysine free, low tryptophan amino acids such as GA·*five* are suitable for all age groups and can be easily added directly to glucose polymer. XLYS TRY Glutaridon could also be used, but does not contain tryptophan. A lysine free, low tryptophan infant formula is used for infants aged 0–1 year. In children aged ≥6 years, there is no consensus about the use of lysine free, low tryptophan amino acids, but it may be advantageous to continue to give if this helps prevent catabolism and limits lysine uptake across the BBB.

- glucose polymer: add to the amino acids to provide a CHO concentration ranging from 10% to 25%, as per standard emergency feeds for age (p. 502).
- fat: is a useful energy source in emergency feeds and can be added but it may not be tolerated during gastrointestinal illness.
- fluid volume: is the same as for standard ER (p. 502).

A calculated example of an ER for a 9-month-old infant who is unwell is given in Table 17.66.

The ER can be implemented at home but patients need to be reassessed by professionals several times per day. Nasogastric feeding can help ensure the full volume of ER is given but parents must be competent in doing this [492]. If the child does not tolerate the ER it is crucial they are admitted to hospital, without delay, for IV therapy of 10% dextrose/0.45% saline and carnitine. The BIMDG provide emergency protocols for IV management and can be accessed at www.bimdg.org. A low volume, continuous tube feed of pure lysine free, tryptophan low/free amino acids (e.g. XLYS TRY Glutaridon, GA·*five*) to provide 1 g protein

Table 17.66 Emergency regimen feed for an unwell infant with glutaric aciduria type 1.

Age 9 months, weight 8 kg, unwell with temperature of 38°C, mild diarrhoea, no vomiting

Aim: provide 1 g protein equivalent/kg/day from lysine free, low tryptophan amino acids and normal energy intake for age

| | Energy | | Protein | Protein equivalent | Lysine | CHO | Fat | Sodium | Potassium |
	kcal	kJ	g	g	mg/day	g	g	mmol	mmol
GA1 Anamix Infant 400 mL	276	1148	–	8	nil	29.6	14	4.8	7.6
Maxijul 100 g	380	1615	–	–	–	95	–	tr	tr
Total volume 1200 mL	656	2763		8		124			
per 100 mL	55	230		0.7		10.4	1.2	0.4	0.6
Intake per kg/day	82	345		1.0					
Aim per kg/day	95*	399*	–	1.0[†]					
Administration	Feed: 100 mL every 2 hours day and night or 50 mL/hour as continuous tube feeds								

Additional glucose polymer can be added up to 12–15 g CHO/100 mL to increase the energy intake provided it does not exacerbate the diarrhoea.
*[389].
[†][481].

equivalent/kg/day can be given along with IV fluids, as tolerated. A concentration of 5 up to 8 g amino acids/100 mL, as necessary, can be given. It may also be possible to add glucose polymer to 10% CHO or higher. In the UK there are no PN solutions designed specifically for GA1. Once the child begins to improve, the usual natural protein intake and diet/feed is reintroduced as for standard ER (p. 504), ensuring an adequate energy intake is given at all times. The GA1 guidelines also provide comprehensive emergency treatment guidelines and detailed strategies to prevent delayed implementation of the ER [481].

Urea cycle disorders

The urea cycle (UC) has two main functions:

- converts toxic ammonia, formed from waste nitrogen compounds, via a series of biochemical steps to form non toxic urea for excretion by the kidney. Waste nitrogen is generated from dietary amino acids and obligatory endogenous protein catabolism.
- the biosynthesis pathway for arginine, which is the precursor for the synthesis of several different important metabolites including nitric oxide (NO), creatine and glutamate.

Normal function of the UC depends on a series of six consecutive enzymatic reactions and inborn errors at each step have been identified (Fig. 17.18): N-acetylglutamate synthetase deficiency (NAGS), carbamyl phosphate synthetase 1 deficiency (CPS1), ornithine transcarbamoylase deficiency (OTC), argininosuccinate synthetase deficiency (ASS) or citrullinaemia, argininosuccinate lyase deficiency (ASL) or argininsuccinic aciduria (ASA) and arginase deficiency. The ASS and ASL enzymes also form part of the overlapping nitric oxide production pathway. Deficiencies of any one of these enzymes reduces flux through the UC blocking normal ureagenesis; consequently waste nitrogen accumulates as ammonia in blood and brain, which is neurotoxic and may cause a severe encephalopathy. Secondary metabolic changes also contribute to central nervous system (CNS) toxicity, such as increased glutamine and deficiency of arginine. The pathology is complex and an overview of current understanding is given by Braissant [493]. Arginine production is reduced except in arginase deficiency where it accumulates. Arginase deficiency is distinct from the other disorders and is discussed separately.

Biochemically, plasma ammonia is raised and can be very high, e.g. in acute neonatal onset patients it can be >1000 µmol/L (normal <40 µmol/L). Also plasma amino acids are deranged, glutamine and alanine accumulate and arginine is low. Additionally, in citrullinaemia citrulline accumulates, and in ASA, argininosuccinic acid accumulates. These are excreted in urine and provide an alternative pathway for nitrogen excretion. These disorders are inherited as autosomal recessive traits apart from OTC deficiency, which is X-linked and the most common of these disorders. There is a wide phenotypic spectrum within each disorder, with some ability to predict the course based on some mutations [494].

There are also disorders of transport proteins of urea cycle intermediates: the aspartate glutamate carrier, known as citrin deficiency (p. 498) and the mitochondrial ornithine transporter, known as hyperornithinaemia, hyperammonaemia, homocitrullinaemia (HHH) syndrome (p. 496). These are discussed separately.

Expanded newborn screening for most urea cycle disorders (UCD) is problematic, suitable screening markers and their specificity being key issues. Worldwide, screening is limited, although ASS, ASL and arginase 1 deficiencies are screened for in some countries [494].

Classification and presentation
These disorders can present at any age from the neonatal period, throughout childhood and in adulthood. Signs and symptoms can be neurological (most frequent) hepatic-gastrointestinal and psychiatric. The clinical presentation may be acute, chronic or, rarely, acute intermittent. Patients with the most severe UCD present acutely with

Legend

	Enzyme	Name of disorder
1.	carbamoyl phosphate synthetase 1	CPS 1 deficiency
2.	ornithine transcarbamoylase	OTC deficiency
3.	argininosuccinate synthetase	ASS deficiency or citrullinaemia type 1
4.	argininosuccinate lyase	ASL deficiency or argininosuccinic aciduria (ASA)
5.	arginase	Arginase deficiency or hyperargininaemia
6.	*N*-acetyl glutamate synthetase (NAGS)	NAGS deficiency
	Transporters	
7.	Mitochondrial aspartate-glutamate carrier (AGC2)	Citrin deficiency
8.	Mitochondrial ornithine transporter (ORT1)	HHH syndrome

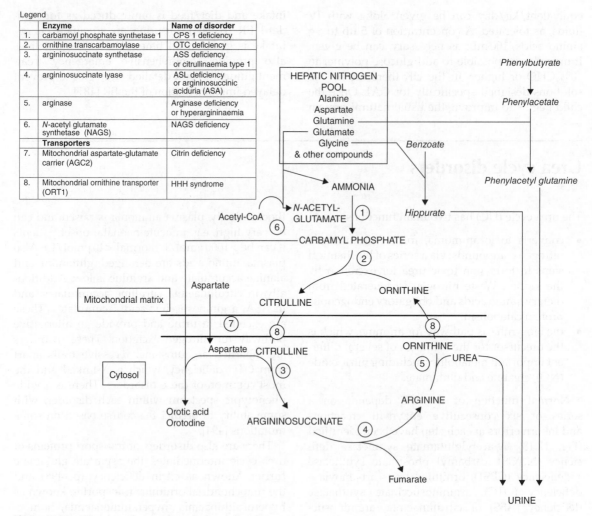

Figure 17.18   Disorders of urea cyle and related disorders.

hyperammonaemia in the neonatal period, most commonly within the first 7 days [495], or later at any age (which may be precipitated by a catabolic event such as an intercurrent infection) and may cause a severe neurological handicap or even death. Loss of appetite, poor feeding, lethargy and vomiting are common in all ages. In the newborn there is often respiratory distress with signs of hyperpnoea, altered level of consciousness and seizures, acute encephalopathy and collapse [496]. A respiratory alkalosis is initially present in about 50% of acute onset patients [497]. In later onset confusion, headache, disorientation, abnormal behaviour, ataxia, focal neurological signs or coma can occur and in some there is also delayed

physical growth and developmental delay [496]. A more detailed review of clinical symptoms and presentation is described elsewhere [494]. Some of these children may have had minor episodes before they present and self-select a low protein diet, due to protein aversion. Heterozygote OTC deficient females can present with postpartum psychosis.

A 'honeymoon period' (a lengthy period between the first episode of hyperammonaemia and recurrence) is reported to occur following an acute neonatal presentation; however, this differs between disorders. Patients with ASA appear to be at lower risk of recurrence during the first year [495].

Outcome and complications

High mortality and morbidity are associated with UCD [495, 497, 498]. The outlook for infants is very poor if the ammonia level is >1000 μmol/L and a decision not to treat may be made [494]. The neurodevelopmental outcome is related primarily to the duration and severity of hyperammonaemia and this can range from mild to profound cognitive deficits [495, 497–499]. In late presenting patients many have some degree of learning and neurological disability [497–500]. Patients with ASL deficiency have poorest cognitive outcome and this supports the idea that toxins other than ammonia may affect this, such as argininosuccinate [495, 501]. Some patients with ASA also develop hepatic complications [501], systemic hypertension [502], GI problems [503] and renal tubulopathy [503, 504]. Possible mechanisms of toxicity include increased concentrations of argininosuccinate or disturbed nitric oxide synthesis [505]. Even patients diagnosed with ASA on newborn screening may still not do well [506, 507].

Liver transplant is successful in preventing further episodes of metabolic decompensation in UCD but cannot reverse any neurological damage. Low protein diet and UCD medicines are not required post transplant [508]. Hepatocyte and stem cell transplants are currently under trial as alternative treatment options.

Treatment guidelines

European treatment guidelines were published in 2012 [494]. The full version of these can be accessed at www.awmf.org. They provide medical and dietetic guidelines on acute and chronic management of UCD patients. The US Urea Cycle Disorders Consortium has also produced guidelines, accessed at www.rarediseasenetwork.epi.usf.edu. An earlier US consensus statement from a conference for the management of patients with UCD was published in 2001 [509].

The aim of treatment of UCD is to reduce waste nitrogen production and prevent hyperammonaemia and consequent neurological sequelae by

- restriction of dietary protein intake, to decrease the nitrogen load on the urea cycle

- provision of an adequate energy intake to prevent catabolism, to reduce production of nitrogen from catabolism
- giving medicines which utilise alternative pathways to the urea cycle for excretion of waste nitrogen
- giving arginine supplements to increase flux through the urea cycle and as substrate for production of arginine metabolites

Medical management – pharmacotherapy

Treatment of UCD with sodium benzoate and sodium phenylbutyrate (phenylacetate) was first described in the early 1980s [510]. Both medicines conjugate with specific amino acids destined for ammonia formation and have the net effect of reducing the nitrogen load to the UC (Fig. 17.18). Phenylbutyrate is metabolised *in vivo* to form phenylacetate which is conjugated with glutamine in liver and kidney to form phenylacetylglutamine. If the reaction were complete then 2 moles of nitrogen would be excreted for each mole of phenylbutyrate given. However, more recent studies indicate only 1 mole is excreted [511, 512]. Sodium benzoate is conjugated with glycine in liver and kidney to form hippurate so that 1 mole of nitrogen is excreted for each mole of sodium benzoate given. These medicines are termed alternative pathway medicines or nitrogen scavengers because of their mode of action. Both can be administered orally or IV and are usually prescribed in doses of up to 250 mg/kg body weight/day, divided between three or four doses to increase effectiveness. Higher doses may be used temporarily during episodes of acute hyperammonaemia. Practices differ with choice of nitrogen scavenger (one or both may be given) and doses vary; this to some extent depends on the severity of the disorder and the patient's tolerance. Doses are individually tailored to optimise management. Both medicines are unpleasant tasting and can cause mucositis and gastritis so it is important they are taken with meals and plenty of fluids to help prevent this. Standard doses provide a significant sodium load, which can be a problem when managing newly diagnosed infants. Some patients have a gastrostomy tube specifically to administer these medicines. Sodium benzoate and phenylbutyrate are available in liquid, granule or tablet format and as an IV preparation.

In the USA, glycerol phenylbutyrate is being investigated as an alternative medicine for UCD. Compared with sodium phenylbutyrate it contains no sodium, is more palatable and similar ammonia control can be achieved [513]. A new sodium phenylbutyrate formulation has also been developed – a 'taste masked granule' – but this is not yet licensed for UCD [514].

Arginine

Arginine becomes an essential or semi-essential amino acid in UCD because its synthesis is greatly reduced [515]. In OTC and CPS deficiencies arginine supplements of 100–200 mg/kg body weight/day are given to replace that which would normally be formed. The aim is to increase the flux through the urea cycle and urea synthesis and to maintain a normal plasma arginine concentration (normal reference range 40–120 μmol/L). Alternatively in OTC, in order to meet the arginine requirements, supplements of citrulline can be given as it is rapidly converted to arginine via the intact part of the urea cycle. Also, citrulline contains one less nitrogen atom than arginine, thereby reducing waste nitrogen production, but it is more expensive than arginine.

In citrullinaemia and ASA deficiency, arginine up to 100–300 mg/kg/day [494] is given to replenish ornithine supply although, traditionally, higher doses have been given. The carbon skeleton of ornithine is needed for the formation of citrulline and argininosuccinic acid which accumulate and are excreted in citrullinaemia and ASA respectively and provide another method for nitrogen removal. Argininosuccinic acid is more effective than citrulline as it carries two waste nitrogen atoms and has a higher renal clearance. Arginine, however, increases plasma concentrations of both citrulline and argininosuccinic acid, the full consequence of which is unknown; concerns have been expressed that high concentrations of argininosuccinic acid in ASA deficiency may have adverse effects on brain and be hepatotoxic [516,517]. A lower dose of arginine, combined with nitrogen scavengers, may reduce production of ASA. In a 1 week cross-over study in ASA patients there was an improvement in liver function tests on low dose arginine plus nitrogen scavengers compared with high dose arginine [518]. Arginine can be administered orally or IV. It is available in liquid, powder or tablet form for oral use. It is given as a divided dose and usually in conjunction with the other medicines.

N-carbamyl-ʟ-glutamate (or carbamylglutamate or carglumic acid)

N-acetylglutamate is the obligatory allosteric activator of CPS1 (first step of the UC). It is formed from glutamate and acetyl-CoA, via NAGS. Defects of this enzyme affect production of N-acetylglutamate. Patients with NAGS deficiency are treated with carbamylglutamate which is an orally active form of N-acetylglutamate. It is sometimes also given during acute neonatal hyperammonaemia as an emergency drug.

Dietary management

Low protein diet

The major route for excretion of waste nitrogen is urea. Its production and excretion are linearly related to increasing protein intake [519]. In UCD the load on the urea cycle can therefore be reduced by limiting protein intake. A low protein diet will reduce the accumulation of waste nitrogen as ammonia, glutamine and alanine. A reduction of 0.1 g/kg/day of protein reduces the nitrogen load on the urea cycle by 16 mg/kg/day [520]. Even on the minimum protein intake for normal growth and maintenance there is always some flux through the urea cycle, as tissue protein is constantly being synthesised and broken down [277]. For those with severe defects the dietary protein intake is reduced to around the safe level of protein intake (Table 17.54) but this needs to be titrated against biochemical parameters (ammonia, glutamine and essential amino acids, see p. 493) [494]. Patients with milder defects will tolerate a higher protein intake.

Protein requirements per kilogram bodyweight are highest during early infancy (at 1 month, 1.77 g/kg) and decrease with age to 0.8 g/kg/day in late adolescence. Neonates may tolerate and need higher protein intakes of 2–2.5 g/kg/day to achieve growth (author's experience). A recent study of 464 UCD patients across central Europe and the UK (nine countries, 41 centres) highlighted a number of differences in dietary treatment practices [521]. Some countries prescribe protein intakes based on safe level of protein intakes (UK and Belgium); others determine protein prescription by biochemical indices (glutamine and ammonia). Consequently a wide variance in prescribed protein intakes was observed across different age groups, particularly in infants and young children. In the UK a higher total protein intake tended to be given to infants.

The practical management of a low protein diet for infants and children is described on p. 456.

Essential amino acid and branch chain amino acid supplements

For some children essential amino acid (EAA) supplements are routinely incorporated as part of the total protein intake. This is considered beneficial because, theoretically, by limiting the intake of non essential amino acids, waste nitrogen is utilised to synthesise these and hence nitrogen destined for excretion as urea will be reduced. This, however, has never been proven in clinical studies. The use and doses of EAA supplements varies widely between countries and centres within countries, providing a range of 0%–90% of total protein intake [521]. In the UK, an EAA supplement is prescribed primarily on a clinical need basis (e.g. low plasma EAA, inadequate natural protein intake and metabolic instability) rather than routinely from diagnosis and typically provides between 20% and 30% of total protein intake [384]. This contrasts with US recommendations of use from diagnosis and to give a higher dose of 25%–50% of total protein as EAA in severe defects [509] and in infancy to give 50% of protein as EAA; as growth rate slows the percentage is decreased [522]. The rationale for use during infancy is not completely clear as protein requirements per kilogram per day are highest and nitrogen retention is at a maximum, but this could be related to using nitrogen scavengers. There are no studies which compare the two methods of management. The European UCD guidelines suggests EAA supplements provide 20%–30% of total protein intake, to be given when natural protein tolerance is too low to achieve normal growth and metabolic stability [494]. EAA supplements may be used:

- if the blood biochemistry cannot be corrected by altering the medicines because the child is either on maximum doses of medicines or refusing to take more and the protein intake is around the safe intake and cannot be reduced further
- to improve the biological value of a low protein diet which may be lacking in one or more EAA, which may occur if the protein is provided from a limited range of LBV protein foods
- temporarily during the stabilisation period in newly diagnosed patients; some centres may continue their use long term
- if natural protein intake is inadequate
- if metabolic control is poor or there are repeated episodes of metabolic decompensation

EAA are generally given as a divided dose between feeds or two or three meals. There are three EAA products available in the UK and they differ in composition and age suitability (Table 17.67). The EAA compositions of EAA mix and Dialamine are the same, but Dialamine is lower in total g EAA/100 g and contains CHO and flavouring to improve palatibilty. It is important to be aware that all EAA provide a source of nitrogen (8.5%–13.7%) but this is lower than the nitrogen content of food which ranges from 13.4% to 19.1% depending upon its amino acid composition [384]. Similar products are available outside the UK (www.abbottnutrition.com, www.meadjohnson.com, www.milupametabolics.com).

Scaglia *et al*. have reported a selective reduction in plasma branched chain amino acids (BCAA) in response to phenylbutyrate therapy, despite an adequate protein intake, and supplementation with BCAA was recommended [523, 524]. A possible mechanism is the ability of phenylbutyrate to cause an enhanced flux through the branched chain α-keto acid dehydrogenase complex activity, which catalyses the reversible oxidative decarboxylation of the BCAA [525]. The effects of lowered BCAA are unknown, but it may cause patients to be less stable [526]. Recent work has shown there is no change in whole body proteolysis or net protein, despite low plasma BCAA [526]. BCAA supplements can be given as single amino acid supplements or a complete supplement (Table 17.67). The use of BCAA supplements in

Table 17.67   Essential amino acid products used in urea cycle disorders.

Product (manufacturer)	Amino acids (g/100 g)	Protein equivalent (g/100 g)	Energy (kcal (MJ) 100 g)	CHO (g/100 g)	Fat (g/100 g)	Vitamins and minerals	Comments
Dialamine* (Nutricia)	30	25	360 (1.5)	65[†]	nil	[‡]	Orange flavoured Suitable from 6 months Can be added to a feed, drink or given as a paste
Essential Amino Acid Mix* (Nutricia)	94.5	79	316 (1.3)	nil	nil	nil	Suitable for infants under 6 months
EAA supplement[§] (Vitaflo)	48	40	288 (1.2)[¶]	31.8	0.1	**	Tropical flavour Suitable from age 3 years 12.5 g sachet. Given as a drink
BCAA supplement Solvil[††] (Vitaflo)	99.4	82.8	337 (1.4)	0	0.6	nil	5 g sachet. Give as a drink or into food

EAA, essential amino acids; BCAA, branched chain amino acids.
*A powdered mixture of essential amino acids (including cystine and histidine). Essential Amino Acid Mix has the same composition as Dialamine without the CHO component.
[†]Contains a mixture of glucose polymer and sugar.
[‡]Contains vitamin C and trace amounts of sodium, potassium, chloride, calcium, phosphorus and magnesium.
[§]A powder mixture of essential amino acids.
[¶] Contains glucose polymer, sugar and sweeteners.
**Contains a comprehensive range of vitamins, minerals and trace elements.
[††]Contains per sachet: L-leucine 2.5 g, L-isoleucine 1.24 g, L-valine 1.24 g.

the UK and Europe appears to be very limited and when given amounts are highly variable [521]. There are no controlled studies related to their use or comparing them with EAA (which also contain BCAA but in lower concentrations g/100 g).

Feeding behaviour and tube feeding

Protein aversion (before and after diagnosis), poor appetite, food refusal and poor variety of foods eaten, frequent vomiting and abnormal eating behaviour are features of some children with UCD [384, 399, 527]. Some children may have an inadequate oral energy and nutrient intake due to mechanical feeding problems and unsafe swallow associated with neurological handicap or severe developmental delay caused by hyperammonaemia or poor appetite. If a child is unable to take sufficient orally, NG or gastrostomy feeding is essential to prevent hyperammonaemia and metabolic decompensation. In the European study

of feeding practices [521] (which included UK data) <20% received enteral feeds and in the UK study, 25% [384]. Tube feeding may also be used specifically for administration of EAA and/or medicines, although the need for this appears to be limited [521]. The provision of a low protein tube feed has been described on p. 467.

Energy intake

A normal energy intake for age is provided to ensure normal growth and to prevent endogenous protein catabolism causing metabolic decompensation. Lower energy intakes will be necessary in children with physical handicaps. Regular feeding and avoidance of prolonged fasts is recommended to help maintain good biochemical control as plasma glutamine and ammonia concentrations will increase with fasting and endogenous protein catabolism. Oral energy supplements are not used extensively in UCD patients, <20% of patients [384, 521].

Nutritional and biochemical monitoring

Clinical and biochemical monitoring are essential to assess metabolic stability and to guide treatment, protein intake and medicine doses, which increase with age during childhood. Nutritional monitoring of a low protein diet has been described (p. 463). The frequency of monitoring depends on the child's overall metabolic stability in relation to treatment and compliance. Younger and more severe patients will need more frequent monitoring, 3–4 monthly being typical for most patients who are stable. Plasma ammonia and quantitative amino acids, including glutamine and arginine, argininosuccinic acid (in ASA) and citrulline (in citrullinaemia) are measured. A 24 hour profile of plasma ammonia and glutamine can be helpful in patients who are difficult to manage. Timing of the blood sample is also important as there is variation in relation to meals and medicines. Ideally, samples should be obtained at the same time and at trough levels 3.5–4 hours post a meal (i.e. pre prandial). This will avoid high concentrations of amino acids (seen following consumption of EAA supplements at mealtimes) and low concentrations

being missed [528]. However, it is not always possible to collect samples under optimal conditions so results need to be interpreted in the light of the conditions. Plasma ammonia may be falsely elevated due to poor or difficult blood sample collection. The overall aim is to maintain plasma ammonia, glutamine (normal range or at least below 1000 µmol/L), arginine and amino acids, particularly BCAA, within normal reference ranges to achieve normal growth and the best possible development [494, 528] (Table 17.68). It is important to be aware that plasma glutamine does not directly influence brain glutamine concentration, as this is synthesised mainly in the brain. It is not known if this is altered if plasma glutamine concentrations are high [528].

Changes to dietary protein, EAA intakes, arginine and medicines (sodium benzoate and phenylbutyrate, and arginine in ASA and citrullinaemia) are based on the results of these investigations and alterations will vary depending on the disorder (Table 17.68). Blood results need to be interpreted carefully (particularly if they are unsatisfactory) because they are influenced by a number of different factors which need to

Table 17.68 Guide to management decisions for urea cycle disorders (excluding arginase deficiency).

All influencing factors should be considered before making changes to diet or medicines.

Ammonia µmol/L, normal reference range <40	Glutamine µmol/L, normal reference range 400–800	Quantitative plasma amino acids	Suggested action
>80–100	>1000	Low EAA/BCAA	Increase medicines in OTC and CPS* Increase medicines in ASA and citrullinaemia[†] Increase natural protein or essential amino acids
>80–100	>1000	Normal	Increase medicines in OTC and CPS* Increase medicines in ASA and citrullinaemia[†] No change to diet
<80	<1000	Low EAA/BCAA	No change to medicines Increase natural protein
<80	<1000	Normal	No change to medicines or diet

EAA, essential amino acids; BCAA, branched chain amino acids.
*OTC and CPS – sodium benzoate and/or phenylbutyrate.
[†]ASA and citrullinaemia – arginine, sodium benzoate or phenylbutyrate. If plasma arginine is high >200 µmol/L (normal reference range 40–120 µmol/L) arginine dose is not increased; sodium benzoate and/or phenylbutyrate would be increased instead. If plasma citrulline or argininosuccinic acid is too high, arginine is not increased; sodium benzoate and/or phenylbutyrate would be increased instead.

be considered before implementing any change to diet or medicines: growth, dietary intake, type and doses (including timings and frequency) of medicines, compliance with diet and medicines, age (puberty can be a difficult time), use of EAA, use of ER, timing of blood sample in relation to foods/EAA intake. Looking for patterns in results over time can be helpful.

High concentrations of glutamine and ammonia in plasma may be caused by

- inadequate medicines, too high or too low a protein intake (causing catabolism); both factors may be a compliance issue. It is also important to ensure that medicines are given as divided doses over the 24 hour day.
- periods of chronic catabolism due to either an inadequate energy and protein intake due to poor appetite or repeated use of ER, so growth and clinical status must always be considered when interpreting the results.

Low plasma BCAA may be due to phenylbutyrate (p. 491). Good biochemical control may be difficult to achieve during periods of slow growth before and particularly after puberty [529]. When the adolescent stops growing there may be a period of instability because protein is no longer needed for growth; protein intake and medicines may require adjustment to restore stability.

Wilson *et al.* [530] have observed that patients with citrullinaemia tend to have higher plasma ammonia concentrations for a given plasma glutamine concentration compared with OTC deficiency. Argininosuccinic acid accumulates in ASA and high dose arginine will also increase its production; the full consequences of this are not known, or if there is a specific plasma concentration that ASA should be kept below. A high plasma arginine may also be harmful by causing an increased cerebral guanidinoacetate concentration [531]; a fasting plasma arginine concentration of up to 70–120 μmol/L is considered acceptable [494]. Liver functions tests (LFT) are routinely monitored in ASA to detect the presence of liver disease early. A lower dose of arginine may help normalise LFT; however, nitrogen scavengers will need to be increased to compensate [518]. Arginine is necessary for the synthesis of creatine (Cr), which is used in energy storage and transmission. Decreased Cr levels have been reported in OTC

deficiency, citrullinaemia and HHH syndrome; in contrast, in ASA and lysinuric protein intolerance (LPI) (p. 507), Cr levels are increased [532]. It is not yet known if altered Cr metabolism effects CNS function in UCD. Monitoring of Cr may help to guide the dose of arginine in UCD as both high or low plasma levels of arginine may have adverse effects [532]. Dietary Cr intake may also be reduced because of the low protein diet as most comes from meat.

Glutamine

Poor appetite is observed in some children [529], with high glutamine levels implicated as a cause. It is thought that glutamine causes an increased influx of tryptophan (the precursor of serotonin) into the brain and promotes serotonin synthesis. Serotonin increases a feeling of satiety [533]. If plasma glutamine is maintained within the normal range then, in some children, appetite may improve.

Initial dietary management of the newly diagnosed child

Patients who present acutely with hyperammonaemia are almost invariably very sick, requiring ventilation and dialysis (to remove ammonia). Haemodiafiltration is recommended [494]. Reversal of catabolism and prevention of hyperammonaemia is a crucial part of the management to help stabilise the child. Treatment must be initiated promptly. The aims are to reduce waste nitrogen production as ammonia by provision of protein free high energy fluids, and to increase excretion of waste nitrogen using IV nitrogen scavengers, arginine and carbaglutamate (in some). Occasionally it can be difficult to reintroduce protein without inducing hyperammonaemia; in these instances an EAA supplement may be used to reduce the nitrogen load to the urea cycle, e.g. Essential Amino Acid Mix (Table 17.67) is given and is replaced with natural protein once the patient is more stable. The dietetic management of a newly diagnosed neonate, infant or child is discussed on p. 463.

Dietary management of illness

During intercurrent illness when oral intake is poor, protein catabolism may cause rapid accumulation of ammonia and glutamine. The standard ER (p. 502) is given to prevent these effects of illness and promote anabolism. Protein intake is stopped temporarily and a high energy intake is given from glucose polymer at regular 2 hourly intervals, either orally as drinks/feeds or via a tube (given continuously if bolus feeds are not tolerated). Rodney and Boneh challenge the need to completely stop protein in UCD patients based on the majority of their patients being protein deficient at admission with hyperammonaemia [534]. However, there are no reports of undertaking this in practice. The usual doses of sodium benzoate, phenylbutyrate and arginine are administered. If necessary during acute illness the dose of both benzoate and phenylbutyrate can be temporarily increased to 500 mg/kg/day. Protein is usually reintroduced within 24–48 hours of starting the ER and over a period of 1–2 days depending on the child's clinical condition. Practical advice on protein reintroduction is given on p. 464. If the child is not improving or does not tolerate oral/enteral ER and medicines, which is common, they should be admitted to hospital without delay for IV 10% dextrose and medicines. The BIMDG (www.bimdg.org) provide emergency protocols for IV management. Oral fluids can usually be recommenced within 24–48 hours, with a gradual changeover from IV to oral, thus always ensuring an adequate energy intake. Plasma ammonia should be measured frequently to help guide protein reintroduction. Once the plasma ammonia is falling and is <80–100 µmol/L, protein is gradually reintroduced usually over the same 24–48 hour period. This should not be delayed as inadequate protein will cause catabolism and increased ammonia. If hyperammonaemia is induced during protein reintroduction an EAA supplement may be used and/or energy intake increased.

Arginase deficiency

Arginase deficiency (Fig. 17.18) is a rare autosomal recessive disorder due to a deficiency of the enzyme arginase 1 (ARG1) which catalyses the conversion of arginine to urea and ornithine. Hyperargininaemia and a mild hyperammonaemia occur due to defective hydrolysis of arginine. Presentation of arginase deficiency is distinct from the other UCD. Patients rarely present in the neonatal period but typically present with first symptoms between 2 and 4 years of age [535]. It is characterised by a progressive spastic paraplegia, seizures or epilepsy in childhood, cognitive impairment (mild to severe mental retardation) which may continue to deteriorate and poor growth [535, 536]. Episodes of hyperammonaemic encephalopathy can occur but are uncommon. Similar to other children with UCD, patients avoid high protein foods. Interestingly, Carvalho *et al.* [536] reported this to be observed in children by their parents only after the age of 5 years. The mechanisms responsible for the neurological damage are not yet completely understood, but arginine and its guanidino metabolites are possible neurotoxins [535, 537].

Management (diet and medicines)

The treatment aims of arginase deficiency are to prevent accumulation of plasma arginine and ammonia by

- a low protein diet (to limit dietary arginine)
- provision of an adequate energy intake (to prevent catabolism)
- nitrogen scavengers (sodium benzoate and phenylbutyrate). These medicines reduce available nitrogen destined for arginine synthesis by increasing its excretion via alternative pathways to the urea cycle.

This treatment should help prevent further neurological damage and may induce a partial recovery of skills over time [535, 538, 539]. Three patients treated from birth are reported to be largely asymptomatic [540]. In patients who already have spastic diplegia dietary treatment will not improve this, but can help prevent hyperammonaemia.

All dietary nitrogen has the potential to be converted to arginine, this source being considerably greater than the small amount of arginine which is naturally present in protein. In the past, in order to restrict the nitrogen intake, diets comprised an EAA supplement with a very limited intake of natural protein. Nowadays, by giving sodium benzoate and phenylbutyrate a more generous intake of natural protein may be possible while still maintaining acceptable plasma arginine and ammonia levels. Protein is restricted to the safe level of intake (Table 17.54) and either is provided by a low protein diet or some of the protein is provided as an EAA supplement, which is a more common practice. In a European study 74% of 23 patients had EAA supplements, ranging from 10% to 50% of protein intake [521]. The precise composition of protein intake must be determined by the balance of requirements for growth and the medicines necessary for good biochemical control. A combination of 50%–75% as natural protein and 25%–50% as EAA has been suggested [540]. The practical management of the low protein diet and EAA supplementation are provided on p. 456 and p. 491. The diet is monitored by regular measurements of plasma ammonia, plasma arginine and the other amino acids quantitatively. The aim is to maintain plasma arginine levels <200 μmol/L (normal reference range 40–120 μmol/L), which is extremely difficult to achieve, and a near normal plasma ammonia (normal range <40 μmol/L).

Management of illness

During intercurrent illness patients are at risk of hyperargininaemia and hyperammonaemia. A standard ER of a protein free, high energy intake, as described for other UCD (p. 502), is given. This should be implemented promptly to prevent irreversible deterioration [538]. Sodium benzoate and phenylbutyrate should be given orally or IV during illness. Hyperammonaemic crisis is rare and this may be because of the activity of a second arginase enzyme. However, episodic hyperammonaemia has been reported in adolescent patients [536, 541] and deaths due to hyperammonaemic encephalopathy triggered by infection [535].

Hyperornithinaemia, Hyperammonaemia, Homocitrullinuria Syndrome

Jacky Stafford

Genetics and biochemistry

Hyperornithinaemia, hyperammonaemia, homocitrullinuria (HHH) syndrome is an autosomal recessive inherited disorder of ornithine transport caused by mutations in the gene SLC25A15 encoding the ornithine transporter protein (ORNT1). To date 22 different mutations have been identified. Other genes coding for additional ornithine transporter proteins (ORNT2 and ORNT3) are thought to mediate residual ornithine transport [542]. Common mutations are found among the French Canadian [543], Japanese and Italian populations [542].

HHH syndrome is due to defective activity of the ornithine transporter across the mitochondrial membrane, which causes a functional deficiency of two mitochondrial enzymes: ornithine transcarbamoylase (OTC) which catalyses the condensation reaction of ornithine and carbamoylphosphate to

citrulline; and ornithine-δ-aminotransferase (OAT) which metabolises ornithine to Δ^1-pyrroline-5-carboxylate and ultimately glutamate and proline (Fig. 17.18). Ornithine accumulates in cytoplasm (3–10 times normal levels) and its depletion in the mitochondrion causes a secondary urea cycle disorder and hyperammonaemia [544]. Carbamoylphosphate accumulates, undergoing secondary metabolism forming homocitrulline from lysine (hence urinary excretion of excess homocitrulline) and orotic acid, secondary to excess flux down the pyrimidine biosynthetic pathway [545, 546]. Despite a functional deficiency of OTC activity, plasma citrulline is normal in HHH syndrome [546]. This triad of hyperornithinaemia, hyperammonaemia and homocitrullinuria is pathognomic. At higher plasma levels of ornithine (>400 μmol/L) raised urinary levels of ornithine and dibasic amino acids (lysine and arginine) are also present [546].

Clinical presentation

Neonatal presentations
These are 12% of reported cases [542]. Symptoms occur 24–48 hours after feeding starts and hyperammonaemia causes lethargy, sleeplessness, refusal to feed, vomiting, tachypnoea with respiratory alkalosis and/or seizures [542, 547].

Late presentations
40% of reported cases before age 3 years; 29% in later childhood; 19% in adolescence or adulthood [542]. They are often diagnosed following an illness or surgery. This may be associated with mild hyperammonaemia, with or without liver dysfunction, e.g. abnormal clotting factors, or may present with fulminant hepatitis like liver failure [544, 545, 547, 548]. Others are diagnosed following an investigation of neurological problems, e.g. developmental delay, recurrent vomiting, ataxia or seizures [542]. On questioning, a history of protein intolerance associated with symptoms of lethargy, nausea, reduced appetite, vomiting or mood changes might be elicited [542]. Plasma ammonia concentrations at diagnosis are significantly less than in classical UCD, even in neonatal presentations [542]. After treatment commences liver function tests (LFT), coagulation factors, orotic acid, ammonia and glutamine levels normalise and episodes of seizures, hyperammonaemia or acute encephalopathy are rare and usually mild. However, despite good metabolic control some patients worsen neurologically with cognitive deterioration, behavioural problems and lower limb spasticity [543].

Dietary treatment

The aim of dietary treatment (as in other UCD) is to prevent hyperammonaemia by use of nitrogen scavengers, a low protein diet (p. 490) and, during illness, an ER (p. 502). Natural protein intakes among treated children are reported to range between 1 and 1.8 g/kg/day [543, 545] and for adolescents and adults to be approximately 40 g protein/day [543]. In two patients aged 1 and 2 years, given 1 g protein/kg, half the protein comprised EAA which was reported to be helpful by normalising ammonia within 24 hours and LFT

within 1 month [544]. Although ornithine levels are significantly reduced by treatment they rarely normalise [542]. The effect of diet on plasma ornithine levels is under-reported in published studies. In one case, after commencing dietary treatment (1 g protein/kg) and arginine (250 mg/kg/day) ornithine levels were reported to be approximately halved to 344 μmol/L [545]. Plasma concentrations of ammonia, glutamine, arginine and EAA should be maintained within normal ranges [494, 542]. The impact of treatment on neurological outcome is uncertain [543]. A long term follow-up (11–38 years) of four patients showed progression of neurological dysfunction despite control of hyperammonaemia [549].

Medicines

Sodium benzoate, a nitrogen scavenger, may be given to reduce nitrogen load to the urea cycle if hyperammonaemia occurs. Arginine may become deficient in disorders of the urea cycle; therefore either arginine or citrulline may be given as a supplement. However, chronic use of arginine may lead to hyperargininaemia (>250 μmol/L) and progression of lower limb spasticity [542, 543]. Secondary creatine deficiency has been reported which may be due to the inhibition of amidinotransferase (the rate limiting enzyme for creatine formation) by increased plasma levels of ornithine and supplementation may be required [543, 548].

Case studies

HHH syndrome – Great Ormond Street Hospital for Children NHS Foundation Trust, London
A 1-year-old boy presented to his local hospital for investigations into lethargy, floppiness, relentless crying, developmental regression and spasticity. He was reported to feed poorly, only managing soft foods and vomiting after most meals, and to be constipated. HHH syndrome was diagnosed by 2 years based on plasma ornithine 780 μmol/L, ammonia 190 μmol/L and homocitrulline in urine. A diet history suggested a protein intake from cow's milk and milk based puddings to be approximately 40 g/day. He was commenced on a low protein diet

and sodium benzoate. On changing from cow's milk to infant formula, to reduce protein intake, the vomiting stopped; addition of glucose polymer helped improve growth. Now 10 years old, he self-selects low protein foods (not measured) often with high energy content and is overweight; increased weight gain started around 5 years. Vitamin and mineral supplements are required. Plasma ornithine levels remain 400–500 μmol/L and EAA levels are often low or low to normal. An EAA supplement had been considered but not implemented as appetite improved. His health is good and ER is rarely needed. He tires easily and walks with a spastic gait using a frame. He continues to make some developmental progress, now managing to form short sentences.

HHH syndrome – Royal Manchester Children's Hospital, Manchester

A child 2 years and 7 months old with global developmental delay, poor fixing and following, poor head control and central hypotonia was referred for metabolic evaluation. Biochemical investigations showed increased urine orotic acid, presence of homocitrulline in the urine, raised plasma ornithine 593 μmol/L and raised glutamine 910 μmol/L, normal ammonia 66 μmol/L and an increased alanine transferase (ALT) level with prolonged clotting. A diagnosis of HHH syndrome was made. She was commenced on treatment with citrulline, a protein restricted diet, 15 g/day (1.4 g/kg/day), and ER for illness. Over time she has had no episodes of hyperammonaemia but has made little developmental progress. Her oral feeding skills deteriorated and she failed to thrive resulting in her being gastrostomy fed. It is unclear if HHH is a contributing factor in her developmental delay as she has a sibling also with global developmental delay but without HHH.

Citrin deficiency

Genetics and biochemistry

Citrin deficiency is an autosomal recessive condition due to mutations in the SLC25A13 gene. The same mutations encode two phenotypes:

a neonatal presentation, neonatal intrahepatic cholestasis caused by citrin deficiency (NICCD); and a late onset citrullinaemia type II (CTLN2). Early case reports come from East Asian populations, especially Japan, but it is now recognised as a worldwide pan ethnic disease [550]. Gene mutations lead to dysfunction of citrin, an isoform of the aspartate-glutamate carrier (AGC2), which is located in the inner mitochondrial membrane of the liver, kidney, heart and small intestine. Aralar, the other isoform, is found in the brain, skeletal muscle, kidney and heart [550]. AGC2 participates in gluconeogenesis, from lactate, transporting cytosolic NADH reducing equivalents into mitochondria as part of the malate-aspartate shuttle, and provides aspartate from mitochondria for the synthesis of protein, nucleotides and urea [550] (Fig. 17.18). Carbohydrate can cause a high cytosolic $NADH/NAD^+$ ratio resulting in a shortage of oxaloacetate and aspartate leading to a blockage of ureagenesis and deranged lipid metabolism. This could explain the toxicity from high CHO treatment and the characteristic aversion to CHO rich foods and self-selection of a high protein diet (which provides a source of arginine and/or aspartate) [550, 551].

Clinical presentation

NICCD presents in the first weeks of life and is characterised by cholestasis, hyperbilirubinaemia, multiple aminoacidaemias (citrulline, threonine, methionine, tyrosine, arginine, lysine and increased threonine/serine ratio), hypoproteinaemia, galactosaemia, hypoglycaemia and growth faltering. Raised LFT, alpha-fetoprotein, lactate and ammonia are reported and low levels of vitamin K dependent coagulation factors [550, 552]. Symptoms usually self-resolve by the first year of life [552] and diagnosis is difficult after this time. Some patients may have a symptom free period of up to several decades before developing severe CTLN2. Regular follow-up of patients with NICCD is essential as adult onset CTLN2 patients present with recurring neuropsychiatric symptoms, citrullinaemia, hyperammonaemia, pancreatitis, disorientation, delirium and seizures. Without liver transplantation, coma and death may result within a few years of onset [553, 554].

Dietary treatment

Case reports describe using lactose free milk, e.g. soya formula, and/or formula supplemented with medium chain triglycerides (MCT) and fat soluble vitamins for treatment of NICCD [555, 556]. While cholestasis persists, lactose should not be reintroduced as it may be toxic [555]. In one case, daily dietary energy intake distributed as CHO 35%, protein 15% and fat 50%, (equating to 4 g protein/kg and 6 g fat/kg) was effective in improving growth and reversing abnormal clotting profile. A reduced protein intake (11% energy intake, CHO 35%, fat 54%) was associated with decreased growth which corrected when protein was increased to previous ratios [551]. In citrin deficient mice, an increase in the proportion of energy from protein (casein) from 14% to 22% was associated with improved appetite and weight gain. This also occurred with supplementation of alanine, sodium glutamate and, to a lesser extent, sodium pyruvate and MCT [557]. From as young as age 1–3 years a preference for protein and fat rich foods has been reported [558] which contrasts with the protein aversion reported in later diagnosed patients with UCD. Aversion to CHO rich, particularly sweet, foods is also described [550, 558]. A study of 18 Japanese patients (age 1–33 years) confirmed a marked decrease in CHO intake compared with controls and a preference for high fat, high protein foods. Their total daily energy intake was distributed as CHO 37% ± 7%, protein 19% ± 2% and fat 44% ± 5% [558].

There is a risk of CHO toxicity in CTLN2. Case reports of glucose and glycerol infusions to manage illness or surgical procedure caused increased ammonia, triglycerides, coma and even death [550]. To prevent this, it is therefore essential that any illness plan avoids excess CHO. Instead of the standard ER based on glucose polymer, the oral illness plan could be based on cow's milk as it has an energy ratio which is high in fat and protein (combined) to CHO and given to meet normal fluid requirements (author's personal practice). If IV fluids are necessary it is suggested these should not contain glucose (www.bimdg.org.uk).

Medicines

In NICCD, vitamin K is given to correct deficiency, to improve low vitamin K dependent coagulation factors or if prothrombin time is prolonged. Bile acids (ursodeoxycholic acid) or bile acid sequestrants (cholestyramine) may be needed if cholestasis continues and biliary secretion is affected. If so, fat soluble vitamins may also be required [552, 555]. Liver transplantation is a promising therapy in CTLN2 with patients becoming metabolically normal and neurological symptoms resolving [559]. An alternative treatment with sodium pyruvate ± arginine has shown clinical and biochemical improvements in patients with CTLN2 [559, 560] and citrin deficient mice [550]. Arginine may facilitate ammonia detoxification via the urea cycle, although the precise mechanism of action in this disorder is unknown. Sodium pyruvate oxidises NADH and provides energy for the tricarboxylic acid cycle, thereby relieving inhibition of glycolysis and activating ureagenesis [560].

Case studies

CTLN2 – Great Ormond Street Hospital for Children NHS Foundation Trust, London

Two asymptomatic siblings (aged 7 and 12 years) were diagnosed with CTLN2 on screening, prompted by the family history of a relative. Dietary assessment revealed that both self-select a high protein (20% of energy intake), low CHO (32% of energy intake) diet and are growing normally. The older sibling has GOR and nausea (treated with ranitidine) and abdominal pain associated with constipation. Ammonia level was increased during one admission for illness when CHO only was given. For treatment of illness, both now have an ER of cow's milk which provides around the same energy distribution as their normal diet (CHO 27%, protein 20%, fat 53%). They remain on their self-selected diet.

NICCD – Great Ormond Street Hospital for Children NHS Foundation Trust, London

A neonate with a possible diagnosis of galactosaemia was commenced on soya formula and then changed to hydrolysed formula with 55% MCT content (Pregestimil) due to liver cholestasis. NICCD was subsequently diagnosed. At age 6 months, when liver function improved the infant was changed to a standard infant formula. The ER plan for illness was initially half strength Pregestimil, then half strength standard formula providing an energy distribution ratio of 10% protein, 50% fat, 40% CHO, similar to the self-selected diet described above. Addition of protein and fat supplements may be required in the future. Weaning advice emphasised the introduction of protein rich foods. Food preferences are being monitored.

NICDD – Birmingham Children's Hospital NHS Foundation Trust, Birmingham

A boy with NICCD self-selected a high protein diet (energy distribution from food being protein 20%, fat 43%, CHO 37%) by 3 years of age and tended to avoid sugary foods. From 4 years he experienced intermittent episodes of abdominal pain with pale stools and ketotic hypoglycaemia which led to frequent hospital admissions. A modified Atkins diet (p. 370) was commenced from 6 years, initially providing 10 g CHO/day, which was then relaxed

over 9 months to 30 g CHO/day (5%–8% energy intake) [561]. Large portions of protein containing foods were eaten at three meals plus a high protein drink to provide energy from protein 30%, fat 65% and CHO 5%. This reduced his abdominal pain, with no reported hyperammonaemia or hypoglycaemic episodes. An emergency drink comprising 4% fat (sourced from Calogen long chain at emulsion) and 3.5% protein (sourced from soya protein) was taken if symptoms reappeared [562].

CTLN2 – Birmingham Children's Hospital NHS Foundation Trust, Birmingham

A boy from consanguineous parents presented in infancy with conjugated neonatal jaundice and episodes of hypoglycaemia. He remained undiagnosed and citrin deficiency was not confirmed until the age of 14 years when he complained of frequent headaches and had developed a profound preference for high protein foods with an aversion to CHO containing foods. All fruits, vegetables and simple CHO were avoided. His headaches resolved after a late evening snack of homemade nut butter mix (high protein and fat) was introduced. He now remains symptom free.

Emergency Regimens

Marjorie Dixon

Background

For some inborn errors of intermediary metabolism (Table 17.69) any physiological stress situation such as intercurrent infection, surgery or trauma combined with a poor oral intake and fasting can precipitate severe metabolic decompensation and possible neurological sequelae. Metabolic decompensation (the accumulation of toxic metabolites, which is disorder specific and causes metabolic encephalopathy) is primarily a consequence of the effects of catabolism, which arises due to fasting and an inadequate energy and nutrient intake. Under normal conditions, as fasting progresses glycogen stores are depleted and hepatic gluconeogenesis and ketogenesis become the main energy

supply. This process occurs more rapidly in infants and younger children. To help prevent catabolism an ER is given during any period when dietary energy intake is reduced, most frequently with illness [563].

The ER provides an exogenous energy source to promote anabolism and

- prevent an energy deficit when energy substrates cannot be produced from the usual metabolic pathways, e.g. glucose from glycogenolysis and/or gluconeogenesis in glycogen storage disorders, ketones in defects of fatty acid oxidation or ketogenesis, glucose via gluconeogenesis in fructose, 1-6 bisphosphatase deficiency

Table 17.69   Disorders requiring an emergency regimen.

Disorder group	Disorder	Emergency regimen and specific therapy: Usual medicines are continued, doses may be increased. Other medicines are given to treat the underlying illness such as antipyretics for fever
Organic acidaemias	Propionic acidaemia	ER*
	Methylmalonic acidaemia	ER* Usual fluids and more Sodium bicarbonate
	Isovaleric acidaemia	ER* Glycine and carnitine
	Glutaric aciduria type 1	ER* Lysine free, low tryptophan amino acids (usual dose or 1 g amino acids/kg) Carnitine double standard dose 200 mg/kg
Amino acid disorders	Maple syrup urine disease	ER* Branched chain amino acids Isoleucine and valine supplements
Urea cycle disorders	NAGS, CPS, OTC deficiencies, ASA, citrullinaemia	ER* Nitrogen scavengers and arginine may be increased or given IV
	Arginase deficiency	ER* Nitrogen scavengers can be given IV
	Hyperornithinaemia, hyperammonaemia, homocitrullinuria (HHH)	ER* Usual medicines such as nitrogen scavengers
	Citrin deficiency	Non standard ER High fat and protein, low CHO IV fluids to be CHO free
Lysinuric protein intolerance	Lysinuric protein intolerance	ER* Usual medicines such as citrulline and any nitrogen scavengers
Disorders of energy metabolism including fatty acid oxidation defects	β-oxidation defects, e.g. LCHAD, VLCAD, MTP deficiencies	ER* No long chain fat
	Carnitine pathway disorders, e.g. CPTI,CPTII, CACT, OCTN2 deficiencies	ER* No long chain fat
	Multiple acyl-CoA dehydrogenase deficiency	ER* No long or medium chain fat
	Malonyl Co-A decarboxylase deficiency	ER* No long chain fat
	Medium chain acyl-CoA dehydrogenase deficiency	ER* Medium chain triglycerides contraindicated
Disorders of ketolysis	HMG-CoA synthase deficiency HMG-CoA lyase deficiency	ER* Avoid medium chain triglycerides
Ketone body utilisation defects	SCOT deficiency β-ketothiolase deficiency	ER* Avoid medium chain triglycerides
Glycogen storage disorders	GSD types 0, I, III, VI, IX, Fanconi Bickel syndrome (Glut 2 deficiency)	ER* to provide at least adequate CHO to meet basal glucose requirements or child's usual requirement Avoid excess CHO, so child does not become hyperglycaemic
Glut-1-deficiency syndrome		Non standard ER CHO free, oral or IV fluids Monitor blood glucose and ketones
Fructose,1-6 bisphophatase deficiency		ER* Avoid fructose, sucrose and sorbitol (drinks and medicines) and fat during acute period
Ketotic hypoglycaemia		ER*
Glycerol kinase deficiency		ER* Avoid fat

*Emergency regimen is the standard emergency regimen shown in Table 17.70.

- reduce production of toxic metabolites from protein and amino acid catabolism, e.g. ammonia in UCD, leucine in MSUD, organics acids in MMA, PA, IVA and GA1
- reduce production of potentially toxic metabolites from lipolysis, e.g. accumulation of long chain acyl carnitines and free fatty acids in long chain fatty acid oxidation disorders

The correct use of ER can be extremely effective and is known to reduce hospital admissions and episodes of metabolic decompensation [477,564].

Composition of emergency regimens

The standard ER is a solution of glucose polymer, which is rapidly absorbed, simple to administer, usually well tolerated and suitable for most disorders. The CHO concentration of the solution given depends upon the age of the child. This ranges from 10% to 25% CHO, with the lowest concentrations given to infants and younger children (Table 17.70). The precise energy requirements to prevent catabolism in patients during illness are not known but are likely to be more than the estimated average requirement (EAR) for energy [389] for healthy children or their usual energy intake, as requirements are known to increase during illness. Bodamer et al. [565] reported that resting energy expenditure was increased by up to 30% in two children with MMA during acute illness. At lower

CHO concentrations standard ER solutions do not provide the EAR for energy for age. Van Hove et al. [564] recommend higher concentrations of glucose polymer solutions be given to younger children to provide more energy. An enteral ER is preferable to IV management as a higher energy intake can be given and it is less invasive. Nevertheless, IV fluids are absolutely essential for certain circumstances, such as vomiting.

Fat

Fat emulsions can be added as an additional energy source, but these may be less well tolerated, particularly in the child who is vomiting as gastric emptying will be delayed. However, fat is often added in the ER for MSUD and some metabolic centres successfully use a protein free feed (which contains fat) such as Energivit in OAA and UCD. Fat (long and/or medium chain) is contraindicated in some disorders of fatty acid oxidation, particularly long chain defects (see Chapter 19).

Oral rehydration solutions

ESPGAN [566] recommends, for oral rehydration in acute diarrhoea, a 4 hour rehydration period, then reassessment, then a return to normal diet, the osmolality of oral rehydration solutions (ORS) to be 200–250 mOsm/kg H_2O. A longer period of rehydration may be necessary. The standard ER

Table 17.70 Standard emergency regimens.

Age years	Glucose polymer concentration % CHO	Energy/100 mL		Osmolality* (mOsm/kg H_2O)	Suggested daily fluid volumes by age and weight
		kcal	kJ		
Up to 1	10	40	167	103	< 6 months 150 mL/kg up to a maximum of 1200 mL 7–12 months 120–150 mL/kg up to a maximum of 1200 mL
1–2	15	60	250	174	11–20 kg: 100 mL/kg for first 10 kg, plus 50 mL/kg for next 10 kg
2–9	20	80	334	245	>20 kg: as above for first 20 kg + 25 mL/kg
>10	25	100	418	342	thereafter up to a 2500 mL maximum

Administration of ER	Divide total volume over 24 hours: give 1–3 hourly orally or via tube (bolus or continuously)

van Hove et al. [564] glucose polymer % CHO: 0–12 months 15%, 1–3 years 20%, 3–6 years 25%, 6–12 years 25% or 30%, 12–15 years 30%, >15 years 30%.

*Data provided by Scientific Hospital Supplies International Limited, *Clinical Paediatric Dietetics*, 3rd edn.

does not provide a source of electrolytes. ORS may be prescribed for the treatment of gastroenteritis in metabolic disorders. As the CHO content of ORS is low (around 2%) they do not provide sufficient energy to prevent catabolism in metabolic disorders. ORS can be supplemented with glucose polymer to provide additional energy, usually to a concentration of 10 g CHO per 100 mL (10%). The osmolality of such feeds needs to be considered [567]; ORS with glucose polymer added to a final concentration of 10% has an osmolality around 320 mOsm/kg H_2O. Van Hove et al. [564] report successful use of such feeds in patients with mild diarrhoea. Too concentrated a solution of glucose polymer will be hyperosmolar, worsen diarrhoea and exacerbate the effects of illness. It is also important to be aware that the child may obtain generous amounts of sodium from standard medicines such as sodium benzoate in UCD and sodium bicarbonate in MMA. Parents need to be informed that ORS alone do not provide adequate energy and be instructed to add glucose polymer. They also need guidance on the number of ORS sachets (with added glucose polymer) to give depending on the severity of diarrhoea and when to return to the child's usual regimen.

Fluids

The fluid volume of glucose polymer solution given depends on age, weight and clinical condition of the child. The suggested figures given are for maintenance fluid requirements (Table 17.70). Higher fluid volumes will be needed in certain circumstances such as dehydration caused by diarrhoea and/or vomiting or increased losses due to high temperature.

Disorder specific therapy

In some disorders the standard ER is combined with additional specific therapy (Table 17.69), e.g. BCAA in MSUD. Normally, the child's usual regular medicines are continued and may be increased temporarily in some disorders to help reduce accumulation of toxic metabolites, e.g. nitrogen scavengers in UCD, L-carnitine in GA1.

The standard ER is not suitable for citrin deficiency (p. 498) or Glut-1 deficiency syndrome (p. 354). Refer to specific disorders for full ER information.

Practical provision of ER drinks and feeds

Glucose polymer is available as a powder (e.g. Maxijul, Polycal, Vitajoule). Liquid glucose polymers in tetrapaks, such as Polycose liquid, are generally not used for ER in children because of their very high CHO content (61.9%). Parents are taught to measure glucose polymer powders using handy scoop measurements or weighing scales, then to add to a measured volume of water. Individual feeds/drinks or larger volume recipes can be made. Pre measured sachets of glucose polymer are available, S·O·S 10, 15, 20, 25 (the number corresponds to the % CHO concentration once prepared and the sachet is colour coded for this). One sachet is added to 200 mL of water in a beaker and dissolves on shaking. These are more accurate than using scoops and weighing [568], are more convenient and are easier to use. To improve palatability the glucose polymer solution can be flavoured with squash, taking care not to greatly exceed the recommended CHO concentration per 100 mL. For children who are unfamiliar with the taste of glucose polymer drinks it is worthwhile having a trial of different drinks when they are well to ascertain what they will take and to familiarise the parents with reconstitution of these in a non emergency situation.

Example emergency regimen for a 4-year-old girl (weight 16 kg) with ketotic hypoglycaemia who is unwell with a sore throat and not eating well.

Use 20% glucose polymer solution. Fluids = 1300 mL/24 hours; ER provides 1040 kcal (4.4 MJ), EAR for energy 1460 kcal (6.1 MJ) [389].

Day and night: 110 mL × 2 hourly × 12 drinks or 160 mL × 3 hourly × 8 drinks

Preparation: 1 sachet of S·O·S 20 (or 4 × 5 g scoops of glucose polymer), add water to 200 mL, flavour with squash as desired

Day 1: give full ER for 24 hours and encourage to eat

Day 2: on recovery, reintroduce usual diet, continue some ER drinks until eating normally again

Commercial drinks

Commercial drinks contain different concentrations of CHO, ranging from 0% to around 17% CHO. Some children dislike the taste of glucose polymer and find commercial drinks to be more acceptable. They can be used, provided glucose polymer powder is added to the required CHO concentration, e.g. to make a 20% CHO ER drink with fruit juice, 10 g glucose polymer (using a scoop to measure) is added to 100 mL fruit juice (10 g CHO/100 mL), final concentration 20 g CHO/100 mL.

It is essential that parents are adept in reading the nutrition information label of the drink for its CHO concentration per 100 mL. They also need to know that CHO concentrations of drinks can change and alternative flavours and formats of the same product can have different CHO concentrations (e.g. the Ribena range), so they must check carefully before use. Parents must be given clear, written instructions on preparation. It is probably best to avoid low calorie, sugar free drinks and no added sugar drinks as they contain very little or no CHO. Commercial drinks can be very convenient because many are ready to use; also these and premeasured sachets are portable and can be stored for use in an emergency situation at nursery or school.

Administration of ER at home

The ER is normally commenced at home at the first signs of illness (e.g. colds, flu, cough, viral infection of the nose, throat, ear, sinuses, any illness associated with fever >37°C, chest infection, tonsillitis, gastroenteritis), particularly if appetite is reduced or usual feeds not tolerated, and may be given orally or enterally. For minor illnesses, a change to ER may not always be necessary and continuation of the normal diet is appropriate. The oral ER is initially fed at frequent 2–3 hourly intervals day and night to optimise energy intake and reduce the period of fasting. In some circumstances, e.g. vomiting, it is better to give small very frequent sips of the ER. Such frequent overnight feeding (2 hourly) can be tiring and difficult to achieve, particularly for patients without a feeding tube, and more realistic targets should be considered, if feasible. Tube feeding should be used if it is not possible to achieve an adequate oral volume. This may necessitate a hospital admission for NG feeding. Continuous NG feeding is generally better

tolerated than bolus feeds. Alternatively, some parents prefer to be taught to do NG feeding at home solely for provision of ER. This may be helpful in young children but may be less well tolerated in older children. As NG feeding may only be used intermittently it is important that parents remain confident and competent in passing an NG tube and administering the ER feed. Alternatively, some children may have a tube passed in the local hospital emergency department, be observed for a few hours and then continue ER treatment at home. Close liaison daily with the metabolic team is essential when a child is unwell at home to assess tolerance, intake of ER and clinical state.

If the child persistently vomits the ER or is obviously not recovering, then an immediate hospital admission for stabilisation with IV therapy is usually necessary. For most disorders glucose 10% and saline 0.45% is given by peripheral drip or more concentrated dextrose can be administered through a central line. The BIMDG provides detailed emergency protocols for IV management of these disorders, available from www.bimdg.org. There are two versions: a short version for immediate use in an accident and emergency department or paediatric assessment unit/ward; and a long version which provides much more detailed information about the disorder and IV and oral ER management.

When oral fluids are reintroduced they are titrated against IV fluids and increased as tolerated, thus ensuring an overall adequate energy intake at all times. If oral or enteral feeds cannot be re-established then an early resort to PN is indicated for some disorders (refer to specific disorders). Placement of a portacath may be considered in those who have frequent episodes of illness and if IV access is difficult. Because of the risk of line infection precipitating metabolic decompensation the benefits of this need to be carefully considered [425].

Reintroducing the normal diet

The standard ER of glucose polymer alone must not be continued for long periods of time (beyond 24–48 hours) because it does not provide adequate nutrition. If prolonged, malnutrition may develop surprisingly rapidly. Severe lactic acidosis caused by acute thiamin deficiency has been reported in two patients with PA who had high energy PN to restore anabolism, but no vitamins were given [569].

As the child improves, their normal diet is reintroduced. With the exception of low protein diets (in OAA and UCD) and MSUD the ER is often just replaced with the child's usual diet within 24–48 hours. During the recovery phase if the child's appetite is reduced it is important to give additional ER drinks or feeds particularly at night to maximise energy intake, reduce the period of fasting and prevent further metabolic decompensation. For patients on low protein diets, the protein intake is stopped for the shortest time possible (24–48 hours). Protein, whether from feed or diet, should be reintroduced: day 1 – provide half the normal allowance; day 2 – return to full allowance, or more rapidly if clinically indicated, taking care to ensure an adequate energy intake is given throughout. It needs to be recognised that this is not always possible in a child who is very sick, metabolically unstable and who may also be in intensive care.

In milder illnesses protein intake is generally not regraded. If on oral diet, additional ER drinks are given throughout the reintroduction period (usually less frequently) to maximise energy intake. Vitamin and mineral supplements should be restarted promptly. If reintroducing feeds, additional glucose polymer is added to the infant formula or low protein tube feed at least to the same concentration as the ER or the usual CHO concentration of the feed, if this is higher. If the feed normally contains fat and vitamins and minerals, these will also be increased over the same 2 days. The child's usual feeding frequency is also gradually resumed as tolerated. Poor growth and nutritional deficiencies will occur in patients on low protein diets who have repeated infections and are frequently on the ER. If so, it may be necessary to increase protein intake temporarily when the child is well to compensate for inadequate intakes of protein while on the ER.

Instructions for parents

Management of intercurrent infections can be an anxious and difficult time for parents, as they know this puts their child at greater risk of metabolic decompensation and/or hypoglycaemia. To make this easier, parents are taught a three-staged plan telling them what to do and when [563]. They are encouraged to phone the metabolic team for advice at an early stage and also to consult their general practitioner for assessment and treatment of common childhood illnesses. This type of approach can help reduce episodes of metabolic decompensation and hospital admissions.

- If the parents are unsure whether their child is showing the first signs of impending illness (pallor, dark eyes, lethargy, irritability, loss of appetite, fever, headache, aches and pain, cough, sore throat or ears) then an ER drink is given as a precaution. Clinical observations are reported to be generally better than biochemical measurements for detecting decompensation; subtle changes in behaviour are usually the earliest signs of this and are most easily detected by carers [570]. The child's clinical state is then reviewed regularly within 1–2 hours.
- If on reassessment the child has improved, the normal diet is resumed; if, however, the child has deteriorated or shown no signs of improvement the full ER is commenced for a period of 24 to a maximum of 48 hours. The parents are instructed how to reintroduce the usual diet.
- If the child is not tolerating the ER (i.e. refusing ER drinks, vomiting, persistently high temperature, not responding or becoming encephalopathic) they should be taken to their local hospital for assessment. Parents are instructed to take all ER information and glucose polymer with them.

Parents are taught to recognise signs of encephalopathy such as disorientation and poor responsiveness, accompanied by a glazed look. Komaromy et al. [571] reported that monitoring of urinary ketones may be useful in deciding when to implement the ER. They observed that ketones were present during times of illness but not in health. This tool would only be suitable for some patients as there is wide variation in how they respond so that each should be assessed individually. Ketone monitoring in MSUD is described on p. 453. For obvious reasons testing for ketones is not to be used in patients with disorders of fatty acid oxidation. Measurement of blood glucose is helpful in some disorders if there is a risk of hypoglycaemia, e.g. glycogen storage disorders, but is not appropriate in disorders of fatty acid oxidation where hypoglycaemia is a late finding and the child may already be very unwell before this develops. Monitoring of temperature is important and should be treated in the normal way.

It is important there is close liaison and good communication between the metabolic centre, the local hospital team and parents to help with the child's management. It is also useful to organise open access to the local hospital's paediatric ward (avoiding the accident and emergency department) and therefore a delay in treatment. Parents are given written instructions on implementation of the ER and practical aspects including recipes, suggested fluid volumes, feeding frequency, contact telephone numbers, an initial supply of glucose polymer and a prescription letter for further supplies. Parents are given laminated 'parent held guidelines'; these are typically a copy of the BIMDG short version emergency protocol. The 'parent held guidelines' are also very useful for families when on holiday. Families can travel abroad, but it is best they go to countries which have expertise in the management of metabolic disease, should the child become unwell. This needs to be discussed with the metabolic team at an early stage. It is essential parents take all ER provisions and up to date medical and dietetic management information with them and know which hospital to go to in the event of an emergency. Sensible precautions need to be taken on holidays abroad, particularly in hot countries, to reduce the risk of infections. ORS should be taken because of risk of gastroenteritis.

Use and understanding of ER, instructions and recipes need to be regularly reviewed with parents in outpatient clinics and updated in accordance with the child's current dietary treatment, age and clinical condition. If a child is reported to be frequently on their ER this warrants further investigation. A Medic Alert bracelet may be useful for some children.

Ketotic Hypoglycaemia

Marjorie Dixon

Ketotic hypoglycaemia (KH) is the most common cause of hypoglycaemia beyond infancy. Children typically present between 18 months and 7 years of age with an episode of hypoglycaemia accompanied by high levels of ketones in plasma and urine, precipitated by a period of prolonged fasting often associated with intercurrent illness. Seizures may occur but neurological sequelae are rare [572]. KH improves with age and rarely manifests beyond about 8 years of age [573]. The prognosis is generally good and some patients never experience a second episode. KH is considered to be due to a failure to sustain sufficient hepatic glucose production [572, 574]. This may, however, just represent the lowest percentile of normative distribution of fasting tolerance in children and as such KH should not be classified as a pathological condition; diagnosis is only made after exclusion of any specific endocrine or metabolic disorder that can cause a ketotic hypoglycaemia [574].

Treatment

Normally the child will present acutely to their local hospital accident and emergency department with a history of being unwell, having gone to bed with a poor food intake the day/evening before and the next morning is pale, floppy and unrousable. On arrival at hospital they are found to be hypoglycaemic. This is treated immediately with either IV glucose, or oral glucose such as Glucogel (a 40% dextrose gel) rubbed into the buccal cavity, or a sugary drink. The child responds promptly to glucose. The BIMDG provides guidelines for IV glucose management, available at www.bimdg.org.

Once the child recovers, and before discharge, it is important the parents are advised on implementation of a standard ER for age (p. 502) to be used during episodes of illness, to help prevent any further episodes of hypoglycaemia. Written instructions and a supply of glucose polymer powder should be given. A supply of a dextrose gel can also be given. General advice on 'healthy eating' with regular meals including complex CHO foods and avoidance of a prolonged overnight fast, with ideas for a starch rich bedtime snack and breakfast, should be given. No other dietary change is necessary in the well child. It is important the ER instructions are given even before the child has been reviewed in a specialist metabolic centre and/or a diagnosis of KH been made or excluded.

Fasting tests are commonly used to help establish the cause of hypoglycaemia and the child's fasting tolerance. The tests are performed under controlled conditions in hospital, usually by a specialist metabolic or endocrine team. Younger children have a faster decrease in blood glucose and faster increase in ketone body levels than older children; thus fasting tolerance improves with age [575]. The results can help establish the diagnosis and determine the maximum safe fasting time for the child at that age. Most children with KH will not develop hypoglycaemia during the fasting test. However, if on fasting the child does become hypoglycaemic further dietary intervention is necessary, usually at night, either

- reducing the length of the overnight fast and giving a starch rich bedtime snack and early breakfast

- the above, plus provision of a high CHO drink (at least 10% concentration) or milk drink in the middle of the night
- a dose of 1–1.5 g/kg of uncooked cornstarch (UCCS) given before bed. Practical aspects of giving UCCS are described on p. 549.

A small number of children complain of hypoglycaemic symptoms even when completely well. Parents often just treat these symptoms with a high CHO drink or food, without knowing the actual blood glucose level. McSweeney et al. [576] reported that a continuous glucose monitoring system (CGMS) over several days at home provided more real time information and helped identify the true incidence of hypoglycaemia in KH children, despite them having normal fasting tests in hospital. CGMS enabled a more individualised treatment plan to be given. Children with KH should be reviewed at outpatient appointments to assess use of the ER, to ensure it is age appropriate, and that parents have written instructions and supplies of glucose polymer as per the standard ER. Follow-up also allows identification of further possible hypoglycaemic episodes necessitating repeat investigation or further dietary manipulation.

Miscellaneous Metabolic Disorders

Jacky Stafford

This section describes mostly rare metabolic disorders where dietary treatment may form part of the overall management.

Lysinuric protein intolerance

Genetics and biochemistry

Lysinuric protein intolerance (LPI) is an autosomal recessive disorder caused by mutations in the SLC7A7 gene encoding for the amino acid transporter y+LAT-1 protein, which transports the dibasic amino acids including lysine (an EAA), arginine and ornithine at the basolateral membrane of epithelial cells in the intestinal and renal

tubules. Lung, liver, immune system, muscle and brain are also affected to varying extents [577]. It has a high prevalence (1 in 60 000) in Finland where a founder effect has been demonstrated, individuals sharing the same homozygous mutation, c.895-2A>T. There is also a high incidence in southern Italy and Japan (1 in 50 000). No genotype–phenotype correlations have been established [577, 578]. Plasma concentrations of lysine, arginine and ornithine are low due to their increased urinary loss and reduced absorption from the intestine. Lysine is lost in massive amounts in urine [579]. Deficiency of arginine and ornithine (urea cycle intermediates) causes dysfunction of the urea cycle with consequent hyperammonaemia if the individual is having a normal protein intake [580].

Clinical presentation

LPI is a multisystem disorder. Patients are usually symptom free when breast or formula fed, only developing symptoms when increased dietary protein is taken, i.e, when weaning onto solid foods or in early childhood. Many have a strong aversion to protein rich foods from an early age [577] and a preference for salty foods [581]. Variable symptoms are reported including recurrent postprandial vomiting, episodes of diarrhoea and an altered neurological status due to hyperammonaemia. Deficiency of lysine may result in growth faltering and short stature [580], hepatosplenomegaly, osteoporosis, osteopenia, muscle hypotonia and bone marrow dysfunction (including anaemia, leukopenia, thrombocytopenia and erythroblastophagocytosis). Patients are predisposed to severe complications such as pulmonary alveolar proteinosis (PAP) and glomerulonephritis [578]. In 10 children with LPI (aged up 16 years) five had proteinuria, two haematuria and three had a GFR <75 [582]. The cause of proteinuria, haematuria and tubular diseases like Fanconi syndrome, which can lead to end stage renal disease requiring dialysis, is not known [583].

Dietary treatment

The primary management is citrulline supplementation and a low protein diet: 0.8–1.5 g protein/ kg/day in children; 0.5–0.8 g protein/kg/day in adults [584]. Citrulline, a urea cycle intermediate with anapleurotic function and is given to correct the urea cycle's lack of arginine and enables an increased protein tolerance. However, a low protein diet remains essential for the management of LPI though it does not correct lysine deficiency [585] and limits, the supply of lysine, arginine and ornithine which are already low in the plasma. During illness patients are at risk of hyperammonaemia and therefore a standard ER of glucose polymer based feeds/drinks is necessary. Those on a self-selected low protein diet may be at risk

of deficiencies including energy, protein, vitamins and minerals [581]. Combined hyperlipidaemia (triglycerides and cholesterol) can develop at an early age. Though dietary intake of total and saturated fat among LPI patients has been reported to be the same as the general population, it may be advisable to limit saturated fat intake and consider medicines (statins) [586] (p. 634). Regular biochemical monitoring is required, aiming for normal plasma levels of ammonia, EAA including BCAA as for other UCD [494], although this is not always possible for lysine, arginine and ornithine. There are recommendations to supplement with lysine to achieve low to normal plasma lysine levels [585, 587].

Medicines

Low dose citrulline is given to treat arginine and ornithine deficiency and enhance the function of the urea cycle. The dose is kept as low as possible, current guidance for upper limits of supplementation being 100 mg/kg/day, to avoid potential trapping of intracellular arginine and consequent excess of nitric oxide (NO) production [578]. Sodium benzoate (100–250 mg/kg/day, four times daily) is given to reduce nitrogen load on the urea cycle [578]. If the patient is hyperammonaemic, the dose is increased and given IV with the addition of sodium phenylbutyrate and arginine.

L-carnitine (25–50 mg/kg/day, twice daily) is recommended as plasma levels can be low due to aversion or restriction of high protein foods containing carnitine, e.g. red meat, poultry, fish, dairy foods. Endogenous carnitine synthesis requires methionine and lysine. As the latter is deficient in LPI, this may also contribute to possible carnitine deficiency. Fanconi-type tubulopathy may further increase carnitine losses [588, 589]. Plasma carnitine levels should be monitored [588].

Low plasma lysine levels in LPI contribute to the chronic symptoms of poor growth and osteoporosis. However, an early report of supplementing the diet with L-lysine described side effects of frequent abdominal cramps and loose stools, possibly due to poor absorption. Also, there was no improvement in plasma lysine levels or growth after 0.5–2 years of supplementation compared with giving citrulline alone [590]. A more recent study reported that low dose lysine supplementation given with meals for 3 days, in addition to usual treatment, did not cause hyperammonaemia or gastrointestinal side effects. Plasma lysine levels normalised in two out of three patients and arginine and ornithine levels normalised in all three patients [585]. Despite the small numbers, this prompted low dose lysine supplementation (20–30 mg/kg, given in three doses) of 27 LPI patients in Finland. After 1 year of treatment plasma lysine reached the lower limit of reference range in 55% of the study group (aged 3–56 years). Other plasma amino acid levels remained unchanged: BCAA were low to normal; ornithine and arginine were not reported. Of five patients aged 3–10.5 years, two received growth hormone treatment, but there was no increased growth in the others; no comment was made about plasma lysine levels in the children [587].

Other medical therapies used in LPI include growth hormone (GH) replacement therapy, if short stature is unresponsive to standard LPI treatment and GH deficiency confirmed [591]; Alendroate (bisphosphonate) to improve bone mineral density in osteoporosis [584]; HMGCoA reductase inhibitors (statins) are prescribed for adults with raised cholesterol (low HDL) and triglyceride levels. Statins are only prescribed in children if they are unresponsive to dietary management. The reasons for combined hyperlipidaemia are not understood but defective endothelial function (due to arginine deficiency) may predispose patients to atherosclerosis and subsequent coronary heart disease [586].

Case studies

Case study 1 Great Ormond Street Hospital for Children NHS Foundation Trust, London

A 3-year-old boy whose parents are first cousins, from North Africa, was diagnosed with LPI. On referral to the specialist centre he had short stature (weight 2nd–9th centile, height 0.4th centile) and was short limbed. As a neonate he had jaundice. During infancy he had a tendency to vomit and refuse breast feeds and later, with introduction of solids, would often vomit within half an hour of meals, this continuing until about 2 years of age. At 8 months he had abdominal distention and hepatosplenomegaly. He met all his developmental

milestones, walking before 1 year. He self-selected a low protein diet, refusing high protein foods, but his appetite was good. His diet was based on starchy foods; he particularly liked crisps and chips but disliked sweet foods. He had frequent loose stools. Due to poor growth, additional energy was given as glucose polymer. Initial blood results showed low plasma concentrations of the dibasic amino acids; other EAA were also low suggesting inadequate protein intake. Low protein dietary treatment was continued and citrulline started. At 4 years he was confirmed to have GH deficiency and commenced on GH injections. Currently at age 13 years he still self-selects a low protein diet, preferring a very limited range of foods. He has citrulline supplements and is also supplemented with glucose polymer drinks, vitamins and minerals. He continues to experience episodes of abdominal pain, vomiting, diarrhoea and lethargy. A 6 week trial excluding milk, egg, wheat and soya made no difference to his gastrointestinal symptoms and so was discontinued. A recent abdominal ultrasound scan showed an echogenic pancreas, cause unknown; however, as there is a risk of pancreatitis this will be monitored. He has shown good catch-up growth on GH injections, height now 2nd–9th centile. His osteopenia is improving on annual DEXA scan. He has consistently low plasma lysine, ornithine and arginine concentrations and normal lipid levels. He is not on lysine supplements. He has an ER for illness.

Case study 2 Birmingham Children's Hospital NHS Foundation Trust, Birmingham

Three brothers of Pakistani origin (current ages 14, 4 and 2 years), born to consanguineous parents, have LPI. They are treated with citrulline, low protein diet (older boy 1 g/kg/day; younger boys 1.5 g/kg/day), overnight enteral tube feeding, comprehensive vitamin and mineral supplements and standard ER for age. They do not take lysine supplements. The index case presented at 2 years of age with poor development, feeding problems, elevated urine levels of lysine, glutamine, alanine, citrulline, ornithine and arginine, and elevated plasma lactate dehydrogenase and ferritin concentrations, with diagnosis later proved by mutation analysis. His younger brothers were diagnosed as high risk sibling screens in the neonatal period.

They all self-select low protein diets, have poor appetites, faltering growth (height and weight), osteopenia, mild developmental delay and hepatosplenomegaly. Their ammonia and glutamine concentrations have remained under good control without nitrogen scavenger drugs. Plasma lysine, ornithine, arginine concentrations vary from low to within normal range. The two younger boys have raised triglyceride levels. They do not have significant lung or renal impairment. The index case attends a mainstream school but with an educational statement. The younger siblings are not yet at school, but receive speech and language therapy support. Both younger boys have episodes of thrombocytopenia.

Gyrate atrophy of the choroid and retina

Genetics and biochemistry

Gyrate atrophy (GA), also known as ornithine amino transferase (OAT) deficiency, is an autosomal recessive disorder caused by mutations in the OAT gene (G91R) with the highest incidence in Finland (1 in 50 000). The gene is highly expressed in the neuroretina as well as the retinal pigment epithelium (RPE) but is universally expressed. It encodes for the mitochondrial matrix enzyme ornithine δ-aminotransferase (OAT) or ornithine-oxoacid aminotransferase [592]. Ornithine is synthesised from arginine in the urea cycle and metabolised by three enzymes, including OAT which converts ornithine into Δ^1-pyrroline-5-carboxylate. Pyridoxal phosphate (vitamin B_6) is the cofactor [592]. Plasma ornithine levels are raised (10–20 times normal) which is specifically toxic to RPE [593]. These high levels also explain the secondary creatine deficiency as ornithine inhibits arginine-glycine amidinotransferase (AGAT), the first enzymatic step in creatine synthesis [594]. High ornithine levels also cause lysinuria ultimately leading to reduced plasma lysine levels [595]. This is due to ornithine being a competitive antagonist for renal reuptake of lysine via the y+LAT-1 dibasic amino acid transporter. The OAT enzyme is also necessary for proline and hydroxyproline synthesis, non essential amino acids which are structural components of collagen [595].

Clinical presentation

Night blindness occurs in early childhood with constriction of visual field due to sharply demarcated round areas of chorioretinal atrophy in the periphery. Visual acuity worsens in the second or third decade of life. Progressive fundus destruction leads to loss of vision by the fifth decade. Cataracts and myopia are also reported [593]. Early diagnosis may allow initiation of treatment before irreversible damage occurs, but hyperornithinaemia is absent in neonates due to reversed enzymatic flux in early infancy in the direction of ornithine synthesis (which causes low plasma ornithine, citrulline and arginine levels and possible impaired urea cycle function); therefore without a strong family history the diagnosis may be overlooked. It often presents non-specifically with vomiting or feeding problems due to raised ammonia [596]. Glutamine, orotic acid and proline are also raised and the proline/citrulline ratio has been proposed for newborn screening to identify GA neonatally [597].

Long term high plasma ornithine levels (>600 µmmol/L) is reported to induce retinal toxicity whereas with mean ornithine levels of 250–400 µmmol/L progression of retinal degeneration is slower. Plasma ornithine levels <250 µmol/L do not produce retinal changes and intermittent or transient high ornithine levels do not lead to lesions [593]. High plasma ornithine also causes selective atrophy in type II skeletal muscle fibrils leading to muscle weakness. Reduced physical activity together with hypolysinaemia (which affects collagen formation and intestinal absorption and renal reabsorption of calcium) may lead to osteoporosis [595]. Developmental delay is also reported, possibly associated with creatine deficiency [594].

Dietary treatment

Arginine is the precursor of ornithine. An arginine restricted diet (by restricting natural protein) has been proposed to lower plasma ornithine levels to <200 µmol/L [598, 599]. It also normalises plasma lysine and may slow or halt the progression of visual loss in GA [600]. To significantly reduce ornithine levels, natural protein intake needs to be severely restricted and an EAA supplement given. In a cohort of 27 patients, 17 adhered to an arginine restricted diet over 15 years. The plasma ornithine levels of the patients on diet were half of those not on diet: 338 μmol/L versus 702 μmol/L. The authors suggested that for older patients who find dietary adherence more difficult, an aim for plasma ornithine levels below an average of 400–500 μmol/L will slow progression of chorioretinal lesions and visual loss [601]. Unfortunately, no dietary details were provided for this study, although an earlier paper by the same group describes the maintenance diet provided for one subject, a 35-year-old female, as 10–20 g natural protein plus 20 g EAA [598].

As Neonatal diagnosis of GA is rare [596], there are only a few case reports describing treatment in young children. One patient diagnosed at 12 years was given 15–25 g natural protein/day and an EAA mix of 55–65 g product/day (the actual amount of EAA not stated). Plasma ornithine levels decreased from >1000 μmol/L to under 100 μmol/L after 2 months [594]. A child (<4 years) with mild developmental delay was prescribed a diet of 0.8 g natural protein/kg which lowered ornithine level (at diagnosis) at nearly 1200 μmol/L to <700 μmol/L, which was maintained over 26 years [602]. Despite raised ornithine levels a delay of the progression in chorioretinal changes, as well as long term stability in the visual field, were reported. Successful long term adherence to dietary management was attributed to the absence of an amino acid supplement, which the child had refused.

The age at which dietary treatment commences is important for dietary adherence [603] and efficacy. Sibling pairs have been described, of whom the younger sibling of each pair was diagnosed earlier (<3 years) and started on the arginine restricted diet at a younger age (no details given). After 16–17 years on diet, each demonstrated a slower progression of lesions compared with their older siblings at the same age, who were diagnosed and started on treatment later (6 and 9 years) [604]. Careful monitoring of the diet to prevent nutritional deficiencies is required, checking growth as well as plasma amino acids (EAA, lysine). Monitoring plasma ornithine levels allows assessment of adherence to diet. A low protein diet is described on p. 456. Outcome data to confirm the efficacy of the treatment are limited due to long term progression of the

disease, the difficulty of adherence to a strict diet that starts from mid teenage years and phenotypic variation. One case diagnosed with ornithine levels <600 μmol/L at 22 years was reported to have very mild progression of visual loss after 17 years, despite never having had dietary treatment [592].

Dietary management is controversial. Treatment is based on case reports and adherence to a strict low protein diet can be difficult due to late diagnosis and introduction of dietary restriction in adolescence or adulthood. Due to the long term progression of the disorder it remains unclear whether lowering ornithine slows retinal deterioration.

Medicines and supplements

Supplementation of the cofactor vitamin B_6, as oral pyridoxine hydrochloride, may be beneficial but only 10% patients are responsive [599]. On diagnosis a 2–4 week trial of a pharmacological dose (300–500 mg/day) is recommended, with no change to dietary protein. Responsiveness is determined by measuring ornithine levels pre and post pyridoxine [599]. Ornithine, arginine, lysine and cysteine share a common renal transport system. Lysine supplements (10–15 g/day) may block ornithine and arginine reabsorption by the kidney, induce renal loss and hence lower plasma ornithine by 30%–39% [605]. This may allow a less strict low arginine diet [605–607]. Ahmet et al. [595] postulate that lysinuria and low plasma lysine levels, a feature of GA, may contribute to increased risk of osteoporosis by affecting cross ligament formation of collagen. Lysine supplements may correct this and in addition stimulate calcium absorption from the intestine and renal conservation of absorbed calcium. Other proposed therapeutic approaches include

- proline supplementation (3 g/day) which prevents ornithine cytotoxicity of cultured RPE cells in vitro but has not proven to be effective in vivo [593]
- creatine supplementation which may improve the neurological course of GA but no benefit has been seen on magnetic resonance imaging (MRI), possibly due to delayed diagnosis and administration in adults or inadequate doses (<2 g/day), equivalent to a normal dietary

intake. The authors question if a more therapeutic dose is indicated (400 mg/kg/day) [594].

The treatment of osteoporosis with calcium, vitamin D and bisphosphonates is described by Ahmet *et al.* [595].

Case studies

Case study 1 Great Ormond Street Hospital for Children NHS Foundation Trust, London

Two adolescent girls (diagnosed with GA at aged 9 and 11 years) were commenced on a very low protein diet (with EAA supplements); at diagnosis ornithine levels were >1000 μmol/L. The younger girl achieved plasma ornithine levels of 400–550 μmol/L on a diet of natural protein (0.4 g/kg/day) plus EAA mix (0.4–0.6 g/kg/day), together with 50 mg pyridoxine four times per day and no lysine supplements. For the older girl, dietary protein was initially restricted to 5 g/day but is now 15 g/day (0.4 g/kg/day), together with EAA mix (0.6 g/kg/day), lysine (10 g twice daily), creatine supplements (4 g twice daily) and pyridoxine (100 mg twice daily). Her plasma ornithine level ranges between 550–760 μmol/L. Both use low protein manufactured foods to achieve adequate energy intake and take vitamin and mineral supplements. Adherence to the strict diet is very difficult. At clinic appointments plasma amino acids including ornithine, lysine and arginine are monitored to assess adherence and nutritional adequacy of the diet. Arginine and lysine levels have been normal for the younger girl, but in the older girl both are usually low.

Case study 2 Royal Manchester Children's Hospital, Manchester

This case was published in 2005 by Cleary *et al.* [596]. Further dietary information is provided from the next 6 years.

A male infant, born to consanguineous Asian parents, developed vomiting, diarrhoea and mild transient hyperammonaemia at 13 days of age. His weight gain was poor and he required transfusions for severe anaemia; following one transfusion he became encephalopathic at 6 weeks. His plasma ammonia level was 812 μmol/L, feeds were stopped and he was treated with IV sodium benzoate and arginine. On reintroducing feeds, protein was restricted to 1.5 g/kg/day. At 7 weeks of age, plasma ornithine level was found to be raised at 680 μmol/L (as a neonate ornithine was found to be low), plasma glutamine and urinary orotic acid were also raised and homocitrulline was detected in the urine, indicating HHH syndrome as the possible diagnosis. However, at 32 weeks OAT deficiency was confirmed. Arginine supplements were discontinued and a low arginine diet given to provide 0.2 g natural protein/kg (4 g/day) supplemented with EAA mix (1 g/kg/day) to achieve the safe level of protein intake for age. For the first 6 years, he maintained plasma ornithine <200 μmol/L. At 14 years, he continues the same low protein diet; quantities are adjusted to meet requirements for weight and age. He has achieved normal growth (weight 10th–25th centile, height 25th–50th centile) and developmental milestones with no further episodes of hyperammonaemia. Plasma ornithine levels have been well controlled with 88% <400 μmol/L (of which 34% <200 μmol/L). His highest ornithine level since diagnosis was 528 μmol/L. He has astigmatism but only very mild retinal changes.

Case study 3 Birmingham Children's Hospital NHS Foundation Trust, Birmingham

A 9-year-old girl of Pakistani origin was diagnosed with OAT after a 4 year history of visual problems. Her plasma ornithine level was elevated at 797 μmol/L. She started a low protein/arginine diet (1 g/kg/day, 25 g protein/day) with 10 g natural protein and 15 g protein equivalent from EAA. For 6 months she was well controlled with plasma ornithine concentrations mainly <200 μmol/L. Dietary adherence then deteriorated and her ornithine increased to >400 μmol/L. Lysine supplementation (12 g/daily) was added. Her initial fasting ornithine concentrations on day 7 and 14 reduced to 179 μmol/L and 119 μmol/L; lysine concentrations increased to 400 μmol/L. No side effects were documented and the lysine was well tolerated. Short term lysine supplementation in combination with the low protein/arginine diet appeared effective in controlling plasma ornithine concentrations. However, at the age of 15 years adherence with lysine and EAA supplements is poor. Ornithine concentrations are mainly 600–700 µmol/L [606].

Guanidinoacetate methyltransferase deficiency

Genetics and biochemistry

Guanidinoacetate methyltransferase (GAMT) deficiency is one of a group of disorders termed creatine deficiency syndromes. GAMT and L-arginine-glycine amidinotransferase (AGAT) are two autosomal recessively inherited enzymatic defects involved in creatine synthesis . SLC6A8 or creatine transporter deficiency (CrT1) is an X-linked disorder of creatine transport. GAMT deficiency is rare and possibly underdiagnosed. In one study of 27 patients with GAMT deficiency the two most common mutations were c59G>C and c327G>A, but there was no obvious genotype–phenotype correlation [608]. Creatine is derived from the diet and endogenous production via AGAT and GAMT [609]. AGAT converts arginine and glycine into ornithine and guanidinoacetate (GAA), then GAMT catalyses the S-adenosyl-L-methionine dependent methylation of GAA to yield creatine [610]. The creatine, phosphocreatine, creatine kinase system maintains a supply of energy for use by skeletal muscle and, to a lesser extent, the brain [611]. A complete absence or a marked decrease of creatine in the CNS is common to all creatine deficiency syndromes. In GAMT deficiency plasma and urine levels of creatine are also low and GAA accumulates in all body fluids [612]. Levels of GAA are raised in plasma (10–20 times normal), urine (2–200 times normal) [613] and cerebrospinal fluid (CSF) (100–300 times) irrespective of phenotype [608, 614].

Clinical presentation

GAMT deficiency is generally more severe than the other creatine disorders [614]. The clinical features are non-specific and have a broad spectrum; the most severe involve basal ganglia changes [613] and may resemble mitochondrial encephalopathies [615]. The pathogenesis of the disorder may involve both creatine deficiency and GAA toxicity which itself is epileptogenic and neurotoxic [610, 611]. In a group of 27 patients onset of clinical symptoms ranged from early infancy to childhood (3–6 months to 3 years) with children presenting with developmental delay, lack of speech, muscular hypotonia, weakness, extrapyramidal movement and epilepsy. Due to the non-specific nature of the presenting symptoms mean age at diagnosis was 12.3 years in this group [608]. This retrospective review highlighted that 78% had severe intellectual disability (hyperactivity, autism, self-injurious behaviour and speech fewer than 10 words). Seizures have been reported from infancy onwards and can be intractable in severe cases [613].

Medicines

The aim of treatment is to increase CSF creatine levels and decrease GAA levels. Therapy can be monitored by measuring both metabolites in plasma and urine while CSF levels can be monitored non-invasively by brain magnetic resonance spectroscopy (MRS) studies [613].

Creatine monohydrate is given in pharmacological doses (300–400 mg/kg in 3–6 divided doses) to replenish the cerebral creatine levels [616] although case reports suggest doses up to 1200 mg/kg may be needed [608, 610, 612]. On creatine supplementation alone cerebral creatine levels normalise, although a much larger increase in plasma levels (20-fold) suggests a limited transport across the BBB [609, 610]. In 18 patients on creatine supplementation alone GAA levels were only partially reduced (creatine regulates GAA synthesis by feedback inhibition of AGAT) [608]. In one patient initial neurological improvements in dyskinesia, muscle hypotonia, seizures, alertness and behaviour were noted. However, these clinical symptoms then deteriorated and seizures recurred [610]. Intellectual disability did not improve in one cohort started on creatine supplementation, possibly due to irreversible brain damage prior to treatment [608, 614]. The reason for this may be only the partial reduction of GAA in CNS serum and urine on creatine supplementation [610]. Raised GAA may contribute to ongoing clinical symptoms, especially epilepsy [612]. In addition to creatine supplementation dietary restriction of arginine and ornithine supplementation is proposed [610], as described below.

Sodium benzoate may contribute to a decrease in GAA formation in two ways: by decreasing arginine formation by reducing the flux through the urea cycle; and by reducing glycine by removing its amino group. Glycine is a substrate in the arginine:glycine amidinotransferase reaction which forms GAA [610].

Dietary treatment

Dietary restriction of arginine, which is the rate limiting substrate for GAA synthesis, further reduced GAA levels in all body fluids and CSF, although not to normal levels, and was found to improve seizures and alertness in one subject [610]. The diet has subsequently been reported with some success in retrospective case reviews and case studies, restricting arginine to 0.2–0.7 g protein/kg/day and supplementing with an arginine free EAA mixture (0.4–1 g/kg/day) [608, 613–615].

In an attempt to further reduce production of GAA, the supplementation of low dose ornithine (100 mg/kg) enabled dietary arginine to be decreased (the rate limiting substrate for GAA synthesis) without compromise of nitrogen detoxification [610]. With this treatment GAA concentration was reduced by about half in plasma, urine and CSF in some patients [608, 610, 614]. Ornithine may have a role in counteracting arginine maintaining mechanisms [610]. In theory a higher ornithine dose (800 mg/kg) may reduce GAA synthesis by two methods: competitive inhibition of AGAT activity, the rate limiting enzyme in GAA synthesis [608], although this did not result in lowering GAA in one subject [616]; or inhibition of renal tubular reabsorption of arginine by competitive inhibition of the dibasic tubular amino acid transporter, e.g. ornithine or lysine [610].

One patient diagnosed as a neonate has received this treatment and shown no symptoms after 14 months. The author suggests that pre symptomatic treatment, preferably in the neonatal period, may prevent symptoms and improve the long term cognitive outcome [614]. In a sibling pair, the second child was treated from 3 weeks of age (400 mg creatine/kg, 400–800 mg/kg ornithine, 100 mg/kg sodium benzoate plus 0.6 g/kg natural protein to restrict arginine and 1 g/kg EAA). She is reported to be developing normally at aged 14 months unlike her older brother who is developmentally delayed and has seizures [614].

Case study

Morris *et al.* [615] reported on a 10-month-old female infant presented with hypotonia and global development delay, poor feeding, poor weight and head growth and nasogastric feeding was required. At 12 months she developed seizures and mild choreoathetoid movements and was unable to sit without support.

On investigation GAMT activity was found to be negligible and she was diagnosed with GAMT deficiency. Treatment with creatine (0.5 g/kg/day) was started at 2 years and the seizures and movement disorder resolved except during febrile illness. Head growth improved and by 3 years she was able to stand and to run at 5 years, but she did not speak and concentration was poor. She continued to be tube fed.

At 6 years, dietary treatment (arginine free EAA mix 0.65 g/kg/day with 0–0.2 g natural protein/kg/day and ornithine supplements 20 mg/kg five times daily) was introduced which partially reduced the GAA levels. This treatment also lowered the plasma arginine levels which were maintained, like ornithine, in the normal range. Clinically, the patient became calmer and responded to simple requests and remained seizure free on clonazepam. However, she still had no expressive language.

An update (given by personal communication, Alder Hey Children's Hospital, Liverpool): she is nearly 15 years old, is mobile but with severe developmental delay and behaviour can be very challenging. Seizures remain a problem to control requiring sodium valproate, clonazepam, leviteracitam and zonisamide. In addition she requires anti-reflux medication and a fibre supplement and lactulose for constipation. Mum has reported that she feels the treatment is beneficial.

GAA levels, creatine and plasma amino acids (ornithine, arginine and EAA in particular) are monitored 4–6 monthly. Raised ornithine levels are seen with higher doses of ornithine (maximum 300 mg/kg/day). Creatine (25 g/day) is given separately. The feed is given via a gastrostomy (EAA mix, Energivit and ornithine) and as dietary intake remains poor (small amounts of crisps, chips and fruit) a dietary arginine restriction of 15 mg/kg/day is easily achieved [615].

Alkaptonuria

Genetics and biochemistry

Alkaptonuria (AKU) is an autosomal recessive inherited disorder caused by mutations in the HGD gene [617] which codes for homogentisate 1,2-dioxygenase (homogentisic acid oxidase, HGO). This enzyme is expressed mainly in the liver and kidneys and is one of six enzymes involved in tyrosine and phenylalanine metabolism, its action converting homogentisic acid (HGA) into maleylacetoacetic acid (Fig. 17.12). The mutation type has no correlation with the level of HGA excretion and/or severity of disease [618].

Alkaptonuria affects 1 in 250 000 to 1 million people worldwide, although the incidence is higher in some countries, e.g. Slovakia and the Dominican Republic [618]. The enzyme defect leads to accumulation of HGA and its oxidation product benzoquinone acetic acid (BQA) in plasma. This causes tissue injury by reducing the cross-linkage of collagen fibres in connective tissue and cartilage resulting in progressive and degenerative changes and accelerated bone loss [617].

Clinical presentation

Increased plasma HGA levels result in homogentisic aciduria which is present at birth. Urine darkens on exposure to air due to the oxidation of HGA to benzoquinones and may enable early diagnosis due to nappy discolouration [619]. In a study of 58 patients with AKU (aged 4–80 years), 21% were diagnosed at <1 year; the mean age at diagnosis of the other 46 patients was 29 years. Plasma HGA ranged from 3.0 to 27.8 µg/mL which is normally undetectable and urine HGA levels were increased by a factor of 300 to over 3 mmol/mmol creatinine (normal <0.01) [618]. Deposition of polymers of oxidised HGA (BQA) in connective tissues leads to melanin like pigmentation (ochronosis) of the skin, sclera and cartilage over 20–30 years. Joint pain which is the main complication is due to degenerative ochronic arthropathies arising in the 3rd–5th decade affecting the spine and large joints of the hips, shoulders and knees. Formation of renal and prostatic stones and calcification of the mitral valves and coronary arteries may also occur [617, 620].

Dietary treatment

A low protein diet, restricting phenylalanine and tyrosine, has been proposed to reduce HGA excretion (an intermediary of tyrosine and phenylalanine metabolism), to decrease deposition of ochronotic pigment and delay arthropathy. However, long term efficacy of the diet in improving symptoms in AKU is unknown. A significant reduction of urinary HGA in six children <12 years was reported when a low protein diet (1 g/kg/day) was followed for 8 days compared with a high protein intake (3–5 g/kg/day), but not in six older patients (>12 years). The author suggests a reduced protein intake (1–1.5 g/kg/day) might be beneficial for younger patients only, particularly as behavioural problems around diet and adherence were reported by the older group [619]. In a 5 month infant treated with a low protein diet, HGA excretion was substantially reduced [621]. This finding was not reported in an adult [622].

A low protein diet may be required in conjunction with low dose nitisinone (see below), which may cause tyrosine levels to rise and lead to corneal erosions, as seen in tyrosinaemia type II (HTII). Adherence to the dietary restrictions may be difficult in adulthood as has been reported in clinical trials establishing nitisinone dosage [623].

Medicines

Symptom control is currently the main treatment for AKU. Nitisinone or NTBC (2-(2-nitro-4-trifluoromethylbenzoyl)-1,3-cyclohexanedione) has been licensed to treat tyrosinaemia type I (HTI) since 1992, and has been proposed as a potential treatment in AKU [624]. Given at low doses, NTBC inhibits the enzyme 4-hydroxyphenylpyruvate dioxygenase, which converts 4-hydroxyphenylpyruvate to HGA (the second step in the tyrosine degradation pathway). Urinary excretion of HGA is reduced by 94%, using a significantly smaller dose of NTBC than in HTI [623, 625]. However, the long term efficacy and side effects of the therapy are not known. In a 3 year randomised controlled trial of nitisinone in AKU patients (adults) in the USA, protein intake was not controlled (70 g/day) and tyrosine levels increased up to 1500 µmol/L (average 800 µmol/L). Side effects were few and only one subject experienced corneal changes. No recommendations were made for a low protein diet or target tyrosine levels but the authors did identify the need to investigate the use of nitisinone in younger patients [625].

A long term clinical trial in the UK is studying efficacy and long term effects of nitisinone as a treatment for AKU and the need for dietary protein restriction. It is funded by the European Commission (www.alkaptonuria.info). The National Alkaptonuria Centre (NAC) opened in June 2012 at the Royal Liverpool University Hospital for patients with AKU aged over 16 years (www.akusociety.org). Patients participating in the trial attend the centre for 4 days for assessment, commencement of nitisinone treatment and dietary advice. The dietary aim at NAC is a moderate protein intake (0.6–1 g/kg/day) initially together with avoidance of aspartame (a source of phenylalanine). No target plasma tyrosine levels have been recommended although clinical signs of high tyrosine are monitored 3 monthly. Tyrosine levels of eight patients treated with nitisinone for 3 months are reported; all have increased from normal levels to 300–950 μmol/L. One patient developed corneal symptoms when plasma tyrosine increased from 47 to 529 μmol/L; in response, protein intake was decreased from 0.8 to 0.6 g/kg/day [626].

Isolated sulphite oxidase deficiency and molybdenum cofactor deficiency

Genetics and biochemistry

Isolated sulphite oxidase deficiency (ISOD) and molybdenum cofactor deficiency are autosomal recessive disorders which affect sulphite oxidase activity. The literature does not always clearly distinguish between the two conditions [627]. The cause of decreased sulphite oxidase (SO) activity can be

- an isolated enzyme defect (ISOD) due to mutations in the SUOX gene, which is very rare. The gene is strongly expressed in the liver, kidney, skeletal muscle, heart, placenta as well as the cerebral cortex [627]
- secondary to defects in the synthesis of its molybdenum cofactor, which is synthesised

from guanosine triphosphate via four enzymatic steps. Patients are classified as type A and B, with about two-thirds of patients being type A [628] who are unable to form cyclic pyranopterin monophosphate (cPMP) [629]. Molybdenum is also the cofactor for two other enzymes, xanthine oxidase and aldehyde oxidase

Sulphite oxidase is a mitochondrial enzyme which catalyses the last step in the oxidation of the sulphur atom of cysteine into sulphate. This involves the transfer of electrons from sulphites into the electron transport chain via cytochrome c. The enzyme oxidises potentially toxic sulphite to sulphate. Catabolism of the sulphur containing amino acids methionine, homocysteine and cysteine contributes to the bulk of the sulphite load in the body. Deficiency of SO results in the accumulation of sulphite and of its detoxification products S-sulphocysteine, thiosulphate and taurine which are excreted in urine, while sulphate production itself is decreased. Plasma levels of total homocysteine and cystine levels are always low [627]. Molybdenum cofactor deficiency, although clinically similar to ISOD, can be differentiated if uric acid is almost undetectable (replaced by hypoxanthine and xanthine) and plasma urate level is low [630] although this may be normal in mild phenotypes [631].

The pathogenesis of both disorders is considered to be due to the accumulation of neurotoxic sulphites and their metabolites, hence the similarity of their clinical picture. *In vitro* studies suggest that endogenous sulphite reduces ATP synthesis in mitochondria and contributes to cerebral infarction or stroke like events [631, 632]. Sulphite accumulation also triggers the reduction of cystine, to cysteine which then forms S-sulphocysteine, a potential agonist of glutamate receptors, possibly explaining the seizures [627, 633]. Progressive white matter loss may be caused by sulphite accumulation and/or decreased synthesis of sulphatides due to deficiency of sulphates affecting myelination in the brain [631, 632]. Early postnatal radiology reports have described chronic changes indicating damage may begin *in utero* despite the protective effects of maternal clearance of sulphites, which appears to protect growth parameters *in utero* [627, 631].

Clinical presentation

Both disorders may present neonatally with severe neurological dysfunction including intractable seizures, hypotonia and respiratory difficulties. Neonates are irritable with high pitched crying and have feeding difficulties. If they survive the neonatal period they often develop progressive hyperkinesia, microcephaly, developmental delay, verbal dyspraxia and additionally are dysmorphic and have visual impairment due to lens dislocation. Premature death may occur in early childhood [627]. Patients with milder symptoms may present later, around 6 months to 2 years of age, possibly triggered by an intercurrent illness. As late onset presentations may not include the characteristic signs of seizures or lens dislocation, diagnosis may be delayed [632]. It is reported that patients with molybdenum cofactor deficiency may survive into the third decade of life [631]. This may be the same for ISOD but reports of long term outcome are not available.

Dietary treatment

In two case reports of neonatal presentations of ISOD, dietary restriction of sulphur amino acids (methionine, cystine) to decrease the toxic metabolites (thiosulphate and S-sulphocysteine) was attempted but neither case showed either biochemical or neurological improvement [627,634]. In another neonatal presentation of ISOD, decreased irritability on dietary treatment was reported but no neurological improvement [635].

In a 3-month-old with molybdenum cofactor deficiency on dietary treatment of a low methionine diet (30 mg/kg/day), supplemented with cysteine (70 mg/kg/day), clinical improvements were noted in head growth, neurodevelopment and decreased irritability. When treatment stopped after 2 months due to parental non adherence to the diet, urinary sulphites, undetectable on treatment, increased to diagnostic levels and clinical deterioration was reported [636]. It was suggested that supplementation of the methionine restricted diet with cysteine was necessary as excessively low cysteine levels, resulting from the diet, may inhibit the excretion of abnormal sulphur containing metabolites to which cysteine can itself bond. This in turn reduces sulphite production seen by the lack of urinary sulphites. However, this finding has not subsequently been repeated [634].

Published case reports in late onset presentations describe clinical improvements in patients given a low protein diet without cysteine supplementation. The low protein diet in these case studies provided 0.9–1.3 g/kg/day natural protein (restricting methionine and cystine) plus a synthetic amino acid product free from methionine and cystine (0.9–1.3 g/kg/day) [627,632,637].

Medicines

Thiamin is destroyed by sulphites *in vitro* and in animal studies and supplementation may be required [627]. Pyridoxine supplementation may be beneficial due to documented low CSF pyridoxal phosphate (PLP) in one patient and sulphite reactivity with PLP [630].

Medicines may be given to control seizures: dextromethorphan to block possible sulfocysteine excitotoxicity at NMDA (N-methyl-D-aspartate) receptors [627].

Injections of cPMP, a precursor of the molybdenum cofactor, may be a potential new therapy for those sufferers of type A molybdenum cofactor deficiency to restore molybdenum cofactor dependent enzyme activities. In studies of a mouse model, affected mice treated with cPMP developed normally, achieved weight gain, adulthood and fertility. On withdrawal of treatment, the mice died within 14 days [633]. In a neonate, all biochemical markers were restored to nearly normal within 2 weeks of commencing daily treatment and they became more alert with reduced convulsions. At 18 months, no evidence of progressive neurological deficit was reported [629]. However, experience suggests that this must be instituted within the first few days of life for a definable improvement in neurological outcome to occur (personal communication).

Glycine encephalopathy or non ketotic hyperglycinaemia

Genetics and biochemistry

Glycine encephalopathy or non ketotic hyperglycinaemia (NKH) is an autosomal recessively inherited disorder of glycine degradation. The genetic defect may be located in one of three genes: AMT (15%–20%), GLDC (75%–80%) or GCSH (very few), which code for the glycine cleavage enzyme system (GCS), a mitochondrial enzyme complex found in the brain, liver, kidney and placenta [638–640]. The prevalence of NKH is estimated at 1 in 60 000 but is higher in Finland (1 in 12 000) due to a founder effect [641]. NKH is due to a deficiency in the GCS which comprises four different protein components [642]. GCS catalyses the oxidative conversion of glycine into carbon dioxide and ammonia. Deficiency of GCS causes raised glycine in plasma, urine and CSF. An increased CSF:plasma glycine ratio (>0.08; normal <0.02) is used as the diagnostic cut-off as elevated plasma glycine may be caused by disorders of organic acids; organic acid analysis is normal in NKH [639]. Carbon dioxide production can also be used to confirm diagnosis by measurement of 13CO-glycine breath tests [643]. Accumulation of glycine in the CNS activates NMDA excitatory receptors in the cerebral cortex brainstem causing seizures and autonomic dysfunction including apnoeas and hiccoughs, while the expression of NMDA receptors in the spinal cord is thought to contribute to hyptonia [640].

Clinical presentation

The most common presenting symptoms are lethargy, hypotonia, myoclonic seizures, progressing to coma and death neonatally in the most severe form, which is more common in girls. Milder variants with various degrees of developmental delay are known. Some neonates make developmental progress [641]. Although severe NKH is often associated with high plasma glycine levels, low levels do not necessarily exclude a severe outcome. A classification system dividing patients into either a severe or attenuated form, based on the historical phenotypes of 45 patients, has been proposed to facilitate prediction of long term outcome and need for counselling in the newborn period [642]. These two groups are further classified by age of onset, i.e. neonatal (<1 week, 39 patients) or infantile (>1 week, 6 patients). 85% neonates had the classic severe form of NKH and two-thirds of all neonatal presentations had apnoeas requiring

ventilatory support. The milder or attenuated form was reported in 15% of neonates and half of the infantile group who presented later in infancy (3–6 months). Prognosis in the severe form is poor and patients die as neonates or by 5 years [642]. Patients with the attenuated form may survive longer [642] and may be associated with developmental progress [638, 641, 642, 644]. A further group have no abnormal symptoms as neonates but may present from 1 year to adulthood with development of varying degrees of neurological symptoms including attention deficit hyperactivity disorder and intermittent lethargy. These have have a far better outcome with some near normal [645].

Medicines

Medical therapy aims to decrease plasma glycine concentrations and block the effect of glycine at neurotransmitter receptors. High dose sodium benzoate (200–750 mg/kg/day) may reduce plasma glycine to a low normal level (100–260 μmol/L) as it conjugates with glycine to form hippurate which is excreted in urine [642]. The CNS glycine level may be reduced but not normalised even when plasma glycine is less than normal [646]. A glycine index or balance was proposed as an outcome parameter measure. The glycine index was calculated by subtracting dietary glycine intake from molar requirement of benzoate dose necessary to normalise glycine. The neurodevelopmental outcome of high index patients was reported to be worse [647].

Some authors report that sodium benzoate is rarely effective [639] but this may be due to inadequate benzoate doses [642]. Benzoate may cause gastrointestinal side effects and doses exceeding 750 mg/kg are associated with toxicity, e.g. renal tubular dysfunction, glycosuria, hypokalaemia, hypocalcaemia which can be fatal [647]. Low plasma carnitine levels were noted with benzoate therapy in three of four patients, possibly due to the formation and excretion of benzoylcarnitine. On supplementation, plasma free carnitine normalised and showed a tendency to increase glycine conjugation of benzoate and reduce the plasma glycine pool. Close monitoring of benzoate, carnitine and glycine is recommended [646]. Treatment with NMDA receptor antagonists, e.g. dextromethorphan, in conjunction with sodium benzoate may decrease seizures and increase alertness, particularly in the newborn period and in the attenuated form of NKH [641,642]. Valproic acid, which can raise glycine levels, is contraindicated [645].

Dietary treatment

There is little evidence to support a low protein diet alone as treatment of NKH; however, it has been proposed that a low glycine (and possibly low serine) intake will reduce the plasma glycine pool and therefore the requirement for benzoate [647]. It was suggested that a glycine free formula might be beneficial; it remains unclear whether this treatment affects outcome. If a glycine free amino acid supplement is given it is essential that it is given in conjunction with an adequate natural protein intake, as there is a risk of amino acid deficiency (the author has experience of one patient on supplements alone who had a low albumin and became oedematous).

A clinical survey of 45 children reported that a reduced plasma glycine was independent of the severity of NKH in a few children on a protein restricted diet. No details of the diet are provided, and as it may have been combined with other medical treatment, e.g. sodium benzoate, it is not possible to make conclusions about its effectiveness. A side effect of the diet was poor adherence, protein deficiency and vitamin B_{12} deficiency [642]. In a single case report, a late onset patient with NKH presented at 2.5 years with behavioural and attention difficulties following an early history of delayed speech and motor skills. Her plasma and CSF glycine were raised and a combination of a low protein diet (1 g/kg/day) and sodium benzoate was reported to lower plasma and CSF glycine levels with some improvement in behaviour. This further improved with the addition of imipramine, an NMDA receptor antagonist. No improvements in behaviour were noted on diet alone [648].

Success of dietary therapy in reducing seizures in a neonatal presentation has recently been reported. A low protein diet and glycine free formula was given, although no details of the diet are provided. L-carnitine (500 mg/day), folic acid, riboflavin and niacin were also given [649]. Giving a classical ketogenic diet (KD) (p. 363) was described in three patients who presented neonatally and a decrease

in seizure frequency was noted. The mechanism of action is not known and the authors hypothesised that the KD may increase the number of mitochondria and so restore hippocampal ATP. This has yet to be confirmed [640].

Nutritional support is likely to be necessary due to lethargy, hypotonia and seizures causing feeding difficulties; high energy supplements are given. Assessment of energy requirements needs to take these symptoms into consideration. Tube feeding may be necessary due to inadequate oral intake or unsafe swallow.

Trimethylaminuria or 'fish odour syndrome'

Genetics and biochemistry

Primary trimethylaminuria (TMAU) is an autosomal recessive disorder caused by mutations in the FM03 (a mixed function oxidase) gene which is located in a cluster of six FMO genes. There are two common mutations reported: P153L and E305X. Homozygosity or compound heterozygosity are associated with moderate or severe TMAU resulting from a significant reduction in the activity of the hepatic enzyme, flavin containing mono-oxygenase type 3 (FM03) [650]. The incidence is thought to be 1 in 100 to 1 in 1000 [651]. TMAU may be due to either

- decreased FMO3 activity due to genetic (primary TMAU), physiological (hormone) or environmental (inhibitory chemicals) factors
- substrate overload of FMO3 activity: excess dietary precursors of trimethylamine (TMA) or variations in gut flora resulting in increased TMA production (secondary TMAU) [652]

FMO3 catalyses the oxidation of TMA to non odorous trimethylamine N-oxide (TMAO) in the liver for excretion in urine. TMA is derived from bacterial degradation of dietary choline, lecithin and TMAO (from seafood and marine fish) in the gut [653]. Individuals with TMAU are unable to oxidise TMA which is very volatile and has a strong ammonia like odour which is excreted in excess in breath, urine, sweat and reproductive fluids. Diagnosis can be confirmed by measuring the urinary ratio of TMA:TMAO of a sample following a high substrate meal [654]. In primary TMAU, the ratio is raised (normal ratio 0.05–0.21). In severe TMAU more than 40% of total TMA is excreted as free unmetabolised TMA; in mild TMAU this percentage is 10%–39%. Unaffected individuals and heterozygotes (carriers) under normal dietary conditions excrete <10% as TMA [654] where normal TMA excretion is 2.5–10.8 μmol/mmol creatinine. In secondary TMAU, both TMA and TMAO excretion are increased and the urinary ratio is normal [655]. A urinary concentration of free TMA of >10 μg/mL (18–20 μmol/mmol creatinine) correlates with a urinary output of TMA of about 15–20 mg/day and represents a threshold for the presence of the odour [655]. The preferred method to measure urine samples for TMA and TMAO is gas chromatography mass spectrometry in specialist laboratories. Choline is required for structural integrity and signalling functions of cell membranes and it directly affects cholinergic neurotransmission, transmembrane signalling and lipid transport and metabolism. It can be produced endogenously and is also derived from dietary sources.

Clinical presentation

Excess TMA is not physically harmful and there are no physical symptoms; however the 'rotting fish smell' associated with TMA, which is not always noticed by the affected individual, can lead to ostracism at school causing social debilitation and psychological problems. In primary TMAU, symptoms have been reported in infancy if a breast feeding mother has recently consumed a choline rich meal [650], on changing formula milk to one with a higher choline content [656] or early in childhood when the child is weaned and foods containing high amounts of choline or TMAO are introduced [653]. Early transient cases are thought to be due to immaturity of FMO3 expression and/or precursor overload and symptoms disappear as children mature [652, 655]. The severity of symptoms may be variable and episodic, commonly becoming more apparent on puberty in females, worsening before and during menstruation. TMAU is likely to be underdiagnosed due to social reluctance to discuss 'personal hygiene' issues, but referrals to specialist centres may increase following enhanced public awareness via media exposure and use of the internet (www.tmau.org.uk).

Acquired TMAU may occur in adults with no history of the disorder as a result of hepatitis, possibly due to altering the expression or activity of the FMO3 enzyme [652]. Transient TMAU may result from substrate overload of FMO3 activity following either excess intake of dietary precursors of TMA and/or excess intestinal TMA production by gut flora. Bacterial overgrowth syndrome, often associated with complications following bowel surgery and other bowel disorders, severe liver disease and chronic kidney disease, can be associated with changed gut flora [652].

Dietary treatment

It is advisable to avoid foods if they are found to exacerbate the odour and may include those rich in choline, TMAO, lecithin or vegetables from the brassica family.

Choline can be synthesised endogenously from phosphatidylethanolamine but it is also an essential nutrient. Dietary deficiency may lead to liver damage, neurological disease and carcinogenesis and dietary reference intakes for choline are based on observed and experimental estimates from the USA [654]. In adult cohort studies, there is a wide variation of choline intake but it is estimated to be about 660 mg for men and 408 mg for women [657].

It is unclear whether a normal dietary choline intake provokes symptoms, as only excess choline passing into the colon is metabolised to TMA by gut bacteria [654]. In TMAU any dietary restriction of choline should aim to minimise the odour without inducing deficiency symptoms. If dietary treatment is successful, assessment of dietary choline intake is recommended to ensure choline requirements for age are met [658]. Adequate daily intakes for choline are: 0–6 months, 125 mg; 6–12 months, 150 mg; 1–3 years, 200 mg; 4–8 years, 250 mg; 9–13 years, 375 mg; boys 14–18 years, 550 mg; girls 14–18 years, 400 mg [659]. There are limited data to assess whether dietary choline is essential at all life stages and if choline requirement may be met by endogenous synthesis at some stages [659].

The USA Department of Agriculture database [660] is a useful resource for the choline content of foods (www.ars.usda.gov/nutrientdata). Using the 2004 edition of this database, Busby *et al.* listed

Table 17.71 Choline content of selected foods reported to be high in choline compared with some similar alternatives [658].

Food (portion size) – reported as high choline sources	Choline content (mg)	Food (portion size) – reported as lower choline alternatives	Choline content (mg)
1 egg (50 g)	125	Egg white (50 g)	0.5
Egg yolk (50 g)	340		
Beef liver (100 g) pan fried	420	Beef mince (100 g)	67
Chicken liver (100 g) pan fried	330	Chicken roasted no skin (100 g)	66
Cod (100 g)*	84	Tuna* canned in water (100 g)	29
Prawns (100 g)*	81		
All Bran, Branflakes (100 g)	49, 31	Cornflakes (100 g)	4
Wholewheat bread (50 g)	13	White bread (50 g)	7
Soya milk, skimmed milk (100 mL)	24, 18	Full fat milk (100 mL)	14
Cheese (100 g): cream, Cheddar	27, 17		
Mayonnaise (30 g)	7		
Fruit, plain or low fat yoghurt (100 g)	15		
Peanuts, peanut butter (50 g)	25, 30	Potato crisps (28 g)	3
Brussels sprouts (50 g)	20	Carrots (50 g)	4
Beans, peas (50 g)	16, 14		
Broccoli (50 g)	20		

*Also source of trimethylamine N-oxide (TMAO).

choline rich foods and some alternative foods, dividing foods into categories based on low, moderate and high choline content [658] (Table 17.71). However, on comparing similar portion sizes, it is unclear why some foods are regularly reported as having a high choline content, e.g. brassicas, peas, dairy products, skimmed milk, peanuts, some wholegrain and soya products.

Other choline sources which may need to be avoided include lecithin or phosphatidylcholine (13% choline by weight) found in emulsifiers (E322) added to mayonnaise, ice cream, chocolate and other manufactured foods. However, the amount of free TMA released from these may be limited [653, 661]. Marine fish and seafood including octopus, squid, lobster, crab, prawns [655] are a moderate source of choline but are of more significance as a rich source of TMAO [661]. In addition, brassicas may inhibit hepatic FMO3 and the effectiveness of the diet may be improved by their restriction [654].

Riboflavin is a cofactor of FMO3 and supplementation may enhance enzyme activity. A pharmacological dose of 90–200 mg/day in adults may reduce the TMA:TMAO ratio [662]. In the author's centre 100 mg/day is given in a single or divided dose. Large doses may cause gastrointestinal upset [655]. Choline is a methyl donor and, together with folate, is required for the methylation of homocysteine to methionine to maintain low homocysteine levels. On a low choline diet, there may be an increased requirement for folate to ensure adequate methyl groups are available [658].

Dietary management of this condition requires a sensible, pragmatic approach, an initial assessment to identify potentially rich sources of choline or TMAO in an individual's diet and advice given to reduce portion sizes of foods if significantly contributing to intake. This dietary treatment may alleviate symptoms in some but not all individuals and not all of the time. A combination of medical and other approaches may be necessary.

Medicines

Metronidazole, amoxicillin and neomycin can be prescribed to eliminate TMA producing bacteria particularly during times associated with increased TMA production (stress, exercise, infection, menstruation or due to dietary relaxation). Neomycin has been reported to be most effective, reducing TMA by 50% [653]. Short courses (1–2 weeks) of antibiotic therapy are given to minimise the development of bacterial resistance [662, 663]. After a course of antibiotics, probiotics may be given to encourage growth of non TMA producing bacteria, e.g. lactobacilli and bifidobacteria, instead of TMA producing bacteria [662]. Other therapies include

- low pH (5.5–6.5) soaps and skin creams to neutralise alkaline TMA and create non volatile salt, which can be washed off
- deodorising tablets or 'internal deodorants', e.g. activated charcoal or copper–chlorophyllin complex (marketed as Nullo) which are not absorbed across the gut and bind irreversibly to TMA in the gut to facilitate its elimination [650]

Hyperinsulinism/hyperammonaemia syndrome

Genetics and biochemistry

Hyperinsulinism/hyperammonaemia (HIHA) syndrome is caused by dominant missense mutations in the GLUD1 gene, which encodes for the intra-mitochondrial matrix enzyme glutamate dehydrogenase (GDH). Most patients are carriers of a *de novo* mutation, but some familial cases show autosomal dominant inheritance [664]. GDH is highly expressed in the liver, pancreatic β cells, kidney and brain [665]. GDH catalyses the reversible oxidative deamination of glutamate to α-ketoglutarate and ammonia, using NAD or NADP as a cofactor. It is a key regulator of amino acid and ammonia metabolism. GDH is allosterically activated by leucine and ADP and is inhibited by guanadino triphosphate (GTP). In HIHA syndrome the sensitivity of the enzyme to allosteric inhibition by GTP and ATP is reduced, leading to a 'gain' in function, with increased leucine induced glutamate oxidation to α-ketoglutarate. In the pancreatic cells, α-ketoglutarate enters the TCA cycle leading to excessive insulin secretion by the β cells, seen clinically as postprandial hypoglycaemia following leucine containing protein rich meals [665]. Unlike urea cycle enzyme deficiency disorders, the mild hyperammonaemia neither falls with fasting nor rises excessively with protein intake [665].

It has been proposed that the mild persistent state of hyperammonaemia may be due to decreased urea cycle activity via two mechanisms: increased GDH activity which causes increased ammonia production from glutamate and the defective regulation of GDH which leads to excessive oxidation of glutamate. By decreasing the glutamate pool and thereby decreasing NAG (*N*-acetyl glutamate) production, the urea cycle is affected. NAG is the activator of carbamoyl phosphate synthase, the first rate limiting step of ammonia detoxification [665, 666]. Treberg *et al.* propose an alternative mechanism of increased renal ammoniagenesis following systemic activation of GDH by a leucine analogue. Mild systemic hyperammonia was demonstrated in Sprague-Dawley rats and, although ammonia levels measured in the hepatic vein were normal, an increased concentration of ammonia was noted in the renal vein *in vivo* [667].

Clinical presentation

HIHA syndrome is the second most common form of congenital hyperinsulinism (CHI). Presentation tends to be later in infancy (mean age 23 weeks) [668]. Once weaning onto solid foods occurs, when fasting times and dietary protein intakes increase, there are recurrent episodes of (postprandial) hypoglycaemia. Plasma ammonia levels are mildly raised (2–5 times upper limit of normal) and plasma amino acid levels, including glutamine, are normal. Older patients do not describe the symptoms of headache, lethargy or nausea often associated with hyperammonaemia [665]. In a study of 16 patients with GLUD1 gene mutations, 15 presented with seizures and 43% of these, all children (aged 1.5–18 years), developed epilepsy [668]. The electroencephalogram (EEG) pattern of generalised epilepsy is thought not to be associated with ammonia toxicity [666].

Dietary treatment

Diazoxide alone is usually effective [667] and dietary treatment is largely unnecessary. Families may be advised to avoid meals containing only protein foods to minimise risk of postprandial hypoglycaemia [665]. A protein restricted diet, limiting daily leucine intake to 200 mg (4 g protein) [669], is not recommended at the author's centre.

Medicine

Diazoxide (5–15 mg/kg/day), a KATP channel agonist, is given to control both fasting and protein induced hypoglycaemia. Alternative therapies for mild hyperammonaemia, sodium benzoate and N-carbamoyl glutamate (carglumic acid), which is a carbamoyl phosphate synthase activator, have not resulted in lowering ammonia levels [666]; management does not include medicines to control hyperammonaemia. Seizure control medicines may be required in patients with epilepsy.

Case studies

Case study 1 Great Ormond Street Hospital for Children NHS Foundation Trust, London

A girl presented at age 7 months with seizures and low blood glucose levels and she was diagnosed to have HIHA syndrome. She self-selected a low protein diet during early childhood and it was often reported to be difficult to achieve the target protein intake (2 g/kg) and plasma EAA were often low. On changing from formula milk to cows milk at around 2 years, her ammonia levels increased. She was treated with diazoxide and nitrogen scavenging medicines. At 10 years of age nitrogen scavengers were stopped because they made no difference to her seizures; the low protein diet was also discontinued. She continued to have severe epilepsy, learning difficulties and challenging behaviour at school and poor weight gain. At age 16 years she is not on a formal protein restriction but self-selects a low protein diet.

Case study 2 Birmingham Children's Hospital NHS Foundation Trust, Birmingham

A girl, born at 38 weeks' gestation, was unsettled during early infancy and breast fed constantly. At 7 months she presented with an episode of floppiness, excessive sleepiness and hypoglycaemia (1.7 mmol/L). HIHA syndrome was diagnosed and she was treated with diazoxide, chlorothiazide and a low protein diet (1.5 g/kg/day). Periodically her parents report episodes of excessive sweatiness and hunger, fatigue, irritability and oedema that resolve with adjustment of medicines and that on eating simple sugars she experiences mild symptoms similar to rebound hypoglycaemia. When unwell, she is given frequent drinks of a low protein milk replacement (Sno-Pro) rather than standard ER based on glucose polymer. On continuous glucose

monitoring using the iPro (Medtronic Ltd) no sign of hypoglycaemia has been demonstrated. At age 7 years, she remains on 1.5 g/kg/day protein (and enjoys protein containing foods), with a high intake of starchy foods. Her height and weight are on the 50th centiles. No epileptiform abnormality has been described, she is active and doing well academically in a main stream school. She has mildly elevated ammonia concentrations but is not treated with nitrogen scavenger drugs.

Glucose-6-phosphate dehydrogenase deficiency and favism

Genetics and biochemistry

Glucose-6-phosphate dehydrogenase (G6PD) deficiency is a recessive, X-linked disorder in the G6PD gene. Worldwide, it is the most common enzyme defect affecting 400 million people [670] and is more prevalent in individuals from most parts of Africa, Asia, Oceania and southern Europe. G6PD is required in the first irreversible and rate limiting step of the pentose phosphate pathway (PPP), which is important in erythrocyte metabolism, and a deficiency makes patients vulnerable to haemolytic anaemia [671]. The G6PD enzyme catalyses the oxidation of glucose-6-phosphate and produces NADPH which is required to maintain glutathione in its reduced form (GSH). GSH acts as a scavenger for oxidative radicals. In G6PD deficiency, NADPH production is decreased making erythrocytes vulnerable to oxidative stress [671].

Clinical presentation

Most people with G6PD deficiency are asymptomatic. In states of oxidative stress the most frequent clinical signs are neonatal jaundice or haemolytic anaemia which can result from infection or taking certain common medicines [672], vitamin K [673] or ingestion of fava beans (broad beans), so-called favism. The exact relationship between increasing oxidative damage and these symptoms is poorly understood [670, 674]. All patients with favism have G6PD deficiency; however, not all G6PD deficient individuals have favism, i.e. symptoms after the ingestion of fava beans. In a study of 757 Saudi men, 42% showed

G6PD deficiency but none reported favism [675]. Indeed favism is thought to be more frequently associated with the Mediterranean variant of G6PD deficiency. Haemolysis is more likely to occur after eating fresh beans and can occur 24 hours post consumption; breast fed babies who have G6PD deficiency are also at risk if their mothers have eaten fava beans [670].

Dietary treatment

Avoidance of fava (broad) beans is advised. Vitamin E and selenium have antioxidant properties and may have some effect on improving red cell half-life [676] but data are inconsistent [670, 676].

Medicines

The British National Formulary (www.bnf.org) outlines drugs which pose a definite or possible risk of haemolysis if taken and so should be avoided. The risk and severity of haemolysis is almost always dose related and varies between individuals [672].

Acknowledgements

Anita MacDonald is grateful to Anne Daly, Sharon Evans, Dr Anupam Chakrapani, Dr Suresh Vijay and Dr Si Santra from the Inherited Metabolic Disorders Team at Birmingham Children's Hospital for their helpful reviews of the section on amino acid disorders.

Fiona White wishes to thank Janine Gallagher and Dr John Walter from the Inherited Metabolic Disorders team and Dr Tara Clancy, Consultant Genetic Counsellor at St Mary's Hospital, Manchester, for their helpful reviews of the section on amino acid disorders.

Marjorie Dixon and Jacky Stafford wish to thank Dr Maureen Cleary, Dr Alex Broomfield, Dr Paul Gissen and Dr Stephanie Grünewald, Metabolic Medicine at Great Ormond Street Hospital for Children NHS Foundation Trust, London, for their constructive reviews of the section on organic acidaemias, urea cycle disorders and miscellaneous metabolic disorders.

Further reading

Salway JG *Metabolism at a Glance*, 3rd edn. Oxford: Wiley-Blackwell, 2004. ISBN 978-1-4051-0716-7.

Salway JG *Medical Biochemistry at a Glance*, 3rd edn. Oxford: Wiley-Blackwell, 2012. ISBN 978-0-470-65451-4.

Greenstein B, Wood D *The Endocrine System at a Glance*, 3rd edn. Oxford: Wiley-Blackwell, 2009. ISBN 978-1-4443-3215-5.

Saudubray JM, van den Berghe G, Walter JH *Inborn Metabolic Diseases Diagnosis and Treatment*, 5th edn. Berlin: Springer-Verlag, 2012. ISBN 978-3-642-15719-6.

Useful websites and addresses

National Genetics Education and Development Centre, http://www.geneticseducation.nhs.uk.

Support groups
National Society for PKU (NSPKU)

PO Box 26642
London N14 4ZF
UK
nspku@ukonline.co.uk
www.nspku.org

European Society for PKU

www.espku.org

National PKU Alliance

PO Box 501
Tomahawk, WI 54487
USA
www.npkua.org

Canadian PKU and Allied Disorders Inc.

260 Adelaide Street East, #180
Toronto, ON M5A 1N1
Canada
www.canpku.org

National Organization for Rare Disorders

55 Kenosia Avenue
Danbury, CT 06810
USA
www.rarediseases.org

National PKU News

www.pkunews.org

Children Living with Inherited Metabolic Diseases (CLIMB)

Climb Building
176 Nantwich Road
Crewe CW2 6BG
UK
steve@climb.org.uk
www.climb.org.uk

MSUD Family Support Group

www.msud-support.org

Professional groups and online resources
British Inherited Metabolic Disease Group (BIMDG)

www.bimdg.org.uk has dietitians subgroup

Society for the Study of Inborn Errors of Metabolism (SSIEM)

www.ssiem.org has dietitians subgroup

EURORDIS Plateforme Maladies Rares

96, rue Didot
75014 Paris
France
eurordis@eurordis.org

PAH/PKU Knowledgebase

www.pahdb.mcgill.ca

Genetics Metabolic Dietitians International

PO Box 33985
Fort Worth, TX 76162
USA
www.gmdi.org

UK Newborn Screening Programme Centre

www.newbornbloodspot.screening.nhs.uk

Manufacturers of low protein foods
Fate Special Foods

Unit B8
Anchor Business Park

New Road
Netherton
Dudley DY2 9AP
UK

Cooking Helpline and General Enquiries

Tel: 01384 233230

First Play Dietary Foods

UNIT 4 Avondale Industrial Estate
Avondale Road
Stockport
Cheshire SK3 0UD
UK
Tel orderline: 0161 429 6847
Queries: 0161 480 4602

General Dietary Limited (Ener-G)

PO Box 38
Kingston-upon-Thames
Surrey ST2 7YP
UK
Tel: 02030 442933

Nutricia Clinical Care

Whitehorse Business Park
Trowbridge
Wiltshire BA14 OXQ
UK
Tel: 01225 711982

PK/Gluten-Free Foods Limited

Unit 270 Centennial Park
Centennial Avenue
Elstree, Borehamwood
Herts WD6 3SS
UK
Tel: 020 8953 4444
Fax: 020 8953 8285

Vitaflo Limited

Suite 1.11 South Harrington Building
182 Sefton Street
Brunswick Business Park
Liverpool L3 4BQ
UK
Tel: 0151 709 9020

18 Disorders of Carbohydrate Metabolism

Marjorie Dixon, Anita MacDonald, Jacky Stafford, Fiona White and Pat Portnoi

An Introduction to Inherited Metabolic Disorders may be found at the beginning of Chapter 17.

Disorders of Galactose Metabolism

Anita MacDonald and Pat Portnoi

Galactose is a monosaccharide that plays an important role in the biosynthesis of complex carbohydrates, glycoproteins and glycolipids [1]. There are three autosomal recessive disorders of galactose metabolism, with variable clinical phenotypes, caused by one of three sequential enzymes in the Leloir pathway: (i) galactokinase, (ii) galactose-1-phosphate uridyl transferase (GALT) and (iii) uridine diphosphate galactose-4-epimerase (GALE), which result in the inability to metabolise galactose (Fig. 18.1).

Galactosaemia

Introduction

Galactosaemia is a multi-organ disorder with wide clinical variability and over 220 different mutations or polymorphisms have been identified [2]. Abnormal glycosylation of glycoproteins and glycolipids may occur [3]. Direct biochemical consequences of GALT deficiency include accumulation of galactose-1-phosphate which, in turn, is metabolised to galactitol and galactonate, both of which accumulate in abnormal quantities in tissues [4]. Three forms of galactosaemia are

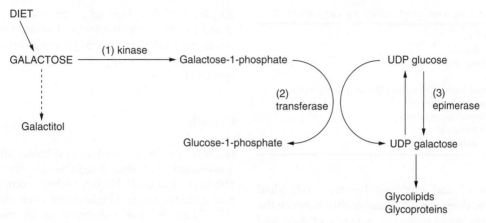

Figure 18.1   Pathways of galactose metabolism.

described: (1) classical galactosaemia, (2) clinical variant galactosaemia and (3) biochemical variant galactosaemia [5].

Genetics, incidence and clinical features

The classical genotype is typified by Q188R/Q188R, the clinical variant by S135L/S135L and the biochemical variant by N314D/QI88R. The incidence in Western Europe is estimated to be between 1 in 16 000 to 1 in 40 000 [6–9]. It is particularly common in the traveller population of the Republic of Ireland where incidence is estimated to be 1 in 480 [10]. The most common mutation in Europe and North America is Q188R [11, 12].

Classical galactosaemia was first described in 1908 [13] and it has been treated by diet since 1935. Homozygosity for the Q188R mutation, associated with substantial or complete loss of GALT activity, causes markedly elevated erythrocyte galactose-1-phosphate concentrations at diagnosis. Many patients are at risk of lethal *Escherichia coli* sepsis, liver disease and cataracts in the neonatal period. In the long term, it is associated with cognitive impairment, language delay, speech deficits and premature ovarian insufficiency [14].

Patients with S135L/S135L may manifest with acute liver disease in childhood but may not show some of the other chronic complications of classical galactosaemia. This is the most frequent mutation in black Africans [15].

The mutation N314D (C940>G; Duarte-I-variant) leads to a residual GALT activity of about 25%. On a galactose containing diet galactose-1-phosphate

concentrations are within target reference range, but there are increased concentrations of other metabolites. These concentrations appear to correlate with galactose intake and do not appear to cause clinical symptoms [16, 17] although long term outcome studies are not reported [5]. This variant of galactosaemia is commonly detected by newborn screening.

Clinical presentation

Classical galactosaemia presents in the neonatal period with life threatening illness after galactose is introduced in the diet. Symptoms and signs include poor feeding, vomiting and diarrhoea, weight loss, jaundice, hypotonia, cataracts, hepatosplenomegaly, hepatocellular insufficiency and encephalopathy [18]. Biochemical findings include abnormal liver function tests, abnormal clotting, hypoglycaemia, raised plasma amino acids and renal tubular dysfunction [19]. Rapid improvement occurs on stopping lactose containing feeds.

Cataracts may develop at the onset of symptoms and result from activation of the aldose reductase shunt, with consequent accumulation of galactitol in the crystalline lens [20]. Rarely, patients may present after the newborn period with faltering growth and developmental delay [15].

Long term outcome

Although serious long term complications may occur (Table 18.1), there is a wide variation in the

Table 18.1   Long term complications in galactosaemia.

Speech defect
Cognitive deficits
Learning problems
Cataracts
Hypergonadotrophic hypogonadism or primary ovarian
insufficiency in females
Reduced bone mineral density
Growth disturbance
Cerebellar ataxia/tremor/dystonia

extent of clinical problems between individual patients with no apparent relationship between the time of initiating treatment, severity of galactose restriction, treatment adherence or monitoring protocol [14]. However, verbal dyspraxia and premature ovarian failure are associated with homozygosity for the Q188R mutation [21, 22].

Cognitive development, executive and neurological function

In many studies of cognitive development, verbal and performance IQ [12, 23–28], memory and executive functions were in the low average range [23], with some children attending special schools [29]. They are more likely to leave school with fewer educational qualifications [30] and less likely to be employed compared with the general population [31]. Nevertheless, there is a range of ability with some achieving university education and attaining higher degrees. Although a decline in intellectual performance with age has been described, evidence from a longitudinal childhood study suggested IQ remains unchanged [32]. Neurological or movement problems (tremor, extrapyramidal motor disturbances) may occur in up to 40% of patients [14]. Neuroimaging studies confirm poor myelination, scattered white matter abnormalities, cerebral atrophy and cerebellar atrophy, as well as abnormalities in glucose uptake and metabolism in many brain regions [33].

Speech

Delayed speech vocabulary and childhood apraxia of speech (CAS) are common [30, 34, 35]. In many cases, impaired speech is related to a decreased

IQ [36]. CAS is a type of motor speech disorder characterised by inconsistent consonant and vowel errors, difficulty transitioning between articulatory movements and inappropriate prosody during speech [35].

Growth

Growth may be delayed in childhood and early adolescence, but final height is usually normal, although decreased height z-scores compared to mid-parental target height have been described [37]. There is also a decrease in fat mass and lean tissue mass compared with actual height z-scores [38].

Bone

Low bone mineral density is evident in male and female prepuburtal and postpubertal children and bone loss is common in adults [37, 39–41]. A correlation was found with the severity of osteopenia, patient age and use of hormonal supplementation, but the exact mechanism is not well understood. There is suggestion of an increase in bone turnover from childhood to adolescence with a possible imbalance between bone resorption and bone formation processes [42], whilst others have suggested a decrease in bone metabolism associated with a low insulin-like growth factor (IGF-1) z-score [37, 40]. Also there may be a possible intrinsic defect in the galactosylation of the collagen matrix of bone resulting in decreased mineralisation [39]. If bone mineral content is low, nutritional intake, physical activity and oestrogen supplementation should be optimised [3]. In a group of children and teenagers receiving a combination of calcium (750 mg/day), vitamin K (1 μg/day) and vitamin D3 (10 μg/day) there was significant improvement in bone formation markers and bone mineral content [43].

Fertility

Primary ovarian insufficiency (POI) occurs in 80% of women with classical galactosaemia despite treatment [18, 44, 45]; the aetiology is unknown.

Most women develop primary or secondary amenorrhoea [46] and premature menopause usually occurs in the third decade [3,47]. Clinical surveillance includes screening for abnormalities in ovarian function at an early age. Treatment consists of age appropriate oestrogen/progesterone supplementation.

Despite the high prevalence of POI several spontaneous pregnancies have been described [6,48,49], particularly in black women with milder mutations. Others have been reported in women homozygous for QI88R mutation [6,49,50]. Pubertal development and fertility are normal in boys, although low semen volume and higher than expected prevalence of cryptorchidism is reported [51].

Pregnancy in women with classical galactosaemia

Only a subtle and clinically insignificant increase of galactose metabolites occurs during pregnancy [52,53] so no additional treatment is required during pregnancy for women with classical galactosaemia. Postpartum there is a transient increase in red blood cell metabolite concentrations and renal metabolite excretion. Normal healthy infant outcome is reported in the few pregnancies documented. A small number of women have successfully breast fed their infants with no adverse effect [52].

Quality of life

A lower health related quality of life has been reported in adults with galactosaemia. Significantly lower scores in cognitive and social domains occur [29], with social difficulties in at least 50% of patients [14]. In particular, the following are described: interpersonal problems, bullying [54], a lower number of friends, boys performing less competitive sports and socialising less [55]. Adults may have shy and timid personalities, being tense, overanxious or oversensitive with poor self-image. They are more likely to remain single [56], live with their parents [30], have delayed psychosexual development [31,55] with men less likely to engage in sexual activities [47]. There is a twofold 'odds' increase of depression for each 10 year age increase in adults [47].

Endogenous production of galactose

Endogenous galactose is thought to originate from the transformation of glucose and from the recycling of glycosylated proteins and lipids [52]. It is considered to be a major cause of late complications [57]. Significant amounts of endogenous galactose is produced in patients with galactosaemia, release rates being several fold higher in infants than in adults [58] with adults producing approximately 13 mg/kg body weight/day compared with approximately 41 mg/kg body weight/day in newborns [59].

It is suggested that long term clinical abnormalities originate from foetal exposure to endogenously produced galactose or its metabolites *in utero* [32,60,61].

Diagnosis of galactosaemia

In many countries, galactosaemia is detected by neonatal screening, but diagnosis requires confirmation by a second independent method, e.g. determination of galactose-1-phosphate uridyl transferase activity in red blood cells or DNA analysis. In non screened populations, infants are diagnosed from clinical presentation. The Beutler test (a fluorescent spot test) may be used as an initial investigation and then diagnosis confirmed by further biochemical and/or molecular testing. Although newborn screening may be life saving through earlier identification it does not appear to change the incidence of long term complications [14].

If galactosaemia is suspected, a low galactose infant formula should be commenced immediately, even before diagnosis is confirmed.

Biochemical monitoring

There is no consensus as to the most relevant biomarker(s) for monitoring patients with galactosaemia. Measurement of red cell galactose-1-phosphate has been widely used to monitor dietary compliance. This is high at diagnosis and falls progressively after the introduction of dietary treatment but it may still take up to 1 year or even longer to decrease to the treatment reference range (laboratories use variable target ranges so a local treatment reference range should be used). Concentrations do not decrease to the levels found in normal, healthy individuals [3]. The units used to express galactose-1-phosphate concentrations vary between different laboratories, usually according to methodology [62].

Galactose-1-phosphate concentrations do not vary greatly in individual patients so frequent monitoring is not indicated [62] (Table 18.2). There is no correlation with clinical outcome [63]. Erythrocyte galactose-1-phosphate is commonly used as a measure of dietary adherence but does not appear to help identify mild dietary indiscretions. Other metabolites such as urinary galactitol and red cell galactonate have been considered. IgG N-glycan profiling may be a more sensitive and informative method of monitoring dietary adherence [63], although further investigation is needed.

Dietary management

Galactose is ubiquitously distributed in animals and plants. It is a constituent of lactose and also certain complex lipids and proteins. Lactose, a β-galactoside in composition, occurs in the milk of mammals and is synthesised in the mammary gland [64].

The immediate and rigorous exclusion of lactose/galactose from the diet is critical in the newly diagnosed infant and should lead to amelioration of symptoms. In the long term, many complications develop despite dietary restriction. There is controversy concerning the optimal strictness and duration of dietary galactose exclusion. In particular, it is unclear how much exogenous galactose patients with classical galactosaemia tolerate and whether galactose tolerance may increase with age.

Table 18.2 Suggested frequency of measuring galactose-1-phosphate concentrations [62].

Age	Frequency of measuring galactose-1-phosphate concentrations
0–1 year	Every 3 months
1–14 years	Every 6 months
Over 14 years	Annually

Acceptable galactose intake on a low galactose diet

There is no consensus on the degree of galactose restriction required for patients with galactosaemia and, unless taking an elemental feed, it would be difficult to have a completely galactose free diet. It has been suggested that infants may tolerate 50 mg galactose/day; toddlers 150 mg/day; children 200 mg/day; adolescents 250 mg/day; and 300 mg/day in adulthood [65]. On a strict lactose free diet (but including five portions of fruit and vegetables daily) galactose intake is calculated at 2–3 mg/kg/day in children aged between 3 and 15 years.

Sources of galactose

Although it is universally agreed that lactose must be avoided, practice regarding restriction of other dietary galactose sources varies widely throughout the world [14].

Lactose

In the UK a lactose free diet only is advocated. Lactose is cleaved into its two components, glucose and galactose, when digested and it is the main dietary source of galactose. Cow's milk contains 4.5–5.5% lactose, i.e. about 23 g of galactose per litre. All milk, milk products and manufactured foods containing milk need to be avoided. Lactose and galactose in milk based foods are shown in Table 18.3 and Table 18.4. Constituents of milk are also likely to be found in foods such as biscuits,

Table 18.3 Lactose and galactose content of foods [67].

Food	Lactose content (g/100 mL or g/100 g)	Galactose content (g/100 mL or g/100 g)
Milk, skimmed	4.4	2.2
Milk, whole	4.5	2.3
Cream, single	2.2	1.1
Yoghurt, low fat, fruit	4.4	2.2
Butter	0.6	0.3
Chocolate, milk	10.1	5.1
Ice cream, dairy	5.2	2.6
Lactofree milk (Arla)*	0.02 g	1.65

*Data analysed by UK Galactosaemia Support Group.

Table 18.4 Milk, milk products and milk derivatives.

Milk and milk products
Cow's milk, goat's milk, sheep's milk
Cheese, cream, butter
Ice cream, yoghurt, fromage frais, crème fraiche
Chocolate

Milk derivatives
Skimmed milk powder, milk solids, milk protein, non fat milk solids, separate milk solids
Whey, hydrolysed whey protein, margarine or shortening containing whey, whey syrup sweetener, casein, hydrolysed casein, sodium caseinate, calcium caseinate
Lactose
Buttermilk, butterfat, butter oil, milk fat, animal fat (may be butter), ghee, artificial cream
Cheese powder

Lactose as a filler may be used in
Flavourings
Table top or tablet artificial sweeteners
Medicines

Table 18.5 Lactose free diet.

Lactose free foods are listed. Manufactured foods which contain or could contain milk or milk derivatives are shown in italics. Food labels should always be checked as constituents change.

Milk, milk products and milk derivatives
These should all be avoided (Table 18.4)

Soya milk and soya products
Infant soya formula
Liquid soya milk – calcium enriched (not before 1 year of age)
Soya cheese, soya yoghurt, soya desserts

Fats and oils
Milk free margarine
Many margarines and low fat spreads contain milk
Vegetable oils
Lard, dripping, suet

Meat and fish
Meat, poultry, fish, shellfish (fresh or frozen)
Ham and bacon (lactose may occasionally be used as a flavour enhancer – see ingredient label)
Fish fingers
Quorn
Tofu
Many meat or fish products such as sausages, burgers, pies, breaded or battered foods or in sauce may not be suitable

Eggs

Cereal, flour, pasta
All grains; wheat, oats, corn, rice, barley, maize, sago, rye, tapioca
Pasta, spaghetti, macaroni, dried noodles, couscous
Tinned pasta such as spaghetti hoops may contain cheese
Flour: plain, self-raising; cornflour, rice flour, soya flour
Custard power, semolina
Carob

Breakfast cereals
Most are suitable, e.g. Weetabix, cornflakes, Rice Krispies
A few cereals may contain chocolate derivatives or milk

Bread and yeast products
Most bread is suitable
Milk bread and nan bread contain milk – avoid
Pitta, chapatti
Muffins, crumpets, teacakes may not be suitable

Cakes, biscuits, crackers
Many cakes, biscuits and crackers contain milk

Desserts
Sorbet, jelly, soya desserts, soya ice cream, soya yoghurt
Homemade soya milk custard or rice pudding
Most desserts contain milk in some form

Fruit
All fresh, frozen, tinned or dried fruit

some sweets and tinned and processed meats (Table 18.5). Many spreads (including reduced fat) and mayonnaise include milk components to improve their flavour. The lactose content of whey derivatives such as whey powder is high, comprising 70% of total solids. In contrast, the lactose content of casein is low, with the Casein and Caseinates Regulations [66] stating the maximum anhydrous lactose content of casein should not exceed 1% by weight [67]. Butter oil and ghee contain only minimal lactose, but the recommendation is to avoid these.

Lactose powder is added to a diverse range of food products including bakery goods, confectionery, dry mixes, dried vegetables and crisps. It is often added to prepared foods to prevent caking or as a coating. It may be used in bakery goods for enhancing browning and, as it has one-sixth the sweetness of sucrose, it is added instead of sucrose to reduce the sweetness. It is commonly used as a filler and flowing agent in seasoning mixes for foods such as instant pot noodles. It may act as a carrier for flavours and seasonings and may be added to ham, bacon and salami. It may also be added to some artificial table top or tablet sweeteners.

Non milk derivatives that may be added to food products are shown in Table 18.6. These do not need to be avoided with the exception of lactitol, a polyol made from galactose. Some residual galactose is left

Table 18.5 *(continued)*

Vegetables
All fresh, frozen, tinned or dried vegetables
Most dried and tinned pulses, e.g. red kidney beans, chick peas, lentils
Baked beans and ready made vegetable dishes such as coleslaw, potato salad may contain milk

Savoury snacks
Plain crisps, poppodom
Nuts, peanut butter
Flavoured crisps may not be suitable because they contain cheese or lactose as a filler in the flavouring
Dry roasted nuts and popcorn may contain milk/butter

Seasonings, gravies
Pepper, salt, pure spices and herbs, mustard
Marmite, Bovril, Bisto
Gravy granules and stock cubes may contain milk

Soups
Tinned, packet, carton soups may contain lactose

Sugar, sweet spreads
Sugar, glucose, fructose
Pure artificial sweeteners
Powdered and tablet artificial sweeteners may contain lactose
Jam, syrup, honey, marmalade, lemon curd

Confectionery
Boiled sweets, most mints, marshmallow, plain fruit lollies, chewing gum
Milk chocolate, most plain chocolate, butterscotch and fudge, toffee contain milk
Plain or carob chocolate may contain milk

Drinks
Soya milk
Milk shake syrup or powders
Fizzy drinks, squash, fruit juice
Cocoa, tea, coffee
Drinking chocolate may contain milk
Instant milk drinks and malted milk drinks – avoid

Miscellaneous – used in baking
Baking powder, yeast, gelatine, marzipan

Flavourings
Lactose may be used as a 'carrier' for flavourings particularly in crisps and similar snack foods. In sweets lactose is rarely used for this purpose except in some dairy flavours

---

after its fermentation in the gut so it is unsuitable in galactosaemia.

Galactosides

The α-galactosides are part of the oligosaccha-rides (raffinose, stachyose and verbacose) and are

Table 18.6   Non milk derivatives.

Lactic acid E270, sodium lactate E325, potassium lactate E325, calcium lactate E327

Lactitol, lactalbumin, lactoglobulin, lycasin, stearoyl lactylates, glucona-delta-lactone, monosodium glutamate, cocoa butter, non dairy cream

Lactitol does not contain lactose but may contain some galactose and should be avoided.

---

a potential source of galactose. They are found in foods such as peas, beans, lentils, cocoa, nuts, wheat, oat flour and vegetables [68] (Table 18.7).

Studies investigating the effects of galactosides in galactosaemia are rare, include limited numbers of subjects, are short term and inconclusive. The α-galactosidase linkage in oligosaccharides is not hydrolysable by the human small intestinal mucosa *in vitro* or *in vivo* [69]. Instead, the galactosides are rapidly degraded and fermented by the caecal microflora to produce volatile short chain fatty acids. Galactoside avoidance is not advocated in galactosaemia in the UK.

Galactose storage organs

Although meats do not contain significant amounts of carbohydrates, small amounts may be present in free form and bound to proteins as glycoproteins and galactolipids. Cell lipids and proteins contin-uously undergo degradation, releasing glycerol, fatty acids, amino acids and their carbohydrate components, including galactose [70]. Offal is a source of galactocerebrosides and gangliosides [3]. These are not avoided in galactosaemia in the UK.

Table 18.7   Dietary sources of galactosides and nucleoproteins.

Galactosides	Peas, beans, lentils, legumes, chick peas, dhals, grams, spinach
	Texturised vegetable protein
	Soya (other than soya protein isolates), soya beans, soya flour
	Cocoa, chocolate
	Nuts
Nucleoproteins	Offal – liver, kidney, brain, sweetbreads, heart
	Eggs

Free and bound galactose

Free galactose has been reported in many fruits, vegetables and legumes [71] (Table 18.8). Free galactose content may vary from <0.1 mg/100 g to 40 mg/100 g [72,73]. In selected plant materials, it ranges from 2 ± 0.1 mg/100 g in red potato to 39.7 mg/100 g in red pepper. Only kiwi fruit and red pepper have galactose contents >20 mg/100 g. Different seasons, variety and storage affect the free galactose content [73]. Generally fruits and vegetables provide nutritional benefit yet induce only a small increase in daily galactose intake (30–54 mg galactose/day) and their intake is not associated with poorer outcome in galactosaemia. In one study, one patient was given a synthetic diet containing <8 mg/day galactose and then challenged with 200 mg/day galactose for 3 weeks. This had little effect on concentrations of metabolic markers [74].

Bound galactose is also present in many plant foods as β-1-4-linked galactosyl residues in chloroplast membranes of green plant tissue. Gums and fibres (carrageenan, locust bean gum, tragacanth gum) are common sources of bound galactose. Whilst mice with galactosaemia are able to hydrolyse bound galactose in mouse chow (the hydrolysis of the bound galactose resulting in excretion of significant amounts of galactose and its metabolites in their urine [75]), in humans there is no evidence that excluding bound galactose is beneficial.

Overall, there are few data to suggest that avoiding galactose from any plant and non milk animal source is helpful. In the UK since 1983, only milk and milk products have been avoided [76] and long term outcome is not dissimilar to other countries where there are more complex and restrictive dietary management guidelines [14].

Table 18.8 Free galactose in fruit and vegetables (mg/100 g).

Food	UK*	USA†
Tomato	10	23
Grape	<10	2.9
Cucumber	20	4.0
Banana	10	9.2
Water melon		14.7
Kiwi fruit		10

*Unpublished. Data analysed by UK Galactosaemia Support Group.
†[40, 41].

Practical management of a lactose free diet

Milk substitutes

Breast feeding and cow's milk based infant formulas are contraindicated because they contain lactose. It is important that infants and young children are given a suitable nutritionally adequate formula. Factors influencing the choice of milk substitute include its nutritional composition, the child's clinical and nutritional status, safety and palatability of the product, ease of preparation, cost and availability.

Soya infant formula

Soya infant formula is commonly the first choice for centres treating babies with galactosaemia [14] and is supported by the European Society of Paediatric Gastroenterology, Hepatology and Nutrition (ESPGHAN) [77] and the UK Galactosaemia Medical Advisory Panel. This is mainly because there are few other safe options to use in infancy. Nutritionally complete soya infant formulas, e.g. InfaSoy, Wysoy, are lactose free and oligosaccharides are removed during manufacture. Estimates suggest that they may contain 1–2 mg galactose per 100 mL [78].

One potential disadvantage of soya infant formula is that it is a rich source of isoflavones, particularly genistein and daidzein. These compounds are structurally similar to the mammalian oestrogen hormone but are much less potent (0.1%–1% of the oestrogenic potential of 17-β-oestradiol [46]). They can bind to oestrogen receptors and act as anti-oestrogenic agents by blocking oestrogen and this was identified as a concern by the UK Food Standards Agency [79] and Department of Health [80]. There is no evidence that the use of soya infant formula is a factor in the fertility problems seen in galactosaemia.

Low lactose and protein hydrolysate formula

Other alternative infant formulas include low lactose formulas and casein hydrolysate formulas (Table 18.9). Medium chain triglyceride (MCT) based casein hydrolysate infant formula, such as

Table 18.9 Low lactose, protein hydrolysate and amino acid formulas for infants with galactosaemia.

Infant formula	Protein source	Lactose content (per 100 mL)
Low lactose		
Enfamil O-Lac (Mead Johnson)	Milk protein (isolate)	<7 mg
Galactomin 17 (SHS/Nutricia)	Caseinate	<10 mg
SMA LF (SMA Nutrition)	60% whey, 40% casein	<10 mg
Casein hydrolysate		
Nutramigen Lipil 1 and 2 (Mead Johnson)	Enzymatically hydrolysed casein	<5 mg
Pregestimil Lipil (Mead Johnson)	Enzymatically hydrolysed casein	<5 mg
Whey hydrolysate		
Pepti-Junior (Cow & Gate)	Hydrolysed whey protein	0.1 g
Meat and soya hydrolysate		
Pepdite (SHS/Nutricia)	Hydrolysed pork and soya amino acids	Nil
Amino acid formula		
Neocate LCP (SHS/Nutricia)	L-amino acids	Nil
Nutramigen AA (Mead Johnson)	L-amino acids	Nil
Neocate Nutra (SHS/Nutricia) *This is not a complete formula. Can be used from 6 months (as a paste) as part of a nutritionally adequate diet*	L-amino acids	Nil

Pregestimil Lipil, may be advantageous when there is significant liver disease and should be administered until this complication has resolved [3].

However, all low lactose and protein hydrolysate formulas based on cow's milk protein will undoubtedly contain some residual lactose and the amounts vary. Manufacturers of these formulas declare their lactose content at <10 mg/100 kcal (420 kJ) as defined by the European Food Safety Authority (EFSA) [81]. A 5 kg infant taking 200 mL/kg of formula would have <10 mg/kg/day (or 50 mg/day) of galactose from this source. However, it is estimated that endogenous galactose production is likely to be at its highest in infancy (calculated at 41 mg/kg body weight/day) [59], so it is probably better to use a formula which contains no source of lactose.

Whey hydrolysate formulas are likely to contain a higher concentration of residual lactose and Pepti-Junior, for example, is likely to contain 100 mg/100 mL of lactose (personal communication) and are unsuitable. Enteral feeds for older children based on whey hydrolysates are unsuitable.

Any formula based on hydrolysed meat and soya should be free of lactose and suitable to use.

Amino acid based formula

This alternative is a suitable lactose free formula and is used by some centres as the first choice in babies with galactosaemia [14]. There have been at least three case reports of infants with galactosaemia given elemental (amino acid based) infant formulas successfully [82, 83] and they may offer an advantage as they are more likely than soya infant formulas to be fortified with novel nutrients such as long chain polyunsaturated fatty acids. The main challenge when using elemental formulas is to ensure infants establish a taste for soya based foods during the weaning period.

Vegetable based milks for children over 1 year of age

A number of commercial nutritionally enriched plant, cereal and nut based drinks (e.g. soya, oat, rice, hazelnut and almond) can be purchased in supermarkets, specialist shops or on the internet. Most of them contain approximately 120 mg/100 mL calcium and 0.8 µg/100 mL vitamin D. There are also nutritionally enriched follow on soya milks designed for children >1 year with added calcium, iron, vitamin D, some B vitamins and an energy profile similar to cow's milk. Calcium absorption from soya drinks is similar to that from cow's milk. Soya beverages made from soya protein isolate contain less free galactose (1.3 ± 0.2 mg/100 g) compared with whole soya beans (4.8–5.3 ± 1.7 mg/100 g) [73]. Rice milk contains traces of inorganic arsenic and it is recommended by the UK Food Standards Agency that children aged between 1 and 4½ years should avoid rice milk.

Unsafe milks

Since lactose is the carbohydrate source in animal milks, e.g. goat's and sheep's milks, these are unsuitable. A low lactose dairy drink, Lactofree (Arla), where about half the lactose is removed by filtration and the remainder is removed enzymatically, is available internationally. However, recent analysis has demonstrated that it contains a significant quantity of galactose, rendering it unsuitable for galactosaemia (Table 18.3) [84]. Lactase enzyme drops, which reduce the lactose content of cow's milk, are also unsuitable.

Cheeses

Hard mature cheeses

A small number of hard mature cheeses are allowed. Most cheese types have high levels of casein (which contains no more than 1% lactose) and low levels of whey (which contains 70% lactose). The lactose content is reduced during the cheese making process: by removal of whey by drainage (during this stage approximately 98% will be removed); type of starter culture and coagulating enzyme can have an effect as can the acid produced – all influence the properties of the curd and the degree of whey expulsion. For harder cheeses the curd is cut into small cubes, which allows fluid to drain from the individual pieces of curd. Any residual lactose in cheese curd is metabolisd during its ripening [85] and, generally, the longer the cheese has matured the lower its lactose content.

In the UK, the following cheeses are allowed: Emmental, Gruyere, Jarlsberg, Parmigiano Reggiano and Grana Padano Italian Parmesans with

an EU PDO (Protected Designation of Origin) seal on the label; also West Country Farmhouse mature Cheddar cheese with an EU PDO seal on the label. All of these cheeses have been extensively tested for their lactose and galactose content [86] and have been shown to contain minimal lactose and galactose on repeated analysis. Information regarding suitable West Country Farmhouse mature Cheddar cheese is available from www.farmhousecheesemakers.com. A PDO seal only guarantees that a food genuinely originates from a region and is produced to a specified quality; it does not indicate that it contains minimal lactose. Many food stuffs carry the PDO seal, e.g. other types of cheese, sausages, hams and regional breads, and these are not necessarily lactose free. However, the PDO seal should always be on the label of any West Country Farmhouse Cheddar cheese or Parmigiano Reggiano and Grana Padano Italian Parmesans to indicate their suitability.

All other cheeses are not permitted. Specific analysis has been commissioned by the UK Galactosaemia Medical Advisory Panel to test Gouda, Edam and some soft and processed cheeses, but all contain lactose and galactose; Mini Emmental Baby Bel contains a mean of 6–7 mg/100 g lactose and so is also unsuitable. The latter cheese is only fermented for 196 days and is usually on the retail market by 32 weeks of age [87].

Enzyme treated cheese products

A Lactofree Cheddar type of cheese has been produced from Lactofree (Arla) milk. Initial findings suggest this is low in lactose and galactose [84], but as there has been only limited analysis it is considered unsuitable in the galactosaemia diet.

Inclusion of cheese in the diet

There are different guidelines in different countries on the inclusion of cheese in the diet for galactosaemia. A survey of European practices [88] found that hard cheese such as Emmental and Gruyere were allowed in 63% of countries. Gouda was allowed in some countries but not others. In Australia and New Zealand some mature Cheddar cheese made by traditional methods are allowed [89]. In the USA some clinics allow mature hard cheese, e.g. Emmental, Gruyere, Tilsider [78].

Acceptability of low lactose/low galactose cheese

For many patients and carers the allowance of low lactose, but milk derived, cheese is a difficult concept to comprehend. However, a recent survey conducted by the UK Galactosaemia Support Group indicated there was a wide acceptance with 76% of patients eating one or more suitable types of cheese. The most preferred of the low lactose/low galactose cheeses were West Country Farmhouse Cheddar (70%), Emmental (31%), Italian Parmesan (24%), Gruyere (18%) and Jarlsberg (14%) [90].

Manufactured foods

Interpreting food labels

European ingredient listing rules [91–93] applied across the EU give clear guidance about food labelling of prepackaged foods that contain intentional milk, milk derivatives or lactose, which have to be clearly identified. Milk or lactose in carry-over additives or flavourings, and any other substances used as processing aids are also acknowledged. This only applies to prepackaged foods, e.g. canned and packet foods and alcoholic drinks, so foods sold loose (i.e. unpackaged), foods served in restaurants and certain fancy confectionery products are exempt.

However, the UK Foods Standards Agency (FSA) [94] has introduced *The Provision of Allergen Information for Non Prepackaged foods – Voluntary Best Practice Guidance*, targeted at food producers. It is requested that food suppliers communicate honestly with customers about the contents of any unpackaged foods that are sold; and that all employees receive training about food allegens (including milk), have up to date knowledge about the ingredient content of foods sold, consider cross-contamination and have an agreed practice for dealing with allergy information. The FSA has also launched a Chef Allergen card. The customer's food allergy requirements are completed on a credit card which is handed to a chef who will then be able to decide if they are able to produce a lactose free meal for the individual. At the end of 2014, new UK legislation will be introduced that will require businesses to provide allergy information on food sold unpackaged in catering outlets, deli-counters, bakeries and sandwich bars.

Cross-contamination of manufactured foods with milk

Both milk free and milk containing foods may be manufactured in the same plant or even using the same machinery. Cross-contamination with milk is always possible and such foods may be voluntarily labelled *may contain milk or milk products*. It is likely that the quantity of milk that such a product would contain if cross-contaminated would be minute. The UK Galactosaemia Support Group Medical Advisory Panel permits foods that only carry a risk of cross-contamination with milk.

Vitamin and mineral supplementation

Many nutrients are involved in optimum bone metabolism, particularly calcium, phosphate and vitamin D. Vitamin K also has an important role to play, acting as a cofactor in the post translational carboxylation of osteocalcin which has a regulatory role in the mineralisation and remodelling of bone [40]. Some recommend routine vitamin K supplementation in addition to calcium and vitamin D in galactosaemia [95]. Maintenance of adequate cellular zinc concentrations is also important for growth and bone metabolism; bone specific alkaline phosphatase and osteocalcin are zinc dependent [37].

It is important to ensure that patients meet the reference nutrient intake (RNI) for all bone related nutrients. Calcium intake is commonly low in galactosaemia [39, 96, 97]. The UK RNI for calcium varies between 325 mg and 1000 mg daily in children and teenagers [98]. Wherever possible, calcium requirements should be achieved by eating foods. Soya infant formula normally provides adequate calcium in the first 1–2 years if sufficient amounts are taken, but it may be necessary to change to a calcium enriched soya drink (preferably supplemented with vitamin D), encourage low lactose cheese, soya yoghurts, sardines, mackerel, sesame seeds, lentils and milk free fortified bread to ensure adequate calcium intake (Table 18.10). Dietary assessment should be performed annually to ensure sufficiency.

If calcium intake is low, it is necessary to give a calcium supplement which may be challenging mainly because of the size, type of presentation (mainly tablets rather than liquid) and nutritional

Table 18.10 Food sources of calcium for galactosaemia [67].

	Calcium (mg)	Vitamin D (µg)
	per 100 mL/100 g	
Calcium/vitamin D enriched soya drinks	100–140	0.8
Soya dairy free yoghurts	120	Variable
Low lactose hard cheese	730	0.3
Whitebait	860	Not available
Sardines in oil/brine	500	5
Pilchards	250	14
Sesame seeds	670	0
Red kidney beans	100	0
Bread	170	0
Spinach	170	0
Apricots	73	0

Table 18.11 Suitable calcium supplements for galactosaemia.

	Presentation	Available calcium (mg)	Vitamin D (µg)
Adcal-D3 (ProStrakan) Calcium carbonate Chewable tablet/ effervescent tablets	Tablet	600	10
Cacit-D3 (Proctor and Gamble Pharm) Calcium carbonate Granules	Sachet	500	11
Calceos (Galem) Calcium carbonate Chewable tablet	Tablet	500	10
Calcichew D3 (Shire) Calcium carbonate Chewable tablet	Tablet	500	5
Calcichew D3 Forte (Shire) Calcium carbonate Chewable tablet	Tablet	500	10
Natecal D3 (Chiesi) Calcium carbonate Chewable tablet	Tablet	600	10
Sandocal+D 600 (Novartis) Calcium lactate gluconate, calcium carbonate Effervescent tablet	Tablet	600	10

Calcium Sandoz Liquid (Alliance) is based on calcium lactobionate. It is contraindicated in galactosaemia because β-galactosidase in human intestinal mucosa hydrolyses lactobionate freeing galactose (Calcium Sandoz Liquid medical information [114]). The amount of galactose released is unknown.

composition of the calcium supplements available for children. Additional vitamin D supplementation will aid calcium absorption, e.g. Healthy Start vitamin drops (p. 20). Alternatively, there are a number of prescribable calcium supplements with added vitamin D (Table 18.11). The latter are mainly chewable or dissolvable in water. They are bulky, unpopular with children and adherence is an issue. There are no suitable liquid calcium supplements listed in the British National Formulary (BNF) for children. If dietary intake is poor, it may be necessary to give a more comprehensive vitamin and mineral supplement in the form of Paediatric Seravit or Fruitivits (suitable from 3 years of age).

There is a suggestion that calcium supplementation may increase the risk of myocardial infarction [99, 100]. This may be related to an acute increase in serum calcium observed after calcium supplements but not dietary calcium [100]. An increase in serum calcium levels has been associated with vascular calcification [101]. Ideally calcium supplements should be co-administered with vitamin D and given as more than one daily dose.

Dietary education

It is important for families to be educated about lactose free food choices and the importance of healthy eating and appropriate nutrition (and exercise) for healthy bones. They also need help with choosing vitamin/mineral supplements. Interpretation of food labelling, suitability of unpackaged food items, lactose free cooking and choice of appropriate school meals are important. Dietary education of children is essential, particularly with the interpretation of food labels to enable them to take control of their own diet and make independent food choices. This will help foster curiosity and a healthy attitude towards their diet.

UK Galactosaemia Support Group

The UK Galactosaemia Support Group produces a wide range of educational materials for parents and carers including a low lactose diet guide for children and adults; a small dietary shopping card; Easter and Christmas lists of suitable lactose free treats; information about healthy bones; picture books of lactose free foods which are particularly useful for carers who cannot read or speak English; and a glossary of food ingredient definitions. It has also commissioned the analysis of a number of foods for lactose and galactose content and employs a dietitian who produces much of the dietary information. The website is www.galactosaemia.org.

Lactose in medications

Lactose is an excipient with properties that make it ideal as a tablet filler or binder and it is found in many medications. For most medications the amount of lactose is unlikely to be significant, particularly if the medication is being used for a short time period [3]. However, it is still important to check the quantity of lactose; e.g. the common laxative lactulose contains high quantities of lactose and galactose: 1 mL contains <100 mg galactose and 67 mg lactose [102] and is contraindicated in galactosaemia.

Contraceptive pills prescribed for oestrogen insufficiency contain lactose as an excipient and provide approximately 20–65 mg lactose/day (manufacturers' data sheets).

Some toothpastes and shampoos may contain milk derivatives. No recommendation is given to avoid these. Although a little may be swallowed by young children, the amount should only be small.

Long term dietary treatment

Although a lifelong lactose free diet is recommended for galactosaemia there is debate about how strict the dietary treatment should be in teenage years and beyond. Historically, some dietary relaxation has been considered in school age children as rigid dietary control did not appear to play a role in intellectual development and there are reports of relaxed dietary approaches, although not all agreed [103]. A follow-up study

of five Estonian patients aged 7–14 years who had followed a lactose restricted diet but had no limitations on eating mature cheeses, fruits or vegetables reported outcomes that were consistent with those experienced by patients maintained on more rigorously galactose restricted diets [104]. There have been at least two case reports of treated patients who discontinued diet at the age of 3 years (both with Q188R homozygosity and severely reduced erythrocyte galactose-1-phosphate uridyl transferase activity) with good long term outcome [105, 106]. The Dublin clinic in Ireland has also reported similar experiences [63]. They increased galactose intake from 300 mg to 4000 mg/day over 16 weeks in five adult patients and compared them with five patients on a galactose restricted diet. IgG N-glycan profiles showed consistent individual alterations in response to diet liberalisation. The individual profiles were improved for all but one study subject. With a galactose intake of 1000 mg/day they had a decrease in agalactosylated, and an increase in digalactosylated, N-glycans. A patient who had self-liberalised his diet to 4000 mg galactose/day pre study had the most favourable IgG N-glycan profile.

Bosch et al. [107] increased oral galactose intake to 600 mg/day for 6 weeks in three adolescent patients homozygous for the Q188R mutation. No significant changes were observed in clinical observations, ophthalmic examination and laboratory measurements of dietary control. Until there is more available evidence it is important that the advice to patients and carers remains that a strict lactose free diet is followed [108].

Follow-up

Dietary intake should be assessed annually, particularly for micronutrient intake. Patients should also be evaluated by a speech and language therapist, focusing on detection of verbal dyspraxia. In addition, all girls with classical galactosaemia should be properly evaluated for primary ovarian insufficiency at approximately 10–12 years of age. Dual-energy x-ray absorptiometry (DEXA) scans should be conducted every 4–5 years after the onset of puberty, but more frequently if the bone mineral content is low [3].

Table 18.12   Case study: clinical presentation of galactosaemia in the neonatal period.

Baby boy, born full term, discharged home from local hospital on day 3
Fully breast fed, birth weight 4.5 kg
Appeared well with the exception of jaundice
Feeding deteriorated and he started vomiting

Admitted to a local hospital, diagnosed with a urine infection and commenced antibiotics. However, he was also found to have liver dysfunction with deranged clotting, intermittent hypoglycaemia, and was transferred to a paediatric liver ward
Galactosaemia was suspected, breast feeding was stopped, soya infant formula given, fluids were restricted

Over the next 3 days, fluid intake was gradually increased to normal requirements, liver function similarly improved, he tolerated the soya infant formula and his clinical symptoms ameliorated within 48 hours
Classical galactosaemia was diagnosed with a galactose-1-phosphate concentration >2000 μmol/L and determination of galactose-1-phosphate uridyl transferase activity. He was homozygous for the Q188R mutation

Discharged home on a lactose free diet only

He drank soya infant formula without difficulty and lactose free solids were introduced at 20 weeks of age
Parents gradually expanded his diet according to his age, introducing low lactose cheese, soya yoghurts and other suitable products
His galactose-1-phosphate concentration only slowly lowered to within treatment range during the first year despite excellent dietary adherence
He continued to feed well and gained weight appropriately

At the age of 2 years, he was changed onto a toddler calcium and vitamin D enriched commercial soya drink. His weight and length were adequate, as were his intakes of calcium and vitamin D

Currently at the age of 3 years, his clinical progress is good, but speech is slightly delayed. His nutrient intake, growth and galactose-1-phosphate concentrations are assessed twice per year

Alcohol

There is no evidence to support the hypothesis that alcohol is more harmful to patients with galactosaemia than to the normal population [62].

Table 18.13   Case study: clinical presentation of galactosaemia in later infancy.

Baby boy, born full term, birth weight 3.5 kg
Demand fed with a standard whey dominant infant formula

At the age of 2 weeks admitted to local hospital with a suspected viral infection. Abnormal liver function was reported, but improved spontaneously

At 4 months of age he had a second hospital admission with recurrent vomiting and faltering growth. This settled without medical intervention but due to poor weight gain, an energy dense cow's milk based infant formula was introduced

By the age of 7 months his development was slow with growth faltering. He had abnormal transferrin electrophoresis. Although this is not a usual test for galactosaemia, abnormal results could suggest a glycoprotein deficient syndrome or galactosaemia

He was transferred to an inherited metabolic disorders unit. Galactosaemia was confirmed by elevated galactose-1-phosphate concentrations and DNA confirmation of heterozygous common Q188R mutation. No galactosuria was detected. Medical examination showed no dysmorphic features, systemic examination was all normal, his liver was slightly enlarged

A lactose free diet with an infant soya formula was started and within 2 weeks there was a significant improvement in his weight. Both weight and height z scores continued to improve:

Age (months)	Weight z score	Height z score
7 (diagnosis)	−2.07	−2.36
12	0.27	−1.53
18	0.31	−0.65

Following treatment, galactose-1-phosphate concentrations were maintained at the lower end of the treatment range

Summary
Atypical presentation. This child was fed on cow's milk based infant formula containing lactose, but did not develop severe liver dysfunction or galactosuria which made diagnosis challenging

Case studies

Two case studies demonstrating the dietary management of an infant diagnosed in the neonatal period and diagnosis in later infancy are given in Tables 18.12 and 18.13.

Galactokinase Deficiency

Galactokinase deficiency is an autosomal recessive disorder which results in the formation of early onset nuclear cataracts. Galactokinase normally catalyses the phosphorylation of galactose with adenosine triphosphate (ATP) to form galactose-1-phosphate (Fig. 18.1). Consequently, the majority of ingested galactose is excreted as such or as its reduced metabolite, galactitol. Galactitol accumulates resulting in osmotic damage to the lens fibre. Hepatic and renal damage and neurological disturbances do not occur.

The incidence of galactokinase deficiency is low and cannot be assessed with any accuracy [3]. In most parts of Europe, in the USA and in Japan birth incidence is of the order of 1 in 150 000 to 1 million. It is higher in the Balkan countries, the former Yugoslavia, Romania and Bulgaria, where it is common in travellers [109, 110]. Over 30 mutations have been described.

Bosch *et al.* [111] reviewed the clinical features of galactokinase deficiency in 55 patients from 25 publications. Cataracts were reported in most patients. In a series of 18 patients diagnosed by newborn screening, slight cataracts without visual impairment occurred in 50% of the patients. Hypoglycaemia, mental retardation, microcephaly and faltering growth were associated with poor dietary adherence [110], but this may not be a consequence of galactokinase deficiency.

Treatment is a low galactose diet [112]. When the diagnosis is made quickly and dietary management is prompt, i.e. during the first 2–3 weeks of life, cataracts mainly clear. When treatment is late and cataracts are dense they will not clear completely (or at all) and must be removed surgically.

UDP-galactose-4-epimerase Deficiency

This is a very rare autosomal disorder and the prevalence varies amongst different ethnic groups. Epimerase deficiency galactosaemia results from the impairment of UDP-galactose-4-epimerase (GALE), the third enzyme in the Leloir pathway of galactose metabolism (Fig. 18.1). The majority of patients have a clinically benign condition (peripheral epimerase deficiency) with enzyme impairment principally in their erythrocytes [3]. Their growth and development is normal. A low galactose diet appears to be unnecessary.

Isolated cases of a severe clinical form and/or biochemically intermediate cases of epimerase deficiency have been reported [113]. The severe form of GALE deficiency resembles classical galactosaemia [18]. It is treated with a galactose restricted diet. Epimerase forms UDP-galactose from UDP-glucose. If epimerase deficiency is absolute, it will result in an inability to form glycoproteins and glycolipids. It has been suggested that it may be necessary to prescribe a small amount of dietary galactose to allow for manufacture of these essential compounds. However, there have been no reports of patients who have total absence of GALE activity [3].

Glycogen Storage Disorders

Marjorie Dixon

Introduction

Glycogen is the storage form of carbohydrates (CHO) and is found predominantly in skeletal muscle and liver; more minor stores are found in heart and brain. It is a large molecule containing up to 60 000 glucose moieties which are linked in straight chains, with α-1,4 glycosidic bonds, and branched, with α-1,6 glycosidic bonds at intervals of 4–10 glucose residues, thus forming a glucose reservoir. Glycogen is a major fuel source. In the fed state glucose forms glycogen (glycogenesis). In the fasting state glycogen is degraded to glucose-6-phosphate (G6P) via a series of enzymatic reactions.

G6P has three fates:

- conversion to free glucose which occurs predominantly in the liver for release into the blood stream. This process from glycogen to glucose is termed glycogenolysis.
- as the initial substrate for energy production via glycolysis, forming pyruvate. Under aerobic conditions pyruvate is oxidised to form ATP; under anaerobic conditions in active muscle tissue it is converted to lactate. Lactate generated from muscle glycogen or glucose can be transported via the blood stream to the liver and, via the gluconeogenic pathway, reform

glucose. This recycling pathway is known as the Cori cycle.

- processed by the pentose phosphate pathway to yield NADPH and ribose derivatives.

Gluconeogenesis is the reversal of glycolysis and is another major pathway for glucose formation via G6P from lactate, pyruvate, gluconeogenic amino acids (p. 381) and glycerol. Fructose and galactose can also enter the gluconeogenic pathway to form glucose or, via glycolysis, to form pyruvate and lactate (Fig. 18.2).

Defects of most of the enzymatic reactions involved in glycogen metabolism have been identified and collectively are known as the glycogen storage disorders (GSD) (Table 18.14). These are notated by a Roman numeral, the deficient enzyme or the person's name who first described the disorder (Fig. 18.2, Table 18.14). In this section mainly the hepatic GSD are discussed as these are treated primarily by diet. Dietary treatment varies between the different disorders and ranges from complex intensive feeding routines with overnight tube feeds to more straightforward treatments of avoidance of fasting and management of illness. Other GSD affect mainly muscle and present with exercise intolerance often followed by rhabdomyolysis; these are not discussed, other than Pompe's disease (GSDII).

Glycogen Storage Disease Type I

Genetics and biochemistry

The glucose-6-phosphatase system has a central role in glucose production. It is the final common pathway reaction for endogenous glucose synthesis from both glycogenolysis and gluconeogenesis (Fig. 18.2). GSDI has two subtypes:

- GSD type Ia due to deficiency of glucose-6-phosphatase which hydrolyses G6P into glucose and inorganic phosphate (gene *G6PC*). It is expressed in liver, renal cortex and intestinal mucosa but not muscle.
- GSD type Ib due to deficiency of glucose-6-phosphate transporter protein (G6Ptranslocase)

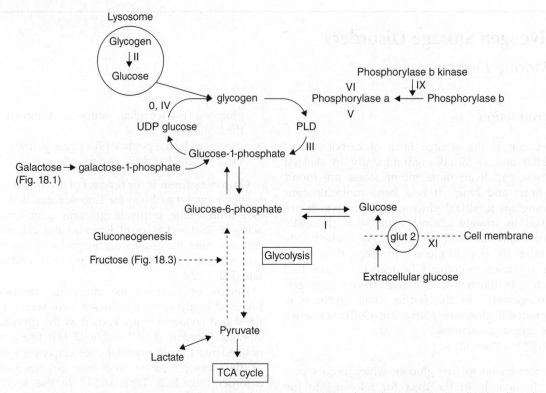

Figure 18.2   Pathway of liver glycogen metabolism. UDP glucose, uridine diphosphate glucose; PLD, phosphorylase limit diatria.

Table 18.14   Selected glycogen storage disorders, nomenclature and main organs involved.

Type	Eponym	Enzyme deficiency	Principal organs involved
0 *		Glycogen synthase	Liver
Ia *	Von Gierke	Glucose-6-phosphatase	Liver, kidney
Ib *		Glucose-6-phosphatase translocase	Liver, kidney and leucocytes
II	Pompe	Acid α-glucosidase	Muscle and heart
III a/b *	Cori, Forbes	Debranching enzyme and subtypes	Liver ± muscle
VI *	Her's	Phosphorylase	Liver
IX *		Phosphorylase kinase and subtypes	Liver and/or muscle
XI *	Fanconi–Bickel	Glut 2	Liver, kidney

*Hepatic glycogen storage disorder.

which transports G6P from the cytoplasm across the endoplasmic reticulum membrane into the lumen for hydrolysis (gene *SLC37A4*) [115]. The transporter is expressed ubiquitously.

Glucose production is inadequate if either enzyme is deficient, as the formation of glucose from both glycogenolysis and gluconeogenesis is blocked. Hypoglycaemia results after relatively short periods of fasting when exogenous glucose sources are depleted, typically around 2 hours.

GSD types Ia and Ib are autosomal recessive inherited disorders. More than 80 mutations have been identified [116]. There are common mutations in different populations such as the p.R83C mutation seen in Caucasian, Tunisian and the Ashkenazi Jewish populations. The estimated incidence is around 1 in 100 000 births [117], although in the Ashkenazi Jewish population a much higher incidence of 1 in 20 000 is predicted, due to increased frequency of the p.R83C mutation [118]. GSDIa occurs more frequently (about 80% of GSDI patients) than Ib and is the most common of the hepatic GSD.

Clinical features

The term GSDI encompasses both types Ia and Ib unless otherwise indicated. GSDI can present in the neonatal period, but more typically occurs later in infancy between 4 and 6 months as periods of fasting are extended, particularly overnight, resulting in a fast induced hypoglycaemic episode which can cause seizures and lactic acidosis [116, 117, 119]. The infant usually wakes for night feeds and may appear sweaty and pale due to low blood glucose levels. The clinical manifestations in untreated patients include growth retardation, truncal obesity and muscle wasting, rounded doll like facies and hepatomegaly (causing a protrudent abdomen) due mainly to fatty infiltration of the liver [116]. These features can also be seen in treated patients, but generally to a lesser extent. As G6P cannot form glucose there is increased glycolytic flux which leads to secondary metabolic derangements of lactic acidosis (with or without hyperventilation), hyperuricaemia and hyperlipidaemia, with triglycerides more markedly elevated than cholesterol [116]. Hyperlipidaemia is considered to be due to increased *de novo* lipid synthesis from excess acetyl-CoA (formed from pyruvate) and decreased lipid serum clearance [120]. Bruising and bleeding can occur due to platelet dysfunction. Hyperuricaemia is caused by decreased renal clearance due to competition with lactate for excretion and increased breakdown of adenine nucleotides to uric acid [116]. Ketone body production, as an alternative fuel during fasting, is reduced because excess acetyl-CoA leads to increased concentrations of malonyl-CoA which promotes lipid synthesis rather than oxidation of fatty acids to form ketones. Additionally in type Ib, there is chronic neutropenia and impaired neutrophil function which increases susceptibility to recurrent bacterial infections, oral and intestinal mucosal ulcerations and a chronic inflammatory bowel disease similar histopathologically to Crohn's disease [116, 119, 121, 122]. Neutropenia is considered to be due to increased

apoptosis of mature neutrophils and the movement of neutrophils from blood to inflamed tissues [123].

Long term complications are reported in both types: renal disease (both glomerular and tubular dysfunction) and also hypertension in some [124]; hepatic tumours (mostly benign adenoma, but with the potential for malignant transformation) which develop predominantly during and after puberty [125]; low bone mineral density and osteopenia [119, 126]; anaemia [127, 128]; and polycystic ovaries in females [119, 129]. Diabetes has been described more recently in both Ia (personal communication) and Ib [130]. Good metabolic control is essential to help delay the onset and severity of these complications.

Dietary management

GSDI is treated primarily by diet. The aims are

- to maintain a constant normal blood glucose concentration without large swings which can cause rebound hypoglycaemia; hypoglycaemia carries the risk of neurological complications [116, 117] and hyperglycaemia can cause hyperinsulinism which, long term, may lead to insulin resistance
- to help correct the secondary biochemical abnormalities (described above) by maintenance of normglycaemia, but it is recognised that these cannot be completely normalised; hyperlipidaemia is frequently observed on treatment [116, 119, 131]
- to promote normal growth and maintain a healthy body mass index (BMI)
- to help delay or prevent long term complications

To maintain normoglycaemia the diet has an increased CHO content compared with the normal population, but the total daily energy intake should be similar. The diet typically provides 60%–70% energy from CHO, 20%–25% from fat and 10%–15% from protein. Maintenance of a normal energy intake is important as overweight and obesity is a problem in some patients [119, 132, 133]. Inactive children should have a lower energy intake. Exercise capacity appears to be reduced in some and this should also be considered [134].

Carbohydrate

Provision of CHO to maintain normoglycaemia in GSDI patients has altered over the years. Traditionally frequent CHO feeding was given day and night. In 1976 Greene *et al.* reported the intensive regimen of regular drinks of glucose polymer by day and continuous nasogastric drip feeding at night [135]. In 1984 Chen *et al.* introduced uncooked cornstarch to the diet to provide a source of slow release glucose to the blood circulation [136].

Infants and children are given a frequent supply of glucose both day and night at least until they have stopped growing. Postpuberty glucose therapy is still needed, but this can generally be given less frequently (p. 549). Growth improves in children on intensive dietary treatment. Glucose requirements are calculated from basal glucose production rates in normal children [137]. It is important to be aware that these glucose requirements (g/kg/hour or mg/kg/minute) decrease with age (Table 18.15). The glucose intakes for children with GSDI can be calculated to be similar to normal hepatic glucose production [135,138] but should be adjusted to achieve good biochemical control (p. 555); more or less glucose may be needed. It is important to ensure that only the required amount of glucose is administered, as excessive CHO intake induces peripheral body fat storage due to glycogen overload and hyperlipidaemia. Large quantities of glucose exacerbate swings in blood glucose levels and make patients more prone to hyperglycaemia and rebound hypoglycaemia [139,140]. Equally important is the need to provide adequate glucose as insufficient amounts lead to high plasma lactate levels and growth retardation. Achieving optimal biochemical control is difficult.

Table 18.15 Glucose requirements based on glucose production rates [137].

Age	Glucose (mg/kg/min)	Glucose (g/kg/hour) Day	Night
Infants	8–9	0.5	0.5
Toddlers and children	5–7	0.3–0.4	0.3–0.4
Adolescents and adults	2–4 at night		0.2–0.25

Glucose is given throughout the 24 hour period as complex CHO and glucose from a combination of food, glucose polymer and uncooked cornstarch. Provision of CHO varies between metabolic centres. For example, in the UK most children are given continuous overnight feeding using glucose polymers and intermittent uncooked cornstarch (UCCS, p. 549) during the daytime, whereas in the USA UCCS is more likely to be given intermittently throughout the 24 hour period with no overnight tube feeds. A systematic review [141] and meta-analysis of these two methods of feeding concluded that UCCS was superior to continuous overnight drip feeding in maintaining blood glucose concentrations, but acknowledged the limitations of the current evidence. Derks *et al.* [142] endorsed the shortcomings of the published evidence, but also highlighted that blood glucose in isolation should not determine this conclusion; all other factors which impact on optimal metabolic control and long term outcome such as plasma lactate and lipid concentrations should also be considered.

Typically around 40%–50% of the CHO energy is provided from a combination of glucose polymer and UCCS, although in some children the percentage may be higher. CHO from foods at main meals will provide more glucose than the basal requirement and this should be taken into account when planning the overall daily CHO and energy intake. Guidance on amounts of CHO to eat and avoidance of foods with high sugar content is necessary to prevent excessive glucose and energy intake and swings in blood glucose. Vitamin and mineral supplements are necessary because of the high energy intake from pure starch and glucose.

Fructose and galactose

Some European and US centres restrict fructose and galactose because these sugars are not converted to glucose but instead lead to increased lactate production via glycolysis [117,143]. However, a mildly elevated blood lactate level of up to 4.0 mmol/L is considered acceptable by some because lactate provides an alternative source of energy to the brain and therefore has a protective effect against fuel depletion [144]. Indeed Melis *et al.* [145] have highlighted the detrimental impact that hypoglycaemia can have on brain function. Lactate may contribute to long term complications but the concentration at which this occurs is not known. There are no published studies to compare biochemical parameters or outcome of patients on restricted or unrestricted intakes of fructose and galactose. Some centres consider that the restriction of these sugars is not essential and ensuring the regular provision of glucose is more important.

The dietary management guidelines from the European Study on GSDI recommends that lactose, fructose and sucrose are restricted, but there is no consensus on the degree of restriction required [139]. The dietary intake of these sugars may inadvertently be reduced because 40% or more of dietary CHO is provided from pure starch and glucose polymer. The author's unit does not routinely limit intake of these sugars. Some children can have near normal plasma lactate levels despite including fructose and lactose in the diet. If plasma lactate is persistently elevated on an unrestricted diet, a trial of reducing fructose and galactose may be warranted. If the diet is restricted this will limit intake of fruit, vegetables, milk and dairy products, and thus vitamin and mineral supplements (specifically calcium and vitamin D) are necessary.

Fat

Fat intake is decreased to compensate for increased CHO intake and to help maintain a normal energy intake. Replacement of saturated with polyunsaturated fats is recommended by some in an attempt to improve the hyperlipidaemia [146], but this is less important than supplying a frequent CHO intake and avoiding overtreatment. Despite persistent hyperlipidaemia, no evidence of endothelial dysfunction or premature atherosclerosis has been observed [147–150]. However, a more recent case control study of 28 GSDI patients (mean age 23 years) from the USA reports arterial dysfunction (based on measurement of surrogate markers for cardiovascular disease, carotid intima media thickness and brachial artery reactivity), thus suggesting that patients may be at increased risk of cardiovascular disease [151]. The publication also debates the previously proposed protective mechanisms against the development of atherosclerosis. In a younger group of 19 GSDI patients, mean age 9 years, plasma levels of asymmetric dimethylarginine levels (ADMA), a biomarker for endothelial

dysfunction and atherosclerosis, were found to be similar to healthy controls and this supports preservation of endothelial function [152]. These studies did not discuss dietary treatments or BMI and this may have had some influence on the findings.

The effects of medium chain triglycerides (MCT), as an energy source, on biochemical parameters has recently been reported in two studies, including six patients (three with mild phenotype) with GSDI [153, 154]. MCT enters β-oxidation bypassing malonyl-CoA and in the liver produces ketone bodies, whereas in GSDI production of ketone bodies is reduced. Use of MCT as a fuel may allow less energy from CHO to be given and help correct the secondary biochemical abnormalities. Both studies report improvements in biochemical control on MCT. Das et al. also reported that CHO energy intake could be decreased with MCT intakes of 15–20 g/day [154]. In the UK, MCT is currently not used in standard dietary treatment of GSDI.

Tube feeding

Continuous tube feeding can be used to provide glucose overnight. Gastrostomy tube feeding is used in preference to nasogastric (NG) feeding in type Ia as it is more acceptable and removes the risk of NG tube displacement or entanglement particularly during the night. GSDI patients have increased risk factors for surgery, such as an increased bleeding tendency and hypoglycaemia, so this requires careful management. Patients should be admitted the day before for assessment and commenced on intravenous (IV) 10% dextrose (ensuring basal glucose requirements are provided) prior to surgery and this is only discontinued once gastrostomy feeds are established. Gastrostomy placement is contraindicated in type Ib because of infection risk and poor wound healing [139].

Careful management of overnight feeding is necessary because there are significant risks. Indeed, fatalities have been reported because of unplanned cessation in delivery of the glucose feed and the failure to switch on the pump delivering the feed [155, 156]. It is therefore essential that the feed pump accurately controls flow rate and alarms if there is electrical or mechanical failure. To prevent any leaks the tubing used for feed delivery must be secure [156]. An enuresis alarm may also be helpful in identifying any leakage of feed into the bed. Some parents use baby alarms to hear if their child is restless or wakens during the night as this can be a sign of problems with the overnight feed or hypoglycaemia. Parents must be well instructed and be adept and confident with the enteral feeding system prior to home use. In the case of pump failure, feeds can be given as 2 hourly boluses in the interim, but rapid access to a functioning pump is essential. An oral or bolus feed is given prior to the commencement of the continuous overnight tube feed if the child has not been fed in the previous 2 hours. On discontinuation of the overnight feed it is extremely important that the child is fed again within 15 minutes to avoid hypoglycaemia [119]. In practice, usually a small bolus feed is given immediately on cessation of the night feed and then the child is fed again within 30 minutes. The pre and post bolus feeds are the same composition as the overnight feed (infant feed or glucose polymer); the amount given is 50% of the volume of 1 hour's worth of the night feed.

Diet for infants

Most patients with GSDI present before 1 year of age [116]. Infants need a frequent supply of glucose both day and night. Regular 2 hourly feeding during the day (although some may need to be fed

more often) and continuous nasogastric feeds by night are needed to maintain normoglycaemia. In infants <4–6 months of age the glucose requirements of around 0.5 g/kg/hour (Table 18.15) can be provided by normal infant formula (from lactose) if fed at normal volumes of 150–180 mL/kg. Both galactose and glucose contribute towards the glucose requirement. If lactose alone does not provide adequate glucose, glucose polymer is added in 1% increments to achieve optimal biochemical control (p. 555), aiming to maintain energy intake around normal for age. Some centres use a soya infant formula to avoid galactose and provide all the glucose as glucose polymer. At night the feed is given continuously via a pump, usually administered for 10–12 hours. At the beginning and end of the night feed, an oral or bolus feed providing sufficient glucose to last for 30 minutes is given (50% the volume given for 1 hour from the night feed). The feeding regimen is established in hospital. Bedside blood glucose monitoring is used to guide dietary treatment, ideally 24 hour blood glucose and lactate profile (1–2 hourly measurements), or continuous glucose monitoring (p. 570) is done prior to discharge once the treatment regimen is established. An example of an infant's feeding regimen is shown in Table 18.16. Breast feeding is possible but experience is very limited. Breast feeding a GSD infant is demanding for a mother:

Table 18.16 Example feeding regimen for an infant with GSDI.

Weight 5 kg   Aim 0.5 g glucose/kg/hour*

	Fluid (mL)	Energy (kcal)	(kJ)	Lactose (g)	Protein (g)	Fat (g)
SMA 1	840	546	2282	60	12.6	30
Amount/kg	170	110	456	12.0	2.5	
Amount/kg/hour				0.5*		
Amount/hour				2.5		

Daily feed distribution

Day: Oral feeds 70 mL
8.30 am, 10 am, 12 noon, 2 pm, 4 pm, 6 pm = 420 mL

Night: Continuous nasogastric feeds 35 mL every hour from 8 pm, finishing at 8 am = 420 mL
Bolus nasogastric feeds 20 mL at 8 pm and 8 am (extra to calculated fluid requirement)

Lactose = 0.25 g glucose and 0.25 g galactose. Glucose polymer can be added to provide more glucose, as indicated by blood glucose and lactate results.

at least 2 hourly daytime feeding is necessary and small volume top-up feeds of 10%–20% glucose polymer solution may be necessary to maintain normoglycaemia. The mother can express breast milk for the continuous overnight feed or infant formula could be given instead.

Weaning is commenced at the normal time around 6 months (26 weeks) of age. Establishing a feeding pattern for solids can be very difficult. Often the infant is not hungry because of the frequent day and overnight feeding and consequently feeding problems are common. Solids should contain complex CHO foods such as baby rice, oat/wheat based cereal, rusk, potato, pasta. As the intake of starchy food increases it can replace the infant feed at main meals as the source of glucose for the following 2 hours. As relatively small quantities of food provide the glucose requirements, a complicated CHO food exchange system is not always necessary. It can sometimes be sufficient just to teach parents which foods provide CHO and to include these at the three main meals. However, if the introduction of solids is difficult a list of quantities of foods which provide the necessary amount of CHO per meal can prove useful. Advantages to teaching parents about food portion sizes include helping to prevent excess CHO and energy intake and to prevent swings in blood glucose. For example, an 8 kg infant requires 0.5 g glucose/kg/hour which equates to 8 g CHO for a 2 hour period; a list of weights of starchy foods which provide around 8 g CHO would be given and/or parents taught to calculate and weigh the amount of food required using the CHO analysis/100 g on the food label, although not all families could cope with this. The CHO content per portion may also be listed and can be used as a guide.

To calculate the amount of food needed to provide a specific amount of CHO:

Example – weight of cornflakes to provide 15 g CHO

Step 1
    Look at total CHO content per 100 g of food (on nutrition analysis label) = 84 g CHO per 100 g
Step 2
    Then 100 ÷ by the CHO content per 100 g of food = 100 ÷ 84 = 1.19
Step 3
    Multiply the answer by 15 (or other amount of CHO required) = 1.19 × 15

This is the weight of food needed to provide 15 g CHO (or other amount of CHO required) = 18 g
Step 4
Weigh out 18 g of cornflakes

Invariably, there is reliance on tube feeding to provide some or even all of the necessary daytime glucose in infants and children with feeding problems and where there is difficulty in establishing a 2 hourly daytime feeding regimen. Feeding problems can begin to improve when UCCS is introduced as the interval between feeding times can be increased.

As more energy is derived from solids, the infant should take smaller daytime feed volumes. However, the daily intake (taking into account the night feed) of infant formula must not fall too low because it continues to provide a major source of nutrients in the older baby's diet. To ensure adequate intake of glucose (0.5 g CHO/kg/hour) from smaller volumes of infant formula, glucose polymer is added to give a final concentration of 10%–15% CHO. The between meal infant feeds should be gradually replaced, ideally by a complex CHO snack (providing the desired amount of CHO) or CHO drinks such as baby juices with added glucose polymer or glucose polymer solution alone, although these are less ideal because they are rapidly absorbed, may cause swings in blood glucose and may not maintain blood glucose for 2 hours in some patients. Care must be taken to avoid giving over concentrated CHO drinks because their osmolality may precipitate diarrhoea. Intermittent diarrhoea or loose stools occurs in some patients, but the cause is not completely understood [157–159]. A maximum concentration of 15% CHO is recommended in older infants.

Infant formula can continue to be given overnight, but for older infants large volumes would need to be given to provide the required amount of CHO, which would compromise the daytime appetite. Therefore, the volume of infant formula is decreased and glucose polymer added to provide around 0.5 g glucose/kg/hour, with the ultimate aim of providing all CHO as glucose polymer from about 1 year of age. It is important to ensure that the daily feeding regimen is nutritionally adequate and contains enough protein as this can be compromised in patients on high CHO diets and who also do not eat well. An example of a weaning diet is shown in Table 18.17.

Table 18.17 Example of a diet for a 10-month-old infant with GSDI.

Weight 8 kg	Aim 0.5 g carbohydrate/kg/hour (4 g CHO/hour)						
Time	Food or drink	Total CHO (g)	CHO g/kg/hour[*]	Protein (g)	Fat (g)	Energy (kcal)	(kJ)
8.15 am	1 Weetabix	10.0	0.9	1.7	0.4	50	210
	100 mL semi-skimmed milk	5.0		3.3	1.6	46	193
10.00 am	15 mL concentrated baby juice diluted to 100 mL	9.0	0.5	–	–	36	150
12.00 pm	Stage 3 pouch – spaghetti bolognese	12.0	1.7	7.4	4.7	125	525
	Small banana	15.3		0.8	0.2	62	260
2.00 pm	2 sponge fingers	10.0	0.8	1.0	0.4	48	200
	Few grapes	3.0			–	11	46
	100 mL water						
4.00 pm	1 potato waffle	9.1	1.6	0.9	4.4	85	360
	1 grilled fish finger	4.6		3.6	2.3	55	230
	30 g soft boiled carrots	2.6		0.2	0.1	10	42
	Small pot low fat yoghurt (60 g)	9.5		3.5	1.7	68	285
6.00 pm	100 mL SMA 2 + glucose polymer to 10% CHO	10.0	0.5	1.5	3.6	79	332
8.00 pm to 8.00 am finish	30 mL hourly for 12 hours SMA 2 + glucose polymer to 13% CHO	47.0	0.5	5.4	13.0	327	1374
8.00 pm and 8.00 am	15 mL bolus SMA 2 + glucose polymer to 13% CHO	3.9		1.0	0.5	27	113
Totals		151		30.3	32.9	1029	4320
% Energy intake		59		12	29		

[*]The portion size of carbohydrate foods (appropriate for age) will make the carbohydrate content of main meals in excess of the specified requirement of 0.5 g/kg/hour (calculated as a combined intake).

Diet for children

In children under 2 years of age a daytime source of CHO continues to be given at 2 hourly intervals either from a meal or snack containing complex CHO or a drink with added glucose polymer. The portion size of CHO foods (appropriate for age) will make the CHO content of main meals in excess of the specified requirement (0.3–0.5 g CHO/kg/hour) so portion sizes may need to be limited. The 2 hourly between meal snacks or drinks should aim to provide only the specified requirement of CHO as excessive amounts may reduce appetite for the main meal. Parents should be given information on different drinks and snacks that supply only the required amount of glucose.

Starchy foods such as potato, rice, pasta, bread and breakfast cereals are encouraged in preference to sugary foods because these are more slowly digested to produce glucose.

From around 1 year of age the night feed is often changed to a solution of glucose polymer. With age, the concentration of glucose polymer solutions is increased up to 15% CHO in 1–2 year olds, 20% CHO in 2–6 year olds, 25% up to a maximum of 30% CHO for older children. A comprehensive vitamin and mineral supplement is needed and is often added to the night feed. Occasionally a paediatric enteral feed is administered at night in preference to glucose polymer alone, particularly if growth and nutrient intakes are inadequate. At night the feed is delivered continuously via an enteral feed pump, usually for 10–12 hours. Pre and post overnight bolus feeds are required, as described for infants. Some children have a starchy snack rather than a bolus feed before the night feed. As many children with GSDI find it very difficult to eat breakfast due to being fed overnight, a CHO or milk drink (plus UCCS) from around age 2 years is usually given 30 minutes after stopping the night feed and giving the bolus feed.

Vitamins and minerals

Children with GSDI can be at risk of vitamin and mineral deficiencies [132,160], particularly as a high percentage of the dietary energy intake is provided as glucose polymer and pure starch. Thiamin is essential for normal glucose metabolism and at least the reference nutrient intake (RNI) for age [98] should be supplied. Excessive intakes of glucose and complex CHO may even increase the requirement of thiamin. Inadequate calcium intakes have been reported and reduced bone mineral density (BMD) has been found [161] although this also occurs in patients reported to have normal calcium intakes [162]. Vitamin D and calcium intakes need to be adequate to optimise bone health [126]. Biotin deficiency causing skin lesions has been reported in a GSDIb child on GSD formula; unfortunately no details were given about the composition of the formula or the actual biotin intake [163]. The vitamin and mineral intakes of children with GSD should be regularly monitored, in particular calcium and vitamin D because of risk of low BMD and osteopenia; supplements are usually necessary. Monitoring of BMD by DEXA scan is recommended [139].

Adolescents

After puberty some form of nocturnal glucose therapy needs to continue to prevent fasting hypoglycaemia and biochemical abnormalities [164]. Adolescents should be reassessed at this time to determine their fasting tolerance as this may differ from that in childhood [132]. Discontinuing the overnight tube feed can be difficult even when growth ceases, as UCCS does not maintain normoglycaemia for sufficiently long periods.

Quality of life

The intensive 24 hour feeding regimen is demanding and time consuming for parents, particularly when managing the young child with a maximum 2 hourly fasting tolerance. It is disruptive to normal living during the day and night for both parents and child, with potentially serious consequences if treatment is not adhered to. Management requires constant watching of the clock and great attention to detail. Feeding problems are common and can manifest as a poor food intake or quality of diet, and overfeeding because of concern about hypoglycaemia. A lower quality of life has been reported in GSDI patients; this study also highlights the burden of care on parents [165]. Support from a paediatric psychologist is valuable.

Uncooked cornstarch

Uncooked cornstarch (UCCS), 'household cornflour', is a branched chain glucose polymer (92% CHO) made up of amylose (linear chain) and amylopectin (branched chain). The ratio can vary; some have a high amylopectin to amylose ratio. Uncooked, it is slowly digested, primarily by pancreatic amylase to gradually release glucose into the circulation. In GSDI it is given to help maintain normoglycaemia. When compared with glucose polymer feeding, a smoother blood glucose profile is produced and less glucose is required [166]. Satisfactory glycaemia has been reported to last from 4 to 9 hours after ingestion [166,167]. However, Lee *at al.* reported only achieving satisfactory glycaemia for a median of 4.25 hours (range 2.5–6.0) [168]. This variation in duration of response may, in some patients, be attributable to malabsorption [169]. A study comparing a novel, uncooked physically modified cornstarch WMHM20 (produced by a controlled heat moisture process) with standard cornstarch in 21 patients (10 subjects >15 years) with GSDI and III reported longer duration of euglycamia, better short term biochemical control and relatively less colonic fermentation [170]. The composition of the two products studied differed in amylopectin and resistant starch content: WMHM20 99.5% and 67.7%, cornstarch 72.8% and 60.5%, respectively. WMHM20 is now marketed as Glycosade. Correia *et al.* [171] conducted a similar study in 12 GSDI subjects, mean age 23 years. The novel starch produced a smoother and more sustained blood glucose response compared with cornstarch; no difference was found in blood lactate concentrations. Further work by the same group on 20 subjects treated with Glycosade showed increased duration of fasting overnight compared with UCCS (on average extended by 4 hours) and after 6 months follow-up subjects were stable or showed improved metabolic control [172]. Glycosade is being used by some patients in the UK. More studies in younger children are needed.

UCCS can obviate the need for 2 hourly feeding. It is administered at regular intervals throughout the day (and night for some patients) in doses which approximate the basal glucose production rate (Table 18.15). In practice the amount of UCCS given per dose is typically 2 g/kg body weight in young children, decreasing to around 1.5 g/kg in older children, 1 g/kg in adolescents who have stopped growing. The dose of UCCS should be tailored to requirements and not necessarily be increased as weight changes, unless blood glucose and lactate control is suboptimal. In overweight and obese children lower doses are given, using ideal weight for height. Usually a dose of UCCS is required every 4–6 hours but this is based on the results of the UCCS load test. UCCS is usually introduced between 1 and 2 years of age. In younger children it may not be adequately digested to maintain normal blood glucose because pancreatic amylase activity only reaches mature

levels between 2 and 4 years of age, although its activity is reported to be induced by oral starch [146]. Success has been reported with UCCS in children <2 years of age using smaller more frequent doses [173–175]. Small doses of UCCS added to 2 hourly feeds has helped to maintain blood glucose levels in children >1 year, rather than by increasing glucose polymer.

Figures 18.3 and 18.4 show results of 24 hour continuous glucose monitoring (p. 570) before and after introduction of small doses of UCCS. A 12-month-old child with GSDIb had 2 hourly feeds of Cow & Gate 1 infant formula with added glucose polymer to 11% CHO, providing 0.45 g glucose/kg/hour during the day and overnight feeds providing 0.41 g glucose/kg/hour. During the day blood glucose levels fluctuated with hypoglycaemia and hyperglycaemia (Fig. 18.3). A dose of 2.5 g of UCCS was added to each 2 hourly daytime feed. Blood glucose results improved with a smoother blood glucose profile and maintenance of normoglycaemia (Fig. 18.4).

Cornflour (cornstarch) is given uncooked; cooking or heating disrupts the starch granules by hydrolysis and thus makes it much less effective. UCCS has a chalky taste. It mixes and dissolves fairly easily in water or milk. To increase palatability it can be added to squash, carbonated drinks but some studies report that mixing UCCS with sugars makes it less effective because of increased insulin production [136, 166, 176]; therefore sugar free options may be best. Less commonly UCCS

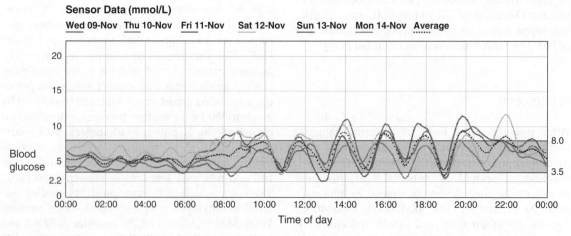

Figure 18.3   24 hour continuous glucose monitoring before uncooked cornstarch. Normoglycaemia is shown by shaded grey band.

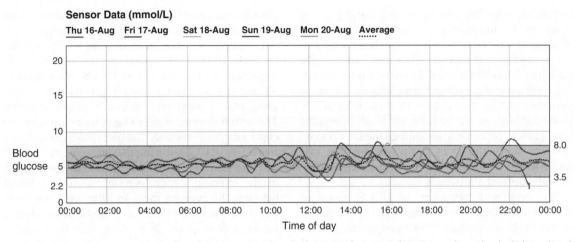

Figure 18.4 24 hour continuous glucose monitoring after uncooked cornstarch. Normoglycaemia is shown by shaded grey band.

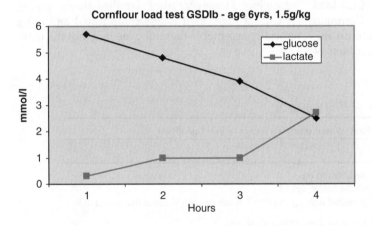

Figure 18.5 Uncooked cornstarch (cornflour) load test.

is given mixed with cold food such as ice cream, yoghurt, fruit purée, thin cold custard or mixed with milk and then poured onto breakfast cereal but this provides more bulk for the child to eat and is also a source of sugars. UCCS settles out on standing and needs to be mixed or shaken prior to consuming. Children taking their UCCS at school, in particular, need to be reminded to do this to ensure the full dose is consumed.

When initiating UCCS treatment, a fasting 'UCCS load test' is done in hospital to assess the child's metabolic response by serial measurement of blood glucose and lactate. The test should be done with the UCCS brand the family use at home as there are differences between brands. The

biochemical test results are used to determine the frequency and quantity of UCCS that should be given. An example of the results of an UCCS load test is given in Fig. 18.5. Over time blood glucose decreases and lactate increases. The test is stopped when blood glucose is <3 mmol/L and/or the child has symptoms of hypoglycaemia. Some children have a poor response to UCCS. In young children the maximum fasting period is usually 3–4 hours but this can improve with increasing age. Prior to the load test, UCCS will have been introduced at home to test its palatability and acceptance; this may be helped by giving a small amount from a young age, around 12–18 months. The dose of UCCS is gradually increased to 2 g/kg at one meal, beginning with 5 g and increasing by 5 g every week to the required dose. Some patients may experience side effects such as diarrhoea, abdominal distention and flatulence but these are usually transient. The child's usual 2 hourly daytime feeding regimen will continue during this introductory period of UCCS. Some children will not take UCCS. Instead it is given via the tube, although it remains important to continue to encourage the UCCS to be taken orally. UCCS can block the feeding tube so it needs to be administered with adequate fluids and the tube flushed afterwards.

The dose and frequency of UCCS needs to be reviewed regularly taking into consideration growth velocity, frequency of hypoglycaemia and biochemical results and should only be increased as indicated rather than routinely based on increasing body weight. Ideally patients should have 24 hour glucose and lactate profiles and UCCS load test repeated every year (Table 18.19) Common times for performing UCCS load test are on initiation of UCCS; increasing age; consideration of

discontinuation of night feed; poor growth or biochemical indices; and starting or changing school. An example of a diet incorporating UCCS is given in Table 18.18. When planning the regimen it is important to be aware that UCCS takes around 30 minutes to start releasing glucose. It is best given after a meal, so it does not reduce appetite. The actual timings need to be planned around the child's daytime routine. The diet usually comprises two doses of UCCS during the daytime, after breakfast and lunch. A third lower dose may be needed in the evening depending on the time interval between the evening meal and the night feed and the child's fasting tolerance. If this is more than 2 hours, a dose of UCCS is given after the evening meal or a CHO snack 2 hours after the evening meal. In children, continuous overnight tube feeding is usually continued until they have stopped growing. However, some families prefer to use UCCS at night as it is less complicated and more socially acceptable than tube feeding, but the main

Table 18.18 Example diet for a 7-year-old child with GSDI.

Weight 25 kg	Aim 0.3 g carbohydrate/kg/hour overnight and cornflour 2 g/kg/dose
Time	Food or drink
8.00 am	**Breakfast** (often refused) including CHO foods, e.g. breakfast cereal, bread 50 g cornflour (2 g/kg) mixed with up to 100 mL water or semi-skimmed/skimmed milk
Mid morning	**Snack** if no breakfast, e.g. semi-sweet biscuit or fruit
12.00 noon	**School dinner** packed lunch including CHO foods, e.g. bread, pitta, wrap as sandwich Fillings, e.g. ham, low fat cheese, egg, chicken, tuna and salad vegetables Fruit, yoghurt
1.00 pm	50 g cornflour (2 g/kg) mixed with up to 100 mL water or semi-skimmed/skimmed milk
5.00 pm	**Evening meal** including CHO foods, e.g. potato, pasta, rice, chapatti Meat, chicken, eggs, fish, dhal Fruit, yoghurt
7.00 pm	**Bedtime snack** including CHO foods to provide 15 g CHO, e.g. toast, crackers, crumpet, muffins, biscuit, cereal
8.00 pm to 7.30 am	20% glucose polymer 40 mL hourly (provides 0.3 g CHO/kg/hour)
8.00 am and 7.30 am	20 mL bolus of 20% glucose polymer

disadvantage of this for young children is the need to wake at around 4–6 hourly intervals, thereby interrupting sleep. Parents also need to wake up to give the UCCS and rely on an alarm clock to do so. Some families routinely give overnight continuous tube feeds but for certain circumstances, e.g. holidays or sleepovers, will instead give UCCS. Cornflour, Glycosade and glucose polymer are approved by the Advisory Committee Borderline Substances (ACBS) for prescription on FP10. Cornflour is usually a shop brand and therefore is food rather than pharmaceutical grade. The dose of cornflour is measured either by scoops or more accurately by weighing. Glycosade is presented in a sachet: each 60 g sachet provides 53 g CHO (which equates to a dose of 55 g UCCS); the required dose is then measured.

Complications of GSD type Ib

Management of type Ib is more complex. Further dietary manipulations may be needed due to additional complications of bacterial infections, oral and intestinal mouth ulcers and, in the majority of children, a chronic inflammatory bowel disease (IBD) of varying severity [116]. Mouth ulcers can make oral feeding difficult and painful. Meals and snacks may need to be temporarily replaced with nutritionally complete fluid supplements and if necessary these can be given via NG tube. Neutropenia is treated with granulocyte-colony stimulating factors (G-CSF); however, there may be complications such as splenomegaly and the IBD continues to occur [116, 121]. In a small study of seven type Ib patients, vitamin E supplementation of 600–900 mg/day, given for its antioxidant properties, was beneficial in reducing infections [177].

Exercise

A major reduction in exercise capacity in adult patients with GSDI has been reported, with mean blood glucose levels for patients showing a progressive decrease throughout exercise and recovery [134]. Children are likely to require additional CHO with prolonged exercise. Parents often report the need to give food or sugary drinks before or after exercise. Pre exercise dietary treatment may need to be adjusted according to the intensity and duration of the exercise being undertaken with complex CHO for low to moderate intensity and sugary snack/drink for high intensity. It is important that children are encouraged to be physically active to help prevent overweight or obesity and associated risks of diabetes and cardiovascular disease.

Hypoglycaemia

Hypoglycaemia occasionally occurs and may be related to delayed meals/drinks/UCCS, illness, poor dietary compliance or prolonged exercise. Parents should contact the metabolic team if there is repeated hypoglycaemia. Parents need to recognise early warning signs such as sweating, pallor, irritability or drowsiness. They should respond to these by immediately giving a sugary or glucose polymer drink orally or via the tube and, on recovery, some starchy foods. Parents need guidance on how much glucose polymer to give as excessive amounts can cause rebound hypoglycaemia; 10–20 g glucose is usually adequate. Dextrose gels such as Glucogel (40% dextrose) can be rubbed into the buccal cavity and is an invaluable treatment for the semiconscious or uncooperative child. If the child is unresponsive or fitting, emergency services should be urgently called. Patients with GSDI do not respond to glucagon (as it normally increases blood glucose via glycogenolysis and gluconeogenesis); IV glucose (10%) or a dextrose gel (as above) is necessary to treat a child with hypoglycaemia who is unconscious.

Illness

During intercurrent infections, the frequent supply of glucose must be maintained to prevent hypoglycaemia and, in GSD type I, lactic acidosis. Parents need to be aware of the different stages of metabolic decompensation from mild to more serious symptoms and the action needed [139]. At least the basal glucose requirement must be given (Table 18.15) and an adequate intake of fluids (similar to standard emergency regimen, ER, volumes). Often a change in dietary regimen is needed because of loss of appetite. During the daytime, 2 hourly glucose polymer drinks or 24 hour continuous tube feeds of glucose polymer will often replace either the usual 2 hourly dietary regimen, or UCCS. Parents are given glucose polymer recipes to provide the basal glucose requirements for age. Some parents use the recipe for the child's usual glucose polymer night feed and this is also appropriate, but more fluid may be necessary. The standard ER concentrations of glucose polymer for age used for management of illness in other metabolic disorders (p. 502) may provide too much glucose, particularly at 20%–25% glucose polymer concentration, resulting in hyperglycaemia and potential rebound hypoglycaemia when discontinued. If the child has diarrhoea and is vomiting, an oral rehydration solution supplemented with glucose polymer to a maximum of 10% CHO is given. It is important to ensure this provides sufficient grams glucose per kilogram per hour for age. If the child does not tolerate the intensive glucose polymer regimen then a hospital admission for IV therapy becomes essential as severe symptomatic hypoglycaemia and lactic acidosis can develop rapidly in this situation. The British Inherited Metabolic Disease Group provides guidelines on IV 10% dextrose therapy (www.bimdg.org.uk).

As the child recovers glucose polymer tube/oral fluids are reintroduced, titrated against IV fluids and increased as tolerated, thus ensuring an overall adequate glucose intake (g/kg/hour) at all times. UCCS and food are usually reintroduced once glucose polymer feeds are re-established, or at the same time.

Example of an illness plan

A 3-year-old girl with GSDIa, weight 14 kg, providing 0.4 g CHO/kg/hour. Calculate the daily amount of glucose = g glucose/kg/hour × kg bodyweight × 24 = 134 g. Recipe for 24 hours: 140 g glucose polymer plus water added up to 1400 mL (10% CHO concentration). Feed 60 mL/hour continuously for 24 hours.

Clinical and biochemical monitoring

Clinical, anthropometric and biochemical monitoring is essential to assess the efficacy of dietary treatment and to guide composition of the diet. Biochemical monitoring is done at home and in hospital. The frequency of monitoring depends upon the child's biochemical results and growth.

Younger and more severe patients will need more frequent monitoring, 3–4 monthly being typical for most patients who are stable.

Growth

Growth measurements are very important as growth retardation occurs with inadequate treatment and even on intensive treatment. Mundy et al. have reported improved growth with intensive dietary treatment but there is a subset within their patient group who, despite therapy, has poor growth. These patients had measured endocrine responses similar to those reported for untreated patients but the reasons for this are not yet clear [178]. Interestingly, the more obese patients were tallest, although as a group they were significantly shorter than average. Melis et al. [179] identified impairment of and differences of the growth hormone insulin-like growth factor (IGF) system between patients with type Ia and Ib and controls and suggest this may account for the differences seen in growth response between patients on similar treatments. They hypothesise that good dietary compliance and metabolic control positively influenced growth due to increased IGF-II and insulin levels. Older studies also report suboptimal growth on different dietary treatments. A comparative study in 1993 of long term management of UCCS versus continuous nocturnal NG glucose feeds reported no significant differences in physical growth and biochemical parameters, but growth in height was still not optimal and obesity was common with both treatments [167]. In 1999 a study of long term continuous glucose therapy with cornstarch or cornstarch alone, mean height standard deviation score was less than target height but within the range of a normal population, but as a group they were overweight for height [175]. Däublin et al. [180] were able to achieve target height in a group of patients by keeping blood glucose in high normal range and blood and urinary lactate fully suppressed in the normal range.

Weight and height should be monitored regularly and BMI calculated. BMI should ideally be in the normal range for age but this can be difficult to achieve in some patients. The suggested aim is to maintain BMI between 0 and +2 standard deviation scores [139].

Table 18.19 Biochemical monitoring for GSDI.

Check at each outpatient appointment unless otherwise indicated

GSD type	0	Ia/b	IIIa/b	VI and IX	Fanconi–Bickel syndrome
CGM	*	*	*	*	*
Glucose ± lactate profiles in hospital	*	*	*	*	*
UCCS load test	*	*	*	*	*
Glucose	√	√	√	√	√
Lactate	√	√		√	√
Ketones	√		√	√	√
Liver profile	√	√	√	√	√
Urate		√			
Triglycerides	√	√	√	√	√
Cholesterol	√	√	√	√	√
Bone profile, vitamin D	√	√	√	√	√
FBC, WBC, iron status	√	√	√	√	√
Renal profile	√	√	√	√	√
Urine protein:creatinine ratio (or equivalent)	√	√			

CGM, continuous glucose monitoring; UCCS, uncooked cornstarch; LFT, liver function tests; FBC, full blood count; WBC, white blood cells.
*Glucose and lactate profiles, CGMS and UCCS are usually performed annually but may vary as clinically indicated.

Biochemical monitoring

Routine outpatient and annual biochemical monitoring are shown in Table 18.19. The biochemical aims of dietary treatment in GSDI are:

- preprandial blood glucose >3.5 mmol/L. Hypoglycaemia is defined as a blood glucose <3.0 mmol/L. Some children may not be symptomatic at these blood glucose levels as lactate may be providing an alternative fuel source. Single blood glucose and lactate levels in a routine clinic appointment are not a good indicator of long term metabolic control.
- plasma lactate <4.0 mmol/L. Some centres aim to maintain lactate in the normal reference range. This can be very difficult to achieve in some patients and a moderately increased lactate may be beneficial as it provides fuel to the brain when blood glucose is low [144]. Lactate can be chronically elevated despite seemingly good dietary treatment. The concentration at which lactate contributes to long term complications is not known.
- plasma triglycerides <6 mmol/L [139]. Triglycerides can be chronically raised.

Other monitoring for GSDI includes DEXA scans, liver ultrasound, markers of renal tubular function. For some patients it may be beneficial to measure blood glucose at home; however, this is not perceived to be essential for daily management. Continuous glucose monitoring is a useful tool for the assessment of management of GSDI patients (p. 570).

Dietary monitoring

The dietary guidelines from the European Study on Glycogen Storage Disease Type I recommend 2–3 monthly dietary reviews for children [139]. The child's dietary regimen needs to be regularly adjusted for age and growth and needs to ensure

- adequate provision of glucose (g glucose/kg/hour) from
  ○ overnight feed and bolus feeds if they are being given pre and post overnight feeds
  ○ 2 hourly daytime feeds or UCCS, and to check dose size, frequency and timing of administration. Adherence may be an issue in some patients; abnormal biochemical results may help reveal this

- nutritional adequacy of vitamin and mineral intake (specifically calcium and vitamin D)

It is also important to regularly check the parents' understanding of

- illness management and that recipes for use during illness are updated regularly for age and weight
- treatment of hypoglycaemia
- wearing a MedicAlert which is useful to alert others to the possibility of hypoglycaemia

Pharmacological treatment

Medicines are prescribed to help correct some of abnormal biochemical results and to help prevent long term complications, e.g. Allopurinol (a xanthine oxidase inhibitor) if plasma urate is raised, an ACE inhibitor if there is persistent microalbuminuria. Both these measures are to help preserve kidney function.

Transplantation

There are reports of successful liver [181, 182] and hepatocyte transplants [183] in GSDI patients. Liver transplant corrects the metabolic derangement, but type Ib patients still experience frequent infections [184]. Post liver transplant dietary treatment is no longer needed but tube feeding may still be necessary because of ongoing feeding problems [185].

Glycogen Storage Disease Type III

Introduction

Glycogen degradation (glycogenolysis) involves both the phosphorylase and debrancher enzymes. Phosphorylase shortens the unbranched outer α-1,4 links of the glycogen molecule to release glucose-1-phosphate and leave four glucosyl units at the α-1,6 branch point (p. 541). The debrancher enzyme then performs two catalytic functions: the transferase component transfers three glucose residues (from the shortened glycogen branch) to the end of a neighbouring glycogen branch, leaving one glucose moiety at the α-1,6 branch point; the glucosidase component releases the glucose moiety thus removing the branch point – hence debrancher enzyme. Glycogen storage disease type III (GSDIII) is due to deficient activity of the debrancher enzyme in various tissues including liver and muscle (Fig. 18.2). Production of free glucose from glycogenolysis is limited and the partially degraded glycogen is stored as an abnormal structure, termed 'limit dextrin'. There are different subtypes of GSDIII: debrancher enzyme deficiency in liver and muscle (GSD type IIIa, 85% of cases); or just in liver (GSD type IIIb, 15% of cases); or, extremely rarely, a selective deficiency in either glucosidase activity (GSD type IIIc, affecting muscle) or transferase activity (GSD type IIId, affecting muscle and liver) [116]. The production of glucose from glycogenolysis is greatly limited due to debrancher deficiency. The gluconeogenic pathway, however, is functional for endogenous glucose production and this prevents the development of profound hypoglycaemia during fasting, although it can still occur. GSDIII is an autosomal recessive inherited disorder with a reported incidence of 1 in 100 000. A high predicted prevalence is reported in the Faroese (approximately 1 in 3100) [186] and North African Jews from Israel (1 in 5400) [187].

Clinical features

Patients can present in infancy and early childhood with predominantly liver related features: hepatomegaly (due to both glycogen and fat accumulation); ketotic hypoglycaemia; markedly elevated liver transaminases; hyperlipidaemia (triglycerides and cholesterol). Lactate is normal. Blood biochemistry improves on treatment. Poor growth can also be seen in childhood, although spontaneous catch-up growth usually occurs during puberty [188]. In type GSDIIIa patients, cardiac manifestations and skeletal myopathy may develop with increasing age. Accumulation of 'limit dextrin' may be involved in the pathogenesis of these. Cardiac involvement is variable, typically manifesting as asymptomatic left ventricular hypertrophy which can progress to symptomatic hypertrophic cardiomyopathy, severe cardiac dysfunction, congestive heart failure and (rarely) sudden death [189–193]. Predictive features for those who have the worst cardiac outcome are not known. Skeletal myopathy presents as weakness and wasting and gradually progresses, being much more of a problem for adults [190, 192]. Many children, however, tire easily with exercise. Skeletal muscle glycogen normally provides an essential energy source to contracting muscle, especially at high intensities. Exercise intolerance in six GSDIIIa patients has been attributed to a block in muscle glycogenolytic capacity [194]. Creatine kinase (CK), as a marker of muscle damage, may increase as children become more active [127]; CK in adult patients, although often still above the normal reference range, is reported to decrease, probably due to progressive muscle loss [190]. Bulbar muscle weakness has been reported in three patients with GSDIIIa [195]. Liver symptoms improve with age; thus hypoglycaemia is less of a problem. A small number of patients develop hepatic cirrhosis and adenomas and, rarely, hepatocellular carcinomas, but this is much less than in type I [192]. Only a few patients have had liver transplant [181, 190, 192]. Bone mineral density is markedly reduced in GSDIII with type IIIa patients being much worse than IIIb [196].

Treatment guidelines

Diagnosis and management guidelines for GSDIII have been published by a multidisciplinary group of experts, mainly from the USA [192], based on current practice and an extensive review of the published literature. They provide recommendations on medical and dietetic management and clinical and biochemical monitoring.

Dietary management

The term GSDIII encompasses GSDIIIa and GSDIIIb, unless otherwise indicated. The main aims of dietary treatment in GSDIII are to

- prevent hypoglycaemia and ketosis in the infant and young child
- promote normal growth and BMI
- help delay onset of cardiac manifestations and muscle myopathy in type IIIa

Dietary treatments – high CHO and high protein diets

Controversy surrounds which dietary therapy is best for patients. Either CHO intake can be increased to provide a continuous supply of glucose (similar to GSDI) or protein intake can be increased to enable gluconeogenesis to provide the main source of glucose. Studies from the early 1980s recommended a high protein diet [197–199]. They suggested an increased demand for gluconeogenesis with loss of muscle amino acids (supported by observations in change of plasma alanine, a major gluconeogenic precursor) and this may be a contributory factor to the skeletal myopathy seen in some patients with GSDIIIa. One of these studies reported a high protein daytime diet and night feed (20%–25% energy from protein) to be beneficial in improving muscle strength in patients with a myopathy but six of seven patients studied were not on any dietary treatment and so perhaps similar improvements could have been achieved with a high CHO diet and night feed [197]. These studies form the basis of current use of high protein diet by some centres. A study of hepatic glucose production and whole body protein turnover using stable isotope techniques in a GSDIIIa patient, compared with control, reported near normal glucose production and unaltered protein turnover; consequently the authors questioned the role of a high protein diet [200].

Three case reports of treatment of cardiomyopathy with a high protein diet (two cases) and a high lipid, low CHO diet and synthetic ketone bodies (one case) have recently been published. The diets had different energy ratios of CHO, protein and fat: case 1, an adult, was given 30% protein (no data were given on CHO and fat) [200]; case 2, an adult, was given 37% protein, 2% lipid, 61% CHO [201]; case 3, an infant, was given 15% protein, 65% lipid, 20% CHO [202]. On treatment, cardiomyopathy improved in all cases, as demonstrated by echocardiography. It is not possible to distinguish which element of the diet was of most benefit. In case 3, ketone bodies and lipid provided the main energy source, and case 2 was obese and had total energy intake reduced to 900 kcal (3.8 MJ)/day. The studies implicate a high CHO diet and UCCS as a possible contributing factor to the development of cardiomyopathy, as excess can cause deposition and accumulation of abnormal glycogen in heart [193, 203].

Provision of a regular high CHO intake using UCCS can be used to maintain normoglycaemia and reduce the need for production of glucose via gluconeogenic substrates [204–206]. Hence this treatment may be as effective as the high protein diet, provided overtreatment is avoided. One small crossover study of five children over a period of 2.5 years compared UCCS diet with a high protein diet and showed unchanged glycaemic control, liver function tests and lipid profiles with both regimens, but better growth and reduced liver spans when using UCCS. Two of the patients with muscle involvement showed increased creatine phosphokinase levels on UCCS diet; no cardiac data were given [207].

Intermittent administration of either UCCS or a high protein supplement is necessary throughout 24 hours with both diets; acceptance of either can be difficult. Achieving a high protein intake from food may be more difficult than a high CHO diet in a young child. Both diets can maintain normo-glycaemia. There are no long term published data to determine which diet therapy is best for patients with myopathy. On current evidence it is not yet clear if a high protein diet is more beneficial than high CHO in treating/delaying onset of cardiac manifestations and muscle myopathy in type IIIa patients. No cohort studies of high protein diets have been reported in infants or young children. Such a high protein intake may not be tolerated or warranted in this age group. A gradual increase in protein intake with age, or if there is evidence of myopathy, may be more appropriate. The final choice of dietary management for children with GSDIII will also vary depending on the severity of the disorder and ultimately what is practically achievable for the child and family. The diet needs to be individually tailored to the child's specific clinical features. A high protein diet in GSD type IIIb patients may not be warranted as they do not develop myopathy.

Practical aspects of dietary treatment

Infants with GSDIII who present early with hypo-glycaemia and poor fasting tolerance require a more intensive dietary regimen with increased CHO, as for GSDI (p. 546). At night, continuous tube feeding is used and regular 2 hourly feeding or UCCS during the daytime. Gastrostomy tube feeding is used in preference to NG (p. 545). Glycosade (p. 553) is used as an alternative to UCCS by some. The suggested energy ratio in GSDI is 60%–70% from CHO, 20%–25% from fat and 10%–15% from protein. In contrast in GSDIII there is greater emphasis on the inclusion of high protein foods in the diet, so protein energy may be greater and CHO less. CHO intake should be provided from complex CHO foods rather than sugary foods. High protein foods are included at each mealtime and UCCS given with skimmed/semi-skimmed milk (to reduce fat intake). Guidelines for provision of a high protein/starch diet are given in Table 18.20. If a higher protein intake is achieved, CHO foods are decreased to prevent overtreatment. It is important to monitor carefully the energy distribution of the diet. Too high an energy intake from CHO can cause rebound hypoglycaemia [208]. If a high percentage of the dietary energy intake is provided as pure starch or glucose polymer, the child will be at risk of vitamin and mineral deficiencies and intakes should be monitored. Calcium and vitamin D intakes are particularly important because of risk of decreased BMD [196].

Children with GSDIII may be able to replace nocturnal feeds with UCCS before they have stopped growing if their fasting tolerance is >6–8 hours. This can happen in late childhood or earlier in some. Fasting tolerance should be assessed in hospital, as described for GSDI. Continuous glucose monitoring (CGM, p. 570) can be used to monitor this change at home.

If a child develops myopathy even more protein should be tried: 20%–25% energy intake from protein, 50%–55% from CHO and 20%–25% from fat [197, 199]. Children who have a good appetite and enjoy milk may possibly achieve a sufficiently high protein intake from protein rich foods, but protein supplements are likely to be necessary. Pure protein powders such as Vitapro, Protifar are versatile and successfully help increase protein intake. They may fully or partially substitute for nocturnal glucose polymer tube feeds and/or

Table 18.20 High starch, normal protein, low fat diet or high protein, normal/reduced starch, low fat diet for glycogen storage disease type III.

Carbohydrate foods (starch and sugar)

Starchy foods At least one serving at three main meals and include at bedtime snack, e.g. bread, chapatti, pitta, cereal, potato, rice, pasta, fruit, plain biscuits or crackers, tea cake, muffins

Sugar and sugary foods These are allowed but should be kept to a minimum, e.g. table sugar, sweets, cakes, ice cream, preserves

* High protein, low fat foods

Milk	Semi-skimmed or skimmed milk, low fat fromage frais or yoghurt
Meat	Lean red meat (<10% fat content), trim off all visible fat
Poultry	
Fish	White fish instead of oily
Cheese	Low fat cheese, e.g. cottage, Edam type, half fat Cheddar, quark
Pulses	Beans, lentils, peas (and sweetcorn)
Eggs	Egg white in preference to yolk
Meat alternatives	Tofu, Quorn

Fats

High fat foods should be used sparingly, e.g. butter, margarine, vegetable oil, animal fats, cream (double, whipping, single), imitation cream, mayonnaise, salad dressings, pastry, batter and breaded foods

Avoid fried or roasted foods. Spread butter or margarine thinly on bread

Snack foods

Most children choose high fat or sugary snack foods, e.g. crisps, nuts, sweets, chocolate. Low fat, high protein or high carbohydrate snack foods should be used instead, e.g. yoghurt, fromage frais, crackers and cheese, glass of milk for the high protein diet or sandwich, plain biscuits, crumpet, fruit for the high starch diet

*High protein diet for GSD III – at least one serving of high protein food at three main meals and bedtime snack. Generous intakes of milk should also be given.

*High starch diet for GSD III – one serving of high protein foods at two meals. Can include milk (or milky foods) in the daily diet.

intermittent UCCS and can be added to daytime drinks. A glucose polymer nocturnal continuous feed can be changed to skimmed milk and protein powder, but this should be instituted in hospital, so blood glucose can be formally monitored. CGM can be used to further monitor this change at home. High protein foods at meals and snack times should be increased (Table 18.20) and parents need guidance on portion sizes. Most high protein drinks or dessert supplements are often too high in energy intake to be very useful. CHO intake will need to be decreased by up to 20% if protein is increased to 25% energy. The overall energy intake of the diet should not increase with changes to the energy ratios. A decrease will be necessary in an overweight child. If a child fatigues and tires early with exercise this should be considered when planning the overall energy intake as overweight and obesity may be a problem for some GSDIII patients [133]. A trial of CHO should be given pre-exercise as this may help prevent symptoms [194].

Children who present later with short stature and hepatomegaly are treated with UCCS or Glycosade which is given to try and improve their growth rate. Symptomatic hypoglycaemia is generally not a problem for these children. Frequency of administration and dose of UCCS (1–2 g/kg/dose) will vary depending on age, growth rate and response. Usually a dose is given before bed and sometimes daytime doses are necessary to improve growth. Children should have regular meals which contain both starchy and protein foods, and a bedtime snack is also important. Fat intake should be decreased to compensate for the increased CHO intake.

Alcohol

Adolescents and adults must be made aware that alcohol is a potent inhibitor of gluconeogenesis and even quite moderate amounts may reduce glucose production. Alcohol intake should be limited and must always be taken in combination with food [209].

Hypoglycaemia

The guidelines given for management of GSDI can also be used for patients with GSD type III (p. 553).

Illness

Children with GSDIII are at risk of hypoglycaemia and therefore during illness a frequent supply of glucose must be maintained. The guidelines given for management of intercurrent illness in GSDI can also be used for patients with GSDIII (p. 553). As not all children with GSDIII are tube fed, glucose polymer feeds are given orally, 2–3 hourly feeds, depending on usual fasting tolerance.

Clinical and nutritional monitoring

Clinical, anthropometric and biochemical monitoring is essential to assess the efficacy of dietary treatment and to guide composition of the diet. Most of the guidelines given for GSDI (p. 554) can be used for GSDIII, taking into account the differences in diet. Table 18.19 provides guidelines for biochemical monitoring. Other recommendations for monitoring in GSDIII include echocardiography to monitor for ventricular hypertrophy, neuromuscular assessment, DEXA scans, liver ultrasound [192].

The Phosphorylase System

Fiona White

Introduction

The phosphorylase system involves two enzymes, glycogen phosphorylase and phosphorylase kinase, which release glucose-1-phosphate from glycogen. Phosphorylase kinase activates glycogen phosphorylase which catalyses the rate limiting step in glycogenolysis, the release of glucose-1-phosphate from the linear chains of α-1,4 linked glucose molecules. Deficiency of either glycogen phosphorylase (GSDVI) or phosphorylase kinase (GSDIX) causes reduced glycogen degradation and consequently decreased glucose production (Fig. 18.2). Gluconeogenesis remains functional for endogenous glucose production.

Glycogen Storage Disease Type VI

Genetics

Glycogen storage disease type VI (GSDVI), first described in 1959, is an autosomal recessively inherited disorder which results from mutations encoding for the enzyme hepatic glycogen phosphorylase (PYGL, EC 2.4.11). The gene is located on chromosome 14 and over 40 mutations have been described [116]. There is a common mutation in the Mennonite population where the incidence is around 1 in 1000 [210].

Clinical presentation and biochemistry

GSDVI usually presents in children around 2–3 years of age with hepatomegaly, due to increased liver glycogen storage, and growth retardation. The clinical presentation is the same as in hepatic forms of GSDIX and similar, but generally milder, to that seen in GSDIII. There may be some muscle or central nervous system involvement with symptoms such as mild hypotonia, delayed motor development, muscle weakness and cramps [211].

Affected children may also present with ketotic hypoglycaemia after an overnight fast or during illness. Blood lipids, particularly triglycerides, are usually raised with a mild increase in liver transaminases and normal uric acid and lactate levels [212]. Large glucose loads may increase postprandial lactate levels; this was seen in 6/6 patients following a glucose loading test [211]. Hypoglycaemia is not always symptomatically obvious and may only become apparent if monitored overnight or after an overnight fast. Therefore it is advisable to do serial blood glucose monitoring, either in hospital or at home, with a period of

CGM (p. 570) and early morning ketone measurement. If hypoglycaemia is present it is usually less severe than in GSDI or GSDIII. Hyperketosis may be present after an overnight fast indicating the occurrence of lipolysis to preserve blood glucose and the need for additional carbohydrate intake overnight even if absolute hypoglycaemia has not occurred. Clinical symptoms generally improve with age, hepatomegaly has usually resolved by puberty [210] and complete catch-up in final height achieved. Osteoporosis is a risk factor if there is chronic ketosis [116].

Glycogen Storage Disease Type IX

Genetics

Glycogen storage disease type IX (GSDIX) or phosphorylase b kinase (PHK) deficiency is one of the most common forms of GSD. The enzyme is composed of four copies each of four subunits encoded by four separate genes and deficiency can be present in the liver, liver and muscle or rarely in muscle only. There are five different subtypes depending upon clinical presentation and mode of inheritance [116, 213].

- X-linked hepatic PHK deficiency, GSDIXa is caused by a wide range of mutations in the PHKA2 gene and is the most frequent form occurring in approximately 75% cases of GSDIX [214], with a mild phenotype which is often thought to be benign, but in some cases there may be a more severe phenotype
- combined liver and muscle PHK deficiency, GSDIXb, results from mutations in the PHKB gene located on chromosome 16, with autosomal recessive inheritance, and is usually a mild phenotype
- autosomal recessive liver PHK deficiency, GSDIXc, results from mutations in the PHKG2 gene located on chromosome 16 and results in a severe phenotype
- X-linked muscle glycogenosis, GSDIXd, is due to mutations in the PHKA1 gene and results in a mild phenotype

- autosomal recessive muscle PHK deficiency, GSDIXe, has a mild phenotype

Clinical presentation and biochemistry

Hepatic forms

The hepatic forms, types IXa, IXb and IXc, present with hepatomegaly, growth retardation, fasting hypoglycaemia, ketosis, hypercholesterolaemia, hypertriglyceridaemia and elevated liver transaminases. Hypoglycaemia may not always be pronounced as both gluconeogenesis and fatty acid oxidation are functional and ketosis may be more significant. Hyperlacticacidaemia, usually postprandial, is also observed in some cases, especially in GSDIXc. They are in general milder disorders than GSDIII [118], but there is wide variation in severity of symptoms. Although hypoglycaemia is usually mild, only occuring after prolonged fasting or infection, in some, particularly GSDIXc, there can be severe hypoglycaemia, ketosis and raised transaminases as seen in GSDI or GSDIII [213, 215]. There is gross accumulation of glycogen in the liver.

The more severe GSDIXc form is associated with liver fibrosis which can progress to cirrhosis and development of adenoma [213, 215]. Uncommonly X-linked GSDIXa has also been associated with liver fibrosis and cirrhosis [214, 216]. Hypertrophic cardiomyopathy has also been reported in a case of GSDIXc [215]. Usually a late growth spurt allows complete catch-up in final height to occur [217–219]. There is usually normalisation of liver enzymes in the majority and most adults will be entirely asymptomatic with a normal life expectancy.

Myopathic forms

The myopathic forms, GSDIXd and GSDIXe, are rare, usually presenting in young adulthood with exercise intolerance, cramps and recurrent myoglobinuria [116,213]. They are normally mild phenotypes.

Dietary management of GSDVI and GSDIX

GSDVI and GSDIX are managed with dietary treatment, aiming to

- maintain a normal blood glucose level and prevent ketosis
- correct hyperlipidaemia
- promote normal growth and maintain a healthy BMI

Advice is based on fasting tolerance and many patients do not require specific dietary treatment. Euglycaemia can be achieved by provision of regular meals high in complex CHO and protein. By maintaining euglycaemia this reduces the need for lipolysis and fatty acid oxidation and so prevents the development of ketosis. It can normally be managed by regular 3–4 hourly meals and a bedtime snack. For some, however, where there is overnight hypoglycaemia or significant early morning ketonuria (>0.5 mmol/L) UCCS should be introduced: 1–1.5 g/kg/dose given at bedtime or late evening (p. 549). A second dose of UCCS may be required overnight to adequately maintain euglycaemia and prevent ketosis. UCCS dosing requirements may be determined by an UCCS load test (p. 551) or by monitoring of early morning (pre breakfast) blood glucose and ketone levels. It is suggested that even where there is no hypoglycaemia or ketosis UCCS at night is beneficial in improving any delayed growth [116]. A few patients, mainly with GSDIXc, in whom hypoglycaemia is particularly severe overnight may require

an even more intensive regimen, as in GSDI, with continuous nocturnal tube feeding to maintain euglycaemia, prevent fasting ketosis and improve growth. This was the case in one of three patients with GSDIXc reported in a retrospective review [215].

During adolescence it is important to discuss alcohol intake as it is a potent inhibitor of gluconeogenesis. The recommendations given in the management of GSDIII can be used (p. 559).

Case study

Case study GSDVI

A 2½-year-old boy presented with hepatomegaly and short stature (height 2nd centile, weight 50th centile). He was eating regular meals and had an overnight fast of up to 12 hours. No symptoms of hypoglycaemia had been recognised. A period of CGM and early morning urine ketone monitoring revealed some overnight hypoglycaemia without significant ketosis (Fig. 18.6). UCCS, 1.5 g/kg, was introduced late evening with resolution of nocturnal hypoglycaemia. The parents have found urine ketones present if UCCS not taken or the child is unwell. There has been some improvement in linear growth to the 9th centile.

Case study GSDIX

A 16-year-old girl with GSDIXc, weight 66 kg (90th centile), height 154.4 cm (10th centile), managed with overnight UCCS, 50 g at 22.30 and 25 g at 05.00, had CGM. She was keen to stop UCCS and as CGM showed no nocturnal hypoglycaemia UCCS therapy was discontinued. At clinic review she reported to be well and had lost weight as a result of decreased energy intake with discontinuing UCCS. However, it became apparent that she craved CHO on wakening. A further CGM profile (Fig. 18.7), with morning urine ketone monitoring, revealed overnight hypoglycaemia (average of 39% daily readings below the lower glucose limit of 3.5 mmol/L) and ketonuria (4–8 mmol/L). She was restarted on 50% (40 g) of her previous total dose of UCCS at 22.00. Repeat CGM assessment showed her improved glucose levels (Fig. 18.8) with just 1% recordings below the lower limit and urine ketones were negative.

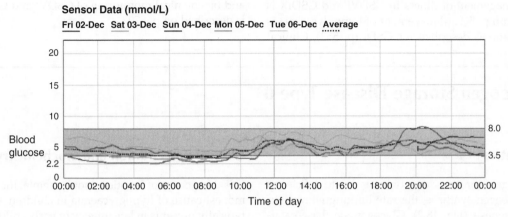

Figure 18.6 Continuous glucose monitoring prior to treatment in GSDVI. The grey shaded band indicates normoglycaemia.

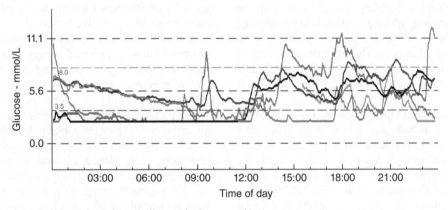

Figure 18.7 Continuous glucose monitoring off uncooked cornstarch.

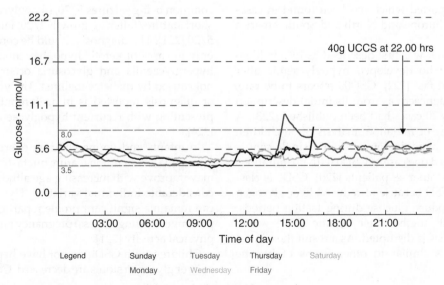

Figure 18.8 Continuous glucose monitoring with uncooked cornstarch restarted.

Management of illness in GSDVI and GSDIX is given on p. 569. Management of hypoglycaemia is the same as described for GSDI (p. 553). Clinical and biochemical monitoring of GSDVI and GSDIX is described on p. 570.

Glycogen Storage Disease Type 0

Genetics

Glycogen storage disease type 0 is due to deficiency of glycogen synthase, the rate limiting enzyme in glycogenesis (Fig. 18.2). Glycogen synthase catalyses the formation of the α-1,4 linkages between glucose molecules enabling the glucose chain to elongate forming glycogen, the body's storage form of glucose, with the major stores being in liver and skeletal muscle. There are two isoforms of glycogen synthase, a hepatic isoform (GSY2) and a muscle isoform (GSY1). Only the hepatic form is discussed.

Hepatic glycogen storage disease type 0 (GSD0), or glycogen synthase deficiency, is an autosomal recessive disorder resulting from mutations encoding for the enzyme glycogen synthase (GSY2, EC 2.4.1.11). The gene is located on chromosome 12. To date 18 mutations have been described [220]. Many of the mutations are unique to particular families and only one common mutation (c.736C>T) has been reported which has been found in cases throughout Europe and North and South America [221].

The disorder was first described in 1963 in identical twins who developed hypoglycaemia after an overnight fast [222]. GSD0 appears to be rare, or under-diagnosed, as from its initial description to 2006 only 20 cases had been published [223]. A recent review of mutation analysis of 50 children with ketotic hypoglycaemia, from a single centre, only identified one case of GSD0 with no mutations found in the other 49 patients [220]. GSD0 is classified as a GSD because of reduced liver glycogen stores to produce glucose during fasting periods; this contrasts to the other hepatic GSDs where glycogenolysis is disrupted. As a result the clinical phenotype is similar to other forms of hepatic GSD [116].

Clinical presentation and biochemistry

GSD0 is a cause of ketotic hypoglycaemia, the commonest cause of hypoglycaemia in children. GSD0 typically presents in late infancy or early childhood with fasting ketotic hypoglycaemia. This is precipitated by an increased length of overnight fast, an intercurrent illness with a lack of dietary intake, or by gastrointestinal symptoms of vomiting and/or diarrhoea causing reduced energy intake. Despite significant hypoglycaemia some patients may be relatively asymptomatic as the high levels of blood ketones can provide an alternative fuel for brain energy metabolism. Seizures are uncommon; developmental delay has only been described in 22% of cases [223] and neurological sequelae appear infrequent [221]. Blood glucose monitoring may reveal postprandial hyperglycaemia. Individuals may have growth retardation due to chronic ketosis. A review of the 20 published cases identified a variety of presenting clinical symptoms, the most common being seizures 5/20, hypoglycaemia 2/20, short stature/faltering growth 2/20, family history 5/20 [221]. The diagnosis should be considered not only in cases of ketotic hypoglycaemia but also if hyperglycaemia and glycosuria occur which are not caused by diabetes mellitus. The youngest age of diagnosis reported is in an 8-month-old child presenting with recurrent hypoglycaemic seizures [224].

In infants and young children overnight hypoglycaemia is a common feature but fasting tolerance may improve with increasing age although there is considerable individual variation. Hypoglycaemia can remain a significant problem particularly with prolonged fasting, illness, pregnancy and increased physical activity [221].

Children with GSD0 do not have hepatomegaly as liver glycogen stores are decreased. Consequently

Table 18.21 Blood glucose and lactate following an oral glucose load in a patient with GSD0.

Time (minutes)	Blood glucose mmol/L (ref range 3.3–5.5 mmol/L)	Blood lactate mmol/L (ref range 0.6–2.5 mmol/L)
0	2.5	1.42
+40	2.6	Haemolysed
+70	7.8	8.15
+120	6.9	8.18

prolonged fasting will result in hypoglycaemia, hyperketonaemia and elevated free fatty acids. In addition low levels of lactate and alanine (skeletal muscle release of alanine is inhibited by high levels of free fatty acids and ketones) reduces precursors for gluconeogenesis exacerbating the risk of hypoglycaemia [221, 225]. Conversely in the fed state, as a result of the reduced ability to produce glycogen in the liver, glucose derived from the diet is mainly channelled into the glycolytic pathway resulting in the postprandial biochemical picture of hyperglycaemia, hyperlactataemia and hyperlipidaemia [226]. A standard oral glucose tolerance test produces an excessive rise in blood glucose and lactate (Table 18.21).

Dietary management

GSD0 is managed with dietary treatment, aiming to

- maintain a normal blood glucose level, preventing both hypoglycaemia and hyperglycaemia
- correct the secondary biochemical abnormalities, of postprandial lactic acidosis and fasting ketosis, by maintenance of normoglycaemia
- promote normal growth and maintain a healthy BMI

Normoglycaemia can be achieved by provision of complex CHO which will minimise the postprandial rise in blood glucose and lactate. Simple CHO may cause a transient sharp rise in blood glucose and an increase in blood lactate; thus their intake should be limited. A high protein intake is beneficial by providing substrate for glucose production via gluconeogenesis. Maintenance of normoglycaemia limits fatty acid oxidation thus preventing free fatty acid and ketone accumulation.

Dietary management is based on fasting tolerance and advice centres on

- regular meals, including a bedtime snack, which contain complex CHO and protein
- restriction of highly refined CHO, e.g. sugary drinks, fruit juice, confectionery, cakes, sweet biscuits, high sugar cereals, if there is a tendency for marked hyperglycaemia
- managing overnight hypoglycaemia or significant early morning ketonuria (>0.5 mmol/L) with UCCS (p. 549) introduced at bedtime/late evening at a dose of 1–1.5 g/kg/dose. One or two doses of UCCS may be required overnight, determined by a UCCS load test (p. 551) or by monitoring of early morning (pre breakfast) blood glucose and ketone levels
- continuous overnight tube feeds if UCCS is not tolerated or fails to maintain blood glucose levels adequately. There is one case report [220] of a child requiring overnight feeds of 25% glucose polymer as 6 hourly UCCS overnight failed to prevent hypoglycaemia
- during adolescence it is important to discuss alcohol as it is a potent inhibitor of gluconeogenesis. The recommendations given in the management of GSDIII can be used (p. 559).

Case study

GSD0

A 6-year-old boy was referred with ketotic hypoglycaemia, hyperlacticacidaemia, postprandial hyperglycaemia and no hepatomegaly. He ate regular meals with complex CHO and had a preference for high protein foods; he fasted for up to 14 hours overnight. CGM was undertaken for 6 days. His usual diet, without any intervention, was continued for the first 2 days following which UCCS, 1.5 g/kg, was started at bedtime. Results showed significant periods (17.5%) in which glucose levels were below the lower limit of 3.5 mmol/L, with morning ketonuria (1.5 mmol/L), before the introduction of UCCS (Fig. 18.9). Glucose control was improved (Fig. 18.10) and ketonuria prevented with UCCS.

Management of illness in GSD0 is given on p. 569. Management of hypoglycaemia is the same as described for GSDI (p. 553). Clinical and biochemical monitoring is described on p. 570.

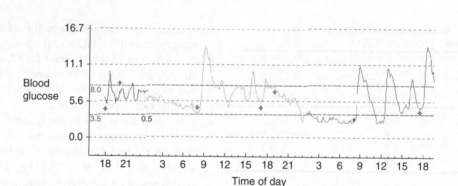

Figure 18.9   Continuous glucose monitoring usual diet.

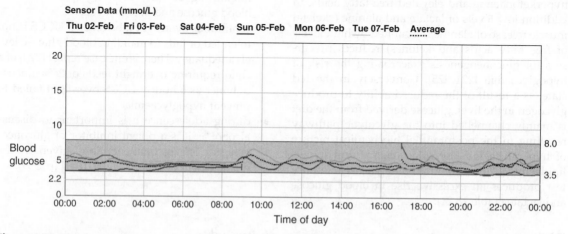

Figure 18.10   Continuous glucose monitoring following introduction of UCCS. The grey band represents normoglycaemia.

Diet for infants with GSD0, GSDVI, GDSIX

GSD0 and GSDVI

It would be unusual for presentation to be in early infancy unless investigated as the result of an affected older sibling; thus there is little experience of the practical management in such situations. In theory, from knowledge of the disorders and their management, cases identified in infancy would require regular feeding at 3–4 hourly intervals throughout the 24 hour period to maintain normoglycaemia and prevent ketosis. A controlled fast, monitoring blood glucose, lactate and ketones, could be used to determine the safe maximum fasting time between feeds. Monitoring of blood glucose, lactate (in GSD0) and ketones could be used to assess the adequacy of the frequency of feeding and volumes taken. Breast fed infants may

need supplementary feeds of infant formula or glucose polymer if breast feeds alone are insufficient to maintain euglycaemia.

Weaning would be advised to start as normal, around 26 weeks of age. As the intake of solids containing complex CHO and protein increase these could replace some of the milk feeds. The frequency of feeding, particularly overnight, would need reassessing regularly throughout infancy, as fasting tolerance may increase.

GSDIX

In mild cases of GSDIX dietary management may be as described above for GSDVI and GSD0. In more severe forms, e.g. GSDIXc, a more intensive dietary regimen will be required to maintain euglycaemia, prevent ketosis and promote growth, similar to GSDIII (p. 558).

Fanconi–Bickel Syndrome

Genetics and biochemistry

Fanconi–Bickel syndrome (FBS) (GSDXI) is due to a defect in the glucose transporter 2 (GLUT2). GLUT2 is a facilitative glucose (and galactose) transporter expressed in pancreatic islet cells, on the basolateral aspect of intestinal epithelial cells, on basolateral membrane of the proximal convoluted renal tubular cells and in hepatocytes. It plays a key role in glucose homeostasis [227] through its involvement in intestinal glucose uptake, renal reabsorption of glucose, glucose sensing in the pancreas, and hepatic uptake and release of glucose (and galactose). It is essential for glucose entry into pancreatic islet cells, a process which is insulin dependent [228].

FBS is a multisystem autosomal recessive disorder caused by mutations in SLC2A2, the gene encoding for GLUT2. The gene is located on chromosome 3; over 70% of cases are in consanguineous families and more than 100 mutations have been described [228, 229], the majority being private, i.e. unique to a single family [230].

FBS was first described in 1949 in a 3-year-old boy with hepatorenal accumulation of glycogen, fasting hypoglycaemia, postprandial hyperglycaemia and generalised renal tubulopathy (Fanconi nephropathy with severe glucosuria and galactosuria) [231]. Prior to this there had been a previous case report in 1921 of a 9-year-old girl with the symptoms of FBS including hepatomegaly, glucosuria and extreme short stature [228].

Clinical presentation

Clinically FBS presents in early childhood with a severe phenotype: hepatomegaly and nephromegaly due to accumulation of glycogen in liver and kidney; growth failure with severe short stature; delayed bone age; hypophosphataemic rickets; and delayed motor development. Bone deformities, including genu valgum and kyphosis, may be present. Malabsorption is not always a presenting feature. In a review of published cases [232] 16% had intestinal symptoms including chronic diarrhoea or failure to thrive in infancy. Cognitive development is normal. Some cases may be identified on newborn screening for galactosaemia with galactosuria. Cataracts, due to hypergalactosaemia, have been seen in a few cases although they were not found in the original patient despite a large milk intake throughout his life [228]. There have been no reports of hepatic adenomas, unlike in other hepatic GSDs [228]. Symptomatic hypoglycaemia in untreated patients is rare, presumably due to increased blood levels of ketone bodies and lactate.

Biochemistry

The biochemical features of FBS are of glucose and galactose intolerance and a Fanconi type nephropathy. Postprandial hyperglycaemia occurs caused by decreased glucose uptake by the liver and low insulin secretion due to impaired glucose sensing by pancreatic β cells (IV glucose loads were shown not to increase serum insulin). There is fasting hypoglycaemia due to altered glucose transport from hepatocytes [231] with ketosis.

Tubular nephropathy results in glycosuria, galactosuria, amino aciduria and increased renal losses of bicarbonate, phosphate, calcium and potassium. Urine testing for amino acids and galactose is usually diagnostic in these patients, in conjunction with the clinical phenotype.

Increased gluconeogenesis increases intracellular glucose, which cannot exit the cells, and inhibits glycogenolysis. This results in glycogen accumulation within the liver, enterocytes and renal tubular cells.

Hydrogen breath tests following a glucose load are normal indicating that intestinal uptake of monosaccharides is not impaired [232]. An additional transport system for glucose, SLGT1 (sodium dependent glucose co-transporter) in the apical membrane and at the basolateral membrane, a vesicle mediated pathway appears to enable intestinal glucose uptake [232].

Intact monosaccharide absorption also has been shown in the mouse model. GLUT2 knockout mice are normal at birth but develop symptoms akin to non insulin dependent diabetes with hyperglycaemia and increased levels of free fatty acids and β-hydroxybutyrate. They die at 2–3 weeks of age with a defect in glucose stimulated insulin release [233]. Re-expression of the GLUT2 transport protein in islet cells enables them to survive, although the GLUT2 defect is still expressed in the gastrointestinal tract and kidneys [234]. Despite lack of GLUT2 in endocytes the mice did not have monosaccharide malabsorption and, as in humans with FBS, it was proposed to be due to another glucose transport system at the enterocytes' basolateral membrane which could compensate for impaired GLUT2 mediated transport [228, 234]. In addition to GLUT2 there appear to be other mechanisms for glucose transport out of the hepatocytes into the circulation [234].

Management

The management of FBS is based on symptomatic treatment. Dietary management is aimed at

- maintaining a normal blood glucose level, preventing both hyperglycaemia and hypoglycaemia
- preventing ketosis
- correcting hyperlipidaemia
- promoting normal growth and maintaining a healthy BMI

Control of blood sugars is managed by frequent intake of complex CHO, UCCS and in some cases continuous overnight feeds. Large intakes of glucose and galactose (including that provided from sucrose and lactose) at a single time should be minimised to help prevent hyperglycaemia. The frequency of feeding can be determined by fasting tests but is usually at least 3 hourly. Fasting tolerance may be improved by using UCCS. Euglycaemia and prevention of ketosis overnight might be possible with several doses of UCCS. If overnight continuous feeding is required the composition of the feed depends on daytime nutritional intake and growth, varying from glucose polymer to a nutritionally complete feed. CGM (p. 570) is an extremely valuable means of monitoring and

improving blood glucose control as shown in the case study below.

There are no definitive recommendations to restrict galactose. Fructose can be tolerated as part of the diet as it is absorbed in the intestine via GLUT5, a transporter specific to fructose which is found in both the apical and basolateral membranes of the enterocyte [228]. Fructose may therefore be useful as an alternative monosaccharide to enable reduction in glucose intake, e.g. in overnight feeds. Fructose does not need to be converted to glucose for release from cells and is released by a different pathway to glucose [234].

Pharmacological treatment

The renal tubulopathy requires renal supplementation of bicarbonate, potassium, phosphate together with calcium and vitamin D supplementation. Adequate fluids must be given because of the polyuria.

Outcome

Despite careful management of symptoms FBS, due to its severe phenotype, is difficult to manage. The clinical symptoms of the original patient described persisted into adulthood and he had severe short stature [235]. Four cases described by Foley et al. had extremely poor linear growth (well below the 0.4th percentile), severe tubulopathy and persistent nephrocalcinosis. Heptomegaly, although reduced in 2/4 cases, remained along with abnormal glucose control, particularly postprandial hyperglycaemia [236]. Similar outcome is seen in cases in the author's unit. Lee et al. [237] proposed the use of UCCS to improve metabolic control and growth; however, the beneficial effects on growth seen in other GSDs with the use of UCCS do not appear to be replicated in FBS.

Recently information on two siblings with a mild phenotype has been published [238]. The elder boy presented with faltering growth and was diagnosed at 9 months of age; his younger sister was investigated in the neonatal period and never had clinical symptoms. They have never had the classic symptoms of hepatomegaly, nephromegaly or hyperphophataemic rickets, and only had mild glycosuria and proteinuria. Both had elevated blood galactose levels. At age $9\frac{1}{2}$ and $4\frac{1}{2}$ years they have achieved normal growth on frequent feeds of a diet restricted in glucose and galactose and avoidance of prolonged fasting. UCCS, 0.5 g/kg, was given at bedtime for the first 2 years. There have not been any other published cases of mild phenotypes with good clinical outcome. Other mild cases may exist as a cause of isolated glycosuria.

Management of illness in GSD0 is given on p. 569. Management of hypoglycaemia is the same as described for GSDI (p. 553). Clinical and biochemical monitoring is described on p. 570.

Case study

FBS

A 14-month-old presented to the local hospital with failure to thrive. By age 7 years he was referred to a nephrologist with poor growth, renal tubular acidosis, asthma and glycosuria. He was found to have a proximal tubulopathy with massive glycosuria and galactosuria and also found to have hepatomegaly. A liver biopsy showed glycogen accumulation. Clinical and biochemical suspicion of FBS was confirmed on mutation analysis. Hypoglycaemia and hyperglycaemia were noted and overnight fasting hypoglycaemia was apparent. A gastrostomy was inserted and overnight feeds (a polymeric feed to provide approximately 0.5 g glucose/kg/hour) were established along with UCCS 1 g/kg/dose 4.5 hourly in the daytime. He continued to have poor weight gain and significant glycosuria. Additional energy was provided as long chain fat emulsion, both to his overnight feed and as a daytime supplement. His overnight feed was also altered to reduce the glucose content and supplemented with fructose in an attempt to provide more usable CHO. Despite maximal nutritional management, including continuous overnight feeds and aggressive supplementation of electrolytes and vitamin D, linear growth failed to catch up and maintenance of normal levels of electrolytes and euglycaemia proved very challenging. His skeletal deformity has progressed and he continues to have overall increasing disability secondary to bone and muscle pain, with background proximal muscle weakness.

A period of CGM showed episodes of nocturnal hypoglycaemia with a daily average of 13% of blood glucose levels <3.5 mmol/L (due to disconnection of pump because of frequent nocturia) and significant periods of daytime hypoglycaemia and hyperglycaemia, due to intake of high sugar drinks. Repeat CGM without prolonged pump disconnection overnight showed hyperglycaemia (28% values >10 mmol/L) overnight and postprandially in the day (he drank high sugar drinks), and episodes of preprandial hypoglycaemia (13% values <3.5 mmol/L). Dietary changes were made including increased UCCS with meals, reduced CHO intake overnight and advice to use sugar free drinks. This resulted in an improved glucose profile with only 1% values <3.5 mmol/L and a reduction of values >10 mmol/L to 21%.

Illness management in GSD0, GSDVI, GSDIX and FBS

Children with GSD0, GSDVI and GSDIX are at risk from hypoglycaemia during periods of intercurrent illness or where there is the need for prolonged fasting, e.g. surgery. An emergency regimen (ER) (p. 502) of 2–3 hourly glucose polymer drinks throughout the 24 hour period should be given providing normal fluid requirements. If the oral ER is not tolerated then hospital admission for IV glucose is required. The British Inherited Metabolic Disease Group provides guidelines on IV 10% dextrose therapy which can be accessed from www.bimdg.org.uk. The child's usual dietary regimen can be reintroduced as they recover. During this time extra glucose polymer drinks may be needed at night until back on full normal diet.

Special considerations:

- In GSDIX patients managed with an intensive dietary regimen, as in GSDI, the ER advice is as for GSDI, based on basal glucose production rather than the standard ER (p. 544).
- In GSD0 the CHO concentration may need to be reduced from the standard age related ER concentrations to prevent hyperglycaemia and maintain blood sugars within a reasonable range (3.5–8 mmol/L).
- In FBS the CHO concentration may need to be reduced from the standard age related ER concentrations to prevent hyperglycaemia and maintain blood sugars within a reasonable range (3.5–8 mmol/L). Additional fluids may be required if there is significant polyuria.

Clinical and biochemical monitoring in GSD0, GSDVI, GSDIX and FBS

Regular clinical and biochemical monitoring is important to evaluate the adequacy and efficacy of current dietary treatment, appraise if any dietary management changes are required and assess parents' understanding and delivery of the management. Monitoring is required to ensure

- adequate provision of CHO and protein from diet

- adequate dosing of UCCS if required (this may be based on results of biochemical monitoring)
- nutritional adequacy of vitamin and mineral intake
- normal growth
- appropriate management of illness and that ER is updated for age and weight
- appropriate management of hypoglycaemia

For further information on monitoring is as for GSDI (p. 554). Routine biochemical and annual monitoring and aims are shown in Table 18.19.

Continuous Glucose Monitoring in Glycogen Storage Disorders

Introduction

Assessment of blood glucose control is pivotal to the management of hepatic GSD and forms an integral part of the broader clinical and biochemical monitoring (Table 18.19). Regular assessment of the child's dietary intake, growth and relevant biochemistry is essential to optimise treatment and outcome, by avoidance of under or over treatment [139].

Practice over the years in assessing appropriateness of treatment regimens, in most UK and European metabolic centres, has been an inpatient admission, usually annually, for a 24 hour blood glucose ± lactate profile, other relevant biochemical parameters and growth measurements. Although such admissions are able to provide true blood glucose ± lactate measurements their benefit is limited due to

- giving only single point in time measurements (typically a maximum of every 1 or 2 hours) with no indication as to whether glucose levels are increasing or decreasing
- the hospital environment differing from home and the inability to reproduce normal home life, e.g. mealtimes and type of food are different, normal activity levels at home and at school cannot be maintained
- changes in dietary regimens may need a further period of inpatient assessment

Continuous glucose monitoring (CGM) is increasingly becoming part of the routine monitoring of GSD patients providing an additional tool in the assessment of metabolic control and appropriateness of the dietary regimen. CGM is a method which allows an individual's glucose levels to be continually monitored over a period of time by use of an indwelling glucose sensor. It is a relatively non invasive technique. CGM has advantages over intermittent glucose monitoring in also providing information on direction, magnitude, duration and frequency of fluctuations in blood glucose levels [239, 240].

The use of CGM in GSD was initially reported in 2001 [241]. It was used in four patients with GSDIa and demonstrated that CGM provided useful longitudinal data on blood glucose concentrations, rather than single time points. A further study in 2004 [242] reported on its use in six patients (GSDIa $n = 4$, GSDIb $n = 1$, GSDIII $n = 1$) aged 10–47 years over a 48 hour period in detecting unrecognised hypoglycaemia, thus enabling appropriate dietary changes to be instituted. In 2011 experience from Manchester, UK, was reported [239] including an audit from 2008–2010 of 55 profiles in 26 patients, of which 95% of profiles produced meaningful data. This study highlighted the usefulness of CGM, in association with diet diaries ± lactate and ketone measurements and growth data in optimising GSD biochemical parameters and nutritional management.

Continuous glucose monitoring systems

Continuous glucose monitoring systems (CGMS) consist of an indwelling glucose sensor which is attached to a wireless data recorder. The sensor, a very fine microelectrode coated with glucose oxidase, is inserted under the skin, usually into the abdomen although other areas can be used, e.g. upper arm, buttock, and connected to a small recorder (www.medtronic.co.uk). The sensor measures glucose levels in the interstitial fluid every 10 seconds and an average reading every 5 minutes is recorded and wirelessly transmitted to the data recorder, producing up to 288 measurements per day. Sensors can remain *in situ* for up to 6 days [243]. The systems are programmed and calibrated using finger stick blood glucose measurements. This is required because CGMS sensor measurements are not as precise as blood glucose meter strip measurements. By calibrating the CGMS with blood glucose meter measurements it allows calculation of the plasma:interstitial fluid gradient which remains valid provided blood glucose meter measurements are taken when blood glucose levels should be stable and not rapidly changing, i.e. in the preprandial period. A major cause of sensor error is calibration with capillary glucose levels that are rapidly changing as there is a lag time between changes in plasma and changes in interstitial glucose levels [244].

Retrospective and 'real time' systems are available. In GSD management the use of 'real time' systems is discouraged as this may result in families making frequent management changes, without discussion, which may not be appropriate [239].

Practicalities of using CGM

The usual practice is to do CGM for up to 6 days. Blood glucose meter measurements are taken four times daily prior to main meals and before a bedtime snack, start of continuous overnight feed or dose of UCCS. Lactate and ketone monitoring, as clinically relevant, is done alongside CGM. Lactate meter measurements are done concurrently with blood glucose measurements. Ketones (urine or blood using a dual purpose blood glucose/ketone meter) are usually measured before breakfast only.

A daily food diary is kept throughout the study and is essential for accurate interpretation of CGM results (Table 18.22).

Measurement of blood lactate is particularly relevant in GSDI. A study by Saunders *et al.* reported validation of use of the Lactate Pro portable meter in GSDIa [245]. They compared intravenous ($n = 166$) and concurrent capillary ($n = 39$) samples from 13 subjects. Intravenous samples were laboratory analysed. Intravenous and capillary samples were simultaneously tested on three different meters. There was minimal inter-meter variability. Correlation between laboratory lactate results and meter readings were reported as very good with meter readings around 0.5 mmol/L higher regardless of lactate concentration. Data from capillary samples were similar to those from intravenous sampling although upward bias of meter readings was greater (1.44 ± 0.2 mmol/L) compared with intravenous samples. Lactate measurements, however, can be inaccurate particularly if the blood sample was not free flowing and thus results should be interpreted with some caution, particularly if they appear unusually abnormal for the child. For example if blood glucose and lactate levels are well controlled a one-off very high lactate level would be unusual, but following a period of hypoglycaemia a high lactate level would be in keeping. Lactate, however, can be high in seemingly well managed patients, despite normoglycaemia; in these cases lactate levels may be more consistently raised.

CGM profiles should be carried out with normal activities (including sports) and no changes to dietary intake unless advised.

Following the monitoring period the sensor data are downloaded using specific computer software

Table 18.22 Home monitoring, indicating the different parameters monitored according to disorder.

GSD type	0	Ia/b	IIIa/b	VI and IX	FBS
CGM	✓	✓	✓	✓	✓
Blood glucose meter levels	✓	✓	✓	✓	✓
Lactate	✓	✓			
Ketones	✓		✓	✓	✓
Food diary • time • quantities	✓	✓	✓	✓	✓

CGM, continuous glucose monitoring.

and the data are then reviewed. Lower and upper limits for glucose levels are defined which the software uses to look at time periods above and below the target range. In the author's unit these are set at a lower glucose limit of 3.5 mmol/L and upper limit of 8 mmol/L, except for Fanconi–Bickel syndrome where the upper limit is set at 10 mmol/L due to the extremes of hyperglycaemia observed in the condition.

Data generated include

- individual daily graph of glucose profile
- overlay of each day's profile on one graph
- data on total number, highest, lowest and average sensor values as well as correlation and calibration data
- excursion summary which describes the number of glucose levels above or below target glucose levels
- duration distribution, giving per cent time below, within and above target in 24 hours

CGM profiles should be reviewed looking at trends and the presence of repeated patterns, rather than relying on single measurements, in conjunction with all other test results to inform management advice.

Summary

CGM is a very helpful tool in the management of GSD. Benefits of CGM include

- avoidance of hospital admissions and associated repeated venepuncture
- may be inserted and removed at home by nurses trained in CGMS
- improved representation of normal lifestyle including dietary intake, activity patterns and adherence to prescribed dietary regimens

- allows comparison of weekend and school day profiles
- profiles provide significantly more information and are more 'visual' than a list of numbers produced during a standard inpatient blood glucose profile
- information gained includes confirmation of the adequacy of the usual dietary regimen or identification of trends indicating regimen changes are needed, e.g. glucose levels falling overnight or before feeds, even if the level is not below the lower target glucose range, indicates the potential for hypoglycaemia and the need to re-evaluate the dietary regimen
- ability to adjust and compare different dietary regimens during a profile period which is valuable in attempting to optimise an individual's treatment without the need for repeated inpatient admissions, over a period of time, to assess different regimens
- glucose profile results are a visual educational tool for families; they can highlight adherence issues which can be addressed to improve biochemical control or illustrate specific foods which may cause high blood glucose levels, typically refined CHO
- increased information on overall dietary intake which can inform targeted advice on improving nutritional adequacy of the diet
- the process is positively accepted by the families
- is well tolerated by all age groups of patients

CGM should normally be done at least annually. In infants and young children with the most severe forms of GSD requiring intensive regimens, or in newly diagnosed or unstable patients, more frequent CGM will be needed to evaluate the effectiveness of management. In very stable or mild patients less frequent CGM may be acceptable.

Glycogen Storage Disease Type II (Pompe Disease)

Genetics

Glycogen storage disease type II (GSDII), or Pompe disease, is a progressive neuromuscular disorder caused by deficiency of the lysosomal enzyme

α-1-4 glucosidase (acid maltase) (Fig. 18.2) and results in glycogen accumulation in the lysosomes which damages muscle cells and impairs muscle function. It is an autosomal recessive disorder. There is a spectrum of phenotypes from the severe infantile form to a more slowly progressing late onset form. The overall incidence is estimated at 1 in 40 000 [246] with the infantile form estimated at 1 in 138 000 [247].

Clinical presentation, treatment and outcome

The severe infantile form of Pompe disease usually presents within the first 2 months of life with progressive cardiac, respiratory and skeletal muscle weakness and feeding difficulties. The later onset form is less severe and progresses more slowly. It is generally characterised by a slowly progressive muscle weakness and respiratory insufficiency. This form can present anytime from childhood through adulthood. The infantile onset form is associated with poor prognosis and early death due to cardiorespiratory failure. Natural history studies indicate ventilator dependency by 4.7 months and death between 6 and 9 months [248].

Nutritional support with tube feeding is usually necessary in the infantile form because of severe muscle weakness and respiratory insufficiency. Later onset forms may also require nutritional support for the same reasons. Historically a high protein diet providing 25% dietary energy was reported to improve muscle strength by reducing protein catabolism, and hence delay the downward course of the childhood form [249, 250]; however, not all patients benefited from this diet [251].

The management of infantile Pompe disease has altered in recent years with the introduction of enzyme replacement therapy (ERT), with Myozyme (alglucosidase alfa). This has improved survival, cardiac, respiratory and motor function [247]. The clinical trial of ERT [251] reported ventilator free survival rate of 88.9% at 1 year of age although this was not sustained (66.7% at 2 years and 49.4% at 3 years).

Twenty reported cases of infantile Pompe disease from the UK have been treated with ERT; 13 (65%) of the cases required nasogastric or gastrostomy feeding. Despite long term ERT tube feeding could not be discontinued in patients requiring enteral feeds [247]. van Gelder *et al.* studied swallowing function (by fibreoptic endoscopic examination of swallowing, FEES) in six of 11 ERT treated children and found 5/6 had dysphagia. Although tube feeding could be discontinued in some during the study, with 5/11 completely orally fed by the end of the study period, four of these still had some signs of dysphagia. FEES examinations had shown bulbar muscle weakness and this was thought to be the reason for continued feeding and swallowing difficulties [253]. Bulbar muscles in Pompe knockout mice have been shown to have significant glycogen storage; although cleared by ERT, there remained residual muscle pathology [253]. In an adult patient treated with ERT for 21 months there was residual glycogen storage in the oesophagus [254]. Bulbar muscles may respond less well to ERT than other muscles and therefore impact on integrity of swallowing function. In addition glycogen storage within the nervous system may also play a part [253]. Input from dietetics and speech therapy is important for regular feeding and swallowing assessments and advice on safe feeding plans.

Hereditary Fructose Intolerance

Jacky Stafford

Introduction

Hereditary fructose intolerance (HFI) is caused by a deficiency of the second enzyme of fructose metabolism, aldolase B (fructose-1,6-bisphosphate aldolase) which is found in the liver, kidney and small intestine. Aldolase B cleaves fructose-1-phosphate (F-1-P) to glyceraldehyde and dihydroxyacetone phosphate, which enter either the glycolytic pathway to form pyruvate and lactate or the gluconeogenic pathway to finally produce glucose (Fig. 18.11).

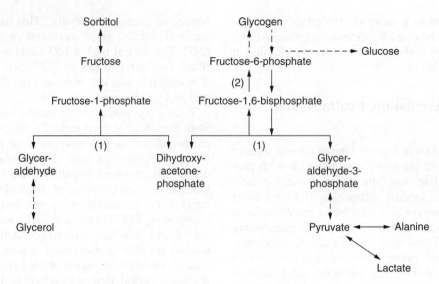

Figure 18.11 Pathway of fructose metabolism.

In HFI, ingestion of fructose causes accumulation of F-1-P, the trapping of phosphate causing decreased intracellular phosphate levels which are central to the metabolic derangement. Glycogenolysis and gluconeogenesis are blocked due to decreased phosphate levels. Glucose production is then limited and causes acute hypoglycaemia. Intracellular ATP production becomes depleted causing hypermagnesaemia, severe hyperuricaemia and other metabolic disturbances. Metabolic acidosis results from the accumulation of alanine, lactate, pyruvate and F-1-P activation of pyruvate kinase. Impaired function of the proximal renal tubule causes hypokalaemia, amino aciduria, phosphaturia and bicarbonate losses leading to metabolic bone disease and poor growth. Accumulation of F-1-P is also reported to affect glycosylation of proteins, e.g. serum transferrin [255–257].

HFI is an autosomal recessive condition. Mutations in the ALDOB gene on chromosome 9q22.3 cause the lack of function of the aldolase B enzyme. The most common mutations are A150P, A175A and N335K, accounting for more than 90% of HFI in some European regions [257, 258]. In the UK the predominance of A149P mutation allowed a predicted incidence of HFI to be reported as 1 in 18 000 [259] and the carrier frequency is 1 in 70 [259, 260]. This incidence figure is comparable to the incidence of PKU; however, many individuals remain undiagnosed and the prevalence of HFI

in adults is unknown [260]. Definitive diagnosis is made by assay of aldolase B activity, mutation analysis or fructose challenge test [260], although this is less reliable and can provoke ill effects [257].

Clinical features

Infants are healthy and asymptomatic until either fructose or sucrose are introduced into the diet. The main presenting symptoms are poor feeding, vomiting, abdominal distention, restlessness, lethargy and growth faltering. These non specific symptoms can lead to an incorrect diagnosis of sepsis, tyrosinaemia or galactosaemia [261].

Diagnosis may be delayed if parents avoid giving fructose containing foods which have been noted to be poorly tolerated. However, acute and severe clinical symptoms of hypoglycaemia, seizures and coma can result from ingestion of fructose, sucrose or sorbitol and in neonates this may lead to liver failure, kidney failure and death [257]. Despite self-imposed dietary restriction of fructose, diagnosis may be made in childhood or adolescence with abdominal pain and vomiting if accidentally exposed to a few grams of fructose [262]. A diagnosis may be made from investigation of symptoms of growth failure, or hepatomegaly due to inadvertent chronic exposure to fructose. If untreated, there may be severe liver failure and proximal renal tubular dysfunction with rickets, jaundice, bleeding tendency, oedema and ascites [257]. The clinical picture and an accurate dietary history, particularly around the time of weaning, should enable a diagnosis of HFI to be made, even if the child is asymptomatic due to the early exclusion of certain foods. In older children and adults, symptoms may be minimal due to aversive behaviour with sweet tasting foods and self-selection of a low fructose diet. Parents may comment that food preferences are very different to their child's peers. HFI is frequently confused with other conditions involving fructose aversion such as fructose malabsorption or fructose 1,6-bisphosphate deficiency (p. 583).

For those who remain undiagnosed until adulthood, the risk of an acute response to fructose remains. In the past, there have been many reports of patients with undiagnosed HFI who, on being given intravenous (IV) fructose and sorbitol preparations during illness or surgery, experienced metabolic acidosis which was reversible on discontinuing the infusion. However, irreversible hepatorenal failure proved fatal in some cases [263–265]. These case reports were mostly from mainland Europe; the need to avoid these IV preparations has been highlighted [262, 264, 266].

In the UK exposure to fructose is uncommon prior to weaning onto solid foods as breast milk is fructose free as are the available first infant formulas. However, the EU directive 2006/141/EC and its amendment allows sucrose to be added to infant formula to a maximum of 20% total carbohydrate content; sucrose, fructose and honey are allowed in follow-on milks with a combined maximum of 20% total carbohydrate content [267]. Ingredients should be checked for these. During the introduction of solid foods, sources of fructose become abundant in the diet: fruits, vegetables and commercial baby foods. The usual intake of fruits and vegetables in infants (aged 4-18 months) is reported to be 100–170 g/day [268].

Outcome and complications

The long term prognosis is good provided a fructose free diet is followed, although hepatomegaly and fatty changes in the liver may persist [269]. The diet needs to be continued for life without relaxation as even small amounts (20 mg/kg in adults) of fructose have been shown to be harmful [270].

Dietary treatment

Sources of fructose

HFI is managed primarily by avoidance of fructose in the diet and in medicines. As well as fructose *per se*, fructose is also derived from sucrose and sorbitol. Fructose is absorbed by a carrier mediated process across the small intestine and then enters the liver to undergo further metabolism (Fig. 18.11). The disaccharide sucrose is cleaved in the small intestine by sucrase-isomaltase to form a molecule each of glucose and fructose. Sorbitol is a sugar alcohol which diffuses slowly across the intestinal absorptive surface with only 10%–30% being absorbed. It does not contain fructose, but in the liver it is rapidly converted via sorbitol dehydrogenase to fructose. This is known as the sorbitol-aldolase or polyol pathway.

The oligosaccharides raffinose (trisaccharide) and stachyose (tetrasaccharide) are composed of fructose and glucose to which galactose is linked in an α-galactosidic linkage; it is thought that in humans these are not hydrolysed due to the absence of α-galactosidase [271]. They are found in small quantities in food: raffinose in sunflower seeds, chicory, onions and other vegetables (about 1 g/100 g food or less); legumes are the richest source of stachyose (1–5 g/100 g food). To assess if these oligosaccharides are hydrolysed, in the diet of six patients with galactosaemia their intake was reduced to 5%–10% and galactose-1-P levels tended to be lower during the test phase. The authors concluded that these oligosaccharides may be absorbed [271] (as this may not be clinically significant galactosides are not avoided in the diet for galactosaemia in the UK, p. 532). However, this suggests that fructose might also be available.

Fructans such as inulin are widespread in various plants, e.g. artichokes and chicory [272], and fructo-oligosaccharides (FOS), also known as oligofructose, are obtained from inulin through enzymatic hydrolysis, producing a mixture of chains of fructose molecules of varying chain length (2 to 20 molecules). Both inulin and these derivative chains are resistant to hydrolysis by digestive enzymes and are not absorbed, but instead are fermented by anaerobic bacteria in the colon. Therefore FOS are primarily sources of dietary fibre. However, as they have an energy value of 1.5–2 kcal (6–8 kJ)/g it is possible that some fructose may be absorbed and that commercial inulin and oligofructose syrups may contain small amounts of fructose and sucrose. Prebiotics, as FOS, are added to some infant formulas, e.g. Aptamil range, Cow & Gate range and the energy dense infant formula Infatrini, to mimic the intestinal flora profile of the breast fed baby [273, 274]. FOS is also added to enteral feeds, e.g. Nutrini and Nutrison Multi Fibre range, Paediasure Fibre and Jevity range, weaning foods and functional foods. The ingredients of special infant formulas and enteral feed products should also be checked for sucrose and fructose. The potential impact of fructose from FOS in HFI was studied in five patients (aged 14–52 years) and a 5-month-old infant. A challenge of oral fructose (4.7 mg fructose/kg/day, 9.7 mg/kg for the infant) was given in the form of FOS. In the two older patients there were slight elevations in plasma uric acid; all other biochemical markers remained normal. The authors concluded that no adverse events would be expected in HFI patients at this level of FOS intake [275]. This study, however, only looked at short term exposure to FOS over 2 days.

Another potential source of fructose is from industrially manufactured polyols (polyhydric alcohols) or sugar alcohols which are produced by the hydrogenation of selected sugars derived from cornstarch. Polyols are sugar free, low energy bulk sweeteners which are used in many foods and medicines. The most widely used and to be avoided in HFI are sorbitol (E420, derived from dextrose), mannitol (E421, derived from fructose), maltitol (E961, derived from maltose) and isomalt (E953, derived from sucrose). Absorption of polyols varies; most are slowly and incompletely absorbed from the intestine and for others absorption is minimal. Nevertheless, they may remain a possible source of fructose or sorbitol [276].

Minimal fructose, sucrose and sorbitol diet

The aim of dietary treatment of HFI is complete elimination of fructose, sucrose and sorbitol. Fructose intake is restricted to <2 g/day from all sources, i.e. the lowest intake that is practically achievable (Table 18.23). On these intakes patients remain symptom free. In adults with long term

daily ingestion of 2.5 g sucrose/day (15–20 mg fructose/kg) symptoms did not develop [275]. In cases where chronic ingestion of fructose has resulted in delayed growth and other abnormal biochemical parameters, an intake of <40 mg fructose/kg is recommended [277].

It is not possible to completely exclude these sugars but, generally, patients who choose to avoid them consume only a few grams fructose per day [277]. This is significantly less than the fructose intake of the normal population. The median intake of non milk extrinsic sugar (NMES) of 4–18-month-old infants in the UK is 7–17 g/day. This does not include fructose from intrinsic sugars (IMS) derived from fruits and vegetables [268]. The UK National Diet and Nutrition Survey (2008–2009) [278] and its update (available online at www.gov.uk) reports that from 4 years to adulthood median daily NMES intakes are 60–85 g, with lower intakes among girls and women. Information on fructose intake only is not available in the UK.

Fructose is the natural sugar present in fruits, vegetables and honey. Sucrose is also found in fruits and vegetables, but a much greater source is from sugar cane or beet. These are refined to produce table sugar which is used extensively in food manufacture as a sweetener and bulking agent. In the USA a large contribution is derived from high fructose corn syrup, used as a sweetener [279, 280]. Sucralose (E955), previously known as Splenda, should be avoided. It is a new intense sweetener which has a potency of about 600 times sucrose and is increasingly used in products including medicines. It is a chlorinated sucrose and reportedly is not hydrolysed in the intestine; however, pharmacokinetic studies in humans have shown an average recovery of radioactive sucralose of 92.8% mostly from faeces (70%–90%) and urine after 5 days. It may therefore be a source of sucrose and fructose [281].

Sugar is a major ingredient in cakes, biscuits, desserts and soft drinks. Many other commercial foods (e.g. stock cubes, tinned meats, bottled sauces and savoury snack biscuits) contain sugar but are much less obvious sources. Indeed, very few manufactured foods are suitable for inclusion in the diet.

There are sugar products regulations (2003) in the UK which provide descriptions and specifications

Table 18.23 Minimal fructose, sucrose and sorbitol diet (aim <2 g fructose/day).

Analysis of fructose and sucrose content of foods [286]

Foods allowed	Foods to avoid
Sugars, sweeteners and preserves Glucose, glucose polymers, glucose syrup, dextrose, lactose, starch, maltose, maltodextrin, maltextract, glycerol Saccharin, aspartame, Acesulfame K, Sweetex (aspartame and saccharin) Polyols: erythritol, xylitol, lactitol	Sugar or sucrose (cane or beet) – white, brown, caster, icing Fruit sugar, fructose, laevulose Honey, treacle, molasses Sucralose Polyols: sorbitol, maltitol, mannitol, isomalt, Lycasin Golden syrup, corn syrup, invert syrup, high fructose or isoglucose syrups, hydrogenated glucose syrup, maple syrup Jam, marmalade, lemon curd
Fruits Avocado, rhubarb (occasionally)	All other fruits and fruit products
Vegetables Seaweed, vine leaves allowed freely See Table 18.24	Beetroot, Brussel sprouts, carrots, gherkins, green beans, kohl rabi, okra, onion, parsnip, peas, pepper, plantain, shallots, spring onion, squash, sweetcorn, sweet potato, tomato, tomato purée Beans – green, French, runner Baked beans, tinned vegetables with added sugar, mayonnaise or salad cream, coleslaw Flavoured crisps Pickles, chutney
Milk and dairy products Infant formula and follow-on milk (check there is no added sucrose, fructose or honey) Cow's milk, unsweetened evaporated milk Coffee mate, dried milk powder Cream Cheese, plain cottage cheese Natural yoghurt	Flavoured milk, condensed milk, milkshake powders and syrups Liquid soya milk Aerosol cream Cheese with added ingredients, e.g. nuts, fruit Fruit and flavoured yoghurt, fromage frais Ice cream
Eggs	
Meat and poultry All fresh meat and poultry Processed meat products (check there is no added sucrose, fructose or honey)	Processed meats which have added sucrose, e.g. meat pastes, frankfurters, salami, paté, sausages, tinned meat Tendersweet meats, e.g. ham, honey cured meats Ready made meat meals (possible sources are gravies, sauces, vegetables, breadcrumbs, batter, pastry)
Meat substitutes Soya products, tofu, Quorn	Ready made meals with these products may contain sucrose
Fish Fresh and frozen fish Shell fish Fish tinned in brine, oil or water	Fish tinned in tomato sauce Fish paste Fish cakes, fish fingers Ready made fish meals (possible sources are sauces, vegetables, breadcrumbs, batter, pastry)
Flour and cereals Flour (white in preference to wholemeal), buckwheat, cornflour, custard powder, sago, semolina, tapioca, oatmeal, barley Flaky pastry, filo pastry, shortcrust pastry (not sweetened)	Bran, wheatgerm Dessert pastry

(continued overleaf)

Table 18.23   (continued)

Foods allowed	Foods to avoid
Pasta and rice	
Spaghetti, macaroni, other pasta (white in preference to wholemeal)	Pasta tinned in tomato sauce
Noodles, egg noodles	Pot savouries, e.g. Pot Noodle
Rice (white in preference to brown)	
Breakfast cereals	
Porridge, Puffed Wheat, Ready Brek, Shredded Wheat	Most manufactured breakfast cereals
Bread and crackers	
White bread (prepacked), tortilla wraps	Wholemeal bread, sweetened breads, e.g. malt bread, soda
Baker's bread (check if sugar is added to dough mixture)	bread, currant bread, malt loaf, brioche, pain au chocolat
Cream crackers, Matzo crackers, water biscuits, Ryvita, plain rice cakes	Savoury snack biscuits
Crumpets (not all are suitable, check label)	
Cakes, biscuits and pastries	
Homemade – using permitted ingredients and sweeteners	All cakes, muffins, pancakes, waffles, biscuits and pastries
Desserts	
Homemade – using permitted ingredients, e.g. custard sweetened with glucose, choux pastry	Most desserts, e.g. jelly, meringue, mousse, gateaux, fruit pie or crumble, ice cream, yoghurts
	Sorbet, ice lollies
Fats and oils	
Butter, margarine, vegetable oils (including olive oil), lard, suet	
Drinks	
Lucozade (not fruit flavour), soda water, mineral water (not fruit flavour)	Fruit juices, vegetable juices, fruit squash, fizzy drinks, diabetic squash containing sorbitol or fructose, tonic water,
Squashes and fizzy drinks flavoured with saccharin or aspartame only (free from sugar, sorbitol, fruit flavourings or comminuted fruits)	fruit ice, Slush Puppy
	Drinking chocolate, malted drinks
	Instant tea mixes, coffee essence
Tea, coffee, cocoa, herbal teas (no sugar)	Fruit teas
Confectionery	
Lucozade Sport Glucose Energy tablets – original	Sweets, chocolate, toffee, jelly, ice lollies, chewing gum, diabetic sweets (sweetened with fructose or sorbitol)
Dextro energy – dextrose and maltodextrin	Flavoured glucose tablets
Glucotabs (BBI healthcare)	
Gravies, sauces and soups	
Marmite, Bovril	Gravy granules, stock cubes
White or cheese sauce made with milk, flour, fat and cheese only	Bottled sauces and dressings, e.g. tomato ketchup, horseradish sauce, mint sauce, soy sauce
	Sauce mixes, e.g. sweet and sour, curry
	Mayonnaise, salad cream
	All soups (packet, tinned or fresh)
Herbs, spices, nuts and seeds	
Pure herbs, mustard and spices, salt, pepper	Nuts, peanut butter, marzipan
Sesame seeds	
Pumpkin and sunflower seeds (maximum of 10 g per day)	
Baking products	
Baking powder, bicarbonate of soda, yeast, arrowroot, food colourings, food essences, gelatine	

Table 18.23 *(continued)*

Foods allowed	Foods to avoid
Alcohol (not suitable for children) Beer – bitter, lager, mild, pale ale, stout (Guinness), strong ale/barley wine	Low alcohol bitter, alcohol free/low alcohol lager, shandy, fruit beers
Note: Sucrose or fructose may be added to bottled, canned or keg beers to adjust the sweetness of the final product	Cider
Sucrose is usually added to cask conditioned beers (sometimes referred to as 'real' beers) to generate secondary fermentation within the container	
Wine – red only	Wine – champagne, mulled wine, rose, white Fortified wines – port, sherry, tonic wine, vermouth
Spirits	Liqueurs Alcopops

- Always read the label of manufactured foods to check for sucrose, fructose, sorbitol, polyols or unsuitable sweeteners.
- Check toothpaste for sorbitol.

for certain types of sugar products and additional labelling requirements. Products covered by these rules include white sugars, dextrose, glucose syrups and fructose. Where a product is labelled to contain 'sugar' this indicates the ingredient is sucrose. In glucose syrup, where glucose syrup or dried glucose syrup contains more than 5% fructose, 'fructose' will be indicated as an ingredient (www.food.gov.uk). Flavourings can be another potential source of sucrose and fructose as these sugars are sometimes used as carriers for flavouring compounds, which will not necessarily be labelled.

Vegetables contain significant amounts of fructose (as fructose and sucrose) so most must be avoided and only vegetables with a very low fructose content, with a predominantly starch content, can be included in the diet but in restricted amounts (Table 18.24). The total daily fructose intake from vegetables should not exceed 1–1.5 g/day as small amounts of fructose from cereals in the diet will increase the total intake to the 2 g/day maximum. As the total fructose content (fructose plus half the sucrose content) varies between different vegetables they have been divided into three groups:

- Group 1 – potatoes
- Group 2 – vegetables containing <0.5 g fructose/100 g
- Group 3 – vegetables containing 0.5–1 g fructose/100 g

Within each group portion sizes are indicated to provide a certain amount of fructose. These can

then be used to calculate daily fructose intake from vegetables.

It is important to note the difference in fructose content between raw and cooked vegetables. Cooking causes a loss of free sugars; consequently cooked vegetables have a lower fructose content and are recommended in preference to raw. The water from boiled vegetables should be discarded and not used to make gravy or sauces. New potatoes have a higher fructose content than old (0.65 g/100 g vs. 0.25 g/100 g). Sucrose content of stored potatoes has previously been reported to both decrease and increase on storage [282, 283]. Information from the Institute of Food Research, Norwich, reports that potatoes in cold storage (<8°C) have a higher fructose content compared with those stored in warm temperatures (>15°C).

Ingredient labels on manufactured foods should be checked for the presence of sucrose, fructose or sorbitol and other polyols, or unsuitable sweeteners (Table 18.23). Wholemeal flour and other wholegrain foods, e.g. brown rice and wholemeal pasta, contain more fructose than white versions because the germ and bran contain sucrose. No accurate analysis for the fructose content of bread is available; however, it would appear prudent to choose white in preference to wholemeal. Bread has previously been restricted in the diets of children with HFI. Nowadays this restriction is probably unnecessary because most flour improvers for bread making do not contain sugar. If the bread does

Table 18.24 Vegetables allowed in a minimal fructose, sucrose and sorbitol diet.

Total daily fructose intake from vegetables should not exceed 1.0–1.5 g per day

Group 1 – potatoes (old)

1 portion = approximately 0.3 g fructose

Boiled – 2 small egg size (100 g)
Jacket (flesh only) – 1 medium (100 g)
Mashed – 2 tablespoons (100 g)
Roast potatoes – 2 small (100 g)
Chips – medium portion (120 g)
Plain crisps – 2 small packets
*Potato waffles (1)
*Potato croquettes (2)

*Check to ensure does not contain sugar

Group 2 - vegetables containing <0.5 g fructose/100 g

1 portion = approximately 0.15 g fructose where a small portion is 1 tablespoon (30 g) unless indicated otherwise

Celery
Globe artichoke (1 globe, 50 g)
Mange tout
Mushrooms
Sauerkraut
Spinach
Watercress (1/2 bunch)
Beans, e.g. haricot, mung, red kidney
Lentils
Yam – boiled or baked (amount = 1/2 small potato)
Dried split peas

Group 3 – vegetables containing 0.5–1.0 g fructose/100 g

1 portion = approximately 0.3 g fructose where a small portion is 1 tablespoon (30 g) unless indicated otherwise

Aubergine – 1 slice (30 g)
Asparagus – 2 spears (50 g)
Beansprouts
Broccoli – 1 spear (50 g)
Cabbage
Cauliflower
Cucumber – 8 thin slices (40 g)
Fennel – (45 g)
Jerusalem artichoke – (40 g)
Celeriac – (35 g)
Leeks – 1/4 medium (30 g)
Lettuce – 4 small leaves (25 g)
New potato – 1 small (50 g)
Pumpkin
Radish (red) × 4 (40 g)
Spring greens
Swede
Turnip
Beans – black eye, broad, butter, soya
Peas – marrowfat, mushy, processed peas in water
Chick peas or hummus

contain sugar it has to be declared on the ingredient label. If there is any doubt about suitability of a particular bread the manufacturer should be contacted. Caution should be applied where richer doughs are used (e.g. in soft rolls) because often the flour improver does contain sugar in these instances. Bread bought from craft bakers may also contain sugar and bakers are under no legal obligation to declare this information to the consumer.

Polyols which are used as low energy bulk sweeteners are potential sources of sorbitol and fructose. Foods and medicines, e.g. sugar free syrups, lozenges, jelly preparations, suitable for children may contain these and need to be checked for suitability. There are different proprietary brands of polyols available, e.g. Lycasin (contains maltitol) and Neosorb (contains sorbitol). Polyols should be declared on the food ingredient and nutritional labels in the UK, therefore making them relatively easy to identify. Parents need to check with a pharmacist about the suitability of medicines as they can contain sucrose, fructose and artificial sweeteners. Some toothpastes contain sorbitol. As a little may be swallowed by young children, these should be avoided.

Starch, glucose and lactose can be included in the diet. Glucose can be used as an alternative sweetener to sucrose and can also provide a useful source of energy. The relative sweetness of glucose is only half that of sucrose, so additional sweetening can be added to baked goods; however, this may not be necessary as children with HFI generally dislike and avoid sweet tasting foods (p. 582). If required, some intense sweeteners, e.g. Sweetex, can be successfully added to cooked food while others which decompose on heating, e.g. aspartame, are not suitable for baking. Glucose is not prescribable on FP10 for treatment of HFI.

Nutritional problems

Children with HFI are at risk of vitamin C and possibly folic acid deficiency due to the exclusion of the major dietary sources of these vitamins, i.e. fruits and vegetables [284]. Pure vitamin C products are available (Table 18.25) and should be prescribed to meet the reference nutrient intake (RNI) [98]; however, the amount that needs to be given is small and powder products may be difficult to measure and tablet preparations provide too

Table 18.25   Vitamin and mineral supplements – sucrose, fructose and sorbitol free.

Name	Manufacturer	Format	Vitamin C	Folate	Additional information	Sweetening agent
Prescribable products						
Paediatric Seravit	Nutricia	Powder Note: flavoured form not suitable	20 mg in 5 g dose	15 µg in 5 g dose	Comprehensive range of vitamins and minerals	Glucose syrup, inositol
Phlexy-Vits	Nutricia	Tablet	50 mg in 5 tablet dose	700 µg in 5 tablet dose	From 11 years Comprehensive range of vitamins and minerals	Dextrose
Phlexy-Vits	Nutricia	Powder (7g sachet)	50 mg	700 µg	From 11 years Comprehensive range of vitamins and minerals	Dextrose
Ketovite	Paynes & Byrne	Tablets Note: liquid is not suitable	16.6 mg in 1 tablet	250 µg in 1 tablet	B vitamins	None
Commercially available products						
Abidec Multivitamin syrup with Omega 3	Chefaro UK		30 mg in 5 mL dose	None	Age 1–5 years Lemon flavour 9 vitamins Can be prescribed	Glycerol
Halib Orange Baby and toddler	Seven Seas		25 mg in 5 mL dose	None	Multivitamin and mineral Orange flavour (orange oil)	Glycerol
Multivitamin Syrup	Boots		25 mg in 5 mL dose	None	Age 4+ months 9 vitamins	Glycerol
Vitamin C	Nature's Best or Lamberts		500 mg, 650 mg or 1000 mg tablets	None		
Vitamin C as ascorbic acid	Nature's Best or Lamberts		Crystals $^1/_4$ tsp = 1 g	None		

large a dose. Any commercial vitamin and mineral preparations should be checked to ensure ingredients do not contain sucrose, fructose, sorbitol or sucralose or other polyols. Very few products are suitable (Table 18.25) and much support is needed to encourage adherence. Some products may contain sucralose or flavouring, e.g. Fruitivits (Vitaflo), suggesting a possible source of fructose; these may be considered to be suitable if all other products are refused. Lack of dietary fibre may also be a problem. This could be overcome by including pulses and oats, which contain only very small amounts of fructose, or inclusion of Resource Optifibre (Nestle); the fibre source is guar gum.

Clinical, nutritional and biochemical monitoring

Clinical, nutritional and biochemical monitoring is essential at all routine outpatient appointments and should include

- liver function tests
- full blood count and plasma folate and iron status (haemoglobin and ferritin)
- clinical assessment of skin and gums, checking for signs of vitamin C deficiency: tissue is swollen, tender and bruises easily and bleeding gums. Vitamin C status can be

measured in white blood cells but analysis is not performed routinely by all laboratories (www.clinbiochem.info). Adult range is 26.1–84.6 µmol/L (there is no paediatric range) and deficiency level is <11.1 µmol/L

- vitamins A and E, vitamin D, selenium and zinc to measure general nutritional status as indicated
- plasma lactate and urate and urinary protein may be assessed

Case studies

Case study 1

A female infant aged 4 months, from consanguineous parents, presented to her local hospital with seizures. She had previously been well, taking infant formula during the day; however, on taking her first fruit juice drink (approximately 50 mL) and rice pudding, she vomited. On taking more juice, she became pale and unresponsive and started to fit on the way to A&E; her blood glucose was unrecordable (0.4 mmol/L). She was found to have fructosuria, 5 mmol/L (normal 0–1 mmol/L), aminoaciduria suggesting proximal renal tubular dysfunction, raised plasma lactate suggesting a disturbance in the gluconeogenic pathway and abnormal urine organic acids suggesting disturbed carbohydrate metabolism. A diagnosis of HFI was suspected and dietary advice was given to avoid sucrose, fructose and sorbitol in weaning foods until diagnosis was confirmed. The common mutation for aldolase B (A149B) was negative, but as the family was of Pakistani origin, further mutational screening was undertaken. She was given a fructose challenge in hospital at about age 1 year, with 130 mL apple juice (providing 10 g fructose); within an hour of the load she vomited and became hypoglycaemic (blood glucose 1.4 mmol/L). Lactate and urate levels increased and phosphate levels decreased which were suggestive of HFI. She was advised to continue avoidance of sucrose, fructose and sorbitol.

On review a year later, parents reported her to be fussy with food, preferring savoury foods and generally disliking sweet foods, very occasionally having a very small quantity of fruits or vegetables. The family reported that they checked all food labels and avoided sucrose, fructose and sorbitol

containing foods. Her growth was good, both weight and height between 9th and 25th centiles and development was normal. Her serum iron levels were low 4.2 (normal range 5–25 µmol/L) and haemoglobin 10 (normal range 11.5–14.5 g/dL) but other parameters including folate, B_{12}, liver function tests and trace elements were normal. A vitamin and mineral supplement (unflavoured Paediatric Seravit) was prescribed to improve iron, vitamin C and folate intake, but not taken. At the next review dad reported her to be pale and often tired; iron deficiency anaemia (Hb 9.0 g/dL, Fe 1.9 µmol/L, ferritin <2, normal range 8.6–74 µg/L) was diagnosed and 25-hydroxyvitamin D (total) levels were insufficient. She had no symptoms of vitamin C deficiency, bleeding gums or skin problems. However, in addition to a suitable preparation of iron (ferrous fumarate), Ketovite tablets were prescribed to provide vitamin C and promote iron absorption. On follow-up, she was encouraged to continue with the new vitamin supplement, as alternative options are limited.

Case study 2

An increased frequency of coeliac disease (CD) has been reported among HFI patients (4% vs. normal population 1%) suggesting a genetic association between these two disorders [285].

A 3-year-old Polish girl presented with hepatomegaly and raised liver function tests to a hospital in Warsaw. She was diagnosed with CD following an intestinal biopsy. However, on commencing a gluten free diet, the clinical features did not improve. Her early history revealed that when fruits and vegetables were introduced at weaning she developed vomiting and abdominal distention. The family tended to retry them at intervals but they were generally refused. A fructose load given in hospital caused dizziness after 30 minutes and the test was stopped; blood glucose was not reported. HFI was suspected based on the clinical history, the hypoglycaemic response to the fructose load and the abnormal glycosylation of transferrin. She was commenced on a formal fructose free diet at 3 1/2 years, in addition to a gluten free diet. She was subsequently diagnosed with HFI on mutational analysis. On relocating to the UK, the parents reported difficulty interpreting labels and keeping to the restricted diet. Her diet was limited and comprised gluten free (GF) bread, GF pancakes, rice, potatoes, dairy foods, eggs, very little meat or fish, and no fruit or vegetables or sweet tasting foods. She was not taking any vitamin or mineral supplements. The family had initially used Polish GF products and so required guidance on accessing suitable prescribable foods in the UK. She was re-investigated to confirm diagnosis of both disorders.

CD was confirmed on biopsy and she has the common mutation for HFI (A149P). In liaison with the local dietetic team, all commercial and prescribable GF foods were checked to ensure they were sucrose, fructose and sorbitol free; this limited the selection of suitable GF foods. The parents requested liaison with school about meals. The family returned to Poland, but re-presented in clinic after 3 years. She was keeping to her strict gluten, sucrose, fructose and sorbitol free diet; she avoided sweet foods. However, she has not been keen to take any vitamin and mineral supplement. Despite this biochemical results including iron, folate and liver function tests were normal although she has an enlarged liver. It is possible that adequate vitamin C is provided by regular potato consumption, but she was advised to recommence unflavoured Paediatric Seravit and if unsuccessful an alternative, e.g. Ketovite tablets, to meet both vitamin C and folate requirements will be considered.

Fructose-1,6-bisphosphatase Deficiency

Anita MacDonald

Introduction

Fructose-1,6-bisphosphatase (FBPase) deficiency is a rare autosomal recessive condition of gluconeogenesis [287]. FBPase is an important gluconeogenic enzyme that catalyses the hydrolysis of fructose-1,6-bisphosphate to fructose-6-phosphate and inorganic phosphate [288] (Fig. 18.11). Its inactivity prevents the endogenous formation of glucose from all its precursors including lactate, glycerol, fructose and gluconeogenic amino acids such as alanine [289]. Instead alanine, lactate, glycerol, glycerol-3-phosphate and/or ketones [290] accumulate. Hypoglycaemia occurs after prolonged fasting when glycogen stores are depleted [288]. Its incidence is unknown, but cases have been reported in Europe [287, 291], Japan [288], USA [292], Israel [293], Turkey [294] and Saudi Arabia [295].

Clinical features

FBPase deficiency may present in the first 4 days of life when glycogen stores are limited, with hypoglycaemia, acidosis, ketonuria and severe hyperventilation [296], and this is associated with a high mortality [291]. Children may experience more than one episode of acute metabolic decompensation before the diagnosis is made. Symptoms usually accompany prolonged fasting associated with illness [297] but they have been reported following ingestion of a large single dose of fructose [257], especially after a period of fasting. Fasting tolerance should improve with age [298, 299] and the frequency of acute metabolic decompensation also decreases with age [257]. However, there have been symptoms reported in adulthood associated with illness and fasting during Ramadan [300] and pregnancy [301].

Generally, once the diagnosis is established the outcome is good, but there should be continued vigilance with avoidance of fasting and use of emergency regimens (ER) during illness, trauma and surgery. The majority of patients have normal growth and psychomotor development [257]. Diagnosis is made by DNA analysis but if the results are inconclusive, determination of enzymatic activity in a liver biopsy could be performed [299].

Dietary treatment

Between episodes of acute metabolic decompensation patients are usually well. Nonetheless there is a dependence on exogenous sources of glucose and the primary dietary goal is to avoid any excessive fasting.

- **Avoidance of prolonged fasting**. An infant ≤4 months of age should be fed at 4 hourly intervals during the day and night. Even when weaning is well established, a late night and early morning feed should be given to reduce the duration of overnight fasting. Children >1 year of age require regular meals containing a complex CHO source to provide 'slow release' glucose. Fasting overnight is usually safe but a bedtime snack containing starchy foods, e.g. bread or cereal, is advisable [302].

- **Uncooked cornstarch** has been advocated late evening (2 g/kg/dose) [294, 303] and should be considered if there is evidence that patients are unable to fast safely overnight (p. 549). In the UK, late evening cornstarch has been given to approximately 17% of children (6/36) with FBPase deficiency [304].

- **Low fructose diet** [294, 303]. The majority of children should keep well without dietary fructose restriction between episodes of intercurrent illness. However, fructose tolerance should be considered on a case by case basis. Children usually tolerate sweet foods (up to 2 g fructose/kg body weight/day when given regularly distributed throughout the day [257]). Fructose loading tests induce hypoglycaemia as in HFI although higher doses are required [305]. This suggests there may be reduced fructose tolerance [257, 294, 299, 303]. It may be advisable for some patients to moderate fructose intake by avoiding an excessive intake of cakes, biscuits, confectionery and sugary drinks. Some UK centres (4/11) routinely restrict fructose and this is mainly by avoiding excess intake of fruit, fruit juice or sugary snacks only [304]. Some patients may self-restrict fructose intake. Some have suggested that fructose, sucrose and sorbitol restriction is only necessary in young children [299] and in the UK no adult patients (six patients from three treatment centres) follow any dietary restriction [304].

- **Teenagers** should take care if alcohol is consumed. Alcohol inhibits gluconeogenesis and if taken in excess it may precipitate hypoglycaemia. If teenagers do drink alcohol it should be in moderation only and always with food [300].

Treatment during illness

Poor appetite, intercurrent infections, vomiting and prolonged fasting can precipitate metabolic decompensation because the gluconeogenic pathway for production of glucose is blocked. During acute episodes there is lactate accumulation, decreased pH and an increased lactate:pyruvate ratio, hyperalaninaemia and glucagon resistant hypoglycaemia [257].

Treatment aims to prevent metabolic decompensation by giving glucose orally or intravenously (IV) [306]. The following guidance during intercurrent illness is recommended:

- An exogenous source of glucose must be supplied. If oral drinks are tolerated ER glucose polymer drinks should be given in the standard concentration and volume for age (p. 502). Fruit juice or squash must not be added as they are sources of fructose. If oral rehydration solution (ORS) is required, glucose polymer should be added to provide an adequate glucose intake. Again, this must not be flavoured with fruit juice or squash. Some patients may not readily accept or refuse to drink glucose polymer solutions (21% or 9/42 of UK treated patients) [304] but any sources of fructose, sucrose and sorbitol must be excluded because these will exacerbate the metabolic derangement [291, 306]. Most low calorie squashes are unsuitable because they still contain some sucrose, fructose or sorbitol or comminuted fruits. Fat should be avoided during decompensation as glycerol may exacerbate the illness.

- Some patients may decompensate rapidly, becoming very ill with marked acidosis. If the child is unwell, a bolus of IV glucose is immediately administered [306] before providing an infusion of IV glucose at maintenance fluid requirements. Metabolic acidosis is treated by giving sodium bicarbonate. Fortunately, this treatment may promptly ameliorate symptoms [307]. In acute metabolic decompensation IV administration of fructose is contraindicated and may lead to death [257].

- All medications must be free of fructose, sucrose and sorbitol.

- Once the child improves a normal diet can be resumed, with a gradual reintroduction of fructose and sucrose. During the recovery period extra glucose polymer drinks should continue to be given, particularly at night.

Case study

Child with FBPase deficiency

An 18-month-old girl of Pakistani origin, born at term of first cousin parents, was admitted to the intensive care unit with life threatening hypoglycaemia and lactic acidosis following a 24 hour gastroenteritis illness. The cause of her symptoms was unknown. Her parents were advised to give an ER (15% CHO) during illness. This episode was followed by two to three further similar acute illnesses per year with intercurrent illnesses always associated with hypoglycaemia and lactic acidosis as the principal features. She disliked the glucose polymer drinks, so they were sweetened with squash containing sucrose/fructose flavouring to improve palatability. She was diagnosed with FBPase deficiency by DNA testing

at the age of 4 years. Although she remained on a normal diet, she was advised to eat regularly during the day with a bedtime snack containing starch each night. She was also given 20% glucose polymer (sucrose/fructose free) drinks for her ER. She is now aged 12 years and remains well. She has normal growth and intellectual ability. She requires her ER (25% unflavoured glucose polymer drinks) for intercurrent infections (about once per year). Although she tries to take her ER drinks (sucrose/fructose free) during illness, she invariably decompensates rapidly requiring an initial IV bolus of glucose, followed by infusions of IV 10% glucose providing maintenance fluid requirements. Bicarbonate is administered to correct metabolic acidosis. She usually responds to treatment within 24 hours and her appetite improves quickly. She is supplemented with glucose polymer drinks until she is fully recovered. As she does not fully comply with her glucose polymer drinks, she also has a 40% glucose gel to take during illness. She has been advised against fasting during Ramadan.

Glut 1 Deficiency Syndrome

Fiona White

Genetics and biochemistry

Glut 1 deficiency syndrome (Glut 1 DS) is predominantly an autosomal dominant disorder caused by mutation in the *SLC2A1* gene located on the short arm of chromosome 1 which encodes for the glucose transporter protein type 1. Many (approximately 90%) are *de novo* heterozygous mutations with neither parent having a mutation [308]. Mutations in the *SLC2A1* gene are not found in all suspected cases [309], with the typical biochemistry and recognised phenotype of Glut 1 DS suggesting that other genes or glucose transporters may be involved. Two families with autosomal recessive inheritance of Glut 1 DS have been described [310].

Glut 1 DS results in defective transport of glucose across blood–tissue barriers including the blood–brain barrier (BBB) due to lack of glucose transporter protein type 1 which is the

exclusive facilitator of entry of D-glucose into the brain [311, 312]. This results in low cerebrospinal fluid (CSF) glucose (<2.5 mmol/L), low CSF glucose:blood glucose ratio (<0.5, the ratio being less reliable than the absolute CSF glucose value) and low to normal or low CSF lactate (<1.6 mmol/L) as neurons can use lactate as an alternative fuel [308] when there is hypoglycaemia.

Clinical features

Glut 1 DS has an expanding clinical spectrum with varying phenotypes seen including

- classical – early onset drug resistant seizures, developmental delay, acquired microcephaly and a complex movement disorder. Hypotonia, ataxia and dystonic features are common together with significant speech problems [313]

- non classical – developmental delay, movement disorder without seizures [314], non epileptic, delayed speech and motor development, unsteady gait influenced by fasting with acute symptoms being carbohydrate responsive [315]
- paroxysmal exercise induced dyskinesia (DYT18) and paroxysmal choreoathetosis/spasticity (DYT9) [316]
- stomatin deficient haemolytic anaemia [317, 318]

There appears to be a genotype–phenotype correlation [319] with those mutations causing the largest disruption to glucose transport being associated with the most severe phenotypes. Even so there is heterogeneity in severity of developmental delay between patients with identical mutations [319].

Treatment

Management with a ketogenic diet (KD) is the first line treatment including cases where there is a strong clinical suspicion and low CSF glucose, but absent *SLC2A1* mutation [309]. The KD produces a consistent state of ketosis. Ketone bodies enter the brain by a different transport mechanism (monocarboxylase transporter 1) and can be used as an alternative energy source to glucose to permit brain functioning and address the neurological symptoms. As not all cases of Glut 1 DS involve epilepsy the positive effects of the KD diet in this disorder on cognition, attention and mood appear to be a primary effect of the diet and not just secondary to improvement in epilepsy [315]. Blood ketones (β-hydroxybutyrate >2 mmol/L) or urine ketones (>4-8 mmol/L) appear in practice to deliver good symptomatic response to the KD. Unlike the treatment of epilepsy with the KD diet where management may be limited to 2 years, the KD in Glut 1 DS is needed for a longer period, at least into adolescence due to continued brain development.

The classical KD remains the first choice [317] with the modified Atkins diet being increasingly used as a practical alternative particularly in adolescents or where adherence is poor, with clinical effectiveness demonstrated with a ketogenic ratio of 2.5–2.1:1 (fat:protein + carbohydrate) [320]. Due to lack of published data on the medium chain triglyceride (MCT) diet, this approach was not recommended. The author's experience, however, is that a modified MCT diet is generally well tolerated with good adherence and positive clinical response. To obtain good levels of ketosis, carbohydrate (CHO) usually needs to be restricted to around 10% energy and total fat (long chain triglycerides, LCT and MCT) increased to provide around 80% energy (ketogenic ratio of approximately 2:1).

A recent email survey of UK practice provided information on 58 patients with Glut 1 DS on KD treatment: 36% were on an MCT diet; 33% on the classical diet with varying ratios; 31% on modified ketogenic diets (modified Atkins diet).

Regular monitoring of dietary tolerance is required. Gastro-oesophageal reflux, particularly with night time vomiting, appears to be a common side effect of the high fat intake. It usually responds to prokinetic agents; in some cases additional treatment with a proton pump inhibitor is needed. Anthropometric, biochemical and haematological monitoring should be undertaken regularly. As the diet is used long term there is increased risk of hyperlipidaemia, which can respond to alterations in types of lipids used [321] and the development of kidney stones. A good fluid intake is recommended as a preventative measure together with management of significant biochemical disturbances, e.g. Allopurinol for hyperuricaemia.

Further details on the practical management of the KD, including monitoring, are given on pages 354-380.

Pharmacological treatment

Supplementation with L-carnitine is essential for the transport of fatty acids into the mitochondria, if plasma levels are low. There has been interest in alternative compounds for the supplementary treatment of Glut 1 DS [322]. Alpha lipoic acid is an antioxidant acting as a co-enzyme in energy metabolism. In cultured muscle cells it improves glucose transport by mobilisation of Glut 4. Currently there is no evidence of similar effects on the Glut 1 transporter. Triheptanoin is a C5 triglyceride which produces five carbon ketone bodies which can cross the BBB and theoretically potentially enhance regular ketone bodies in providing alternative brain fuel. There is currently no clinical evidence to support its use in Glut 1 DS.

Outcome with treatment

In most patients the KD completely controls or markedly reduces the frequency of seizures [323] and the severity of the movement disorder [314]. Behaviour, alertness, activity and psychomotor development frequently improve [313, 323]. A retrospective study of 44 individuals with Glut 1 DS treated with the KD [319] showed that in the classical phenotype (37 individuals) total or partial seizure reduction occurred in 86% of cases; 48% had improvement or resolution of the movement disorder and 51% showed subjective improvement of cognitive function. Those with non classical phenotype (seven individuals) showed 71% reduction in the movement disorder and 29% had subjective improvement of cognitive function.

Acknowledgement

Marjorie Dixon and Fiona White thank Dr Elaine Murphy, Consultant Inherited Metabolic Disease, Charles Dent Metabolic Unit, London, for her comments on the Glycogen Storage Disorders section.

Useful addresses

The European Galactosaemia Society (EGS)

www.galactosaemia.eu
c/o Jeroen and Maaike Kempen
Zandoogjelaan 4
NL-5691 RJ Son

The UK Galactosaemia Support Group

www.galactosaemia.org
c/o Sue Bevington
31 Cotysmore Road
Sutton Coldfield
West Midlands B75 6BJ

Association for Glycogen Storage Disease (UK)

Old Hambledon Racecours
Sheardley Lane
Droxford SO32 3QY
www.agsd.org.uk

19

Disorders of Mitochondrial Energy Metabolism, Lipid Metabolism and Other Disorders

Marjorie Dixon, Jacky Stafford, Fiona White, Nicol Clayton and Janine Gallagher

An Introduction to Inherited Metabolic Disorders may be found at the beginning of Chapter 17.

Disorders of Mitochondrial Fatty Acid Oxidation and Related Disorders

Marjorie Dixon

Introduction to mitochondrial fatty acid oxidation

Mitochondrial fatty acid β-oxidation is the primary breakdown pathway of fatty acids to generate energy. Fatty acids are a major fuel source for most tissues of the body, especially during fasting, when glucose supply is limited. They are the principal energy source for cardiac muscle and skeletal muscle in the resting state and during prolonged exercise. Fatty acid oxidation is also important for the production of ketone bodies; these are another important fuel which can be used by all tissues and particularly by the brain during prolonged fasting as it cannot use fatty acids to generate energy.

Fatty acids consist of a hydrocarbon chain with a carboxylic acid group at one end. Most naturally occurring fatty acids have a chain length of 16–18 carbon atoms and are referred to as long chain fatty acids. Fatty acids are stored in adipose tissue as triglycerides, in which the carboxylic acid groups of three fatty acids are esterified to glycerol. Fat metabolism begins in adipose tissue as a response to falling levels of blood glucose. Insulin activates hormone-sensitive lipase which promotes the release of free fatty acids from triglycerides into the blood stream. The fatty acids are then transported to the tissues bound to albumin. In tissues where they are used, fatty acids enter the mitochondria bound to carnitine. This pathway is called the carnitine cycle or shuttle.

Clinical Paediatric Dietetics, Fourth Edition. Edited by Vanessa Shaw.
© 2015 John Wiley & Sons, Ltd. Published 2015 by John Wiley & Sons, Ltd.
Companion Website: www.wiley.com/go/shaw/paediatricdietetics

Carnitine cycle/shuttle

The carnitine cycle involves three enzymes which transport long chain fatty acids into the mitochondria. The first step occurs at the outer mitochondrial membrane where long chain fatty acids are activated to a coenzyme A ester, then to an acylcarnitine by the action of carnitine palmitoyl transferase I (CPTI); next it is transported by carnitine acylcarnitine translocase (CACT) into the mitochondria where it is converted back to an acyl-CoA ester by carnitine palmitoyl transferase II (CPTII), ready to undergo mitochondrial β-oxidation (Fig. 19.1). Carnitine is required in this process; it is transported inside the cells by an organic cation transporter (OCTN2) present in the heart, muscle and kidney. CPTI is the regulatory step for fatty acid oxidation. Malonyl CoA is involved in the regulation of CPTI, so indirectly controls fatty acid oxidation [1]. Circulating levels of malonyl CoA are high during the fed state and inhibit CPTI; conversely in the fasting state they fall and activate CPTI.

Mitochondrial β-oxidation

Within mitochondria, fatty acids are broken down by the spiral pathway of β-oxidation (Fig. 19.1). Every turn of the spiral involves four steps, catalysed by several enzymes of different chain length specificities. The first step, for example, is catalysed by very long chain, medium chain and short chain acyl-CoA dehydrogenases (VLCAD, MCAD, SCAD). The third step in the β-oxidation spiral is another dehydrogenation reaction and is catalysed by long and short chain 3-hydroxyacyl-CoA dehydrogenases (LCHAD, SCHAD). Both of these dehydrogenation reactions release energy which can be harnessed for use by the cell. This is achieved by passing electrons to the mitochondrial respiratory chain, either directly or via electron transfer flavoprotein (ETF) and ETF ubiquinone oxidoreductase (ETFQO). In addition to producing energy, each turn of the β-oxidation spiral releases a molecule of acetyl-CoA and shortens the fatty acid by two carbon atoms. Acetyl-CoA can be metabolised in the tricarboxylic acid cycle, but in the liver it is converted to ketone bodies via 3-hydroxy-3-methylglutaryl-CoA (HMG-CoA)

synthase and lyase. A more detailed description of the biochemical basis of mitochondrial fatty acid oxidation is described elsewhere [2, 3].

Overview of disorders of mitochondrial fatty acid oxidation, ketogenesis and ketolysis

A number of disorders of the mitochondrial fatty acid oxidation pathway have now been described. These vary in severity and may present at any time from the neonatal period to adulthood [2, 3]. The clinical features associated with fatty acid oxidation disorders (FAOD) probably result from the failure of the production of energy and accumulation of toxic intermediates [4]. The commonest disorder is medium chain acyl-CoA dehydrogenase deficiency (MCADD). Typically, this presents in early childhood with hypoglycaemia and acute encephalopathy brought on by fasting or an acute infection. The fatty acid oxidation defect impairs the production of ketone bodies and the hypoglycaemia is therefore 'hypoketotic'. Most other defects affect long chain fatty acid oxidation, either because they involve long chain specific β-oxidation enzymes, e.g. very long chain acyl-CoA dehydrogenase deficiency, or because they affect the carnitine mediated entry of long chain fatty acids into mitochondria, e.g. carnitine palmitoyl transferase deficiency type I. Defects of ETF and ETFQO cause multiple acyl-CoA dehydrogenase deficiency (MADD); in this condition there is impaired oxidation of long chain, medium chain and short chain fatty acids and various other substrates. Patients with long chain fatty acid oxidation defects may present with hypoglycaemia and encephalopathy, as in MCADD. They may often have additional problems such as cardiomyopathy, weakness or episodes of muscle breakdown (rhabdomyolysis).

The synthesis of ketone bodies occurs via the intermediate HMG-CoA and depends primarily on the enzymes HMG-CoA synthase and HMG-CoA lyase. Deficiencies of these enzymes are known as the disorders of ketogenesis and present with 'hypoketotic' hypoglycaemia. There are also defects in the utilisation of ketone bodies; the enzymes involved are succinyl-CoA 3-oxoacid-CoA transferase (SCOT) and 2-methylacetoacetyl-CoA thiolase (MAT). Deficiencies of these enzymes are known as the disorders of ketolysis or ketone body utilisation defects. They present primarily with a severe ketoacidosis.

Disorders of fatty acid oxidation and ketone bodies are treated primarily by diet. Some aspects of management are universal but others vary with the underlying disorder, age at onset and severity. The main aim is to minimise the oxidation of fatty acids by using an emergency regimen during illness and avoiding fasting. Additionally in severe defects of long chain fatty acid oxidation the intake of dietary fat is limited and medium chain fats may be used.

Medium chain acyl-CoA dehydrogenase deficiency

MCADD is the commonest of the fatty acid oxidation defects, with an incidence of 1 in 10 000 to

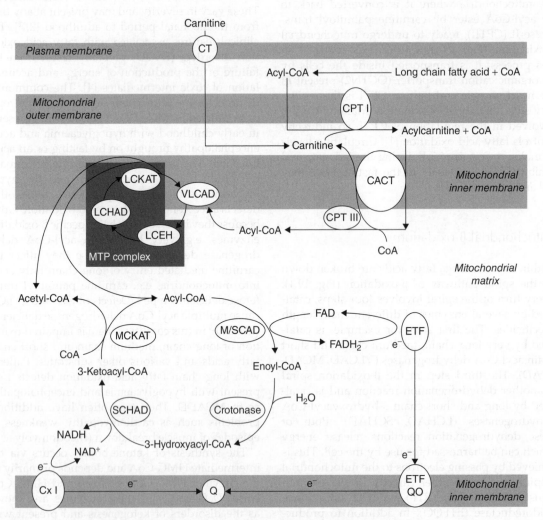

Figure 19.1   Biochemical pathways of mitochondrial fatty acid oxidation (permission to reproduce)
Enzymes involved: CT, carnitine transporter; CPTI, carnitine palmitoyltransferase I; CACT, carnitine acylcarnitine translocase; CPTII, carnitine palmitoyl transferase; VLCAD, very long chain acyl-CoA dehydrogenase; LCEH, long chain enoyl Co-A hydratase; LCHAD, long chain 3-hydroxyacyl-CoA dehydrogenase; LCKAT, long chain ketoacyl-CoA thiolase; MTP, mitochondrial trifunctional protein; M/SCAD, medium or short chain acyl-CoA dehydrogenase; SCHAD, short chain acyl-CoA dehydrogenase; MCKAT, medium chain ketoacyl-CoA thiolase; CxI, complex I of respiratory chain; Q, ubiquinone; e⁻, electrons; ETF, electron transfer flavoprotein; ETFQO, electron transfer flavoprotein ubiquinone oxidoreductase. Reprinted with permission of Springer.

27 000 in babies of Northern European descent. MCADD is due to a deficiency of the enzyme medium chain acyl-CoA dehydrogenase which is necessary for the oxidation of medium chain fatty acids (carbon chain length C6–C12). Ketone body and energy production is reduced and there is accumulation of medium chain fatty acids, specifically octanoyl carnitine (C8), which are considered to be responsible for the clinical sequelae. Clinically, MCADD usually presents between 6 months and 4 years of age but neonatal and adult onset can also occur. Some patients remain asymptomatic throughout life. The typical picture is of encephalopathy with 'hypoketotic' hypoglycaemia, precipitated by metabolic stress such as fasting, gastrointestinal illness or respiratory infections [5–7]. Alcohol intoxication is another precipitating cause seen in adult patients [8]. Without prompt treatment there is a high morbidity and mortality; some patients die suddenly, probably due to cardiac arrhythmias [5–7]. Between episodes patients are usually completely well because, under basal conditions, oxidation of medium chain fatty acids is near normal [9]. Once diagnosed the outlook is much improved [10].

Genetics

MCADD is inherited as an autosomal recessive disorder, so a baby has a 1 in 4 chance of inheriting the disorder from its parents. Due to a founder effect the c.985A>G mutation is common in Northern Europeans and is associated with classical clinical disease. Screening has resulted in the identification of further mutations, some of which have never been reported in clinically presenting patients [11]. Currently, in the UK all babies are treated irrespective of mutation.

Expanded newborn screening for MCADD

MCADD is part of the existing blood spot newborn screening programme in the UK (since 2009 for England, all of the UK since 2012). In England newborn screening identifies about 60 babies per year, with a prevalence of about 1 in 10 000 [12]. For this a heel prick blood sample is collected between 5 and 8 days of age on the standard newborn screening collection cards. MCADD screening uses the quantitative assay of C8 and decanoylcarnitine (C10).

More details on screening, diagnostic and clinical management protocols in the UK can be found at www.newbornbloodspot.screening.nhs.uk/mcadd and www.bimdg.org.

Dietary management

At risk neonate with a family history of MCADD

Neonatal deaths have been reported in MCADD in breast and formula fed babies [13, 14]. Newborns are at greatest risk during the first 72 hours of life, especially if they are being breast fed (see below). Therefore it is essential that at risk infants who have a family history of MCADD receive adequate feeds during the first few days of life. The 2012 UK guidelines for managing at risk babies for MCADD can be accessed from the above websites and are as follows:

- any at risk babies should be screened at 24–48 hours and results made available, promptly
- the baby should be fed regularly, a term baby at least 4 hourly and preterm 3 hourly day and night until a diagnosis of MCADD is confirmed or excluded
- breast fed babies are at particular risk because the energy content of breast milk is low for the first few days and only small volumes of breast milk are available and initially consumed; top-ups of formula milk are therefore recommended
- a volume of 60 mL/kg/day of standard infant formula is advised for the first three complete days (72 hours); ideally this should be divided evenly between 6 to 8 feeds and given after the breast feed
- if there are concerns about the baby or they are taking inadequate volumes of feeds they should be transferred to the neonatal unit and fed by nasogastric tube or given an intravenous infusion containing 10% glucose

Dietary management overview

Normal diets contain predominantly fatty acids with a chain length of C16 and C18. These long chain fatty acids undergo β-oxidation to release energy and the carbon chain length is progressively shortened to a medium, then short chain length. Under basal conditions, the oxidation of medium chain fatty acids has been reported to be near normal in patients with MCADD due to overlapping enzyme substrate specificity [9]. This only becomes a problem when there is an increased demand for fatty acids to provide energy such as during fasting or illness. The well child can therefore have a normal diet without restriction of long chain fat. It is important, however, to avoid prolonged fasts as fatty acid oxidation rates increase with fasting. In infants, fatty acid oxidation rates rise after a shorter duration of fasting and frequent feeding is therefore recommended. There are few published data on the safe duration of fasting in MCADD. Derks *et al.* have suggested treatment guidelines based on data from the literature and Dutch MCADD patients, but they note the paucity of data in the first 6 months of life [15]. Compared with the UK guidelines (Table 19.1) the fasting times are more restricted in younger children. Illness in any child is usually associated with loss of appetite and prolonged fasting; fatty acid oxidation rates increase to provide essential energy sources. In MCADD this process is limited and the child is at risk of encephalopathy. To prevent encephalopathy an emergency regimen (ER) of frequent feeding of high carbohydrate (CHO) drinks/feeds needs to be given. This will provide energy, stimulate insulin secretion and thereby minimise lipolysis and fatty acid oxidation.

Children with MCADD need to avoid medium chain triglycerides (MCT). Medium chain fatty acids can enter mitochondria without being bound to carnitine, so bypassing the step at which fatty acid oxidation is normally regulated (CPTI). MCT ingestion could therefore lead to a more severe metabolic disturbance than with long chain fats.

Table 19.1 Medium chain acyl-CoA dehydrogenase (MCAD) deficiency: guidelines for 'maximum safe fasting times' for the well child.

Age	Time in hours
*Positive screening result to 4 months of age	6
From 4 months	8
From 8 months	10
From 12 months onwards	12

*Around 2 weeks of age.
Source: www.bimdg.org.

Dietary guidelines and information leaflets (e.g. MCADD is Suspected, MCADD and Your Child) for screened patients have been developed and can be accessed from www.bimdg.org.uk and www.newbornbloodspot.screening.nhs.uk. There are dietary information sheets for use at specified ages, from a positive screening result throughout childhood; they can also be used for clinically presenting patients. Information on suggested safe fasting times and ER for management of illness is included. Another useful educational tool is an e-learning resource on MCADD which is specifically designed for dietitians and midwives, accessed from www.geneticseducation.nhs.uk.

Dietary management during illness

If a child with MCADD is unwell (particularly if there is fever, vomiting and/or diarrhoea) and has a reduced appetite they should be given the standard ER of at least 3 hourly drinks containing glucose polymer, day and night (p. 502). The ER needs to be implemented at an early stage to prevent metabolic decompensation and risk of sudden death. Fat is usually excluded during the acute period, although there is little evidence to support if this is essential. As the child improves, the normal diet can be resumed but extra ER drinks should be given, particularly during the night, until the child is fully recovered and eating well. If the ER is refused or vomited the child should have rapid access to their local paediatric services, avoiding a wait in the accident and emergency department, so there is no delay in starting an intravenous (IV) infusion containing glucose; 10% glucose, 0.45% saline is generally suitable but electrolytes should be monitored. Management decisions should be based on the child's clinical state. Monitoring of blood glucose at home is not recommended because precision is poor at low concentrations and hypoglycaemia is a relatively late finding during illness in MCADD [16]. If for any reason the child needs to be commenced on a special infant formula or paediatric enteral feed during illness, it should not contain added MCT (see below). Emergency regimen guidelines (IV and oral) for hospital use can be accessed from www.bimdg.org.uk Although newborn screening has markedly improved the outcome for children with MCADD [17], there is still a risk of sudden death, specifically associated with vomiting [18].

The child who is vomiting should therefore be managed with extra vigilance.

Dietary management of well infants

With the introduction of newborn screening for MCADD in the UK it was important to set 'maximum safe fasting times' (Table 19.1). These were based mainly on feeding practices used in screened populations elsewhere in the world that had proven successful in avoiding symptomatic episodes. A review of these guidelines are planned

Infants can be breast or bottle fed with a normal infant formula and weaned onto a normal diet without restriction of long chain triglycerides (LCT), but it is important they are fed at regular intervals day and night. Small amounts of MCT are present in the vegetable oils of normal infant formulas, but the quantities are not sufficient to cause a problem. However, MCT are added to some special infant formulas and energy supplements and these should not be given. It is important to check the current composition of all such products for added MCT. Examples include hydrolysed infant formulas Pregestimil Lipil, MCT Pepdite, Pepti-Junior; high MCT special infant formulas Monogen, Lipistart; high MCT energy supplements MCT Duocal, MCT Procal. Low birthweight infant formulas should also be checked for added MCT.

The following dietary guidelines should be followed when treating an infant with MCADD:

Infants (under 1 year of age)

- breast feeding or normal infant formula is suitable
- avoidance of long fasts (Table 19.1)
- demand feeding every 3–4 hours throughout the day
- night feeds according to guidelines for 'maximum safe fasting times' (Table 19.1)
- weaning is commenced at the normal time around 6 months (26 weeks) of age
- weaning onto a normal diet and encouragement of regular starchy foods as weaning progresses
- restriction of LCT is *not* necessary
- avoidance of special infant formulas which contain added MCT

Note that newborn infants at risk for MCADD because of family history must receive adequate feeds (as described above).

Dietary management of well children

Children with MCADD should be encouraged to adopt a 'healthy lifestyle' through diet and exercise. Some parents worry their child may not be eating enough but they need to be reassured that not always finishing a meal can be normal; if necessary a snack can be offered later. There may be a risk of overweight or obesity due to parental anxiety surrounding feeding [19, 20]. Children with MCADD should be encouraged to exercise as normal. The need for provision of additional CHO pre-exercise should be individually monitored as muscle pain and/or reduced exercise tolerance has been reported in some patients [19]. All children, including those with MCADD, can feel hungry after exercise and a CHO snack should be given to help replenish glycogen stores.

From 1 year of age children can fast for 12 hours at night. In the author's centre a minority of patients are not able to fast all night as they develop early morning symptoms; these symptoms have been resolved by being given either a night feed or uncooked cornstarch before bed as it is slowly digested to release glucose.

It is not necessary to restrict dietary fat. MCT, C8 and C10, occur in only a few foods and in small amounts, e.g. in butter, cow's milk, and these can be included in the diet. Coconut is the only exception where 5% of the fatty acids have a chain length of C8 or C10; for coconut oil, the figure is 13%. Precautions should be taken in countries, such as the Philippines, where coconut oil is used as the main cooking oil. Pure coconut and coconut oil may be best avoided as the effect of large amounts of these in children with MCADD is not known. Theoretically there is risk of accumulation of toxic medium chain fats. Coconut products such as coconut milk and coconut paste may be suitable (provided the C8 and C10 content is low) and small amounts of coconut as an ingredient in food are acceptable in healthy children with MCADD. MCT are added to some special paediatric feeds and energy supplements and these should not be given. It is important to check the current composition of all such products for added MCT. Examples include hydrolysed paediatric feeds Peptamen Junior, Paediasure Pepdite; paediatric enteral feeds Paediasure, Frebini Energy; high MCT energy supplements MCT Duocal, MCT Procal.

The following dietary guidelines should be followed when treating a child with MCADD:

Children (from 1 year of age)

- regular meals (three main meals daily, including breakfast which must not be missed)
- a bedtime snack containing starchy foods such as bread, crumpets, muffins, rice cakes, crackers, biscuits, pitta bread, chapatti or cereals
- missed meals can be replaced with a starchy snack if necessary
- avoidance of special dietetic products which contain added MCT
- a maximum fasting interval of 12 hours overnight (Table 19.1)
- encouragement of a 'healthy lifestyle' and maintenance of normal body mass index
- restriction of LCT is *not* necessary.

Alcohol

Adolescents (and adults) need to know that an excessive alcohol intake is hazardous. Alcohol intoxication with resultant vomiting has been a cause of presentation in adults [8]. Vomiting and loss of appetite associated with excessive alcohol intake can be particularly dangerous. Alcohol inhibits gluconeogenesis so both fatty acid oxidation and gluconeogenesis which provide fuel during fasting are impaired. Moreover, the symptoms of hypoglycaemia might be attributed to inebriation rather than MCADD. Teenagers and adults need to be educated about the risks associated with excessive alcohol intake. A sensible approach is to advise that alcohol intake is limited and must always be taken in combination with food.

Carnitine

Plasma carnitine concentrations are often below the normal range in patients with MCADD, particularly after illness. The consequences of this are not clear. Carnitine supplements are given by some but this is not universal [21]. Maintenance of free carnitine levels (albeit at the lower end of normal range) has been reported in 46 patients from one centre not receiving carnitine supplementation; no patient experienced significant episodes of rhabdomyolysis or decompensation [22]. In the author's centre, a trial of carnitine is given to a minority of children who complain of muscle symptoms and also have low plasma carnitine levels. There is conflicting evidence concerning the beneficial effect of carnitine on exercise tolerance [23, 24].

Disorders of long chain fatty acid oxidation

The long chain fatty acid oxidation disorders include:

- *Defects of the carnitine cycle.* Carnitine palmitoyl transferases I and II (CPTI and CPTII), carnitine acylcarnitine translocase (CACT) deficiencies and defects of the transporter for uptake of carnitine across the cell membrane (OCTN2 or CT) (Fig. 19.1).
- *Defects of β-oxidation.* Very long chain acyl-CoA dehydrogenase deficiency (VLCADD), mitochondrial trifunctional protein deficiency (MTPD) which encompasses the three MTP enzymes LCHAD deficiency (LCHADD), due to an isolated deficiency of LCHAD enzyme within the MTP complex (Fig. 19.1).

For a description of the biochemical pathway of long chain fatty acid oxidation refer to Introduction to Inherited Metabolic Disorders (p. 383), page 589 and Fig. 19.1.

Overview of clinical presentation

Long chain fatty acid oxidation disorders (LC-FAOD) vary in severity and may present at any time from the neonatal period to adulthood. The organs affected are heart, liver and skeletal muscles. The clinical presentation for all disorders commonly includes one or all of these problems:

- an acute 'hypoketotic' hypoglycaemia and encephalopathy with associated liver failure and hyperammonaemia
- cardiomyopathy and arrhythmias (often in infancy)
- myopathy presenting as weakness or episodes of muscle breakdown (rhabdomyolysis) induced by illness in early childhood or more commonly by exercise in older children or adults (as seen in patients with partial deficiency of CPTII); additionally some patients

with CPTI deficiency have renal tubular acido-sis during infancy

- most patients with LCHADD or MTPD develop pigmentary retinopathy and/or peripheral neuropathy as long term complications
- patients with partial deficiencies (e.g. VLCADD) often remain asymptomatic throughout childhood and sometimes throughout life

A review of 187 patients with LC-FAOD identified hepatic symptoms (hepatomegaly, increased blood alanine transaminase (ALT) and steatosis), hyperammonaemia and hyperlactacidaemia as being the most predominant clinical and biochemical features at diagnosis, irrespective of the underlying defect [25]. More details of the clinical presentation of the individual disorders are described elsewhere [26]. Inadequate energy production from fatty acids and ketones and the accumulation of toxic intermediates (such as long chain acylcarnitines) are probably responsible for the clinical features [4]. Many of these symptoms are reversible with the provision of adequate, appropriate energy.

Genetics

All LC-FAOD are autosomal recessive inherited disorders. In all, there is molecular heterogeneity but prevalent mutations have been identified in some, e.g. CPTI (Inuit population only) and CPTII, LCHAD deficiencies. In different LC-FAOD the genotype and phenotype relationship varies, e.g. in VLCADD homozygous nonsense mutations are generally associated with severe early onset disease; the c.848T>C mutation has only been found in mildly affected or asymptomatic patients. A more detailed description of genetics for different LC-FAOD is found elsewhere [26, 27].

Expanded newborn screening

A number of countries worldwide such as Germany, Australia and the USA undertake expanded newborn screening for LC-FAOD, using tandem mass spectrometry. Expanded newborn screening for VLCADD has identified a common milder phenotype for which less dietary modification is required (see below). A pilot project of expanded newborn screening has been under way since July 2012 in parts of England; LCHADD is one of the disorders being evaluated. Screening is by measurement of hydroxypalmitoyl (C16-OH) carnitine in dried blood spots using tandem mass spectrometry. More information on the screening, diagnostic and clinical management protocols can be accessed at www.expandedscreening.org. LCHADD is not part of the national screening programme in England.

Principles of dietary management

Treatment of LC-FAOD disorders is primarily by diet with the exception of defects of the transporter for cellular carnitine uptake (OCTN2). Although they are different disorders the principles of dietary treatment are similar. The prescribed dietary treatment will vary depending on the severity, age at onset and underlying disorder. The main aims of dietary treatment are to prevent an energy deficit and, at the site of the defect, the accumulation of potentially toxic acyl-CoA intermediates and acylcarnitines (formed from these) by minimising fatty acid oxidation and provision of adequate energy. The abnormal metabolites which accumulate are disorder specific and present in higher concentrations during times of metabolic stress such as illness. Abnormal plasma acylcarnitines are not seen in CPTI or OCTN2 [26].

Long chain fatty acids for oxidation are derived from both dietary fat and adipose tissue. Dietary treatment therefore involves avoiding long fasts (especially during illness), exercise management (when energy needs are increased) and additionally in severe defects restricting the intake of dietary fat and instituting more frequent feeding with an increased CHO intake and supplements of MCT. The response to dietary treatment is mainly good. Cardiomyopathy (if present) will resolve and hypoglycaemia and major metabolic decompensations can be prevented. Muscle pain with exercise may still occur in some disorders, despite good dietary management. Patients with LCHADD and MTPD have specific long term complications, particularly a pigmentary retinopathy and progressive peripheral neuropathy (which is more of a problem in MTPD). It is reported that diet may help delay the onset and progression but not prevent retinopathy [28–30]. Frequent decompensations, late diagnosis with severe symptoms and hypoglycaemia may increase the progression of pigmentary retinopathy [29]. The pathogenesis of retinopathy remains to be fully elucidated.

During illness patients are at risk of metabolic decompensation due to increased lipolysis and fatty acid oxidation. Provision of glucose using a standard ER is needed to help prevent this.

Treatment recommendations have been published for β-oxidation defects based mainly on expert opinion from a European workshop [31, 32] and 'A Delphi clinical practice protocol for the management of VLCADD' from the USA [33]. Genetics Metabolic Dietitians International (GMDI) has also produced guidelines for management of VLCADD which can be accessed at www.gmdi.org. There are no such publications for defects of the carnitine cycle.

Long chain triglycerides

The safe upper limit for long chain fat intake is unknown and varies with the severity of the disorder. Normalisation of acylcarnitine profiles is observed in LCHADD and MTPD when LCT intake is <10% total energy and MCT are given [34]. Recommendations from published guidelines suggest for severe VLCADD to limit LCT to 5%–10% total daily energy intake [32, 33]. This is also recommended by GMDI. For severe defects of LCHADD and MTPD it is recommended to restrict LCT to as low as practically possible (5%–10% energy intake) but in practice it is typically more likely to be <15% (including 3%–4% from essential fatty acids) [32, 34]. Importantly, in those presenting with a milder myopathic form of the disorder, as can be seen in VLCADD and CPTII deficiency (CPTIID), such restriction of LCT may not be necessary [32].

Medium chain triglycerides

Dietary MCT are absorbed through the hepatic portal vein; they pass directly into the mitochondria primarily independent of the carnitine cycle and are then rapidly converted to ketone bodies, bypassing the long chain β-oxidation enzymes. Ketones inhibit the mobilisation of fatty acids from adipose tissue and the oxidation of fatty acids by cardiac muscle [35]. In patients with VLCADD, MTPD and LCHADD, MCT (C8, C10) can provide

a useful energy source, 8.3 kcal (35 kJ)/g, and may have other beneficial effects. MCT have led to the resolution of cardiomyopathy in patients with VLCADD and LCHADD deficiencies [36, 37]. Medium chain fatty acids may also suppress long chain fatty acid oxidation without being converted to ketone bodies; they have been shown to inhibit the accumulation of potentially toxic long chain intermediates in cultured skin fibroblasts from LCHAD and MTP deficient patients [38]. It has been suggested that patients should maintain a high intake of MCT throughout life (10%–20% energy intake) [34]. The optimal amount or ratio of C8, C10 fatty acids to provide is not known. Skin fibroblast studies have shown that C10 undergoes elongation prior to oxidation, so it has been suggested that C8 may be preferable [39, 40]. Recommendations from published guidelines from GMDI and other authors [32, 33] suggest 20%–25% total daily energy intake be provided from MCT for severe LCHADD, MTPD and VLCADD. In the UK, infant formulas which can be prescribed for LC-FAOD provide either 17% or 30% total energy intake as MCT (Table 19.2).

The role of MCT is less clear in defects of the carnitine cycle. In several infants with CPTI deficiency, renal tubular acidosis has only resolved when they have been changed to an MCT based feed [41]. MCT has also been used with apparent benefit in patients with mild CACT deficiency (CACTD). In cases of severe CACTD and CPTIID, MCT has been reported to have caused markedly abnormal blood acylcarnitines and dicarboxylic aciduria [42, 43]. They suggest the amount of MCT, may need to be limited because it may in part enter the mitochondria by a carnitine dependent mechanism.

MCT is found in insignificant amounts in normal diets. Although MCT have benefits in LC-FAOD, their long term use in humans has never been systematically studied, so it is not known if there are any detrimental effects.

MCT and exercise

In the normal population the primary fuel source during low intensity prolonged exercise is fatty acids, and for high intensity exercise CHO (glucose and glycogen stores). Glucose is also the initial fuel during any exercise. Patients with VLCADD, LCHADD, MTPD and CPTIID can experience

Table 19.2 Low LCT infant formulas per 100 mL.

		Monogen (SHS)	Lipistart (Vitaflo)	Basic-f (Milupa)	Low Fat Module (SHS)
Dilution		17.5%	15%	13%	18%
Scoop size		5 g	5 g	4.3 g	6 g
Energy	kcal	73.5 (310 kJ)	68 (282 kJ)	49 (207 kJ)	67.3 (286 kJ)
Protein	g	2.2	2.1	1.8	1.6
Carbohydrate	g	12	8.3	10.2	14.9
Fat	g	1.9	3.1	<0.1	0.14
- MCT	g	1.52	2.5	Nil	Nil
	% fat energy	80%	80%		
	% total energy	17%	30%		
- C8	g	0.83	1.5		
- C10	g	0.6	0.93		
- LCT	g	0.38	0.57		
	% fat energy	20%	20%		
- Linoleic acid	mg	90	259	Nil	Nil
	% total energy	1.1%	3.4%		
- α-linolenic acid	mg	10	36.3	Nil	Nil
	% total energy	0.17	0.5%		
- DHA	mg	Nil	30.3	Nil	Nil
- AA	mg	Nil	15.2	Nil	Nil
Vitamins					
- E	mg	0.5	1.7	0.3	0.4
- A	μg	56.9	69.9	52	71.3
- D	μg	1.2	1.4	0.9	1.2

Reconstitution: Monogen 1 scoop added to 25 mL water
Lipistart 1 scoop added to 30 mL water
In UK only Monogen and Lipistart are prescribable.
SHS, Scientific Hospital Supplies International; MCT, medium chain triglycerides; LCT, long chain triglycerides;
DHA, docosahexaenoic acid; AA, arachidonic acid.
Source: Manufacturers.

muscle pain and rhabdomyolysis with exercise. This may be due to their limited ability to oxidise long chain fatty acids as a fuel source for exercising muscle or the accumulation of toxic intermediates. Supplements of MCT pre-exercise have been reported to improve exercise capacity although only very small numbers of patients of varying ages and disorders have been studied [44–46]. In patients with the myopathic form of CPTIID and VLCADD there appears to be sufficient enzyme activity for fatty acid oxidation at rest, but not for the increased requirement of exercise [47, 48]. Some patients with CPTIID appear to benefit from taking a diet rich in polysaccharides pre-exercise [49]. As yet, no treatment has conclusively been shown to prevent rhabdomyolysis.

The effect of diet on exercise capacity has also been studied in the VLCADD knockout mouse. This has reduced exercise intolerance which is not improved by a low fat, CHO enriched diet [50]. Exercise capacity was improved by an MCT bolus prior to exercise but not by long term use of an MCT based diet. Moreover, long term use of MCT caused severe hepatic steatosis and increased long chain acylcarnitine accumulation [51] which was not seen following an MCT bolus [52]. Although these results are interesting it is not yet clear how they relate to human patients.

Triheptanoin

Triheptanoin, an oil containing C7 fatty acids, has been substituted for conventional MCT in a number of patients with LC-FAOD. Use of MCT leads to the production of acetyl-CoA but it is hypothesised that a shortage of oxaloacetate prevents this from being oxidised in the citric acid cycle. Triheptanoin generates acetyl-CoA and also propionyl-CoA.

The latter can be converted to oxaloacetate, which acts as an 'anaplerotic' substrate for the citric acid cycle. Improved cardiac function and/or muscle weakness has been reported in three patients with VLCADD [53] and seven patients with myopathic CPTIID [54] given triheptanoin. However, triheptanoin was not compared with MCT in a controlled manner, so it is impossible to be certain if it conferred any specific benefit. Triheptanoin is not yet widely available outside the USA.

Frequency of feeding

Frequent feeding is recommended to reduce lipolysis. The safe duration of fasting for different disorders and ages has not been well defined and practices differ between countries and centres. Treatment recommendations from Spiekerkoetter *et al.* suggest a maximum safe fasting time at night of 8 hours from 6 months of age and 10 (–12) hours from 12 months in VLCADD, MTPD and LCHADD during stable metabolic condition [32]. In the USA no consensus on overnight feeding could be reached by an expert panel using the Delphi method [33]. The GMDI guidelines (www.gmdi.org) for VLCADD are similar to those of Speikerkoetter *et al.* In the UK, fasting is more severely limited to help reduce the risk of cardiomyopathy and onset of long term complications of retinopathy and neuropathy (although this has never been proved). Children with severe defects are fed 3–4 hourly during the day and by continuous nasogastric or gastrostomy feeding overnight (or the child is woken for feeds during the night). Overnight feeding is not standard practice but the literature suggests that some other countries do this, such as Scandinavia.

Questionnaire surveys have shown that uncooked cornstarch (UCCS) is used by some centres to provide a source of 'slow release glucose' [31, 55]. In older children continuous tube feeding overnight may be replaced with UCCS (personal practice). This may be a better option than stopping overnight feeds completely. Before use, the metabolic response to UCCS should be assessed since this varies between patients [56]. However, there are no published studies comparing the metabolic profiles of patients on overnight feeds, UCCS and those who fast overnight or the outcome between those given long term overnight feeding or not. Patients with milder defects are likely to tolerate overnight fasting without problems.

Prevention of deficiencies on a low LCT diet

Patients on minimal LCT diets require supplements of fat soluble vitamins, essential fatty acids (EFA) and long chain polyunsaturated fatty acids (LCPUFA). In the UK at least 1% total energy intake from linoleic acid and 0.2% from α-linolenic acid are recommended [57]. Others recommend a much higher intake of 4.5% daily energy intake in infants <4 months of age, decreasing to 3% from age 4 years [32]. The joint FAO/WHO 2008 report recommended an adequate daily intake for children >6 months to be linoleic acid 3%–4% and α-linolenic 0.4%–0.6% of daily energy intake [58]. Most sources of EFA (such as walnut oil) do not provide LCPUFA, such as arachidonic acid (AA) and docosahexaenoic acids (DHA), but these are expected to be synthesised from the EFA that are provided. In the author's experience, deficiency is rare if patients are receiving adequate EFA in the form of walnut oil [59].

It has been suggested that DHA deficiency may contribute to the pathogenesis of chorioretinopathy of LCHADD [60], although this is not prevented by supplementation. Nevertheless supplements of DHA at a dose of 60 mg/day in children <20 kg and 120 mg/day in children >20 kg are recommended in MTPD and LCHADD [32]. FAO/WHO recommends an adequate daily intake of DHA for normal children to be

- the amounts found in breast milk for infants
- 100–150 mg for children aged 2–4 years
- 150–200 mg for children aged 4–6 years
- 200–300 mg for children aged 6–10 years [58]

Fat soluble vitamin supplements (A, D, E) are essential for those on reduced LCT intake. Vitamin E deficiency is associated with a peripheral neuropathy which is one of the long term complications of MTPD and LCHADD. It is therefore essential that vitamin E is provided in normal requirements for age, at least.

Carnitine

It remains uncertain whether carnitine supplements should be given to patients with long chain fatty acid oxidation disorders. Plasma free carnitine concentrations are often below the normal range, particularly after episodes of illness, but tissue levels are probably not low enough to affect fatty acid oxidation. Supplements may facilitate the excretion of metabolites but, by increasing the level of long chain acylcarnitines, it is possible that they may increase the risk of arrhythmias [61].

Energy distribution of the diet

As LCT is restricted more energy needs to be provided from CHO and supplements of MCT. The optimal distribution of energy intake from CHO and MCT is not known. The following provides a guide to the typical energy distribution and long chain fat intake of the diet in severe defects (based on personal practice):

- 60%–65% energy from CHO
- 10%–15% energy from protein
- 20%–25% energy from medium chain fat (depending on the disorder)
- 1.2%–2% energy from EFA (based on FAO/ WHO [58] higher intakes may be appropriate)

Long chain fat

During infancy, total LCT intake will vary depending on the choice of low LCT infant formula as the percentage energy from LCT varies (Table 19.2): Monogen 4.5%, 0.5 g LCT/100 kcal (420 kJ); Lipistart 6.9%, 0.8 g LCT/100 kcal (420 kJ). However, a source of LCPUFA needs to be given with Monogen, so the overall LCT intake will increase. The LCT intake from formula could range from 2 to 7 g/day in infants aged <6 months. In children, it is possible to restrict intake of long chain fat to provide ≤ 6% total energy intake, ≤7 g LCT/1000 kcal (4.2 MJ), excluding EFA. Similar dietary practices are reported to be used by others [28, 32].

The suggested percentage of energy from protein is based on typical intakes in the normal UK population. Due to concerns about excess weight gain over time in their cohort of LCHADD and MTPD patients, Gillingham et al. trialled a high protein diet providing 30% energy intake in an attempt to lower energy intake, without loss of metabolic control [62]. Short term, the diet was reported to achieve this and increase resting energy expenditure. Longer term studies are needed to see if this can be sustained.

Minimal long chain fat diet

Infants

Infants with severe long chain defects need a minimal LCT feed supplemented with MCT and frequent feeding. This could be provided by Monogen or Lipistart; both are nutritionally complete infant formulas with minimal LCT (Table 19.2). Exclusive breast feeding is contraindicated except for asymptomatic VLCADD infants diagnosed on newborn screening. Compared with Monogen, energy from MCT is higher in Lipistart and energy from CHO is lower; it also contains LCP-UFA and provides more vitamin E. It is important to establish if MCT can be oxidised before using either of these formulas. If MCT is considered inadvisable because of a possible diagnosis (as in, perhaps, severe CACTD or CPTIID), a modular feed without fat (long or medium chain) may need to be used during the initial stages of management until the diagnosis is established. Skimmed milk powder or whey protein powder, although they do contain small amounts of LCT, can be used as the protein base with glucose polymer and additional minerals and vitamins to provide recommended intakes. EFA and LCPUFA should also be provided if the infant remains on a modular feed for several days. Suitable commercial minimal fat feeds with no added MCT are Low Fat Module (0.14 g fat/100 mL) or Basic-f (<0.1 g fat/100 mL), although the latter is generally not available in the UK (Table 19.2).

Clinically diagnosed infants are likely to be very sick, managed in intensive care and receiving IV 10% dextrose. Once stabilised, nasogastric (or oral) feeds should be introduced and titrated against IV fluids so that an adequate energy intake is maintained and further metabolic decompensation is prevented. The initial feeds given may vary depending on the clinical situation but should, if possible, provide 10 g CHO/100 mL (10% CHO) to maximise energy intake and reduce lipolysis. Once the infant is well and established on full feeds these should be given 3 hourly during the day and night, or 3 hourly during the day with a continuous feed overnight. The overnight feed can be commenced 2 hours after the last 3 hourly day feed and can probably be stopped 2 hours before the first day feed in the morning. The amount of glucose required overnight to minimise lipolysis is not known. For infants, practice is to provide a minimum of 0.5 g CHO/kg/hour which will equal basal glucose production rates (p. 544) and should therefore minimise lipolysis. When babies are just on infant formula the feed is distributed evenly over the 24 hours, e.g. a 6 kg infant fed 150 mL/kg (900 mL) would have 120 mL 3 hourly × 5 feeds during the day (at 8 am, 11 am, 2 pm, 5 pm, 8 pm) with 300 mL given at 40 mL/hour continuously overnight for 8 hours from 10 pm to 6 am. At this volume Monogen provides 0.8 g CHO/kg/hour and Lipistart 0.5 g CHO/kg/hour (but provides more energy from MCT than Monogen).

Infants diagnosed on newborn screening Treatment recommendations have been given by Spiekerkoetter *et al.* for infants diagnosed on expanded newborn screening [32, 61]. The dietary treatment advised for VLCADD depends on the clinical presentation and biochemistry. Asymptomatic infants with a normal creatine kinase and liver transaminase levels can be fed normally, either breast fed or with standard infant formula. In symptomatic infants, or those with abnormal creatine kinase or transaminases, the diet should contain greater amounts of MCT formula and less or no breast milk. If cardiomyopathy is present then feeding should proceed as for the clinically presenting patient. Asymptomatic infants should continue to have clinical and biochemical follow-up.

For LCHADD (MTPD) dietary treatment should proceed as for the clinically presenting patient, even if the infant is asymptomatic. There is some evidence that this may delay the onset and progression of the long term complications of peripheral neuropathy and retinopathy.

Weaning Weaning is commenced at the normal time around 6 months (26 weeks) of age. An example of a suggested menu plan for infants is provided in Table 19.3. Solids should have a minimal fat content and be high in CHO. Rice cereal, potato, fruit and vegetables are suitable as first

Table 19.3 Minimal long chain fat weaning diet: sample menu.

8 am Breakfast	*Commercial baby cereal mixed with Lipistart or Monogen
11 am	Infant feed
1 pm Lunch	Purée turkey, chicken (white only), white fish or lentils Purée or mashed potato, sweet potato Pasta, rice Purée or mashed vegetables *Commercial baby savoury foods
4 pm Tea	Purée or mashed fruit and sugar or *commercial baby fruit dessert Very low fat yoghurt or fromage frais Milk pudding (custard, cornflour, ground rice) made with infant feed or skimmed milk
7 pm	Infant feed
9 pm to 6 am	Continuous overnight feed for a 7 kg infant: Monogen – 30 mL/hour provides 0.5 g CHO/kg/hour (197 kcal, 825 kJ) Lipistart – 40 mL/hour provides 0.5 g CHO/kg/hour (245 kcal, 1025 kJ, provides) Lipistart provides more MCT so a lower volume could be considered
	Extra feeds or baby juice can be given with meals
	Finger foods may be introduced from 6–9 months: soft cooked vegetables, soft ripe fruit (pasta, bread and cereals may also be suitable but LCT content must be checked first)

*Commercial baby foods.
Allow freely: wet baby foods ≤0.5 g fat/100 g and dried baby foods ≤2 g/100 g.
Wet baby foods 0.5–1.0 g/100 g or dried baby foods 2–5 g/100 g may also be suitable but counted as part of total fat intake.
Baby foods with a higher fat content are best avoided.
Walnut oil dose (p. 601).

weaning foods. Once these have been introduced low fat, high protein foods can also be given, e.g. turkey, white fish, lentils, very low fat cottage cheese and yoghurt. Commercial baby foods can be included in the diet but need to be limited to those with a low fat content. Wet baby foods (fat content <0.5 g/100 g) and dried baby foods (fat content <2 g/100 g) can be given freely. Baby foods with a higher fat content need to be counted as part of the daily fat intake. Parents can be taught how to calculate the amount of fat a food provides from the nutritional labelling (p. 602). As the amount of starchy solid food begins to increase, this should replace some of the 3 hourly day feeds, ensuring it provides at least the same amount of energy, e.g. an 8 kg infant fed 150 mL 3 hourly × 5 daytime feeds (8 am, 11 am, 2 pm, 5 pm, 8 pm) and 50 mL/hour continuous overnight feeds from 10 pm to 6 am. Each 150 mL of minimal fat feed provides 110 kcal (460 kJ) so the replacement solids should provide the same energy. Alternatively this can be calculated as follows:

- energy requirements are 95 kcal (400 kJ)/kg = 760 kcal (3.2 MJ)
- provide 60% of daily energy requirement from CHO = 460 kcal (1.9 MJ) = 5 g CHO/hour = 15 g CHO for 3 hours (0.6 g CHO/kg/hour)

Infants who eat well will easily exceed this amount of CHO in a meal but the amount of solids taken needs to be checked in those who feed poorly. MCT oil (p. 602) can be incorporated into the diet of older infants who are eating well. The infant formula can continue to be given overnight, but with increasing age larger volumes are needed to provide the required amount of CHO; this may interfere with the daytime appetite or lead to excessive weight gain. Therefore as the amount of solids progresses the volume of feed should be decreased and glucose polymer added to provide the required amount of CHO (0.5 g CHO/kg/hour = 2 kcal (8 kJ)/kg/hour). It is not yet clear whether the overnight feed should be changed to glucose polymer or whether it is helpful to continue some MCT at night [63]. In this case it may be more appropriate to base the overnight feed on a total energy intake per kilogram per hour from CHO and MCT, although this is not current practice.

Fat soluble vitamin supplements will be required once the daily intake of certain infant formula falls below 600 mL (Table 19.2. p. 602).

EFA intake differs depending on the formula used (Table 19.2). Once weaning is commenced and volume of formula decreases and no longer provides the sole source of nutrition, an additional source of EFA is needed. Walnut oil provides a good source of EFA and allows a minimum amount of LCT to be given (Table 19.4). To provide the UK suggested requirement of EFA the dose of walnut oil needed is 0.1 mL per 56 kcal (235 kJ) of the estimated average requirement (EAR) of energy for age [57], subtracting the energy provided by the feeds. If the infant is on Lipistart >1% of energy intake from linoleic acid will be given. The walnut oil is administered as a single dose and given as a medicine from a spoon or via the feeding tube. In the UK, walnut oil can be purchased from most large supermarkets. It should be stored as recommended to avoid peroxidation. Other oils such as sunflower, safflower (mainly linoleic acid), soya and flax are also rich sources of EFA and a combination of these can be used to give the required EFA intake if walnut oil is disliked.

LCPUFA are added to Lipistart; 400 mL provides the suggested intake of 60 mg/day advised for LCHADD [32]. Monogen does not contain added DHA or AA, so additional supplements are necessary. These can be added as KeyOmega (p. 630): one sachet provides 100 mg DHA and 200 mg AA.

Children

Long chain triglycerides Children should remain on a minimal LCT diet with an energy distribution as previously outlined (p. 599). Inevitably, daily intake of long chain fat increases with age. The

Table 19.4 Walnut oil – essential fatty acid composition.

1 mL walnut oil provides	
Energy	8.4 kcal
	35 kJ
Fat	0.93 g
Linoleic acid	0.58 g
α-linolenic acid	0.12 g
Ratio n6:n3 fatty acids	4.5

For analysis of other oils see Fatty acids, 7th Supplement to *McCance and Widdowson's The Composition of Foods*, 5th edn. Cambridge: Royal Society of Chemistry and London: Ministry of Agriculture, Fisheries and Food, 1992 and p. 754.

figures quoted are based on the lowest possible long chain fat intake that is practicably achievable for a given age, as the safe upper limit for long chain fat intake is not known. Ideally, the increased CHO intake should be derived from starchy foods (e.g. rice, pasta, potato, bread, cereals) because these are more slowly digested than sugary foods. It is recognised, however, that some children cannot manage such a bulky diet and sugar containing foods such as low fat ice cream, cake or biscuits should form part of their diet. The diet should contain very low fat sources of protein, such as white fish, white chicken or turkey meat, pulses (Table 19.5). There are many very low fat alternatives to regular high fat foods such as crisps, sauces, desserts, ice cream and cheeses which can also be incorporated into the diet. To allow a greater variety of manufactured foods to be included in the diet, parents need to be given guidance on interpreting food labels for fat content and on understanding the many and potentially misleading wordings used to describe the fat content of food, e.g. reduced fat, low fat, virtually fat free, 90% fat free. The different types of fat, e.g. saturated, mono-unsaturated and polyunsaturated, can cause confusion and it is helpful to explain that total fat should be used when calculating fat intake. Nutritional labelling expresses the total fat content as grams of fat per 100 g and often grams of fat per portion. To help parents work out if a food is suitable they can be taught to calculate and then weigh the amount of food which provides a certain amount of fat. This also makes it easier to monitor the daily fat intake. For example,

$$\text{weight of food to provide 1 g fat} = \frac{100}{\text{fat content per 100 g of food}}$$

Manufactured foods which have a fat content <0.5 g/100 g can generally be allowed in the diet freely, unless large amounts are being consumed.

Medium chain triglycerides The intake of MCT naturally falls as less infant formula is consumed. Alternative sources of MCT should be incorporated into the diet because of the potential beneficial effects discussed above. A daily intake of 20%–25% of total energy intake is suggested which equates to 2.5–3 g/100 kcal (420 kJ) consumed. The optimal timing of administration has not been defined;

however, it is common practice to divide the dose and give 3–4 times a day, as it is rapidly absorbed and used.

MCT can be added to the diet as an oil, emulsion or powder. These products vary in C8, C10 fatty acid composition (Table 19.6). MCT oil can increase the palatability of the diet. It has a low smoke point compared with other cooking oils. Care must be taken when cooking foods in MCT oil to ensure it does not burn or become overheated as it develops a bitter taste and an unpleasant odour. The optimum cooking temperature for MCT is 160°C. MCT oil can also be used in baking, e.g. cakes, biscuits and pastry, and can be added to a variety of foods such as pasta, soups. MCT emulsion such as Liquigen may be more acceptable as it can be easily mixed into skimmed milk without separating. It can also be added to other liquids or foods and used in baking. MCT Procal powder can be added to hot or cold food or drinks (not fruit juice as it curdles). MCT Procal comes in a convenient sachet form, making it easy to use away from home (p. 632). Recipes are available for all products from their manufacturers.

Table 19.7 gives an example of how to provide the daily intake of MCT.

Other nutrients EFA need to be provided in the diet and can be added from walnut oil or combinations of other oils as described for infants. LCPUFA can be given as one sachet of KeyOmega, 100 mg DHA and 200 mg AA, which is more than the suggested intake of 60 mg DHA/day for young children with LCHADD or TFPD. In children weighing >20 kg more DHA is needed to provide the suggested intake of 120 mg/day [32]. One sachet of DocOmega provides 200 mg DHA.

Supplements of fat soluble vitamins (A, D and E) are needed unless the child is still taking around 600 mL infant formula. Intakes of iron, zinc and B_{12} should be regularly calculated as these can also be low in minimal LCT diets. The choice of supplement will depend on need, age and desired format: powder, tablets or soluble tablets are available. Ketovite tablets and liquid provide an adequate intake of fat soluble vitamins and are suitable for all ages. Alternatively, more complete vitamin and mineral supplementation can be provided: Fruitivits (from age 3 years), Paediatric Seravit (all ages), Phlexyvit sachets or tablets (from age 10

Table 19.5 Minimal long chain fat diet.

	Foods allowed	Foods to avoid
Milk	Skimmed milk, condensed skimmed milk Natural yoghurt, very low fat yoghurt and fromage frais (<0.2 g/100 g) Low fat cottage cheese (<0.5 g/100 g) *Very low fat cheeses Quark (skimmed milk soft cheese) Low fat ice cream	Full fat and semi-skimmed milk. Cream (all types) Full fat yoghurt and fromage frais Full and half fat cheeses †Ice cream
Egg	Egg whites, egg white replacer, meringue	Egg yolks
Fish	White fish (no skin), e.g. haddock, cod, sole, plaice Crab, crabsticks, tuna, prawns, shrimps, lobster Tinned: tuna in brine or water, crab, prawns, shrimps	Oily fish, e.g. sardines, kippers, salmon, mackerel Fish in breadcrumbs, batter, sauces, pastry Tinned: fish in oil
Poultry	*Chicken,*turkey (white breast meat, no skin)	Chicken, turkey (dark meat and skin), basted poultry, duck, goose Chicken in breadcrumbs, batter, sauces, pastry
Meat	*Lean red meat (<5% fat content)	Fatty meat, sausages (normal and low fat), burgers, meat paste, paté, salami, pies
Meat substitutes	Soya mince, *Quorn, *tofu	
Pulses	Peas, e.g. chick peas, split peas Beans, e.g. red, white, borlotti, black-eyed	None, unless in made-up dishes containing fat
Fats/oils	Medium chain triglyceride oil as advised	Butter, margarine, low fat spread, vegetable oils, lard, dripping, suet, shortening
Pasta and rice	Spaghetti, macaroni, other pasta, noodles, couscous, rice (white)	Wholemeal pasta, pasta in dishes, e.g. macaroni cheese, carbonara Brown rice, egg noodles
Flours and cereals	Flour (white), cornflour, custard powder, semolina, sago, tapioca	Flour (wholemeal), soya flour, oats, bran Foods made with flour which contain fat, e.g. pastry, sauces, cake, biscuits, batter, breadcrumb coatings
Breakfast cereals	Many are suitable Wholewheat cereals, e.g. Weetabix branflakes are higher in fat content than non-wholewheat cereals , e.g. Rice Krispies, cornflakes	Cereals with nuts and chocolate, e.g. muesli All-bran, Ready Brek
Bread and crackers	*White bread, white pitta, crumpets, muffins Some crackers have a low fat content, e.g. rice cakes, Matzos, Ryvita (not sesame)	Wholemeal, wholegrain breads, nan bread, chapatti made with fat, croissants, oatcakes, cheese crackers, †crackers
Cakes and biscuits and pastry	Only those made from low fat ingredients 95% fat free cakes and biscuits	†Cakes, †biscuits, buns, pastry for sweet and savoury foods, e.g. apple pie, quiche
Desserts	Jelly, meringue, sorbet, very low fat ice cream, skimmed milk puddings, e.g. rice, custard	Most desserts, e.g. whole milk puddings, trifle, cheesecakes, gateaux, †mousse, fruit pie or crumble
Fruit	Most varieties – fresh, frozen, tinned, dried	Avocado pears, olives, yoghurt/chocolate covered dried fruit, banana chips
Vegetables	All vegetables and salad Very low fat crisps	Chips, †crisps, †low fat crisps, roast potato, potato or vegetable salad in mayonnaise or salad dressing, †coleslaw

(continued overleaf)

Table 19.5   *(continued)*

	Foods allowed	Foods to avoid
Herbs and spices	Pickles, chutney Herbs, spices, salt, pepper	
Nuts Seeds		Nuts, peanut butter, seeds, e.g. sesame, sunflower
Sauces and gravies	Tomato ketchup, brown sauce, soy sauce, Marmite, Oxo, Bovril, very low fat gravy mixes Fat free dressings and mayonnaise Minimal fat sauces (jars, tins, packets)	†Gravy granules, †stock cubes Salad cream, mayonnaise, oil and vinegar dressings †Sauce mixes (jars, tins, packets)
Soups	Some low calorie and 'healthy eating type' soups are very low fat	Most soups, cream soups
Confectionery	Boiled sweets, jelly sweets, fruit gums, pastilles, marshmallow, mints, ice lollies	Chocolate, chocolate covered sweets, toffee, fudge, butter mints
Sugars and preserves	Sugar, golden syrup, jam, marmalade, honey, treacle	Lemon curd, chocolate spread
Baking products	Baking powder, bicarbonate of soda, yeast, arrowroot, essences, food colouring	
Drinks	Fruit juice, squash, fizzy drinks, milkshake flavourings, tea, coffee	†Instant chocolate drinks, cocoa, malted milk type drinks, e.g. Horlicks

*Intake of these foods may need to be restricted because of their fat content.
†These foods in the 'avoid list' often have very low fat equivalents which can be included in the diet.

Table 19.6   Medium chain triglyceride products.

Product	Energy kcal (kJ)	MCT	MCT g/100 g fatty acids			Other nutrients
			C8	C10	C12	
MCT oil (Nutricia)	855 (3.6 MJ)/100 mL	94 g/100 mL	58	38	1.7	Nil
Liquigen emulsion (Nutricia)	450 (1.9 MJ)/100 mL	50 g/100 mL	82.1	15.9	1.3	Nil
MCT Procal (Vitaflo)	657 (2.7 MJ)/100 g 105 (440 kJ)/16 g sachet	62.2 g/100 g 10 g/16 g sachet	54	39	–	Per sachet: 2 g protein, 3.3 g CHO

MCT, medium chain triglyceride.
Other MCT products such as MCT margarine can be sourced from www.ceres-mct.com or www.drschar.com. These
are not prescribable in the UK.

Table 19.7   Example providing daily medium chain triglyceride intake.

Daily MCT intake for a 4-year-old girl

Estimated average requirement for energy for age = 1400 kcal (5.9 MJ)/day [57]
Provide 20%–25% energy from MCT = 280–350 kcal (1.2–1.5 MJ) ÷ (8.3 kcal, 35 kJ/g MCT) = 34–42 g/day

Breakfast	20 mL MCT emulsion (10 g MCT) added to breakfast cereal
Lunch	1 sachet MCT Procal (10 g MCT) added to very low fat yoghurt at school
Evening meal	10 mL MCT oil (10 g MCT) added to cooked pasta

Another 10 g of MCT could be added to the night feed (Table 19.8) from MCT emulsion

MCT, medium chain triglyceride.

years), Forceval Soluble Junior (from age 6 years) and Forceval Soluble (from age 12 years) (p. 21).

Frequency of feeding Lipolysis can be minimised by 3–4 hourly feeding during the day and continuous overnight tube feeds. It is difficult to be sure, however, whether overnight feeding is necessary, particularly in older children who have larger glycogen stores. In LCHADD it may help delay the onset of retinopathy or neuropathy. If overnight feeding is used the amount of glucose given overnight should equal basal glucose production rates for age (around 0.3–0.4 g CHO/kg/hour) (p. 544). It is not yet known whether the addition of MCT to the night feed is helpful [63]. Less CHO energy may be needed if MCT is added to the night feed. Table 19.8 gives examples of overnight feeds.

Fasting tolerance increases with age; therefore in older children it may be possible to stop the overnight feeds completely or substitute with one or more doses of UCCS. Before changing management, it is the author's and others' practice [56] to assess the child's metabolic response by serial measurement of plasma free fatty acids, blood glucose and long chain 3-hydroxyacylcarnitines on their usual regimen and after a dose of UCCS. This needs to be done in hospital under controlled conditions, ensuring the child is not fasted for longer than planned. If UCCS is to be used the results of these studies are used to plan how frequently a dose of UCCS needs to be given. Doses of cornflour used

are 1–1.5 g/kg/dose in older children. UCCS is generally introduced at home to test its palatability and tolerance. It should be given raw because cooking or heating disrupts the starch granules and thus makes it much less effective. It is usually mixed with skimmed milk. The dose of UCCS is gradually increased, starting with 5 g and increasing in 5 g increments every few days/week to the full amount.

Exercise management Patients with VLCADD, LCHADD, MTPD and CPTIID can experience episodes of rhabdomyolysis, with myalgia, elevated creatine kinase levels and, in severe cases, myoglobinuria. These episodes are sometimes triggered by infection but more often they are induced by exercise in children or young adults as they become more active and play sports for longer periods. Rhabdomyolysis can be the only clinical symptom in patients with partial deficiencies of CPTII or VLCAD and management can be difficult. Under normal circumstances CHO is the main fuel used for moderate to high intensity exercise such as sprinting, whereas fatty acids are the main fuel for low to moderate intensity exercise. Thus 'short burst exercise' may be more suitable for these patients than prolonged low intensity exercise because CHO will be used in preference to long chain fatty acids. Several papers suggest that dietary modification may reduce the risk of rhabdomyolysis. In one study patients with partial CPTIID tolerated exercise better on a CHO rich diet

Table 19.8 Examples of an overnight feed for long chain fatty acid oxidation disorders.

Overnight feed for a 6-year-old boy, weight 22 kg

25% CHO from glucose polymer, administered at 25 mL/hour from 10 pm to 6 am via gastrostomy
Fluid 200 mL
Energy 200 kcal (840 kJ)
Glucose polymer 53 g (95% CHO)
CHO 0.3 g CHO/kg/hour

or

Glucose polymer and MCT feed, administered at 25 mL/hour from 10 pm to 6 am via gastrostomy
Fluid 200 mL
Energy 200 kcal (840 kJ)
Glucose polymer 30 g (95% CHO) = 114 kcal, 479 kJ
MCT = ¼ of daily dose (10 g MCT) as 20 mL Liquigen (=5 g MCT/100 mL) = 90 kcal, 370 kJ

MCT, medium chain triglyceride.

than on a fat rich diet [49]; a bolus of glucose before exercise did not help [64]. In contrast pre-exercise boluses of MCT (0.3–0.4g/kg/dose) have been reported to improve exercise capacity in patients with various fatty acid oxidation disorders [65]. Pre-exercise dietary treatment may need to be adjusted according to the intensity and duration of the exercise being undertaken. MCT can be given as a prescribed dose of Liquigen, or MCT Procal, and CHO can be given from food such as a low fat cereal bar, banana, bread or high CHO drink such as Lucozade. Some children may not be able to do prolonged periods of exercise without developing muscle pain, so this must be avoided. In some patients, drug treatment with bezafibrate may also be helpful [66].

If a child develops rhabdomyolysis and muscle pain during or following exercise they may find it very difficult to walk for 24–48 hours. These episodes must be treated promptly as there is a risk of acute renal failure. An emergency regimen using the standard glucose polymer ER (p. 502) and extra fluids (determined on an individual basis), is implemented and may help reduce the risk of worsening rhabdomyolysis. MCT can be added to the ER (personal practice with a few patients). The ER feed should aim to provide at least the normal energy intake for age. The feed can be given orally but if there is associated loss of appetite then it should be given via a tube to ensure the full amount of fluid and energy is taken. Rest is important until symptoms resolve. It is essential parents and patients know to look for signs of myoglobinuria (dark, cola coloured urine) and make immediate contact with their metabolic team as a hospital admission may be necessary. Plasma creatine kinase can be markedly elevated during episodes of rhabdomyolysis and may be helpful in determining the extent of muscle damage and management needed.

Feeding problems Feeding problems are common in children with LCHADD, particularly in early childhood, and they occur despite good metabolic and clinical condition [67]. With age these problems either improved or resolved in this cohort. However, early recognition and management of feeding problems remains important and newborn screening may help prevent the development of these.

Monitoring

Dietary monitoring

Once an infant or child is established on dietary treatment, families need continued support and advice. Regular monitoring of this complex diet is essential to

- ensure the diet is nutritionally adequate, in particular intakes of fat soluble vitamins, EFA and LCPUFA
- ensure the overnight feeds provide adequate CHO (or energy) for age
- check the intake of long and medium chain fat
- provide new ideas and information on low fat manufactured foods
- assess exercise tolerance and provide advice on CHO/MCT intake
- check the ER for CHO concentration and volume and parents' understanding of its use

Clinical monitoring

This should include a review of weight, growth and development. There has been little documented on the growth of children with LC-FAOD. Gillingham *et al.* reported excess weight gain with time in most of their LCHADD and MTPD patients [62] but others have not observed this, including the author's centre [56]. If a child is overweight this needs to be managed carefully as weight loss could precipitate metabolic decompensation. A gradual reduction in energy intake is needed. If a child develops muscle pain with exercise this can make weight management difficult. Cardiomyopathy usually resolves on institution of a minimal LCT diet supplemented with MCT. Thereafter cardiac function (echo and electrocardiogram) should be monitored annually. Liver ultrasound is also performed annually to assess for steatosis. In LCHADD and MTPD annual ophthalmological (electrophysiology) and neurophysiological follow-up is important. For LCHADD an ocular examination is suggested within the first month of diagnosis as changes have been documented as early as 4 months of age [30].

Biochemical monitoring

Blood acylcarnitine concentrations may correlate with outcome in these disorders, but this is not certain. For example in LCHAD deficient patients cumulative long chain 3-hydroxyacylcarnitine concentrations appear to correlate with the progression of retinal disease [30]. Monitoring of acylcarnitines may therefore be useful in guiding dietary management. Plasma free carnitine levels should also be monitored, although there is dispute about supplementing carnitine if levels are low (p. 598), except in OCTN2. Plasma transaminases and creatine kinase are helpful markers of clinical status. Creatine kinase increases markedly during episodes of exercise induced rhabdomyolysis and returns to normal once treated. Fat soluble vitamins, EFA and LCPUFA concentrations should be monitored annually and more often if there are concerns about dietary deficiencies. Erythrocyte measurements are a better marker of long term nutritional status than plasma. Other nutritional markers such as iron and B_{12} status may also be necessary if there are concerns about nutritional adequacy of the diet.

Emergency regimen for treatment of illness in LC-FAOD

If the child becomes unwell and is unable to take their usual regimen the standard ER of very frequent feeds of glucose polymer, day and night, should be given (p. 502). In mild illnesses it will probably not be necessary to implement the ER. In patients with a gastrostomy or nasogastric tube, the drinks can be given via the tube if refused orally. The ER needs to be started promptly to inhibit the mobilisation of fatty acids as decompensation may be rapid. Long chain fat is strongly contraindicated. The role of MCT during acute illness is not clear. As the child improves, the normal diet can be resumed. While this is being reintroduced it is essential to maximise energy intake and continue with frequent feeding, usually 2–3 hourly by day and continuous tube feeds overnight. If the child does not tolerate the ER enterally they need to be admitted to hospital for an IV infusion containing glucose; 10% glucose, 0.45% saline is generally suitable but electrolytes should be monitored. Emergency regimen guidelines (IV and oral) for hospital use can be accessed from www.bimdg.org.uk. IV carnitine should not be given because long chain acylcarnitines may be arrythmogenic.

Patients with cardiomyopathy should probably be admitted during any intercurrent illness since there is a risk of deteriorating cardiac function. Families should also be warned to look for dark urine since illness (or exercise) can precipitate rhabdomyolysis with myoglobinuria. If there is myoglobinuria it is essential that the child is admitted to hospital for further management because of the risk of acute renal failure. A high fluid intake is recommended to increase myoglobin excretion and help prevent renal failure. Blood glucose monitoring by parents is not recommended as a marker of metabolic status, since hypoglycaemia is a relatively late finding and treatment should be initiated long before this develops [16].

Carnitine transporter deficiency

Patients with carnitine transporter deficiency (CT or OCTN2, Fig 19.1) have low plasma and intracellular concentrations of carnitine, which can impair fatty acid oxidation as carnitine is necessary for the transport of long chain fatty acids into the mitochondria. Patients generally present between 1 and 7 years of age with the typical features of an LC-FAOD; other patients remain asymptomatic [26]. Heart failure is a common presentation which can rapidly deteriorate with risk of death if patients are not treated with carnitine (around 100 mg/kg/day divided into two or three doses). Doses are adjusted according to plasma carnitine level. When given carnitine, generally no dietary treatment is necessary except during illness when there is a risk of metabolic decompensation. The standard ER of frequent glucose polymer drinks day and night should be given to prevent increased lipolysis (p. 502). A more detailed overview of clinical manifestations, diagnosis and management is described elsewhere [26, 68].

Electron transfer defects

Multiple acyl-CoA dehydrogenase deficiency (MADD), also known as glutaric aciduria type II is caused by defects of electron transfer flavoprotein (ETF) or ETF ubiquinone oxidoreductase (ETFQO, fig 19.1). These molecules pass electrons from a number of flavin adenine dinucleotide (FAD) containing dehydrogenase enzymes to coenzyme Q in the mitochondrial respiratory chain. The dehydrogenases include the acyl-CoA dehydrogenases of β-oxidation and also enzymes involved in choline metabolism and the breakdown of several amino acids (lysine, tryptophan and the branch chain amino acids).

MADD has a wide range of clinical severity. All forms of the disorder can cause hypoglycaemic encephalopathy. The most severely affected patients present with congenital malformations, such as renal cystic dysplasia leading to pulmonary hypoplasia (Potter's syndrome). Less severely affected patients may present with cardiomyopathy (usually as neonates) or with muscle weakness (at any age). Sudden death can occur in these patients. Some mild cases show a clinical and biochemical response to riboflavin (100–200 mg/day), the co-factor for these enzymes and the acyl-CoA dehydrogenases [69]. These patients usually present with progressive muscle weakness as young adults although other symptoms such as cyclical vomiting may have occurred in childhood. Riboflavin responsiveness is usually associated with mutations affecting ETFQO. Patients with late onset ETFQO deficiency have also been shown to have a secondary coenzyme Q10 (CoQ10) deficiency and supplements are recommended [70]. A more detailed description of the biochemical and clinical presentation of the individual disorders is described elsewhere [26,71].

Dietary management

In patients with severe congenital malformations, no treatment is effective or appropriate. At the other end of the spectrum, some patients respond completely to riboflavin and CoQ10 and no dietary modification is necessary.

There are very few publications concerning dietary treatment. Designing an appropriate diet can be difficult and the degree of restriction needs to be tailored to the individual patient. Most patients with MADD are commenced on a low fat diet as the acyl-CoA dehydrogenases of β-oxidation are affected. Severely affected patients may also benefit from a modest protein restriction because MADD affects the breakdown of some amino acids (see above) in addition to fatty acids. Regular feeding

with a high CHO intake is necessary to provide an adequate energy intake and to reduce lipolysis. Overnight fasting should be avoided in patients towards the severe end of the spectrum. A late night snack may be sufficient in some patients but others require a continuous overnight feed. Uncooked cornstarch could be substituted in older children to provide a 'slow release' source of glucose. It is essential to assess tolerance individually. It is advised that MCT should be avoided in MADD as it has appeared to have precipitated problems in some patients [72]. Medium chain fatty acids can enter the mitochondria independent of carnitine bypassing CPTI, the step at which β-oxidation is normally regulated. High concentrations of toxic metabolites may therefore be generated. At the author's centre MCT has been given in small amounts to two patients, without any obvious problems.

The following provides a guide to the typical energy distribution of the diet in severe defects (based on personal practice):

- 65%–70% energy from CHO
- 8%–10% energy from protein (at least the safe level of protein intake for age [73])
- 20%–25% energy from fat (use of MCT is probably best avoided)
- frequent feeding

Some patients with severe MADD have deteriorated despite the above dietary measures. Oral treatment with the ketone body, sodium-D,L-3-hydroxybutyrate, has led to sustained clinical improvement in a few such patients [74]. It is important to take account of the sodium provided by this medicine when planning therapeutic feeds.

Monitoring

Regular monitoring of this complex diet is essential to ensure nutritional adequacy and normal growth. There is no useful biochemical marker to determine the response to diet. Routine biochemical nutritional monitoring should be undertaken for patients on low fat diets similar to LC-FAOD (p. 606). If the child is on a very low protein diet, monitoring of plasma amino acids may be indicated.

Emergency regimen for use during intercurrent illness

During illness the standard ER of very frequent feeds, day and night, of glucose polymer should be given to minimise endogenous protein catabolism and lipolysis (p. 502). These should be given via a tube if not managed orally. Fat should be avoided during the acute period. The normal diet can be introduced during the recovery period, but it is important to continue with frequent feeding and additional glucose polymer feeds until the normal diet is resumed.

Malonyl-CoA decarboxylase deficiency or malonic aciduria

Malonyl-CoA decarboxylase (MLYCD) catalyses the reaction of malonyl-CoA to form acetyl-CoA and regulates the intracellular concentration of malonyl-CoA, which is involved in the regulation of fatty acid oxidation through inhibition of CPTI [75]. Deficiency of MLYCD is recognised as having phenotypic overlap with LC-FAOD. It is a rare, autosomal recessive disorder with variable presentation and severity of developmental delay, seizures, cardiomyopathy (around 40% of cases), hypoglycaemia and acidosis [76]. The pathogenesis of all the clinical features seen in MLYCD deficiency have yet to be elucidated.

Biochemically there is raised malonylcarnitine in blood and increased urinary excretion of malonic and methylmalonic acids. Patients are treated with carnitine as total and free carnitine concentrations in plasma are low. Use of a low fat/high CHO diet and MCT supplements has been reported in individual cases as being of possible clinical benefit including the improvement of cardiomyopathy [76–79]. A biochemical response to diet has not been seen in all reported cases. There is limited detail and description of the diet for many of the published cases. The author's centre reported improvement of cardiac function in a child when MCT provided around 25% of energy intake and LCT was minimal; she was also on an angiotensin-converting-enzyme (ACE) inhibitor [77]. MCT was given as these enter mitochondria directly, bypassing CPT1, and provide an alternative fuel for the heart. Prada *et al.* reported

development of cardiomyopathy in a 5-month-old infant whose fat intake had been altered to provide 50% as LCT and 50% as MCT (combined fat intake 32 g). On altering the fat ratio further to 30% LCT and 70% MCT and commencing an ACE inhibitor her cardiac condition stabilised [78]. A trial of a low fat, MCT supplemented diet may be indicated in MLYCD deficiency patients who have cardiomyopathy. As yet there is inadequate evidence to know if diet may help in the prevention of onset of cardiomyopathy in patients diagnosed early or through expanded newborn screening. It is not yet known at the molecular level which patients may develop cardiomyopathy [76]. During illness the standard ER (p. 502) of very frequent feeds, day and night, of glucose polymer should be given to prevent metabolic decompensation.

Disorders of ketogenesis and ketone body utilisation

Ketones are an important fuel source which can be used by all tissues and particularly for the brain during prolonged fasting. They are also the preferred fuel for the heart. Ketones are formed from acetyl-CoA, produced mainly from the oxidation of fatty acids but also from the ketogenic amino acids leucine and isoleucine. Patients can present in the early neonatal period or later in childhood precipitated by prolonged fasting, intercurrent illness or other metabolic stress.

The disorders of biosynthesis of ketones (ketogenesis) and ketone body utilisation (ketolysis) include the following.

Defects of ketogenesis: 3-hydroxy-3-methylglutaryl-CoA (HMG-CoA) synthase deficiency and HMG-CoA lyase deficiency. The latter enzyme is also involved in the formation of ketones via the leucine degradation pathway (Fig. 19.2). The typical initial presenting symptoms include vomiting and lethargy which can progress to coma, with 'hypoketotic' hypoglycaemia, acidosis and hepatomegaly.

Defects of ketolyis: succinyl-CoA 3-oxoacid-CoA transferase (SCOT) deficiency and 2-methylacetoacetyl-CoA thiolase (MAT) deficiency (commonly known as beta-ketothiolase deficiency, abbreviated to T2). The latter enzyme is also involved in the isoleucine degradation pathway (Fig. 19.2).

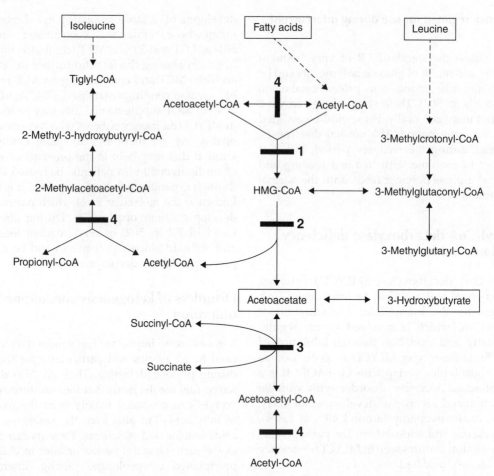

Figure 19.2 Biochemical pathways of ketogenesis and ketolysis. HMG-CoA, 3-hydroxy-3-methylglutaryl coenzyme A. 1, Mitochondrial(m) HMG-CoA synthase; 2, HMG-CoA lyase; 3, succinyl-CoA 3-oxoacid CoA transferase (SCOT); 4, mitochondrial acetoacetyl-CoA thiolase (T2). Reprinted with permission of Springer.

Patients typically present with vomiting and high levels of ketones (as they cannot utilise them) which can cause a severe ketoacidosis, a reduced level of consciousness and dehydration.

A more detailed description of the clinical and biochemical features for these disorders can be found elsewhere [80,81]. The disorders are all inherited as autosomal recessive traits.

Dietary management during illness

During illness the standard ER (p. 502) of very frequent feeds/drinks, day and night, of glucose polymer should be given to minimise lipolysis and

endogenous protein catabolism (specifically the ketogenic amino acids).

In defects of ketogenesis provision of glucose will help prevent hypoglycaemia and limit the production of potentially toxic metabolites. Blood glucose monitoring by parents is not recommended as a marker of metabolic status, since hypoglycaemia is a relatively late finding and treatment should be initiated long before this develops. In defects of ketolysis, providing glucose will prevent illness from leading to ketoacidosis. Patients can become anorexic at an early stage, refusing ER drinks. It is essential feeds/drinks are therefore given via a nasogastric tube. In the event of persistent vomiting or the child not improving a hospital admission is needed for IV 10% glucose. Sodium bicarbonate may also be necessary to correct acidosis. Extra fluids will be needed if the child is dehydrated, which is common in the ketone body utilisation defects. Emergency management guidelines for use in hospital can be accessed at www.bimdg.org.uk.

As the child recovers and begins to eat again it is important that additional ER drinks of glucose polymer are given until the normal diet is fully resumed, particularly if they have not eaten well for several days. This needs to be managed carefully to prevent subsequent hypoglycaemia. If for any reason the child needs to be commenced on a special infant formula or paediatric feed during the recovery phase these should not contain added MCT which, once absorbed, are rapidly converted to ketones. In these disorders where there is a defect in either formation or utilisation of ketones, MCT may be of potential harm. Theoretically in SCOT and beta-ketothiolase deficiency MCT may increase concentrations of ketones (which cannot be utilised) and inhibit long chain fatty acid oxidation, thus contributing to the energy deficit. In the defects of formation of ketones, the conversion of MCT to ketones may be limited and so will not provide an energy source.

Dietary management – long term

There is little published information on the detailed dietary management of these disorders. Between episodes of metabolic decompensation patients are likely to be clinically asymptomatic. In the well child avoidance of prolonged fasts and provision of adequate energy is important. There are no published guidelines on safe fasting times for any of these disorders. In infants regular feeding, day and night, is important and it seems reasonable to continue a night time feed until the age of 1 year. Older children should tolerate overnight fasting (10–12 hours) without problems but they should be given a bedtime snack containing starch. Missed meals should be replaced with a high CHO drink if there is any risk of impending illness. MCT are theoretically best avoided as either they cannot be used to form ketones or they will add to the total ketone load which cannot be utilised.

A moderate protein (leucine) restriction (1–2 g protein/kg/day) is recommended for HMG-CoA lyase and beta-ketothiolase deficiency because these enzymes are involved in the catabolism of the ketogenic amino acids [82–84]. Also, in HMG-CoA lyase deficiency this has been combined with a modest fat restriction in some cases [82, 83]. However, opinions differ about the necessity of these dietary manipulations. Stable isotope studies suggest that protein catabolism contributes little to the abnormal metabolites in HMG-CoA lyase deficiency and fatty acid catabolism may be more important [85]. In the well child it is reasonable to suggest a generous CHO intake and avoidance of a high protein and fat intake.

Mild protein restriction (1.5–2.0 g/kg/day) has been described in SCOT deficiency (probably to limit increased concentrations of ketones being formed from the ketogenic amino acids) and avoidance of a fat rich diet which would cause ketosis [86, 87]. In the well child it is reasonable to suggest a generous CHO intake and avoidance of a high protein and fat intake.

A recent publication highlighted the potential foetal and maternal risks to women with HMG-CoA lyase deficiency, particularly the risk of metabolic decompensation associated with nausea and vomiting which needs careful management at an early stage [88].

Future research needs/unanswered questions

With the exception of MCAD deficiency, most disorders of fatty acid oxidation are rare and have only been described since the late 1980s; therefore long term experience of dietary treatment is limited and there are many unanswered questions about treatment. Moreover, in the long chain defects, treatment needs to prevent or delay long term complications such as retinopathy in long chain 3-hydroxyacyl-CoA dehydrogenase deficiency. Some aspects of dietary treatment are the same worldwide; however, other aspects such as 'safe fasting times', use of overnight feeds and prescription for LCPUFA vary. Comparisons of different cohorts and further animal studies may begin to answer some of these questions. Proper evaluation of dietary treatment will require long term controlled studies in which other aspects of management are unchanged, but this can be very difficult to do.

Disorders of the Mitochondrial Respiratory Chain

Jacky Stafford

Introduction

These are a heterogeneous group of disorders characterised by impaired energy production. They are caused by mutations in either mitochondrial or nuclear DNA which directly or indirectly affect the oxidative phosphorylation (OXPHOS) system. The mode of inheritance is variable due to the large number of genes that encode respiratory chain proteins and ancillary factors: autosomal recessive, dominant, X-linked, maternal or sporadic. Mitochondrial disorders are estimated to affect 1 in 5000 children but this may be an underestimate [89].

Biochemistry

One of the major functions of mitochondria is the generation of ATP via the OXPHOS system which catalyses the oxidation of fuel molecules by oxygen into ATP, transferring electrons to oxygen via these complexes. Primary mitochondrial disorders are genetic disorders affecting any of the OXPHOS complexes, which are five functional enzyme complexes embedded in the inner mitochondrial membrane. Deficiency of any one of the enzymes will affect all cells containing mitochondria. Mitochondrial disorders may be classified by phenotype or enzyme deficiency which may be an isolated enzyme complex deficiency, e.g. commonly complex I or IV (cytochrome oxidase (COX) deficiency) or defects affecting several enzyme complexes [90,91].

Disorders of OXPHOS affect the citric acid cycle due to excess NADH and lack of NAD. Ketone bodies increase particularly after meals due to channelling of acetyl-CoA towards ketogenesis. The blood lactate and lactate/pyruvate ratio is raised.

Clinical picture and treatment

Mitochondrial disorders may present at any age and certain clinical features are more frequent at certain ages. Complex I and IV deficiencies are more common (approximately 50%) among those disorders presenting in childhood [90]. Gastrointestinal symptoms and growth faltering are more often described as presenting features in infancy. Seizures may occur in 35%–60% of patients although clinical histories reveal they are preceded by other symptoms such as developmental delay and poor growth. Consistent factors are the increasing number of unrelated organs affected with time and the rapid progression involving the central nervous system at a later stage. The overlap of clinical features leads to difficulties in classification [92].

There is no satisfactory medical or dietetic therapy available; any treatment options are unproven and the prognosis is very poor [90,93,94].

Oral intake is poor and energy and/or nutrient dense supplements or supplementary feeds are used to support growth. Poor feeding is often associated with dysphagia and textural changes may be required. Continuous tube feeding may be necessary to manage gastrointestinal problems of nausea or early satiety (Table 19.9). A protein hydrolysate or amino acid based feed may be necessary if the child has diarrhoea. As the disorder progresses the feed may become the sole source of nutrition.

Ketogenic diet in mitochondrial disorders

Ketone bodies can form ATP via the Krebs cycle and the OXPHOS system and may partially bypass complex I, thus potentially providing an alternative energy source for the brain and other tissues. In mitochondrial disorders a ketogenic diet (KD), high fat and low carbohydrate, may be beneficial to treat epilepsy in some specific subgroups. Complex I and IV deficiency represent a significant proportion of the group of patients with mitochondrial epilepsy: in a study of 48 children, 73% and 23% respectively [100]. KD was trialled in 24 of those children; 50% became seizure free and seizures were reduced by up to half in 25%. Kang *et al.* [95] reported safe

Table 19.9 Mitochondrial disorders whose syndromic presentations in infancy or childhood can require dietary management [89, 92].

Name of disorder	Enzyme complex affected	Age of presentation	Symptoms and disorder specific treatment
Leigh syndrome (subacute necrotising encephalomyelopathy)	I, II, III, IV, V (singly or in combination); pyruvate dehydrogenase deficiency (PDH) is the most dominant phenotype (p. 614) [92]	Infancy (but can be later in childhood or occasionally in adulthood)	Vomiting, feeding difficulties Seizures; ketogenic diet tried but efficacy unclear [95]
Pearson syndrome	I, III, IV and V (all enzymes with mtDNA encoded subunits)	Infancy	Pancreatic insufficiency (requiring enzyme replacement therapy), diarrhoea, enteropathy Diabetes mellitus (may require insulin)
Alpers syndrome (progressive neuronal degeneration of childhood with liver disease)	I, III, IV and V (all enzymes with mtDNA encoded subunits)	Infancy	Bowel obstruction and perforation Seizures; ketogenic diet tried (one case report) but efficacy unclear [96] Liver failure (may be precipitated by sodium valproate) [89]
MELAS (mitochondrial encephalomyopathy, lactic acidosis and stroke like episodes)	I, III, IV and V (all enzymes with mtDNA encoded subunits)	Late in first decade	Anorexia, vomiting, poor feeding, enteropathy, abdominal discomfort, constipation, diarrhoea, gastroparesis, pseudo-obstruction and recurrent pancreatitis Stroke like episodes may be due to decreased vasodilation capacity in small arteries which may be improved by supplementation with L-arginine [97]
MERRF (myoclonus epilepsy, ragged red fibres)	I, III, IV and V (all enzymes with mtDNA encoded subunits)	Childhood onset in ~30% of cases	Rarely swallowing problems, gastrointestinal dysmotility [98]
MNGIE (mitochondrial neurogastrointestinal encephalopathy)	I, III, IV and V (all enzymes with mtDNA encoded subunits)	Generally between 10 and 30 years of age (average 18 years; can occasionally present in infancy)	Abdominal cramps, bloating due to gut dysmotility (dysphagia, nausea, vomiting, early satiety, abdominal pain, pseudo-obstruction and bloating)
Coenzyme Q_{10} deficiency (multisystem disease: nephropathy, encephalopathy including seizures, hearing loss)	Combined deficiency of I and III or II and III	Infancy (adult presentations include ataxia and myopathy)	Feeding difficulties and faltering growth related to nephropathy Response to replacement coenzyme Q_{10} to help restore electron transfer flow and antioxidant function is variable [99]
EME (ethylmalonic encephalopathy)	IV (COX)	Infancy	Diarrhoea

and effective use of the classical KD in treatment of intractable epilepsy in 14 patients mostly complex I or IV, with seizure reduction (3/14) or seizure free (7/14). The same group describe better tolerance and adherence with use of the modified KD

in 14 patients; 3/14 were seizure free and 5/14 had >50% seizure reduction [101]. However, it is unclear whether the KD affects disease progression in different mitochondrial subgroups and formal clinical trials are necessary [90,95,96,101].

Pyruvate Dehydrogenase Deficiency

Fiona White

Introduction

Pyruvate dehydrogenase (PDH) deficiency is an inherited mitochondrial disorder of brain energy metabolism and is a major cause of primary lactic acidosis. The PDH enzyme is a complex comprising multiple copies of three subunits: pyruvate dehydrogenase (E1, consisting of two α and two β subunits), dihydrolipoamide (E2), dihydrolipamide transacetylase (E3) and E3 binding protein (E3BP). In addition there are two regulatory enzymes associated with the complex, PDH phosphatase and PDH kinase [102]. The majority of cases are due to mutations in PDHA1 which is an X-linked gene encoding the E1α subunit. A recent review of 371 patients reported 76% of cases resulted from deficits in the E1α subunit [103]. All other forms of PDH deficiency are autosomal recessively inherited [102] with the majority of cases having parents who are consanguineous, and often with several affected children in one family [103].

Biochemistry

The PDH complex is essential for the aerobic oxidation of glucose which is normally the obligate pathway for energy metabolism in the brain [102]. The PDH complex catalyses the rate limiting conversion of pyruvate, derived predominantly via glycolysis from glucose to acetyl-CoA. Pyruvate accumulates and is reduced to lactate in the cytoplasm. Pyruvate is in equilibrium with lactate and in PDH deficiency both blood and CSF lactate are elevated. The resulting lack of acetyl-CoA affects the availability of precursors feeding into the tricarboxylic acid (TCA) cycle and as a result limits mitochondrial energy production.

Clinical picture and treatment

PDH deficiency is a heterogeneous condition. The clinical spectrum is broad [103] ranging from severe neonatal presentation with overwhelming lactic acidosis, refractory to treatment and resulting in death in the neonatal period [104] to a more benign onset. Those with mild to moderate deficiency usually present in infancy with varied symptoms including developmental delay, seizures, hypotonia, failure to thrive, microcephaly, motor dysfunction [103,105] and structural brain abnormalities as seen in Leigh syndrome [102].

In general, treatment is not very effective and prognosis is poor [106]. Sodium bicarbonate is used during periods of metabolic decompensation to manage lactic acidosis. Unlike in some other disorders, where lactic acidosis is a feature of metabolic decompensation and for which a high glucose emergency regimen may be used, this is not the case in PDH deficiency. A high glucose intake would result in further accumulation of pyruvate and lactate thus exacerbating the lactic acidosis. Chronically, a number of treatments are used although these rarely influence the course of the disease [104]. Supplementation with pharmacological doses of the cofactor thiamin is advocated as there is a rare cohort with the thiamin responsive form [104] where the mutation affects the interaction between thiamin pyrophosphate and the E1α subunit [103]. Dichloroacetate, a structural analogue of pyruvate, inhibits E1 kinase so improving activity of PDH complex and decreasing lactate levels and may benefit some patients [106]. Ketogenic diet (KD) treatment is employed in some cases as a means of providing an alternative energy source of acetyl-CoA, particularly for use by the nervous system [102]. Wexler *et al.* [107] reported the effectiveness of KD in E1 deficiency, improving cognitive development and survival. Response to KD therapy has also been reported by others in cases of E3BP deficiency [102] and E1 mutations [106]. Current practice in the author's unit is to try KD treatment only in milder presenting patients, aiming to slow down the clinical progression. The outcome of KD treatment is variable with some patients having further metabolic decompensations and others either remaining static or making some developmental progress. A recent email survey of UK practice provided information on 22 patients on KD treatment; three were on MCT diet, 17 on classical diet and two on modified Atkins diet. Further details on the practical management of the KD, including monitoring, are given on p. 363.

Smith-Lemli-Opitz syndrome

Introduction

Smith-Lemli-Opitz syndrome syndrome (SLO) is an autosomal recessively inherited disorder of sterol biosynthesis caused by mutations on chromosome 11q13. More than 130 mutations have been described. The severe IVS8-1G>C is the most common among Caucasians (a third of reported cases) [108–110]. The incidence of SLO is reported to be 1 in 15 000 to 1 in 60 000, with highest prevalence in Caucasians [110].

SLO is due to a deficiency of 7-dehydrocholesterol reductase (DHCR7) which reduces the C7–C8 double bond in the sterol B ring, converting 7-dehydrocholesterol (7DHC) to form cholesterol, the final step of its biosynthesis.

Biochemistry

Patients with SLO have raised plasma 7DHC, the precursor of cholesterol. 8DHC, the isomer of 7DHC, is also raised and is probably synthesised from the accumulating 7DHC [110]. Plasma cholesterol is low or low to normal [111] but total cholesterol values may be in the normal range if they include significant amounts of 7DHC and 8DHC [109]. In SLO, the different fractions can be measured by specialist laboratories.

Clinical problems may be caused by the deficiency of cholesterol or total sterols, or the toxic effects of 7DHC and 8DHC and their derivatives, or a combination of all of these [108, 109]. Cholesterol is an important structural component of cellular membranes and myelin and a precursor of bile acids, steroid hormones, neuroactive steroids and oxysterols [109]. It has a role in signalling and defects in cholesterol metabolism affect the structure and function of the central nervous system. In the SLO affected pregnancy, mother to foetus cholesterol transport is limited and efficiency of transfer may affect severity of the disorder postnatally [108]. Clinical severity appears to correlate best either with absolute cholesterol levels or with the sum of 7DHC and 8DHC expressed as a fraction of total sterol [110].

Clinical picture and treatment

SLO is a multiple malformation syndrome with a wide phenotype ranging from a severe infantile presentation with early or perinatal death due to organ malformations, to minimal facial abnormalities and behavioural and learning difficulties [109].

Patients with SLO have a distinctive facial appearance, and typical craniofacial features include microcephaly, small upturned nose, ptosis, micrognathia, cleft palate (cleft lip is not common) or bifid uvula. Structural abnormalities are also observed: syndactyly of the second and third toes is the most common finding (95%) and in males genital abnormalities are frequently reported. In more severely affected patients there are often structural abnormalities of the heart, lungs, brain, limbs and kidneys and gastrointestinal tract, e.g. Hirschsprung's disease, pancreatitis [108, 109].

Infants show growth faltering attributed to poor sucking and swallowing and a lack of interest in feeding [111]. They may also have psychomotor retardation, photosensitivity, behavioural abnormality, irritability, autistic tendencies and prefer not to be held [109]. An older child will demonstrate various degrees of hyperactivity, self-injurious behaviour, sleep disturbances and temperament deregulation [109].

As cholesterol is required for adrenal steroid and bile acid synthesis deficiencies of both may occur. The latter can cause a reduced ability to absorb cholesterol and fat soluble vitamins and bile acid supplementation may be required [100,108] although a multicentre trial of 14 patients demonstrated no benefit of bile acid supplementation [112]. 7HDC and 8HDC may be monitored, but may have limited value for ongoing management.

Cholesterol supplements

A cholesterol supplement is given to raise plasma cholesterol. It may also decrease 7DHC and 8DHC synthesis via a feedback inhibition effect of plasma cholesterol on HMG-CoA reductase, diminishing endogenous cholesterol synthesis [108,113]. Its effectiveness may be limited once normal cholesterol levels are achieved [114]. It also restores both adrenal and bile salt deficiencies [108].

Crystalline cholesterol in oil or aqueous based suspension and egg yolk cholesterol, in varying doses, has been reported to have different degrees of biochemical effectiveness [113,115]. This may be due to the fact that cholesterol does not cross the blood–brain barrier and cannot treat the biochemical defect in brain [113]. Also, if 7DHC levels remain raised, detrimental effects may persist [109].

Clinically, the beneficial effects of cholesterol supplementation are not established as no controlled clinical trials have shown improvements in central nervous system function, i.e. behaviour and development [113]. A double blinded placebo crossover controlled trial showed no significant difference in short term behaviour over 2.5 months, using a placebo (egg substitute) or pasteurised egg yolk [116]. A standardised study of 14 patients indicated that cholesterol supplementation had little effect on developmental progress over a 6 year period [117]. There are anecdotal reports of better behaviour within days or weeks particularly in sleep disorders, irritability responding more quickly than other issues, e.g. tactile sensitivity [116], and improved growth with cholesterol

supplementation [113]. It is also reported that behavioural abnormalities return when cholesterol therapy is interrupted [116]. It is generally considered that availability of cholesterol during foetal development is a major determinant in phenotypic expression of SLO. Most anomalies are of early embryonic origin and it is not feasible for treatment to cure patients postnatally [110].

HMG-CoA reductase inhibitor

Simvastatin reduces endogenous cholesterol synthesis by blocking the cholesterol biosynthesis pathway proximally at the first rate limiting step. It is proposed that this therapy may also reduce the levels of 7DHC and 8DHC in SLO. Simvastatin may also upregulate residual DHCR7 activity to increase cholesterol and decrease 7DHC and 8DHC [113]. Its use may be detrimental in subjects with little or no DHCR7 activity [114]. It can cross the blood–brain barrier and may have an effect on the central nervous system. A retrospective study of 39 patients showed no benefit with simvastatin on anthropometry or behaviour [114]. Clinical trials are needed to assess suitability of statins in SLO patients [109].

Nutritional support

Nutritional support is necessary in patients with postnatal growth failure and poor feeding [109,111]. Growth charts for SLO have been produced from longitudinal data from 78 patients (0.1–16 years); 43% of patients were receiving treatment (nutritional support ± cholesterol) and showed growth restriction of 2 SD below norms for age [111].

Cholesterol supplementation of 60–100 mg/kg/day is given as divided doses twice or three times per day. It is preferred to a high cholesterol diet because achieving the recommended intake from diet would be difficult, particularly in those with poor oral intake. This may be administered via the feeding tube or taken orally. Different preparations are available.

Preparations used at the author's centre include

- cholesterol suspended in Ora-Plus and flavoured with blackcurrant syrup (150 mg cholesterol/mL) (Cardiff and Vale NHS Trust). This

Table 19.10   Nutritional and gastrointestinal characteristics of 26 patients with SLO from three metabolic centres.

Metabolic centre	Number of patients	Number of patients requiring tube feeding	Reasons for tube feeding	Cleft palate	Number of patients requiring nutritional support	Number of patients with vomiting	Number of patients with constipation/loose stools
Birmingham Children's Hospital NHS Foundation Trust, Birmingham	7 (<17 years)	n = 2 (1 tube now removed)	Feeding difficulties		n = 3 high energy tube feeds or ONS n = 3 described as fussy eaters	n = 1 periodic vomiting but eats well	
Central Manchester University Hospitals NHS Trust, Manchester	7	n = 1 with gastrostomy	Faltering growth, feeding difficulties	1	n = 4 sip feeds n = 2 poor appetite All described as fussy eaters		Most with constipation
Great Ormond Street Hospital for Children NHS Foundation Trust, London	12	n = 4 with gastrostomy n = 8 orally fed (n = 2 had nasogastric tube previously)	Feeding difficulties: slow to feed, vomiting, slow to suck, not interested in feeding, spitting out food, growth faltering	n = 5	n = 8 require high energy feeds and/or energy supplements (2)	n = 5 n = 2 required anti-reflux medicines n = 1 had Nissen fundoplication n = 3 had vomiting controlled by slow feed delivery	n = 4 n = 1 required lactulose n = 2 improved with solids n = 3 reported loose stools n = 2 improved with fibre containing feeds

ONS, oral nutritional supplements.

product has a shelf life of 3 months and is stored in the fridge. It can be given orally or via a feeding tube.

- cholesterol powder (100 g tub) (Mawdsley Brooks Unlicensed Division). The powder is difficult to dissolve; in the past it was prepared in olive oil which had a very limited shelf life. It is now provided in powder form for addition to food or drinks.

Characteristics of patients with SLO are given in Table 19.10.

Glycerol Kinase Deficiency

Introduction

Glycerol kinase deficiency (GKD) is an X-linked recessive disorder with mutations within or deletions on the GK gene in the Xp21 region. There is no genotype–phenotype correlation in isolated GKD [118]. Patients with complete deletions are symptomatic. Those with mutations resulting in residual GK enzyme function may be symptomatic or asymptomatic [119].

Glycerol kinase catalyses the phosphorylation of glycerol by ATP to yield glycerol-3-phosphate (G3P) and ADP. After phosphorylation 10%–30% G3P combines with free fatty acids to form triglycerides. The remainder is oxidised to dihydroxyacetone phosphate and enters the glycolytic or gluconeogenic pathway [120].

Biochemistry

GKD is characterised by hyperglycerolaemia and glyceroluria. Normal plasma glycerol levels (<0.2 mmol/L) may increase to 8 mmol/L resulting in urine levels >150 mmol/L (normally undetectable in urine) [120, 121]. In non fasting situations glycerol (via gluconeogenesis) contributes little to hepatic glucose production. In prolonged fasting conditions its contribution increases to about 20% energy as gluconeogenesis and fatty acid oxidation become essential for energy [122].

Clinical picture and treatment

There are three clinical forms based on phenotype [123]. Complex GKD is an Xp21 contiguous gene deletion syndrome involving GK locus together with congenital adrenal hypoplasia (CAH) and/or Duchenne muscular dystrophy loci. It usually presents neonatally and the clinical features depend on the loci involved [122]. Symptoms of isolated GKD may occur in addition to those of adrenal insufficiency, salt wasting, developmental delay and muscular dystrophy. Early diagnosis and prompt treatment to prevent hypernatraemic dehydration are required [122, 124, 125].

There are two forms resulting from isolated GK deficiency; the juvenile or benign adult form with pseudohypertriglyceridaemia [119, 123]. The juvenile form occurs in the first few years of life and is often precipitated by catabolism due to illness or poor feeding and can include episodic vomiting, metabolic acidosis, ketotic hypoglycaemia, lethargy, hypotonia, seizures and unconsciousness. Patients are at risk of insulin resistance, glucose intolerance and type 2 diabetes [118].

Avoidance of prolonged fasts is crucial [121, 123]. During illness an emergency regimen (p. 502) is necessary to prevent hypoglycaemia due to limited capacity to convert glycerol to glucose via gluconeogenesis. If IV fluids are required only glucose should be given and not lipids [123]. There are anecdotal reports that low fat diet (i.e. low in glycerol) may be beneficial for those experiencing symptoms of vomiting, acidaemia and stupor associated with GKD [126]. However, the mechanism for this is unclear. In the adult form, lipid lowering management is not reported to affect raised triglycerides [119]. At three main metabolic centres in the UK the standard emergency regimen during intercurrent illness is the only dietary treatment.

Barth Syndrome

Nicol Clayton

Introduction

Barth syndrome is an X-linked recessive genetic disease caused by defective remodelling of cardiolipin in the mitochondrial inner membrane due to mutations in the taffazzin (TAZ) gene [127]. Cardiolipin is the major phospholipid in mitochondria and has an important role in maintaining mitochondrial structure, the activity of the electron transport chain and other elements of the mitochondrial energy generating system [128]. The disorder was first described in 1983 [129] and the main characteristics are dilated cardiomyopathy, skeletal myopathy, growth retardation, neutropenia and 3-methylglutaconic (3-MGC) aciduria [130].

Epidemiology

Fewer than 200 living male patients have Barth syndrome worldwide and the Barth Syndrome Trust estimates the prevalence to be 1 in 300 000 to 1 in 400 000 live births. However, evidence is growing that the disease is significantly under-diagnosed [131].

Presentation

Boys with Barth syndrome typically present with symptoms of cardiac dysfunction or recurrent bacterial infections. Registry data show that 68% of patients develop cardiomyopathy in the first year of life [132]. Although neutropenia occurs in most patients with Barth syndrome, it is often intermittent and unpredictable and therefore might not be recognised when the cardiac disease is diagnosed. Increased concentrations of 3-MGC may be found by urine organic acid analysis. However, this is not a universal occurrence and levels can occasionally be normal [133], particularly in the newborn period. Other less specific presentations include faltering growth, feeding difficulties, biochemical disturbances such as hypoglycaemia or lactic acidosis (especially in neonates [134, 135]), episodic diarrhoea and delayed motor milestones; there are also characteristic facial features with a cherubic appearance (chubby cheeks and deep-set eyes) and prominent ears [136].

Diagnosis

Confirmation of a clinical diagnosis of Barth syndrome can be made either by mutation testing of the TAZ gene or by cardiolipin analysis using whole blood or stored blood or tissue, such as Guthrie cards or skin fibroblasts. Abnormal results of cardiolipin testing are followed up with mutation analysis to confirm the genetic diagnosis. Diagnostic testing by cardiolipin analysis is free of charge at the NHS Specialised Services Barth Syndrome Service, Bristol Royal Hospital for Children (see Useful addresses). Due to the variable nature of the neutropenia and levels of 3-MGC, all boys with idiopathic dilated cardiomyopathy should be screened for Barth syndrome.

Medical treatment

Historically, most boys with Barth syndrome died during infancy due to either heart failure or sepsis. However, advances in early diagnosis and treatment have reduced mortality significantly, although there is evidence that Barth syndrome is a cause of miscarriage and stillbirth [137, 138]. After diagnosis, patients are treated for their cardiac failure and given prophylactic antibiotics and granulocyte colony-stimulating factor (G-CSF) when significant neutropenia is present. The Bristol NHS Specialised Services Barth Syndrome Service runs bi-annual clinics and offers multidisciplinary care from specialists in haematology, cardiology, psychology, nursing, dietetics, genetic counselling, physiotherapy, speech therapy and occupational therapy.

Biochemistry

Cardiolipin deficiency alters the functioning of proteins within mitochondria [139]. Ongoing studies on the intermediary metabolism of Barth syndrome suggest that abnormalities of the cardiolipin-deficient, inner mitochondrial membrane lead to a disordered flow of substrates through the citric acid – or tricarboxylic acid (TCA) – cycle. This in turn reduces the complete oxidation of acetyl-CoA from the breakdown of glucose and fat and increases the catabolism of those glucogenic amino acids that enter the TCA cycle at or after alpha-ketoglutarate, a process termed 'anaplerosis'. The diversion of specific amino acids is thought to be sufficiently great to lower plasma amino acid levels and impair muscle protein synthesis. Thus, whereas there is sufficient anaplerosis to maintain normal or near normal energy metabolism, this occurs at the cost of wasting of muscle, potentially including cardiac muscle. Of particular interest are the amino acids arginine and cysteine, as children with Barth syndrome often have fasting levels in the lower range of normal [140].

Growth delay

Growth delay is common in Barth patients [141] and the growth pattern is consistent with constitutional growth delay with late onset puberty. Delayed bone age, with a range between 8 months and 2 years 6 months, has been seen in all boys attending the author's Barth syndrome clinic. Reduced nutritional intake due to cardiomyopathy, sore mouth/gums and recurrent infections may also contribute to poor weight gain.

Boys with Barth syndrome are typically normal size at birth, but their growth rate progressively decelerates in the first 2–3 years. Height usually falls to the 2nd centile, and often well below the 0.4th centile, by the third year with a concurrent deceleration in rates of weight gain. Until onset of a late puberty, height remains on or below this centile, although the trajectory of growth remains parallel to the centile. Because of the almost universal muscle hypoplasia seen in Barth syndrome, weight centile can be 1 to 2 standard deviations below height centile. Using data from the Barth syndrome registry, Spencer et al. [142] showed that 58% of patients under 18 years of age were 5th centile for weight and at or below the ≤5th centile for height. However, once boys reach puberty at 15–18 years of age, they grow rapidly, achieving their predicted adult height by their late teens or early 20s. The average centile reached after 18 years is the 50th centile, although some boys exceed this and reach above their mid-parental height centile.

In line with constitutional growth delay, mildly to moderately depressed levels of insulin-like growth factor 1 (IGF-1) and growth hormone may be found in Barth syndrome. Because most boys have bone ages in accordance with height age and low growth velocities, the low hormone levels are likely to be a reflection of the slow growth pattern rather than a sign of an underlying endocrinopathy.

Not all children with Barth syndrome display poor weight gain. Although just over half of boys have a weight <5th centile, nearly 25% of boys younger than 18 years have a weight >20th centile and more than 50% have normal or increased body mass index (BMI) [142]. Data from the Bristol UK clinic show an increasing trend of boys becoming overweight for their height and body composition measurements, using dual X-ray absorptiometry and bioelectrical impedance, and show that even when weight and height are on similar centiles the boys have higher body fat percentages and lower muscle mass. As a result, an appropriate healthy BMI in Barth syndrome will be at or below the 25th centile for age. Boys with BMI >25th centile have markedly abnormal, often truncal, adiposity, possibly aggravated by misconceived overfeeding to achieve normal weights for age (unpublished observations). However, in view of the marked deficiency of oxidative metabolism in muscle, where most dietary fat is metabolised, a propensity to excess adiposity is to be expected and needs to be addressed in the dietary management of Barth syndrome.

Dietary management

There are few published data on nutritional requirements. Dietary management is individualised, based on maintaining growth within appropriate parameters. The key nutritional aims are to

- provide adequate but not excessive energy to maintain appropriate growth and keep the weight centile within 2 centiles of the height centile. Energy requirements start to decrease after infancy and by the age of 5 years are likely to be around 70% of the estimated average requirement (EAR) for chronological age depending on activity.
- provide sufficient protein to promote muscle protein synthesis and mitochondrial anaplerosis with an even and regular distribution of protein throughout the day. A higher than usual percentage of energy as protein should be given with a protein intake up to 2 g/kg/day.
- limit fasting to reduce muscle proteolysis, thereby preserving muscle mass. A regular intake of low glycaemic index (GI) carbohydrates should be given throughout the day with cornstarch therapy or a carbohydrate rich snack before bed (p. 622).
- encourage low fat food options, particularly dairy products and between meal snacks, if the weight centile is at or above the height centile.
- supplement vitamin and mineral intake to ensure 100% of the reference nutrient intake (RNI) is achieved, particularly with respect to vitamin B_6.

Infancy

Infants with Barth syndrome often have difficulty feeding and maintaining sufficient feed volumes to allow for growth. This is due in part to low muscle tone and early fatigue with feeding, but may also be secondary to cardiac dysfunction in more severe cases. Infants typically take very small amounts and feed frequently throughout the day and night, often feeding during the night until after their second year.

Whereas energy requirements during the first 6 months are usually normal for weight and chronological age, energy requirements reduce to around 90% of the EAR as growth slows towards the end of the first year. Nutrition should be targeted at maintaining an appropriate weight velocity, with a weight centile that is likely to be within one to two centiles of the height centile. Protein requirements are increased in Barth syndrome and unless a high protein diet is otherwise contraindicated, the aim is to give up to 2 g/kg/day throughout childhood.

Although a small number of infants with Barth syndrome have successfully breast fed, due to the low volumes taken and the need to ensure an adequate protein intake, supplemental feeding with high energy formulas or nasogastric feeding can be necessary. However, tube feeding can cause infants to become rapidly overweight and have a negative impact on oral feeding, so regular monitoring is required. Caution should also be exercised if a high target for energy intake, e.g. 120–150 kcal (500–630 kJ)/kg, is used in an attempt to achieve catch up weight after a period of faltering growth as this can cause vomiting and exacerbate diarrhoea.

Hypoglycaemia and (usually mild) lactic acidosis has been reported, particularly in the first year, although this usually resolves after infancy. However, unresponsive hypoglycaemia following 24 hours of fasting during a period of acute illness has been seen in a 2 year old (personal observation). The reasons for hypoglycaemia in Barth syndrome are not fully understood and families are encouraged to ensure that infants do not go for long periods without feeds; early admission to hospital is advised if intercurrent illness substantially limits feeding.

Weaning can commence at the normal time around 6 months of age, although progression onto a full diet is often slow paced and parents should expect a marked delay, with infants at 1 year still depending on regular small milk feeds and tolerating only smooth textures. As many Barth infants have poor muscle tone, care must be taken to ensure that they are able to sit up and support their heads in order to reduce the risk of choking. Gagging is commonplace and this often precipitates vomiting. Moving onto stronger tasting food and encouraging bite and dissolve finger foods when safe to do so can help make weaning more enjoyable. Delayed physical maturation and often repeated hospitalisations during infancy can also compound weaning being delayed and critical developmental stages being missed. If transition to solid food is not possible at 6 months, families should be encouraged to offer very small amounts of foods, such as puréed fruits and vegetables, yoghurts and cheese sauces, given from finger tips or the tip of a spoon to expose the infant to a variety of tastes until full weaning can commence.

Childhood

Many boys continue their slow transition to solid food during the first 3 years and will continue to have a degree of oromotor weakness and sensory issues. A sensitive gag reflex and poor chewing skills can lead to extended mealtimes and small portion sizes should be expected. Some boys continue to receive supplemental feeding and moving onto a solid diet can be problematic, especially when excessive energy is being given by tube feeding or supplement drinks. A slow approach is the most successful including sensory play with food (cooking, tasting, playing), involving the boys in mealtimes (particularly with their peers) and being positive and encouraging about their preferred food choices, which may be unusual (see below). The amount of tube feeds or oral nutritional support should be reviewed frequently to ensure that appetite for food is not being suppressed by excessive energy intake from feeds.

Restricted variety in the diet is commonplace and boys favour milk, cheese, crisps and toast (Bristol Clinic data). There is a propensity for food fads, especially for unusual savoury foods. A patient list-serve email discussion on food fads (December 2011) described boys having cravings for pickles, hot/chilli sauce, olives, mayonnaise, ketchup, soy sauce, cheese, milk and especially salt. Behaviour ranged from adding salt to food through to drinking the brine from feta cheese to eating salt by itself. There is no current evidence for a salt wasting state or any other explanation for this almost universal craving for salt. Judicious use of salty tasting sauces and dips when offering new foods can help encourage boys to expand the range of foods that they will eat. Limiting high fat foods, such as crisps and full fat dairy products, is sensible if they are overweight.

Energy requirements reduce throughout childhood as a consequence of reduced physical activity, slower growth and a lower muscle mass. By the age of 5 years, energy requirements can drop to 70% of the EAR so if boys are tube fed their weight gain must be carefully monitored to make sure they are not overfed. Protein requirements remain high at up to 2 g/kg/day and additional protein, vitamin and mineral supplements may be required if feed volumes are low.

Children who do eat are encouraged to have regular small meals and snacks and where possible, each containing a source of protein and carbohydrate. The diet should start to contain more complex low GI carbohydrates such as multigrain bread, pulses, wholegrain cereals and oats. A lower fat diet should be encouraged for those whose weight is on a higher centile than their height; for all other boys fat intake should be in line with current UK guidelines for children over 5 years of age, i.e. no more than 35% of total dietary energy. As most boys have low arginine and cysteine levels, foods with a higher content of these amino acids (such as nuts, lentils, sunflower seeds, tuna, chicken, salmon, prawns, dairy products and eggs) may be helpful.

Adolescence

Boys with Barth syndrome have delayed puberty, typically with onset between 15 and 18 years of age. When this later pubertal growth spurt does occur it is often without a significant increase in food intake, with the result that many previously slim boys may become abnormally thin. This, together with a worsening of cardiac function to some degree during puberty, may indicate a need for supplemental feeding via nasogastric or gastrostomy tubes.

Vitamins and minerals

Vitamin and mineral requirements are often not met due to small portion sizes, restricted range of foods taken and lower energy requirements. There is a potential increased need for vitamin B_6 due to increased amino acid catabolism; low functional levels of B_6 may contribute to poor plasma cysteine levels, although serum B_6 levels in all boys tested at the author's clinic were within the normal range. Evidence of B_6 insufficiency has been seen as a block in the transsulfuration pathway, manifested as inappropriately high levels of plasma methionine that normalise immediately with B_6 supplementation

(unpublished observations) and further investigation of this is under way. A number of the boys have low vitamin A levels which do not respond to supplementation; toxicity may occur with continued high doses. Vitamin D levels can be low, although the trends and percentage of boys who have suboptimal vitamin D status are the same as those seen in the general population (UK Bristol Clinic data 2010–2013). To ensure an adequate intake of all vitamins, it is recommended that boys taking diet alone have a multivitamin and mineral supplement that provides up to 50% of the RNI. Those receiving oral nutrition supplements (e.g. Paediasure, Fortini, Ensure) which are fortified with vitamins and minerals may require a lower dose.

Carnitine and coenzyme Q_{10}

A number of mitochondrial cocktails have been tried in Barth syndrome, including giving L-carnitine [143] and pantothenic acid [144]. With the exception of one isolated success, these results have not been favourable [145]. Although some benefit from treating carnitine deficiency (total plasma carnitine level <20 µmol/L) is possible in Barth syndrome, any high dose carnitine treatment (e.g. 50–100 mg/kg/day) given in the absence of deficiency, as used in some metabolic disorders, can precipitate cardiac failure and muscle weakness and should be avoided (patient registry, Barth Syndrome Foundation, 2011). There is no evidence that coenzyme Q_{10} is beneficial in Barth syndrome.

Omega-3 fatty acids

The anti-arrhythymic effects of fish oils has led to the suggestion that supplementation could be beneficial in Barth syndrome. Early work has established that neutrophil counts are not altered by docosahexaenoic acid (DHA) supplementation (personal communication). Until more investigations are undertaken, current recommendations are to have two portions of fish per week, one of which should be oily fish, in line with current UK guidelines [146].

Cornstarch therapy

During an overnight fast, degradation of muscle and other body protein occurs to release amino acids for gluconeogenesis when liver glycogen stores have been exhausted. This small muscle loss can be significant in Barth syndrome, where muscle mass is already reduced and the ability to rebuild it during the daytime is diminished due to hypotonia and decreased physical activity. Supplementary cornstarch at bedtime provides a slow release of glucose overnight and is a protein sparing treatment aimed at reducing overnight fasting time.

Cornstarch therapy can be started once overnight feeding has stopped at about the age of 2–3 years. The dose is built up to a maximum of 2 g/kg (as tolerated) and mixed into milk or yoghurt and given before bed. If cornstarch therapy is rejected, it is beneficial to offer a small snack close to bedtime, ideally containing protein and low GI complex carbohydrate, such as yoghurt or milk with a small oat biscuit or wholegrain cracker, multigrain toast or cereal.

Dietary management of illness

Careful attention is necessary during any intercurrent illness especially where there is a reduced or no intake of feed or food, such as vomiting. During this time children should be given an oral rehydration solution (p. 106) supplemented with glucose or glucose polymer up to 10% carbohydrate concentration. This should be offered frequently throughout the day to reduce the risk of hypoglycaemia. Drinks and emergency regimens containing higher concentrations of glucose, and extended periods of receiving carbohydrates only, should be avoided as the effect is to lower amino acid levels which may depress TCA cycle activity further. A source of protein should be introduced as soon as tolerated.

If fasting exceeds 24 hours, or the child is less than 1 year old, hospital admission is recommended for early treatment with intravenous (IV) glucose at 10% concentration. If feeding cannot be restarted within 48 hours of admission, and consequently protein intake is minimal, enteral or parenteral nutrition should be considered.

Diarrhoea

Diarrhoea may occur as a persistent or intermittent feature; it is not clear whether this is caused by viruses or abnormal smooth muscle function. Although most children with Barth syndrome do not have fat malabsorption this has been occasionally reported.

A possible contribution to diarrhoea is overproduction of acetylcholine, a neurotransmitter that increases contractility of smooth muscle in the intestine, via shunting of citrate (a TCA cycle intermediate and precursor of acetylcholine) out of the TCA cycle (personal communication). Citric acid is found naturally in many fruits and vegetables, and is most concentrated in oranges, lemons, lime, grapefruit, berries and tomatoes. Some cheeses (especially mozzarella) contain citric acid and it is added to foods (as the preservative E330) in particular to soft drinks, jams and preserves, fruit yoghurts, tinned tomatoes, sweets, sherbet, some ice creams and some flavoured crisps. Although there is no evidence that citrate or citric acid should be completely excluded from the diet, some patients have experienced improvement in symptoms when citric acid is reduced; therefore a trial reduction may be helpful.

During prolonged diarrhoea low muscle mass, and therefore lower potassium stores, can result in a more rapid depletion of potassium so electrolytes should be closely monitored. Care is also needed with IV fluids containing potassium, as patients may become hyperkalemic more quickly than would be expected.

Ongoing work

Specific amino acid supplementation

A number of boys in the USA, Europe and Australia have received amino acid supplementation with combinations of arginine, citrulline, cysteine and methionine to normalise fasting blood levels of these amino acids and in turn enhance muscle protein synthesis. The amounts and combinations are individually titrated. This work is being undertaken by Dr Richard Kelley, Professor of Paediatrics, Johns Hopkins School of Medicine, Baltimore, USA. Evidence based guidelines for amino acid supplementation will be produced from this work. Early reports include improvements in weight gain, appetite and cardiac function. There is ongoing work into the efficacy, tolerance and safety of this treatment.

Lipid Disorders

Janine Gallagher

Introduction

There are three main pathways responsible for the production and transport of lipids in the body: the exogenous pathway; the endogenous pathway; and the reverse cholesterol transport (Fig. 19.3 and Table 19.11). There are three main types of lipids: triglycerides, cholesterol and phospholipids. Lipids are transported in plasma as lipoproteins; these have a core of hydrophobic lipids (triglycerides and cholesterol esters) with amphiphilic molecules on the surface (phospholipids, cholesterol and proteins known as apolipoproteins). There are four

main classes of lipoproteins (Table 19.11) which are categorised according to their density.

Disorders of lipid metabolism which are managed by dietary intervention can be classified into those in which the serum lipoproteins are deficient or absent, hypolipoproteinaemia, or in which they are increased, hyperlipoproteinaemia.

Hypolipoproteinaemias

Abetalipoproteinaemia, hypobetalipoproteinaemia and chylomicron retention disease are rare genetic

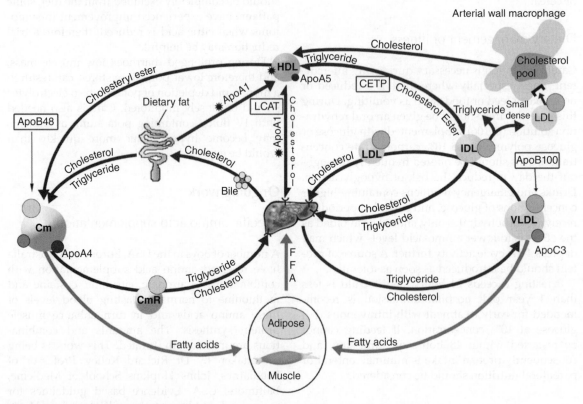

Figure 19.3   Lipid transport [147].
Cm, chylomicron particles; CmR, chylomicron remnant particles; VLDL, very low density lipoproteins; HDL, high density lipoproteins; LDL, low density lipoproteins; IDL, intermediate density lipoproteins; CETP, cholesterol ester transfer protein; FFA, non esterified fatty acids; LCAT, lecithin-cholesterol acyltransferase; Apo, apolipoprotein. Reprinted with permission of Oxford University Press.

Table 19.11   Lipoprotein composition and function [148].

Lipoprotein	%wt TG	%wt PL	%wt C+CE	Apoproteins	Function
Cm	90	5	4	Apo B-48, C-I, C-II, Apo A-I, A-IV, C-III, E	Transport of absorbed TG from intestines and hydrolysed by endothelium-bound LPL in adipose tissue and muscle. CmR taken up by liver (exogenous pathway)
VLDL	55	19	20	Apo B-100, C-I, C-II, C-III, Apo A-I, A-II, E	Transport of TG synthesised in liver to adipose tissue and muscle (endogenous pathway)
LDL	5	20	55	Apo B-100, Apo C-I, C-II, C-III, E	Transport of cholesterol from liver to peripheral tissues (endogenous pathway)
HDL	5	27	21	Apo A-I, A-II, Apo C-I, C-II, C-III, E	Transport of cholesterol from peripheral tissues to liver (reverse cholesterol transport)

Cm, chylomicrons; CmR, chylomicron remnants; VLDL, very low density lipoproteins; HDL, high density lipoproteins; LDL, low density lipoproteins; TG, triglyceride; PL, phospholipid; C+CE, sum of cholesterol and cholesterol ester; LPL, lipoprotein lipase.

diseases which cause malnutrition, growth failure and vitamin E deficiency [149].

Abetalipoproteinaemia

Abetalipoproteinaemia (ABL) is an autosomal recessive disorder, incidence <1 in 100 000, caused by mutations in the microsomal triglyceride transfer protein (MTP) gene resulting in the absence of plasma apolipoproteins (apo), B-containing lipoproteins, chylomicrons, VLDL and LDL [150]. MTP facilitates the transfer of lipids onto apo B. Presenting features are given in Table 19.12.

The onset of neurological symptoms usually begins in the first or second decade of life [153]. Prior to the use of high dose oral fat soluble vitamin treatment, neurological complications developed before the second decade and in some cases survival was not past the third decade [154]. Ophthalmic involvement is variable and covers a wide range of symptoms and manifestations [155]. The neurological and ophthalmic manifestations appear to be secondary to deficiency of vitamin E; vitamin A deficiency may also contribute to retinopathy.

Dietary management

Treatment involves reduction of dietary fat to prevent steatorrhoea and supplementation with tocopherol to prevent progression of the neuromuscular and retinal degenerative disease [156]. Fat restriction is determined by individual tolerance

Table 19.12   Presenting features of abetalipoproteinaemia.

Diarrhoea, steatorrhoea
Faltering growth due to fat malabsorption
Fat soluble vitamin deficiency (A, D, E, K)
Low plasma lipids and apolipoprotein B levels
Low plasma levels of essential fatty acids
Liver function tests may reveal elevated serum transaminases with hepatomegaly due to hepatic steatosis [151]
Acanthocytosis
Anaemia due to iron and folate deficiencies secondary to fat malabsorption [152]
Elevated prothrombin time and in severe cases gastrointestinal bleeding associated with vitamin K deficiencies [151]
Ophthalmic involvement, predominantly retinitis pigmentosa
Neurological manifestations including areflexia, ataxia, dysarthria and possibly cognitive decline
Muscle involvement including myopathy

(monitoring gastrointestinal, GI, symptoms) which increases with age and can vary from 5 g fat/day in infants up to 20 g/day in the older child. In the author's centre fat intake has been maintained at 10 g/day, not inclusive of fat derived from walnut oil, which is given to provide essential fatty acids (EFA). Despite the inability to secrete chylomicrons, there does appear to be some absorption of long chain fatty acids [157]. These are probably transferred to the liver as free fatty acids. Dietary treatment should aim to alleviate GI symptoms and increase energy intake to allow for catch up growth.

Medium chain triglycerides

The fatty acids derived from medium chain triglycerides (MCT) (C:8, C10:0, C12:0) do not require chylomicrons for their absorption as they are transported directly from the intestine to the liver via the hepatic portal system. The use of MCT as an energy source in ABL is controversial. There have been several reports of hepatic fibrosis with the use of MCT [158, 159], but there have also been reports of children who developed cirrhosis independent of the use of MCT oil [160, 161]. There are case reports of the benefit of MCT [162] and absence of adverse effects with its use [163]. Historically, MCT has not been used in the treatment of ABL, but some metabolic centres have started to use it; regular liver ultrasound scans and biochemical monitoring of liver function is required.

Infant feeds

An example of a minimal fat modular feed is outlined in Table 19.13. The feed requires a minimal fat protein source (e.g. Protifar, Vitapro, skimmed milk powder), a carbohydrate source as glucose polymer (e.g. Polycal, Vitajoule), electrolytes, a source of EFA (e.g. walnut oil), vitamins and minerals (e.g. Paediatric Seravit). Long chain triglycerides (LCT), given as a fat emulsion, e.g. Calogen, are added gradually to the feed as tolerated. LCPUFA can be given as KeyOmega. Consideration could be given to the use of Walnut oil as a LCT source if EFA remain low.

An extremely low fat infant formula, Basic-f (Milupa), is available providing, per 100 mL (13% dilution), 49 kcal (207 kJ), 10.2 g CHO, 1.8 g protein and <0.1 g fat (p. 597). A source of EFA must be added together with LCT (to tolerance) and glucose polymers to provide adequate energy.

Historically breast feeding has been considered to be contraindicated in ABL; however, partial breast feeding may be possible [164] in combination with a minimal fat feed. Close monitoring is required and the ratio of breast feeding to formula feeding altered according to biochemical parameters, clinical symptoms and growth.

Weaning

At the usual time for weaning, around 26 weeks of age, minimal fat foods can be commenced, e.g. baby rice mixed with the minimal fat feed, fruits and vegetables (except avocado pears and olives), pulses, meats and fish naturally low in fat (Table 19.14). As a guide for using commercial baby foods, wet baby foods and dried baby foods containing ≤0.5 g fat/100 g and ≤2 g fat/100 g, respectively, are allowed freely if given in usual portion sizes. Other baby foods with a higher fat content would need to be counted as part of the total daily fat allowance.

Table 19.13 Minimal fat feed (<5 g fat) for use in abetalipoproteinaemia.

16-week-old boy, prior to weaning, weight 5.4 kg (2nd centile), length 60 cm (9th centile)

Daily requirements:

fluid 150 mL/kg, energy 95 kcal (400 kJ) to 130 kcal (545 kJ)/kg, protein 1.6 g to 3 g/kg

EFA given as walnut oil to provide 0.1 mL/56 kcal (235 kJ) of the estimated average requirement (EAR) for energy for age [57]

This can be given as 180 mL × 6 feeds

	Energy (kcal)	Protein (g)	CHO (g)	LCT (g)	Na+ (mmol)	K+ (mmol)
Vitapro 15 g	54 (225 kJ)	11.3	1.4	0.9	2.0	2.7
Polycal 115 g	442 (1850 kJ)	–	110.4	–	0.2	0.1
Paediatric Seravit 15 g	45 (190 kJ)	–	11.3	–	0.1	–
Calogen 6 mL	27 (115 kJ)	–	–	3.0	–	–
Walnut oil 1 mL	8.4 (35 kJ)	–	–	0.9	–	–
KCl 6 mL (2 mmol/mL)	–	–	–	–	–	12.0
NaCl 1.5 mL (5 mmol/mL)	–	–	–	–	7.5	–
Water to 840 mL						
Total	576 (2415 kJ)	11.3	123.1	4.8	9.8	14.8
Per 100 mL	69 (285 kJ)	1.3	14.6	0.6	1.2	1.8
Per kg	107 (445 kJ)	2.1	22.8	0.9	1.8	2.7

Table 19.14   A sample minimal fat weaning menu.

On waking	Minimal fat feed
Breakfast	Suitable commercial baby cereal* mixed with minimal fat feed
Mid-morning	Minimal fat feed
Lunch	Purée turkey, chicken (white only), white fish or lentils
	Purée or mashed potato/sweet potato/pasta/rice (white)
	Purée or mashed vegetables
	Suitable savoury commercial baby food*
	Purée fruit or suitable commercial baby fruit dessert*
	Very low fat yoghurt/fromage frais
	Milk pudding (custard, ground rice) made with minimal fat feed or skimmed milk
Mid-afternoon	Minimal fat feed
Evening meal	As lunch
Bedtime	Minimal fat feed
Extra feeds or water can be given with meals	
Suitable finger foods from 6–9 months: fingers of toast (white bread)* (no spreading fat), soft cooked broccoli florets/carrots, soft pear/mango, banana slices	

*Check fat content of product.

Families can calculate the fat content of baby foods from nutrition labels so that higher fat foods can be counted in the total daily fat intake.

To calculate 1 g fat from a food product:

$$1\text{ g fat} = \frac{100\text{g}}{\text{grams of fat}/100\text{ g of food}}$$

Older children and adolescents

In order to achieve an adequate energy intake on a minimal fat diet, glucose polymers (e.g. Maxijul, Polycal, Vitajoule) may need to be used. Manufactured low fat foods are readily available in the supermarkets, but their fat content per portion needs to be assessed before including in the diet. Standard recipes (e.g. for biscuits, cakes and savoury foods) can be adapted to make low fat versions. Ongoing dietary assessment is required to ensure the diet remains nutritionally adequate. During adolescence, non adherence with diet and treatment may occur, so growth velocity, plasma levels of EFA and fat soluble vitamins need to be monitored closely.

As a guide for achieving a minimal fat diet in children, the aim in the author's centre is for main meals to contain ≤3 g fat per meal; snacks ≤0.5 g fat per item; and desserts ≤0.5 g fat per portion. The LCT content of foods is given in Table 13.11. A sample menu providing ≤10 g fat/day is given in Table 19.15.

Essential fatty acids

In ABL, plasma EFA levels tend to be low and so must be provided from the diet. Normal recommendations for linoleic acid (C18:2) and α-linolenic acid (C18:3) are that they should provide at least 1% and 0.2% of total energy intake, respectively [57]. These are minimum requirements for EFA and their absorption will be impaired in ABL. There are currently no specific guidelines for EFA supplementation in ABL and individual tolerance of dietary fat limits the amount of supplement that can be given. Regular monitoring of EFA is essential with biochemical analysis of red blood cell membrane (RBC) fatty acids, rather than plasma fatty acids. RBC fatty acids reflect the long term fatty acid balance in the tissues and are not influenced by recent dietary fat intake [165].

Fat soluble vitamins

The plasma transport and delivery of these vitamins to tissues depends almost exclusively (for vitamin E and beta-carotene) or in part (for vitamins A, D and K) on intact synthesis and secretion of apo B containing lipoproteins [150]. Supplementation with high doses of vitamin E increases serum vitamin levels but they tend to remain low, often <30% of the lower limit of normal. In contrast, high doses of vitamin A therapy can normalise serum levels. Although there is impaired absorption and

Table 19.15   A sample minimal fat menu providing ≤10 g fat/day.

Quantities will vary according to age and appetite	
Breakfast	Low fat cereal (<2 g fat/100 g, per 30 g serving = 0.5 g fat) e.g. cornflakes, Rice Krispies with minimal fat feed/skimmed milk/very low fat yoghurt (<0.2 g fat/100 g)
	White bread* toast (no spreading fat) and jam/honey/marmalade
	Fruit juice
Lunch	Sandwich made with bread*/bread roll*/tortilla wrap* with filling of chicken/lean ham/tuna in brine or spring water/salad/low fat cottage cheese
	OR baked beans and jacket potato
	OR egg white omelette with peppers and mushrooms
	Fruit/jelly/very low fat yoghurt
Snack	Fruit/vegetable sticks/suitable low fat snack items
Evening meal	Chicken/turkey (light meat)/very lean beef (with fat drained)/white fish
	Vegetables or salad
	Boiled/jacket/mashed potato or boiled pasta/rice/chapattis (no fat)
	Meringue and very low fat yoghurt/milk pudding made with skimmed milk
Bedtime	Skimmed milk to drink, toast and jam (no spreading fat)/low fat cereal with skimmed milk

*Check fat content of product.

transport from the intestines, subsequent transport of vitamin A by retinol binding protein is not impaired [150]. Vitamin D follows a different pathway; plasma levels need to be monitored but it may not be necessary to give supplements. Vitamin K is monitored by checking clotting times and prothrombin levels. High dose oral vitamins are considered to bypass the intestinal chylomicron assembly pathway via the portal circulation. The recommendations for supplementing vitamins A, E and K first proposed in 1983 are still used [166]:

- vitamin A: 7000 µg/day to maintain normal plasma concentrations
- vitamin E: 100 mg/kg/day (water soluble form available)
- vitamin K: 5–10 mg/day (water soluble form available)

In the author's centre, higher doses of vitamin E have been given up to 340 mg/kg/day. High doses of vitamin E (150 mg/kg/day) have been associated with increased tissue levels of α-tocopherol [150].

Chylomicron retention disease

Mutations in the SAR1B gene have recently been identified as responsible for chylomicron retention disease (CRD) [167]. The SAR1B protein is involved in transporting chylomicrons within enterocytes and mutations impair the release of chylomicrons into the bloodstream. CRD is an autosomal recessive disorder and only 40 cases have been described [149]. The presenting clinical signs are given in Table 19.16.

Dietary management

A minimal LCT diet, to tolerance (monitoring GI symptoms), is required with an adequate energy intake achieved by supplementation with glucose polymers and MCT. This leads to improvement in GI symptoms [168]. The following doses of oral fat soluble vitamins in early diagnosis have been recommended [149]:

- vitamin E: 50 IU (33.5 mg)/kg/day (water soluble form)
- vitamin A: 15 000 IU (4500 µg)/day (adjusted according to plasma levels)
- vitamin D: 800–1200 IU (20–30 µg)/kg/day
- vitamin K: 15 mg/week (adjusted according to international normalised ratio (INR) and plasma levels)

Table 19.16   Presenting clinical signs of chylomicron retention disease [149]. Reprinted wtih permission of Peretti *et al.*

Gastrointestinal symptoms: diarrhoea, steatorrhoea, vomiting and abdominal swelling
Hepatomegaly with steatosis
Neurological, muscular and ophthalmic manifestations
↓ total cholesterol, LDL and HDL and normal TG
Elevated CK levels
Acanthocytosis is rare
EFA deficiency
Vitamin E deficiency
Endoscopy: white duodenal mucosa

LDL, low density lipoprotein; HDL, high density lipoprotein; TG, triglycerides; CK, creatine kinase; EFA, essential fatty acids.

Infants
Initially a minimal fat modular feed (Table 19.13) maybe required with further LCT added to tolerance. Alternatively a high MCT, low LCT formula feed containing vitamins, minerals and EFA can be given, e.g. Monogen (17.5% normal concentration) or Lipistart (15% normal concentration). For infants between 0 and 6 months the aim is to meet their fluid requirements of 150 mL/kg/day. The compositions of these two formulas are compared in Table 19.17.

Monogen is usually introduced at 15% concentration. If well tolerated there can be an increase to the standard concentration of 17.5%. Feeds containing MCT should always be introduced slowly and care taken to ensure the feed provides sufficient EFA [169].

If an infant is showing faltering growth the concentration of both these formulas can be increased gradually by 1% increments depending on fat tolerance; close biochemical monitoring is required. The energy density of the feeds can be increased further with the addition of glucose polymers and/or MCT emulsion, but this will reduce the protein:energy ratio of the feed.

At the usual time for weaning, minimal LCT baby foods can be given (Table 19.14) with suitable finger foods as weaning progresses. In addition, MCT oil can be considered for cooking foods and can be incorporated into recipes. It is a good source of energy providing 855 kcal (3.57 MJ)/100 mL.

Children and adolescents
If children are achieving good growth through having an adequate intake from their minimal LCT diet (Table 19.15), the MCT formula feed can be discontinued. It can be replaced by skimmed milk and a source of EFA, given as walnut oil (p. 601), and LCP-UFA, given as KeyOmega (Table 19.18).

The dose of walnut oil is 0.1 mL/56 kcal (235 kJ) of the estimated average requirement (EAR) for energy for age [58]. The dose of KeyOmega depends on age and red blood cell membrane EFA levels. Ongoing growth monitoring is essential.

Table 19.17 Comparison of two minimal LCT formulas.

Lipistart	Per 100 g	Per 100 mL (15% dilution)
Energy	450 kcal (1880 kJ)	68 kcal (285 kJ)
Protein	13.7 g	2.1 g
Carbohydrate	55.3 g	8.3 g
Fat	20.6 g	3.1 g
of which LCT	3.8 g	0.57 g
of which MCT	16.5 g	2.5 g
of which linoleic acid	1728 mg	259 mg
of which α-linolenic acid	242 mg	36 mg
of which AA (C20:4)	202 mg	30 mg
of which DHA (C22:6)	101 mg	15 mg
Sodium	11.1 mmol	1.7 mmol
Potassium	12.6 mmol	1.9 mmol
Calcium	12.3 mmol	1.8 mmol
Monogen	Per 100 g	Per 100 mL (17.5% dilution)
Energy	420 kcal (1755 kJ)	73.5 kcal (310 kJ)
Protein	12.5 g	2.2 g
Carbohydrate	68 g	12 g
Fat	11 g	1.9 g
of which LCT	2.2 g	0.38 g
of which MCT	8.8 g	1.52 g
% energy linoleic acid	1.1	
% energy α-linolenic acid	0.17	
Sodium	8.7 mmol	1.5 mmol
Potassium	9.2 mmol	1.6 mmol
Calcium	6.4 mmol	1.1 mmol

LCT, long chain triglycerides; MCT, medium chain triglycerides; AA, arachidonic acid; DHA, docosahexaenoic acid.

Table 19.18 Nutritional composition of KeyOmega.

	Per 100 g	Per 4 g sachet
Energy	476 kcal (1990 kJ)	19 kcal (79 kJ)
Protein (g)	4.37	0.17
CHO (g)	70.5	2.8
Fat (g)	19.6	0.8
of which AA (mg)	5000	200
of which DHA (mg)	2500	100

AA, arachidonic acid; DHA, docosahexaenoic acid.

Additional energy is encouraged as MCT oil, refined carbohydrates and glucose polymers. In adolescence, good quantities of complex carbohydrates are recommended; in younger children a high intake may be too bulky and increase levels of satiety. Good dental hygiene needs to be encouraged. Adherence with the diet may be difficult in adolescence and good support is required at this time. Haemoglobin and ferritin levels need to be monitored as minimal LCT diets tend to be low in haem iron.

Familial hypobetalipoproteinaemia

Familial hypobetalipoproteinaemia (FHBL) is an autosomal dominant disorder usually due to mutations in the gene for apoB [149]. Heterozygotes are generally asymptomatic, they have low plasma apo B and LDL cholesterol concentrations [170, 171] and a reduced risk for premature atherosclerosis [171]. The incidence is approximately 1 in 2000 [172]. In contrast, homozygotes have clinical manifestations indistinguishable from ABL: acanthocytosis, fat soluble vitamin deficiencies and fat malabsorption and, without treatment, long term neurological and ophthalmological complications [156].

For infants with symptomatic homozygous FHBL, the dietary management is as previously described in ABL. Dietary supplementation with MCT can be considered although there would be concerns about hepatic fibrosis. Large doses of vitamin E are effective in preventing neurological complications in homozygotes [170]. Vitamin E doses (100–300 mg/kg/day) have been shown to normalise adipose tissue levels of vitamin E, although serum levels often remain low [173]. Modest doses of vitamin E (200 mg/kg/day) may be given to heterozygotes, even though asymptomatic,

as there have been reports of neurological complications [171]. High doses of vitamin A have been recommended (200–400 IU (60–120 µg)/kg/day) to restore normal serum levels [173]. Vitamin K should be supplemented if bruising, bleeding or hypoprothrombinemia are present [171]. Vitamin D needs to be monitored and supplemented if levels are low.

Hyperlipoproteinaemias

The classification of familial hyperlipidaemias is summarised in Table 19.19. Primary hyperlipidaemias are due to genetic disorders, while secondary hyperlipidaemias occur due to an underlying disease. In childhood the two most prevalent hyperlipidaemias are familial lipoprotein lipase deficiency (type I hyperlipidaemia) and familial hypercholesterolaemia (type IIa). The other disorders are rare in childhood and treatment has not been described.

Familial lipoprotein lipase deficiency

This is an autosomal recessive disorder with an incidence of 1 in 1 000 000 [172]. It is characterised by absence of lipoprotein lipase (LPL) activity and an accumulation of chylomicrons in plasma and a corresponding increase of plasma triglyceride concentrations [175]. Hypertriglyceridaemia often ranges between 5000 mg/dL (57 mmol/L) and 10 000 mg/dL (114 mmol/L) [172], normal fasting levels being 0.5–2.2 mmol/L. Patients may present with acute abdominal pain, recurrent episodes of pancreatitis, eruptive xanthomas and hepatosplenomegaly but more often the diagnosis is made incidentally when a routine blood specimen is lipaemic, or hepatomegaly is found in an older child. Premature atherosclerosis is uncommon [172]; however, pancreatitis maybe life threatening.

Dietary management

The aim of dietary treatment is to relieve the symptoms. Restriction of LCT to 5 g/day will result in optically clear fasting serum and lowering of serum triglycerides. This severe fat restriction is difficult to maintain in the long term and fat intake is determined by individual tolerance. A restriction of dietary fat to 20 g/day or less is usually sufficient to reduce plasma triglyceride levels and keep

Table 19.19 Classification of familial hyperlipidaemias [174]. Reprinted with permission of Cambridge University Press.

Primary defect	Type	Lipid abnormality
Familial lipoprotein lipase deficiency Apo C-II deficiency	I	Exogenous hyperlipidaemia ↑↑ chylomicrons
Familial hypercholesterolaemia Familial combined hyperlipoproteinaemia	IIa	Hypercholesterolaemia ↑↑ LDL
Familial combined hyperlipoproteinaemia	IIb	Combined hyperlipidaemia ↑LDL + VLDL
Familial dysbetalipoproteinaemia	III	Remnant hyperlipidaemia β-VLDL
Familial hypertriglyceridaemia Familial combined hyperlipoproteinaemia Tangier disease	IV	Endogenous hyperlipidaemia ↑ VLDL
Familial hypertriglyceridaemia Familial lipoprotein lipase deficiency	V	Mixed hyperlipidaemia ↑ VLDL and chylomicrons

LDL, low density lipoproteins; VLDL, very low density lipoproteins.

the patient symptom free [175]. Triglycerides will remain above the normal range but as the condition is not associated with premature atherosclerosis there is no need for severe dietary restriction. Ideally triglycerides should be maintained at <10 mmol/L but a more realistic target is <20 mmol/L. A few LPL deficient patients respond to therapy with MCT oil or omega-3 fatty acids by normalising fasting plasma triglycerides [176].

Acute episodes

During episodes of acute abdominal pain, a strict minimal LCT diet providing <5 g/day should be implemented (Tables 13.9, 13.12). This will produce a rapid decrease in serum triglyceride levels within 5–7 days. In addition frequent high carbohydrate drinks, e.g. 20% glucose polymer, should be given. If an older child requires enteral tube feeding then a modular LCT feed can be given (adapting the feed given in Table 19.13) or 'juice' style oral nutritional supplements, e.g. Paediasure Plus Juce, Ensure Plus Juce, Fortijuce, Fresubin Jucy; these are fat free. EFA (counting their fat content within the LCT allowance) and electrolytes need to be added to provide complete nutrition. Total parenteral nutrition may need to be considered if feeds or diet are not tolerated.

For infants, a minimal LCT feed (Tables 19.13, 19.17) and minimal LCT weaning diet is recommended (Table 19.14).

Long term management

Fat There seems to be individual tolerance of fat intake ranging between 20 and 30 g/day. Recommended treatment is with a very low fat diet (10%–15% of energy) [176]. Based on the EAR for age and sex with fat providing 10% energy, this gives a range for boys from infants to 15–18 years of 6–30 g fat/day and for girls 6–23 g fat/day. Serum triglyceride levels need to be monitored if fat intake is increased; this level of fat restriction should be sufficient to avoid acute episodes of pancreatitis or development of xanthomas. Fat should be equally distributed between meals.

Infants A minimal LCT formula with MCT can be used as shown in Table 19.17. These feeds contain EFA and fat soluble vitamins so additional supplements should not be needed. Partial breast feeding may be possible in combination with a minimal LCT formula. When weaning is commenced, a minimal LCT diet should be followed (Table 19.14). Monogen and Lipistart can continue during infancy and EFA and fat soluble vitamins should continue to be monitored to ensure dietary adequacy.

Children and adolescents In this age group it is important to ensure adequate energy intake is achieved to support growth and development.

Table 19.20 Nutritional content of MCT Procal.

	Per 100 g	Per 16 g sachet
Energy	657 kcal (2742 kJ)	105 kcal (439 kJ)
Protein (g)	12.5	2
CHO (g)	20.6	3.3
Fat (g)	63.1	10.1
of which MCT	62.2	10
of which LCT	0.9	0.14

Energy requirements can be met by the use of MCT oil and emulsions, glucose polymers and refined and complex carbohydrates. The introduction of MCT oil will help to improve the palatability and the energy density of the diet. Families can use MCT oil in recipes, e.g. MCT oil margarine, cakes and biscuits. MCT Procal is an MCT supplement, suitable from 12 months (Table 19.20) that can be added to minimal LCT foods, e.g. very low fat yoghurts.

Suitable minimal LCT diets are outlined in Tables 13.12 and 19.15. Educating families to identify and calculate the fat contents of foods from nutrition labels will allow the inclusion of low fat manufactured foods. Advice should be given to families about minimal LCT choices when eating out. EFA will need supplementing as previously described.

Fat soluble vitamins will need to be monitored and, depending on individual fat tolerance, may require supplementation. In order to achieve adequate calcium intakes, minimal fat calcium sources should be encouraged in the diet, e.g. skimmed milk and very low fat yoghurt. Haemoglobin and ferritin levels should be monitored in view of the low haem sources in the diet.

Adherence can be difficult with a restricted diet and families need ongoing support. In transition clinics teenagers need to be educated to understand and manage the diet themselves in order to ensure suitable dietary choices and dietary adherence as they move to adult care.

Familial hypercholesterolaemia

Familial hypercholesterolaemia (FH) type IIa is the most common primary lipoprotein disorder of childhood with an estimated incidence of 1 in 500 for heterozygous FH and 1 in 1 000 000 for homozygous FH [177]. It is inherited as an autosomal dominant trait; homozygotes are more severely affected than heterozygotes. FH is characterised by an elevated plasma low density lipoprotein (LDL) concentration and deposition of LDL cholesterol in tendons and skin (xanthomas) and in arteries (atheromas) [177]. FH is due to a mutation in the LDL receptor gene; more than 900 different mutations have now been reported [178]. This mutation reduces the rate of removal of LDL from plasma and cholesterol is then deposited in cells, producing the xanthomas and atheromas.

FH is completely expressed at birth and in early childhood [172]. Heterozygous FH will lead to a greater than 50% risk of coronary heart disease by the age of 50 years in men and at least 30% in women by the age of 60 years [179]. Homozygotes usually develop coronary artery disease in the second decade and virtually all have planar xanthomas by the age of 5 years [172]. Homozygous FH presents with a four to eight fold increase in LDL cholesterol levels and heterozygotes present with a two to three fold elevation in the plasma levels of total and LDL cholesterol [172]. Cholesterol levels change during childhood due to the influence of growth and puberty. The aim of treatment for both heterozygotes and homozygotes is to lower plasma LDL levels and reduce the risk of ischaemic heart disease. This is managed by dietary treatment, medications, in particular statins (HMG-CoA reductase inhibitors), and lifestyle advice. More aggressive treatment, such as plasma LDL apheresis or liver transplantation, may need to be considered for homozygous FH.

Screening

The National Institute for Health and Care Excellence (NICE) published the *Identification and Management of Familial Hypercholesterolaemia* guidelines in 2008 [179]. A diagnosis of FH should be made using the Simon Broome diagnostic criteria for index individuals [180], which include a combination of family history, clinical signs (xanthomas), cholesterol concentration and DNA testing. A definite diagnosis of FH is defined as

- total cholesterol >6.7 mmol/L or LDL cholesterol >4.0 mmol/L in a child aged younger than 16 years

  or

- total cholesterol >7.5 mmol/L or LDL cholesterol >4.9 mmol/L in an adult

plus

- tendon xanthomas in patient or in first-degree relative or in second-degree relative

or

- DNA based evidence of an LDL receptor mutation, familial defective apo B-100, or a PCSK9 mutation

In children at risk of FH due to an affected parent, diagnostic tests should be carried out before 10 years of age. A screening strategy for FH based on a meta-analysis carried out by Wald *et al.* [181] revealed that screening by measurement of serum cholesterol is most effective if done in early childhood after the first year of life, between 1 and 9 years, when a high detection rate can be achieved with a false positive of only 0.1%. The NICE guidelines recommend that all children with FH should be referred to a specialist centre with expertise in FH with this age group.

Lifestyle advice

It is important that families are given information about exercise, smoking, alcohol and weight management alongside lipid modifying dietary intervention. In this chapter the focus will be on the dietary intervention in FH. Further details of the lifestyle interventions can be found in the NICE guidelines [179].

Dietary management and intervention

Evidence for current dietary recommendations
The NICE guidelines [179] reviewed evidence of randomised controlled trials [182–185] and recommended a lipid modified diet for managing FH. A review of the guideline in 2011 showed no new evidence to change the 2008 recommended dietary advice:

- total fat intake 30% or less of total energy intake
- saturated fats 10% or less of total energy intake
- intake of dietary cholesterol <300 mg/day
- saturated fats replaced by increasing the intake of mono-unsaturated and polyunsaturated fats

In addition recommendations were given to include at least five portions of fruit and vegetables a day and two portions of fish a week, one of which should be oily fish. If food products containing plant stanols and sterols are consumed, these products need to be taken consistently to be effective.

Total fat intake
Assessing each child's diet individually is essential. Some families may already be following a healthy eating plan and achieving the recommended guidelines for total fat intake. Other families will require help to be able to identify foods which have a high fat content in order to achieve this target. Education is required to interpret food nutrition labels. As a guide, a high fat food contains ≥20 g fat/100 g and a low fat food contains ≤3 g fat/100 g [186]. In order to achieve this, simple adjustments in the diet can be made, e.g. encouraging the use of low fat dairy products. Full fat milk can be replaced with skimmed milk (0.1% fat), 1% fat milk or semi-skimmed milk (1.7% fat). Decreasing the intake of hidden sources of fat in manufactured foods, such as cakes and biscuits, will help in achieving the target fat intake. In the author's centre it is advised that lean red meat is only eaten two to three times per week and is replaced with alternative protein sources such as beans, pulses, poultry (light meat, no skin), soya protein and white fish (not fried). Oily fish such as pilchards, mackerel or salmon should be included in the diet at least once a week. Eggs may be included as part of the total fat allowance. Suggestions for making suitable food choices when eating out can be given to the family.

Saturated fatty acids
There is substantial evidence to support a reduction of saturated fatty acids (SFA) in the diet [178]. A high intake of SFA raises plasma levels of total and LDL cholesterol. As a guide, foods high in SFA contain ≥5 g/100 g, e.g. fatty cuts of meat; meat products including sausages and pies; butter, ghee and lard; cheese, especially hard cheese; cream, soured cream and ice cream; some savoury snacks and chocolate confectionery; biscuits, cakes and pastries. Foods low in SFA contain ≤1.5 g/100 g [186].

Dietary cholesterol
Dietary cholesterol is found in eggs, high fat dairy products, shellfish and offal. In the author's centre foods containing dietary cholesterol are not

restricted unless they also have a high SFA content. Epidemiological surveys of coronary heart disease (CHD) risk report no consistent independent relationship between dietary cholesterol/egg consumption and CHD risk [187]. Reducing the SFA in the diet, e.g. high fat dairy foods, will lead to a decreased intake of dietary cholesterol. Some centres exclude foods low in SFA but high in dietary cholesterol (e.g. prawns and liver).

Increasing mono-unsaturated fats and polyunsaturated fats

Mono-unsaturated fats (MUFA) are found in olive oil, rapeseed oil and fat spreads made from these oils. Rapeseed oil is a cheaper alternative to olive oil. Polyunsaturated fats (PUFA) are found in sunflower oil, corn oil and soya oil. These can be incorporated into the diet and used in cooking. MUFA have been shown to have a hypocholesterolaemic effect when substituted for SFA in the diet.

Plant stanols and sterols

Plant sterols and stanols reduce the absorption of cholesterol from the intestines. The incorporation of plant stanol/sterol containing foods into the diet of children with FH has been shown to reduce total cholesterol by 9.1% and LDL cholesterol by 11.4% [188]. This was achieved by taking an average intake of 1.2 g plant sterol a day. In the NICE guidelines no evidence was identified to demonstrate that the use of plant sterols or stanols in children was associated with vitamin deficiencies [179]. There is a wide variety of products now available from the Flora Proactiv and Benecol ranges providing varying amounts of plant sterols or stanols. These products need to be taken consistently to be effective. However, they can be expensive for some families to use in the daily diet.

Fruit and vegetables

Families should be encouraged to increase their intake of fruit and vegetables, fresh, frozen or tinned. The aim is for five portions a day, eating a wide variety [186]. For children, as a guide, a portion is the amount that fits in the palm of their hand. Fruit juice (150 mL) counts as one portion a day.

Complex carbohydrates

Starchy foods such as cereals, bread, pasta, rice, chapattis, noodles and potatoes should be included at most meals. Encouraging wholemeal or wholegrain products is beneficial, e.g. porridge, popcorn, rye crackers and brown rice. The soluble fibre, beta-glucan, found in oats has been shown to lower cholesterol by the formation of a gel in the digestive tract which binds to cholesterol and bile salts, preventing absorption. This results in the body then utilising the cholesterol from the blood to make more bile salts. Weight needs to be monitored because starchy foods, which potentially can be bulky and increase satiety levels, affect overall energy intakes.

Weight maintenance

Advice and support should be given to individuals about weight reduction to achieve a healthy weight as obesity is a further risk factor for CHD. The primary goal of diet therapy should be to reduce weight initially and then to focus on a lipid modifying diet.

Monitoring

Clinic reviews should include fasting total cholesterol, LDL cholesterol, HDL cholesterol and triglycerides. Families may choose to go to their GP for fasting lipid levels prior to clinic review. If a modified lipid lowering diet is followed, fat soluble vitamin supplements should not be required; however, it is beneficial to check fat soluble vitamin levels annually. If lean red meat is restricted, then iron stores need to be monitored. Calcium intakes should be assessed and supplements given if there is poor intake of low fat dairy products.

Adherence

Adherence with dietary intervention is variable because patients with FH do not experience any symptoms during childhood. It is difficult to be motivated to avert symptoms that will present later in life. Adherence is better in families with a history of parental death from CHD due to heightened anxiety levels.

Table 19.21 gives a suggested meal plan for a 10-year-old boy with newly diagnosed FH.

Drug therapy

The NICE guidelines highlight the need for lifestyle advice as a component of medical management and not as a substitute for lipid modifying drug

Table 19.21 A suggested meal plan for a 10-year-old boy newly diagnosed with familial hypercholesterolaemia.

Weight 31 kg (50th centile) Height 143 cm (75th centile)

Breakfast	Large bowl of porridge with skimmed milk, chopped banana and maple syrup Wholemeal toast/bagel – 'light' olive oil margarine/plant stanol/sterol margarine and honey Fruit juice
Mid-morning snack Lunch	Low fat crisps* Tuna in spring water (drained) with 'extra light' mayonnaise and cucumber slices Tortilla wrap* Small pot low fat hummus and carrot sticks Cereal bar* Low fat yoghurt Juice or water
Mid-afternoon snack	Jam sandwich – 1 slice white/wholemeal bread Skimmed milk, milkshake using milkshake syrup
Evening meal	Chicken curry (using light meat) with vegetables, olive oil and tomato based sauce and rice (white or brown) ± fat free chapatti **or** Grilled salmon and new potatoes with steamed vegetables Meringues and low fat yoghurt with chopped strawberries **or** Stewed fruit and low fat custard made with skimmed milk
Bedtime	Suitable crackers* and very low fat cheese spread **or** Cereal* and skimmed milk Hot chocolate using low fat drinking chocolate and skimmed milk and topped with marshmallows

*Check nutrition label for fat content.

therapy which should be considered by the age of 10 years; treatment should be lifelong. In short term studies, statins have not been associated with significant adverse effects in children aged 8–18 years [179] in terms of growth rate or pubertal development. There are no longer term studies. Statins (HMG-CoA reductase inhibitors) should be the initial treatment. If children are intolerant of statins, other lipid lowering drug therapies should be offered, e.g. bile acid sequestrants, fibrates or ezetimibe. If bile acid sequestrants are used in the long term, then supplementation with fat soluble vitamins and folic acid should be considered.

Future research

Further long term studies are required to demonstrate the effectiveness of lifestyle interventions with children and young people with FH. In addition the effectiveness of a cholesterol lowering diet needs to be monitored and long term studies are required. Children and young people with FH should ideally be seen in family clinics to ensure lifestyle advice is incorporated into the family's routine. Emphasis should be focused towards lifestyle changes in order to reduce the risks for CHD.

Acknowledgements

Marjorie Dixon would like to thank Dr Andrew Morris, Royal Manchester Children's Hospital, for his invaluable contribution and review of the section on disorders of mitochondrial fatty acid oxidation, ketogenesis and ketolysis.

Nicol Clayton would like to thank the following for kindly contributing to the section on Barth syndrome: Dr Richard Kelley, Professor of Paediatrics, Johns Hopkins School of Medicine, Director, Clinical Mass Spectrometry Laboratory, Kennedy

Krieger Institute, Baltimore, USA; Dr Colin Steward, Clinical Lead Barth Syndrome Service, Bristol Royal Hospital for Children, UK.

Janine Gallagher would like to thank Fiona White, Chief Metabolic Dietitian, and Dr Andrew Morris, Royal Manchester Children's Hospital, for their contribution to this chapter. She would also like to thank Marjorie Dixon, Principal Paediatric Dietitian, Great Ormond Street Hospital for Children, for the discussion on the dietary management of ABL.

Further reading

Clarke SLN, Bowron A, Gonzalez IL *et al*. Barth syndrome review. *Orphanet J Rare Dis*, 2013, 8 23.

Useful addresses

The Children's Mitochondrial Disease Network

EMDN
Mayfield House
30 Heber Walk
Chester Way
Northwich CW9 5JB
www.emdn-mitonet.co.uk

Children Living with Inherited Metabolic Diseases

Climb Building
176 Nantwich Road
Crewe CW2 6BG
www.climb.org.uk

NHS Specialised Services Barth Syndrome Service

Bristol Royal Hospital for Children
General enquiries: Dr Colin Steward, Clinical Lead, Barth Syndrome Service
Telephone: 0117 342 8044
www.barthsyndromeservice.nhs.uk

Barth Syndrome Trust

www.barthsyndrome.org.uk

Heart UK

www.heartuk.org.uk

British Heart Foundation

www.bhf.org.uk

20 Peroxisomal Disorders

Anita MacDonald and Eleanor Baldwin

Introduction

Peroxisomal disorders are a group of inherited metabolic heterogeneous disorders resulting from dysfunction of either peroxisomal biogenesis or peroxisomal functions [1, 2]. Peroxisomes are cellular organelles that have an important role in at least eight different metabolic pathways [1] including the β-oxidation of very long chain fatty acids (VLCFA); the production of plasmalogens (a class of phospholipids); and the synthesis of bile acids [3]. Peroxisomes normally metabolise as much as 20% of cellular oxygen [4].

Peroxisomal disorders are divided into two main categories:

- single peroxisomal (enzyme) protein deficiency, e.g. X-linked adrenoleukodystrophy and Refsum's disease
- peroxisome biogenesis disorders (PBD) including Zellweger syndrome, neonatal adrenoleukodystrophy, infantile Refsum's disease and rhizomelic chondrodysplasia punctata [3, 5] (Table 20.1). They vary in their age of onset, clinical symptoms, tissues affected and pathology.

X-linked Adrenoleukodystrophy

Anita MacDonald

Genetics

X-linked adrenoleukodystrophy (X-ALD) is a rare, severe, neurodegenerative, X-chromosomal disorder with reduced peroxisomal VLCFA β-oxidation activity [6, 7]. It causes progressive brain and peripheral demyelination and adrenal insufficiency in males [8, 9]. It is characterised by accumulation of saturated and mono-unsaturated VLCFA, especially hexacosanoic acid (C26:0) and tetracosanoic acid (C24:0), primarily in the nervous system, adrenal cortex and testis [8]. It produces wide ranging and unpredictable clinical phenotypes with members of the same family presenting with different phenotypes [10].

It is estimated that 93% of X-ALD cases are caused by mutations in the *ABCD1* gene [11, 12], encoding the peroxisomal protein ATP binding

Clinical Paediatric Dietetics, Fourth Edition. Edited by Vanessa Shaw.
© 2015 John Wiley & Sons, Ltd. Published 2015 by John Wiley & Sons, Ltd.
Companion Website: www.wiley.com/go/shaw/paediatricdietetics

Table 20.1 Peroxisomal disorders.

Group 1: Single peroxisomal enzyme (transporter)
deficiencies
X-linked adrenoleukodystrophy; (X-ALD/AMN)
Refsum's disease
Rhizomelic chondrodysplasia punctata (type 2) (DHAPAT
 deficiency)
Rhizomelic chondrodysplasia punctata (type 3) (alkyl-DHAP
 synthase deficiency)
D-Bifunctional protein deficiency
α-Methylacyl-CoA racemase deficiency
Glutaryl-CoA oxidase deficiency

Group 2: Peroxisomal biogenesis disorders
Zellweger syndrome
Infantile Refsum's disease
Neonatal adrenoleukodystrophy
Rhizomelic chondrodysplasia punctata (type 1)

AMN, adrenomyeloneuropathy
DHAPAT, dihydroxyacetone phosphate acyltransferase;
DHAP, dihydroxyacetone phosphate.

cassette transporter D1. It is suggested that this plays a crucial role in transporting VLCFA, or their CoA derivatives, into peroxisomes in humans [7]. More than 1000 distinct mutations in the defective gene are described [13]. The remaining 7% of cases are caused by a *de novo* mutation [14]. The disorder has been reported in all races and geographical locations. Estimates of the incidence of X-ALD are 1 in 15 000 [15] in males and 1 in 14 000 in females [16]. As females have two X chromosomes they don't usually show the clinical features of X-ALD. There is no correlation between X-ALD phenotype, *ABCD1* gene mutations [13] and concentrations of VLCFA in the plasma and fibroblasts [17], although a combination of genetic and environmental factors may modulate the outcome of the condition [18, 19].

Clinical features

There are at least six known clinical phenotypes which vary greatly with respect to expression, age of onset, rate of progression and therapy (Table 20.2). Pre-symptomatic boys may progress to one of several phenotypes between the age of 3 and 50 years. Presentation ranges from the rapidly progressive childhood cerebral form to the more slowly progressive adult form (adrenomyeloneuropathy, AMN) and variants without neurological involvement even within the same family.

Cerebral X-ALD (childhood or adulthood)

This causes a rapidly progressive inflammatory demyelination of the white matter within the brain [19, 20] and may involve autoimmune mechanisms [21], mostly causing severe disability. It usually occurs between 4 and 12 years [21] with a peak at 7–8 years, and less frequently in teenagers and adults [22]. Early symptoms in children are behavioural changes (withdrawn or hyperactive behaviour) and visual impairment. Brain magnetic resonance imaging (MRI) abnormalities precede symptoms [16], but unfortunately in many cases diagnosis is made only after significant deterioration in neurological function. In some cases the demyelinating process can stop spontaneously without further progression when it is not associated with disruption of the blood–brain barrier [23]. Death may occur within 5 years of the onset of neurological symptoms [24] but some patients survive for several years with severe neurological impairment and are bed ridden, blind and unable to eat or speak [25].

Symptoms in adults include psychosis, mania, depression, spastic paraparesis, epilepsy, optic atrophy and adrenal insufficiency [26]. It may be mistaken for a psychiatric disorder such as schizophrenia with dementia [27]. Addison's disease may precede overt neurological involvement in about 80% of males [23]. The mechanisms leading to neuroinflammation are unknown but data suggest there may be a relationship between the expression of inflammation mediators, impairment of peroxisomal function and accumulation of VLCFA in the cerebral ALD brain [28]. Oxidative stress appears to play a role in the neurodegenerative features [29].

Adrenomyeloneuropathy

This is the slightly more common adult form with symptoms and signs of spinal cord involvement usually occurring between the ages of 30 and 40 years [30]. It causes a non inflammatory, slowly progressive distal axonopathy in the spinal cord tract and peripheral nerves, with patients surviving to their eighth decade [13]. About 80% of men with AMN have impaired adrenocortical function at the time neurological symptoms are first noted [23].

Table 20.2   Clinical phenotypes of X-linked adrenoleukodystrophy.

Clinical phenotype	Age of presentation (years)	Relative frequency (%)	Features	Progression
Childhood cerebral ALD	3–10	31–57	Progressive behavioural, cognitive and neurological impairments resulting in total disability within 2 years. Addison's disease. Behavioural changes, school failure, dementia, psychoses, paralysis, epilepsy, loss of vision, loss of speech	Rapid, rarely slowly
Adolescent ALD	11–21		Similar to childhood cerebral ALD. Resembles cerebral childhood ALD but with slower progression	Rapid, rarely slowly
Adult cerebral ALD	>21	1–3	Similar to childhood cerebral ALD. Symptoms resemble schizophrenia with dementia. Addison's disease	Rapid, sometimes slowly
AMN	>18	25–40	Symptoms include leg stiffness, clumsiness, progressive spastic paraparesis (stiffness, weakness and/or paralysis) of the lower extremities, ataxia, impotence. Primary adrenal failure	Slowly, sometimes rapidly
Addison's disease only	>2	8–14	Fatigue, hypotension, diffuse or focal bronzing of skin. May occur at any age	–
Pre- or symptomatic ALD	–	4–10	Genetic and biochemical disorder without any evident neurological involvement. Risk of developing neurological symptoms high, but some patients remain asymptomatic for many years	–

AMN, adrenomyeloneuropathy.
Source: adapted from van Geel *et al.* [87].

Approximately half the patients have normal MRI results although they are at risk for developing the cerebral form of X-ALD.

Addison only phenotype

These are male patients who have primary adrenocortical insufficiency without clinical or MRI evidence of neurological involvement [16].

Asymptomatic/normal MRI phenotype

These are males commonly diagnosed by family screening and they have the biochemical and gene abnormality of X-ALD. They are at high risk of developing one of the other phenotypes at a later stage.

Heterozygous females

Neurological symptoms may occur in up to 50% of women [31] and vary in severity from mild hyperflexia and vibratory sense impairment, with little or no functional disability, to severe paraparesis in middle age or later [13]. Cerebral involvement is rare and adrenal insufficiency occurs in less than 1% [23]. There is no correlation between clinical severity and VLCFA blood levels [9].

Diagnosis

The diagnosis of X-ALD is made with clinical findings, brain MRI, plasma concentrations of VLCFA and molecular genetic testing of *ABCD1* gene [14]. 99.9% of hemizygous males and 85% of heterozygous female carriers will have increased levels of VLCFA in plasma [32], but a normal result does not exclude carrier status [33].

X-ALD is probably underdiagnosed [25] and may be misdiagnosed as attention deficit hyperactivity disorder in boys and as multiple sclerosis in men and women [31]. In female carriers, molecular analysis of the *ABCD1* gene should provide a reliable diagnosis [33].

Genetic counselling of family members is essential [34] and molecular genetic testing has been used primarily to determine carrier status in at risk female relatives and for prenatal diagnosis when the nature of the familial mutation is known.

Treatment

Adrenal insufficiency is treated with appropriate steroid replacement therapy. The prognosis for patients with symptomatic childhood cerebral X-ALD is poor and specific treatment options are limited. For boys with asymptomatic childhood cerebral X-ALD treatment options include

- Lorenzo's oil
- bone marrow transplant before the onset of neurological symptoms

The inability to predict the future clinical course in individual patients is a major problem when considering the choice of appropriate therapy.

Dietary treatment

Although VLCFA are obtained from dietary sources they are mainly derived from endogenous synthesis through elongation of medium and long chain fatty acids [6]. Consequently, diet therapy has been designed to limit the intake of C26:0 fatty acids and to decrease their synthesis [35] by competition for the microsomal elongation system. The diet is based on Lorenzo's oil and a moderate fat restriction. The aim is to achieve normal plasma C26:0 concentrations [10]. The diet is summarised in Table 20.3.

Table 20.3 Summary of diet therapy used in adrenoleukodystrophy.

Lorenzo's oil	Glyceryl trioleate oil (GTO)	Moderately low fat diet	Vitamin and mineral supplementation	Essential fatty acids	Energy supplements
Description 4 parts GTO: 1 part GTE	**Description** Rich in oleic acid, free of C26:0	**Description** Give 15% of dietary energy as fat (try not to exceed 35% energy from fat)	**Description** Diet is low in fat soluble vitamins and commonly trace elements	**Description** Diet is low in essential fatty acids Lorenzo's oil leads to reduced levels of omega 6 and omega 3 fatty acids	**Description** Energy intake may be low
Dose 20% of energy intake Some boys need less than this to normalise C26:0 levels.	**Dose** No set dose	Note: No other dietary restrictions are necessary	**Type of supplements** Give comprehensive vitamin and mineral supplement, e.g. Fruitvits or Paediatric Seravit	**Type of supplements** Give 1%–2% of total energy from essential fatty acid supplement It should provide a source of linoleic acid and α-linolenic acid in the ratio 4:1 to 10:1, e.g. walnut oil	**Type of supplements** Useful ACBS energy supplements include glucose polymers, glucose drinks (liquid Polycal) and fortified fat free fruit 'juice' drinks (Fortijuce, Paediasure Plus Juce)
Administration Give 2–3 times daily Give neat as a medicine, or mixed with skimmed milk and flavouring or fruit juice Can also be mixed with very low fat yoghurt	**Administration** Use for frying potatoes, fish and meats, salad dressings		**Monitoring** Vitamin and mineral status must be monitored annually		
Not ACBS prescribable	Not ACBS prescribable				

ACBS, Advisory Committee on Borderline Substances; GTE, glyceryl trierucate oil.

Table 20.4 Composition of Lorenzo's oil.

Nutritional information	Composition (per 100 mL)
Energy kcal	807
kJ	3320
Protein g	Nil added
Carbohydrate g	Nil added
Fat g	89.7
Typical fatty acid profile	g/100 g fatty acids
C16:0	0.8
C17:0	0.16
C17:1	0.16
C18:0	2.4
C18:1	73
C18:2	3.25
C18:3	0.16
C20:1	0.48
C22:0	0.02
C22:1	19.1
C24:1	0.36
Other	0.14

Table 20.5 Suggested daily dosage of Lorenzo's oil.

Age (years)	Estimated average requirement for energy kcal (kJ)/day [88]	Daily requirement Lorenzo's oil (mL) (20% of energy intake)
1–3	1230 (5150)	30
4–6	1715 (7160)	45
7–10	1970 (8240)	50
11–14	2220 (9270)	55

Lorenzo's oil

Lorenzo's oil (Table 20.4) is a blend of four parts glycerol trioleate (GTO) and one part glycerol trierucate (GTE) (the triacylglycerol forms of oleic acid C18:1n-9 and erucic acid C22:1n-9). It is therefore high in mono-unsaturated fatty acids. It was developed by Augusto and Micaela Odone to treat their son, Lorenzo, after he was diagnosed with ALD in the 1980s [36].

How does Lorenzo's oil work?

Fatty acid synthesis and elongation are complex highly regulated processes. Endogenous VLCFA are synthesised in microsomes by a series of elongation steps [37] with mono-unsaturated and saturated VLCFA sharing the same microsomal enzyme system [38]. As Lorenzo's oil contains a high proportion of long chain mono-unsaturated fatty acids it probably works by competitive inhibition of the elongation of the saturated docosanoic acid (C22:0) to hexacosanoic acid (C26:0) [39]. In untreated patients the rate of synthesis of C26:0 is increased and the ability to degrade saturated VLCFA is impaired [40] but, when Lorenzo's oil is administered, sustained lowering of plasma C26:0 is achieved.

Dosage and use of Lorenzo's oil

It is recommended that 20% of total energy intake is given from Lorenzo's oil [41]. Examples of calculated daily dosage is given in Table 20.5. Lorenzo's oil is 90% fat providing 8 kcal (34 kJ)/mL. Although this dose normalises plasma C26:0 levels, the figure of 20% is arbitrary. Because of an apparent dose–response effect of Lorenzo's oil on lowering C26:0 concentrations, it has no benefit unless substantial and sustained lowering of C26:0 concentrations are achieved [10, 42]. The GTE component is a solid fat at room temperature. It is about 93% erucic acid which is purified from rapeseed oil. When GTO and GTE are combined a clear yellow liquid is produced, although the GTE can solidify and form white sediment at ambient temperatures.

- Lorenzo's oil should be left at room temperature for 1 hour before use but otherwise should be stored in a refrigerator.
- The bottle should be shaken very well until the white sediment of GTE is evenly distributed throughout the oil so that a homogeneous dose of oil can be given.
- The daily amount of oil should be divided into two or three doses throughout the day. There is no evidence to suggest that its efficacy is affected if taken at different times to meals or in a single dose, although children may develop diarrhoea if the oil is taken in one dose.
- It is difficult to disguise the oily taste or consistency of Lorenzo's oil. Many children take it as a medicine direct from a spoon or by syringe. Some prefer to take it mixed with skimmed milk and milk shake flavouring or fruit juice; unfortunately, it does not mix well with either.
- It may be easier to take the mixture in a covered cup or beaker to help mask the smell and the poorly dispersed fat. Others mix the oil with yoghurt or other low fat desserts.
- It is not recommended to cook with the oil.

Lorenzo's oil is not recommended before 18 months of age because it may lower levels of

Table 20.6   Composition of glyceryl trioleate oil.

Nutritional information	Composition (per 100 mL)
Energy kcal	819
kJ	3367
Protein g	Nil added
Carbohydrate g	Nil added
Fat g	91
Typical fatty acid profile	g/100 g fatty acids
C16:0	1
C17:0	0.2
C17:1	0.2
C18:0	3
C18:1	91
C18:2	4
C18:3	0.2
C20:1	0.4

Table 20.7   Guidelines on daily dietary fat intake.

Age (years)	Estimated average requirement for energy kcal (kJ)/day [88]	Approximate fat intake from food (g/day) (15% of energy intake)
1–3	1230 (5150)	20
4–6	1715 (7160)	30
7–10	1970 (8240)	35
11–14	2220 (9270)	40

docosahexaenoic acid (DHA) which plays an important role in early retinal and brain development [42]. It is unclear at what age Lorenzo's oil therapy could be discontinued in patients who remain neurologically normal and there are no recommendations about stopping diet. There is some evidence of benefit in adult patients with AMN [43] and heterozygous female carriers. It is not available on prescription (Advisory Committee on Borderline Substances, ACBS).

Glyceryl trioleate oil

Glyceryl trioleate oil (GTO) is often used in addition to Lorenzo's oil, specifically as cooking oil. It is a pale yellow oil free of C26:0 and rich in oleic acid (Table 20.6). It is 90% fat providing 8 kcal (34 kJ)/mL. It is useful in the preparation of salad dressings, cakes and biscuits and for frying potatoes, crisps, fish and meats. It should be stored at 4°C under dry conditions. It is not currently available on ACBS prescription and is quite expensive to buy.

Moderately low fat diet

Although the VLCFA that accumulate in X-ALD are mostly of endogenous origin [6], it is recommended that the intake of other dietary fats should be reduced to 15%–20% of total energy [27]. Guidelines for daily fat intake are given in Table 20.7. Moser has suggested that a total fat intake in excess of 30%–35% of total energy (from Lorenzo's oil and dietary fat) may counteract or nullify the C26:0

reducing effect of Lorenzo's oil. Table 20.8 gives examples of permitted foods on a moderately low fat diet. Children soon become bored with such a limited diet and imaginative use should be made of all freely allowed foods to try to prevent anorexia or non adherence.

Energy supplementation

Although the aim is for 20% of total energy intake of the diet to be from Lorenzo's oil, appetite and energy from food is sometimes poor and growth may be affected. It is essential that both nutritional intake and status of patients are assessed at regular intervals and energy supplements given if needed. These include glucose polymers; glucose drinks such as Polycal; milk shakes made from skimmed milk, glucose polymer and low fat milk shake flavourings; or fat free fortified 'juice' drinks such as Paediasure Plus Juce or Fortijuce (Table 11.3). Fortunately, with increasing public awareness of healthy eating, the number of suitable commercially available low fat products has greatly increased which can be incorporated into the diet.

Vitamin and mineral intake

The fat soluble vitamins A, D and E may be low in the diet, and also vitamin C and folic acid. If appetite is poor a comprehensive vitamin and trace mineral supplement such as Paediatric Seravit or Fruitivits (Table 1.23) is advocated. If a child is eating well a fat soluble vitamin supplement may be all that is needed. The dose and type of vitamin and mineral supplement should be determined for the individual child.

Essential fatty acid supplementation

An essential fatty acid (EFA) supplement is recommended for all X-ALD patients, providing linoleic

Table 20.8 Moderately low fat diet.

	Foods allowed	Foods not allowed
Meat and poultry	Extra lean beef, lamb, turkey, chicken, pork; lean ham, bacon	Fatty meat, sausages, salami, black pudding, corned beef
Fish	White fish, e.g. haddock, sole, plaice, whiting; prawns, shrimps; tuna; fish fingers	Oily fish, e.g. sardines, mackerel, kipper, fish canned in oil
Milk	Skimmed milk, low fat yoghurt, Quark, 'diet' low fat cheeses <3% fat	Whole milk, semi-skimmed milk, cream, full fat yoghurt, full fat cheese
Eggs	Egg in moderation	
Pulses, nuts, seeds	Peas, beans, lentils, dhal	Nuts, seeds
Fruit	All fruits (except those on not allowed list)	Avocado, olives
Vegetables	All vegetables (except those on not allowed list) Low fat crisps (<5 g fat per bag): 1 bag per day	Chips, roast potatoes, regular crisps
Fats	Scraping of very low fat margarines Use GTO for cooking	All other fats, oils, butters and margarines
Bread, pasta, rice, cereals and breakfast cereals	All bread, chapatti, pasta, rice, tinned pasta, flours, most breakfast cereals	Breakfast cereals with nuts
Cakes and biscuits	Low fat cakes/biscuits cereal bars (but providing no more than 3 g fat/day in total)	Any other cakes, biscuits, pastries
Puddings and desserts	Jelly, sorbet, meringues, skimmed milk puddings, skimmed milk custard	Ice cream, milk puddings and desserts not made with skimmed milk
Sugar, preserves and spreads	All kinds of sugar Jam, marmalade, honey, syrup	Chocolate spread, peanut butter
Confectionery	Boiled sweets/lollies, gummy sweets, pastilles, jelly beans, marshmallows	Chocolate, toffee, fudge, carob
Soups	Low calorie and 'healthy eating' soups	Cream soups
Beverages	Fruit juice, squashes, tea, coffee, milkshake flavouring, low fat drinking chocolate	Malted milk drinks, cocoa, regular drinking chocolate

GTO, glyceryl trioleate oil.

acid (C18:2ω6) and α-linolenic acid (C18:3ω3) in a ratio of between 4:1 and 10:1. Although GTO contains some linoleic and α-linolenic acid and Lorenzo's oil contains some linoleic acid, the overall quantity of EFA obtained from a moderately low fat diet and Lorenzo's oil is estimated to be approximately only 2% of total energy intake. It is recommended to give a further 1%–2% EFA from supplements such as walnut oil, although Moser recommends 5% [25]. It has been demonstrated that Lorenzo's oil therapy causes reduced levels of omega 6 and omega 3 fatty acids in red blood cells [44, 45].

Some have suggested that a DHA supplement is given in addition to Lorenzo's oil. DHA has an important role in brain development and myelination; it may also lead to an increase in eicosapentaenoic acid (EPA), via a negative feedback mechanism, and EPA and DHA are incorporated into inflammatory cell phospholipids exerting an anti-inflammatory effect [46].

Effectiveness of Lorenzo's oil

A summary of the clinical studies describing the effectiveness of Lorenzo's oil is given in Table 20.9.

Table 20.9   Summary of clinical studies using Lorenzo's oil or GTE ± GTO.

Authors	Trial design	Phenotype of patients	Outcome
Rizzo et al. 1989 [47] USA	Double blind crossover of erucic acid with oleic acid for 2–19 months	12 boys with mild, moderate or severe disease	Mean plasma C26:0 returned to normal in 4 weeks 6 boys with moderate/advanced disease deteriorated 2 with mild disease remained stable at 10 and 19 months follow-up
Uziel et al. 1991 [51] Italy	Erucic acid therapy administered	20 patients with X-ALD 6 severely affected 9 mild neurological disease 5 pre-symptomatic boys	C26:0 returned to normal target ranges in almost all subjects Pre-symptomatic patients remained free of symptoms after 1 year of treatment Symptomatic patients clinically deteriorated
Aubourg et al. 1993 [89] France	Lorenzo's oil given for 18–48 months GTO (1.7 g/kg/body weight) and GTE (0.3 g/kg/body weight)	14 men with AMN 5 symptomatic heterozygous women 5 pre-symptomatic boys	C26:0 returned to normal target ranges in all subjects within 10 weeks 9 of 14 AMN patients clinically deteriorated 1 of 5 pre-symptomatic boys developed myopathy No change in heterozygous women
Korenke et al. 1995 [90] Germany	GTO/GTE given for 19 months	6 X-ALD with symptoms 3 AMN 2 Addison's variant only 5 pre-symptomatic boys	C26:0 returned to normal target ranges in all subjects 7 patients without neurological involvement remained stable 6 of 9 patients with symptoms deteriorated
Di Biase et al. 1998 [91] Italy	GTO/GTE given for 1–9 years	68 subjects 38 with symptomatic X-ALD 15 with AMN 15 pre-symptomatic boys	18 of 38 symptomatic ALD boys clinically deteriorated 5 of 15 AMN men clinically deteriorated 4 of 15 pre-symptomatic boys clinically deteriorated
van Geel et al. 1999 [53] Netherlands	Lorenzo's oil given for 1–6 years	22 patients adults 2 pre-symptomatic 4 Addison's variant only 13 AMN 3 symptomatic carriers	C26:0 returned to normal/almost normal target ranges in 86% of the patients Disability increased in 11 patients and improved marginally in 2
Moser et al. 2003 [42] USA and Europe	Lorenzo's oil given to 2 pre-symptomatic boys for mean of 2.6 years (USA) and 4.3 years (Europe) Aged 2–10 years	69 pre-symptomatic patients USA 36 pre-symptomatic patients Europe Lorenzo's oil provided 20% energy intake	Subjects were divided into two groups according to lowering of plasma VLCFA: group 1 lowered mean annual plasma C26:0 concentrations within 2 SD of normal and group 2 subjects, who were less adherent with diet, failed to do so. A positive association between the degree of lowering of C26:0 concentrations and clinical outcome was observed. The effect was only partial as 24% of group 1 patients developed neurological or MRI abnormalities. Delay in initiating the therapy increased the possibility of neurological involvement

Table 20.9   (*continued*)

Authors	Trial design	Phenotype of patients	Outcome
Moser *et al.* 2005 [10] USA	Lorenzo's oil given for 6.9 ± 2.7 years	89 pre-symptomatic boys with mean age 4.7 ± 4.1 years	24% developed MRI abnormalities and 11% developed neurological and MRI abnormalities. Significant associations occurred with MRI abnormalities and plasma ↑ in C26:0. A 0.6 µg/mL reduction in plasma C26:0 concentration was associated with a twofold reduction in the risk of developing MRI abnormalities. Boys with neurological involvement did not normalise plasma C26:0 concentrations
Kohler *et al.* 2005 [43]	Lorenzo's oil given at 1 mL/kg for 6.3 years (range 2–12.8 years)	47 AMN adults	45 of 47 patients normalised C26:0 levels for at least 2 years 48% remained stable 84% were clinically better than expected based on their own natural history data 6.5% developed progressive cerebral leukodystrophic lesions Lorenzo's oil appeared to slow neurodegeneration

GTE, glyceryl trierucate oil; GTO, glyceryl trioleate oil; AMN, adrenomyeloneuropathy; X-ALD, X-linked adrenoleukodystrophy; MRI, magnetic resonance imaging; VLCFA, very long chain fatty acids.

Early studies demonstrated that Lorenzo's oil could normalise C26:0 concentrations within 4–6 weeks in X-ALD [6,47]. It reduces C26:0 concentrations in the plasma, adipose tissue and liver [48]; however, there has been no increase in brain erucic acid in postmortem samples of Lorenzo's oil treated patients [49].

Lorenzo's oil does not halt the neurological degeneration in the cerebral form of childhood X-ALD [47,50–52] but there is evidence supporting the use of dietary therapy in asymptomatic boys. Indications for treatment with Lorenzo's oil and a moderately low fat diet are given in Table 20.10.

Table 20.10   Indications for treatment with Lorenzo's oil and moderately low fat diet in X-linked adrenoleukodystrophy.

- Offer to male patients with ALD who are neurologically asymptomatic, have normal brain MRI results and are at risk of developing cerebral ALD
- No benefit in X-ALD boys with neurological symptoms
- Lorenzo's oil may delay neurodegeneration but evidence limited
- No benefit in female carriers

MRI, magnetic resonance imaging.

Complications associated with Lorenzo's oil

A number of side effects have been noted with Lorenzo's oil including mild increases in liver enzymes, gastrointestinal complaints and gingivitis [53]; thrombocytopenia [54–57]; decreased membrane anisotrophy [25]; and a reduction of plasma EFA [44,45]. Platelet reduction has been noted in about 30%–40% of patients [10,25] but is not severe enough to warrant discontinuation of diet therapy in the majority, although careful monitoring is recommended. Some suggest discontinuing Lorenzo's oil when platelet count falls unacceptably low, but maintaining patients on GTO as an alternative. This usually results in restoration of platelet count to pretreatment levels when Lorenzo's oil is then resumed but at a lower dose [10].

Other dietary factors that may enhance effectiveness of Lorenzo's oil

There is some evidence that added conjugated linoleic acid (a group of isomers of linoleic acid) could act synergistically with Lorenzo's oil and induce peroxisomal β-oxidation. When administered with Lorenzo's oil to five heterozygous women, it crossed the blood–brain barrier and lowered both saturated C26:0 and C26:0/C22:0 ratio in plasma; the combined supplement also improved somatosensory evoked potentials [39].

Other treatments

- Eighty per cent of asymptomatic patients with ALD develop evidence of adrenal insufficiency [58] and it is essential that corticosteroid replacement treatment be provided. This does not change the neurological progression of the disorder [22].
- Haematopoietic stem cell transplant (HSCT) is the only effective treatment option once there is inflammatory cerebral involvement [24] providing it can be performed at an early stage of brain lesions [59]. Beyond a certain stage, demyelination cannot be arrested and it is not recommended for patients with advanced disease. In patients with early neuropsychological deterioration, it has been shown to reverse or stabilise abnormalities on cerebral MRI [60, 61] and may result in stability of mental ability. Evidence suggests that the 5 year survival for boys absent of clinical disease at HSCT was 91% whereas that for boys with neurological dysfunction was 66% [62]. It is limited by donor related constraints and carries a considerable risk of mortality [59].
- Haematopoietic stem cell gene therapy has recently been reported in patients with ALD and may be of clinical benefit [59] providing it is conducted before the onset of neurological damage.
- Cell transplantation of myelin producing exogenous cells is being extensively explored as a means of remyelinating axons in X-ALD [63].

- Antioxidants have been considered as an adjuvant therapy as Lorenzo's oil does not prevent free radical generation in X-ALD [64].

Monitoring

Regular monitoring of the following is important.

- *Neurological function*: for detecting early deterioration so boys who are potential candidates for HSCT are identified. Asymptomatic boys should be monitored serially for the earliest evidence of demyelination. Monitoring should include brain MRI, neurological examination, neuropsychological evaluation and evoked potentials.
- *VLCFA levels*: to monitor the effect and compliance with Lorenzo's oil. Ideally, these should be checked every 3 months. Most laboratories measure the absolute concentration of C26:0 as well as the C24:0/C22:0 and C26:0/C23:0 ratios [32].
- *Platelet counts and liver function.*
- *EFA and long chain polyunsaturated fatty acids.*
- *Adrenal function.*

Other issues

In boys, once clinical neurological deterioration is evident, further deterioration is usually rapid and it may be only a matter of months before the child is unable to eat or drink adequate amounts to sustain nutrition. Home nasogastric or gastrostomy feeding is usually required with a standard enteral feed; their nutritional management should be similar to other children with severe neurological impairment. Parents provide the majority of care which may lead to physical and psychological stress including a high risk of them developing depression and neurosis [65].

Peroxisomal Biogenesis Disorders

Peroxisomal biogenesis disorders (PBD) are autosomal recessive disorders due to a failure of protein import into peroxisomal matrix or membrane. This results in multiple peroxisomal enzyme deficiencies leading to developmental defects and progressive

neurological involvement [66]. PBD are classified into two diagnostic groups:

- Zellweger spectrum disorders which include the phenotypes of Zellweger syndrome (ZS),

Table 20.11 Biochemical markers in peroxisomal biogenesis disorders.

	Zellweger spectrum disorders		Rhizomelic chondrodysplasia punctata 1
	Severe	Mild	
Very long chain fatty acids	↑↑	↑	Normal
Phytanic acid	↑	↑	↑
Pristanic acid	↑	↑	Normal
Plasmalogens	↓	↓ Normal	↓↓
Pipecolic acid, plasma	↑	↑↑	Normal
Pipecolic acid, urine	↑↑	↑	Normal
Bile acid metabolites	↑↑	↑	Normal

Source: adapted from Steinberg *et al.* [70].

neonatal adrenoleukodystropy (NALD) and infantile Refsum's disease (IRD)
- Rhizomelic chondrodysplasia punctata 1 (RCDP1). Abnormal biochemical findings are outlined in Table 20.11.

Zellweger spectrum disorders (ZSD) have clear clinical similarities and they represent a disease spectrum with varying degrees of overlapping symptoms and outcomes [5]. ZS is the most severe disorder and infants rarely survive beyond the first year. Infants present in the neonatal period with dysmorphic features, severe neurological abnormalities (muscular hypotonia, faltering growth and seizures), psychomotor dysfunction, retinal degeneration, hepatomegaly and multi-organ dysfunction [67–70] and inability to feed. Sensorineural hearing loss may be present. ZS is pan ethnic with an overall estimated incidence of 1 in 50 000 births in the USA to 1 in 500 000 in Japan [71].

In NALD, abnormal clinical features are present at birth and include muscle hypotonia, severe psychomotor disability and faltering growth. These infants are generally blind and deaf with seizures developing during the first few weeks [72]. They usually die by late infancy [1]. Patients with IRD do not have progressive white matter disease and neuronal migration [73]. There is little or no facial dysmorphia and early developmental milestones are usually normal before psychomotor disability develops between 1 and 3 years of age [74]. Most survive into childhood and some reach adulthood.

The symptoms found in RCDP1 include disproportionally short stature with severe shortening and disturbed ossification of the proximal long bones (rhizomelia), typical dysmorphic face and profound psychomotor dysfunction [68, 75]. Most patients present with cataracts and ichthyosis is quite common. Lifespan is variable, with some children dying in the first year and others surviving into young adulthood [70]. Only a few patients with milder forms of RCDP1 have been described [76].

Treatment

There is no effective treatment for PBD. In the severe PBD, including ZS and RCDP1, abnormalities develop *in utero* which consequently limits postnatal treatment. Treatments are mainly for symptom alleviation and support, e.g. anticonvulsants for seizure control, fat soluble vitamins for cholestasis, enteral nutrition for feeding difficulties and aspiration, ophthalmological and auditory interventions, physical and orthopaedic therapy [77].

With the recognition of a larger number of PBD patients with milder phenotypes, a number of experimental diet therapies have been tried [70, 73]. Dietary treatments have targeted individual biochemical defects, e.g. high phytanic acid, low erythrocyte DHA concentrations, high C26:0 concentrations, but the outcome of such interventions is mainly reported in case studies only.

DHA supplementation

Several studies have explored the effect of supplementing with DHA. This is thought to play an important role in membrane integrity. Tissue concentrations are markedly reduced in ZSD due to impaired peroxisomal synthesis, with brain DHA concentrations reduced to as little as 20% of normal and the retina has less than 1% DHA [77].

Preliminary studies demonstrated that oral DHA supplementation increases erythrocyte DHA and there has been reported improvement in clinical status, particularly growth and vision [77–83], but due to variation and severity of ZSD, results are difficult to interpret. However, in nine patients with NALD/IRD it was demonstrated that retinal appearance remained stable in all but one and visual acuity remained stable [77]. Some recommend early supplementation with DHA before any irreversible damage occurs [83].

The Kennedy Krieger Institute, Baltimore, gave 100 mg/kg/day DHA in a randomised, double blind controlled trial to 50 patients aged 1–144 months with ZSD. Supplementation was well tolerated and it increased DHA blood concentrations. However, there was no difference between treated and untreated groups in biochemical outcome, electroretinogram or growth [84]. Some improvements in vision, weight and height were observed but were unrelated to DHA as they occurred in both control and treatment groups [84].

Low phytanic acid diet

A low phytanic acid diet (p. 651) has been recommended for RCDP1 to avoid the longer term consequences of phytanic acid accumulation, particularly in milder forms of RCDP1 [76]. Others have recommended a low phytanic acid diet in milder forms of ZSD [73]. There are no outcome data reported on the use of low phytanic diets in these disorders.

Lorenzo's oil

A combination of Lorenzo's oil (2 g/kg/day) and DHA was given to four patients with ZS. Although Lorenzo's oil lowered plasma C26:0 in two patients and DHA concentrations increased in erythrocyte lipids, all patients died [85]. A further case study of an infant with classical ZS given a combination of Lorenzo's oil, DHA, lunaria oil (rich in nervonic acid) and medium chain triglyceride (MCT) formula found on postmortem that organ VLCFA was reduced and DHA increased in frontal cortex, liver and kidney [86].

Other treatments

Oral bile acid administration has been shown to improve hepatobiliary function in infants with ZS.

Adult Refsum's Disease

Eleanor Baldwin

Genetics

Adult Refsum's disease (ARD) is a rare, autosomal recessive disorder of fatty acid metabolism. ARD is genetically heterogeneous. Two Refsum's disease genes have been identified: phytanoyl-CoA hydroxylase (PhyH) and peroxin-7 (PEX7) [92–94]. Most cases appear to be caused by mutations in the enzyme phytanoyl-CoA hydroxylase which catalyses the second step in the breakdown of phytanic acid to pristanic acid using the CoA derivative as a substrate. 5%–10% of cases seem to be a mild phenotypic variant of RCDP [95] caused by defective import of PhyH through the peroxin-7 PTS-2 transporter system [96].

An enzyme defect in the α-oxidation pathway involving α-methyl-acyl-CoA racemase (AMACR) can mimic adult Refsum's disease, but is associated with elevated pristanic acid levels and much lower levels of phytanic acid than in ARD [92,94,97]. AMACR deficiency has a variable presentation: as a neonate with coagulopathy, possibly a leukodystrophy syndrome and mild cholestasis; or as an adult with late onset sensorimotor neuropathy. The predominant mutation c.154T>C, found in six of seven reported cases, is inherited in an autosomal recessive fashion.

A further Refsum like disorder has been identified, PHARC, characterised by polyneuropathy, hearing loss, ataxia, retinitis pigmentosa and cataract [98]. It is caused by mutations in α/β-hydroxylase-12 (ABDH12), involved in the metabolism of the endocannabinoid 2-arachidonyl-glycerol. It presents with similar symptoms to ARD but patients do not have anosmia and plasma phytanic acid and peroxisomal function are normal.

Biochemistry

ARD is a fatty acid oxidation disorder. Most fatty acids are oxidised in the mitochondria by β-oxidation. However, complicated fatty acids with a methyl or other functional group on carbon 3 can only be broken down by α- or ω-oxidation in the peroxisome [92, 94]. The fatty acid phytanic acid (3,7,11,15-tetra-methyl-hexadecanoic acid) is a common fatty acid in the diet. It is completely exogenous in origin and is derived from microbial breakdown of the chlorophyll molecule to phytol in ruminant animals. Phytol is oxidised to phytanic acid and on ingestion is normally rapidly degraded through α-oxidation so that <10 μmol/L is usually detected in the plasma (Fig. 20.1).

In ARD, there is a block in this metabolic pathway resulting in the accumulation of phytanic acid in the liver, plasma and all fat containing tissues. Plasma concentrations at diagnosis may range from 100 to 6000 μmol/L. There is a much lower capacity secondary pathway for the metabolism of phytanic acid, ω-oxidation [94, 99] (Fig. 20.2). The ω-oxidation pathway in adults may metabolise 6.9–30 mg of phytanic acid per day [99]. Published estimates of phytanic acid intake in adults suggest western diets provide a daily intake of 50–100 mg [100, 101]. Diet plans are usually calculated to provide <10 mg of phytanic acid to allow a gradual

reduction in plasma phytanic acid concentrations and a gradual depletion of phytanic acid stores in fat containing tissues.

Reference values for plasma phytanic acid:

Normal	0–20 μmol/L (usually <10 μmol/L)
Peroxisomal disease	0–320 μmol/L
ARD after 1 year of treatment	20–1000 μmol/L
ARD untreated	100–6000 μmol/L
ARD stable on treatment diet	0–400 μmol/L

Diagnosis

Clinical presentation with acute ARD typically occurs in the second to fifth decade of life [92]. Early features such as night blindness and retinitis pigmentosa are often present in early adolescence and ARD needs to be considered in the differential diagnosis of all adolescent onset night blindness [93, 102]. Earlier presentation with the full syndrome is much less common because a build-up of

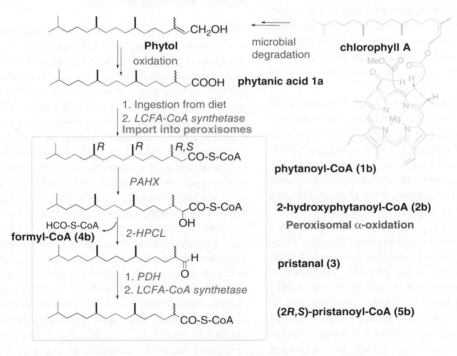

Figure 20.1 Metabolism of chlorophyll to phytol and metabolism of phytanic acid by α-oxidation.

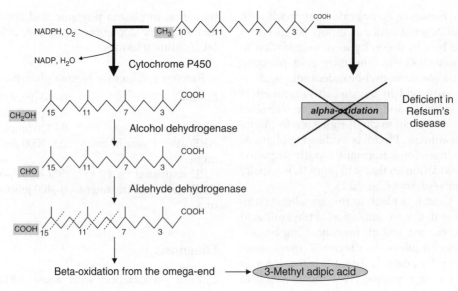

Figure 20.2 ω-oxidation of phytanic acid.

the neurotoxic fatty acid, phytanic acid, takes time as it derives from sources in the diet.

Clinical features of the full syndrome are retinitis pigmentosa, anosmia/hyposmia, peripheral neuropathy, deafness, icthyosis and cerebellar ataxia. Skeletal abnormalities are also common; short third or fourth fingers and toes may be present. When phytanic acid levels are very high icthyosis, acute neuropathy and cardiomyopathy may be present.

Initial presentation is usually in adolescence with night blindness, which progresses to retinitis pigmentosa. Anosmia, though difficult to diagnose, is often present at this stage [103]. Hearing loss occurs progressively from middle age. Symptoms of the full syndrome (peripheral neuropathy, ichthyosis) may be present at diagnosis if the plasma phytanic acid levels are very high, i.e >1000 μmol/L.

A child or adult presenting with acute ARD may be anorexic and experiencing vomiting, making it very difficult to establish feeding. Marked weight loss is likely. If the phytanic acid level is very high plasmapheresis or apheresis (removal of lipoproteins by plasma exchange/filtering) may be important to give some symptomatic improvement so that feeding can be established. It is important to arrest weight loss because a catabolic state increases the acute mobilisation of phytanic acid from body fat and stores in the liver, with a phytanic acid doubling time of 29 hours [99].

Nutritional requirements

There is no evidence that the nutrient requirements of children or adults with ARD are different from the general population. The Chelsea and Westminster Hospital Adult Refsum's Clinic is conducting a study to assess nutritional intake and biochemical micronutrient status of adults with ARD. In general, micronutrient status seems adequate but there may be deficiencies in iron, fat soluble vitamins and EFA based on individual clinical data. In the absence of systematic data, assessment of intake and feeding targets should be compared with dietary reference values [88], allowing for growth or weight gain as appropriate. If the child or adult is anorexic or vomiting enteral feeding may be appropriate using proprietary formulas. Most enteral feeds and oral nutritional supplements do not contain ruminant animal fats and are therefore not a source of phytanic acid, but some do contain fish oil which is also a concentrated source of phytanic acid. The ingredients label should be studied to establish suitability, but it may be wise to contact the feed manufacturer to check that the ingredients are fully declared.

General dietary principles

A dietary aim of providing <10 mg phytanic acid daily (taking into account that the ω-oxidation pathway in adults may metabolise 6.9–30 mg of phytanic acid per day) may be achieved by the following dietary manipulations:

- *Avoidance of foods with a high phytanic acid content.* These foods are listed in Table 20.12. Foods with no or only trace amounts of phytanic acid are listed in Table 20.13.
- *Avoidance of rapid weight loss or fasting.* Nutritional support needs to be aggressive during intercurrent illness, surgery or any other circumstances where food intake is reduced in order to avoid an acute exacerbation in symptoms. A rapid rise in plasma phytanic acid levels due to the liberation of phytanic acid stores in the liver and adipose tissue will occur.
- *Appropriate growth and frequent dietary review.* A review of ARD cases following the dietary advice advocated by the author's hospital for more than 10 years (Chelsea and Westminster Hospital, London, as described in Tables 20.12 and 20.13) revealed flavour fatigue was common [104]. This may reduce dietary compliance, reduce intake and affect growth.
- *A good fruit and vegetable intake.* Fruit and vegetables are rich sources of lutein and zeaxanthin, carotenoids which are believed to protect the eye by acting as blue light filters and antioxidants. Some studies have shown there may be an improvement in vision in people with retinitis pigmentosa when given an oral supplement containing 10–30 mg of lutein [105, 106]. A good intake of lutein and zeaxanthin can be obtained by eating a variety of fruits and vegetables every day. Dark green leafy vegetables are the richest sources of lutein and zeaxanthin and one (250 ml capacity) cup daily provides sufficient quantities. Eggs are also a good source [107]. Caution should be exercised on the promotion of oral supplements of these substances because of the lack of long term data or information on toxicity. Caution should also be exercised on the promotion of a high fruit and vegetable intake where appetite is poor or there are difficulties attaining and maintaining an adequate energy intake. The diet for adult Refsum's disease is essentially a low fat diet which can make it difficult to achieve an adequate energy intake. Achievement of this dietary recommendation regarding fruit and vegetables is therefore very much a lower priority.
- *Limited caffeine intake.* A high intake of caffeine can increase the concentration of phytanic acid in the blood by increasing peripheral and hepatic lipolysis [108], thus increasing the release of phytanic acid from fat containing tissues. Whilst the quantity of caffeine required to produce this effect may be high, some children and adolescents regularly consume large amounts of caffeine in the form of energy drinks. The risks of caffeine abuse and toxicity in children who do not have ARD have been described [109, 110]. Sports and energy drinks are not recommended for children, adolescents or adults with ARD.
- *Supplementation with EFA.* Fish and oil rich fish are significant sources of phytanic acid and as such are excluded from the diet for ARD. In order to ensure that EFA requirements are met, supplementation is required. The phytanic acid content of Omacor, a supplement of eicosapentaenoic acid (EPA) and docosahexaenoic acid (DHA), is very low. The optimum dose is unknown, but it is the practice at the author's hospital to prescribe 1 capsule (1000 mg) Omacor daily.

Monitoring and follow-up

It is important to have regular follow-up to ensure that growth is adequate, nutritional intake meets requirements and dietary compliance is good. Nutritional support should be aggressive during periods of intercurrent illness to minimise any rise in plasma phytanic acid concentration due to catabolism or rapid weight loss. Most oral nutritional supplements and enteral feeds are suitable, but the ingredients should be checked to ensure that fish oils and ruminant animal products are not present. Dietary management should generally suffice, but where the phytanic acid concentration is very high (800–1000 µmol/L) and the patient is symptomatic plasmapheresis/apheresis may be necessary to remove phytanic acid from the plasma.

When the plasma phytanic acid concentration is reasonably controlled (<200 µmol/L) cardiac symptoms, peripheral neuropathy and ichthyosis resolve. No further progression of hearing loss

Table 20.12 Foods containing phytanic acid.

Foods rich in phytanic acid – avoid	Foods low in phytanic acid – eat instead
Meat products Beef, beefburgers, cottage pie Calves liver and kidneys Duck Goose Lamb, mutton, shepherd's pie Rabbit	**Meat and meat substitutes** Bacon Chicken, chicken liver Eggs Ham Pork, pork liver and kidneys Turkey Bean curd, tofu Quorn Soya meat substitutes, e.g. soya mince, soya sausages
Dairy products Cheese made from cow, sheep or goat milk Cream Cow's milk (full cream or semi-skimmed) Goat milk Sheep milk Ice cream Yoghurt (full cream or Greek style) Butter, ghee, suet	**Dairy products** Cheese substitutes made from soya (e.g. PURE soya cheese spread, Redwood soya cheeses, Bute Island Foods soya cheeses) Cream substitute (e.g. Alpro Soya single cream, Soya Too dairy free spray cream, Soya Too cooking cream, Soya Too topping cream) Skimmed cow's milk Soya milk Swedish Glace ice cream substitute Fat free or virtually fat free yoghurt Soya yoghurt style puddings Low fat spreads made only from vegetable oil (e.g. the PURE range) Vegetable ghee, vegetable suet, lard
Fish Fish, especially oily fish (e.g. herring, salmon, sardines) Shellfish: clams, mussels, octopus, prawns, shrimps Fish oil	**Fish substitutes** Soya or pulse based fish substitutes (e.g. Redwood fish style fingers, fish style steaks, scampi style pieces, Thai fish style cakes)
Nuts Walnuts, peanuts	**Nuts** Very few nuts have been analysed
Bread and baked goods Brioche, croissants, shortcrust pastry Biscuits and cakes made with butter, suet or fish oil	**Bread and baked goods** Filo pastry, e.g. Jus-rol All bread, biscuits and cakes which do not contain butter, suet or fish oil
Breakfast cereals Tesco Chocosnaps	**Breakfast cereals** Breakfast cereals that do not contain milk powder (skimmed milk powder is allowed) Small portions only of cereals containing nuts, e.g. muesli
Confectionery Milk chocolate	**Confectionery** Dark chocolate, carob, chocolate that does not contain milk fat or butter Fat free sweets, e.g. boiled sweets
Alcoholic drinks Any drinks containing cream (e.g. Bailey's Irish Cream)	**Alcoholic drinks** Any alcoholic drink that does not contain cream

Data on manufactured foods is not available as food products are not routinely analysed for their phytanic acid content. Any recommendation for using manufactured foods can only be based on the published data above or by scrutinising ingredient labels.
Source: Brown *et al.* [112].

Table 20.13 Foods known to contain no or only trace amounts of phytanic acid.

Any foods which are fat free
Most breakfast cereals (for exceptions see Table 20.12)
Safflower oil, corn oil, olive oil, sunflower seed oil
Bread, rice, pearl barley, pasta
Jelly
Honey
Tea, coffee
Cooked green vegetables, carrots, mushrooms, onions, potato and swede
Salad vegetables
Fruit

or anosmia occurs. However, retinitis pimentosa continues to progress, but may be stable for some time before a stepwise deterioration occurs. Visual deterioration can occur at different rates in siblings within an affected family; some may be blind by their 40s, others may retain some vision past this time. Depression, particularly associated with visual loss, can be a significant management problem.

Future research areas

Some case reports suggest that the prescription of a gastric lipase inhibitor, Orlistat, which is licensed for weight loss may improve plasma phytanic acid levels by reducing absorption of fat from the diet. However, the exact balance between Orlistat improving adherence to dietary treatment and any direct effects on phytanic acid absorption remain to be clarified. This medication needs to be used

carefully in order to avoid acute weight loss which can raise phytanic acid levels [111].

Medications which upregulate the ω-oxidation pathway of phytanic acid are an avenue for current research following the development of a mouse model for ARD.

The role of EFA supplementation in increasing phytanic acid metabolism, or whether it directly protects the retina in the eye, needs to be explored.

The potential role of autologous stem cell retinal pigment epithelium transplantation in the treatment of the disorder and the prevention of recurrence of deterioration is a further research area.

The food composition data on which the dietary management for ARD is based is out of date and very narrow in scope [112]. There are applications in process for research funding to analyse foods to update dietary data.

Useful resource

The Chelsea and Westminster diet sheet includes the information shown in Tables 20.12 and 20.13, together with guidance on the avoidance of fasting, managing intercurrent illness and restricting caffeine intake. This diet sheet is currently available in English and French from www.dietetics@chelwest.nhs.uk free of charge.

Dietary information for the management of ARD developed by the Chelsea and Westminster Dietetic Department is also published on the Refsums network www.health.groups.yahoo.com/group/refsums_discussion.

21

Childhood Cancers

Evelyn Ward

Introduction

With advances in the treatment of childhood cancers achieving an overall cure rate that now exceeds 70% in developed countries, with figures up to 80% now being quoted [1, 2], the role of nutrition has become essential in terms of treatment, supportive care and treatment related morbidity. Childhood cancers are rare and currently in the UK 1 in 600 children under the age of 15 years develops a cancer, equating to approximately 1700 newly diagnosed children each year [3]. Childhood cancers generally refer up to the age of 15 years. These cancers are different from cancers affecting adults in terms of appearance, location and response to treatment. However, older adolescents and young adults who develop paediatric type malignancies are generally treated on the same treatment protocols as younger children. There are 21 Children's Cancer and Leukaemia Group (CCLG) principal treatment centres in the UK with many having dedicated Teenage Cancer Trust Units where adolescents are treated. Many of the 21 principal treatment centres have shared care facilities with local district general paediatric wards.

As survival rates from childhood cancers increase the need to maintain growth and development is paramount. Both advances in the use of multimodal therapy and combination chemotherapy and/or the primary diagnosis frequently result in nutritional depletion. It is well documented that malnutrition is a common complication of paediatric malignancy and its treatment.

The consequences of malnutrition are multiple and include a possible influence on outcome, with children who are underweight at diagnosis having a poorer outcome compared with those who are adequately nourished at diagnosis [4, 5]. Malnutrition contributes to a reduced tolerance to therapy and protein-calorie intake may affect the sensitivity to chemotherapy agents [6–10]. Malnutrition may contribute to problems of drug toxicity due to altered pharmokinetics secondary to changes in body composition and relationship between body surface area and lean body mass [7, 11]. The relationship between malnutrition and increased risk of infection is well documented in the child with cancer [10, 12]. However, the evidence of malnutrition at diagnosis or during treatment on overall survival is controversial and may depend on the disease and its extent [10, 13, 14].

The provision of safe, appropriate and effective nutritional support for the child undergoing treatment for cancer is well recognised as an important part of supportive care in order to enhance therapy, decrease complications, improve immunological status and improve quality of life.

Types of cancers seen in childhood

The types of cancers seen in children can be divided into three main groups:

- leukaemias
- lymphomas
- solid tumours

Leukaemias

Leukaemia is the most common malignant disease in infancy and childhood and accounts for one-third of all childhood cancers. Acute lymphoblastic leukaemia (ALL) is the most common form of the disease in childhood with its incidence highest at 3–7 years of age, falling off by 10 years [15]. Boys are affected more than girls. Approximately 80% of ALL in children is of precursor B-cell origin, about 15% is T-cell and 5% is more mature B-cell derived. Acute myeloid leukaemia (AML) is the second most common leukaemia in childhood accounting for 10%–15% of leukaemias, with 15%–20% of the cases occurring in patients with predisposing conditions that include certain congenital syndromes such as Down's syndrome, Li –Fraumeni syndrome or DNA instability syndromes such as Fanconi anaemia [16]. Although rare, accounting for 15% of leukaemias, chronic myeloid leukaemia (CML) can occur in older children.

Five year survival rates are around 87% in children with ALL and 65% for those with AML [17]. It should be noted, however, that prognosis in infants with ALL is poor.

The leukaemias are fatal unless treated and clinical features at presentation include bone marrow failure, anaemia (pallor, lethargy), neutropenia (fever, malaise), thrombocytopenia (bruising, purpura, bleeding gums, nose bleeds) and organ infiltration; tender bones; lymphadenopathy; splenomegaly; hepatomegaly.

Diagnosis is by blood test usually showing the total white cell count to be decreased, normal or increased to 200×10^9/L. Blood film examination typically shows a variable number of blast cells. A hypercellular bone marrow aspirate with >20%

leukaemic blasts confirms diagnosis. A lumbar puncture is performed to confirm any leukaemia cells in the spinal fluid. Biochemical tests may show raised serum uric acid and serum lactate dehydrogenase (LDH) levels [15].

Current treatment for ALL includes initial induction chemotherapy aimed at achieving remission. The protocol is graded as regimen A for those children with standard risk disease; regimen B for those children with intermediate risk disease; and regimen C for those children with high risk disease who have not responded to initial treatment, or those with poor cytogenetics: Philadelphia chromosome t (9;22); near haploidy (<44 chromosomes); iAMP21 t (17;19); and MLL gene arrangement. All of these are rare.

Following induction the next phase of treatment is consolidation (intensification) and central nervous system (CNS) treatment aimed to completely reduce or eliminate the tumour burden and to prevent or treat CNS disease. There are one to two intensification treatment blocks in children depending on the presence of any minimal residual disease (MRD) detected after induction chemotherapy.

Maintenance chemotherapy is then given for up to 2 years in girls and up to 3 years in boys. Children with CNS disease at diagnosis may need to have cranial radiotherapy.

Intensive chemotherapy is primarily the treatment for AML, generally given as four blocks of chemotherapy 3 weeks apart, but may be delayed if the patient has not recovered their neutrophil and platelet counts to an acceptable level before commencing the next course of chemotherapy. Bone marrow transplant (BMT) is used for children with ALL or AML which is likely to recur, or for those who have relapsed disease.

Lymphomas

Lymphomas account for approximately 10% of all childhood cancers and can be divided into two main groups:

- non Hodgkin's lymphomas (NHL) account for 60% of lymphomas and are a large group of lymphoid tumours. Those most commonly seen in children include B-cell NHL and T-cell NHL. The majority of patients present with asymmetric enlargement of lymph nodes in one or more peripheral lymph node regions. Those with diffuse bone marrow disease present with anaemia, neutropenia or thrombocytopenia. Diagnosis is made by a variety of investigations including biopsy of a swollen gland, x-rays, ultrasound scans (USS), computerised tomography (CT) scans and biochemical tests. Serum LDH levels are raised in more rapidly proliferating and extensive disease. Five year survival rates are around 85% [17]. Chemotherapy is the most important treatment for children with NHL. High dose chemotherapy and autologous stem cell transplant is sometimes used in relapsed disease.

- Hodgkin's lymphoma accounts for 40% of lymphomas. Presenting symptoms are usually painless cervical and/or mediastinal adenopathy. Symptoms also generally include fever, night sweats, weight loss, fatigue and anorexia. Hodgkin's disease is more common in adolescents than younger children. Diagnosis is made by biopsy of a swollen lymph gland, x-rays, CT scan, magnetic resonance imaging (MRI) and in some cases positron emission tomography (PET) scans. Biochemical tests include erythrocyte sedimentation rate (ESR) and C-reative protein (CRP) which are usually raised and are useful in monitoring disease progression. Serum LDH levels are increased in 30%–40% of cases. Five year survival rates are around 95% [17]. Treatment is by chemotherapy, with radiotherapy restricted to those with extended disease or lack of response to chemotherapy. Some relapsed patients may require high dose chemotherapy and autologous stem cell transplant.

Solid tumours

Solid tumours account for approximately 45% of all malignant disease in children. Diagnostic tests for most solid tumours include tumour biopsy, x-rays, USS, CT and MRI scans and in some cases PET scans and bone scans. The most common solid tumours seen in children are as follows.

- *Brain tumours.* Brain and spinal CNS tumours are the most common solid tumours. Medulloblastoma is the most common CNS tumour in children. Signs and symptoms of CNS tumours are generally caused by increased intracranial pressure and include headaches, vomiting, drowsiness, irritability, fits and diplopia. Other symptoms may include weakness or unsteadiness on walking. Treatment varies depending on the underlying tumour but surgery, radiotherapy or chemotherapy may be used alone or in combination. Steroids may be given to reduce swelling around the brain and a ventriculoperitoneal shunt may need to be inserted. Five year survival rate for medulloblastoma is around 80% for children with standard risk disease and between 40% and 60% in those with high risk disease, i.e. those with disseminated disease or who have undergone a subtotal resection [18].

- *Neuroblastoma* is the most common tumour before the age of 5 years and accounts for 8% of all childhood cancers. It arises from the neural crest tissue in the adrenal medulla and elsewhere in the sympathetic nervous system; therefore it most frequently occurs in one of the adrenal glands but can also occur alongside the spinal cord in the neck, chest, abdomen or pelvis. Most children present with an abdominal mass, loss of appetite, lethargy and bone pain. At presentation the tumour mass can often be large and complex. A variety of tests and investigations are undertaken to confirm diagnosis including meta-iodo-benzyl guanidine (mIBG) scan. Urinary catecholamine levels are raised in neuroblastoma. Chromosomes and biological markers are also examined following tumour biopsy and the presence of one of the markers, MYCN, in a certain amount in the cells (known as MYCN amplification) suggests more aggressive disease and treatment is more intensive. Treatment and survival depends on the stage of the disease. In those with high risk disease treatment involves chemotherapy, surgery, radiotherapy and in some cases high dose chemotherapy and autologous stem cell transplant. 1-*cis*-retinoic acid is being used as a differentiating agent to reduce the risk of relapse in high risk patients. The use of the monoclonal antibody anti-GD2, with or without interleukin-2 alongside, is currently being investigated for high risk disease. Five year survival rate is currently around 64% [17].

- *Wilms' tumour* is a congenital malignant kidney tumour, which can be bilateral. It is most commonly seen in children under the age of 5 years with the majority presenting with a large abdominal mass. Other symptoms may include poor weight gain and loss of appetite, blood in the urine and high blood pressure. Children with the WT1 gene or WT1 syndromes have an increased risk of developing a Wilms' tumour. Treatment depends on histology and stage of the tumour but usually involves surgery, chemotherapy and occasionally radiotherapy. Prognosis for Wilms' tumour is good with 5 year survival rates around 90% [17].

- *Rhabdomyosarcoma* is the most common type of soft tissue sarcoma in children which develops from muscle or fibrous tissue. It can develop at any age but is more common in children under 10 years. There are two main subgroups: embryonal (80%) and alveolar (20%). Rhabdomyosarcoma occurs at a wide variety of primary sites but is most common around head and neck sites. Other sites include genito-urinary and occasionally limb, chest or abdominal wall. Treatment depends on tumour size, position and whether or not metastatic disease is present but involves chemotherapy, surgical resection and sometimes radiotherapy. Five year survival rate is around 65% [17].

- *Ewing's sarcoma and peripheral primitive neuroectodermal tumour (pPNET)*. Ewing's sarcoma is a type of bone tumour. Any bone can be affected but it is more common in the pelvis, femur or shin bone. It can occur in the teenage years but is also seen in younger children. Persistent localised bone pain is a characteristic symptom that usually precedes the detection of a mass. Treatment involves chemotherapy followed by surgery, usually limb sparing but sometimes amputation is unavoidable followed by further chemotherapy and radiotherapy especially if surgical resection is impossible or incomplete. Poor responders may receive high dose chemotherapy and autologous stem cell transplant. Five year survival rates are around 65% [17]. pPNET is a soft tissue sarcoma of neuroepithelial origin which can be thought of as being similar to a Ewing's sarcoma.

- *Osteosarcoma* is a high grade bone tumour which is more commonly seen in older children and teenagers and is more common in boys. It often occurs at the end of bones where new bone tissue is forming, predominantly in the arms or legs, particularly around the knee. Pain and swelling around the affected bone are the most common symptoms. Treatment depends on factors including size, position and stage of the tumour and initially involves chemotherapy. Surgery may be amputation or limb sparing surgery. Further chemotherapy is then given and treatment lasts for about a year. Radiotherapy may occasionally be given. Five year survival rates are around 50%–60% [17].

- *Retinoblastoma* is the commonest malignant eye tumour in children, accounting for around 3% of childhood cancers with most occurring under the age of 5 years. All bilateral tumours are thought to be hereditary due to the RB1 gene in 40% of cases, as are 15% of unilateral cases. Children of affected families are screened from birth. Diagnostic tests include an eye examination under anaesthetic and a blood test to look for the RB gene. Treatment options include local treatment with cryotherapy, laser therapy, external beam therapy, chemotherapy and plaque brachytherapy and in some cases enucleation is necessary. Five year survival rates are over 90% [17].

- Additional information on rarer tumours, e.g. hepatoblastoma and germ cell tumours, can be obtained from the Children's Cancer and Leukaemia Group (CCLG) website [3].

Aetiology of malnutrition in children with cancer

The incidence of malnutrition in paediatric oncology at diagnosis is variable partly due to the variation in studies conducted on different types of paediatric malignancies and variation in nutritional assessment parameters used [10]. The estimated incidence of malnutrition ranges from 6% to 50% depending on the type, stage and location of the disease [4, 19, 20]. It is estimated that malnutrition is present in <10% of children with standard risk ALL but the prevalence increases to 50% in children with advanced solid tumours such as neuroblastoma, Wilms' tumours and sarcomas [20, 21]. Malnutrition is more severe with aggressive tumours in the later stages of malignancy, occurring in up to 37.5% of newly diagnosed patients with metastatic disease [22]. The risk of nutritional morbidity is higher in patients with a greater tumour burden and higher treatment intensity. The initial nutritional problems resulting from the tumour are soon compounded by iatrogenic nutritional abnormalities, the consequence of the treatment and its complications. Metabolic and psychological factors also have a role [23–25].

Metabolic factors

Cancer cachexia is complex and multifactorial marked by early satiety, weight loss, organ dysfunction and tissue wasting. Changes in the metabolism of fat, carbohydrate and protein have been demonstrated in the cancer bearing host [26, 27]. In children with cancer the result is a cascade of metabolic events, which are typically characteristic of the acute metabolic response. In addition to glycogenolysis and lipolysis this response includes a marked increase in energy expenditure, proteolysis and gluconeogenesis. This response results in an accelerated depletion of endogenous energy and substrate stores in the face of decreased exogenous fuel substrate provision [6].

Cachexia is more common in children with solid tumours at diagnosis (33%) and during treatment (57%) compared with children with leukaemia (12% and 38%) respectively [28]. Severe weight loss in children with leukaemia appears to be associated with more intensive treatment regimens such as those for AML and children treated on regimen C.

With the ever increasing intensity of treatment regimens and treatment of relapsed patients there is a greater number of children at risk of the metabolic demands of their disease and treatment.

Complications of the disease and treatment

Anorexia, mucositis, vomiting, diarrhoea and alterations in taste are important contributory factors to the weight loss seen in children undergoing treatment for cancer [29]. Nutritional status can deteriorate rapidly, particularly during the initial intensive phases of treatment if nutrition support is not provided [30]. Table 21.1 shows the side effects relating to drugs commonly used in treatment of paediatric malignancies.

Table 21.1 Side effects relating to treatment seen in paediatric oncology patients.

Side effect	Causative drug
Infection	Both chemotherapy and radiotherapy are known immune depressants
Diarrhoea	Actinomycin, doxorubicin, methotrexate, cytosine, interleukin-2
Nausea and vomiting	Actinomycin, carboplatin, cisplatin, cyclophosphamide, doxorubicin, ifosfamide, cytosine, etoposide, methotrexate, procarbazine, thioguanine, interleukin-2
Stomatitis mucositis	Actinomycin, adriamycin, daunorubicin, doxorubicin, epirubicin, bleomycin, melphalan, methotrexate
Renal damage and nutrient loss	Cisplatin, cyclophophamide, ifosfamide
Constipation	Vincristine
Weight gain and raised blood glucose levels	Dexamethasone, prednisolone
Hypoalbuminaemia	L-Asparaginase
Pancreatitis	L-Asparaginase
Weight loss	α-Interferon
Bone morbidity	Dexamethasone, prednisolone, methotrexate, ifosfamide Vincristine (due to reduced physical activity) L-Asparaginase ? associated with osteonecrosis

Psychological factors

Learned food aversions, nausea and vomiting associated with foods consumed close to chemotherapy administration have been demonstrated in children with cancer along with the phenomenon of anticipatory vomiting [31]. Food is one area of treatment that both the child and parent can try to control resulting in increased tension and anxiety around food, which can lead to negative feeding behaviour and eating becoming an unpleasant experience for both the child and their family.

Identification of nutritional risk and assessment

Assessment of nutritional status is a vital component of supportive care and is essential for monitoring the need for nutritional intervention. Nutritional status indices may be useful prognostic markers of response to therapy or toxicity [32]. Accurate height and weight measurements are the mainstay of nutritional assessment in children with cancer [33]. However, the reliability of weight related indices is reduced in children with solid tumours, particularly those with large abdominal tumours, e.g. neuroblastoma, hepatoblastoma, Wilms' tumour, and therefore a measurement independent of tumour mass, such as mid upper arm circumference or triceps skin fold thickness, should be undertaken.

It is well documented that the nutritional risk of the child with cancer is associated with the diagnosis of certain tumours and stages of the disease, either as a result of the underlying disease and/or as a result of the anticipated toxicity from the current treatment protocol (Table 21.2) [34, 35]. Recently new paediatric, nurse administered nutrition screening tools have been developed and validated [36, 37]. They are not specific for children with cancer as, due to the scoring systems used, the vast majority of children on active treatment would score as being high risk. A recent study highlighted that no simple methods were found to accurately identify poor nutritional status in children treated for malignancy [38]. There is also inconsistency between treatment centres [39]. As a result the UK Royal College of Nursing (RCN) has produced a guideline in which nutritional assessment is based on the Screening Tool for the Assessment of Malnutrition in Paediatrics (STAMP) [36], but also uses the criteria in Table 21.2 [35]. This tool, however, has not yet been audited and validated.

Given the potential impact nutritional status and intervention can have on children undergoing treatment for cancer nutritional assessment and early identification for nutrition support is crucial.

Table 21.2 Types of childhood cancers associated with high or low nutritional risk.

High nutritional risk	Low nutritional risk
Advanced disease during initial intense treatment	ALL regimen A patients
High risk neuroblastoma	Non metastatic solid tumours
Stage III and IV Wilms' tumour	Retinoblastoma
High risk rabdomyosarcoma	Hodgkin's disease
Ewing's sarcoma/pPNET	Germ cell tumours
Osteosarcoma Medulloblastoma/CNS PNET	Advanced disease in remission during maintenance treatment
B-cell NHL	
AML	
Some ALL – infants and teenagers regimen B and C patients relapsed ALL	
Bone marrow transplant patients – allogeneic autologous	

pPNETnet, peripheral primitive neuroectodermal tumour; CNS PNET, central nervous system primitive neuroectodermal tumour; NHL, non Hodgkin's lymphoma; AML, acute myeloid leukaemia; ALL, acute lymphoblastic leukaemia.

Nutritional requirements and feeding

Aiming for the estimated average requirement (EAR) for energy and the reference nutrient intake (RNI) for protein, vitamins and minerals is a useful starting point for the non catabolic, low nutritional risk child with cancer [40]. An estimation of the protein and energy requirements for sick children is given in Table 1.13 and can be useful when determining requirements for the catabolic child with cancer, based on actual body weight and not expected weight. Consideration of requirements and method of nutrition support must be individualised taking into account the child's age, weight and clinical condition. The RCN guideline includes a useful algorithm for nutritional intervention for the child with cancer (Fig. 21.1).

Oral feeding

Advice should be given routinely about

- the impact of cancer and its treatment on nutritional status
- eating problems related to the side effects of treatment
- food safety
- use of high energy foods and small frequent meals and snacks [41]

Oral feeding is the best method of nutrition support in patients with a low nutritional risk if they are able to consume enough food. However, some will require oral nutritional supplements, e.g. Frebini, Frebini Energy, Fortini, Fortini Energy, Paediasure, Paediasure Plus, Paediasure Plus Juce, Resource Junior (Table 11.3), and advice on how to modify them in order to improve their palatability. Many children often have good intentions to comply with taking dietary supplements but this is often hindered by the taste abnormalities associated with treatment so limiting their usefulness in this patient group. Fresh milk based supplements have been shown to be more acceptable [42], e.g. Calshake, Scandishake. Low volume energy supplements can be more acceptable, e.g. Pro-Cal Shot, Calogen, Fresubin 5 kcal SHOT and glucose liquid added to drinks, e.g. Polycal liquid, liquid Maxijul. The aim in feeding these children should be to provide the right food at the right time by taking a

flexible approach tailored to the individual needs of the child, with less reliance on dietary supplements [35, 43]. With this is mind some treatment centres have the facility for meals to be prepared at ward level and there is currently a national campaign in the UK by one of the leading childhood cancer support charities, CLIC Sargent, to encourage all centres to provide a more flexible meal service.

Enteral nutrition

Children at higher nutritional risk due to their disease and/or treatment should be identified early in treatment and enteral nutrition (tube feeding) instigated; early intervention can prevent nutritional decline during treatment [30]. Enteral nutrition has been successful in reversing malnutrition and maintaining adequate nutritional status. Studies report that nasogastric feeding during intensive treatment results in improved nutritional status with minimal complications, and improves energy intake and wellbeing [44–46].

The advantages of enteral nutrition over parenteral nutrition (PN) are well documented [34, 45, 46]. Enteral feeding also has the advantage of offering an alternative route for administration of medication and additional fluids, and can help to reduce both parental and child anxiety related to achieving an adequate nutritional intake by mouth.

Whilst nasogastric feeding is effective, when there is a need for long term nutrition support the child may find it psychologically unacceptable, especially if going to school and participating in normal activities. Other problems such as vomiting, thrombocytopenia, mucositis and dysphagia also result in a reduced acceptance of nasogastric feeding. Studies have demonstrated that gastrostomy feeding is a safe and effective method of delivering nutrition support in terms of cost and nutritional status. It was only associated with minor complications such as inflammation, minor infections and over-granulation of the gastrostomy site that required topical or systemic antibiotics [47–49]. Table 21.3 gives criteria for gastrostomy tube placement in children with cancer. Nasojejunal or jejunostomy feeding should be considered in children with prolonged vomiting or gastric dysmotility associated with treatment in whom antiemetics and prokinetics have had a limited

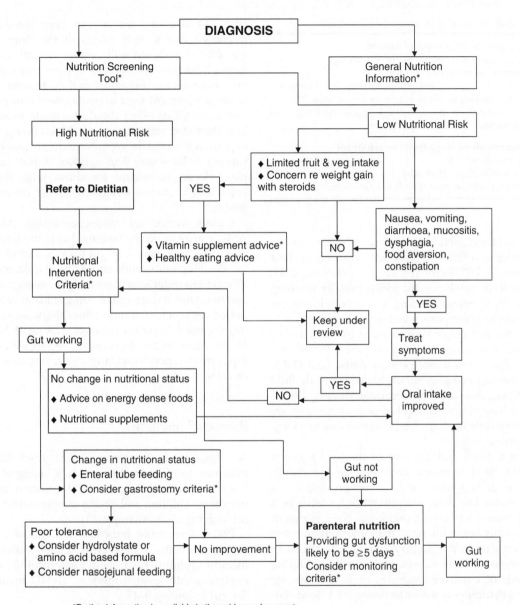

DIAGNOSIS

Nutrition Screening Tool*

General Nutrition Information*

High Nutritional Risk

Low Nutritional Risk

Refer to Dietitian

♦ Limited fruit & veg intake
♦ Concern re weight gain with steroids

YES

Nausea, vomiting, diarrhoea, mucositis, dysphagia, food aversion, constipation

♦ Vitamin supplement advice*
♦ Healthy eating advice

NO

Nutritional Intervention Criteria*

YES

Keep under review

Gut working

Treat symptoms

No change in nutritional status
♦ Advice on energy dense foods
♦ Nutritional supplements

NO

YES

Oral intake improved

Change in nutritional status
♦ Enteral tube feeding
♦ Consider gastrostomy criteria*

Gut not working

Poor tolerance
♦ Consider hydrolystate or amino acid based formula
♦ Consider nasojejunal feeding

No improvement

Parenteral nutrition
Providing gut dysfunction likely to be ≥5 days
Consider monitoring criteria*

Gut working

*Further information is available in the guidance document.

Algorithm reproduced from *Nutrition in children & young people with cancer*, RCN guidance [35]

Figure 21.1 RCN pathway for nutritional management of paediatric oncology patients. Reprinted with permission of Springer.

effect. Jejunal feeding has been particularly useful in weaning children with poor gastric motility off PN.

The choice of enteral feed depends on the child's age, gastrointestinal function and, to some degree, their treatment protocol. Generally an age appropriate standard nutritionally complete enteral feed will be tolerated in children with a normal gastrointestinal function. Children at risk of constipation due to vincristine treatment should routinely receive a fibre containing feed. Following chemotherapy a protein hydrolysate or amino acid based feed (Table 7.11) may be more appropriate if there is malabsorption and should

Table 21.3   Indications for gastrostomy placement.

Indications for gastrostomy placement
Patients treated on intensive protocols with high
emetogenicity or risk of mucositis
Patients requiring long term nutritional support ≥ 3 months
Patients unwilling to accept or tolerate a nasogastric tube
Adolescent patients should routinely be offered the choice of
a gastrostomy

Contraindications for gastrostomy placement
Poor anaesthetic risk
Short term feeding < 3 months
Abdominal disease present (individual assessment)

be considered in children with lower gut mucositis, radiation enteritis and those with graft versus host disease (GvHD) involving the gut following BMT. These feeds can be useful whilst initially weaning from PN to enteral feeding. Children with cancer may develop temporary lactose intolerance due to their chemotherapy, compounded by rotovirus or norovirus infection, and then require a lactose free feed. The use of a more energy dense feed (Table 3.3) should be considered in children who are fluid restricted due to veno-occlusive disease (VOD) of the liver, large drug volumes or those who are unable to tolerate high feed volumes due to a large abdominal mass.

The volume and delivery of the feed regimen should be determined according to the child's normal daily routine and can be provided as a continuous infusion, intermittent bolus feeds or a combination of both. Continuous feed regimens are usually better tolerated than intermittent bolus feeding due to the gastrointestinal side effects of treatment such as nausea and vomiting. During periods of intensive treatment or admissions for febrile neutropenia it may be necessary to feed continuously 20–24 hours in order to achieve tolerance and maximum nutrient intake. Children prone to vomiting and those with large abdominal masses tolerate continuous feeding with frequent breaks by feeding in cycles of say 5 hours with 1 hour rest.

Children on treatment frequently require additional electrolyte supplementation of potassium, phosphate, magnesium or calcium; an enteral tube *in situ* can help with their administration and subsequently improve compliance.

Frequent monitoring is essential to provide effective nutrition support as feed (type, volume,

delivery) and oral intake can vary throughout treatment due to side effects of the drugs. The majority of children will require enteral feeding throughout their intensive treatment protocol, but once treatment is completed or they go onto maintenance treatment their appetite usually improves and a conscious effort should be made to reduce and then stop enteral feeding. Maintaining some oral intake whilst being tube fed can make this process a lot easier and quicker. Input from a psychologist is helpful for those with feeding behaviour problems struggling to get off enteral feeding.

Infants treated for cancer, especially ALL or AML, can be more challenging due to the length of treatment, problems with gut toxicity and stomatitis. Weaning onto solids should be started around 17 weeks in order to achieve a higher energy intake and to establish some oral feeding skills in between periods of severe oral mucositis; otherwise feeding development becomes delayed making it harder for the infant to develop normal feeding skills [50]. Input from a speech and language therapist should be considered.

Parenteral nutrition

A recent Cochrane review highlighted limited evidence from individual trials to suggest that PN is more effective than enteral nutrition in well nourished children and young people with cancer undergoing chemotherapy [51].

PN is commonly indicated for children with severe mucositis and enteritis. Other indications include typhlitis, neutropenic enterocolitis, ileus, chylous ascites post surgery or GvHD involving the gut following BMT.

Careful consideration should be given before commencement of PN and it is of limited nutritional benefit if given for less than 1 week [52]. The child's clinical condition may also limit the effectiveness of PN where fluid from medications and blood products need to take precedence over nutritional fluids. The majority of children with cancer will have central venous access so more concentrated solutions can be prescribed in order to maximise protein and energy intakes.

Metabolic complications of PN are well documented [53] and are not significantly different between children with malignancies and other children requiring PN. However, it is important that electrolyte levels are monitored closely, particularly in children with severe diarrhoeal losses or those receiving chemotherapy drugs that impair renal function. Chemotherapy drugs such as cisplatin and ifosfamide can cause renal tubular damage associated with excess losses of magnesium, potassium, phosphate and calcium. Frequently children with large diarrhoeal losses and/or renal tubular dysfunction require electrolyte additions above those normally recommended [53]. The use of the antifungal amphotericin can result in hypokalaemia requiring a higher potassium intake from PN. Care should be taken if the potassium sparing diuretics amiloride, spironolactone or potassium canrenoate are subsequently used to counteract this effect.

Parenteral iron should not be routinely given as the majority receive frequent blood transfusions and hence there is a potential risk for iron overload. Trace element levels should routinely be monitored if PN is required for longer than 2 weeks and then monthly thereafter, as children with cancer receiving PN frequently require extra additions of zinc and selenium.

Nutrition and the child with cancer undergoing bone marrow transplant

BMT is widely used in children with malignancies. Allogeneic transplant is indicated for patients with high risk leukaemia or patients with leukaemia who have disease recurrence. Some children with solid tumours, e.g. high risk neuroblastoma, rhabdomyosarcoma and Ewing's sarcoma may undergo autologous stem cell transplantation.

The priming chemotherapy causes severe nausea, vomiting, mucositis, diarrhoea and protein losing enteropathy. Transient intestinal failure is common. Nutrition support is provided to minimise the morbidity of both the conditioning regimens and complications resulting from the procedure such as GvHD or VOD of the liver.

PN continues to have a role in children who develop severe gastrointestinal toxicity or GvHD. Children on PN receiving steroids as part of their management of GvHD can experience hyperglycaemia and hyperlipidaemia; it may be necessary to use intravenous insulin infusions to manage the hyperglycaemia where a reduction in glucose intake is inappropriate as it would compromise nutritional intake. Children who develop VOD often require a fluid restriction and concentrated PN solutions should be considered to maximise nutrition; sodium additions should be kept to a minimum to prevent/treat ascites.

Adequate nutrition support can be provided enterally [54] and during periods of gut toxicity an amino acid or hydrolysed protein based feed is recommended. Some centres use a graded dietary guideline for children with GvHD consisting of five phases relating to the grade of GvHD:

- phase 1 – gut rest (Grade IV GvHD)
- phase 2 – clear liquid diet and amino acid based enteral feed (Grade III GvHD)
- phase 3 – low fat, low fibre, low acid, low irritant, lactose free diet (Grade III–II GvHD)
- phase 4 – continuation of low fat, low fibre, low acid, low irritant, lactose free diet (Grade II GvHD)
- phase 5 – lactose free diet (Grade II–I GvHD) [55, 56]

Children who receive a cord blood stem cell transplant may have prolonged diarrhoea which is distinct from GvHD and if all other causes have been excluded cord colitis syndrome may be considered [57]. Treatment involves a 10–14 day course of metronidazole alone or in combination with a fluoroquinolone.

In addition patients undergoing BMT are severely neutropenic and need to have a 'neutropenic' or 'clean' diet in order to prevent gastrointestinal infection from food borne pathogens. The provision of a neutropenic/clean diet is described elsewhere (p. 30).

Steroid induced diabetes

Children treated for ALL regularly receive the corticosteroid dexamethasone as part of their treatment. Dexamethasone has potent lymphocytotoxic activity causing lymphoblast lysis. Side effects include an increased appetite and raised blood glucose levels. Hyperglycaemia is usually only transient whilst the child is receiving the dexamethasone; however, in some cases it may be permanent. Children who appear more susceptible to hyperglycaemia include those with a family history of diabetes, those overweight at diagnosis and older children/adolescents.

Sliding scale intravenous insulin is given until blood sugar levels are controlled. Subsequently an alteration in diet may be all that is necessary to control blood sugar levels; however, a twice daily injection of premixed analogue and isophane insulin may be advised, or a basal bolus regimen. Using basal and rapid acting analogue insulins allows greater flexibility with regard to mealtimes as there is no need to adhere to rigid meals and snacks as a bolus of insulin is injected prior to food. Children treated for ALL can have variable appetites and food intakes and hence a basal bolus regimen allows for this variation.

Dietary advice should be simple: the avoidance of rapidly absorbed carbohydrate with suitable alternatives and snack suggestions. Restriction of high fat foods and increased fibre intake may not be appropriate in children who have poor appetites and who would be unable to achieve an adequate energy intake.

Late effects of childhood cancer

The development of curative therapy for the majority of paediatric cancers has resulted in a growing population of childhood cancer survivors who are at an increased risk of various health problems [58, 59].

Bone morbidity

Bone morbidity in children with cancer both during and after completion of treatment is increasingly recognised as both a short term and long term problem [60, 61]. This is especially the case in children who receive large cumulative doses of glucocorticosteroids and methotrexate for treatment, such as ALL. Peak bone mass is attained by late adolescence or early adulthood with approximately 40% of total bone mass accumulated in adolescence. Any interruptions to the normal process of bone mass accretion during childhood and adolescence may impact on skeletal fragility in adulthood [62]. Hence children and adolescents treated for cancer potentially miss the opportunity for skeletal maturation. Other risk factors include reduced physical activity, calcium and vitamin D

deficiency and genetic factors [63]. Other patients at risk include those treated for Ewing's sarcoma and osteosarcoma who have received methotrexate and ifosfamide [58, 64].

Correction of bone mineral loss may be possible by correcting dietary deficiencies including those of calcium and vitamin D; however, in some cases bisphosphonates such as pamidronate or alendronate are given. Advice on improving diet and physical activity should be recognised as a strategy for amelioration and prevention [64].

Obesity

Another well reported effect in childhood cancer survivors is the prevalence of obesity, particularly in children treated for ALL and brain tumours [7]. The majority of studies have looked at ALL survivors where, as well as obesity, there is a high prevalence of endocrine and metabolic disorders such as growth hormone deficiency, hypothyroidism, insulin resistance and hyperlipidaemia [65, 66], being most detrimental in those patients treated with BMT and total body irradiation [66].

The mechanism for the onset of obesity following treatment for ALL may be partly due to a sustained imbalance between energy expenditure and energy intake. Lack of physical activity, high energy intake and metabolic changes following prolonged courses of chemotherapy may all play a part in altering body composition in ALL survivors [59, 61, 67]. Thought should be given to routinely giving 'healthy eating' advice to children treated for ALL and perhaps this should be at the start of or during long term maintenance therapy.

Complementary and alternative diets

Increasing awareness amongst families with regard to the role of alternative or complementary nutritional therapies prompts them to seek information on food choices, dietary supplements and complementary nutritional therapies in a bid to improve quality of life and increase chances of survival [68]. The majority of such diets are made up of components which claim to have three major functions: detoxification, strengthening of the immune system and specific therapies to attack the cancer cell [69].

These diets generally advocate a strict vegetarian or vegan regimen and restrict animal products, salt and refined carbohydrates and only allow small quantities of fat. Many are high fibre, high fruit/fruit juice and vegetable diets and may involve additional detoxification in the form of fasting as well as the use of laxatives and enemas. Some involve the addition of different supplements to the basic diet, which can be in potentially toxic doses. Diets where fruit juice must be taken frequently can result in early satiety and diarrhoea [70] which will be more pronounced in children, leading to weight loss. Malnutrition can occur due to the high fibre content of the diet, the low energy density and low protein content which in turn can result in a reduced immune function, increased toxicity from conventional treatment and therefore a poorer response [69].

High doses of vitamins and minerals may be harmful to children as well as there being a risk of interaction with conventional treatment. With a current 80% cure rate of childhood cancer by conventional treatments it is imperative to ensure nothing is given which has a negative interaction with treatment [69]. It is essential that any parent contemplating the use of an alternative diet seeks appropriate advice from their child's physician or dietitian. Those health professionals treating the child should enquire non-judgementally about their use.

Areas requiring further research

Vitamin supplementation

Parents frequently ask if it is necessary for their child to take vitamin supplements, especially the antioxidant vitamins A, C, E and beta carotene, whilst being treated for cancer. Certain chemotherapy agents' mode of action involves the generation of free radical oxidants to cause cellular damage and necrosis/apoptosis of malignant cells, such as alkylating agents, antitumour antibiotics and platinum compounds. The formation of free radicals, leading to oxidative stress, is one of the main pathogenic mechanisms for toxicity with toxicity being a dose limiting factor for treatment.

Currently there are very few studies looking at changes in antioxidant status and oxidative stress in children undergoing treatment for cancer

and studies generally tend to only involve small patient numbers. It is clear that further studies are required and until then the UK Paediatric Oncology Dietitians' Interest Group (PODIG) advise the following for children with cancer: that supplementation of vitamins and minerals above the RNI is not recommended because of potential toxicity and interactions with the efficacy of conventional treatment [71]. Children receiving enteral feeds or oral nutritional supplements should not need additional vitamins and minerals. Children not receiving nutrition support, but who have a limited fruit and vegetable intake, may benefit from a general multivitamin supplement; they should also be given advice on how to incorporate more fruit and vegetables into their diet. As children undergoing treatment for cancer frequently require blood transfusions it is advisable that they take a supplement which does not contain any iron, or only a small amount of iron (maximum of 15% RNI).

Glutamine

Many chemotherapy drugs, in particular anthracyclines, actinomycin and high dose methotrexate, result in both structural and functional injuries to the gastrointestinal tract resulting in mucositis severe enough to prevent an adequate oral intake. It is well documented that glutamine is a major fuel and important nitrogen source for enterocytes and plays a key role in maintaining mucosal cell integrity and gut barrier function [72]. Whilst there have been several studies looking at the role of both enteral and parenteral glutamine in adult oncology patients, there are very few published studies looking at glutamine in children with cancer. An oral dose of up to 0.65 g/kg has been shown to be safe and acceptable to use in paediatric oncology patients [73]. A significant reduction in the severity and duration of stomatitis using a smaller dose of oral glutamine in children has been demonstrated [74]. Although no significant difference in oral mucositis was observed, significant reductions in number of children requiring PN and duration of PN have been demonstrated in other studies [75,76], perhaps reflecting the role of glutamine in improving lower gut mucositis.

Evidence for the use of glutamine in PN given to children with cancer is weak. One randomised study in children following stem cell transplantation found no significant difference in the incidence of mucositis [77]. Evidence in other patients groups, adult BMT patients and young infants with severe gastrointestinal disease is not clear due to poor study designs making conclusions difficult [78, 79].

Although oral glutamine has been shown to be safe to use in paediatric oncology patients further larger multicentre studies are still required to determine its effect, in particular regarding use in children undergoing high dose chemotherapy and stem cell transplantation.

Bone morbidity and vitamin D

Bone morbidity has been well reported in survivors of childhood cancer; however, there is now a growing awareness of poor bone health at diagnosis and during treatment, particularly in children with ALL and following haematopoietic stem cell transplant [80]. Predictors of poor bone health include certain drugs (Table 21.1), disease process, vitamin D, body mass composition, nutritional problems, mineral abnormalities and physical inactivity.

Studies have highlighted lower vitamin D status in survivors compared with controls with the majority either insufficient or deficient [81]. Audits are being undertaken looking at vitamin D status of newly diagnosed patients, both haematological malignancies and solid tumour patients. Vitamin D supplementation during treatment is now being advised by some centres in line with current national guidelines [82] (Table 21.4). The longer term effects of vitamin D supplementation on bone health in children treated for cancer continues to be researched.

Eicosapentaenoic acid

Eicosapentaenoic acid (EPA) derived from fish oil has been studied in adult cancer patients with cachexia. EPA may modulate aspects of the inflammatory responses implicated in the metabolic changes associated with weight loss and muscular atrophy. EPA may downregulate production of pro-inflammatory cytokines and attenuate progression of the acute phase protein response. A recent Cochrane review looking at EPA supplements in

Table 21.4 Serum 25-hydroxyvitamin D concentrations, health and disease [82]. Reprinted with permission of BMJ Publishing Group Ltd.

Serum 25-OHD nmol/L	Vitamin D status	Manifestations	Management
<25	Deficient	Rickets	Treat with high dose calciferol
25–50	Insufficient	Osteomalacia Associated with disease	Vitamin D supplementation: 400 IU (10 µg)
50–75	Adequate	Healthy	Lifestyle advice
>75	Optimal	Healthy	None

adult studies highlighted insufficient data to define the optimal dose of EPA, insufficient data to establish if EPA was better than placebo and insufficient evidence that EPA improved symptoms associated with cancer cachexia often seen in patients with advanced cancer [83].

One study in paediatric oncology patients demonstrated that the percentage of weight loss was significantly lower in children receiving a protein energy supplement providing a total of 2.18 g EPA daily for 3 months compared with a control group [84]. There were drawbacks to the study [85]. The control group was not given an equivalent protein energy supplement without EPA. It is hard to interpret the data as overall the results were mainly derived from the group of patients with leukaemia, where significant weight loss during treatment is not usually expected due to their increased appetite and intake whilst on steroids and less incidence of severe mucositis. Cachexia is more common in solid tumour patients at diagnosis and during treatment, but no significant reduction in weight loss in the solid tumour patient group was seen compared with the control group. For the study to be more convincing as to the benefits of EPA in reducing weight loss there would need to be a significantly lower percentage of weight loss in the solid tumour patient group compared with the control group.

Whilst some paediatric enteral feeds have EPA added, e.g. Nutrini, Nutrini Multi Fibre, Nutrini Energy, Nutrini Energy Multi Fibre, Peptamen Junior Advance, there is still insufficient information to determine the ideal amount of EPA that would be effective in children [86]. There are also lipid solutions containing fish oils for use in parenteral nutrition, e.g. SMOFlipid, Omegaven, and further studies are required to determine their safety and benefits for the child with cancer. Despite concerns regarding interaction of EPA with ciclosporin and platelet function in cancer patients there is no strong evidence of this in studies involving other patient groups [87–89]. However, some centres are using fish oil containing lipids if the clinical need arises, e.g. where there are increasing conjugated bilirubin levels or increasing abnormal liver function tests.

Useful addresses/resources

Paediatric Oncology Dietitians Interest Group (PODIG)

Evelyn.Ward@leedsth.nhs.uk for information about PODIG

Information available:
Consensus statement vitamin supplements

Dietary management of gut graft-versus-host disease – the Leeds experience
Indications for gastrostomy feeding in paediatric oncology
Addenbrookes algorithm nutritional intervention for paediatric oncology
Guidelines for nutritional support in children treated for medulloblastoma – CCLG

Children's Cancer and Leukaemia Group (CCLG)

University of Leicester
3rd Floor, Hearts of Oak House
9 Princess Road West
Leicester LE1 6TH
www.cclg.org.uk
Information available:
Helping your child to eat

Cancer BACUP

3 Bath Place
Rivington Street
London
EC2A 3DR
www.cancerbacup.org.uk

22 Eating Disorders

Graeme O'Connor and Dasha Nicholls

Introduction

Eating disorders are psychiatric disorders with diagnostic criteria based on psychological, behavioural and physiological characteristics. Eating disorders comprise anorexia nervosa (AN), bulimia nervosa (BN) and associated eating disorders. Detailed classifications and treatment methods of eating disorders can be found in the Diagnostic and Statistical Manual of Mental Disorders 4th edition (DSM IV) [1] and the International Classification of Diseases 10th revision (ICD-10).

AN has a point of prevalence of 0.48%–0.7% in adolescent females, with diagnosis peaking between 16 and 17 years of age. The incidence begins to increase around the age of 10 years [2] and has been reported in children as young as 7 or 8 years [3]. BN occurs in approximately 1%–2% of the adolescent population while clinically significant bulimic behaviours occur in an additional 2%–3% [4]. BN is rare below the age of 13 years [3].

Disturbances in nutrition may be particularly harmful during vulnerable periods of brain development and physical growth, resulting in excessive and potentially permanent physical and psychological consequences [5]. Nutritional intervention in the treatment of eating disorders is an essential component and therefore the dietitian is an essential member of the multidisciplinary team, drawing on specialist skills in areas of nutrition, physiology and behaviour change. Dietitians should not treat eating disorders as sole practitioners and must work within a multidisciplinary team [6].

Screening and diagnosis

Paediatricians and general practitioners often refer young people with a history of weight loss to the dietitian. It is therefore not unusual for dietitians to be the first health professionals to identify or question a possible eating disorder.

Anorexia nervosa – clinical features

AN is a psychiatric disorder that predominately affects females. It varies in severity, with extreme nutritional restriction accompanied by other associated behaviours such as binge eating, self-induced vomiting, purging, over-exercising and self-harm [7]. Whether the incidence of AN is increasing is a matter of some debate but there is consensus that the mortality rate is amongst the highest of all psychiatric disorders [8]. The cognitive distortion associated with AN results in dieting behaviour and an intense fear of weight gain and fatness. Generally there is no loss of appetite, but satisfaction in feeling 'empty' and hungry overrides the need to eat, and weight loss is viewed as an achievement; thus sufferers have limited desire to change [9].

Identifying an eating disorder in the early stages is difficult due to the deceptive nature of the disease, especially when presentation is atypical. In addition, lack of awareness that AN can occur in children and boys may lead to a delay in referral, diagnosis and treatment [10], although this may be changing. Clinical signs of AN include

- *Weight loss* – in AN body weight is maintained at least 15% below that expected. The World Health Organization (WHO) definition of underweight and the diagnostic criterion for AN is a percentage body mass index (%BMI) below 85% (where %BMI is BMI/median BMI for age and gender). For the majority of the population a healthy %BMI will fall between 95% and 105% [1, 11]. A consequence of low weight is that pubertal development is halted, resulting in either a delay in reaching menarche or secondary amenorrhoea, which can have implications on bone health. Physical signs of poor nutrition and low weight include sunken cheeks, temporal lobes and eyes; dull thinning hair; lanugo hair; cold extremities and feeling cold; and delayed puberty [12].
- *Avoidance of food* – this can occur gradually over time, with subtle restriction of nutritional intake including eliminating snacks, reducing portion sizes, hiding food and missing meals. Furthermore, avoidance of food can transfer into the social setting: the young person will avoid eating out due to a lack of control over food preparation, or it may interrupt rigid exercise routines or other 'rules'. Conversely, the young person can be overly involved with food shopping, meal preparation and baking but will avoid eating themselves. Patients will often have an extensive knowledge about the calorie content of food but this is often the limit of their understanding about food and nutrition. It is a common misconception that young people with AN have a good comprehension of nutrition but they are often unable to understand information or interpret it correctly; hence the importance of nutrition education for them [13].

- *Morbid preoccupation with weight and/or shape* – energy dense foods are avoided through fear of gaining weight or a change in body shape that may accompany it. Girls perceive their stomach and thighs as particularly fat, whereas boys may be more concerned about musculature and are more likely to exercise excessively.
- *Poor self-esteem* – feelings of ineffectiveness are extremely common and often married with depressive and anxiety features, impaired concentration and obsessional symptoms. Social interests decline as patients lose weight and most become socially withdrawn. Many of these features reverse with weight gain [9]. Perfectionism is a trait that can converge with poor self-esteem, resulting in extreme competitiveness, asceticism and the need to please; subsequently young people with AN tend to be high achievers and can be perceived by peers and family as flourishing.

Bulimia nervosa – clinical features

In BN there is a persistent preoccupation with eating, with craving and consequent binges, associated with a feeling of loss of control. Weight is usually maintained within the normal range by compensatory exercise, vomiting or purging. In BN a preoccupation with weight, comparable to that seen in AN, leads to attempts at weight control with a characteristic cyclical pattern of missing meals which is not sustained as hunger reinforces a propensity to binge eat, often followed by compensatory behaviours and guilt [9]. A patient with BN is more likely to be depressed than one with AN, although there is enormous overlap between the disorders and a patient with features of BN who is also underweight would be diagnosed with AN using current diagnostic criteria.

There are well validated treatments for BN that are effective in over 60% of patients. However, BN is less obvious than AN to recognise and may only come to light through suspicion of a family member or friend [14]. Clinical signs of BN include

- irregular menses
- Russell's sign – callouses on the knuckles of forefingers due to abrasions from self-induced vomiting

- dental erosion from damage to teeth enamel from stomach acid
- depression/low mood

Binge eating disorder – clinical features

In binge eating disorder (BED) the patient has binge episodes, a sense of loss of control over food intake and a preoccupation of weight and/or shape but does not utilise compensatory behaviours following a binge episode [1]. Consequently they are often overweight. To be clinically significant the behaviours must be frequent and cause the patient distress or impairment.

Screening

There are questions that the dietitian can ask the patient to ascertain whether a referral to child and adolescent mental health services (CAMHS) is warranted:

- Would it be OK if we discussed your eating habits?
- You seem to have excluded fats/carbohydrates from your diet. Is there a reason for this?
- Have you been a vegetarian/vegan for long? What made you decide to change?
- Is there any reason why you do not eat after a certain time?
- Do you like the feeling of having an empty stomach? What do you do when you feel hungry?
- How many times a week do you miss a meal?
- If you miss a meal do you find it difficult to control the amount you eat at the next sitting?
- How often do you exercise a week? (Try to gain a sense of intensity and duration)
- When was the last time you ate out with friends/family?

Assessment of eating disorders

Medical

Although medical investigations may be necessary to rule out organic aetiology responsible for weight loss or food avoidance, eating disorders are much more common than most possible differential diagnoses for weight loss: hyperthyroidism, type 1 diabetes, inflammatory bowel disease (IBD), coeliac disease or neoplastic disease (tumour); food avoidance may be a result of achalasia. Amenorrhoea may result from ovarian or pituitary disease, or following use of the contraceptive pill. Clinical assessment should focus on determining the severity of malnutrition as well as possible causes, and should include hydration status, temperature, muscle wasting and cardiovascular status with particular attention to heart rate and orthostatic blood pressure. The sit up, squat, stand (SUSS) test is a useful clinical sign to monitor the clinical status of malnourished patients [15].

Anthropometric

The use of simple weight or BMI has limited use in young people owing to the normal changes in weight, height and BMI in childhood and through puberty. Weight and BMI can be used to track changes in an individual but any comparison of weight against population norms needs to take account of height, sex and age. It is perfectly correct to use BMI centile charts and to report BMI centile in young people. However, for patients below the 0.4th BMI centile, there is a need to quantify the degree of underweight. Using %BMI (BMI/median BMI for age and gender) instantly provides information about a patient's nutritional status without the need to refer to a chart. Patients and parents understand the concept of %BMI.

Mid upper arm circumference (MUAC) is a simple and effective additional anthropometric measure; its use can eliminate some of the methods employed by AN patients to mislead practitioners about their true weight, such as water loading and attaching weights to various parts of the body [16].

Nutritional

Acquiring an accurate diet history from young people with an eating disorder has the added barrier of intentional overestimation and underestimation of intake; therefore it is essential to have input from families along with a 3 day food record. Nutritional assessment should expand on the history of food restriction and other self-imposed nutritional 'rules' such as exclusion of a food group (fats and/or carbohydrates), vegetarianism/veganism, daily calorie limits, ritualistic behaviours or even a limit to the number of spoonfuls of food the young person will allow themselves to eat each day. Additionally, when reviewing young people with binge eating tendencies the dietitian will need to ascertain if there is a specific binge food/food group, specific binge time, cyclical pattern to binges and which meals are missed.

Exercise routines should form part of the nutritional assessment and be taken into account when estimating nutritional requirements. An in-depth nutritional assessment also allows the dietitian to gauge the extent of the young person's nutritional knowledge.

Biochemical

The initial consultation should include a detailed laboratory assessment to rule out any organic cause of weight loss and to obtain baseline biochemistry. Additional markers that should be monitored include vitamin B_{12}, folate, zinc, fat soluble vitamins A, D and E, and ferritin [15,17]. Biochemical monitoring for patients at risk of refeeding syndrome is given on p. 674.

Dietetic management

Dietitians working in eating disorders must have an understanding of the underlying dynamics [18] and be aware of their professional boundaries when treating these complex patients. It is important to highlight the possible synergy between psychological and nutritional factors; without psychological understanding and support, nutritional rehabilitation is likely to be ineffective. Conversely, malnutrition will impact cognitive function and behaviour, including increasing preoccupation with food and eating in a way that mirrors the eating disorder itself.

Dietitians are recognised as important members of the eating disorders multidisciplinary team, providing a specialist role assisting patients to

- restore a healthy body weight
- achieve a dietary intake that meets the nutritional requirements of a growing child/adolescent

- meet the nutritional requirements of those with additional dietary needs (e.g. diabetes, food allergies, gastroenterological disorders)
- restore normal eating patterns
- provide sound and current evidence based nutritional education to patients and the team

Most patients with eating disorders can be treated in an outpatient setting and will not require an inpatient stay. The Junior Management of Really Sick Patients with Anorexia Nervosa (MARSI-PAN) guidelines provide guidance on the most appropriate treatment setting taking into account cardiovascular parameters, %BMI, rate of weight loss, vomiting, purging, exercise and self-harm [19].

Nutritional requirements

Energy requirements for patients at risk of the refeeding syndrome are given on Table 22.3.

For patients who are prepubertal, or in early puberty, malnutrition will delay puberty and marked stunting is often present. It is therefore essential to use height age when calculating estimated average requirements (EAR) for energy and reference nutrient intakes (RNI) for micronutrients if the patient's height is less than the second percentile. If there is no evidence of stunted growth (i.e. the patient's height falls within the normal percentile ranges) then requirements for chronological age should be used.

Additional energy will need to be factored in for those patients exercising above expected healthy daily activity. Table 22.1 provides guidance on appropriate physical activity levels based on intensity and duration of exercise. Activity levels will normally be curtailed as part of the therapeutic treatment and restored gradually, with guidance from the dietitian on the energy compensation required [20].

Meal planning

If a meal plan is used, this should be devised and agreed with the eating disorders team and family, minimising communication errors and avoiding discussions around anorexic preoccupations and concerns at the point of eating a meal or snack. It

Table 22.1 Exercise energy requirements (EER).

Exercise/activity	Duration/intensity	EER = EAR × (PAL × time spent)
Seated jiggling/swinging legs	4 hours/day	EAR × (1.4 × 4/24)
Walking/jogging	2 hours/day	EAR × (1.8 × 2/24)
Competitive training (gymnastics/dance/swimming)	High intensity 2 hours/day	EAR × (2.4 × 2/24)

EAR, estimated average requirement for energy; PAL, physical activity level.
Adapted from [21].

Worked examples

A 10-year-old girl spends 5 hours seated jiggling per day. EER = 1790 kcal (7510 kJ) × (1.4 × 5/24) = 520 kcal (2180 kJ)
Total daily energy requirements = 1790 kcal (7510 kJ) (EAR) + 520 kcal (2180 kJ) (EER) = 2310 kcal (9690 kJ)

A 7-year-old boy spends 2 hours jogging per day. EER = 1890 kcal (7900 kJ) × (1.8 × 2/24) = 285 kcal (1185 kJ)
Total daily energy requirements = 1890 kcal (7900 kJ) (EAR) + 285 kcal (1185 kJ) (EER) = 2175 kcal (9085 kJ)

A 14-year-old girl spends 2 hours swimming per day and 1 hour jogging. EER = 1845 kcal (7710 kJ) × (2.4 × 2/24) + 1845 kcal (7710 kJ) × (1.8 × 1/24) = 505 kcal (2110 kJ)
Total daily energy requirements = 1845 kcal (7710 kJ) (EAR) + 505 kcal (2110 kJ) (EER) = 2350 kcal (9820 kJ)

is important that the family's usual diet is accommodated as much as possible, including medically proven specialist diets [21] (e.g. food allergies, coeliac disease, inflammatory bowel disease, diabetes) and cultural or religious needs. It is essential that a regular pattern of meals and snacks is established with the focus on when, rather than what, the patient eats [15, 22]. A written prescriptive outline of several meal and snack options can be helpful for some patients and reinforces healthy eating patterns [23].

Initially, the devised meal plan may be low in or devoid of energy dense foods to help reduce anxiety and to promote adherence with the meal plan and regular eating pattern. However, it is essential to let the patient know that fat (and hence essential fatty acids) and energy dense foods will be introduced into the meal plan. It is reasonable to allow the patient to have three to five foods omitted from the diet if they truly dislike them [24].

The meal plan should ideally comprise solid food. If meals are not completed then the patient can have the option to make up lost energy with high energy oral complete nutritional supplements (e.g. Ensure TwoCal, Fortisip Compact). It is important that these complete supplements are used rather than juice style or carbohydrate energy modules (powders or liquids) as initially these sip feeds may constitute the predominant intake. It is important that the meal plan is reviewed regularly and is easily adaptable to suit the needs of the patient and team.

Meal supervision

Meals and snacks should be provided under supervision ideally by someone who can demonstrate empathy and understanding, while setting firm boundaries about what is expected, i.e. how much is to be consumed in a set period of time [25]. It is essential that appropriate observations are in place at mealtimes, i.e. consideration is given to who is present at each snack and mealtime, and who has the responsibility for observation and documentation of the food and fluid consumed and the time limits for snacks and meals. Time limits for eating, e.g. 15 minutes per snack and 30 minutes per meal, all need to be agreed and documented. Support and supervision is recommended for 1 hour after each meal and has been shown to reduce the need for nasogastric feeding [25]. Additionally, meal supervision is a good opportunity to explore and discuss normal hunger and feelings of satiety.

Any actions to be taken if a meal is not completed need to be agreed and documented in advance, e.g. volume of feed to be given instead of the incomplete meal. Individual circumstances will help to dictate the exact needs of the young person and any help that may be needed with respect to helping them eat the required amount of food.

Nutrition education

Patients may have entrenched beliefs about nutrition, especially about energy dense foods. Therefore, the Socratic style can be adopted to help the patient question their own beliefs about nutrition [26]. This encourages patients to test their beliefs as a hypothesis, for instance a patient may hold the fear that eating a forbidden food will result in substantial weight gain or body shape change. By using anthropometric measurements as part of behavioural experiments these fears can be challenged, providing compelling evidence to the patient.

A growing body of evidence is supporting the importance of a structured nutrition education programme that covers basic topics such as food groups, portion sizes, metabolism and exercise [27], but this may be more appropriate for parents or older/adult patients than young people.

Nasogastric/jejunal feeding

The preferred option for feeding is oral food and fluid. Exclusive enteral feeding should be avoided as it is notoriously difficult to reinstate food once excluded from the diet. Some young people prefer nasogastric feeding because it relieves them of the responsibility of eating [28], but it also reduces opportunities to eat meals/snacks and may occasionally be used for self-harm. Nasogastric feeding is usually a short term measure, tailed off as oral intake improves. Nasojejunal feeding may be necessary in patients who persistently vomit (>3 times a day) which can compromise serum potassium levels.

Expected weight gain

If the patient is at risk of the refeeding syndrome see Table 22.4 for expected weight gain.

Weighing in the same way and at the same time of day will help to minimise fluctuations in weight from non-nutritional reasons, e.g. the patient should be weighed on the same scales in the morning before breakfast and after emptying their bladder, in underclothes only (bearing in mind that items can be hidden in these). Access to the ward or family weighing scales may need to be restricted to decrease the likelihood of frequent weighing by the individual.

Consideration needs to be given to water-loading by the patient in order to produce a gain in weight. This may necessitate restricted access to fluids and the team need to be aware that other patients' drinks may be consumed. Water may be drunk from taps, toilets, showers; access to these facilities may need to be restricted.

Assuming the patient is medically stable, weight restoration at a rate of 0.8–1.0 kg per week for inpatients and 0.3– 0.5 kg in an outpatient setting [6, 15, 17] is safe. Initially weight restoration can usually be achieved by meeting the EAR for energy for height age. However, sometimes this is not adequate and daily increments of 200–300 kcal (840–1255 kJ) are required until sufficient weight gain is achieved.

It is not uncommon for a member of the psychiatric team to request that the dietitian put a hold on weight gain once the young person is out of the high risk category (once their %BMI is >85%) to allow for directed therapy around anxiety which has resulted from the weight gain.

Complications

Chronic fasting, malnutrition and low weight, along with compensatory behaviours, have profound effects on all of the body's physiological systems [29]. However, bone health is of particular importance in adolescents as it is a time when linear bone growth and mineralisation is rapid and when bone formation should normally exceed bone reabsorption in order for peak bone mass to be acquired [30]. Impaired linear growth and possible permanent short stature are significant medical problems in adolescents with AN [31]. Invariably, short stature in AN is due to delayed growth, the result of delayed puberty as a consequence of having a low weight [32]. With a few exceptions patients with AN ultimately reach their expected height [33]. Furthermore, low levels of insulin-like growth factor-1 (IGF-1), as seen in adolescents with AN, have been linked with low bone mineral density (BMD) [34]; other factors associated with the uncoupling of bone turnover in AN include low levels of oestrogen (amenorrhoea), testosterone, dehydroepiandrosterone and leptin, and high levels of cortisol, ghrelin and peptide YY.

All contribute to low BMD and susceptibility to the development of osteopenia, osteoporosis and increased fracture incidence [35].

Transfer of care

Transfer between Child and Adolescent Mental Health Services (CAMHS) and adult services can be problematic. Often there is a significant cultural difference between these services. Whilst most CAMHS emphasise the responsibilities of the parents, adult services focus on individual responsibility. Without a careful transition, making sure that the young person is indeed capable of taking responsibility or that their capacity to make decisions about their treatment is clarified, a sudden change of approach can cause confusion and dissatisfaction at best and tragedy at worst. Ideally, there should be joint protocols between services to ensure the safe transfer and optimal transition between services of young people with severe anorexia nervosa. If this is not possible, when a patient is transferred from one service to another there should be a properly conducted and recorded meeting between representatives of the two services, usually including the patient and family.

The refeeding syndrome

The refeeding syndrome was originally described in prisoners of war. It is a physiological phenomenon driven by insulin resulting in biochemical and cardiovascular abnormalities when refeeding a malnourished individual. During starvation, insulin concentrations decrease and glucagon levels rise in response to depleted glucose. Glucagon breaks down glycogen forming glucose, rapidly depleting muscle and liver glycogen stores [36]. As glycogen stores are depleted, gluconeogenesis is activated utilising lipids and proteins as metabolic substrates to form glucose. However, gluconeogenesis has a limited capacity to support the body's energy requirements. Therefore, during this period of low serum insulin, hormone sensitive lipase is activated and breaks down adipose tissue to form fatty acids and glycerol; the fatty acids are transported to the liver to be converted to ketones. Ketones now replace glucose as the body's major energy source during acute starvation [37, 38].

Complications manifest with the introduction of carbohydrates, triggering a metabolic sequence of events due to a switch from ketone to glucose metabolism. The subsequent insulin surge that occurs in response to rising serum glucose levels causes a rapid intracellular movement of glucose, fluid and electrolytes (namely phosphate, potassium and magnesium). This intracellular movement results in hypophosphataemia, hypokalaemia, hypotension, oedema, cardiac arrhythmias and, if not identified and treated, potentially death [39, 40].

Table 22.2 outlines a guide to identify patients who are at increased risk of developing the refeeding syndrome. However, all malnourished patients should be closely monitored.

Monitoring

Baseline biochemical and cardiovascular parameters are paramount. Invariably, pre-refeeding biochemistry is unremarkable due to increased renal tubular reabsorption, tissue breakdown

Table 22.2 Risk factors for developing the refeeding syndrome.

Patient group	Anorexia nervosa Gastroenterology (inflammatory bowel disease, fistulae and short bowel) Neoplastic (tumours) Alcoholics Elderly
Body mass	Percentage median BMI <70% (approximates to <0.4th BMI centile) Rapid weight loss
Biochemical	Deranged electrolytes prior to refeeding
ECG abnormalities	QTc >460ms with evidence of bradyarrhythmia or tachyarrhythmia (excludes sinus bradycardia and sinus arrhythmia) ECG evidence of biochemical abnormality
Hydration status	Severe dehydration (10%)
Temperature	<35.5°C (tympanic) or 35.0°C axillary A result of extremely low % body fat

BMI, body mass index; ECG, electrocardiogram.

Table 22.3 Refeeding phases in high risk patients [45].

Refeeding phase	Target energy requirements and weight gain
Primary Days 1–2	• Commence at 40 kcal (167 kJ)/kg/day • Increase 200 kcal (840 kJ)/day until secondary refeeding phase reached • Correct deranged electrolytes; do not stop refeeding • Weight loss/maintenance likely during this primary refeeding phase • Consider oral thiamin 100–200 mg twice a day, continue for 10 days
Secondary Days 2–4	• Basal metabolic rate (BMR) × physical activity level (PAL) • Maintain secondary refeeding phase if adequate weight gain (0.5–1.0 kg/week) • Once weight gain reduces, increase 200–300 kcal (840–1255 kJ)/day until tertiary refeeding phase reached
Tertiary Days 7–14	• Estimated average requirement (EAR) energy for height age • Maintain tertiary phase if adequate weight gain (0.5–1.0 kg/ week)
Progression	• If sufficient weight gain not achieved with EAR continue to increase energy intake 200–300 kcal (840–1255 kJ) every 4 days until weight increase of 0.5–1 kg/week
Maintenance	• Once weight is >85% median BMI, weight gain can be slowed or maintained depending upon the therapeutic plan as discussed with the multidisciplinary team

and dehydration. It is essential that biochemistry is monitored daily for the first 72 hours after commencing refeeding.

If biochemical anomalies occur it is crucial that nutrition is not withdrawn, but that electrolytes are replaced orally or intravenously:

• oral phosphate 2–3 mmol/kg
• oral potassium chloride 0.5–1 mmol/kg
• oral magnesium sulphate 4 mmol/kg

(refer to the British National Formulary for further information)

Cardiovascular anomalies are generally corrected with nutrition and weight gain [41]. Any abnormalities need to be closely monitored.

Thiamin is often depleted in malnourished patients and is essential for effective utilisation of the newly introduced glucose. Thiamin forms a cofactor needed to transport pyruvate, the end product of glycolysis, from the cytosol into the mitochondria for energy metabolism. This reduces the risk of metabolic acidosis and non-diabetic ketone acidosis (NDKA) as a result of hyperglycaemia.

Energy requirements and expected weight gain for at risk patients

The refeeding of malnourished patients needs to be gradual and closely monitored and must increase in controlled phases in order to avoid further weight loss, which has been termed 'under-feeding syndrome'. Table 22.3 outlines the refeeding phases that can be adopted to promote appropriate weight gain in a timely and safe manner. A worked example of a phased refeeding regimen is given in Table 22.4.

Carbohydrates and the refeeding syndrome

Despite low energy intakes in the secondary phase of refeeding, weight gain is often achieved due to the rapid replenishment of glycogen stores. However, the refeeding syndrome is driven by insulin and therefore the carbohydrate intake should not exceed the recommended amount of 60% of dietary energy [42]. Most oral nutritional supplements and enteral feeds contain 42%–46% energy from carbohydrates, regardless of whether they are standard or high energy formulas. However, the total energy load from high energy formulas is higher than that from standard formulas, which may have an overall deleterious effect [43].

Future directions

The recommendations in this chapter are largely drawn from accumulated consensus opinion and some limited research evidence. There have been

Table 22.4   Worked example of a phased refeeding regimen.

14-year-old girl with anorexia nervosa, weight 30 kg. She is restricted to limited activity on the ward giving her a physical activity level (PAL) = 1.2. Her basal metabolic rate (BMR)* = 1223 kcal (5112 kJ)

Day (refeeding phase)	Target energy requirements and weight gain
Day 1 (primary phase)	It has not been possible to elicit an accurate reliable diet history: Start a meal plan at 40 kcal (168 kJ)/kg = 1200 kcal (5040 kJ)/day Now calculate the secondary phase energy intake target: BMR × 1.2 PAL [(17.686 × 30 kg) + 692.6] × 1.2 PAL = 1468 kcal (6165 kJ)/day
Day 2	Increase meal plan by 200 kcal (840 kJ) = 1400 kcal (5880 kJ)/day
Day 3	Increase meal plan by 200 kcal (840 kJ) = 1600 kcal (6720 kJ)/day
Day 4 (secondary phase energy intake target should have been met)	Halt energy increments and monitor weight gain From this point weight gain target 0.6–1.0 kg/week (0.1 kg/day)
Day 7–14 (tertiary phase energy intake target)	If weight gain is <0.6 kg/week, calculate the tertiary phase energy intake target: EAR for energy [39] = 1845 kcal (7750 kJ) Increase meal plan by 300 kcal (1260 kJ) = 1800 kcal (7560 kJ)/day Tertiary phase energy intake target has been met Halt energy increments and monitor weight gain From this point weight gain target 0.6–1.0 kg/week (0.1 kg/day)
Progression	If sufficient weight gain is not achieved with EAR for energy continue to increase energy intake by 300 kcal (1260 kJ) every 4 days until weight gain target of 0.6–1.0 kg/week (0.1 kg/day) is achieved

EAR, estimated average requirement for energy.
*Schofield equation for calculating BMR can be found in Table 5.6.

few clinical trials to date in the areas of refeeding or dietetic involvement in the care of children and young people with eating disorders. Trials which evaluate the effectiveness of structured nutritional sessions in conjunction with psychological input would help elucidate the most effective method of working with young people with eating disorders from a nutritional perspective. Furthermore, research evidence is needed to support the reintroduction of carbohydrates into the diet and the safest refeeding procedure to ensure adequate weight gain without the complications associated with the refeeding syndrome.

23

Autistic Spectrum Disorders

Zoe Connor

Introduction

Autistic spectrum disorders (ASD) are common, comprising a range of complex and heterogeneous developmental disabilities that affect the way a person communicates and relates to people around them. Dietitians from all disciplines need an awareness of the challenges faced and posed by children with ASD. The typical characteristics of rigid thinking and resistance to change, combined with common sensory processing issues, make feeding problems, undereating and overeating common and traditional approaches to changing dietary behaviours are often inadequate.

Diagnosis and terminology

Diagnosis of ASD involves trained professionals marking a child (or adult) in three main areas of functioning, known as the 'triad of impairments':

- social interaction (difficulty with social relationships, e.g. appearing aloof and indifferent to other people and difficulty with understanding others' viewpoints and intentions)
- social communication (difficulty with verbal and non verbal communication)
- imagination (difficulty with interpersonal play and imagination, e.g. having a limited range of imaginative activities, possibly copied and pursued rigidly and repetitively)

For a diagnosis of ASD, there must be impairments in each of these three areas, i.e. functioning falls below a threshold at which it interferes with day to day living [1]. Diagnostic criteria are taken from either the international or US diagnostic manuals ICD-10 [1] or DSM-4 [2]. In addition to this triad, repetitive behaviour patterns and resistance to change in routine are often present.

ASD is an umbrella term for three diagnoses:

- autism, also known as classic autism and Kanner's autism
- pervasive development disorder not otherwise specified (PDDNOS), sometimes known as atypical autism
- Asperger's syndrome

Two rarer diagnoses are sometimes included under the ASD umbrella, but are not covered specifically in this chapter:

- Rett syndrome, which affects primarily girls and is characterised by severe mental and physical regression (Table 29.1)
- childhood disintegrative disorder (CDD), which is characterised by 3 years of normal development followed by regression to display severely autistic characteristics

Clinical Paediatric Dietetics, Fourth Edition. Edited by Vanessa Shaw.
© 2015 John Wiley & Sons, Ltd. Published 2015 by John Wiley & Sons, Ltd.
Companion Website: www.wiley.com/go/shaw/paediatricdietetics

The differentiation between autism, PDDNOS and Asperger's syndrome depends on the number and distribution of impairments within the triad as specified by descriptors in the diagnostic manuals [1, 2]. As a crude generalisation children with Asperger's have developed speech by the age of 3 years and are seen as the more able end of the spectrum; autism is often seen as the less able end of the spectrum; and PDDNOS falls in between the two. The National Institute for Health and Care Excellence (NICE) has published guidance on recognition, referral and diagnosis of ASD [3].

Fifty per cent of children with ASD have learning difficulties and 70% have psychiatric disorders [4] including depression, anxiety, attention deficit hyperactivity disorder (ADHD) and behavioural or conduct problems. Other common coexisting conditions are motor coordination problems and epilepsy. These often multiple conditions further impair social and psychological functioning and increase the need for medical and dietetic input.

Genetics, prevalence and causes

ASD was once thought of as an uncommon disorder, but prevalence is increasing and it now occurs in at least 1% of children in the UK [5–7]. Boys are affected four times more than girls [8]. The increase is partly but not wholly due to increased recognition. For the majority of cases of ASD, the cause is unknown and is likely to be varied and multifactorial; 10% have underlying medical causes including at least 60 different metabolic disorders, neurological disorders and complex chromosomal abnormalities [9]. Genetic studies have failed to find any single 'autism gene', but genes that are linked to higher risks of autism are being identified. For families with a child diagnosed with ASD, the likelihood of having another affected child is increased by five to ten times [10]. It is thought that for idiopathic cases of ASD there could be an inherited predisposition which is triggered by some as yet unidentified environmental factor such as an infection, immunological reaction or toxin during pregnancy or early life [11] or, indeed, maternal nutrition. A large US population based case control study found that women who reported not taking prenatal vitamins (containing folic acid) before and

during the first month of pregnancy were twice as likely to have a child with ASD as women who did not take supplements. The same study identified particular maternal gene variants which made the likelihood of having a child with ASD seven times as likely when not taking vitamins [12].

There is much research into the biochemistry of children with ASD in the hope it will give a clue as to cause, enabling better sub-typing and treatment. Published research reports low serum iron [13], zinc to copper ratios [14, 15], magnesium [16], calcium and vitamin D [17]; increased plasma vitamin B_6 [18]; abnormal plasma essential fatty acids [19] and amino acids [20], markers of reduced sulphation capacity [21–23], urine peptides; increased urine homocysteine; various other abnormal vitamin, oxidative stress, energy transport, sulphation and detoxification markers [24–28]. The quality and size of these studies vary, the dietary intake of the subjects tested is rarely taken into account and the clinical relevance and robustness of some of the methodology and results are yet to be clarified.

Management of ASD

ASD is seen as a lifelong condition; however, 4%–40% of children lose their diagnosis as they get older [29–33]. Loss of diagnosis is more common for those more 'mildly' affected, or without other coexisting conditions. Whether these changes are due to some sort of 'recovery' or just a shifting of how much underlying ASD traits impede 'normal' life is not known.

Management, with specialised education and structured support, aims to help children maximise their skills and achieve their full potential as adults. Many individuals who were 'disabled' as children can get to the point where they will 'function normally' socially and find work, have a family and live independently.

Medical treatment is usually focused on managing common comorbidities such as ADHD, anxiety, sleep problems or epilepsy. Other treatments focus on the early implementation of education and behaviour interventions where these services are available, teaching the individual (or helping parents to teach the individual) appropriate responses to social situations they struggle with, and on developing communication.

Table 23.1   Considerations for dietetic consultations.

Setting

- A quiet and not too brightly lit consultation room and equally appropriate waiting area
- Child safe consultation areas
- Minimising the occasions parents need to bring their child to clinic
- Consideration of home or school visits instead of clinic attendance

Organising appointments

- Appointments that start on time to reduce anxiety of waiting, e.g. by giving the first appointment of the day or clinic
- Giving a clear explanation of what to expect, with visual cues when possible, e.g. the appointment letter including a picture of the clinic, clinic room and dietitian
- Allowing extra time for an effective consultation

Communication

- Use of clear, simple language with short sentences
- Avoidance of idioms, irony, metaphors and words with double meanings
- Avoiding use of body language, gestures or facial expressions without verbal instructions
- Awareness that dietary instructions may be misinterpreted or taken literally, e.g. 'avoid fatty foods' without clarification of what this means could result in an able young person with ASD checking labels and refusing to eat anything with a fat content
- When needing to give instructions, e.g. for weighing or measuring, do not assume that a non verbal patient cannot understand what is being said
- Explain what you are going to do clearly before doing it and if possible show a picture or doll to explain what you are going to do, or demonstrate on a parent or yourself
- Give direct, clear requests with as few words as possible, e.g. sit here, stand here
- Awareness that a person with ASD may not make eye contact and may invade your personal space and climb over you; they may also use self-stimulating behaviour such as flapping their hands, making noises or putting their hands over their ears to relax themselves when overwhelmed by noises, lights, new surroundings or other non obvious stressors

Consider involving an education or speech and language specialist to aid more effective communication with the child

Key strategies commonly advocated for individuals with ASD are

- creating a structured routine, which reduces the anxiety a person may feel at the unpredictable environment around them
- care with use of verbal communication. People with ASD are likely to take things literally and so may misunderstand idioms (e.g. 'I'll be back in a second', 'Eating that will put hairs on your chest'). It is recommended to use simple language and positive commands rather than negative (e.g. 'Sit down there' rather than 'Don't stand over there')
- using visual tools to complement any verbal instructions, e.g. signing, the use of objects or (commonly) the use of picture cards (see www.do2learn.com)

The National Autism Plan [34] recommends that all professionals working with children have training in ASD awareness and that additional training should be provided for all staff delivering specific ASD interventions. Desirable changes to dietetic consultations for children and young people with ASD are given in Table 23.1.

Nutritional management

Sensory processing difficulties

Impairment in perception of sensory stimuli is commonly reported in children and people with ASD. The reasons for this are not understood. Under-sensitivity in ASD may result in an increase in behaviours such as fidgeting, spinning, rocking or hand flapping which are forms of self-stimulation. Other children may demonstrate over-sensitivity by being aversive to touch, light and/or sound. Assessment of sensory issues and advice on management is best

Table 23.2   Examples of sensory issues that could affect food preferences and mealtime behaviour.

Sense	Hypersensitivity	Hyposensitivity
Taste	Strong preference for bland tasting foods Aversion to spicy foods/many foods	Preference for strong tasting spicy foods Licking objects
Smell	Distracted or disturbed by food smells Ability to detect smells that others may not, e.g. protein foods	Preference for strong smells
Visual	Distracted by lighting, movement or colours at mealtimes Preference for bland coloured foods Preference for different foods to be presented separately Disturbed by foods not presented in the usual way Aversion to certain coloured foods	
Auditory	Dislike of crunchy foods Distracted or disturbed by background sounds some of which may not be obvious, e.g. fluorescent light tubes	Preference for foods that make sounds when eaten, e.g. crunchy ones
Touch	Dislike of mixed textures in mouth Dislike of hot or cold foods and drinks Dislike of some cutlery in mouth Dislike of tooth brushing	Preference for lumpy or crunchy foods Preference for very hot or very cold foods and drinks (possibility of burning self as hyposensitive to pain) Tendency to frequently put foods and other objects to the mouth
Proprioception	Alterations can contribute to clumsiness in eating or drinking or being distracted by arm movements during eating	
Vestibular attention	Alterations can cause child to be distracted by moving or not moving self or by body position during a meal	

undertaken by an occupational therapist or other healthcare professional trained in sensory integration therapy (dietitians can access this training). Simple and practical help like wearing specially designed weighted clothing, having a discrete object to fiddle with, changing lighting, or reducing noise can sometimes have very significant effects on concentration and reduction in undesirable behaviours. Table 23.2 shows examples of sensory issues which could affect food intake and mealtimes.

Selective eating

Children with ASD have been shown to have significantly more feeding problems (around 60%) than children without autism and they also eat a significantly narrower range of foods. This is

not associated with the severity of ASD [35–38]. Commonly reported aspects of selective eating in ASD are

- texture preferences/difficulty with transition to textured foods
- food neophobia, i.e. significant distress at trying new foods
- strong preference for foods of a particular colour
- acceptance only of foods with familiar packaging
- distress in some mealtime environments, e.g. it may be too noisy; too quiet; too bright; distressed by smells or look of other people's food; distressed by being around other people
- demands that food is presented in a consistent way, e.g. same plate and cutlery, positioning of food on plate
- seeming not to recognise their own thirst or hunger

Nutritional assessment of a child with selective eating

As for any child with eating problems the assessment includes growth monitoring, assessment of nutritional adequacy of diet through diet history and recommendation of dietary changes to ensure adequacy, including supplements where needed. Additional areas to consider

- underlying factors causing the selective eating
- helping parents and other carers to understand the characteristic features of ASD that make selective eating more common
- strategies to help change their child's diet, both generic and specific for ASD
- coordinating a multidisciplinary approach to changing the child's dietary intake
- requesting blood tests to check nutritional status

Continued refusal of family foods can cause great distress to families. Often one of the key things parents seek from a dietetic consultation is reassurance that their child is growing well and that their problem is not unique.

Risk of deficiencies

Children with ASD and selective eating are significantly more likely than typical controls to be at risk of at least one serious nutrient deficiency [39]. There are a number of case reports of severe nutritional deficiencies including scurvy presenting as muscle atrophy [40, 41], concurrent vitamin A and D deficiency presenting as a limp and periorbital swelling [42], three cases of vitamin B_{12} deficiency presenting as partially reversible optic neuropathy [43], three cases of vitamin A deficiency presenting as vision loss [44–46] and two cases of severe malnutrition, one involving a rash resolving with zinc supplementation [47].

Strategies for dealing with selective eating

Typically, parents with children with ASD and chronic selective eating will report that they have tried standard behavioural advice for toddlers with faddy eating and not found this to be helpful. Parents often need individualised advice to deal with the specific needs of their children or need intensive interventions such as those offered by multidisciplinary feeding clinics to see even small progressions with their child's diet.

Parents find the following strategies useful.

Make mealtimes more predictable

- establishment of a structured eating routine
- use of visual timetables – detailing when and where they will eat and what will be eaten. The timetable can be supplemented with picture symbols or photographs
- use of visual schedule – written or picture symbol schedules detailing behaviour expected at mealtimes or foods to be tried at a mealtime

Deal with underlying issues that may be exacerbating eating problems

- medical problems which may reduce appetite, such as pain, dental problems and medications such as methylphenidate
- problem behaviours at mealtimes can be a marker of undiagnosed underlying constipation, gastro-oesophageal reflux, intestinal inflammation, malabsorption, maldigestion, irritable bowel syndrome or functional abdominal pain [48]
- positioning at mealtimes, swallowing problems and sensory issues – occupational therapy, speech and language therapy or physiotherapy interventions may involve special seating, messy play and other activities such as massage and touching around the mouth and face to desensitise to different foods
- food phobia – may need a slow step-by-step programme for introducing new foods which minimises anxiety

Find ways to motivate
This can be extremely difficult with some children as praise, affection and star charts may not have any effect. Parents and other carers can be helped to think of things that have motivated other changes, e.g. toilet training. Some things that have been found to help:

- 'eat it up' books. A written list or picture symbol list of foods liked, foods parents want the child to try and the foods the child is going to try next. Foods can be moved gradually up the lists

- use of 'social stories'. A specially written story in simple language explaining how and why to do something (see www.thegraycenter.org/Social_Stories.htm)
- using 'special interests' to motivate. Children with ASD often have 'obsessive' interests, e.g. watching the same part of a particular popular children's DVD story. Restricting access to a special interest to 'reward' times can be effective
- modifying a favourite game to include activities to taste new foods, e.g. snakes and ladders – trying a new food to prevent going down a snake. An example of clinical use of a specially devised board game is listed in the references [49].

Excessive weight gain

The prevalence of overweight and obesity in children and adolescents with ASD (up to 2002) was found to be similar to that of the general population in the USA [50]. However, a more recent US study found levels in 12–19-year-olds to be two to three times that of the general population, with 50% overweight [51]. Useful strategies for managing overeating include

- using a visual timetable to dictate set snack and mealtimes
- helping parents to find strategies to say no to their child's demands
- keeping tempting foods out of the house or locked away
- getting other carers and school staff to give consistent messages
- considering potential gastrointestinal or sensory issues which may drive overeating

Gastrointestinal issues and ASD

The reported prevalence of gastrointestinal symptoms in children with ASD ranges from 9% to more than 70% [48, 52, 53]. An expert US multidisciplinary group consensus statement recommends that 'individuals with ASD who present with gastrointestinal symptoms warrant a thorough evaluation, as would be undertaken for individuals without ASD who have the same symptoms or signs' [48]. Behaviours and symptoms that can be

markers of abdominal pain or discomfort include irritability, agitation, aggression, constant eating, pica, unusual posturing and unexplained repetitive behaviours, aggression and sensitivity.

Coeliac disease

With coeliac disease having up to a three times increased prevalence in ASD [54], together with the possibility that coeliac disease can present atypically as neurological symptoms including autism [55] and with the frequent use of therapeutic gluten exclusion in ASD it is surprising that there is no recommendation to routinely screen children with ASD for coeliac disease. NICE guidance advises that serological coeliac screening be offered to anyone with unexplained gut problems, including those with ASD; it should also be considered for a number of conditions that often occur along with ASD: fatigue, depression, epilepsy or iron deficiency [56].

ASD specific gut inflammation

There is ongoing research to elucidate whether specific gastrointestinal disturbances occur in ASD. Famously an association between ileocolitis and developmental regression was claimed in 1998 in a paper that, controversially, has been retracted due to concerns regarding the ethics of the data collection [57]. Similar results have been found in neurotypical children as well as children with allergies and immune deficiencies; therefore the significance of the findings is not clear [48]. Increasing links are being made between gut inflammation in children with ASD and resultant inflammatory responses in the brain which could elicit autistic behaviours or impair neurodevelopment [48].

Intestinal permeability ('leaky gut')

Studies have found altered intestinal permeability in 43% (9/21) of children with ASD versus none of 40 healthy age matched controls [58] and in 37% (33/90) of children with ASD versus none of the 69 controls [59]. Increased permeability did not, however, correlate with gastrointestinal symptoms or inflammation markers. Those on a gluten and casein free diet had significantly lower levels of permeability. Another study of intestinal permeability in 14 children with ASD showed no difference compared with controls [60]. Further studies of prevalence of altered intestinal permeability and its clinical relevance are needed.

Altered intestinal flora

Two studies report significant alterations in the upper and lower intestinal flora of children with 'late onset' autism, with particular increase in clostridial species [61, 62]. The clinical significance of this dysbiosis is yet to be clarified.

Mitochondrial disorders

Disturbance in mitochondrial energy production is an underlying pathophysiological mechanism in a subset of individuals with autism. Mitochondrial disorders have been identified in as many as 7% of 69 adolescents with ASD [63]. Constipation is an indicator for mitochondrial disorder, caused by gut dysmotility. Guidelines for recognition, diagnosis and management of mitochondrial disease are listed in [64].

Constipation, gastro-oesophageal reflux, diarrhoea and functional abdominal pain

In children with any of these symptoms it may be necessary to give advice on adjusting fibre and fluid intakes, the use of prebiotics and/or probiotics, and food exclusions and challenges where food intolerance or allergy is suspected.

Therapeutic diets for treating children with ASD

There is much anecdotal evidence, spanning the last 50 years, for the improvement of behaviour, communication and learning in children and adults with ASD who have followed various regimens, dietary exclusions and/or nutritional supplements, with sometimes near miraculous results. A survey of 325 parents of children with ASD

in England reported that up to 29% had tried or were on an exclusion diet, and up to 52% were on micronutrient supplements [65].

In theory, dietary changes could have a large impact on the functioning of a child with ASD or any other neurodevelopmental disorder: diet can directly affect brain structure and neurotransmitter activity via sub-clinical deficiencies of essential nutrients such as omega-3 fatty acids or via dietary manipulation to cause ketosis. Indirectly, dietary changes that remove pain or discomfort due to deficiencies, reactions to foods or gut fermentation can improve ability to concentrate and learn thereby overcoming communication difficulties.

Despite anecdotal evidence and widespread use, there is a paucity of quality evidence to confidently recommend any particular dietary interventions for treating ASD. However, some children show clear improvement with dietary interventions. With appropriate support, exclusion and other diets are relatively safe and inexpensive. A trial diet may be advised in some cases, e.g. in those with gastrointestinal problems, or in those whose symptoms have been linked to particular dietary components. Dietitians who are confident in supporting exclusion diets are best placed to help parents navigate safely through the 'trial and error' aspect of diet therapy in ASD. Left unsupported, parents are at risk of putting their child on more and more restricted and imbalanced diets, accompanied by expensive and often excessive supplements. Table 23.3 compares the ease, supporting evidence and potential risk to health when using therapeutic diets for the treatment of ASD.

Exclusion of gluten and milk

The most popular and best known dietary intervention for ASD is a gluten and/or casein free diet (GFCF). It is more accurately a gluten and milk free diet; all mammalian milks and milk products are avoided. ASD is not an indication for prescribing gluten free products and therefore the cost of this diet is completely borne by the family, although some GPs will prescribe products at their discretion. It is good practice to consider serological coeliac screening before undertaking gluten exclusion.

A popular theory for the mechanism of action of this therapeutic restriction is the 'opioid theory'.

Table 23.3 Qualitative comparison of therapeutic diets used in ASD.

Intervention	Difficulty in following intervention	Supporting evidence	Negative impact on nutrition/health
Exclusion of gluten and/or milk	Moderate*	Some	Insufficient calcium, iodine, fibre and energy intakes possible but minimised with dietetic support
Other exclusion diets	Moderate*	None	Possible dietary deficiencies but minimised with dietetic support
Ketogenic diet	High*	Some	High risk of dietary deficiencies and growth faltering but minimised with dietetic support
Other named diets	Moderate*	None	Risk of dietary deficiencies but minimised with dietetic support
Individual vitamin and mineral supplementation	Low*	None/some for vitamin B_6	Possible side effects at high doses, e.g. neuropathy in high dose vitamin B_6, possible antagonistic effect for other vitamins and minerals
Multivitamin and mineral supplement (standard levels)	Low*	None (some for supplements with high doses of some nutrients)	Unlikely (possible side effects of high doses)
Fish oil supplements	Low*	Some	Unlikely
Probiotics	Low*	Some	Unlikely
Digestive enzymes	Low*	Very little	Unlikely

*Ease of intervention is greatly decreased if child is resistant to changes in diet/resistant to taking supplements.
Note: Improvement when on dietary modifications may mask underlying disorders (e.g. coeliac disease, metabolic disorders, epilepsy); therefore continued communication with patient's doctor is key.

Opioid-like peptides that are known metabolites of casein and gluten (similarly to many other dietary proteins) are absorbed into the blood stream through an abnormally permeable or 'leaky' gut and then cross the blood–brain barrier where they interfere with various neurological processes in a similar way to opioids [66]. The ability for these large peptides to enter the blood stream and subsequently the brain is yet to be proven. Urine tests are available privately which some parents use to guide their choice in undertaking a gluten and milk free diet. These tests check for peptides, particularly indolyl-3-acryloylglycine (IAG), which have been proposed as biomarkers for those with ASD who would benefit from a gluten and/or casein free diet [67]. Other research refutes this work [68–70].

Some theorise that a particular form of casein present in some milks, A1 casein, is particularly harmful to general health and could cause or exacerbate autism (and many other chronic diseases).

Most milks in the UK contain predominantly A1 casein, with the exception of milk from Guernsey cows, goat and sheep ('A2' milks). The European Food Safety Authority did not establish any cause and effect relationship [71], but this has not been enough to reassure many parents and organisations who prefer to limit children with ASD to the alternative 'A2' milk.

In a survey of parents of children with ASD in England, 19% had tried a gluten and/or milk free diet; 43% of these had never seen a dietitian [65]. A majority of these parents reported significant improvements in various aspects of their child's wellbeing on a gluten and/or milk free diet with significant improvements in bowel habits (65%, $n = 54$); general health (87%, $n = 55$); sleeping patterns (60%, $n = 31$); concentration (74%, $n = 42$); and social communication (72%, $n = 38$). Parents of two children reported significant 'recovery' from autism on the gluten and/or milk free diet [65]. These results are consistent with other anecdotal reports and surveys worldwide. Published studies also show some positive outcomes in communication and behaviour but are of varying quality [72–75]. Research has yet to prove that the effect of these diets goes beyond the possibly large placebo effect of submitting a child to any significant dietary change. A Cochrane review [76] concludes that there is insufficient evidence to recommend GFCF diets in the treatment of ASD.

Exclusion of phenolic compounds and salicylates

Some children with ASD have impaired sulphation capacity which is purported to result in reduced detoxification ability [77–79]. Some organisations advocate the avoidance of foods high in compounds broken down by sulphur dependent enzymes, as their consumption may inhibit the body's usual sulphation detoxification pathways [80] and lead to raised levels of neurotransmitters such as serotonin. Foods that are often excluded are cheese, chocolate, tomatoes, oranges, bananas, yeast extract, some food colourings and foods high in salicylates. Salicylates are found naturally in fruit and vegetables and levels vary according to varieties and growing conditions. Lists of the foods to avoid are often obtained from the organisations which advocate their use. Some self-help organisations also advise on sulphur supplementation either orally or transdermally using magnesium sulphate (Epsom Salt) baths; more research is needed.

Exclusion of various food additives

There has been little good quality research on the affect of food additives in children with ASD, although the avoidance of particular substances is very common. Although all food additives in the UK must pass legislative safety tests, there is evidence that some people find approved additives problematic. A double blind placebo controlled trial of 400 healthy preschool children found an increase in hyperactive behaviour when they were given a drink of sunset yellow (E110), tartrazine (E102), carmoisine (E122), ponceau 4R (E124) and sodium benzoate (E211) compared

with placebo drink [81]. A meta-analysis of 15 double blind placebo controlled crossover trials reported that removing artificial food colours is 30%–50% as effective in improving ADHD symptoms as stimulant medication, without side effects [82]. Since July 2010 the UK government has required that foods containing the colours E102 (tartrazine), E104 (quinoline yellow), E110 (sunset yellow FCF or orange yellow S), E122 (azorubine or carmoisine), E124 (ponceau 4R or cochineal red A) or E129 (allura red AC) must bear the warning statement 'may have an adverse effect on activity and attention in children'.

Additionally, the sweetener aspartame has been linked to depression [83], altered brain activity in people with epilepsy [84] and migraine [85–87]; the flavour enhancer monosodium glutamate (MSG, E621) has been linked to migraine [88]. A trial period of excluding aspartame, MSG, artificial food colours and benzoate preservative has little effect on the nutritional quality of the diet (and is in line with healthy eating guidelines) so could be recommended as first line advice for any children, including those with ASD, with behavioural problems.

Yeast free diet with antifungal treatment

It has been proposed in a popular autism treatment manual published by a commercial laboratory that yeast proliferation in the gut following antibiotic use causes 'leaky gut' syndrome, behavioural and allergic reactions and a greater susceptibility to food allergies [89]. This manual recommends antifungal treatment in the form of metronidazole, vancomycin or grapefruit seed extract, followed by 'dietary control of yeast overgrowth', i.e. elimination of natural and refined sugars (including all fruit for a month), with the simultaneous use of antifungals, vitamin B_6 and magnesium supplementation. It is reported that a 'die-off reaction' may occur in the first 3–7 days after antifungal treatment commences and can include heart palpitations, fever and extreme tiredness; it is suggested that these reactions are due to the release of toxins from Clostridia. Yeast free diets are not generally used in dietetic practice as evidence for their use does not exist.

Other dietary manipulations

Ketogenic diet

A pilot study of 30 children with ASD found improvements on the Childhood Autism Rating Scale in all 18 who tolerated the diet. For 10 children, the improvement was average to significant [90]. Further research is needed. Ketogenic diets are described in Chapter 16.

Feingold diet

This involves the elimination of artificial colourings, flavourings and preservatives, aspartame and salicylates [91]. Beyond the above mentioned research regarding some additives and behaviour, there is no evidence for its use.

The Body Ecology Diet™, Specific Carbohydrate Diet™ and the Gut and Psychology Syndrome Diet™

The Body Ecology Diet (BED) involves eating a diet of foods that are kept as close to their natural state as possible, with gluten excluded and including a number of special foods that are purported to re-establish the intestinal flora and heal the body, such as fermented coconut juice and raw butter [92]. The Specific Carbohydrate Diet (SCD) involves the elimination of grains, sucrose and lactose with the theory that this will modify intestinal bacteria growth [93]. The Gut and Psychology Syndrome (GAPS) diet is a modification of SCD, designed by a Russian neurologist based in the UK who makes claims for its use in many different disorders [94]. The first stage of the GAPS diet involves a limited range of broths and fermented foods, and claims to heal the gut. BED, SCD and GAPS have similarities to other more traditional dietetic approaches; they are modified few foods diets and may also be ketogenic. However, the basis for a food being on the allowed or disallowed lists for each diet is sometimes unclear and often not based on any clear criteria for food composition. These diets can be very restrictive and GAPS, for example, advocates following stage one for as long as it takes for diarrhoea to settle – over a year if necessary. The risks of dietary deficiency are therefore high. There are anecdotal reports that these diets can cause great improvement in symptoms related to ASD but there are no published reports or studies.

Therapeutic supplementation

Some organisations advocate high doses of individual vitamins and minerals due to proposed metabolic and biochemical abnormalities. Sometimes the suggested doses exceed the safe upper limit for adults and little is known about long term high doses in children [95]. Advice on vitamin and mineral supplementation to meet the reference nutrient intake (RNI) when dietary intake is insufficient is appropriate in children with ASD. Pharmaceutical doses for corrections of deficiencies normally fall under medical rather than dietetic scope, and appropriate referrals and requests when deficiencies are suspected should be made.

- **Multivitamin and mineral supplementation** – 24% of parents surveyed in England reported giving their child combined vitamin and mineral preparations [65]. In a randomised, double blind placebo controlled 3 month study with 20 participants, vitamin and mineral supplementation was associated with significant improvements in sleep and gastrointestinal problems in children with ASD compared with control subjects given placebo [96]. The study used a supplement with doses of B_6 and zinc that were well above the RNI. Another randomised double blind placebo controlled 3 month study involving 141 children and adults with autism, by the same author, saw a significant improvement in parent reported global autism symptoms, hyperactivity, tantrums and language, and significant improvement in markers of metabolic status in those taking a vitamin and mineral supplement compared with control. The supplement used in the study contained high doses of B vitamins, no iron, and most notably a sub-clinical dose of lithium. More research is needed in this area.
- **Vitamin B_6 and magnesium** – several investigators have reported significant improvement in behaviour following doses of 15–30 mg/kg/day pyridoxine (700–1000 mg/day) and 10–15 mg/kg/day magnesium (380–500 mg/day) [97, 98]. A Cochrane review concluded that these studies were inadequately designed

and too small to make any recommendations [99]. The usual doses used in these reports exceed the safe upper limit for vitamin B_6 (10 mg/day). Long term doses >200 mg/day have been associated with neuropathy, low serum folic acid, night restlessness and rashes, and >2000 mg/day can cause nerve damage. In most but not all reported cases, the damage has been reversible [100]. Advocates of vitamin B_6 therapy purport that the side effects of neuropathy are rare and the concurrent use of magnesium is protective against this. They hypothesise that the therapeutic effect of B_6 and magnesium is due to an abnormal metabolism or a deficiency and advise that, if no improvements are seen within 4 weeks, therapy is unlikely to help and should be stopped. It is particularly important to advise parents who are considering this intervention to consider whether their child would be able to let them know if they experienced the side effects of neuropathy.

- **Vitamin C** – researchers in the USA reported improvement in sensory motor symptoms in a double blind placebo controlled trial of 20 children with autism given extremely high doses of ascorbic acid (8 g/70 kg/day) [101]. The researchers proposed a dopaminergic mechanism of action.
- **Vitamin A** – two case studies report improvements of social skills after treatment with natural *cis* forms of vitamin A in cod liver oil [102]. The author hypothesises that autism 'may be a disorder linked to the disruption of the G-alpha protein, affecting retinoid receptors in the brain'. At a cost this protocol can be obtained from the website for use by paediatricians [103].
- **Iron** – an open-label treatment trial found that iron therapy significantly improved sleep in many children with ASD [104], many of whom had low serum levels.
- **Zinc** – reduced autism symptom severity was seen in children with abnormal zinc:copper ratios after zinc and vitamin B_6 supplementation [105, 106].
- **Dimethylglycine (DMG)** – sometimes known as pangamic acid, calcium pangamate or 'vitamin B_{15}', this non-essential amino acid is anecdotally reported to improve behaviour and communication in some children and adults

with ASD in doses of 60–600 mg/day. A double blind placebo controlled crossover pilot study of low dose DMG and placebo in eight autistic males did not find any significant differences [107].

- **Fish oil and other fat supplements** – fish oil supplements are used by 28% of children with ASD in England [65]. Evidence to support their use is encouraging; a recent randomised control trial in 27 children found a decrease in hyperactive behaviour in the supplemented group [108]. A number of small studies have had similar encouraging results, but larger scale research is needed [109, 110]. The evidence for the use of omega-3 fatty acids for other disorders commonly associated with ASD, such as depression and ADHD, is also promising [111]. A trial of increased omega-3 intake via supplements or food sources (plus reduction in antagonistic omega-6 intake) seems a sensible and safe intervention to trial, and is in line with healthy eating guidelines. As it is hypothesised that the mechanism of action of omega-3 intake is the improved composition of brain cell membranes and subsequent effect on nerve transmission and brain function [112], it is wise to trial this intervention for 3 months, the suggested time it takes for cell membrane composition to change. Some organisations advocate the use of hemp oil rubbed into the skin as a therapeutic option, but there is no evidence for this.
- **Probiotics** – are taken by 10% of children with ASD in England [65]. A double blind placebo controlled trial of *L. plantarum* WCFS1 showed improvements in stool consistency and behaviour in children with ASD, but the drop out rate was high and resulted in only 17 out of 62 completing the 3 week trial [113]. More research is needed, and use of different probiotics strains for help with gastrointestinal symptoms should be considered on an individual basis.
- **Digestive enzymes** – numerous digestive enzyme products containing peptidases aimed at children with ASD are available, and are taken by 3% of children with ASD in England [65]. A double blind placebo controlled trial, using crossover design over 6 months for 43 children, saw no clinically significant improvement in behaviour or gastrointestinal

symptoms, but a small significant improvement was seen in food variety eaten [114].

Practicalities of implementing and monitoring dietary interventions

Monitoring symptoms before, during and after any dietary intervention can help a family to be objective about any perceived outcomes and help them to convince any sceptical professionals of any improvements they have seen. It can be useful to spend some time helping parents draw up an objective list of symptoms to monitor that are pertinent to their child. Another checklist which could be used is the autism treatment evaluation checklist (ATEC), a tool that has been developed by the Autism Research Institute in the USA and can be accessed and scored via their website. The scoring is of 77 items, split into four subgroups. Scoring is quite crude, e.g. constipation – not a problem/minor problem/moderate problem/serious problem. ATEC score changes are sometimes used

as outcome measures in research; the nearer to zero, the more neurotypical the result. A preliminary study on validation found high internal consistency, but more work is needed for it to be accepted as a valid tool [115].

Parents can be advised to undertake any desired intervention objectively by establishing baseline behaviours and symptoms, implementing the chosen intervention strictly for a set time and then reintroducing the baseline diet. Reintroduction is the key step to determine whether an intervention has been effective. Parents who have seen improvements in their child are often very reluctant to take this step and those who have seen no, or only subtle, changes are often keen to continue as organisations report that it can take up to a year to see any improvements.

Transition to adult care

Access to 'ASD friendly' adult services varies and in some areas is non-existent. In England the

Table 23.4 Suggested good practice for dietetic care of children and young people with ASD.

Make necessary changes to clinic setting and appointment times

Initially aim for intake in line with healthy eating guidelines, aiming for intake to meet the RNI for the full range of vitamins and minerals using a supplement if unachievable with diet modification. Particularly consider iron supplementation if sleep problems are present

Be proactive in requesting vitamin and mineral tests for children with restricted diets. Consider seeking local consensus that this is automatically included (plus coeliac screen) when blood is drawn for genetic screening after initial diagnosis to minimise stress on child

In children with restricted diets for whom advice about faddy eating has not been successful, assess contributing factors which may include sensory issues and food phobia; advise appropriately on strategies for overcoming these. Involve other professionals in the assessment and management of identified problems where possible

Consider avoidance of food additives and sweeteners, and inclusion of omega-3 rich foods or supplements with concurrent reduction of omega-6 intake, particularly if ADHD also present

If there are signs of any otherwise unexplained gastrointestinal problems, refer to paediatrician or gastroenterologist for coeliac screen and further investigation

If indicated by gastrointestinal symptoms, or behaviour that may be caused by gastrointestinal distress, consider trial exclusion of gluten and/or milk and/or soya and/or fermentable carbohydrates and/or any foods suspected by parents to be troublesome; and/or trial of prebiotics or probiotics

If epilepsy is present consider trial of classic or modified ketogenic diet, in conjunction with neurologist, or referral to a centre which is experienced in this approach

If parents are keen to try therapeutic doses of supplements advise them to seek supervision from a doctor and to consider monitoring serum vitamin and mineral levels government published the Adult Autism Strategy in 2010 as a requirement of the Autism Act 2009. It sets out key actions and recommendations for central government, local authorities and the NHS to improve services. Transition is particularly stressful for individuals with ASD who generally dislike change and therefore clear preparation and good handover of care is important.

Good practice

The rapid rise in cases of ASD and the cost of this little understood condition is leading to much research into its causes and effective management internationally. The interest in and evidence behind diet in the management, and even prevention, of ASD is certain to increase. It is an area in which dietetic input will become increasingly important and dietitians should identify gaps in their knowledge and skills for working with this group of patients and seek out training opportunities to fill them. Suggested good practice for the dietetic care of a child or young person with ASD is set out in Table 23.4. Dietitians should ensure that commissioners and service managers are aware that additional funding may be needed in order to provide good dietetic care for children and young people with ASD, in light of the increase in patient numbers, the need for longer consultations and additional training.

Appendum

The National Institute for Health and Clinical Excellence (NICE) published *Autism – Management of Autism in Children and Young People (CG170)* in August 2013, available at http://guidance.nice.org .uk/CG170. This guidance highlights eating problems as common and recommends that diet should not be used as a treatment for core autism features. The NICE Autism Quality Standard QS51 was published in January 2014 and includes standard 2: "people having a diagnostic assessment for autism are also assessed for coexisting physical health conditions and mental health problems". Available at http://publications .nice.org.uk/autism-qs51

The fifth version of the American Psychiatric Association Diagnostic and Statistical Manual of Mental Disorders (DSM5) was published in 2013 and sets out new criteria for the categorisation of autism spectrum disorders – see www.dsm5.org /Documents/Autism%20Spectrum%20Disorder %20Fact%20Sheet.pdf

Acknowledgements

This chapter is a significant revision of the chapter in the third edition of this book, which was written with the kind help of members of the UK group Dietitians in Autism (then known as DASIG) and numerous other colleagues experienced in working with children with ASD. A major contribution to the section on dietary interventions was drafted by David Rex RD. Additional thanks to current members of Dietitians in Autism for feedback on this revised chapter.

Useful addresses

Dietitians in Autism is part of the Paediatric and Mental Health Groups of the British Dietetic Association. Membership is open to dietitians who are members of either of these BDA groups and who have an interest in autism. For more information see the BDA website, www.dietitiansinautism.org.uk or info@dietitiansinautism.org.uk.

24 Epidermolysis Bullosa

Melanie Sklar and Lesley Haynes

Introduction

Epidermolysis bullosa (EB) comprises a group of rare genetically determined skin blistering disorders characterised by extreme fragility of the skin and mucous membranes.

Types

The most recent classification [1] separates EB into four main types which are further divided into subtypes:

- Simplex (EBS) – suprabasal and basal, including EBS-Dowling Meara and EBS-Localised (previously known as EBS-Weber Cockayne)
- Junctional (JEB) – Herlitz (HJEB) and others, including non-Herlitz JEB (NHJEB)
- Dystrophic (DEB) – dominant (DDEB) and recessive (RDEB)
- Kindler syndrome – has recently been added to this classification

The first three types are illustrated in Fig. 24.1.

The classification of each EB type and subtype is based on genotype, phenotype and mode of inheritance. All types result from genetic mutations which cause a defect in, or absence of, a structural protein in the dermal–epidermal basement membrane zone or, in the case of suprabasal EBS, between adjacent keratinocytes. The resultant defective adhesion means that minor knocks or friction can cause the skin to blister. Currently, 14 different genes encoding these proteins have been implicated in different types of EB. In many instances, the exact nature of a mutation and its position on the gene will determine the phenotypic characteristics. Mutations are identified by screening the child's DNA. This helps to confirm the diagnosis, may be useful for genotype–phenotype correlation and may determine the mode of inheritance.

Mode of inheritance

EB is usually inherited either dominantly or recessively; it may also result from a spontaneous genetic mutation with no previous family history [2]. In dominant inheritance, the affected parent (who has EB) passes on the faulty gene to their child. There is a 1 in 2 chance with each pregnancy that a child will inherit the affected gene. The more severe forms, where each parent carries the affected gene (but does not have EB), are generally recessively inherited. In each pregnancy with two carrier parents, there is a 1 in 4 chance of an affected child being conceived.

Clinical Paediatric Dietetics, Fourth Edition. Edited by Vanessa Shaw.
© 2015 John Wiley & Sons, Ltd. Published 2015 by John Wiley & Sons, Ltd.
Companion Website: www.wiley.com/go/shaw/paediatricdietetics

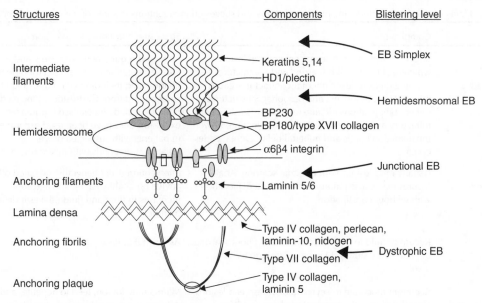

Structures   Components   Blistering level

Intermediate   Keratins 5,14   EB Simplex
filaments   HD1/plectin

                                                                        Hemidesmosomal EB

                                                    BP230
Hemidesmosome   BP180/type XVII collagen

                                                    α6β4 integrin

                                                                        Junctional EB

Anchoring filaments   Laminin 5/6

Lamina densa

Anchoring fibrils   Type IV collagen, perlecan,
                                                    laminin-10, nidogen
                                                                        Dystrophic EB
                                                    Type VII collagen

Anchoring plaque   Type IV collagen,
                                                    laminin 5

Figure 24.1 Schematic representation of the dermal-epidermal basement membrane zone. This shows the position of specific structural proteins relevant to EB. Image reprinted with permission from Medscape.com, 2012. Available at http://emedicine.medscape.com/article/1062939-overview.

Diagnosis

A history is taken and physical examination performed; this may be followed by a skin biopsy. Non molecular techniques that are used to examine the skin biopsy include

- immunofluorescence microscopy and antigen mapping – these determine the expression of different EB associated proteins in the skin and the level of blistering by the use of antibodies [3]
- transmission electron microscopy – this determines the level of blistering and other ultrastructural clues to aid diagnosis. This is the gold standard for EB diagnosis; however, it requires great expertise and special equipment which many laboratories worldwide lack [4]

Prevalence

Prevalence is difficult to assess as mild cases may go undiagnosed, while the severely affected may die before a diagnosis is confirmed. In the UK, prevalence of all types of EB and all ages in late 2010 was estimated at 15 per million of the population [5]. EB affects the sexes equally and occurs in all races. The consequences of different EB types vary greatly in their impact, ranging from death in infancy to relatively minor handicap with normal life expectancy. Mental development is normal.

Management

Some types of EB remain the most physically disabling and disfiguring of all diseases and nutritional status is severely compromised (Table 24.1). These include RDEB, HJEB and the Dowling-Meara subtype of EBS where nutritional intervention is generally required from birth. There is currently no cure for any type of EB. A claim that one can be effected by giving an exclusion diet combined with topical and systemic treatments (the Kozak regimen) was disproved in an open evaluation [6]. Management is geared towards supportive care and prevention, or minimisation, of complications where possible. This includes control of infection, wound management, pain relief, promotion of optimal nutritional status, surgical intervention and provision of best possible quality of life (QoL) [7]. These should be addressed in a multidisciplinary team setting.

Research is currently under way into new therapies which provide longer lasting improvement in

Table 24.1 Main complications influencing nutritional status and suggested interventions in some of the main types of EB.

EB type	Complications	Suggested nutritional intervention
RDEB Severe Generalised	Recurrent moderate to severe generalised lesions which heal poorly with scarring and contractures (causing digits to fuse). Internal contractures cause microstomia, dysphagia and oesophageal strictures. Other complications include osteoporosis/osteopenia, refractory anaemia, anal fissures, constipation, bowel inflammation/colitis and pubertal delay. Dental caries common	Increased requirements of energy and protein. Supplementation of certain micronutrients may be indicated including vitamins C and D, zinc, calcium and iron. Gastrostomy tube feeding often indicated. Specialised formula feeds and exclusion diets have been used experimentally in patients with suspected bowel inflammation/colitis with mixed results
DDEB Generalised	Usually mild lesions with minimal scarring. Anal fissures may cause painful and reluctant defaecation with/without constipation	Intervention is not generally indicated other than advice on healthy eating and age appropriate increases in fibre and fluid intakes if defaecation painful
NHJEB Generalised	Recurrent mild to severe lesions heal without scarring, but often very slowly. May be genito-urinary involvement	As for RDEB, if severe
HJEB	Recurrent moderate to severe and widespread lesions. Dental pain due to abnormal tooth composition. Laryngeal and respiratory complications. Initial weight gain usually followed by profound, intractable growth failure, possible protein losing enteropathy and diarrhoea. Death usually within first year or two of life	Maintain hydration, feed to appetite, address deficiencies within terminal care framework. Experimentally, minimal fat diet with medium chain triglycerides has been used. Gastrostomy placement not recommended as laryngeal/respiratory issues greatly complicate general anaesthesia and healing around exit site is very poor. Regular weighing to be undertaken only to determine best regimen for pain relief. Emphasis to be placed on quality of life
EBS Dowling–Meara	Wide range of severity in this type of EB. Feeding difficulties often severe in infancy including gastro-oesophageal reflux and oropharyngeal blistering. Problems generally lessen in late infancy/early childhood. Catch-up growth often occurs around adolescence. Sedentary lifestyle during adolescence tends to promote overweight as blistering becomes more confined to hands and feet. Anal fissures frequently cause painful defaecation with/without constipation	As for RDEB in early years, but gastrostomy placement is rarely necessary. Fibre, iron, zinc and vitamin supplementation may be indicated. Advice on healthy eating and weight maintenance/reduction may be indicated
EBS–Localised	Lesions usually confined to hands and feet, especially in hot weather, often severely limiting mobility. Frequently painful defaecation with/without constipation	Intervention is generally not indicated other than advice on healthy eating and age appropriate increases in fibre and fluid intakes if defaecation painful. Due to compromised mobility, advice on weight maintenance/reduction may be indicated
Kindler syndrome	Photosensitivity. Thin papery skin with variable tendency to develop lesions which predominantly affect limbs and fingers (which may fuse). May also be involvement of oesophageal, laryngeal, urethral and anal mucosa. Colitis has been documented. Gingival fragility and inflammation with poor dentition. Blistering tendency may lessen around adolescence	Intervention not generally indicated unless growth falters and/or gastrointestinal complications necessitate relevant management

EB, epidermolysis bullosa; RDEB, recessive dystrophic EB; DDEB, dominant dystrophic EB; NHJEB, non Herlitz junctional EB; HJEB, Herlitz junctional EB; EBS, EB simplex.

patients' conditions and, ultimately, a cure. These include [8]

- therapies which target local healing such as grafting with genetically corrected skin or injections into the skin of collagen or fibroblasts
- systemic therapies aimed at whole body healing using intravenous (IV) injections of bone marrow or other stem cells

Whilst some interventions aim for temporary improvement (collagen or fibroblast therapy) others aim for a permanent cure (grafting with genetically corrected skin or bone marrow transplant).

Nutrition support

Current practice relies on retrospective studies of small numbers of children, expert clinical experience and extrapolation from other conditions affecting the skin such as burns and pressure ulcers. Published work suggests that early, proactive intervention has the best chance of optimising nutritional status, wellbeing and wound healing in the longer term [9–12].

Breastfeeding should always be encouraged; however, rooting at the breast may cause or exacerbate facial lesions and suckling may lead to blistering of the mouth, tongue and gums. This can be eased by applying white soft paraffin (white petroleum jelly) to the lips and to the nipple to reduce friction. Except in mild cases, breast milk alone fails to meet increased nutritional requirements and it should be supplemented with standard age appropriate infant formulas either mixed with expressed breast milk (EBM) (p. 17) or given in addition to direct breast feeding. Alternatively, if formula feeding, the nutrient density of a standard age appropriate formula can be increased by concentrating the feed, or a proprietary formula with increased nutrient density can be used (Table 1.18). It is essential that any feed modifications and their rationale are explained to parents and community medical and nursing personnel to avoid misunderstandings and conflicting advice.

Feeding teats should be moistened with cooled, boiled water before feeding to avoid the teat sticking to the lips and causing damage when it is removed. A specialised teat and bottle such as the Special Needs Feeder (www.medela.com) is extremely useful as it minimises trauma to the gum

margin and its internal valve and long shaft allow the carer to control the flow of feed so that even a weak suck will deliver a satisfactory milk flow. Alternatively, the hole in a conventional teat can be enlarged using a sterile needle. Care is required to ensure that the hole is not so large that milk flow causes gagging and possible feed aspiration. Babies who cannot suck may need to be fed from a spoon or dropper, but this is time consuming for regular use.

Weaning foods can be offered at the usual time of around 6 months of age using a shallow soft plastic spoon with rounded edges. Carers will need continual reassurance if progression to solids is slow and babies with an extremely fragile mouth may feed more confidently from the carer's fingertip. Reluctance to try new foods is often due to previously, or ongoing, poorly controlled gastro-oesophageal reflux (GOR) [13], a very fragile painful mouth or previous nasogastric tube feeding. Scarring and tongue tethering can cause an uncoordinated swallow with the risk of aspiration [14].

There is often early aversion to food composed of mixed textures (such as the soft lumps within a more liquid matrix found in many commercial baby foods) whereas uniform textures tend to be accepted with more confidence. Hard or sharp foods such as baked rusks or crisp bread crusts are unsuitable as they damage the fragile mucosa of the mouth and gums. Although there is no evidence to suggest that long term adherence to puréed or very soft foods necessarily influences the course of dysphagia and oesophageal strictures, babies who demonstrate swallowing problems from early on may be best to remain indefinitely on such textures. The expertise of a speech and language therapist is invaluable in recommending appropriate feeding utensils and promoting confidence in feeding. Practical information for carers and community personnel can be found in the booklets *Nutrition for Babies with Epidermolysis Bullosa* and *Nutrition in Epidermolysis Bullosa, for Children over 1 Year of Age* published by the Dystrophic Epidermolysis Bullosa Research Association (DEBRA) and downloadable from www.debra.org.uk/publications.

The complications of RDEB in particular begin in infancy and, except in mild cases, progressively increase as the child gets older [11, 15]. The causes and effects of severe generalised RDEB on

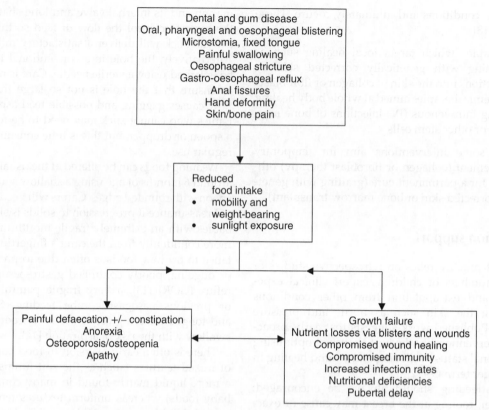

Figure 24.2 Causes and effects of nutritional problems in severe generalised recessive dystrophic epidermolysis bullosa.

nutritional intake are shown in Fig. 24.2. Factors such as painful defaecation (with or without constipation), extensive non healing lesions, chronic infections, general skin and bone pain, anaemia, malaise and refusal of oral medications and supplements all contribute significantly to the potential for profound nutritional compromise.

Nasogastric tube feeding

Despite taking great care, nasogastric (NG) tubes can cause external and internal trauma and should not be placed routinely. Externally, NG tubes should be secured with only non adhesive dressings or silicone tapes that are recommended for fragile skin. Internally, NG tubes may cause damage to the nasal tissues. In addition, they may traumatise or scar the pharynx and oesophagus interfering with oral feeding and compromising a safe swallow. Circumstances in which NG feeding

may be indicated as a temporary measure include when

- a baby's mouth becomes excessively traumatised by suckling
- satisfactory volumes of oral nutrition are not taken at any age
- gastrostomy placement is considered appropriate but evidence of the effects of improved nutrition are needed before surgery can be agreed

A 4–6 week period of NG feeding should be sufficient to show benefit.

Gastrostomy tube feeding

Publications documenting gastrostomy tube feeding (GTF) describe differing outcomes. While it has been associated with minimal complications and improved growth and bowel function, it has also been linked to pain; intractable leakage; infection and excoriation around the gastrostomy tube (G tube) insertion site; gastrointestinal (GI) problems such as severe abdominal bloating, diarrhoea, colitis, feed and food intolerance, worsening of GOR disease; abnormal body composition and central obesity [16–23]. However, in all cases, parents have expressed great relief in the stresses surrounding feeding and administration of supplements and medications, highlighting the value of GTF as a management choice and the importance of determining best practice.

The reasons for conflicting outcomes are currently unidentified, but several potential factors have been suggested including malnourished state when placement is delayed; constipation; GOR; poor placement technique of G tube and its aftercare; chronic inflammation; polypharmacy [19]. Pro-inflammatory cytokines are thought to play a critical role in GI complications and the central obesity, increased fat mass and poor linear growth seen in some G tube fed children with EB [22]. After G tube placement some children develop an aversion to oral intake, preferring to rely almost entirely on gastrostomy feeds. This may reflect previous long term negativity about eating and relief at having an alternative route for nutrition. The general consensus is for G tube placement to be undertaken before complications allow malnutrition and growth retardation, with their many sequelae, to become established. With early intervention, the child is more likely to continue with oral nutrition, albeit in small and varying amounts. This is important in relation to the potential to minimise volumes of feed given overnight which impacts on tolerance of feed volumes and the need to pass urine during the night, as well as the social aspects of eating.

Oesophageal stricturing is a major reason for reduced food intake in RDEB and oesophageal dilatation (OD), singly or in series, can ease dysphagia. However, OD cannot guarantee a sufficiently increased oral intake to reverse nutritional deficits and promote catch-up growth so is not a substitute for GTF. Further work is needed to identify best practice in GTF (probably in tandem with OD) as these are currently the only practical interventions available to address nutritional compromise in the longer term [19].

Various methods of G tube placement in EB are used including open surgical gastrostomy, laparoscopically assisted endoscopy, modified laparoscopic gastrostomy and endoscopic and non-endoscopic percutaneous gastrostomy [22, 23].

The tube may be replaced by a low profile device 10–12 weeks postoperatively [23]. It is important that all internal securing material is soft or deflatable to minimise local irritation or damage to the fragile tract during change or removal. The device must be neither too loose nor too tight and the site measured each time it is changed to ensure a continuing good fit. Local policies vary regarding whether the device should be rotated. G tube feeds are generally begun within 4–6 hours of surgery, initially using sterile water, to ensure absence of leakage; discharge is usually within 48–72 hours (personal communications).

In children with impaired gastric emptying, intractable GOR or feed aspiration it may be advantageous to feed lower into the gut via a gastrojejunal or jejunal tube. As with any other child, this has implications for the rate at which feeds can be given, their volume and composition (Table 3.4).

Parenteral nutrition

Parenteral nutrition (PN) has been used in EB children with profound malnutrition or when oral intake has been severely limited by painful oral ulceration [18]. However, indwelling intravenous lines pose significant risks of septicaemia which limits their usefulness; therefore PN should be reserved for cases refractory to enteral feeding [24].

Nutritional assessment

Measurements of weight and height velocity are currently the most practical means of assessing growth. Weight and if possible height (length) should be measured regularly. Downward deviation from the birthweight centile in the first year is common in severe types of EB despite proactive nutritional interventions.

Weight measurements should ideally be performed directly after a dressing change as wound exudates in the dressings could lead to overestimation. Although nude weight is ideal, the skin damage incurred during handling usually precludes this.

Due to pain and contractures around joints, height measurements are impractical in severely affected children. A supine stadiometer or measuring mat may provide greater accuracy. If neither of these is possible, segmental measurements using specialised calipers or a metal tape may be used [11].

Other anthropometric measurements are difficult to perform as dressings impede access to desired areas and measuring instruments may damage the skin.

Despite proactive nutritional intervention, growth retardation often occurs early in the course of severe EB [20, 21]. Since complications increase in number and severity over time, it is difficult to judge whether growth and overall nutritional status are optimal. The traditional 'rule-of-thumb' that disparity between weight and height should not be greater than two major centiles is generally applicable. Although body mass index (BMI) does not differentiate between lean and fat tissue, data from a centre with good outcomes following G tube placement suggests it as a reliable means to monitor growth and predict optimal timing for placement [25].

Regular nutritional assessment (Table 24.2) is important not only to address ongoing problems but also to anticipate them. The proforma in Table 24.2 can be used to record relevant information.

THINC, a Tool to Help Identify Nutritional Compromise (currently unvalidated), has been developed as a comprehensive method of assessing the risk of actual or potential nutritional compromise in EB children under and over 18 months of age and forms part of nutrition clinical practice guidelines written for EB [26]. It has been developed to aid, not replace, clinical judgement and its scoring charts rate the three key aspects of the child's state: weight and height; gastroenterology and feeding; dermatology. The higher the score, the greater is the likelihood of nutritional compromise. According to the total nutritional compromise score, algorithms suggest varying courses of action.

Biochemistry and haematology

Interpretation of laboratory results in EB children is difficult because of the inflammatory nature of the condition. Table 24.3 [27] lists investigations that should be carried out with suggested sampling

intervals. Frequency depends on disease severity, the need to evaluate an intervention or to modify management.

Nutritional requirements

Two main factors potentially compromise nutritional status in EB:

- the hypercatabolic state in which open skin lesions with consequent losses of blood and serous fluid, increased protein turnover, heat loss and infection all contribute to increased requirements
- the degree to which oral, oropharyngeal, oesophageal and GI complications limit intake

It is difficult to quantify nutritional requirements due to [11]

- the diversity of disease severity of patients even with the same EB type
- the variability over time of individual patients' requirements
- the difficulties associated with estimating desirable weight gain when height is compromised
- the location and presence of infection which complicates the interpretation of laboratory results
- the chronic inflammatory nature of EB characterised by continued expression of pro-inflammatory cytokines [19]

Energy

Energy requirements can be estimated using the following formula [15]:

$$\text{weight (kg)} \times \text{(kcal/kg for height age)}$$
$$\times [1 + (\text{sum of 3 additional factors})]$$

Additional factors:

1 Ratio of blisters to body surface area (BSA): 20% BSA = 0.19, 40% BSA = 0.5, 100% BSA = 0.95
2 Sepsis: mild = 0.2, moderate = 0.4, severe = 0.8
3 Catch-up growth: 0.1 to 0.2

An example calculation using this formula is given in Table 24.4. Although this method provides a working figure, the scoring of skin involvement is

Table 24.2   Suggested proforma for recording nutritional intake and other relevant information.

NAME:	DOB:	HOSPITAL NUMBER:	DATE:

WEIGHT:	kg	centile	**HEIGHT:**	cm	centile

CONSISTENCY OF FOOD: Normal   Soft   Purée   Fluid

REASON(S)	Oral blistering	Microstomia	Fixed tongue
	Dental caries	Dysphagia	Oesophageal stricture
	Regurgitation of mucus/pooled secretions		Gastro-oesophageal reflux

TYPICAL BOWEL HABIT: BO   × day   × week

Pain   Bleeding per rectum   Stool consistency

LAXATIVE(S), PREBIOTIC(S), PROBIOTIC(S) etc.   *Record name(s), dose, frequency

Lactulose   Movicol   Sodium picosulphate   Other*

Resource Optifibre   Other prebiotic*   Probiotic*

TYPICAL	Breakfast:
	Snack:
MEAL	Lunch:
	Snack:
PATTERN	Evening:
	Bedtime:

Time taken over an average meal: minutes   Finishes amount offered?

FEEDING TUBE *in situ*?   Type (including make, shaft length)

NUTRIENT DENSE/ENERGY DENSE SUPPLEMENT(S)/GASTROSTOMY FEEDS:

Record name(s), dose, frequency

OTHER SUPPLEMENT(S):   Record name(s), dose, frequency

Iron	Zinc	Fluoride	Calcium	Vitamin D_3
Other vitamins		Selenium	Other	

APPROX. DAILY INTAKE: Protein   g (/kg)   Normal DRV =   g (/kg)

Energy   kcal (/kg)   Normal DRV =   kcal (/kg)

COMMENTS/ACTION

DRV, dietary reference value for age and gender matched healthy child.

Table 24.3 Laboratory investigations.

Investigation	Suggested sampling intervals
Urea and electrolytes: Sodium, potassium, urea, creatinine	6 monthly unless abnormal
Liver function tests: Total bilirubin, albumin, alkaline phosphatase, alanine aminotransferase, aspartate aminotransferase	6 monthly
Bone profile: Calcium, phosphate, alkaline phosphatase, vitamin D	6 monthly
Trace elements: Zinc, selenium, vitamin B_{12}, vitamin A, vitamin C, folic acid	Annually
Iron studies: Total iron binding capacity Serum iron Ferritin	3–6 monthly depending on degree of anaemia and if having iron infusions
Full blood count (FBC)	3–6 monthly depending on degree of anaemia
Red cell folate	Annually

Table 24.4 Case study: high energy and protein requirements in EB.

A 6-year-old boy with severe generalised recessive dystrophic EB (RDEB)
Weight 13 kg (<0.4th centile) Height 107 cm (2nd centile) Height age 4.7 years
He is on iron supplements twice a day and suffers from constipation. He has 20% body surface area (BSA) blistered, with mild sepsis. He has microstomia and after two oesophageal dilatations within a year a gastrostomy was placed. He continues to manage small amounts of food orally

Daily requirements
Fluid requirement based on actual weight 1150 mL

Energy requirement calculated by applying the formula (p. 696): $13 \times 90 \times [1 + (0.19 + 0.2 + 0.2)] = 1860$ kcal (7.8 MJ) or 143 kcal (595 kJ)/kg

Energy requirement based on 130–180 kcal/kg = 1690–2340 kcal (7.1–9.8 MJ)

Protein requirement based on 2.5–4 g protein/kg = 33–52 g

Fibre requirement = 11–16 g

Gastrostomy feeds
1150 mL high energy paediatric fibre containing formula, e.g. Paediasure Plus Fibre: 150 kcal (630 kJ), 4.2 g protein and 1.1 g fibre per 100 mL
Energy = 1725 kcal (7.2 MJ)   Protein = 48 g   Fibre = 12.7 g

Feeding plan
100 mL/hour × 10 hours continuously overnight or 2 × 500 mL boluses morning and late evening depending on tolerance and family's preference
150 mL orally or given as a bolus through the gastrostomy at lunch or mid-afternoon
Continue to offer oral intake of foods with the textures altered accordingly. Foods such as fruit and vegetable purées should be particularly encouraged due to their fibre content

Follow-up
Initially monthly to assess feed tolerance and weight gain and then every 3 months

subjective and the formula is complex. A simpler method is to use 115%–150% of the estimated average requirement for energy [28] in order to provide sufficient energy to promote weight gain and wound healing: 130–180 kcal (545–750 kJ)/kg actual body weight per day. Requirements can be as high as 225 kcal (940 kJ)/kg if the skin is septic or growth failure is profound.

Protein

Protein plays a most important role throughout the entire wound healing process. Collagen is the protein that is produced mainly in the healing wound of normal skin; therefore a lack of protein decreases the synthesis of collagen and the production of fibroblasts [29]. Protein requirements in EB are estimated to be approximately 10%–15% of energy intake, extrapolated from the recommendation of 9% energy intake for catch-up growth in children with normal skin [30]. Children with extensive lesions will require an intake at the higher end of the range, especially where there is associated sepsis. Protein requirements tend to be 2.5–4 g/kg (115%–200% reference nutrient intake [28]), based on chronological age.

Micronutrients

Micronutrients are known to play essential roles in metabolism, wound healing, cellular immunity and antioxidant activity. Research in burns and pressure ulcers suggests that it may be beneficial to supplement certain micronutrients in EB [31] since deficiencies of specific micronutrients including iron, selenium, zinc and vitamins A, B_6, B_{12}, C and D have been identified [15, 17, 32]. However, the role of increased intakes of single or multiple micronutrients is unclear even in individuals with normal skin, and more work is required to identify both the clinical conditions and the doses of individual micronutrients that actively promote or accelerate healing [33, 34]. Severely affected EB children are often prescribed multiple supplements and medications, many of which are co-administered with feeds for reasons of practicality. This raises questions of nutrient bioavailability and drug–nutrient interactions which are poorly understood even in

healthy individuals [35] and even less so when body composition is disordered [36].

Vitamins

It is likely that severely affected children need increased amounts of all vitamins [32]. Babies taking concentrated or nutrient dense feeds receive correspondingly increased amounts of all vitamins. Older children consistently consuming significant volumes of nutritional supplements receive corresponding amounts of vitamins from these. If, however, a satisfactory vitamin intake is in doubt at any age, an age appropriate multivitamin supplement should be recommended. The provision of 150%–200% of the RNI of all vitamins ensures intakes are still within safe limits.

Vitamin C enhances iron absorption and promotes collagen synthesis [37]. It also plays a role in the immune response [29] through its antioxidant properties where it limits tissue damage and prolonged inflammation [38]. Children with EB often avoid the main food sources of vitamin C due to their tendency to irritate the mouth and pharynx, so supplementation is recommended.

Zinc

Zinc is an essential cofactor for more than 200 enzymes and plays vital roles in growth, wound healing, immune function and membrane stability where its antioxidant properties are crucial [39, 40]. However, the degree of desirable supplementation in EB is unclear. Intakes of more than 200% of the RNI are probably unnecessary because improvement in wound healing may only occur in previously deficient states, if at all. Excessive intakes have been reported to impair the immune response in adults [41] and may interfere with copper and iron absorption [29, 42].

It is not appropriate to supplement zinc routinely or solely on the basis of blood tests as these are not dependable measures of zinc status; dietary assessment is a far superior means of estimating potential deficiency. Blood tests are unreliable as inflammation and infection sequester zinc within the liver and, when plasma levels of albumin are low (often the case in EB), plasma zinc levels will also be reported as low [43]. In this situation, body tissues are saturated and supplementary zinc is simply excreted in the urine. This is not only uneconomical but, more importantly, zinc frequently causes nausea, abdominal pain and even vomiting, major causes of non-compliance with nutritional treatment.

If supplementation is considered necessary, flavoured zinc lozenges (not prescribable) may be better tolerated than liquid or effervescent preparations. These dissolve slowly in the mouth, but their chalky mouth feel is unacceptable to some children and their texture may irritate the fragile oral mucosa. To optimise absorption and minimise nausea, the daily dose should be divided into two.

Iron and zinc have the potential to interact, leading to potentially reduced absorption of both [29]. It may be prudent to advise giving zinc supplements, if not on different days from iron supplements, then at least at different times of the day, although no trial has yet shown clearly the merits of either regimen.

Immune enhanced formulas

'Immune enhanced' formulas containing nutrients such as arginine, glutamine and essential fatty acids are marketed for adults as promoting healing, optimising immune status and exerting a beneficial effect on inflammatory conditions [38, 44]. These properties would be highly advantageous in EB, but as yet their efficacy has not been tested.

Calcium and vitamin D – osteopenia and osteoporosis

A number of mechanisms are thought to contribute to the observed low bone mineral density (BMD) for chronological age seen in RDEB and JEB [24, 45–47]. These include reduced mobility, poor nutritional intake, reduced sunlight exposure (from restricted outdoor activities and extensive bandaging), chronic inflammation (pro-inflammatory cytokines increase osteoclastic activity) and pubertal delay. In addition, GI complications may affect absorption of relevant nutrients [11].

Annual monitoring of all children with RDEB and JEB from 5 years of age is recommended. Dual energy x-ray absorptiometry (DEXA) scan and lateral x-rays of the lumbar and thoracic spine and ankles are suggested to detect clinically significant osteoporosis and fractures respectively. Annual bone age assessment for adolescents, specifically those with pubertal delay, should also be undertaken [48].

Intravenous pamidronate and oral risedronate have been used to address bone pain associated with osteopenia, osteoporosis and fractures. However, information on their effects on BMD in this group of patients is lacking. If osteoporosis, fractures and/or low serum levels are detected, calcium and vitamin D should be supplemented and the serum bone profile monitored (p. 704).

Iron and anaemia

Children with severe EB are at risk of iron deficiency through reduced dietary intake, increased iron losses (through blood and skin) and possibly reduced GI iron absorption. Due to inflammation, a degree of 'anaemia of chronic disease' accompanies iron deficiency changes. Although iron's participation as a cofactor for antioxidants and collagen synthesis has been demonstrated, causal links between iron supplementation and improved wound healing have not been identified [38].

Haemoglobin (Hb) levels correlate very poorly with measures or markers of iron status in EB. Hepatic mechanisms respond to inflammation by decreasing intestinal uptake and release of iron into plasma. In addition, transferrin levels decrease in response to inflammation and ferritin levels can increase. Therefore currently there may be little value in routine iron evaluation; rather it may be assumed that all children with severe EB are likely to be iron deficient. There is no clear consensus regarding timing of anaemia treatment especially as the relative inactivity of many children allows them to tolerate low Hb levels before becoming symptomatic [19].

Oral iron supplements are widely used, although compliance is often poor because of the association with constipation and gastric irritation. IV iron supplementation may be necessary in children refractory to, or unable to tolerate, oral supplements. An Hb level of <8 g/dL or symptoms such as shortness of breath are taken as a signal to intervene with blood transfusion. However, this provides only temporary improvement and carries the risk of iron overload [19].

The limited data on the use of erythropoietin (EPO) (or an analogue) in EB, either alone or in conjunction with IV iron, indicate that such treatments result in improvement in Hb levels and general wellbeing. However, the need for regular injections of EPO and its high cost limits its usefulness in routine practice for children with EB [19].

Selenium and carnitine – dilated cardiomyopathy

No clear cause of dilated cardiomyopathy (DC) in children with EB has yet been identified [49] but poor global nutritional status, chronic iron overload from repeated transfusions [50], low carnitine and selenium levels [50,51], concomitant viral illness, chronic anaemia, coexistent renal failure and medications (amitriptyline and cisapride) [52] have been proposed as possible contributors to its development. Most reported cases have been fatal and to date there is no evidence that the underlying genetic mutations in RDEB have a role in the pathogenesis of DC. Annual cardiac assessment (echocardiogram and electrocardiogram and referral to a cardiologist if either of these is abnormal) should be performed in all children with severe RDEB and JEB to identify early changes leading to DC.

Selenium supplementation reverses cardiomyopathy if started early in the disease process [50]. Pure selenium is currently available in the UK as a 50 μg/day tablet which must be prescribed and dispensed from a hospital pharmacy (it cannot be prescribed by a GP). If it is to be given via an NG feeding tube or gastrostomy, it must be crushed finely and carefully mixed with water. This is time consuming and any undissolved pieces can block the device. A liquid formulation of selenium is more practical (e.g. Selenase Oral Solution) and provides 500 μg/10 mL. This is prescribable but contains no preservative and therefore has a very short shelf life which restricts its use.

When total plasma carnitine is normal, any decrease in free carnitine should not be considered as a real deficiency and does not represent a risk for the development of DC [17]. Carnitine supplementation does not reverse cardiomyopathy, but it can prevent its progression. Carnitine deficiency should be addressed by giving 50–100 mg/kg/day Carnitor Paediatric Solution.

Painful defaecation with or without constipation – fibre

Painful defaecation with or without constipation is one of the most common and under-recognised GI problems associated with EB and is seen in all major subtypes, especially RDEB. Constipation results from straining to defaecate leading to painful perianal blistering and fissures or faecal retention due to pain or fear of defaecation. Disordered food intake due to oral lesions, dental problems and dysphagia is not conducive to a regular bowel pattern and iron supplements cause constipation in some children. This situation is exacerbated by reduced physical activity [18].

Measures to normalise bowel habit include increasing intake of fluid and fibre in the form of age appropriate fibre rich foods and fibre containing feeds, pure fibre supplements such as Resource Optifibre and/or softeners/laxatives [53]. In the absence of UK recommended intakes of fibre for children and adolescents, the US formula of age (years) plus 5–10 g/day is a useful guideline [54].

For babies, extra fluid in the form of water is recommended or, if this is refused, one teaspoon of fresh fruit juice diluted in 100 mL water or ready-to-feed baby juice diluted with an equal volume of water should be offered.

A stool softener such as lactulose should be prescribed, starting with 2.5 mL once daily to 2.5 mL twice daily or a polyethylene glycol formulation such as the Movicol range. Resource Optifibre can be introduced at 6–9 months of age and, because constipation is such a likely complication of all types of EB, it is prudent to introduce an age appropriate fibre source proactively from about 12 months of age, whether the infant is constipated or not [11].

Mineral oil may be useful as a softening agent to lubricate the stool, but should be avoided if there is any risk of aspiration. Fragility of the anal mucosa means that suppositories and enemas should never be given. If clearance of faecal impaction or preoperative bowel preparation is required an osmotic agent, given orally or via feeding tube, is preferred

[24]. In the older child, overflow incontinence can be mistaken for diarrhoea, and carers often reduce or stop the prescribed laxative therapy, inadvertently exacerbating the situation. Children with faecal impaction demonstrable on abdominal radiograph must have their bowel evacuated before the introduction of a further fibre source. If such preparations are introduced while the child remains faecally loaded, abdominal pain, GOR and vomiting will ensue and compliance will be jeopardized [11].

Prebiotics and probiotics

These have been shown to enhance immune function, improve colonic integrity, reduce incidence and duration of intestinal infections, downregulate the allergic response and improve digestion and defaecation; all very desirable for children with EB. Although probiotics have been shown to favourably influence immune status and improve GI tolerance to antibiotic therapy, they have also been associated with adverse effects such as bacteraemia, sepsis and endocarditis [11]. It would be prudent to advise their use only in selected and carefully monitored EB children.

Other issues

Bowel inflammation (colitis)

The precise mechanisms responsible for the colitis seen in EB are not yet understood, but absence of type VII collagen which is normally expressed in the colonic mucosa has been implicated. There have been reports of children almost exclusively with RDEB presenting with diarrhoea which was often explosive in nature. Histological features ranged from absence of abnormality to moderately severe inflammatory changes. The mechanism underlying these changes is uncertain but the defective cell adhesion may result in altered epithelial cell turnover and abnormal mucosal permeability stimulating an inflammatory response [55, 56].

Improvement in symptoms has been documented in children treated with sulfasalazine and occasionally prednisolone. Suspicions that colitis is exacerbated by food antigens have led to regimens excluding milk, egg, wheat and soya [56] (Table 7.10). In two RDEB patients (one adult and one child), exclusion of gluten with concomitant low dose cortisone is reported to have reversed compromised renal function and proteinuria [57]. In addition, both patients reported a reduction in spontaneous skin blistering, general pain and itching and an improvement in mobility. The imposition of stringent dietary restrictions can only be justified if significant benefit can be expected to result and more research is required to investigate this.

Protein losing enteropathy

Protein losing enteropathy (PLE) and diarrhoea have only been described in JEB [56]. It has been reported in both NHJEB and HJEB children, but mostly in those with JEB with pyloric atresia. Alpha-6-beta-4 deficiency has been shown in an infant with total GI mucosal separation and intractable diarrhoea [58]. Hydrolysed protein feeds or whole protein feeds containing mainly medium chain triglycerides (MCT) as the fat source have been used empirically. As in intestinal lymphangiectasia (p. 126), the use of predominantly MCT decreases lymphatic flow and its use has been suggested to improve hypoalbuminaemia and to reduce levels of stool alpha-1-antitrypsin in JEB [56].

Gastro-oesophageal reflux disease

Gastro-oesophageal reflux usually manifests itself in infancy as effortless vomiting. In older children, it may be asymptomatic or cause dyspeptic symptoms. Recurrent oesophageal scarring by acidic gastric contents may cause shortening of the oesophagus, which may predispose to gastro-oesophageal reflux disease (GORD) and to stiffening of the lower oesophageal sphincter, fixing it in an open position, worsening reflux [59]. GORD may be exacerbated by oesophageal dilatation which allows freer reflux of stomach contents into the oesophagus, or by the introduction of gastrostomy feeding [24, 60].

When vomiting and poor weight gain are observed, GOR should be investigated and managed in accordance with age and symptoms as in the child without EB (p. 136). Nissen fundoplication (p. 148) has been used for refractory GOR in children with EB, but there was only a temporary

(<1 year) reduction of symptoms [56]. The surgery is believed to have failed owing to abnormal structure and fragility of the gastric mucosa.

Oesophageal strictures

Oesophageal strictures and dysphagia are almost exclusively seen in RDEB. Lower oesophageal strictures are likely to be precipitated or exacerbated by GORD, whereas upper strictures probably arise from blistering related to ingestion of food. The latter tend to impose ever greater restrictions on the textures of foods that the child is able to swallow, showing dysphagia with hard or bulky foods initially, then with softer foods and eventually with liquids [24].

Initially, food consistency should be modified to tolerance with nutritional supplementation. Moist foods of soft consistency are often preferred but, if swallowing problems are more severe, foods should be puréed [15]. Sips of water between mouthfuls are helpful. Drinking while food is still in the mouth risks gagging and aspiration. When these measures alone are insufficient to ensure adequate nutritional intake, oesophageal dilatation (OD) should be considered.

In the past, OD was performed blindly by bougienage. This technique applied longitudinal shearing forces affecting the entire length of the oesophagus and carrying significant risk of oesophageal perforation. More recently, balloon dilatation (which applies mainly radial forces) either endoscopically or fluoroscopically has been used very successfully. Endoscopic dilatation techniques all carry the inherent risk of oropharyngeal and oesophageal trauma, potentially resulting in strictures which worsen over time. Fluoroscopic guided balloon dilatation uses larger balloons that can achieve a greater dilatation diameter. Once children are awake and alert post procedure, they can drink. When they are comfortably able to swallow (usually within 2–4 hours) a soft diet can be given with most resuming a normal diet within 24 hours of the procedure. One potential disadvantage of this procedure lies in the repeated exposure to radiation. This is particularly significant for children with RDEB who are known to be predisposed to aggressive squamous cell carcinoma of the skin in late teenage or adulthood [61].

When oesophageal strictures are too tight to allow antegrade passage of a guide wire or if oral contractures severely limit mouth opening, a retrograde approach through a gastrostomy may be successful. If OD is unavailable or strictures have not responded satisfactorily to this procedure, surgical interventions including colonic interposition and the resection of localised oesophageal strictures with end-to-end anastamosis (oesophago-colonoplasty) have been used. However, these procedures involve highly complex surgery and have high rates of morbidity and mortality [24]. They therefore remain the last resort for those whose nutritional status cannot be maintained by any other means.

Oral manifestations

Oral manifestations in EB children vary markedly depending on the specific EB type. Features include microstomia (reduced mouth opening), trismus (spasm of the jaw muscles), ankyloglossia (fixation of the tongue to the mouth floor), malocclusion, blistering and scarring which all compromise mouth opening and the normal cleansing action of the tongue. Teeth can be structurally defective, having little or poor quality enamel which erodes easily, rendering them more prone to decay and gum disease [19].

Other factors contributing to increased dental caries include consumption of a diet high in fermentable carbohydrate, slow and frequent eating, ineffective use of a toothbrush due to extreme fragility of the oral mucosa and poor manual dexterity, side effects of some medications which cause a dry mouth or necrosis of the jaw, GORD and carers' capabilities [19, 62].

Dental reviews should be scheduled according to caries risk. Caries prevention is the dentist's approach of choice. This includes [19, 63]

- Diet control by modifying and manipulating what, when, how often and how sugar containing foods are eaten; safer alternatives and dietary regimens can be developed to help prevent tooth decay. High sugar foods should ideally be restricted to the end of mealtimes and continuous sipping of sugary drinks outside mealtimes discouraged. To avoid families being given confusing or contradictory advice, it is important that dentists and dietitians work together on well planned programmes for each patient.

- Mechanical plaque/substrate control by brushing (using appropriate equipment and techniques), flossing, rinsing (with alcohol free mouth washes) and chewing sugar free gum.
- Adjuvant therapies which include fluoride (in toothpaste or supplement) and chlorhexidine (in mouth washes, swabs, sprays, gels or topical varnish).
- Protective covering of teeth using fissure sealants and stainless steel crowns.

Exercises for maintaining mouth opening by using 'mouth expanding devices' as well as for the tongue to maintain mobility for adequate swallowing and intelligibility of speech can be provided, but evidence for the effectiveness of these exercises in these children is lacking [64].

Pubertal delay

Malnutrition can affect the entire hormonal system (involving insulin, thyroid hormones, cortisol and growth hormone (GH) and the hypothalamic-pituitary-gonadal axis) and is a well known cause of pubertal delay [65]. Chronic inflammation mediated by cytokines causes disturbances in the pathway involving GH and insulin like growth factor 1 (GH/IGF-1) and the hypothalamic-pituitary-gonadal axis [66, 67]. Improving nutrition and growth with the use of GTF and OD may facilitate attainment of puberty. However, the introduction of such measures after adolescence may mean that catch-up growth is not possible. Radiographs of the left hand and wrist to evaluate bone age can assess skeletal maturation and help to confirm the picture of delay (p. 700). In girls a pelvic ultrasound scan is helpful to assess uterine development and ovarian activity. Induction of puberty with appropriate hormonal intervention is necessary from a psychological point of view as well as to optimise peak BMD. This may present particular problems for boys, in whom intramuscular testosterone injections may be painful and in whom buccal preparations may be difficult to take when microstomia has led to obliteration of the buccal sulci [68].

Reduced mobility

Mobility in severe EB is frequently reduced due to complications such as fixed flexion contractures, bone and skin pain and fatigue secondary to anaemia [19, 69]. When longitudinal growth falters such that weight centile deviates upwardly by more than two centiles from height, wheelchair dependency is more likely. Consequent lack of weight bearing compounds, low BMD and an increased tendency to experience bone pain and fractures leads to further immobility. Maintenance of a balance between mobility, growth and nutritional status is challenging [47]. Regular review and close liaison between dietitian and relevant multidisciplinary team members (especially physiotherapy and endocrinology) is essential.

Psychological and psychosocial issues and QoL

The psychological and psychosocial issues affecting both children with severe EB and their parents can pose significant challenges to dietitians. The drive to nurture a child is primal and, for mothers especially, failure to achieve this can be demoralising and irreparably damaging, overlaid as it frequently is by guilt arising from the knowledge that their child's incurable and life limiting condition is genetic in origin. This may lead to denial of feeding difficulties and/or inability to comply with dietetic advice. Increased tension is caused if other parties (partners, family members, other professionals) are unsupportive or undermine agreed feeding strategies. Balancing the care of a partner and healthy siblings with the care of an EB child can greatly increase family stresses, interpersonal problems and likelihood of depression [70]. Frequent dietetic follow-up with sensitivity, empathy and good communication is essential.

When parents must undertake unpleasant procedures such as lancing of blisters and painful dressing changes, they often feel compelled to compensate with rewards that entail significant amounts of sweets. Intake at mealtimes is then compromised and oral hygiene may deteriorate. In such a distressing and life limiting condition, short term gratification is hard to deny in favour of indefinite longer term benefits. Realistically, it is parents who prioritise the numerous aspects of daily care and that may mean the time involved in coaxing the child to drink a nutritional supplement is deemed to be better spent changing dressings or simply being 'normal' for a few hours.

Multiple factors affect QoL in EB. These vary not only with the degree of severity, but also with age. Although a validated tool to assess QoL specifically in EB adults is available [71], there is nothing similar yet for children. A study [72] found that children with severe EB express five main areas of distress: continually itchy skin, pain, difficulties in participation with peers, lack of understanding by others and being different. All these can impact on nutritional intake, either directly or indirectly, and it is important that dietitians are aware.

Transition from paediatric to adult care

For young people with any severe form of chronic illness, transition to adult services is a major life event involving the loss of trusted professional carers [73]. In EB, increasing age and transition may be perceived as moving a step closer to increasing and worsening of complications, the potential development of terminal metastatic squamous cell carcinoma [74] and death [70], highly sensitive issues that are openly discussed nowadays. Such issues are highly relevant to EB, since parents' long term and close rapport with key EB professionals often starts very soon after the birth of an extremely fragile baby.

Awareness of potential transition related problems is paramount and protocols should be in place to minimise them [75]. EB clinical nurse specialists are key in liaising between parents, patients and healthcare professionals in the hospital and community settings, and good communication between all concerned should ease the transition process.

It is important that a comprehensive history is provided by the paediatric dietitian at the time of transition. Much of the necessary information for this can be recorded on a proforma for recording nutritional intake (Table 24.2). The following information is also extremely helpful:

- summary of relevant medical history, including oesophageal dilatations, bowel pattern, iron, bone, mobility and dental status
- growth chart, ideally from birth, details of supplements tried and rejected

- If G tube fed, details of make, size (including shaft length), reordering procedure, recent problems encountered. Details of current feeds, feeding regimen and home delivery arrangements
- Current medication regimen including vitamins and minerals, orally or via gastrostomy
- Contact details of GP and other relevant community health professionals, especially if the child has a G tube *in situ*
- Social details – family dynamics, educational stage, career ambitions, hobbies

Future research needs

There are now several specialist EB centres worldwide. Establishment of collaborative studies between them would greatly facilitate improved practice in several areas:

- nutrient requirements for children with severe EB and appropriate biochemical and haematological monitoring in order to implement and evaluate nutrition support
- reasons for the various complications experienced by some EB centres in G tube placement and gastrostomy feeding. Complications may be reduced by changes in surgical technique, type of device and/or aftercare. Placement of devices lower down in the GI tract, modified feed composition and reduction in polypharmacy are all areas that should be investigated further
- validation of THINC (p. 696)
- ways in which to minimise the adverse effects of the inflammatory process in EB as chronic inflammation is increasingly suspected of playing a major role in complications such as anaemia, osteoporosis and abnormal body composition
- the role of exclusion regimens in the potential reduction of bowel inflammation and other sequelae
- the role of probiotics in promoting optimal gut health and immune status as EB is a condition for which antibiotics are regularly prescribed

Acknowledgements

The authors are greatly indebted to Siphosami Msebele for retrieval of online references and to

Dr Jemima Mellerio for advice regarding aspects of genetics and medical management.

Useful addresses

Dystrophic Epidermolysis Bullosa Research Association (DEBRA UK)

www.debra.org.uk

DEBRA International

www.debra-international.org

EB Medical Research Foundation

www.ebkids.org

EB Nurse

www.ebnurse.org

25 Burns

Helen McCarthy

Introduction

It has been estimated that approximately 250 000 people suffer from a burns injury each year in the UK with only a small number being admitted to hospital [1, 2]. The 2008 International Burn Injury Database (iBID) report estimated that 18 600 (44%) of those admitted to hospital are children with the majority (75%) being under the age of 5 years [3]. These figures have generally remained unchanged over the past 10 years.

Assessment of injury

Thermal injury can be classified in a number of ways but include contact, flame, electrical and chemical burns as well as scalds [4]. The main causes and types of thermal injury in children and adolescents are listed in Table 25.1. The most common injury reported in children is a scald (61%) with contact burns accounting for 21% and 8% of injury being as a result of a flame burn [3].

It is well documented that the size and depth of a thermal injury has a direct impact on morbidity and mortality [5, 6]. Burns are dynamic injuries that are rarely uniform in depth and therefore require continual reassessment [4, 7].

Burn depth is generally classified as partial or full thickness. Partial thickness injuries are further subdivided into superficial, where only the epidermis is affected; superficial dermal, where the injury extends through the epidermis into the dermis and blistering is observed; deep dermal where the injury extends through the dermis but does not infiltrate the subcutaneous tissue [7].

Burn size relates to the surface area affected by the injury. There are a number of ways to assess burn size. The simplest method is the 'palmar surface', which is based on the palm of the patient's hand (including fingers) being approximately 0.8% of the total body surface area (TBSA) [7]. This method works well with small injuries but with increasing wound size becomes less so. In adults the Wallace 'rule of nines' is commonly used, and this has been adapted for children (Table 25.2) [7]. The most common method for determining burn size in children is using the Lund and Browder charts which have been reproduced in many formats since originally proposed in 1944 [7–10].

The severity of an injury combines the depth, size and other factors. In children the types of burn are

- a major burn, defined as a full thickness burn covering an area of >10% TBSA
- a partial thickness burn of >20% TBSA

Table 25.1 Causes and types of burn injury.

Type of burn	Cause of burn
Water	Kettle, teapot, cup, mug, bath, saucepan
Contact	Radiator, iron, oven, hot water bottle
Flame	House fire, chip pan, electric/coal fire, barbecue
Fat	Chip pan, oven trays
Chemical	Cement, hair dye, cleansing agents, cytotoxic drugs
Electrical	Electrical appliances, overhead and underground cables
Other	Overexposure to radiotherapy, frostbite, animal manure

- burn injuries to the eyes, ears, face, hands or feet or other areas that are likely to result in functional impairment
- burns complicated by another major trauma or inhalation injury [6]

Metabolic response to burn injury

Thermal injury results in a marked change in metabolism that is reported to last up to 12 months or longer depending on the severity of the original injury [11–14]. Initially there is a reduction in metabolic rate that lasts 3–5 days. This is the 'ebb phase'. During this period there is evidence that the requirements of the child fall below the estimated average requirements (EAR) for age [15]. This is then followed by the hypermetabolic 'flow phase' which is associated with physiological, endocrine and immunological changes [11–14, 16, 17]. The exact cause of the hypermetabolic response remains poorly defined; however, catecholamines, corticosteroids and inflammatory cytokines are primary mediators with raised levels being observed for an extended period post injury [16].

Modern medical and nursing management has had the effect of moderating the hypermetabolic response to the burns injury [12, 16]. These include early excision and grafting; increased use of artificial skin and other novel wound coverings; regular analgesia; control of ambient temperature; and nutritional intervention [17–19]. Nonetheless the metabolic response remains elevated and evidence clearly links this to the extent of the injury, and in children their age and gender [20–22].

Aim of nutritional support

The aim of nutritional support in a child with a thermal injury is to provide appropriate intervention in order to moderate the hypermetabolic response, promote optimal wound healing and maintain normal growth. It is well documented that improved nutritional status in the critically ill patient reduces the likelihood of complications

Table 25.2 Methods of quantifying burn surface area.

	Wallace 'rule of nines'		Lund and Browder					
	Adult	Child	< 1 year	1 year	5 years	10 years	15 years	Adult
Head (front and back)	18%	9%	19%	17%	13%	11%	9%	7%
Neck (front and back)			2%	2%	2%	2%	2%	2%
Chest/trunk (front)	18%	18%	13%	13%	13%	13%	13%	13%
Back/trunk (back)	18%	18%	13%	13%	13%	13%	13%	13%
Arm (front and back)	9%	9%						
Upper arm (front and back)			4%	4%	4%	4%	4%	4%
Lower arm (front and back)			3%	3%	3%	3%	3%	3%
Hand (front and back)			3%	3%	3%	3%	3%	3%
Perineum	1%	1%						
Genitalia			1%	1%	1%	1%	1%	1%
Buttocks (both)			5%	5%	5%	5%	5%	5%
Leg (each)	18%	13.5%						
Thigh (front and back)			5.5%	6.5%	8%	9%	9%	9.5%
Lower leg (front and back)			5%	5%	5.5%	6%	6.5%	7%
Foot (top and bottom)			3.5%	3.5%	3.5%	3.5%	3.5%	3.5%

Adapted from Hettiaratchy and Papini [7].

Table 25.3 Factors influencing nutritional requirements.

Age
Sex
Weight
Height/length
Pre injury nutritional status
Current nutritional status
Percentage burn surface area
Thickness of burn
Grafted area
Extent of healing
Comorbidities

Table 25.4 Formulas for energy requirements.

Hildreth/Galveston equations

Infants <1 year	2100 kcal (8.8 MJ)/m² TBSA + 1000 kcal (4.2 MJ)/m² BSA
Children <12 years	1800 kcal (7.5 MJ)/m² TBSA + 1300 kcal (5.4 MJ)/m² BSA
Children >12 years	1500 kcal (6.3 MJ)/m² TBSA + 1500 kcal (6.3 MJ)/m² BSA

Curreri Junior equations

Infants <1 year	RDA + 15 kcal (0.063 MJ)/m² BSA
Children 1–3 years	RDA + 25 kcal (0.105 MJ)/m² BSA
Children 4–15 years	RDA + 40 kcal (0.167 MJ)/m² BSA

TBSA, total body surface area; BSA, burn surface area; RDA, recommended dietary allowance.

(e.g. infection, poor wound healing) and length of stay in hospital [23–25].

Nutritional requirements

Factors influencing the nutritional requirements of a child with a thermal injury are listed in Table 25.3. A full assessment of nutritional requirements should be made taking these and any additional factors, such as surface area used as donor sites for skin grafts, into consideration.

Energy requirements

Several researchers have investigated energy requirements in children with thermal injuries. Although the gold standard method for estimating energy requirements would be to measure them daily using indirect calorimetry and adjusting all nutritional support to meet these figures, this is often impractical. Calculations have been proposed to estimate energy requirements and, while these are commonly used in clinical practice, there is some evidence to suggest their accuracy is limited [26, 27].

Energy requirements in children with burns rarely rise above the EAR in the first 24 hours post burn injury [15, 28]. Therefore it may be reasonable to aim for the EAR for age initially for all injuries, particularly those classified as minor or of a small surface area. Commonly used formulas for estimating energy requirement for children are detailed in Table 25.4. These include the Curreri Junior formula and the Galveston or Hildreth formula [29–33]. These formulas require an estimate of body surface area and burn surface area. There are a number

of equations to aid with this estimation, but the simplest is probably the Mosteller formula [34]:

$$\text{total body surface area} = \sqrt{[(\text{weight} \times \text{height})/3600]}$$

where weight is in kilograms and height is in centimetres.

Any formula is only a guideline and provides a starting point for estimating requirements. As already stated thermal injuries are dynamic and require frequent reassessment and amendment of nutritional requirements.

Protein requirements

Protein requirements for children with burns injuries remain unclear, but it is evident that these will be increased above the recommended nutrient intake (RNI) for age [28]. The hypermetabolic response to the thermal injury results in an upregulation of protein turnover with both protein catabolism and synthesis being increased. Losses of lean muscle mass and negative nitrogen balance have both been recognised in studies investigating the nutritional needs of this patient group [35, 36]. Cunningham *et al.* suggest that appropriate wound healing is achievable in children receiving 2–3 g protein/kg/day [32]. It has also been suggested that higher protein intakes may have beneficial outcomes in thermally injured children [33, 37]. However, a recent review by Herndon and Tompkins states that protein intakes of 3 g/kg/day may raise urea production without improvement in muscle protein synthesis [12].

Protein synthesis, as well as wound healing, does appear to be improved when relatively higher protein provision is made in combination with anabolic agents such as growth hormone and oxandrolone [16, 17, 38]. Studies have reported improvements in lean muscle mass, wound healing and scarring at 2 years post injury when recombinant human growth hormone (rhGH) is administered during the hospitalisation although its use is not without side effects [17]. Oxandrolone has similarly been shown to have beneficial effects on lean muscle mass, muscle strength and bone mineral density [38].

Several amino acids become conditionally essential following trauma, particularly burn injuries, including glutamine, arginine, histidine and cystine [25]. Most of the research into supplementation of specific amino acids has focused on glutamine and arginine [39–41]. Current evidence suggests that while there are benefits to supplementation of major burn injured patients with glutamine, supplementation with arginine does not appear to provide any benefits despite the role it plays in wound healing [42]. Recommended levels of supplementation for glutamine have not been established for children although deficiency has been reported, and further research is required in this area [43].

Moderate hypoalbuminaemia is common in children with thermal injuries and this can be well tolerated. Increasing protein provision above that recommended in the literature has little impact on this. However, it has been suggested that if the serum albumin level falls to <25 g/L then albumin infusions should be considered [25, 44].

Vitamin and mineral requirements

Vitamin and mineral requirements at the varying stages of recovery from a thermal injury are still very much under debate and very few studies specifically look at the requirements for vitamins and minerals in children. Animal models and studies in adults suggest that requirements are increased for certain vitamins and minerals due to their role in the metabolic pathways of the body. When assessing the nutritional requirements in burns patients the following should be considered.

- Deficiency in Vitamins A, E and C has been reported [45]. This deficiency would appear

to respond well to enteral supplementation. The benefits of routine supplementation over and above meeting the dietary reference values when deficiency is not present has yet to be proven, with the evidence presently equivocal in this area [46].
- B group vitamins are required proportional to energy intake; however, little research has been undertaken so there are no clear recommendations other than ensuring nutritional adequacy.
- Low levels of serum iron in most cases are not diet related and may have a protective effect against infection. Supplementation should be closely monitored in relation to transfusions and status [47].
- Both zinc and copper have been shown to be depleted in serum following thermal injury. Copper supplementation can result in increased urinary losses; similarly the role of zinc in the upregulated inflammatory processes suggests that redistribution rather than deficiency may explain low serum levels [47, 48].

In recent years an increased incidence of fractures has been reported in children post burns injury raising awareness of vitamin D deficiency in this group. It has been suggested that risk factors for vitamin D deficiency include lack of sunlight exposure, reduced intake and poor absorption post injury, coupled with a pre injury insufficiency [49, 50]. Current evidence suggests that standard supplementation of vitamin D is not sufficient to correct deficiencies seen in burn injured children; however, the provision of therapeutic doses routinely has not been proven [51].

Before a vitamin and mineral supplement is considered it is important to check the nutritional composition and bioavailability of enteral and/or parenteral nutrition intervention, in conjunction with the biochemical status of the child. Excessive routine supplementation with a multivitamin and mineral preparation may result in a nutritional imbalance and potential toxicity, as well as interfere with the utilisation of other nutrients.

Novel substrates

These include immune enhancing nutrients such as antioxidants, omega-3 fatty acids, glutamine, arginine and nucleotides. The limited number of

Table 25.5 Factors influencing the achievement of nutritional requirements.

Percentage burn surface area
Site of injury
Pre-existing clinical conditions
Previous nutritional status
Special dietary needs
Gastrointestinal function
Pain management and sedation
Pyrexia
Periods of fasting
Psychological distress

studies has focused on use in adults and much of the available research has used heterogeneous intensive or critical care unit patient groups, which include a small number of thermal injury patients [52]. As such the current recommendation is that immunonutrition is not used in children [53].

Antioxidant therapy (vitamins A, C, E) has been shown to reduce burn and burn sepsis mortality in adult burn patients [54]. Omega-3 fatty acids may impact on immune response and wound healing, although the anti-inflammatory properties have lead to confounding results in some studies [52, 55]. The potential therapeutic benefits of specific amino acids (glutamine and arginine) have been addressed (p. 57, 79).

These substrates are usually provided in combination rather than individually, and early studies have suggested some benefits both in terms of the immune enhancing nutrients included and in the ratio that they are present alongside macronutrients [56, 57].

Meeting nutritional goals

This has been covered in detail in Chapter 1. Additional factors need to be considered in a child with a thermal injury and these are listed in Table 25.5. The size and depth of the injury will have a direct impact on the hypermetabolic inflammatory response and therefore the nutritional requirements of the child. The position and the psychological impact of the injury, including the cause, can have a significant effect on compliance with dietary management strategies.

Minor burns (<10% body surface area)

A 'food first' approach should be taken with minor injuries of <10% surface area, not including the face, and if the child does not have a compromised nutritional status pre injury. The child should be encouraged to start eating and drinking as early as possible and every effort should be made to provide familiar foods in order to promote appetite. Nutritious drinks such as milk and milkshakes, in preference to juice or fizzy pop, should be encouraged.

Daily food and fluid intake should be accurately recorded by nursing staff. If this highlights difficulties in meeting the dietary targets alternative nutritional intervention may be necessary. A multivitamin supplement or a proprietary dietary supplement may be beneficial in this group if acceptance of hospital food is limited.

Major burns (>10% body surface area)

In a major thermal injury an enteral feeding tube should be passed during the resuscitation period, and also where the injury is complicated by smoke inhalation, the injury is extensively to the face or where additional trauma has been incurred. Many studies report that early enteral feeding of burns patients (within the first 6 hours) reduces the incidence of paralytic ileus and may moderate the hypermetabolic response [58–60]. However, a Cochrane review on early versus later initiation of enteral feeding concluded that the benefits were inconclusive as only three studies met their inclusion criteria [61]. Other benefits of early enteral feeding include maintenance of gut integrity and a reduction in bacterial translocation, as well as improvements in immune status and wound healing [58–60].

Current practice in most UK centres is to commence continuous enteral feeding at a low rate and increase as tolerated, aiming to achieve full requirements within the first 24–48 hours post injury. This should be done cautiously and be guided by the severity of the thermal injury. While published studies have failed to demonstrate irrefutable evidence of the benefits of early feeding, there are reports of feed related intestinal necrosis and thus for more severe injuries just trophic feeding in the early phases may be indicated [62].

Nasogastric feeding is routinely used in many centres but where this is poorly tolerated, as demonstrated by increased gastric aspirates, transpyloric feeding should be considered [63,64]. Delayed gastric emptying and gastric aspirates in excess of the hourly feed rate are closely correlated with ileus, infection and sepsis [65]. Diarrhoea occurs frequently in children with burn injuries, but appears to be more closely related to the use of broad spectrum antibiotics rather than feed osmolality or volume [66]. It has been suggested that the use of prebiotics and probiotics may have a beneficial effect on gut flora thus reducing the incidence of diarrhoea; however, the timing and dose, as well as the most effective strain, remains unclear [67].

Optimising nutrient provision via enteral feeding can prove difficult as feeding regimens must take into account fasting periods related to surgical intervention, dressing changes, physiotherapy and medications. Several studies within a critical care environment have demonstrated suboptimal provision of nutrition support; therefore effective communication and team working is imperative to the nutritional management of children with thermal injuries [68].

Parenteral nutrition (PN) should only be considered when there is prolonged paralytic ileus or where poor tolerance of enteral feeding prevents nutritional requirements from being met by this route alone. Where possible, trophic enteral feeds should continue to be infused at a very low rate (as little as 2 mL/hour) to maintain the brush border integrity of the gastrointestinal tract [25,69,70]. The complications of PN are well recognised and as infection risks are already high in burns patients special care must be taken when considering PN. Other issues, such as electrolyte imbalances and hyperglycaemia, also require particularly close monitoring. Further guidance on enteral and parenteral nutrition support in children may be found Chapters 3 and 4.

Choice of oral and enteral feeds

The choice of feed will vary depending on the age of the child, the calculated requirements, any unrelated medical condition and the clinical course during admission. There is some evidence to suggest that the use of high carbohydrate feeds may improve protein synthesis and muscle mass accretion, although such feeds are not routinely used in the UK at the present time [12,71]. A recent Cochrane review concluded that there were limited randomised controlled trials on optimal feed composition and further research is therefore required [72].

As the child's condition improves the move from enteral feeding to oral diet, with or without supplementation, should take place as a managed process. Weaning from enteral feeding is challenging requiring team work and clear communication between the healthcare professionals, the family and the child. Much of the published work on weaning from enteral to oral nutrition is related to children with longstanding feeding aversion and not shorter term nutrition support [73]. Enteral feeds should be reduced gradually to encourage oral intake, but nutritional requirements should continue to be met; simply stopping the enteral feed without adequate oral intake being established increases the risk of nutritional deficiency and wound breakdown.

Monitoring

Burns injuries are dynamic and this patient group has constantly changing nutritional needs related to the healing of their wounds. As the percentage burn surface area changes so the nutritional requirements should be reassessed.

- Regular weights (without dressings) should be recorded and plotted on appropriate centile charts. These should be compared with pre admission measurements where available. It is important to remember that oedema may mask true weight early in the clinical course.
- Routine biochemistry should be monitored. Frequency will vary depending on the child's clinical course. Vitamin, mineral and trace element status should also be monitored in extensive burns injuries as evidence of deficiency has frequently been reported in the literature [45–51]. Raised serum levels of C-reactive protein (CRP) predict sepsis in children with burns injuries [74]. Guidelines for monitoring blood parameters in burns patients have been developed by several of the regional

burn networks and local policy should reflect these.

- Changing clinical condition, including aspects such as burn area and healing, temperature, infection and sepsis, ventilation issues and rehabilitation programmes, should all be closely monitored and requirements recalculated on the basis of these changing factors.
- Feed intake and tolerance should be closely monitored. Prescribed versus actual intakes can vary for a number of reasons and under delivery of nutrition is a commonly recognised problem [68]. Aspirate volumes and bowel motions (frequency and consistency) should be recorded accurately. Adjustments to feeding regimens, including rate, type of feed and route of administration, may be beneficial. As the child moves from enteral to oral nutrition intakes should be recorded accurately to ensure adequate nutritional intake is being achieved.

Monitoring of nutritional intake and overall nutritional status should continue post discharge. Changes in the medical management of burns patients have resulted in earlier discharge home, with follow-up being provided within the community or at outpatient clinics. The hypermetabolic response has been demonstrated to continue for 12 months or more following a burn injury [11–14, 75], putting these children at risk of longer term nutritional deficiencies and growth failure [75–78]. It should also be noted that even with adequate nutritional intake, poor growth often continues to be an issue. In these circumstances children exhibit increased body fat stores but no significant increase in lean body mass [14, 78].

Specifically with major burn injuries, bone health should be reviewed longer term with studies reporting significant increases in long bone fractures post injury [49]. Long term follow-up and monitoring of nutritional status and intake should be integral to the dietetic management of burn injuries, particularly those falling into the major burn classification.

Case study

A 3-year-old girl has sustained a 12% mixed thickness scald (7% full thickness, 5% partial thickness) to the lower legs and feet as a result of being placed in a bath of hot water.

Weight on admission 12.85 kg (25th centile), estimated height 92 cm (25th centile).

Blood results are within the normal range and there is no history of iron deficiency anaemia.

She eats three meals plus supper daily and has no noted dislikes or food intolerance. Usual dietary intake is reported to be 'children's food' such as chocolate based breakfast cereals, ham or cheese sandwiches, chicken nuggets and chips or sausage and mash. Reported portion size appears appropriate for age. Drinks are mainly diluted juice or fizzy pop. No additional vitamin or mineral supplements are taken.

Calculating requirements

Total body surface area (TBSA)

$$= \sqrt{[(\text{weight} \times \text{height})/3600]}$$
$$= \sqrt{[(12.85 \times 92)/3600]} = 0.57 \text{ m}^2$$

Burn surface area (BSA)

$$= 12\% \times 0.57 = 0.068 \text{ m}^2$$

Energy: 1800 kcal (7.5 MJ)/m^2(TBSA)

$$+ 1300 \text{ kcal } (5.4 \text{ MJ})/\text{m}^2(\text{BSA})$$
$$= (1800 \times 0.57) + (1300 \times 0.068)$$
$$= 1114 \text{ kcal } (4.6 \text{ MJ})$$

Protein: 2–3 g protein/kg = 26–39 g protein

Fluid: 1140 mL

Achieving requirements

The following need to be considered:

- site of injury – lower legs therefore not likely to directly compromise dietary intake
- percentage burn area – this is >10% and is therefore a major burn
- there is no previous medical history of note
- previous nutritional status – reasonable, possibility of vitamin insufficiency, particularly vitamin D
- no gastrointestinal problems
- pain management – as a result of the injury the child will be in a great deal of pain and will be commenced on pain relief. This should be considered when planning intervention
- pyrexia – none noted yet
- the child is scared and unsure of what is happening to her

Method of feeding

An enteral feeding tube should be passed during the resuscitation period. Enteral feeds should commence within 6 hours of admission via this route, until such time as the child is able to feed orally. Enteral feeds should gradually be replaced by oral intake to meet full nutritional requirements. Good oral hygiene should be maintained throughout.

Choice of feed

- A standard 1 kcal (4 kJ)/mL paediatric enteral feed. The advantage of this option is a nutritionally complete feed that should meet all nutritional requirements without modification. The use of fibre containing feed could be considered. The final feeding regimen should be planned in conjunction with medical and nursing management taking account of times of dressing changes, physiotherapy sessions and other interventions.
- If taking anything orally or as oral intake begins encourage nutrient dense foods that are familiar and acceptable to the child. Encourage high protein foods. Avoid diluted juice and fizzy drinks; encourage milk based drinks or oral nutritional supplements instead.

Monitoring

- Dressings are changed twice weekly. The child should be weighed and the degree of healing assessed on each of these occasions. Nutritional support should be reassessed according to these criteria.
- Nutritional biochemical markers should be requested and monitored weekly in the early stages of recovery and then as necessary to 'fine tune' dietetic intervention and promote a positive outcome.
- A possible side effect of analgesia is constipation; bowel habits should be monitored closely and fibre enriched feeds considered.
- Following discharge on oral diet, the child should be monitored at the first review appointment to assess intake and weight change at home. Input should be guided by progress but at every appointment with a team member a weight and height should be recorded and dietary intake should be considered. Longer term use of a multivitamin and mineral supplement, particularly if the oral diet is limited, should be recommended.

Acknowledgement

Thanks to the co-authors of previous versions of this chapter Dearbhla Hunt and Claire Gurry.

Part 4

Community Nutrition

26 Healthy Eating

Judy More

Introduction

Infants, toddlers and school children need to satisfy their energy and nutrient requirements for normal growth, development and activity through eating a varied and balanced diet. The UK Department of Health's Dietary Reference Values [1] and the Scientific Advisory Committee on Nutrition's (SACN) energy recommendations [2] can be used as a guideline for the healthy child (Tables 1.9–1.11). In addition the Food Standards Agency has set maximum guideline daily amounts of sodium and salt consumption for babies and children [3] in order to tackle the longer term problems of hypertension and cardiovascular disease found in the adult population (Table 26.1). However, these are not evidence based for children and at only 50% above the reference nutrient intake (RNI) for sodium they are difficult to achieve in practice, despite a reduction of approximately 15% of the salt content in some commercial foods over the last few years.

UK Government policies emphasise healthy eating for children through a number of initiatives:

- promoting breast feeding
- broadening the nutritional support given to low income families through the Sure Start and Healthy Start schemes
- Healthy Child Programmes [4, 5]

Table 26.1 Guideline daily amounts of sodium and salt.

Age	Reference nutrient intake [1] Sodium g/day	Daily recommended maximum intake [3] Sodium g/day	Daily recommended maximum intake [3] Salt g/day
0–12 months	0.21–0.35	0.4	1
1–3 years	0.5	0.8	2
4–6 years	0.7	1.2	3
7–10 years	1.2	2.0	5
11+ years	1.6	2.4	6

- widening children's exposure to fruit and vegetables through the School Fruit and Vegetable Scheme
- voluntary guidelines on food to be served to children in Early Years settings
- nutritional standards for school meals and food available in state schools including vending machines and tuck shops
- promoting initiatives to combat obesity [6]

Infants

Breast milk and infant formula are the only two options of milk drink throughout the first 6 months of life. Both are nutritionally adequate but breast

Clinical Paediatric Dietetics, Fourth Edition. Edited by Vanessa Shaw.
© 2015 John Wiley & Sons, Ltd. Published 2015 by John Wiley & Sons, Ltd.
Companion Website: www.wiley.com/go/shaw/paediatricdietetics

milk is the preferred option as it additionally provides protection against illness [7].

Breast feeding

Colostrum is the breast milk produced in the first few days after birth and is particularly high in proteins, especially immunoglobulins, which confer maternal immunity against infection. It is low in fat and energy and newborn babies generally take very small volumes infrequently [8]. Over the first few days infants have a net weight loss, which is mostly fluid, of up to 10% of their birthweight. From about days 2–3 postpartum the composition of breast milk changes to transitional milk which has a higher water content and coincides with the infant demanding feeds more frequently. Mature breast milk is produced about 3 weeks postpartum.

The average energy composition of mature breast milk has been estimated to be 69 kcal (289 kJ)/ 100 mL [9]. A recent systematic review of data from 1088 samples of mature breast milk showed an energy content of 65.2 ± 1.1 kcal/100 mL (273 ± 4.6 kJ)/100 mL [10]. The energy content varies throughout the feed: at the beginning of the feed the milk is low in fat and higher in lactose and satisfies the infant's thirst; as the feed progresses the fat and energy content increases and the high fat milk towards the end of a feed satisfies the infant's hunger.

Mothers should be encouraged to let their infant drink as much as desired from the first breast before offering the second breast; this way the infant gets the higher energy milk at the end of the feed. Less milk (or none at all) may be taken from the second breast offered. At each feed the first breast offered should be alternated so that both breasts receive equal stimulation and drainage. Young infants may need to be woken by cuddling them upright and changing their nappy after finishing at the first breast before being offered the second breast.

Provided there is no restriction on how much an infant can breast feed (i.e. demand feeding is practised) no extra water is needed, even in very hot weather, as the infant will simply feed more frequently to obtain more fluid when thirsty.

Breast feeding offers the infant several advantages over formula feeding [7, 11–13]:

- optimal growth and development
- reduced incidence of gastrointestinal, urinary tract and respiratory infections
- reduced risk of otitis media until the age of 5–7 years
- reduced incidence of both insulin and non insulin dependent diabetes
- growth factors, which enhance the infant's gut development and maturation
- reduced risk of constipation
- reduced incidence of some childhood cancers (leukaemia and lymphomas, e.g. Hodgkin's disease)
- reduced risk of sudden infant death syndrome (SIDS)
- fewer visits to the doctor in the first 2 years of life

Evidence is controversial around whether breast feeding reduces

- risk of childhood obesity [14, 15]
- severity of the allergic conditions asthma and eczema [16, 17]

Benefits of breast feeding for the mother include [12, 16]

- delay in return to menstruation allowing maternal iron stores to replenish following pregnancy and childbirth
- reduced risk of breast and ovarian cancer [18]
- helps the return to pre pregnant weight
- lower risk of postnatal depression
- women over the age of 65 years who have breast fed show a lower incidence of osteoporosis and hip fractures

There are some contraindications to breast feeding:

- the baby has classical galactosaemia, a long chain fatty acid oxidation defect or glucose-galactose malabsorption
- the mother is taking certain medications, receiving radiotherapy or chemotherapy, is a drug abuser or takes excessive alcohol
- HIV positive status of the mother as HIV transmission from mother to infant can occur via breast milk; however, in developing countries, where formula feeding may greatly increase the risk of gastrointestinal infections and mortality, breast feeding is preferable

Health professionals can support and promote breast feeding through policy development, through the provision of environments conducive to breast feeding and by having the knowledge and skills to give consistent practical advice and support to breast feeding mothers.

Factors which improve rates of breast feeding include the following.

- *The UNICEF Baby Friendly status of the maternity unit where the baby is born.* The UNICEF UK Baby Friendly Initiative provides a framework for the implementation of best infant feeding practice in maternity units and is represented by the *Ten Steps to Successful Breastfeeding* (Table 26.2). Accredited units which have successfully implemented all 10 steps have increased breast feeding rates.
- *Early contact between mother and baby.* Healthy infants should be placed and remain in direct skin-to-skin contact with mother immediately after delivery until the first feeding is accomplished [19]. Putting the baby to the breast immediately after birth assists in developing the suckling reflex which is particularly strong for a short while after delivery.
- *Extra support by trained professionals with special skills in breast feeding* to help with good positioning and technique [20]. A good understanding of the physiology of lactation is essential for all who are involved in the care of breast feeding mothers and can be achieved with training. The UNICEF Baby Friendly Initiative has

developed an accreditation system for assessing higher education institutions in the UK based on the training they provide to midwives and health visitors on breast feeding.

- *Peer support.* Local peer support groups are particularly effective [21]. In the UK, the large nationally organised groups which provide peer support and training for counsellors are
  - Association of Breastfeeding Mothers
  - Breastfeeding Network
  - La Leche League
  - Multiple Births Foundation
  - National Childbirth Trust
- *Family support and encouragement.*
- *Supportive communities where breast feeding is seen as the norm* and facilities are available for women to breast feed. Both England and Scotland have legislated against discrimination towards mothers feeding infants in public places. The UNICEF Baby Friendly Initiative also accredits community settings if they are implementing the Seven Point Plan for the Protection, Promotion and Support of Breastfeeding in Community Health Care Settings.

Perceived barriers to breast feeding may include

- *Too much demand on the mother's time.* Family members can provide invaluable support by helping with other children or taking over household duties.
- *Embarrassment.* Some mothers are embarrassed to breast feed even within the home, particularly those in lower socioeconomic groups [23]. Many women find that the attitude of other people to breast feeding in public, coupled with the frequent lack of facilities to feed in private, make prolonged excursions outside the home difficult.
- *Jealousy and lack of support from other family members.* Husbands, relatives and siblings may resent the exclusive role of the mother in breast feeding. Involving everyone in all other aspects of caring for the infant can help alleviate this problem.
- *Incompatibility with work.* Women in the UK are entitled to 12 months maternity leave (9 months of this paid). However, many return to work within 12 months and unless there are suitable facilities for child care or expressing breast milk, continuing with full breast feeding can

Table 26.2 The 10 steps to successful breast feeding [22].

1	Have a written breast feeding policy that is routinely communicated to all healthcare staff
2	Train all healthcare staff in the skills necessary to implement the breast feeding policy
3	Inform all pregnant women about the benefits and management of breast feeding
4	Help mothers initiate breast feeding soon after birth
5	Show mothers how to breast feed and how to maintain lactation even if they are separated from their babies
6	Give newborn infants no food or drink other than breast milk, unless medically indicated
7	Practice rooming-in, allowing mothers and infants to remain together 24 hours a day
8	Encourage breast feeding on demand
9	Give no artificial teats or dummies to breast feeding infants
10	Identify sources of national and local support for breast feeding and ensure that mothers know how to access these prior to discharge from hospital

be difficult. Partial breast feeding (e.g. in the mornings and evenings) is often possible on return to work and should be encouraged.

Initiating, establishing and maintaining breast feeding

Breast feeding is not an entirely instinctive process and most new mothers need support and advice. The 2010 Infant Feeding Survey (Table 26.3) reported that 81% of UK mothers initiate breast feeding soon after birth; however, exclusive breast feeding declines rapidly with only 46% mothers doing so at the end of the first week, 23% at 6 weeks and 1% at 6 months [24]. This decline is often due to lack of support to address common problems and difficulties. The National Institute for Health and Care Excellence (NICE) recommends that when mothers leave a maternity unit they should be given contact details of breast feeding counsellors and information on local peer support groups [25].

Good positioning and attachment is essential for successful breast feeding. Infants should be held so that

- they are close and facing the mother with their tummy towards her
- the baby's back, shoulders and neck are supported
- they can easily tilt their head back
- their head should be in line with the body so that the neck is not twisted

The baby's mouth will gape wide open in response to the rooting reflex to accept the nipple and it is important that the baby takes in the nipple and much of the areola. The lower lip should be turned out and the tongue under the mother's nipple.

During the first few days infants take minimal amounts of colostrum (21.5 ± 4.2 mL on day 1

[10]) and its provision is under hormonal control (Table 1.15). After day 3 postpartum the supply of transitional, and later mature, breast milk is determined largely by demand and is stimulated by regular, rather than prolonged, suckling. During the early weeks of demand breast feeding mothers may need to feed every 2–3 hours or 8–12 times a day. Once lactation has become fully established after about 3–4 weeks, the time between feeds usually increases although some infants continue to prefer smaller more frequent feeds.

If the baby is unable to suckle at birth, the mother can express her milk. Expressing 8–12 times a day will be necessary to establish a good milk supply and considerable practical and emotional support is important for these mothers.

Complementary and top-up feeds

Complementary formula feeds usually hinder breast feeding by decreasing the demand and hence supply of breast milk. Very occasionally when an infant is not gaining sufficient weight, a complementary feed after the breast feed may be recommended.

Problems and difficulties with breast feeding

Some problems and difficulties with breast feeding are shown in Table 26.4.

Expressing breast milk

Once breast milk supply is established it can be expressed using one of three methods:

- by hand
- using a hand pump
- using an electric pump

Table 26.3 Incidence and prevalence of breast feeding in the UK.

Age of infants	% of infants in the UK receiving some breast milk				% of infants in the UK being exclusively breast fed	
	1995	2000	2005	2010	2005	2010
At birth	66	69	76	81	76	81
1 week	56	55	63	69	45	46
6 weeks	42	42	48	55	21	23
4 months	27	28	34	42	7	12
6 months	21	21	25	34	<1	1
9 months	14	13	18	23	–	–

Table 26.4 Common breast feeding problems and suggestions for their management.

Concern	Background	Action
Perceived inadequate supply A common reason cited by mothers and may be due to persistent crying or fussing of infants that are not necessarily signs of hunger	Crying in a baby does not always signal a demand for food. It may be because the baby is uncomfortable, needs a nappy change, is overtired, or just bored and lonely A breast fed baby having an adequate intake will • be alert, responsive, and have a healthy appearance • have 6+ feeds in 24 hours during the day and night • have 6+ wet nappies daily • have 2+ yellow stools daily	Check the baby is feeding for as long as s/he wishes on both breasts. More frequent breast feeds may help establish a better supply or suit a mother who produces low volumes of breast milk. Check mother's diet and fluid intake are adequate and that she is getting enough rest Check medications
Sore nipples	Some tenderness is normal but breast feeding should not be painful. Pain is usually due to poor attachment and positioning. However, in some cases it may be due to thrush (*Candida albicans*). In rare cases it may be due to Reynaud's syndrome, where nipples become blanched due to poor blood supply	Treatment from a GP is necessary to resolve thrush in both the mother and infant Heat treatment and feeding in a warm room may help in Reynaud's syndrome
Cracked nipples	Usually due to poor attachment	With improved attachment and positioning nipples will begin to heal
Engorgement Oedema caused when the breast is full of milk and the blood and lymph flows are slow and seep into breast tissue	Usually due to poor drainage of the breast as a consequence of poor positioning and attachment and can occur when feeds are missed	Hand expressing before the feed can make it easier for the infant to suck efficiently. Advice may include • use of warm compresses or taking a warm shower before feeding • frequent breast feeding (every 1–2 hours) and encouraging the infant to suckle from both breasts • applying an ice pack to breast and under-arm after feeding until swelling decreases can also be helpful • seek expert advice if the problem persists
Mastitis Swollen, inflamed or infected area in breast	Usually a result of engorgement or poor drainage of the breast so it is important not to stop breast feeding	Advise rest, frequent breast feeds and that the mother should drink plenty of fluids. Antibiotics may be needed
Baby has poor weight gain	Less emphasis is now placed on frequently weighing healthy infants as small variations in weight centiles can cause considerable parental stress. Weight gain is not expected to be regular: • infants often cross centiles in the first 6–8 weeks to adjust for the intrauterine environment • thereafter variations of up to 1 centile space are normal	Check the weight chart carefully and reassure the mother if possible. Check position and feeding technique. Check the number of feeds being offered and if necessary advise an increase to 2 hourly feeds during the day. If top-up formula feeding is necessary, advise the mother to give the bottle at the end of each breast feed to encourage stimulation of breast milk with the goal of fully resuming breast feeding Refer to the GP for assessment if growth is faltering
Tongue tie	If severe can limit the infant's ability to suckle effectively	Refer for an assessment. Surgery resolves the problem.

NICE recommends that all mothers are taught to hand express their milk [25]. Expressed breast milk (EBM) can be given to the baby via a spoon, cup or a bottle, although not all babies are happy to accept an occasional feed in this way. Bottles, containers for storage and other utensils must be sterilised until the infant is 1 year of age. EBM should be labelled and stored correctly to minimise the risk of infection. The Department of Health recommends that EBM is stored:

- in the refrigerator for up to 5 days if parents are confident that the fridge remains at 4°C or lower. It should be stored at the back of the fridge where it is colder. A domestic fridge that is opened frequently may not maintain a low enough temperature; it is preferable to freeze EBM if it is not going to be used within 48 hours
- in the freezer compartment of a fridge for up to 2 weeks
- in a domestic freezer at −18°C for up to 6 months

Frozen EBM should be thawed in a fridge and then used within 24 hours. It must not be reheated in a microwave oven because of the risk of 'hot spots' occurring and causing burns [26]. Standing the bottle in warm water is a suitable way of reheating milk if necessary; some babies will drink it cold from the fridge.

Nutrition for lactating mothers

The nutritional quality of breast milk is only affected if the mother is undernourished. To support lactation higher requirements for energy, thiamin, riboflavin, niacin, vitamin B_{12}, folate, vitamins C, A and D, calcium, phosphorus, magnesium, zinc, copper and selenium are set [1]. The increased energy requirement is usually met through utilising the adipose stores deposited during pregnancy. Eating a balance of the five food groups (Table 26.5) will meet the increased nutrient requirements with the exception of vitamin D, where a daily supplement of 10 µg is recommended [1].

Vegan mothers need to plan their diets carefully and may need additional supplements of calcium and vitamin B_{12}.

Foods to be limited or avoided

To ensure a good intake of omega-3 long chain polyunsaturated fats (LCP), mothers should be encouraged to include fish in the diet, but oily fish should be limited to no more than two servings per week; marlin, swordfish, shark and tuna should be avoided [27].

Alcohol and caffeine both readily pass into breast milk and high intakes of either should be avoided during lactation. The highest level of alcohol in milk will occur between 30 and 90 minutes after ingesting alcohol; mothers should not ingest alcohol for about 2 hours before breast feeding and should keep alcohol intake to a minimum, e.g. 1–2 units once or twice per week. Regular or binge drinking should be avoided. Caffeine in tea, coffee, chocolate and energy drinks does not need to be

Table 26.5 Recommended intakes from the five food groups for lactating mothers.

Food group	Recommended daily intake
Bread, rice, potatoes and pasta and other starchy foods	Base each meal and some snacks on these foods. Use wholegrain varieties as often as possible
Fruit and vegetables	Include one or more of these at each meal and aim for at least five portions per day
Milk, cheese and yoghurt	2–3 portions of milk, cheese, yoghurt. Use low fat varieties if weight needs to be managed
Meat, fish, eggs, beans and nuts	2–3 portions. Two servings of fish per week are recommended, one of which should be oily fish
Foods and drinks high in fat and/or sugar	Limit these to small quantities and not to be eaten in place of the other four food groups. For those trying to lose weight limit them to 2 small portions per day
Fluid intake	To satisfy thirst but at least 6–8 drinks per day (1 1/2–2 litres). This includes all drinks: water, tea, coffee, milk, soup, fruit juices, squashes and fizzy drinks. More drinks may be needed in hot weather and after physical activity

avoided, but some mothers find large amounts of caffeine unsettle their baby.

Breast milk is believed to be flavoured by foods eaten by the mother. There are reports that highly spiced or strong tasting foods can unsettle the infant.

Infants may be sensitised to antigens in breast milk, e.g. cow's milk protein, eggs or nuts (p. 322). If the infant reacts to the presence of these antigens in breast milk, the mother needs to avoid these foods. If dairy products are avoided she will need advice on dietary adequacy which may need to include a calcium supplement.

Formula feeding

Until 12 months of age the only nutritionally adequate alternatives to breast milk are infant formula from birth, and from 6 months either infant formula or follow-on milk. The composition of these two types of feed must comply with government regulations according to European Union (EU) Directives. These Directives are based on expert advice from the EC Scientific Committee for Food and the European Society of Paediatric Gastroenterology, Hepatology and Nutrition (ESPGHAN), and also implement the 1981 World Health Organization International Code of Marketing of Breastmilk Substitutes as appropriate to the EU [28].

Recent research suggests that infant formulas may contain too high an energy level for normal growth. The energy content of breast milk may be lower than current accepted estimations and the higher energy density of infant formulas may account for the different growth patterns seen between breast fed and formula fed infants (Table 26.6) [10, 29].

Table 1.14 lists the infant formulas available in the UK. The whey dominant formulas (whey:casein ratio of 60:40) have a protein ratio that is similar to that found in mature breast milk; those with a lower whey:casein ratio (20:80) are more similar to the protein ratio found in cow's milk. The energy and nutrient contents are similar in both types of feed, although the casein dominant formulas are marketed as more suitable for hungry babies; this is simply because the curd formed by the higher casein level slows gastric emptying.

Formula fed babies should be demand fed just as breast fed babies are and offered adequate feed to satisfy their hunger and growth needs. This will approximate to a total daily intake of around 150 mL/kg body weight/day, although it varies with each baby. The number of feeds per day and the volume taken at each feed will vary as in breast feeding.

Follow-on milks

These milks (Table 1.14) are only recommended from 6 months of age as they have higher levels of protein, minerals and some vitamins than the infant formulas designed for feeding from birth. Some mothers choose to use them but it is not generally necessary. They can be used to give additional nutrients to children who do not eat solids very well and they have been shown to reduce iron deficiency anaemia in inner city deprived populations [30–34].

Making up infant formula from powder

Tap water or bottled waters which comply with EU standards for tap water [35] may be used for making up infant formula. Up to 200 mg/L sodium is allowed in tap water which will add 0.9 mmol sodium/100 mL feed. This extra sodium will not matter for most infants and powdered feeds on sale in the UK will still comply with the EU Directive's acceptable sodium content if made up with water containing this level of sodium. Bottled mineral waters may contain excess amounts of sodium or other electrolytes and should not be used for making up infant formula. Just as tap water must be

Table 26.6 Energy densities of breast milk.

per 100 g/100 mL	Hester et al. 2012 [10]	Hosoi et al. 2005 [29]	McCance and Widdowson 1991 [9]
Colostrum	53.6 kcal (224 kJ)	57 kcal (238 kJ)	56 kcal (236 kJ)
Transitional milk	57.7 kcal (241 kJ)	63 kcal (263 kJ	67 kcal (281 kJ
Mature breast milk	65.2 kcal (273 kJ)	64 kcal (268 kJ)	69 kcal (289 kJ)

boiled before being used for reconstituting formula feeds, so must any bottled water. Carbonated fizzy water is not suitable for making up formula feeds.

Infant formula powder is not sterile and may contain microorganisms such as salmonella and *Enterobacter sakazakii* (now known as *Cronobacter sakazakii*). Neonates, particularly those who are preterm, of low birthweight or immunocompromised, are most at risk. To minimise the risk of gastroenteritis from these bacteria:

- feeds should be made up using boiled water >70°C (that has been left to cool in the kettle for no more than half an hour)
- this water is measured into a sterile bottle and the appropriate number of scoops of powder added (1 level unpacked scoop of powder per 30 mL/1 fluid ounce water)
- the bottle should then be sealed with a sterilised cap and shaken to mix the powder
- the feed must be cooled (by holding the sealed bottle under cold running water) and the temperature tested before giving to the baby
- bottles should be made up freshly for each feed
- any left over milk at the end of the feed should be thrown away
- parents who require a feed for later are advised to keep water they have just boiled in a sealed flask and make up fresh formula milk when needed [36]

If parents choose not to follow this advice and make up feeds for up to 24 hours in advance, the bottles of formula should be cooled quickly and stored in a fridge at <5°C. These feeds can be warmed just before use by standing the bottle in a container of hot water. Microwave ovens must not be used as the milk is not uniformly heated and hot spots in the milk could burn the baby's mouth [26].

Feeds should be made up using boiled water and sterile bottles or cups until 1 year of age because of the potential for bacterial growth. This is enhanced if bottles, teats and cups are not cleaned properly.

In the case where a baby is prescribed a multi-ingredient feed the dietitian may deem it safer, from the point of view of accuracy of feed reconstitution, for the parent to make up 24 hours' worth of feeds at one time. It is incumbent on the dietitian to give advice about scrupulous hygiene, rapid cooling and safe storage at <5°C if feeds are to be made up in advance. Any remaining milk

not completed after 1 hour of feeding should be discarded.

Bottle feeding

Feeding position
Bottle fed babies should be held in a supportive, semi-upright position, which encourages eye contact and bonding with the caregiver. The bottle should be angled so that the teat is always full of milk thus minimising the amount of air consumed. It is usual to 'wind' bottle fed babies half way through and after a feed.

Feeding equipment
Various types of bottles are available, some with air release devices to reduce colic. Different teats have varying flow rates according to the size and number of holes and they also vary in size and shape.

Problems preparing feeds
Lucas *et al.* [37] measured the energy content of infant formulas made up by a group of bottle feeding mothers and found the energy content ranged from 41 to 91 kcal (171 to 380 kJ)/100 mL whereas the manufacturer's intended energy content was 68 kcal (284 kJ)/100 mL. One-third of feeds contained less than 50 kcal (210 kJ)/100 mL and around half the feeds over 80 kcal (335 kJ)/100 mL. These discrepancies may arise from

- compression of the powder in the scoop or by using heaped scoops
- miscounting the number of scoops
- adding an extra scoop mistakenly thinking it will be more satisfying for the baby

Overconcentration of the feed may lead to hypernatraemia with consequent dehydration and possible severe brain damage or death, or to hypercalcaemia and hyperphosphataemia. Much of this potential danger has been reduced following compositional changes to modern infant formulas and the redesign of packaging to improve standards of hygiene and accuracy of mixing. The use of ready to feed (RTF) liquid formulas ensures the correct concentration is always given.

Overdilution of feeds may lead to excessive volumes being ingested in order to meet energy needs and this can cause vomiting and hyponatraemia. Faltering growth and malnutrition may ensue because the capacity of the young infant's stomach cannot cope with the much larger volumes of feed required to meet nutritional requirements.

Additional fluids

Formula fed infants may become thirsty between feeds in very hot weather and additional drinks of cooled boiled water can be given so long as these do not interfere with the required intake of formula. Fruit juices are not necessary as formula milks contain adequate vitamin C.

Infants with fever, diarrhoea or vomiting can dehydrate quickly and need additional fluids, and possibly electrolytes, to replace losses.

Weaning

When to start

The age of introduction of solid foods has become a controversial area. In 1994 the UK Department of Health (DH) recommended that weaning should begin between 4 and 6 months [38]. In 2001 the World Health Organization (WHO) recommended exclusive breast feeding until 6 months (26 weeks) of age because of the afforded protection against gastroenteritis. Because SACN advised that breast milk is nutritionally adequate for most babies until 6 months in the UK [39], the DH changed its recommendation on weaning to: exclusive breast feeding (or formula feeding) is ideal until 6 months and solids should be introduced at around 6 months; should parents choose to introduce solids earlier than this then weaning should not commence before 17 weeks (4 calendar months). Both DH and WHO have advised that these ages for the introduction of solids are population recommendations and each infant should be considered individually.

Subsequently, other publications have highlighted that there is no harm in beginning solids between 4 and 6 months of age and that some infants may be at risk of nutrient deficiencies if weaning is delayed until 6 months [40–42].

Infants should therefore be considered individually and the following developmental stages indicate readiness for solids:

- putting toys and other objects in the mouth
- chewing fists
- watching others with interest when they are eating

- seeming hungry between milk feeds or demanding feeds more often even though larger milk feeds have been offered

These developmental signs are generally seen between 4 and 6 months and from this age infants learn to accept new tastes and textures relatively quickly [43].

Around 4–6 months infants may start to sleep less and begin to wake again during the night. Night-time waking and crying are not necessarily signs of hunger at this age. Unfortunately many parents hope that weaning onto solid food will help their infant sleep through the night.

The 2010 Infant Feeding Survey (IFS) showed that 30% of infants are weaned onto solid food before 4 months and 75% were having solid food by 5 months, 94% by 6 months and 5% after 6 months [24]. The Diet and Nutrition Survey of Infants and Young Children in 2011 reported 42% of infants receiving solid food by 4 months but similar figures to the IFS at 5 and 6 months [44].

During the weaning period infants learn new skills and will progress through the developmental stages of weaning as they are given the opportunities to learn. Some progress faster than others. Table 26.7 gives a rough guide.

What to give

Weaning usually begins with 1–2 teaspoons of a smooth purée or mashed food being offered at just one meal a day. The addition of solids to bottles of milk is not advised in the UK; however, this is accepted practice in other European countries.

As the baby learns to manage solid food and begins to take a larger quantity, a second meal and then a third meal can be introduced. Once three meals are established, a variety of foods from the four main food groups should be included [38]. Table 26.8 shows the food groups and recommended servings. Meals should be nutrient dense and contain iron rich foods. Foods high in fat and sugar do not have a place in the early weaning diet. It is recommended that [38]

- salt and sugar should not be added to baby foods although a small amount of sugar can be added to make tart or sour fruits palatable
- honey should not be given before 12 months as there is a small risk of infant botulism

Table 26.7   Developmental stages of weaning.

Stage	Age guide	Skills to learn	New food textures to introduce
1	6 months, but not before 4 months (17 weeks) if parents choose to begin earlier	• taking food from a spoon • moving food from the front of the mouth to the back for swallowing • managing thicker purées and mashed food	Smooth purées Mashed foods
2	6–9 months	• moving lumps around the mouth • chewing lumps • self-feeding using hands and fingers • sipping from a cup	Mashed food with soft lumps Soft finger foods Liquids in a lidded beaker or cup
3	9–12 months	• chewing minced and chopped food • self-feeding attempts with a spoon	Hard finger foods Minced and chopped family foods

There is no evidence to support delaying any foods before 6 months to reduce the incidence of allergy [45] although advice may differ where there is a family history of food allergy (p. 814). SACN has reviewed the evidence on the age of introduction of gluten containing foods and concluded: 'Overall currently available evidence on the timing of introduction of gluten into the infant diet and subsequent risk of coeliac disease and T1DM [type 1 diabetes mellitus] is insufficient to support recommendations about the appropriate timing of introduction of gluten into the infant diet beyond 3 completed months of age, for either the general population or high-risk sub-populations' [46].

Responsive feeding allows the baby to decide how much solid food is eaten and how much milk is drunk. Parents should be encouraged to recognise their infant's signal when s/he indicates s/he has had enough of either solid food or milk feed. Parents should not coerce their infant to eat or drink more when they have indicated they have had enough. Force feeding is counterproductive to developing a positive attitude to food. Offering finger foods at each meal in addition to spoon feeding allows the infant to develop self-feeding skills.

Milk based desserts can be given to replace the milk feed at one and then two meals as the baby takes more food and two courses are offered at each meal time. The amount of breast milk or infant formula consumed by the infant will gradually reduce to about 500–600 mL/day towards the end of the first year. The pattern of feeding during weaning is shown in Table 26.9.

The majority of infants will try a wide variety of tastes and textures and they learn to like the foods they are offered [47]. The frequency with which they are offered a food, rather than the amount they eat, determines how quickly they will learn to like it. By the end of their first year infants should be eating family foods and the more variety they have been offered by around 12 months the wider the range of foods they will be familiar with and accept before food neophobia begins in their second year (p. 732).

Commercial weaning foods

The energy density and composition of homemade weaning foods varies widely [48] as does the taste and texture. By contrast commercial weaning foods are uniform in their texture and must conform to EU Directives which govern their composition [49]. The regulations governing pesticide residues in all commercial weaning foods are very strict; however, many parents choose to use commercial organic baby foods which allow no pesticides to be used in their culture and preparation. Organic food regulations prohibit iron fortification and consequently organic savoury baby foods are much lower in iron content than non organic savoury baby foods, which are usually fortified with iron sulphate:

• iron fortified non organic savoury jar 1.4 mg/100 g
• organic savoury jar 0.6 mg/100 g [50]

Table 26.8 Food groups and recommended servings.

Food group	Foods included	Main nutrients supplied	Recommendations			
			Infants 6–12 months [36]	Toddlers and preschoolers 1–4 years	School children 5–18 years	
1. Bread, other cereals and potatoes	Bread, chapatti, breakfast cereals, rice, couscous, pasta, millet, potatoes, yam, and foods made with flour such as pizza bases, buns, pancakes	Carbohydrate B vitamins Fibre Some iron, zinc and calcium	3–4 servings a day	Serve at each meal and some snacks	Serve at each meal and some snacks	
2. Fruit and vegetables	Fresh, frozen, tinned and dried fruits and vegetables. Also pure fruit juices	Vitamin C Phytochemicals Fibre Carotenes	3–4 servings a day	Offer at each meal and aim for about 5 small servings a day	Aim for 5 servings a day	
3. Milk, cheese and yoghurt	Breast milk, infant formulas, follow-on milks, cow's milk, yoghurts, cheese, calcium enriched soya milks, tofu	Calcium Protein Iodine Riboflavin	Demand feeds of breast milk or infant formula as main drink (about 500–600 mL/day) Some yoghurt and cheese	3 servings a day 1 serving is • 120 mL milk in a beaker or cup • 1 pot yoghurt or fromage frais • a serving of cheese in an sandwich or on a pizza • a milk based pudding • a serving of tofu	3 servings a day 1 serving is • 1 glass milk 150–250 mL • 1 pot yoghurt or fromage frais • a serving of cheese in a sandwich or on a pizza • a milk based pudding • a serving of tofu	
4. Meat, fish and alternatives	Meat, fish, eggs, pulses, dhal, nuts, seeds	Iron Protein Zinc Magnesium B vitamins Vitamin A Omega-3 long chain fatty acids: EPA and DHA from oily fish	1–2 servings a day 2–3 for vegetarians	2 servings a day 3 for vegetarians Fish should be offered twice per week and oily fish at least once per week*	2 servings a day 3 for vegetarians Fish should be offered twice per week and oily fish at least once per week*	

(continued overleaf)

Table 26.8 (continued)

Food group	Foods included	Main nutrients supplied	Recommendations		
			Infants 6–12 months [36]	Toddlers and preschoolers 1–4 years	School children 5–18 years
5. Foods high in fat and/or sugar	Cream, butter, margarines, cooking and salad oils, mayonnaise, chocolate, confectionery, jam, syrup, crisps and other high fat savoury snacks	Some foods provide: vitamins D and E omega-3 fatty acids – α-linolenic acid		In addition to but not instead of the other food groups	In addition to but not instead of the other food groups
Fluid	Drinks	Water Fluoride in areas with fluorided tap water	Water or well diluted fruit juice with meals and milk feeds	6–8 drinks per day and more in hot weather or after extra physical activity	6–8 drinks per day and more in hot weather or after extra physical activity
Vitamin supplements			Vitamins A and D for breast fed infants and formula fed infants drinking less than 500 mL formula milk/day	Vitamins A and D up to 5 years	Folic acid for adolescent girls who could become pregnant. Vitamin D for pregnant teenagers

Serving sizes of food and drinks will increase as children grow. Examples of average portion sizes for different ages are shown in Table 2.1.
*See p. 742.

Table 26.9 Pattern of feeding during weaning.

Stage	Age guide	Milk feeds	Meals	Variety of foods
1	6 months, not before 4 months	5–4	1–2	From 1 or 2 food groups
2	6–9 months	4–3	3	3 different meals from 4 nutritious food groups 1–2 courses per meal Vitamin A and D supplement for breast fed babies
3	9–12 months	3–2	3	3 different meals from 4 nutritious food groups 2 courses per meal Vitamin A and D supplement for breast fed babies

Fluids

Once weaning is established water should be offered from a cup or beaker with meals. This water does not have to be boiled for babies over 6 months old but can be freshly drawn tap water or bottled water given from a clean cup.

Juices

Infants do not need fruit juices or baby fruit juices as

- both breast milk and infant formula are nutritionally complete until 6 months and contain adequate vitamin C
- a balanced weaning diet for infants over 6 months will include fruit and vegetables

Many parents give baby fruit juices which are sold in a concentrated form or pre-diluted and ready to feed. All fruit juices (including baby juices) even when diluted are acidic and contain non milk extrinsic sugars. They can cause dental erosion so if offered

- should be well diluted
- should be served only at meal times in a cup or beaker, never a bottle
- drinking times should be kept short
- they should not be given at or after bedtime
- infants should never be left alone with juices as they may choke

Other fluids

Tea and coffee should not be given as they contain caffeine and the tannins and polyphenols in them inhibit iron absorption. Sugary drinks should not be given as they cause dental caries especially when taken frequently from a bottle.

Vitamin supplementation

The DH recommends a supplement of vitamins A and D for

- breast fed infants from 6 months (or from 1 month if there is any doubt about the mother's nutritional status during pregnancy)
- formula fed infants over 6 months when they are taking <500 mL/day of formula

Vitamin drops should always be given from a spoon, not added to bottles, to ensure the full dose is taken.

This recommendation is particularly important for infants at risk of low vitamin D status and includes those living in northern areas of the UK and those of Asian, African and Middle Eastern origin [38]. In areas of high incidence of vitamin D deficiency some NHS trusts and boards now have a policy of recommending that supplementation begins at birth or within a few weeks.

Toddlers and young children under 5 years of age

The diets of toddlers and preschool children should be based on a combination of foods from the five food groups in Table 26.8. Although the Public Health England Eatwell Plate [51] is not designed for the under 5s, children in this age group do grow satisfactorily on the same percentage energy contributions from the macronutrients as discussed below for school age children. However, under 5s are growing rapidly and therefore need a nutrient rich diet that is based mainly on the first four food groups, with very small amounts of foods from the fifth food group (foods high in fat and sugar).

The diet of this toddler and preschool group differs from that of the infant or that of older children and adults:

- less milk than the infant diet

- less fibre than the healthy eating recommendations for older children over 5 years and adults
- a meal pattern of three meals with two to three planned nutritious snacks per day, as toddlers may only take small quantities of food at any one time

Two courses at each meal, a savoury course followed by a sweet course, ensure a wider variety of foods and nutrients will be offered. Parents should be encouraged to think of the sweet course as a second opportunity to offer energy and nutrients and should not offer it only as a reward for finishing the savoury course.

The food groups

Bread, rice, potatoes, pasta and other starchy foods

A mixture of some white and some wholegrain varieties should be offered as the fibre load from only wholegrain cereals may be too high for toddlers. Excess fibre can fill up the stomach and reduce food intake thereby restricting energy and nutrient intake. Phytates in fibre reduce the absorption of certain nutrients and excess fibre may exacerbate loose stools in some toddlers.

Fruit and vegetables

Fruit and vegetables should be offered at each meal and some snacks. Toddlers may be averse to the bitter taste of some vegetables and may eat a limited variety. This should not be a cause for concern as this age should be seen as a time for learning to like fruits and vegetables and parents should encourage their toddlers to eat these foods by setting an example and eating and enjoying these foods themselves.

Milk, cheese and yoghurt

Milk intake should reduce from 12 months of age. During the preschool years three servings of milk, yoghurt and cheese per day will ensure calcium requirements are met. An excess of milk in the diet usually means less iron rich foods are eaten and iron deficiency and anaemia are associated with toddler diets where there is excessive milk drinking [52, 53].

Toddlers up to 2 years of age should have whole (full fat) milk for the extra vitamin A it contains. After 2 years toddlers can change to semi-skimmed milk if they are eating well and growing normally.

Follow-on and toddler milks marketed for this age group are enriched with more iron, zinc and vitamin D than that found in cow's milk. They can provide a nutritional safety net for toddlers who are not eating well, but a cheaper option is to give the toddler a vitamin and mineral supplement. These milks are lower in certain nutrients than cow's milk: calcium, phosphorus, iodine and riboflavin.

Meat, fish, eggs, nuts and pulses

Many toddlers do not like the texture of chewy meat and prefer soft tender cuts of meat products made from minced meat such as sausages, burgers and meatballs. As long as these foods are made from good quality ingredients with a high lean meat and low salt content they will make a valuable contribution to a healthy diet. Chicken, which often has a softer texture than red meat, is popular with this age group.

Fish should be offered twice a week and one portion should be oily (p. 742). Most toddlers enjoy fish when served as fish cakes or fish and potato pie.

Dhal is commonly used by some Asian cultures and a variety of other pulses can be used in soups and stews. Hummus and nut butters can be used as spreads.

Foods high in fat and/or sugar

These high energy foods add flavour and enjoyment to meals. Small amounts of them can be given in addition to the other food groups, but not instead of them. An excess of these foods will increase the likelihood of obesity which is increasing in this age group.

Drinks

Bottles for milk or other drinks should be discontinued around 12 months as sucking on a bottle can become a comfort habit that is hard to break. Children who drink sweet drinks from bottles have a higher risk of dental caries [54]. Water and milk are preferred drinks and should be given in a cup, beaker or glass. Six to eight drinks of about 100–120 mL can be offered throughout the day, with meals and snacks. More may be needed in very hot weather or after a lot of physical activity. Drinks containing artificial sweeteners should be kept to a minimum and be well diluted.

Portion sizes

The under 5s eat more on some days and less on other days; hence set portion sizes are not useful for them. The midpoints of the portion size ranges in Table 26.10 meet the RNI for nutrients and average energy requirement for children 1–4 years when combined according to the specified number of daily servings [55]. They can be used both to reassure parents of young children who eat small

amounts and to limit overeating particularly of food group 5.

Vitamin supplements

A supplement of vitamins A and D is recommended for children up to the age of 5 years [38]. As for infants this recommendation is particularly important for children at risk of low vitamin D status and includes picky fussy eaters, those living in northern areas of the UK and those of Asian, African and Middle Eastern origin.

Nutrients at risk in the preschool diet

The first three years of the rolling programme of the National Diet and Nutrition Survey (NDNS) has

Table 26.10 Portion size ranges for children aged 1–4 years.

Food group	Foods	Range of portion sizes
• Bread, rice, potatoes, pasta and other starchy foods ○ *5 servings per day*	Bread Mashed potato Pasta (cooked) Rice	$1/2$–1 medium slice 1–4 tbsp 2–5 tbsp 2–5 tbsp
• Fruit and vegetables ○ *3 servings fruit and 3 servings of vegetables per day*	Apple/pear/peach Broccoli/cauliflower Clementine/tangerine/mandarin Sweet corn	$1/4$–$1/2$ medium fruit 1–4 small florets or $1/2$–2 tbsp $1/2$–1 fruit $1/2$–2 tbsp
• Milk, cheese and yoghurt ○ *3 servings per day*	Cow's milk Grated cheese Yoghurt	100–120 mL or 3–4 fluid oz 2–4 tbsp 1 average pot or 125 mL
• Meat, fish, eggs, nuts and pulses ○ *2 servings per day*	Baked beans in tomato sauce Chicken drumsticks Peanut butter Scrambled egg Tinned fish	2–4 tbsp $1/2$–1 drumstick $1/2$–1 tbsp 2–4 tbsp $1/2$–$1 1/2$ tbsp
• Foods high in fat and sugar *Divided into 4 subgroups:* • *2 servings per day of fats and oils* • *1 serving per day of puddings and starchy snacks* • *1 serving per day of sauces, or sweet/savoury spreads* • *1 serving per week of confectionery, savoury snacks and sweet drinks*	Fruit crumble (e.g. apple or rhubarb) Ice cream Plain biscuits Honey/jam Butter/oil Sugar Crisps	2–4 tbsp 2–3 heaped tbsp 1–2 biscuits 1 tsp Thinly spread or 1 tsp $1/2$–1 tsp 4–6 crisps

tbsp, tablespoon (15 mL); tsp, teaspoon (5 mL).
Adapted from More & Emmett 2014 [55].

Table 26.11 Percentage of population groups with nutrient intakes from food and supplements below the LRNI [56].

Nutrient	Age groups				
	1½–3 years	4–10 years		11–18 years	
	Girls and boys	Girls	Boys	Girls	Boys
Vitamin A	8	4	5	14	9
Riboflavin	0	0	0	20	8
Folate	1	1	1	6	2
Iron	7	1	1	45	6
Calcium	1	2	0	18	7
Magnesium	1	3	0	50	27
Potassium	1	0	0	31	16
Zinc	5	8	5	19	11
Selenium	1	1	0	44	22
Iodine	1	3	2	20	8

LRNI, lower reference nutrient intake [1].

only surveyed 303 preschool children aged 1½–3 years but results indicate that their mean intake is above the RNI for all nutrients except iron and vitamin D. Less than 50% of this population met the RNI for iron and the mean intake of vitamin D was 34% RNI. More than 3% of this population did not meet the lower RNI (LRNI) for iron, vitamin A and vitamin C [56] (Table 26.11).

Developmental changes in preschool children

How easily parents manage to feed their young children depends to some extent on parental knowledge and parenting skills. At the same time developmental changes in toddlers affect how they respond to food and meals.

Neophobia

During their second year toddlers develop a neophobic response to food which means they become wary of trying new foods. The origin of this may be a survival mechanism to prevent the mobile toddler from poisoning themselves. This neophobic response usually peaks around 18 months and is more evident in some toddlers than others. If toddlers are being offered a wide variety of foods by around 12 months then they will enter their second year with a wider range of foods they recognise, like and readily accept [57].

Disgust and contamination fears

Between 3 and 5 years young children may develop disgust fears and stop eating foods they may have previously enjoyed [58]. They will refuse a food on sight if it resembles something they find disgusting, e.g. they may find spaghetti suddenly looks like worms. Contamination fears occur around the same time: if a disliked food is put on a plate next to a liked food the toddler may refuse both foods.

Learning to like new foods

The neophobic response dissipates slowly throughout the rest of childhood and adolescence [59, 60]. Toddlers and young children can be helped to pass through this stage by eating in social groups, as they learn by copying adults and other children. It is therefore important that families eat together as often as possible and that toddlers are praised when they eat well. Toddlers may also learn to eat new foods when eating with other children at nursery or with friends. Some toddlers need to be offered a new food more than 10 times before they accept it as a liked food [57, 61].

Some toddlers have more problems than others [62] and there are two main reasons for this in healthy individuals:

- Some become very rigid about the foods they will eat. They tend to be more emotional and more stubborn about what they will or will not do. They do not copy other children and so will not copy other people's eating behaviour.
- Others may be more sensory sensitive and have extreme reactions to touch, taste and smell. They may have problems with different textures of food and may have taken longer to progress from purée to lumpy food and onto more difficult textures. They may worry about getting their hands and face dirty and find it difficult to handle food and feed themselves.

Toddlers who experience faltering growth as a result of this will need to be referred to specialists who can assess and advise.

Exacerbating food refusal

Parental anxiety when toddlers only eat a limited variety of foods can exacerbate the problem, especially if parents try to coerce or force feed the child with food they are wary of or dislike. Until 4–5 years young children's appetites are determined mainly by their energy and growth needs. They eat well at some times and less so at other times and should always be allowed to decide the quantity they eat themselves.

Some parents expect their toddlers to eat more than they need and coerce or force feed when the toddler is signalling they have had enough food. As mealtimes develop into a battle ground between toddler and parent, the toddler can lose their appetite just by becoming anxious as the mealtime approaches. Toddlers may exhibit the following signals to indicate that they have had enough food:

- saying 'no'
- keeping their mouth shut when food is offered
- turning their head away from food being offered
- pushing away a spoon, bowl or plate containing food
- holding food in their mouth and refusing to swallow it
- spitting food out repeatedly
- crying, shouting or screaming
- gagging or retching
- trying to escape from the meal by climbing out of their chair or highchair

Around 5 years of age children learn to modify their eating according to social rules and will learn to finish what is on their plate, eat when others are eating even if they are not hungry, and they will also begin to comfort eat.

Social support for toddlers in low income families

Healthy start

Families who qualify for this scheme are those in receipt of certain benefits. Under the scheme they are entitled to vouchers that can be exchanged for cow's milk, fresh fruit and vegetables and infant formula (Table 26.12). Children up to 4 years in these families are also entitled to free vitamin drops containing vitamins A, C and D. Details of entitlement and how to access the scheme can be found on the Healthy Start website [63].

Table 26.12 Voucher entitlement for infants and children through Healthy Start.

	No. of vouchers valued at £3.10/week*
Term infants up to 12 months	2
Preterm infants up to 12 months after EDD	2
Children 1–4 years	1

EDD, estimated date of delivery.
*Voucher value as defined in 2014.

Nursery milk

Children under 5 years are entitled to $\frac{1}{3}$ pint (189 mL) milk per day if they attend a nursery or are with a registered childminder for more than 2 hours per day [64].

Sure Start Children's Centres

Sure Start is a government programme which provides services for preschool children and their families, bringing together early education, childcare, health and family support. Services include advice on healthcare and child development, play schemes, parenting classes, family outreach support and adult education and advice. One aim is to help overcome the barriers to feeding young children a healthy diet and dietitians have been involved in

- training Sure Start workers, community food assistants and play workers about weaning and healthy eating messages
- developing food policies with parents and staff
- developing resources with parents
- education sessions for parents on cooking, shopping, weaning. Cook and eat sessions are popular and developing literacy skills has become part of some shopping and cooking sessions
- holiday play schemes
- clinical input and home visits

Current schemes and activities can be accessed on the Sure Start website [65].

Primary and secondary school children

From around the age of 5 years the principles of healthy eating which are recommended for the adult population should be introduced:

- at least 50% of energy from total carbohydrates
- a maximum of 11% of energy from non milk extrinsic sugars
- a maximum of 35% of energy from fat
- a maximum of 11% of energy from saturated fat
- about 15% energy from protein [1]

Combining the five food groups in the proportions represented in the Eatwell Plate underlies the basis of healthy eating (Fig. 26.1). In order to satisfy the nutrient requirements of children the recommendations need to be more specific than those given by the DH for the general population. Table 26.8 is based on recommendations from the Paediatric Group of the British Dietetic Association.

A vegetarian diet is based around the same food groups shown in Table 26.8. Within the milk, cheese and yoghurt group calcium enriched soya milk, soya yoghurts and tofu can be substituted for cow's milk and its products. Within the meat, fish and alternatives group eggs, nuts, pulses and seeds will be eaten. At least three servings are needed each day to provide an adequate iron intake as the bioavailability of iron from eggs and plant sources is much lower than that of haem iron found in meat and fish.

During childhood many children remain neophobic, preferring to eat foods they are familiar with. They must be motivated to taste new foods. Work in this field continues to show that the number of times children are exposed to food increases the likelihood they will try the food and then learn to like it [66].

The food intakes of primary school children are fairly closely controlled by their parents and the most recent NDNS showed that the 'at risk' nutrients for primary age school children (4–10 years of age) are zinc and vitamin A (Table 26.11) [56]. In stark contrast older children (11–18 years) who are making more of their own food choices are more likely to have inadequate nutrient intakes, particularly girls.

Adolescent growth spurt

The adolescent growth spurt lasts approximately 2 years and takes place, on average, around 12 years of age for girls and 14 for boys, but can be 2 years earlier or later. The peak height velocity can be up to 13 cm/year for boys and 10 cm/year for girls [67]. Growth rate then declines until full

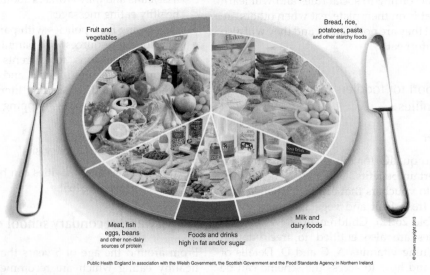

The eatwell plate

Use the eatwell plate to help you get the balance right. It shows how much of what you eat should come from each food group.

Fruit and vegetables

Bread, rice, potatoes, pasta and other starchy foods

Meat, fish eggs, beans and other non-dairy sources of protein

Foods and drinks high in fat and/or sugar

Milk and dairy foods

© Crown copyright 2013

Public Health England in association with the Welsh Government, the Scottish Government and the Food Standards Agency in Northern Ireland

Figure 26.1   The eatwell plate (Copyright: Public Health England).

height is reached. During this time adolescents' energy requirements will be noticeably higher and appetite may be larger. Extra snacks often make up this increase in food intake, but the NDNS in 2000 showed that snacks were often from food group 5, the high fat high sugar foods, rather than food groups 1 to 4 [68] which would enhance their nutrient intakes.

Good choices for snacks

These snack ideas are suitable for all children from 1 year of age, not just adolescents:

- fresh fruit (dried fruit can be cariogenic when eaten as a snack so it is not advised)
- vegetable sticks, e.g. carrot, cucumber, pepper, baby corn and dips based on yoghurt, low fat cream cheese or pulses such as hummus
- wholegrain breakfast cereals with milk
- cheese cubes and crackers or chapatti
- unsalted nuts
- sandwiches, filled rolls and pitta breads
- French toast or toast with a range of spreads, used sparingly
- slices of pizza with a plain dough base that has not been fried
- yoghurt and fromage frais
- crumpets, scones, currant buns, teacakes, Scotch pancakes, fruit muffins and plain biscuits
- homemade plain popcorn
- cakes containing dried fruit or vegetables, e.g. fruit cake and carrot cake

Suitable healthy drinks for meal and snack times include

- water
- milk (plain or flavoured)
- vegetable juices
- no added sugar (sugar free) squashes

Emotional changes in adolescents

During adolescence teenagers develop their own autonomy, rejecting their parents' values and developing their own. Values around food and meals are no exception to this and many teenagers change their eating habits so that they are different from the rest of their family [59]. Their choices include a lot of high fat high sugar foods [68].

Hill [59] suggested adolescents may

- eat more and more food outside the home and convenience may be influential in choices made
- eat according to personal ideology such as the use of vegetarian diets
- begin slimming or weight control (whether justified or not)
- choose less healthy foods as an act of parental defiance and peer solidarity
- consume certain foods or brands due to peer group pressure
- follow specific diets to enhance sporting prowess

Understanding why adolescents choose the foods they do is crucial when developing health education programmes for this age group.

Nutritional initiatives in schools

Food and drinks taken at school can make a large contribution to a child's nutrient intake. The School Food Trust, a national charity and advisor to Government on school meals, published nutrient based standards for school meals and foods sold on school premises in 2007 [69]. From 2008/2009 the nutrient and food based standards became mandatory for all local authority maintained primary, secondary, special and boarding schools and pupil referral units in England. The newly formed academies are not required to follow these standards. Scotland and Wales also have nutrient and food based standards. Northern Ireland has food based standards.

School meals

The content of school dinners/lunches is based on the reference nutrient intakes and estimated average requirement for energy for children [2] and in England and Wales the midday meal must provide

- 30% estimated average requirement for energy
- not less than 50% energy from carbohydrate
- not more than 35% energy from fat nor 11% energy from saturated fat

Minimum and maximum values of key nutrients are specified and listed in Table 26.13.

Table 26.13   Energy and key nutrients that an average school lunch must provide [69].

	Maximum or minimum amount	Primary school lunch	Secondary school lunch
Energy (kcal)		530 ± 26.5	646 ± 32.3
		(2215 ± 110 kJ)	(2700 ± 135 kJ)
Protein (g)	Minimum	7.5	13.3
Carbohydrate (g)	Minimum	70.6	86.1
Non milk extrinsic sugars (g)	Maximum	15.5	18.9
Fat (g)	Maximum	20.6	25.1
Saturated fat (g)	Maximum	6.5	7.9
Fibre	Minimum	4.2	5.2
Sodium (mg)	Maximum	499	714
Vitamin A (µg)	Minimum	745	245
Vitamin C (mg)	Minimum	10.5	14
Folate (µg)	Minimum	53	70
Calcium (mg)	Minimum	193	350
Iron (mg)	Minimum	3	5.2
Zinc (mg)	Minimum	2.5	3.3

The Scottish standards introduced in 2004 [70] are very similar specifying

- minimum 30%–40% of RNI for fibre, protein, iron, calcium, vitamin A, folate, vitamin C (these nutrients are least likely to be consumed in sufficient amounts in Scottish diets)
- maximum levels of fat, saturated fat, sugar and sodium are given for some groups of manufactured products

Food based standards for school food other than lunches

This applies to all food and drink provided by local authorities or school governing bodies to pupils on and off school premises, during an extended school day (up to 18.00) and covers

- breakfast clubs
- mid morning break services
- vending machines
- tuck shops
- after school snacks and meals

Guidelines on permitted food and drinks are given in Table 26.14.

School breakfasts

Many schools have begun offering breakfasts and anecdotal claims have been made that school attendance, behaviour and performance have improved. However, a systematic review found that although a school breakfast is better than no breakfast, this only makes a difference in children who are malnourished. Furthermore they found that any improved academic performance may be due in part to the increased school attendance that a school breakfast encourages, rather than the food itself [71]. Children say they enjoy the social side of school breakfasts.

Packed lunches

Many children bring a packed lunch rather than have school meals they dislike or that their parents either cannot afford or of which they disapprove. Packed lunches can be of poor nutritional content; a Food Standards Agency (FSA) survey of school lunchboxes showed that 74% failed to meet the food based standards for school meals [72]. Typically, a packed lunch comprised sandwiches, a chocolate bar, savoury snack and sweetened drink. Fresh fruit was often absent.

Suggestions for healthy lunchboxes, including guidance on food safety, can be obtained from the FSA website [73]. The aim should be to include foods from each of the food groups and include a drink (Table 26.15). A small ice pack or a frozen drink will keep a closed lunchbox cool for a few hours.

Table 26.14 Guidelines for food and drinks allowed or restricted (other than lunches).

Foods encouraged	Fruit and vegetables must be provided in all school food outlets
	These can include fresh, dried, frozen, canned and juiced varieties
	Nuts, seeds, vegetables and fruits with no added salt, sugar or fat
	Free, fresh drinking water (still or carbonated) should be provided at all times
	Fruit juice, vegetable juice, low fat milk (milk with a fat content of not more than 1.8%), plain soya, rice or oat drinks enriched with calcium and plain yoghurt drinks
	Combinations of water (still or carbonated) and fruit and/or vegetable juice, containing at least 50% juice and no added sugar, and may contain vitamins or minerals
	Combination drinks:
	• milk (low fat or lactose reduced), or plain yoghurt, water, fruit or vegetable juice • plain soya, rice or oat drink, water, fruit or vegetable juice • milk (low fat or lactose reduced), plain yoghurt or plain soya, rice or oat drinks (with or without plain water) with cocoa
	Restrictions for these drinks:
	• The milk, yoghurt or soya, rice or oat drink must be at least 50% by volume • May contain vitamins and minerals • Less than 5% sugar or honey may be added
	No colourings are permitted
Foods restricted	Condiments such as ketchup and mayonnaise must only be available in sachets or individual portions of not more than 10 g or 1 teaspoonful
	Cakes and biscuits must not be provided at times other than lunch
	Starchy food cooked in fat or oil must not be provided more than three times a week across the school day
	No more than two deep-fried food items such as chips and batter coated products can be provided in a single week across the school day
	Meat products (manufactured or homemade) are divided into four groups. A meat product from each of the four groups may be provided no more than once per fortnight across the school day
Foods not allowed	Confectionery such as chocolate bars, chocolate coated or flavoured biscuits, sweets and cereal bars
	Snacks such as crisps
	Salt must not be provided at tables or service counters

Other issues around food eaten by school children

There are further schemes to support the nutritional intakes of school children:

• *The national fruit and veg scheme.* All 4–6-year-old children in Local Education Authority (LEA) maintained infant, primary and special schools are entitled to a free piece of fruit or vegetable each school day [74].
• *Subsidised school milk.* This is available for primary school children. In England schools choose whether they wish to offer it, but in Wales children up to 7 years of age are entitled to 1/3 pint (189 mL) milk free per day [75].

Foods eaten on the way to and from school are also a significant part of school children's nutrient intake. A survey produced by a large international school caterer [76] reported that in 2005

• £519 million was spent by school children on their way to and from school
• main purchases were sweets, crisps and savoury snacks, chocolate, canned fizzy drinks, chewing gum, other soft drinks, cigarettes, bottled water, chips and ice cream

Nutritional problems in children

There are a number of common nutritional problems in children that are discussed elsewhere:

Table 26.15 Suggestions for packed lunchboxes.

Food group	Suitable foods
Bread, other cereals and potatoes	This should be the base of the lunch: • Breads, rolls, wraps and pittas can be filled or used for sandwiches • Crispbread or bread sticks • Pasta, rice or cooked potatoes as the base for a salad or soup
Fruit and vegetables	• Sliced in sandwiches • Combined in a salad • Sticks of raw vegetables (celery, carrots, cucumber) or small tomatoes as finger foods or crunchy alternative to crisps • Pieces of fruit or small packets of dried fruit
Milk, cheese and yoghurt	• Cheese is a popular sandwich filling • Cubes or triangles of cheese as finger foods • Pots of yoghurts, fromage frais or rice pudding are popular desserts • Cartons of milk or flavoured milk as the drink
Meat, fish and alternatives	• Cold meats or flaked fish can be included in sandwiches or salads • Chicken drumsticks or cold sausages
Combined food group foods	• Slices of quiche or pizza • Soups
Food high in fat and sugar	• Fun sized chocolate bars or small cakes or muffins • Buns, scones, tea breads are a lower fat alternative • Fruit juice or smoothies can be included as the drink

obesity (Chapter 30), faltering weight (Chapter 28), constipation and diarrhoea (Chapter 7), food allergy (Chapter 14).

Dental caries

Children, particularly the under 5s, are more susceptible to dental caries than adults although the incidence of caries in children in the UK decreased following the introduction of fluoride toothpaste in the 1970s. However, the current high and frequent consumption of sugary foods and sugary acidic drinks contributes to

- 31% of 5 year olds having at least one decayed, missing or filled tooth, but this ranged from 17.7% to 53% in different Primary Care Trusts [77]
- 33.4% of 12 year olds having experience of caries, having one or more teeth which were decayed to dentinal level, extracted or filled because of caries [78]

The incidence of dental disease is lower in children who brush their teeth twice a day and limit sugary and acidic food and drinks to four eating episodes per day, e.g. three meals and one snack [79]. DH recommendations on toothpaste use are [80]:

- teeth should be brushed twice daily, once in the morning and last thing at night
- use a smear of paste containing 1000 ppm of fluoride up to the age of 3
- use a pea sized amount of 1350–1500 ppm of fluoride paste over the age of 3

Iron deficiency anaemia

Iron deficiency is associated with frequent infections, poor weight gain, developmental delay and behaviour disorders. It is more common in preschool children than those over 5 years of age and is usually of dietary origin and seen more in socially disadvantaged groups and in the immigrant population.

Depletion of iron stores in the second half of infancy occurs when the iron content of the weaning diet is poor, even though deficiency may not be evident until after 12 months of age. The early introduction of cow's milk as a main drink before 12 months of age is a risk factor [81, 82]. The lack of commercial halal meat based weaning foods may be partly responsible for the low iron intakes commonly found in infants of Asian families [83]. A range of halal baby foods is now available in the UK.

Overdependence on milk in toddlers and preschool children, where it replaces iron rich or iron enhancing foods, is another common cause [84, 85].

In older children deficiency occurs more commonly in teenage girls who have begun menstruating and in children who are vegetarian or from minority ethnic groups who do not eat a balanced diet.

Prevention of iron deficiency

The use of iron fortified infant formulas or follow-on milks, rather than cow's milk, into the second year of life has been shown to reduce the prevalence of iron deficiency anaemia in inner city deprived populations [30–34]. Toddler milks produced for 1–3 year olds are also higher in iron than cow's milk and, if parents can afford them, may be useful for those eating poorly.

Dietary advice should emphasise the importance of regularly consuming iron rich foods (food group 4, Table 26.8) along with iron fortified breakfast cereals and dried fruit. Liver and liver products, although a very rich source of iron, contain very high levels of vitamin A and should be limited to one serving per week. Haem iron in meat and fish is absorbed much more efficiently than non haem iron from eggs, nuts, pulses, cereals, fruit and vegetables. Simultaneous consumption of fruits, vegetables and drinks rich in vitamin C will enhance non haem iron absorption [86]. This is a particularly important measure in vegetarian children. Iron uptake can be maximised by avoiding drinking tea which hampers absorption at meals.

Vitamin D deficiency

Infants and children with rickets and hypocalcaemic seizures resulting from extremely low levels of vitamin D are rising in the UK [87]. The main source of vitamin D in the UK is not the diet, as oily fish is the only significant source, but cutaneous synthesis when outside with bare skin exposed in the summer months. Children with pigmented skins are at higher risk of deficiency as cutaneous synthesis is less efficient. When body stores are low and cutaneous synthesis and dietary sources of vitamin D are limited, vitamin D deficiency develops in those with high requirements such as rapidly growing infants, toddlers and adolescents.

Epidemiological studies report associations between low vitamin D levels and higher rates of inflammatory and autoimmune diseases and other chronic diseases in children [88] including type 1 and type 2 diabetes, allergy, upper respiratory tract infections and wheeze including asthma, infectious diseases. In addition the risk of severe pre-eclampsia in pregnant women is higher in those with low levels of vitamin D [89, 90].

The main cause of deficiency in infants and toddlers is the low vitamin D status of women of child bearing age. Infants whose mothers entered the pregnancy with low vitamin D levels and who did not take the recommended supplement are likely to be born with low levels of vitamin D and poor stores [91–93]. Exclusively breast fed infants born with low stores of vitamin D are at risk as the vitamin D content of breast milk is normally low. It is lower still in the milk of mothers who are vitamin D deficient [94]. Although infant formulas are fortified with vitamin D the level appears to be inadequate for an infant born with very low stores; formula fed infants have been diagnosed with hypocalcaemic seizures, cardiomyopathy and rickets [95, 96].

Dietary requirements

The UK RNI for vitamin D is set to guarantee sufficiency in age groups whose needs may not be met by sunlight alone, i.e. infants, toddlers, pregnant and breast feeding mothers. However, very few foods naturally contain vitamin D: oily fish is the most significant source; eggs and meat provide very small amounts; breast milk provides extremely small amounts and this varies depending on the mother's own vitamin D status.

A few foods in the UK are fortified with vitamin D: margarine, evaporated milk, all formula milks and some brands of breakfast cereals and yoghurts. Some countries fortify other foods with vitamin D, e.g. fresh cow's milk, some fruit juices and other foods in Finland, the USA and Canada.

The most recent UK NDNS [56] reports that

- very few preschool children consume the RNI through food alone: the mean daily intake of 1$^1/_2$–3 year olds is about 20% RNI
- the mean plasma levels of vitamin D in women of childbearing age is <50 nmol/L indicating insufficiency and 20% have levels <25 nmol/L indicating deficiency

The RNI for young children can only be guaranteed by taking vitamin D supplements. The UK policy for vitamin D supplements for under 5s and pregnant and breast feeding women is given in Table 26.16. Most multivitamin supplements for infants, children and pregnant and breast feeding women sold over the counter in the UK include vitamin D of varying quantity. Supplements containing vitamin D only are available in some retail outlets. The Healthy Start vitamins (Table 1.22) are the most cost effective supplement, but they are only available in some NHS clinics. Although NHS trusts and health boards are expected to provide them free of charge to beneficiaries of the Healthy Start scheme and sell them to other clients, not all do this.

Table 26.16 Recommendations for vitamin D supplementation for mothers and children in the UK [25, 97].

Group	Recommended supplement
Pregnant and breast feeding women	10 µg/day
Breast fed infants from 6 months or from 1 month if the mother's nutritional status in pregnancy was in doubt	7.5 µg/day
Formula fed infants who are drinking less than 500 mL formula milk	7.5 µg/day
Toddlers 1–4 years	7.5 µg /day
Breast fed preterm infants	A vitamin supplement that includes vitamin D is usually prescribed

Children 4–18 years

There is currently no RNI for children over 4 years of age as it is expected that cutaneous synthesis of vitamin D will suffice. This is a subject of much debate as low blood levels of vitamin D are found in significant numbers of children and adolescents in the UK [56, 68].

Other countries do set dietary recommendations for older children, e.g. 5–10 µg/day for children in most European countries and 15 µg vitamin D for all children in the USA. The European tolerable upper intake level for vitamin D for infants and children up to 10 years is 25 µg/day [98] and the USA Institute of Medicine considers it to be 50 µg/day for infants and 100 µg/day for toddlers and older children [88].

Cutaneous synthesis of vitamin D

Cutaneous synthesis is the main source of vitamin D in the UK. The critical wavelength for synthesis does not pass through glass so one must be outside for vitamin D synthesis to occur. The ideal time to spend outside each day to ensure adequate vitamin D levels is not easy to define as skin synthesis depends on

- season – the critical wavelength only reaches the UK between April and September; it is absorbed by the atmosphere during winter months
- latitude – less vitamin D is made in the north of the UK than in the south where more of the UVB rays are present
- weather – on a cloudy day less vitamin D is made than on a bright sunny day
- pollution in the air – reduces the critical UV light waves
- time of day – more vitamin D is synthesised when sunlight is most intense in the middle of the day compared with early morning and late afternoon
- skin type – darker skins require more time in the sun to produce the same amount of vitamin D [99]
- lifestyles – time spent outside in April to September
  – bare skin exposure when outside; cutaneous synthesis is extremely limited when most skin is covered as dictated by religious and cultural traditions
- use of sunscreen – it blocks cutaneous synthesis

Cutaneous synthesis is regulated and shuts off when a particular plateau is reached so excessive amounts are not synthesised [100]. Vitamin D is stored in the body when cutaneous synthesis and dietary intakes exceed daily requirements and these stores can be used during the winter months.

Conflicting advice on the use of sunscreen

Concern over the balance between having sufficient sun exposure to produce vitamin D and overexposure leading to burning of the skin and an increased risk of skin cancer has led to confusion in public health messages. To provide unified, evidence based advice on the subject, a consensus statement on vitamin D was agreed in 2010 by several organisations with an interest in this area [101]:

The time required to make sufficient vitamin D varies according to a number of environmental, physical and personal factors, but is typically short and less than the amount of time needed for skin to redden and burn. Enjoying the sun safely, while taking care not to burn, can help to provide the benefits of vitamin D without unduly raising the risk of skin cancer. Vitamin D supplements and specific foods can help to maintain sufficient levels of vitamin D, particularly in people at risk of deficiency. However, there is still a lot of uncertainty around what levels qualify as 'optimal' or 'sufficient'.

Inappropriate dieting

Girls as young as 9 years old, and some younger, indicate body dissatisfaction and a desire to be thinner. Similar aged boys aspire for a more muscled body, but overweight boys and girls both desire weight loss and are unhappy with their body shape [102]. Hill suggested this body dissatisfaction was a result of picking up on parental attitudes to weight and shape, the idealisation of thinness promoted in the media and peer behaviour.

Implications of poor teenage diets on future risk of osteoporosis

Even after the growth spurt calcification of bones continues as peak bone mass is not reached until the early 20s. Three large servings of milk, cheese or yoghurt will ensure that calcium and phosphorus requirements are being met to ensure bone deposition [103]. This applies for Caucasian teenagers but not necessarily for other minority ethnic groups [104]. Adequate calcium intakes at this age may protect against osteoporosis in later life [105].

Sports nutrition

Meeting the higher energy needs for adolescents undertaking sports training is essential and may require specialist input from a registered sports dietitian. Energy requirements should be calculated to support the training programme using basal metabolic rate and physical activity level and adding in 60–100 kcal (250–420 kJ)/day to allow for extra growth [1]. Monthly height measurement can be used to assess when the growth spurt is taking place. Adolescents in sports training should eat a high carbohydrate snack or meal, containing some protein, within an hour of finishing training to ensure good glycogen stores within muscles (as should any other athlete).

Teenage girls of child bearing age

All women of childbearing age should have a nutritious diet with adequate folate. The DH recommends a supplement of 400 μg folic acid for any woman or teenager who could become pregnant. Since most teenage pregnancies are unplanned, a diet rich in folate should be recommended to all teenage girls.

Pregnancy

Pregnancy during the teenage years places extra nutritional needs on girls who may not have finished growing themselves and who will not have attained their peak bone mass. Nutrient requirements have not been specified for these young mothers but a healthy balanced diet with folic acid and vitamin D supplementation would be a minimum requirement. For those eating poorly a multivitamin and mineral supplement (not containing vitamin A) could be recommended. Under the Healthy Start scheme all pregnant girls under 18 are entitled to benefits regardless of their financial circumstances [63].

Food safety

Good food hygiene and storage is extremely important for young children, particularly infants and children under 5 years. To offset any risks of bacterial food poisoning meat, fish, shellfish and eggs should be well cooked right through [106].

Dioxin levels in oily fish

Varying levels of dioxins accumulate in the fatty tissues of oily fish and to limit their intake the FSA recommends that boys have a maximum of four portions of oily fish per week. A maximum limit of two portions is set for girls to reduce the amounts they will have accumulated in their tissues as they enter their childbearing years [107].

Mercury levels in large fish

Large fish (shark, swordfish and marlin) live for many years and can accumulate high levels of mercury in their flesh. The FSA recommends that pregnant women, babies and young children under 5 years do not eat these fish [107].

High vitamin A levels in liver

Although liver is a very good source of several nutrients, particularly some 'at risk' nutrients discussed above, e.g. iron and zinc, it contains very high levels of vitamin A. SACN has recommended that no-one should increase their consumption of liver beyond one portion per week [108]. Although no recommendations were made for young children and babies it would be prudent to avoid giving liver to babies who are weaned early, before 6 months, and to limit it to once per week in older infants and young children.

Organic foods

Many parents choose to buy organic food for their babies and children despite the extra expense; the majority of commercially prepared baby foods sold are now organic. Parents do this to avoid the possible detrimental effects that pesticide residues found in foods from non organic sources may have on the developing organs and systems of babies and children. This remains a controversial issue as food safety bodies in the UK and Europe only allow pesticides at levels that are judged to be non harmful in conventional baby foods. However, advocates of organic food point out that there may be toxic effects of ingesting combinations of several different chemicals which may have been harmless when tested individually. Many of these chemicals are new, having only been synthesised in the last few decades, so their potential cumulative effects are unknown.

Studies linking pesticide or synthetic chemical exposure in children with an increased incidence of cancer [109] and impaired cognitive function [110] have been published. *In utero* exposure of the foetus to these chemicals may be the most damaging [111].

Controversial issues around nutrients and foods

Omega-3 fatty acids and learning skills

Optimum brain functioning and sight are dependent on an adequate intake of the omega-3 long chain polyunsaturated fatty acids (LCP), eicosapentaenoic acid (EPA) and docosahexaenoic acid (DHA), during foetal growth and early infancy [112]. They are present in breast milk and are added to all whey dominant and casein dominant infant formulas (Table 1.14). Whether their presence in food or supplements for older infants and children influences brain function, behaviour or the risk of atopy remains controversial.

A weekly serve of oily fish will ensure an adequate intake of omega-3 LCPs. Walnuts and linseeds as well as rapeseed, walnut, linseed and soya oils are good sources of the omega-3 essential fatty acid, α-linolenic acid. Current research has not shown that children with adequate dietary intake of omega-3 fats will benefit from extra supplements. However, omega-3 supplements and foods that have been enriched with omega-3 fats are now subject to high level marketing following anecdotal evidence of children's learning skills improving with supplementation [113].

Food advertising

Media messages about food are targeted at children through

- television, radio and internet advertisements
- in store displays
- child friendly packaging including familiar cartoon characters on the packaging
- stealth marketing techniques such as embedding products in the programme content in films, online and in video games

The majority of foods advertised are high fat, high sugar and low fibre foods. These advertisements often feature messages implying that low nutrient foods are desirable or beneficial. These implications may confuse children and their parents about what makes a particular food a healthy choice.

Marketing experts know that toddlers and children have considerable purchasing influence and successfully negotiate purchases through 'nag factor' or 'pester power'. Requests are often for brand name products and food accounts for over half of total requests, with parents honouring these 50% of the time [114]. The most requested item is breakfast cereal, followed by snacks, drinks and toys. Children younger than 8 are especially vulnerable to these marketing strategies because they lack the cognitive skills to understand the persuasive intent of television and online advertisements [115]. Older children exposed to advertising choose advertised food products significantly more often than those who are not exposed [114].

Several studies point towards the contribution of food marketing to rising levels of childhood obesity [116–118].

Genetic modification

The long term effects of genetic modification (GM) are as yet unknown and remain controversial. The nutritional content of GM and non GM foods sold in the UK are comparable and therefore do not affect a baby or child's nutritional intake. Many parents choose not to give GM food to their children, but they may not always be aware of the extent to which GM ingredients are used in processed foods.

Further reading and information

More J *Infant, Child and Adolescent Nutrition: a Practical Handbook*. Boca Raton, FL: Taylor and Francis, 2013.
Studies from the Avon Longitudinal Study of Pregnancy and Childhood www.alspac.bris.ac.uk.

Hall DMB, Elliman D *Health for All Children*, 4th edn. Oxford: Oxford University Press, 2003.

Infants and preschool children

Healthy Child Programme – e-learning programme www.e-lfh.org.uk/projects/healthychild/index .html
Morgan J, Dickerson JWT *Nutrition in Early life*. Chichester: John Wiley, 2003.
Unicef Babyfriendly Initiative: www.babyfriendly.org .uk
National Childbirth Trust www.nctpregnancyandbaby care.com
The Association of Breast Feeding Mothers www.abm .me.uk
La Leche League www.lalecheleague.org
The Breast Feeding Network www.breastfeeding.co.uk
Infant and Toddler Forum www.infantandtoddler forum.org
Eat Better Start Better Voluntary Food and Drink Guidelines for Early Years Settings in England – A Practical Guide School Food Trust 2012: Available at www.schoolfoodtrust.org.uk/eatbetterstartbetter
Nutritional Guidance for Early Years: Food Choices for Children Aged 1–5 Years in Early Education and Childcare Settings. Scottish Executive, 2006. Available at www.scotland.gov.uk/Publications/ 2006/01/18153659/0
Nutrition matters for the early years: Guidance for feeding the under fives in the childcare setting. Public Health Agency for Northern Ireland, 2012. Available at http://www.publichealth.hscni.net/ publications/nutrition-matters-early-years-guidance-feeding-under-fives-childcare-setting
Eating Well for 1-4 Year Olds Practical Guide, The Caroline Walker Trust, 2010. Available at http://www .cwt-chew.org.uk/
Crawley H *Eating Well for Under-5s in Childcare*. London: Caroline Walker Trust, 2006.
Crawley H *Eating Well for Under-5s in Childcare: Training Materials*. London: Caroline Walker Trust, 2006.

School children

The School Food Trust www.schoolfoodtrust.org.uk
The Health Education Trust www.healthedtrust.com
British Heart Foundation www.bhf.org.uk
School Fruit and Vegetable Scheme http://www.nhs .uk/Livewell/5ADAY/Pages/Schoolscheme.aspx

Adolescents

Adolescent health http://www.e-lfh.org.uk/projects/ adolescent-health/
Eating Disorders Association www.b-eat.co.uk

27

Children from Ethnic Groups and those following Cultural Diets

Eulalee Green

Introduction

The UK is the home to a multicultural and multi-ethnic society. Immigration during the late 1950s and early 1960s was in response to labour shortages. Since the 1980s conflict in Africa and Europe has led to further immigration and, together with movement of people from newly joined European Union countries, the diversity of the UK has increased. As with the early migrations, ethnic communities have remained near large industrialised cities. These ethnic groups have introduced a wide variety of cultures, including dietary beliefs and practices, which have had to fit into their new lifestyles. Achieving nutritionally adequate diets became a challenge with people finding themselves in an environment very different from their homeland.

The top 15 countries of last residence of migrants to the UK in 2005–2006 are shown in Fig. 27.1 and Table 27.1. Table 27.2 shows the percentage of ethnic groups in England and Wales in 2011.

Infants and children of any age have special dietary requirements. It is therefore essential that healthcare professionals understand religious and cultural attitudes towards diet when they are initiating any dietary intervention, in order to achieve optimal growth and development in these children.

Assessment of intake must be accurate and any advice given must be relevant to dietary custom so that it is both realistic and achievable.

Children are subject to many outside influences and often start to develop westernised dietary ideas. With time, these ideas are taken home and adopted by other members of the family. The extent of adoption of dietary practices which differ from traditional customs is variable; therefore all diets must be individually assessed.

Table 27.3 shows the religions practised in the UK and Table 27.4 gives a guide to religious and cultural influences on the diet.

Vegetarian and vegan diets

Vegetarianism and veganism are common dietary practices among many religious and ethnic groups. In addition, increasing numbers of the indigenous population are restricting their intake of meat and animal products for either humanitarian, ethical or health reasons. Table 27.5 gives a classification of vegetarian and vegan diets. Providing careful attention is given to ensuring nutritional adequacy, these diets will support normal growth and development [4–6]. In general the greater the degree of dietary restriction, the greater is the risk of

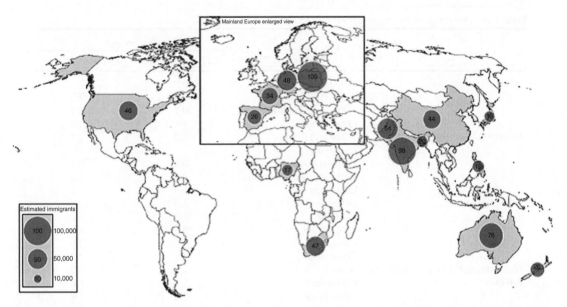

Figure 27.1   Immigrants to the UK in 2005–2006: top 15 countries of last residence. Source: Office of National Statistics [1].

Table 27.1   Top 15 countries of last residence of all migrants 2005–2006 combined.

Ranking	Country of last residence	Thousands of immigrants
1	Poland	109
2	India	98
3	Australia	76
4	Pakistan	54
5	Germany	48
6	South Africa	47
7	USA	46
8	China	44
9	France	34
10	New Zealand	26
11	Spain	26
12	Bangladesh	20
13	Philippines	19
14	Nigeria	17
15	Japan	16

Source: Office of National Statistics [1].

nutritional deficiency [7]. The vegan diet is most restricted; Table 27.6 gives dietary sources of the nutrients most at risk.

Infant feeding

The current recommendation is for infants to be exclusively breast fed until 6 months of age. Solids should be introduced at around 6 months of age; breast feeding should be continued during this time [8]. There is a higher proportion of women from minority ethnic groups who choose to breast feed their babies up to 6 months (Table 27.7).

All breast fed infants and infants having less than 500 mL of infant formula should be given a vitamin D supplement which should continue until 5 years of age [10]. Suitable vitamin drops include Healthy Start, Abidec and Dalivit (Table 1.22).

If the infant is not breast fed an infant formula must be given. Table 27.8 shows normal infant formulas and special therapeutic formulas which are suitable for vegetarian and vegan families and for those who require a Halal formula. Some families will accept 'unsuitable' formulas if there is a clinical need.

Some vegetarian families choose to give their babies goat's milk or ewe's milk in the belief that these confer health benefits and are preferable to cow's milk. These milks are contraindicated because of their nutritional inadequacy, high renal solute load and doubtful microbiological safety [11, 12]. The European Food Safety Authority considers that protein from goat milk can be suitable as a protein source for infant formula provided the formula complies with the compositional criteria laid down in Directive 2006/141/EC [13];

Table 27.2   Percentage of ethnic groups in England and Wales, 2011

		Percentages	
		Total population	Ethnic population
White	White British	80.5	
	Irish	0.9	4.6
	Gypsy or Irish traveller	0.1	0.5
	Other White	4.4	22.5
Mixed/multiple ethnic groups	White and Black Caribbean	0.8	4.1
	White and Asian	0.6	3.1
	White and Black African	0.3	1.5
	Other mixed	0.5	2.6
Asian/Asian British	Indian	2.5	12.8
	Pakistani	2.0	10.3
	Bangladeshi	0.8	4.1
	Chinese	0.7	3.6
	Other Asian	1.5	7.7
Black/African/Caribbean/Black British	African	1.8	9.2
	Caribbean	1.1	5.6
	Other Black	0.5	2.6
Other ethnic group	Arab	0.4	2.1
	Any other ethnic group	0.6	3.1

Source: Office of National Statistics [2].

Table 27.3   Percentage of the UK population belonging to a religion, April 2011–March 2012.

Religion	Population percentage	Number (thousands)
Christian	62.0	37 191
Islam/Muslim	4.6	2755
Hindu	1.4	860
Sikh	0.6	350
Jewish	0.5	287
Buddhist	0.4	246
None or undeclared	29.9	17 927

Source: Office of National Statistics [2].

however, goat's milk formula has no health benefits over normal infant formulas.

Providing the maternal diet is adequate, breast milk will be nutritionally adequate for the first 6 months of life for most infants. Specific attention must be paid to the mother's vitamin D, calcium and iron intakes. Vegan mothers may require supplementation with additional vitamin B_{12} [11]. Vitamin B_{12} deficiency resulting in neurological damage [14], irritability, faltering growth, apathy, anorexia and developmental regression has been reported in breast fed infants of vegan mothers [12]. Some algae (e.g. spirulina) and seaweeds (e.g. nori) contain natural compounds that are similar to vitamin B_{12}; however, the human body cannot use these nutrients. Furthermore, because they are so similar to B_{12} they compete with it and can be the cause of B_{12} deficiency in people who do not eat animal products. Vegetarian sources of iron and vitamin B_{12} are given in Table 27.9.

Weaning

At around 6 months of age solids should be gradually introduced to the infant's diet, increasing flavours and textures with time. Only a small number of women choose to introduce solids before their child is 4 months old, but only 10% of women wait until their child is 6 months old. Table 27.10 shows the age of introduction of solids by ethnic group.

Fruit, vegetables and pulses should be cooked with the skin on to preserve nutrients. This should then be removed to avoid an excessive fibre intake, which adds too much bulk to the diet and may bind certain trace minerals, inhibiting their absorption [15]. Pulses must be thoroughly cooked to destroy toxins such as trypsin inhibitors and haemaglutinins which may cause diarrhoea and vomiting [11]. Breast feeding or infant formula should be continued until 1 year of age. As the

Table 27.4 A guide to religious and cultural influences on diet.

Food	Buddhist	Christian	Hindu	Jewish	Muslim	Rastafarian	Seventh Day Adventist	Sikh
Eggs	Acceptable to some	Acceptable	Acceptable to some	No blood spots	Acceptable	Acceptable to some	Acceptable to most	Acceptable
Milk, yoghurt	Acceptable	Acceptable	Acceptable to some	Acceptable	Acceptable to some	Acceptable to some	Acceptable to most	Acceptable
Cheese	Acceptable	Acceptable	Not with rennet	Not with rennet	Not with rennet	Acceptable to some	Acceptable to most	Acceptable to some
Pork	Acceptable to some	Acceptable to most	Rarely acceptable	Not acceptable	Not acceptable	Not acceptable	Not acceptable	Rarely acceptable
Beef	Acceptable to some	Acceptable	Not acceptable	Kosher	Halal	Acceptable to some	Acceptable to some	Not acceptable
Lamb	Acceptable to some	Acceptable	Acceptable to some	Kosher	Halal	Acceptable to some	Acceptable to some	Acceptable
Chicken	Acceptable to some	Acceptable	Acceptable to some	Kosher	Halal	Acceptable to some	Acceptable to some	Acceptable to some
Fish	Acceptable to some	Acceptable – some only fish with fins and scales	Acceptable – with fins and scales	Acceptable – with fins, scales and backbone	Acceptable – with fins and scales	Acceptable – with fins and scales	Acceptable – with fins and scales	Acceptable to some
Shellfish	Not acceptable	Acceptable to most	Acceptable to some	Not acceptable	Acceptable to some	Not acceptable	Not acceptable	Acceptable to some
Animal fats	Acceptable to some	Acceptable	Acceptable to some	Kosher	Halal	Acceptable to some	Not acceptable	Acceptable to some
Alcohol	Not acceptable	Acceptable to most	Not acceptable	Acceptable	Not acceptable	Not usually wine	Not acceptable	Acceptable
Cocoa, coffee, tea	Acceptable	Acceptable	Acceptable	Acceptable	Acceptable	Not acceptable	Decaffeinated are suitable	Acceptable
Fasting		Good Friday and Ash Wednesday	3 days a year or 1–2 days every week	Yom Kippur 1 day of atonement (no food or liquid for 25 hours)	Ramadan 1 month fasting (no food or liquid during daylight)			

(continued overleaf)

Table 27.4 (continued)

Food	Buddhist	Christian	Hindu	Jewish	Muslim	Rastafarian	Seventh Day Adventist	Sikh
Other comments	Most Buddhists are vegetarians or vegans, although some may not be		Certain foods are taken during prayers. Some Hindus may be vegetarians or vegans (Jains)	Kosher (food fit to eat), i.e. meat from animals slaughtered by a Kosher butcher. Meat and dairy products are not consumed within 3 hours of each other	Halal, i.e. the meat must be from animals that have been bled to death and the phrase 'in the name of God' is said	Processed, preserved or tinned foods may be avoided. Most only eat Ital foods, i.e. in a whole and natural state. No fruits of the vine, e.g. sultanas, grapes, currants	Some are vegetarians	Some are vegetarians
Black and minority ethnic groups	Chinese, Vietnamese	Afro-Caribbean, Chinese, Greek, Greek Cypriot, Ugandan, Vietnamese, West African (e.g. Nigerian and Ghanaian), Indian	Gujarati, Punjabi, Indian	Jews of all nationalities	Arab, Bangladeshi, Pakistani, Gujarati, Somali, Turkish, Turkish Cypriot, Ugandan, West African (e.g. Nigerian and Ghanaian), Indian	Afro-Caribbean	Afro-Caribbean	Indian

Source: Adapted from British Dietetic Association Community Nutrition Group [3].

Table 27.5 Classification of vegetarian and vegan diet.

	Foods excluded	Animal protein source	Non animal protein source	Nutrients at risk of deficiency
Partial vegetarian	Red meat Offal	Poultry Fish Milk Cheese Yoghurt Eggs	Beans Pulses Nuts Seeds	Iron
Lacto-ovo vegetarian	Red meat Offal Poultry Fish	Milk Cheese Yoghurt Eggs	Beans Lentils Nuts Seeds	Iron
Lacto vegetarian	Red meat Offal Poultry Fish Eggs	Milk Cheese Yoghurt	Beans Lentils Nuts Seeds	Iron Vitamin D
Vegan	Red meat Offal Fish Poultry Eggs Milk Cheese Yoghurt		Beans Lentils Nuts Seeds	Protein Energy Iron Fat soluble vitamins Vitamin B_2 Vitamin B_{12} Calcium Zinc

Table 27.6 Sources of nutrients at risk of deficiency in a vegan diet.

Nutrient at risk of deficiency	Suitable dietary alternative sources
Protein	Pulses (soya, tofu, tempeh, beans and lentils), grains (wheat, rice, rye, millet), seeds, groundnuts*, nuts* and nut spreads*. Meals should have a combination of grains with seeds or grains with pulses to get the right balance of essential amino acids
Energy	Vegetable oils/margarines, ground nuts*, nut spreads*
Iron	Iron fortified breakfast cereals, wholegrain cereals, wholemeal bread, pulses, dried fruit, nuts*. Dark leafy green vegetables are not a good source of iron for infants and young children as the portion size is so large (120 g for 2 mg iron). Foods rich in vitamin C, such as fruits and vegetables, aid the absorption of non animal sources of iron
Fat soluble vitamins	In England, white Caucasians will make enough vitamin D for the year from 30 minutes/day of moderate sunlight exposure from April to October. Black and Asian people living in England will not make enough and must rely on dietary sources or supplements: vegetable oils/margarines, fortified soya milk and fortified breakfast cereals
Essential fatty acids	Whole grains, nuts, seeds and seed oils
Vitamin B_2	Wheat germ, almonds, green leafy vegetables, yeast extract (e.g. Marmite, Tastex†), avocado, soya beans, fortified soya milk
Vitamin B_{12}	Fortified yeast extract (e.g. Marmite, Tastex†), fortified cereals, fortified soya milk, tofu
Calcium	Fortified soya products (milk and yoghurt), seaweed products (kombu, wakame, nori), nuts* and seeds. Other sources (bread, leafy green vegetables, pulses) are not good sources of calcium for infants and young children as the portion size is so large (>120 g for 100 mg calcium)
Zinc	Some soya products (flour, miso, cheese and tempeh), nuts*, seeds, wheat germ, wholemeal bread, fortified breakfast cereals, seaweed and hard cheeses
Iodine	Whole grains, seaweeds and vegetables

*Nuts should be introduced with care if there is history/evidence of nut allergy and nuts should not be given to children under 2 years of age unless finely ground due to choking risk.
†Yeast extracts should be used with care in children under 2 years of age due to the high salt content.

Table 27.7   Prevalence of breast feeding at ages up to 6 months by mother's ethnicity in Great Britain, 2010.

	Total Great Britain %	White %	Mixed %	Asian or Asian British %	Black or Black British %	Chinese or other ethnic group %
Birth	82	79	87	96	95	96
2 days	77	75	81	88	90	94
3 days	75	73	80	86	90	93
4 days	73	71	80	85	90	93
5 days	72	69	79	84	90	93
6 days	71	68	79	83	90	93
1 week	70	67	79	83	90	92
2 weeks	66	63	79	81	89	87
6 weeks	56	52	75	73	85	82
4 months	43	39	60	58	73	76
6 months	35	32	49	49	61	66

Source: Data.Gov.UK [9].

Table 27.8   Infant formulas suitable for Halal, vegetarian and vegan diets.

Cow's milk based formulas	Suitable for Halal	Suitable for vegetarian
Abbott Similac	X	√
Cow & Gate First Infant Milk	√	X
Cow & Gate Infant Milk for Hungrier Babies	√	X
Cow & Gate Follow-on Milk	√	X
Milupa Aptamil First Infant Milk	√	X
Milupa Aptamil Hungry Milk	√	X
Milupa Aptamil Follow-on Milk	√	X
Milupa Aptamil Growing-up (1+)	X	√
Milupa Aptamil Growing-up (2+)	X	√
SMA First Infant Milk	√	X
SMA Extra Hungry Infant Milk	√	√
SMA Follow-on Milk	√	√

At the time of printing, there were no formulas suitable for vegan diets. In addition, there were no amino acid, peptide or soya based infant formulas that were suitable for Halal, vegetarian or vegan diets, based on their ingredients. However, some manufacturers have statements to the effect that their formula is acceptable for certain cultural and religious groups – check with the manufacturer.

child gets older he or she should be encouraged to take 500 mL/day full fat cow's or approved fortified soya milk, or the equivalent in cheese or yoghurt, in order to provide enough calcium [11]. Suitable weaning foods for vegetarian and vegan diets are given in Table 27.11.

Children

Vegan diets are typically high in fibre and low in fat, so care must be taken to ensure an adequate energy intake to support growth. There have been many conflicting studies examining the dietary intake and growth of vegan children [16, 17]. To provide optimal nutrition a vegetarian or vegan diet should be well balanced, containing two or three helpings of protein foods daily plus cereals, vegetables, fruits and fats (Table 27.12). Vegetable and pulse proteins have a lower concentration and range of essential amino acids than protein from animal or fish sources. Therefore, careful planning of menus with pulse and cereal combinations is necessary to provide sufficient protein of high biological value

Table 27.9 Sources of iron and vitamin B_{12} suitable for vegetarians.

Source	Iron mg	B_{12} µg
Infant formula, 200 mL	1.4	0.4
Milk (all types except UHT), 200 mL	0.06	1.8
Yoghurt full fat (1 medium pot), 150 g	0.15	0.3
Cheddar type cheese (1 slice), 40 g	0.12	1.0
Fromage frais (1 medium pot), 100 g	0.06	0.5
Soya cheese (1 slice), 40 g	0.44	1.0
Spinach boiled (1 average serving), 90 g	1.44	0
Fenugreek/methi seeds (1 tbsp), 11 g	2.56	0
Watercress (1 cup), 35 g	0.77	0
Broccoli/peas (1 average serving), 45 g	0.45	0
Dried apricots (6)/figs (3), 60 g	2.46	0
Raisins/sultanas (1 tablespoon), 30 g	1.0	0
Bread wholemeal (2 slices), 60 g	1.44	0
Bread white (2 slices), 60 g	0.8	0
Bran flakes (3 tbsp), 30 g	7.29	0.5
Fortified breakfast cereals, e.g. Special K, Cheerios (3 tbsp), 30 g	6.99	0.5
Weetabix (2 biscuits) 40 g	4.76	0
Lentils (dhal), green/brown (2 tbsp) 80 g	1.92	0
Black-eyed beans/kidney beans/chickpeas boiled (2 tbsp), 80 g	1.52	0
Baked beans (1 small can), 200 g		
Hummus, (1 average serving), 60 g	1.14	0
Tofu, fried (1 average serving), 60 g	0.72	0
Vegeburger (soya mince) (1 burger), 60 g	2.7	0.2
Nuts, e.g. almonds, cashew, brazil, (1 average serving), 40 g	1.7	0
Seeds, e.g. melon, pumpkin, sesame (1 average serving), 40 g	4.0	0
Curry powder (1 teaspoon), 3 g	1.75	0
Plain chocolate (1 bar), 54 g	1.24	0
Yeast extract (1 spread on 1 slice), 2 g	0.06	0.01

Tbsp, tablespoon.
Source: Extracted from DietPlan 6 Nutritional Database produced by Forestfield Software Ltd, based on *McCance and Widdowson's the Composition of Foods* and UK Nutrient Databank, Crown copyright, reproduced under licence from the Controller of Her Majesty's Stationery Office.

[11]. The protein and energy content of the diet can be increased by the use of nuts, beans and oils [11].

The main micronutrients at risk of deficiency in the vegan diet are shown in Table 27.5. In addition, vegan children may require a daily supplement of $1-2$ µg vitamin B_{12} [11]. The increased intake of phytate containing legumes and whole grains may lead to poor bioavailability of zinc [18] and iron [19]. It is important to ensure that a food or drink rich in vitamin C is given alongside iron containing foods to increase bioavailability. When considering recommendations for dietary fat [20], a vegan diet is often regarded as 'healthy'. However, the vegan diet, as well as being low in total fat and hence energy, may also contain very poor quality fat. The essential fatty acid, docosahexaenoic acid, DHA (22: 6n-3), has been found to be absent from vegan diets [4]. DHA has an important role in growth, the health of the retina, central nervous system and skin. Vegans should therefore use oils with a low linoleic:α-linolenic acid ratio such as rapeseed, flax and linseed oils [16] (Table 27.13).

Sources of vitamin D and calcium are shown in Tables 27.14 and 27.15.

Zen macrobiotic diets

The Zen macrobiotic principle originates from Japan and is based on the correct balance between Yin (positive) and Yang (negative) foods. This balance is believed to keep spiritual, mental and physical wellbeing. There are 10 levels of dietary elimination. Animal products, fruits and vegetables are gradually removed from the diet until the ultimate goal is achieved of consuming only brown rice. Fluids are also severely restricted [21]. This type of diet is nutritionally inadequate for a child of any age. Marked growth retardation, associated with muscle wasting and a delay in gross motor and language development, has been documented in infants fed macrobiotic weaning diets [22, 23]. Growth failure [24] and reduced bone mass [25] have also been documented in older children. Deficiencies of vitamins B_{12}, D and thiamine and of calcium and iron have also been observed [26, 27]. Improved growth has been reported following the addition of fatty fish and dairy products to the macrobiotic diet [28].

Fruitarian diets

Fruitarian diets are based on fruit and uncooked fermented cereals and seeds. These diets are nutritionally inadequate for children of any age and can

Table 27.10 Age of introduction of solids by mother's ethnicity, 2010.

	% White	% Mixed	% Asian or Asian British	% Black or Black British	% Chinese or other ethnic group	% Great Britain total
6 weeks	1	4	2	5	1	2
8 weeks	2	4	3	5	1	2
3 months	5	4	4	9	1	5
4 months	30	24	22	33	19	29
5 months	77	69	62	65	65	75
6 months	95	90	90	90	83	94
9 months	99	99	97	99	–	99

Source: Data.Gov.UK [9].

Table 27.11 Suitable vegetarian and vegan weaning foods.

Age	Foods
Around 6 months Initially foods may need to be puréed or mashed	Baby rice Cooked fruits and vegetables Weetabix Cooked pulses and lentils with rice or wheat foods Pudding or custards made with cow's milk or calcium fortified soya milk
7–9 months Introduce lumps and soft finger foods	Whole grains Bread Pasta and rice Cooked pulses or lentils with rice or wheat foods Finely ground nuts Dried fruits Cheese made from cow's milk or calcium fortified soya curd Egg Tofu and Quorn
9–12 months Minced and chopped textures	As above

lead to severe protein energy malnutrition, anaemia and multiple vitamin and mineral deficiencies.

South Asian subcontinent

The communities from the South Asian subcontinent include those from India, Pakistan, Bangladesh, Sri Lanka and those who came to the UK via East Africa [28]. Migrations to the UK began in the seventeenth century when the British East Indian Company first began trading with India. Today the Asian community represents 38.5% of the ethnic groups in the UK [2]. Traditional dietary

Table 27.12 Sample vegetarian or vegan meal plan for young children.

Breakfast	Cereal with milk or milk substitute Wholemeal or white bread, margarine, peanut butter or yeast extract *Egg
Midday meal	Bean, dhal, lentil, soya, nut based dish, *egg based dish, or *cheese based dish Bread, chapatti, pasta, potatoes or rice Fruit or fruit based dessert
Evening meal	Alternative choices from above
Drinks	Dilute fruit juice (not squash, cordial or juice drink) Cow's milk* or recommended milk substitute Water
Snacks	Nuts, dried fruit, toast, fruit

*Not suitable for vegans.

customs are largely based on the religious and cultural beliefs of the three main religious groups: Hindus, Muslims and Sikhs. Dietary variance has been observed within these groups, as income and geographical area have an influence on the diet.

Dietary customs of Hindus

Approximately 1.4% of the UK population are Hindu [2]. The majority originally came from the Gujarat region of India, although some are from the Indian Punjab and East Africa [29, 30].

Hindus classify foods into three groups [31]: sattvik (nutritious foods) such as milk, fruit, vegetables, nuts, whole grains; rajasi (foods of strong emotions) such as meat, eggs, fish, spices, onions, garlic, hot peppers, pickles and other pungent or spicy

Table 27.13   Vegetarian and vegan sources of essential fatty acids.

	Energy kcal (kJ)	α-linolenic acid g	Linoleic acid g
Nuts and seeds			
Walnuts – 6 nuts	138 (575)	1	8
Sunflower seeds – 1 tablespoon	96 (400)	0	4
Brazil nuts – 3 nuts	68 (285)	0	3
Sesame seeds – 1 tablespoon	72 (300)	0	3
Pumpkin seeds – 1 tablespoon	91 (380)	0	3
Peanut butter (smooth) – thin spread on 1 slice of bread	73 (305)	0	2
Peanuts (groundnuts) – 10 nuts	73 (305)	0	2
Almonds – 6 nuts	80 (335)	0	1
Hazel nuts – 10 nuts	65 (270)	0	1
Oils (1 tablespoon or 11 g)			
Safflower	99	0	8
Evening primrose	99	0	8
Grape seed	99	0	7
Sunflower	99	0	7
Soya	99	1	6
Walnut	99	1	6
Wheat germ	99	0	6
Corn	99	0	6
Cottonseed (linseed or flaxseed)	98	0	6
Sesame	99	0	5
Peanut (groundnut)	99	0	3
Rapeseed	99	1	2
Hazelnut	99	0	1
Palm	99	0	1
Olive	99	0	1

Source: Extracted from CompEat Nutritional Database produced by Forestfield Software Ltd, based on *McCance and Widdowson's the Composition of Foods* and UK Nutrient Databank, Crown copyright, reproduced under licence from the Controller of Her Majesty's Stationery Office and USDA Databases.

Table 27.14   Vegetarian sources of vitamin D.

Non animal foods (1 average portion)	Vitamin D (µg)	Non animal foods (1 average portion)	Vitamin D (µg)
Special K 30 g	2.49	Bran Flakes 30 g	1.26
Shreddies 45 g	1.26	Sultana bran 45 g	0.94
Ricicles 45 g	1.26	Nutri-Grain 40 g	1.12
Weetos 45 g	1.26	Fruit-n-Fibre 30 g	0.63
Rice Krispies	0.63	Coco Pops 30 g	0.63
Frosties 30 g	0.63	Non-dairy margarine	0.87
All-Bran 40 g	1.24	(1 filling) 11 g	

Source: Extracted from DietPlan 6 Nutritional Database produced by Forestfield Software Ltd, based on McCance and Widdowson's *the Composition of Foods* and UK Nutrient Databank, Crown copyright, reproduced under licence from the Controller of Her Majesty's Stationery Office.

Table 27.15 Vegetarian sources of calcium.

Foods	Calcium (mg)	Foods	Calcium (mg)
Milk, cheese, yoghurt and alternatives			
Milk, all types, 200 mL	240	Soya milk, calcium enriched, 200 mL	240
Hard cheeses (1 slice), 40 g	290	Water/orange juice enriched with calcium, 200 mL	180
Fruit yoghurts, 150 g	200		
Whole milk yoghurt, 150 g	300	Soya yoghurt, calcium enriched (1 average pot), 150 g	134
Milk pudding (e.g. kheer/rice pudding) (1 average serving), 200 g	240		
Rice dessert (1 pot), 150 g	180		
Bread, cereals and alternatives			
Nan bread (one), 160 g	300	Fortified breakfast bar (1 bar), 37 g	180
Chapattis (one), 55 g	33	Gluten free bread (2 slices), 50 g	180
Brown bread (2 slices), 60 g	60	Swiss style muesli (1 average portion), 50 g	60
White bread (2 slices), 54 g	60		
White flour self-raising (1 tbsp), 30 g	105		
Meat alternatives			
Nuts, e.g. almonds, brazils, pistachios (1 medium packet), 40 g	38	Baked beans (1 average portion), 135 g	72
Sesame seeds (1 tbsp), 16 g	107	Bombay Mix (1 medium packet), 100 g	58
Sunflower seeds (1 tbsp), 16 g	18		
Fruit and vegetables			
Spinach boiled (1 average portion), 90 g	135	Figs (1 ready to eat), 55 g	127
Okra boiled (1 average portion), 90 g	108	Orange (1 medium), 160 g	75
Spring greens (1 average portion), 75 g	56	Sultanas (1 tbsp), 30 g	19

tbsp, tablespoon.
Source: Extracted from DietPlan 6 Nutritional Database produced by Forestfield Software Ltd, based on *McCance and Widdowson's the Composition of Foods* and UK Nutrient Databank, Crown copyright, reproduced under licence from the Controller of Her Majesty's Stationery Office.

foods; and tamsai (left overs producing negative emotions), i.e. foods which are stale, overripe, spoilt or imperfect. Fasting is common among Hindus to help reinforce control over the senses and to achieve closeness to God. Fasting occurs for a few days during holy days, new moon days and festivals.

A restriction on eating beef was introduced between 1500 and 500 BC because Hindus regard the cow as sacred. It is also unusual for pork to be eaten as the pig is thought to be unclean. Devout Hindus believe in the doctrine of Ahisma (not killing) and are vegetarian. Some will eat dairy products and eggs, while others refuse eggs because they are potential sources of life. A minority of Hindus practise veganism. Wheat is the staple food eaten by Hindus in the UK. It is used to make chapattis, puris and parathas. Oil and ghee (clarified butter), which is believed to sanctify food, are used extensively in cooking [29]. Most Hindus fast on 3 days a year to celebrate the birthdays of the Lords Shiva (March), Rama

(April) and Krishna (August). Orthodox Hindus may also fast once or twice every week (often on Tuesdays and Fridays). Fasting lasts from dawn to dusk and varies from avoiding all foods except those considered pure (e.g. rice, fruit and yoghurt) to total food exclusion [29, 31].

Jainism has its roots in Hinduism. Jains practise non violence to all living creatures and their diet is a form of lacto vegetarianism that includes the avoidance of root vegetables, with the exception of ginger and turmeric.

Dietary customs of Muslims

Approximately 4.6% of the UK population are Muslim. With the majority originating from Pakistan and Bangladesh, more recently they have been joined by Muslims from African countries such as Somalia, Yemen, Sudan, Morocco, Syria and Lebanon [2].

The Koran provides Halal guidelines [31]. Acceptable animal foods are beef, sheep, lamb, goat, deer, poultry and fish prepared and stored under Halal conditions. Unclean foods are carnivores (except fish), pork, birds of prey, reptiles, amphibians, rodents, insects and maggots. Wheat, usually in the form of chapattis, is the staple cereal eaten by Muslims from Pakistan, whereas those from Bangladesh eat more rice. Cooking oil is used in preference to ghee.

Fasting for Ramadan occurs during the ninth lunar month of the Islamic year. Muslims fast between sunrise and sunset. The purpose is to purify oneself both spiritually and physically and to share the experiences of the poor and hungry. Children under the age of 12 years (puberty) and the elderly are exempt from fasting. People who are ill, pregnant, menstruating or on a long journey are also excused but are expected to fast later. Unfortunately, many pregnant women fast with the rest of the family during Ramadan as they find it more convenient. The Koran also dictates that children should be breast fed up to the age of 2 years.

Dietary customs of Sikhs

Approximately 0.6% of the UK population are Sikhs. Sikhism is a relatively new religion, originating as a reformist movement of Hinduism in the Indian Punjab in the sixteenth century [2].

Non practising Sikhs are not usually vegetarian, but they will usually avoid beef, pork and their products. They will also avoid Halal meats preferring animals that have been killed with a single stroke, i.e. the Jatka method. Sikhs who have undergone the Amrit ceremony are usually lacto vegetarians avoiding meat, fish, eggs and their products [31].

Punjabi food customs include a wide range of milk dishes from cream, white cheese, butter, ghee and yoghurt that include maize flat bread (roti), spinach, dhal and chickpeas.

Common South Asian dietary habits

Common dietary patterns across the three main groups (Table 27.16) include alcohol abstinence and the hot and cold properties of foods. Many of the Asian people in the UK share dietary customs, despite their varying religious and geographical background. Older members of the Asian community tend to retain traditional dietary customs while second and later generations are consuming more westernised foods, especially convenience foods. The extent of adoption of these foods is variable, tending to be greater in the younger generations who were born in the UK and in those who have lived in the UK for some time [29], although they may continue to eat traditional meals in the evening [32].

The traditional breakfast includes chapattis, parathas, bread and occasionally hard boiled or fried eggs are traditionally eaten. The two main meals are based on staples, usually served with a vegetable, pulse or nut based curry [21, 30]. Most foods, including spices, are usually fried before adding to the curry, which is then served with homemade chutneys, side salads of tomatoes and onions and yoghurt [21]. Very little hard cheese is eaten; paneer, an Indian soft curd cheese, is preferred [21]. Meals are usually served with tea, which is made with hot milk and sugar, although English tea is becoming popular [21]. Traditionally, Asians rarely eat snacks, although western snack foods are increasing in popularity. Traditional Asian savoury snacks (usually reserved for celebrations only) are high in fat and the sweets are often very high in refined sugar. Many Asians believe that foods have heating and cooling effects on the body. These hot and cold foods should be eaten in the correct balance to achieve a healthy state. Certain hot foods cause symptoms such as constipation, sweating and body fatigue, while certain cold foods lead to strength and happiness. Foods may also be used to treat a condition, e.g. hot foods should be avoided during pregnancy and cold ones avoided when breast feeding [21].

Infant feeding

Early studies reported lower breast feeding rates among Asians in the UK compared with the Caucasian population [33, 34] and Asians in the Indian subcontinent [35]. However, high incidences of breast feeding among Asian mothers (49% at 6 months) compared with white mothers (32% at 6 months) have more recently been reported in the 2010 Infant Feeding Survey [9]. Interestingly, of

Table 27.16 Foods commonly eaten by the Southern Asian population in the UK.

Food	Nutrient	Method of cooking
Cereals Breakfast cereals, wheat, bread, rice, semolina, ground rice, bajri (millet flour), puffed rice, rice flakes	Energy B vitamins	Baked, boiled or fried: chapatti, paratha, poppodom, bhagi, poori, pakora, porridges, samosa, sweetmeats
Tubers Arvi/colocasia root, cassava, taro tuber, yam	Energy	Boiled, fried, curries
Vegetables Ackee, amaranth (tanjurdo), aubergine (ringun), colocasia leaves, mustard leaves, radish leaves, cluster beans, mint leaves, fennel leaves, okra, bringal, pepper, cho cho/chayote, fenugreek leaves, bitter gourd (darela/dudhi/turia/gulka), kantola, patra leaves, spinach (palak), leeks, tomatoes	Vitamin A Riboflavin Folic acid Vitamin C Iron Calcium Fibre	Boiled, fried, curries, chutneys, pickles
Pulses Peas, beans, balor/valor/urad gram, chickpeas (channa dhal), lentils (masoor), black-eyed beans dhal, whole urad dhal (black gram), whole mung dhal, sprouted pulses	Energy Protein B vitamins Iron Fibre	Curries, fried snack
Seeds and nuts Sesame seeds, peanuts, dried coconut, pistachios, almond, cashew nuts	Energy Fibre Iron Essential fatty acids	Fresh, fried
Fruits Banana, citrus fruits, unsweetened juices, dates, blackcurrants, figs, raisins, apricots, prune/prune juice, guava (jamphal), mango, sapodilla (sapato/chikku)	Vitamin A Vitamin C Fibre	Raw, curries, chutneys
Milk products Milk, yoghurt, cheese/paneer	Energy Protein Vitamin A	Milk drinks: boiled, fresh Cheese: fresh, fried
Eggs	Protein Riboflavin Nicotinic acid Vitamin D	Fried
Fats and oils Ghee/clarified butter Vegetable oil Margarine	Energy Essential fatty acids	Frying, spreading

mothers who were born outside the UK, 30%–40% who bottle fed initially or who stopped breast feeding to bottle feed reported that they would have fed their babies differently had the babies not been born in the UK. Unfortunately, for some bottle feeding is perceived as the western ideal and therefore better for the baby. This problem is compounded by communication difficulties and

overcrowded housing [11], making it difficult for a mother to breast feed in privacy.

Weaning

Social disadvantage, the varying quality, expense and availability of familiar Asian weaning foods and the pressures of westernisation may compromise good weaning practice [36]. Late weaning and prolonged breast feeding are common in infants who are born on the Indian subcontinent and those who have only been in the UK for a short time [33, 34, 37]. In the UK, late weaning may be partly because of the poor availability of suitable foods and the lack of adequate and appropriate advice [38]. Some Asian infants born in the UK are weaned earlier [34, 35], but are commonly given sweet commercial weaning foods that are low in protein and iron [33, 34, 36, 37]. This mainly occurs because many mothers do not know the composition of savoury weaning products and will not use them unless they are vegetarian [29]. Because of these problems, mothers should be encouraged to cook savoury weaning foods at home. Suitable homemade Asian weaning foods are given in Tables 27.11 and 27.12.

The practice of sweetening milk and adding foods such as rusk, honey, Weetabix and baby rice to bottles is common [29, 34, 38] and should be discouraged. Many Asian infants are given cow's milk from the age of 5 months [29, 38]. This results in a higher saturated fat and salt intake and a reduced vitamin D and iron intake than if breast milk or infant formula were continued [15]. Feeding development is often delayed because of late conversion from bottle to cup and very late progression onto family foods [29, 34, 37, 38]. It is not unusual for a 2 year old to derive the majority of their nutrition from bottles of cow's milk and sweetened fruit drinks. Very few differences have been reported between the diets of first and second generation Asians [39]. It has been suggested that this may be because of the cohesive nature of the community and because all young children are subject to similar dietary and cultural expectations and pressures. Therefore, infant feeding practices among the Asian population can still be improved.

- The teaching curriculum of all catering and health related training should include ethnic cultures, food and diet, so that effective advice can be given [37]. This training should be updated regularly [34].
- Practical demonstrations, the use of bilingual interpreters and written advice in the Asian languages should be available [29, 34, 37].

- Education promoting breast feeding should reach the parents before pregnancy, and support should be given while breast feeding [34].
- Breast or formula milk should be given up to 1 year of age [34].
- Sugary drinks should be avoided [34].
- Infants should be weaned around 6 months of age.
- Weaning advice should include the use of appropriate family foods in addition to commercial baby foods [29, 34].
- Salt, sugar, honey or hot spices should not be added to bottles or weaning foods.
- Advice should be given on foods rich in vitamin C, vitamin D and iron, as these nutrients may be at risk of deficiency [34].
- The cup should be introduced between 6 months and 1 year of age [34].
- Vitamin drops should be given up to 5 years [40].

Nutritional problems commonly found in Asian children

Faltering growth

Dietary intake, family income, housing standards, maternal education, psychological distress and morbidity all influence growth [29, 33]. Low birthweight has been reported in the Asian population, both in this country and in the homeland [33, 35]. Birthweight has increased recently, however, with longer birth intervals, fewer teenage pregnancies and improved nutrition thought to be contributing factors [29]. Despite lower birthweights, some studies show that Asian babies and children grow as well as the indigenous population [29, 33, 35, 38, 41, 42]. Table 27.17 shows birthweight by ethnic group in 2005.

Iron deficiency anaemia

Iron deficiency anaemia has been described in Asian infants [44, 45]. Contributing factors include maternal iron deficiency during pregnancy, premature delivery and low birthweight. Inadequate dietary intake of iron is commonly related to the early introduction and excessive use of unfortified

Table 27.17   Birth weight by ethnic group, 2005.

Birthweight	Asian			Black		White	
	Bangladesh %	Indian %	Pakistani %	African %	Caribbean %	White British %	White other %
<2.5 kg	10.0	10.6	9.9	7.4	11.0	5.5	4.9
2.5–3.4 kg	71.5	69.6	66.6	56.4	60.4	50.5	51.5
3.5–4.4 kg	18.1	19.6	23.0	34.8	27.8	42.0	41.9
>4.5 kg	0.4	0.3	0.6	1.4	0.8	2.0	1.7
Mean birthweight at 95% confidence interval (g)	3075	3082	3130	3288	3162	3393	3393

Source: Office of National Statistics [43].

cow's milk [29]. Prolonged use of a baby bottle and the mother being born outside the UK have also been shown to have a negative influence on the iron status of Asian children [45]. Advice should include information on the use of foods rich in iron and vitamin C [38].

Megaloblastic anaemia

Megaloblastic anaemia resulting from vitamin B_{12} deficiency has been observed in some strict vegetarian and vegan Asians [46]. Education regarding vitamin B_{12} sources in the vegetarian diet is required and supplementation may be needed in the vegan diet.

Rickets

The steady decline in rickets in the UK was halted in the late 1960s and early 1970s when a number of cases appeared in immigrant families, mainly of Asian origin [37, 47, 48]. There is now evidence that the incidence is in decline again following large scale vitamin D supplementation [29]. However, low plasma vitamin D levels are still observed in some members of the Asian population, especially those of Pakistani origin and those who do not take routine vitamin supplements [49, 50]. In addition to the dietary intake of vitamin D, other factors such as low sunlight exposure, skin pigmentation, late weaning, high fibre and high phytate intakes may also contribute to the development of rickets in Asian children [29]. The weaning diets of infants should include foods rich in vitamin D such as milk, milk products, eggs, oily fish, liver, fortified

breakfast cereals and margarine [11, 51, 52]. Vitamin D supplementation is advisable for infants, young children and deficient pregnant women to prevent neonatal hypocalcaemia and rickets [11, 29, 51]. In addition, children should be encouraged to play outside [52].

Dental caries

Traditionally, sugary foods are reserved for celebrations and therefore do not have a major role in Asian diets. However, with increasing westernisation, over consumption of refined sugar leading to a high incidence of dental caries has been observed in Asian preschool children [53]. Asian mothers often add sugar to babies' bottles and give sweetened drinks via the bottle for prolonged periods. These drinks, as well as having high sugar content, are acidic which can lead to tooth decay [34]. Education regarding infant feeding with the restriction of quantity and frequency of sugar intake, the use of fluoride containing drops and toothpaste and frequent dental visits will help to reduce the incidence of dental caries.

Obesity and diabetes

With the increasing consumption of high sugar and high fat foods, the prevalence of obesity is increasing. The incidence of obesity and diabetes is now higher in Asian children than in Caucasian children. In addition to restricting these foods, advice on acceptable Asian food alternatives and appropriate cooking techniques must be given. The dietary fat intake can be reduced by avoiding deep fried foods, reducing the amount of oil or ghee used in cooking and restricting or not adding fat to chapattis. Avoiding the popular sweet sugary tea and Asian sweetmeats will reduce dietary sugar.

Afro-Caribbean communities

Migration from the Caribbean to the UK began in the eighteenth century, with small communities settling around the major British port cities of Cardiff, Liverpool and South Shields [54]. The largest phase of migration from the Caribbean occurred in the 1940s and 1950s [55]. Most were recruited to re-staff national transport and health services [56]. Today the Afro-Caribbean community is 1.1% of the UK population and 5.6% of minority ethnic groups in the UK [2].

Dietary customs

Most Afro-Caribbeans are Christians (such as Seventh Day Adventists, Pentecostals, Baptists) and Rastafarians. A higher proportion of Afro-Caribbeans living in the UK have adopted the dietary patterns of the wider UK population than other ethnic groups. However, a small group retain traditional meal patterns.

Seventh Day Adventists and Pentecostals aim to eat foods that are natural and abstain from eating pork, fish without scales and other foods considered 'unclean'. Alcohol, caffeine and high intakes of sugar and salt are discouraged. Some Seventh Day Adventists may also be lacto vegetarians. Rastafarians aim to eat food in their natural states (Ital foods). Some avoid meat completely to obey the commandment 'thou shalt not kill' and follow a lacto-ovo vegetarian or vegan diet [57]. Vinegar, raisins, grapes and wine are also avoided by some Rastafarians as the Nazarite law states that fruits of the vine should not be eaten.

The two main meals are taken at breakfast time and in the evening [58]. Traditional breakfasts include fried plantain, cornmeal dumplings and fried dumplings. However, many dietary practices have now been adopted from British culture, with toast and cereals largely replacing these foods. The evening meal is more likely to contain traditional foods, especially with the younger generation who seem keen to retain their identification and culture. Cereals and tubers such as rice, green banana,

yam and sweet potato form the main part of the diet [59]. These starchy foods are served with small amounts of meat or fish [58]. The tropical climate in the homeland makes it difficult to keep foods fresh and therefore preserved meat, fish and milk are eaten [59]. Peas, beans, nuts and green leafy vegetables are widely used, often being made into homemade soups and stews, which are well seasoned with herbs and spices [29].

Infant feeding

Infant feeding is mainly influenced by the place of birth, knowledge of traditional practices and advice from relatives. Ninety five per cent of women breast feed their babies initially and 61% are still exclusively breast feeding or mixed feeding when their child is 6 months old [9].

Weaning

Infants use to be traditionally weaned as early as 1 month of age and 45% have been reported to be receiving food by 3 months [58, 59]. The 2010 Infant Feeding Survey indicates that most black and black British women now delay the introduction of solids to between 4 and 6 months [9]. Late weaning occurs in <10% of babies from this group. Common weaning solids include high starch foods with a low nutrient density such as cornmeal, oats or rice porridge. This practice may lead to energy, protein, vitamin and mineral deficiencies if continued for a long time [11, 21, 60, 61]. The common practice of adding thin porridge to bottles should be discouraged as it can lead to a delay in the weaning process. It is common for infants to be given bush teas (infusions of herbs and leaves) as a cure for minor ailments [58]. Care should be taken to ensure that these are not given instead of milk. By the age of 9 months, most infants are eating family foods with the diet having both traditional and western influences [58].

Nutritional problems found in Afro-Caribbean children

Obesity and diabetes

With the adoption of British dietary customs, there has been an increase in the consumption of high sugar and high fat convenience foods and drinks. This has led to an increased prevalence of obesity and diabetes in Afro-Caribbean children compared with Caucasian children.

Iron deficiency anaemia

Iron deficiency anaemia has been observed in Afro-Caribbean children living in the UK. The main causes are thought to be prolonged bottle feeding, late weaning onto foods with low iron content and the early introduction and excessive use of cow's milk [29].

Megaloblastic anaemia

There have been reports of megaloblastic anaemia in Rastafarian children living in Jamaica [62,63]. Vegan children may require vitamin B_{12} supplementation.

Rickets

Rickets is common amongst Afro-Caribbean children and vitamin D supplementation is beneficial.

Lactose intolerance

There is a high incidence of lactose intolerance because of hypolactasia among the Afro-Caribbean population. A reduction in, and occasionally the avoidance of, the consumption of milk and other foods containing lactose will usually reduce symptoms (p. 124).

Chinese communities

Today Chinese people represent 0.7% of the UK population and 5.6% of ethnic groups in the UK [2], with roots from the Caribbean, Hong Kong, Taiwan, China, Malaysia, Vietnam and Singapore [64].

Dietary customs

Dietary habits vary according to the country and region of origin. The common religions include Buddhism, Confucianism, Taoism and Islam.

Very few foods are avoided, with the exception of pork not being eaten by the Chinese Muslim population. Eggs are highly valued as they are regarded as food for the brain. Northern China has a cool climate favouring the growth of wheat, maize, sorghum and millet. These staples are often made into steamed bread, dumplings, pancakes or noodles [21,64]. Meals are often based on root vegetables such as sweet potato and turnip, with very little meat being eaten. In contrast, because of its high rainfall, rice is the staple in southern China. Fresh vegetables and fruit are also found in abundance [64]. In the east, because of the long coastline, fish and shellfish are plentiful. In the west, livestock are reared and therefore the consumption of meat, milk and cheese is much higher [64].

Traditional breakfasts include rice porridge (congee), served either plain or with liver, meat, salted fish, salted eggs or Chinese cheese, and a soup made from rice and meat [21,64]. These traditional foods are slowly being replaced by western alternatives, however. The midday and evening meals consist of boiled rice or noodles and a variety of highly seasoned dishes such as fried or steamed meat and fish and stir fried vegetables. Raw food is rarely eaten, as fertiliser in China commonly contains human manure. Meals are usually served with either China tea or a thin soup and then followed with fruit. Sweet foods are usually reserved for special occasions [21,64]. The main health concern is the high salt intake associated with many of the preserved foods, seasonings and soya sauce. A high fat and refined sugar intake associated with the increasing consumption of western foods, especially by the younger generation, is also of concern [64]. A high incidence of lactose intolerance, because of hypolactasia, is also becoming apparent with the increasing consumption of milk and other dairy products [64].

Yin and Yang foods

To Chinese people health is perceived as the maintenance of a sound body and mental state, rather than absence of disease. Traditional Chinese medicine states that good health relies on the body's balance of two opposite elements, Yin (cold) representing female energy, and Yang (hot) representing male energy [21,64]. In illness the balance becomes disturbed and the body becomes either too hot or too cold. Tolerance of Yin and Yang increases with age. Thus, an adult can eat a much wider variety of foods than can a child. The classification of foods varies: in general meat, duck, goose, oily fish, potatoes, coffee, chocolate, sugar, nuts, herbs, spices, alcohol and fats are regarded as hot foods; chicken, milk, rice and some vegetables are neutral foods; fish, shellfish, soya beans, certain fruits and vegetables and barley water are cold foods. Stewing, deep fat frying, grilling and roasting make foods hotter, steaming neutralises and boiling and stir frying have a cooling effect [21, 64]. The Chinese believe that a healthy diet should be three parts Yang and two parts Yin. The balance should be changed for certain illnesses (e.g. for hyperactivity more Yin foods should be eaten than Yang foods).

During pregnancy and after childbirth the woman's body is thought to become cool and therefore cold foods are avoided. Alcohol, ice cream, mutton, beef and fizzy drinks are also avoided. In addition, if the woman is breast feeding, green vegetables and fruit are avoided because of concern that they may give the baby diarrhoea. Consequently, breast feeding mothers often have a high protein intake [64].

Infant feeding

In the UK, Chinese women often return to work soon after childbirth which has led to a decrease in the rate and duration of breast feeding. Low breast feeding rates in the Chinese population living in other countries have also been observed [65, 66]. Soya bean oil, which is a poor source of essential fatty acids, is a major source of fat in the Chinese diet. Because of this, breast milk has been found to have a low concentration of docosahexaenoic acid (DHA) and arachidonic acid (AA) [67]. It has therefore been suggested that mothers who are breast feeding should supplement their diet with a good source of DHA and AA such as fish oil. Because infant formula is regarded as hot, bottle fed babies are often given frequent cooling drinks such as water and barley water.

Most infants are weaned at 3 months of age. Traditionally, rice based porridges are introduced

but commercial baby foods are being used [64]. A study examining westernisation of the nutritional pattern of Chinese children living in France reported that at 1 year of age Chinese children mainly consumed a traditional diet. The intake of dairy products and fresh fruit was very low and that of soft drinks high, resulting in suboptimal calcium and vitamin C intakes [65]. In general, infants are thought to have a hot equilibrium and therefore neutralising or cooling foods are considered best for them. It is common practice for children to be given afternoon tea consisting of cooling foods such as bread, biscuits, cake, barley water and herb teas to counteract the heating effect of school meals [64].

Vietnamese communities

Some 75% of Vietnamese settlers in the UK are ethnic Chinese and therefore share many of the Chinese traditions [64]. Most arrived in the UK during the 1970s. Common religions among Vietnamese are Buddhism, Roman Catholicism and Confucianism.

Dietary customs

The Vietnamese diet is typically high in carbohydrate and low in fat [68]. Vietnam borders the ocean and has an extensive river system and therefore fish and shellfish are staple parts of the traditional diet. There are no forbidden foods; however, certain unfamiliar foods such as lamb, ox liver, tinned or cooked fruit and some root vegetables may be avoided [21]. Rice is the main staple food and is served either boiled or fried with small amounts of meat or fish. Like Chinese food, main dishes are often heavily seasoned and vegetables are lightly steamed or stir fried in oil or lard. The resultant high sodium intake is the main health issue. Very little fresh milk, butter, margarine and cheese are used, because of their lack of availability in Vietnam and the high incidence of lactose intolerance. Snacks of roasted nuts, sweet potatoes, rice or noodle soup, spring rolls and fresh fruit are frequently eaten. Common beverages include tea, coffee and fruit juice and alcohol is taken on special occasions [21].

With increasing westernisation, the intake of high sugar and high fat snack foods is increasing, especially in the younger generation. This has led to an increase in dental caries and obesity in the Vietnamese population, both in the UK [69] and other countries [70]. Unfortunately, obesity is traditionally seen as a sign of prosperity. The Vietnamese people observe hot and cold food principles, similar to the Chinese. In contrast to the Chinese, however, pregnancy is regarded as a hot condition and therefore women eat less red meat and fish. A traditional stew called Keung Chow, made from pigs' trotters, boiled eggs, vinegar and ginger, is given to women after childbirth to help recovery and to celebrate the birth of the child. After childbirth, women are encouraged to eat hot foods to regain their strength [21].

Infant feeding

Since their arrival in westernised countries, including the UK, Vietnamese mothers have abandoned traditional infant feeding practices in favour of more modern bottle feeding methods [70–72]. In addition, many Vietnamese women believe that breast feeding will cause their breasts to sag. Hence, the incidence of breast feeding is low and there is a need for culturally sensitive health education programmes to support breast feeding in this group. Infants are typically given a rice based porridge at around 6 months, minced meat and vegetables are given at 9 months and more solid food at 1 year.

Nutrients at risk of deficiency

Iron

There is an increased risk of iron deficiency in young Vietnamese children [73]. This is particularly associated with a high milk intake and poor body weight.

Calcium

Children are at risk of calcium deficiency, especially if minimal milk and associated products are eaten [21]. The rice traditionally grown in Vietnam is a good source of calcium, but is unavailable in Britain. Traditional Vietnamese fruits and

vegetables also contain more calcium than British varieties [21].

Vitamin D

Deficiency of vitamin D has been noted in Vietnamese children and a vitamin D supplement may be needed [21].

Somalian communities

Somalis first settled in the UK in 1914 when they were recruited to fight in the First World War. They are now thought to be the oldest African community in London. Later arrivals included Somalian asylum seekers who fled the civil unrest in their country and settled around the main cities in the UK. Today there are second, third and fourth generation Somalis living in the UK.

Dietary customs

Somalis are of Arab-African ethnicity and their faith is Islam. They therefore share many of the Islamic (Muslim) dietary customs. Somalia was formed in 1960 from a British Protectorate and an Italian Colony. As a result, many Southern Somalis eat Italian food and spaghetti is a national dish. The Somalian diet tends to be relatively high in protein.

Breakfast usually consists of two to three pieces of injera (fermented pancake like Somali bread made from corn and wheat) with ghee or butter and tea. Lunch is the main meal and usually consists of spaghetti or rice with a meat sauce (beef or goat) and mixed vegetables. Food is often flavoured with aromatic spices (cumin powder, cinnamon, cloves, cardamom, garlic, cilantro, parsley). Pork is avoided and chicken, fish and eggs are not usually eaten. The evening meal consists of injera or bread with butter and jam, or a traditional meal of rice, beans, butter and sugar. Desserts and snacks are not considered as part of the daily diet. Sweets are usually given to children but are not usually eaten by adults. Children usually drink cow's or goat's milk three times or more each day. From the age of 3 years, sweetened tea is usually added to the milk. During pregnancy, Somali women tend to decrease their meals to ensure an easier delivery. They believe that too much food will make the baby grow too big and it will be hard to deliver normally. The diet usually improves during the third trimester although most women do not take prenatal vitamins.

Infant feeding

Almost all women breast feed, often for 2–3 years. Breast milk is not offered in the first 24 hours when infants may be given sugar water or fresh cow's or goat's milk. Colostrum is thought to have a poor nutritional value or to be unhealthy, and it is often expressed and discarded. A mixture of rice and cow's milk is introduced at 6 months of age and drinks from a cup are offered at 6–8 months.

Calcium and vitamin D

The traditional Somalian diet is low in vitamin D and calcium and could give rise to poor bone mineralisation and the development of osteoporosis [74]. Vitamin D deficiency has been reported in 82% of Somalis living in Liverpool [74]. Advice should therefore focus on improving the intake of these nutrients from dietary sources and consideration should be given to additional supplementation with vitamin D where appropriate.

Further reading

Thaker A, Barton A *Multicultural Handbook of Food, Nutrition and Dietetics*. Chichester: Wiley-Blackwell, 2011.

28 Faltering Weight

Zofia Smith

Introduction

The term 'failure to thrive' was once used to describe infants and young children who failed to reach their expected growth. Over the last 15 years, more has been understood about poor weight gain and the term has been criticised for being pejorative [1]. The term 'faltering weight' has now been accepted as the term for infants who show a fall in weight or poor weight gain. However, some of the literature still refers to the term 'failure to thrive' (FTT).

Earlier definitions also focused on whether the cause of faltering weight was 'organic', with a medical diagnosis, or 'non-organic', related to unknown psychosocial factors. It is now clear from research that only 5% of cases of faltering weight have an underlying medical problem. The two categories are not mutually exclusive and undernutrition is recognised as the primary cause of poor weight gain in infancy [2].

Identification and prevalence of faltering weight

Faltering weight is identified in the main from interpretation of growth charts which show accurate weight and height measurements; this is still the most reasonable marker for diagnosis [3]. Guidelines on the 2009 UK-WHO growth charts suggest that a sustained drop of weight through two or more centile spaces is unusual (fewer than 2% of infants) and should be carefully assessed by the primary care team [4]. Several other patterns of faltering weight have been identified which suggest undernutrition (Table 28.1).

As well as weight and height, head circumference is a most useful indicator in the first 2 years. Height centile should be compared with the parental height as weight gain has been shown to correlate with parental height, suggesting that smaller parents have infants with poorer weight gain [5]. Mid upper arm circumference (MUAC), which indirectly assesses nutritional status by estimating body fat and muscle bulk, is also a useful measurement for children under 5 years (Table 28.2).

Although growth charts are the most likely way of identifying faltering weight, the following features may also be linked with poor weight gain:

- muscle wasting, poor skinfold thickness
- thin, wispy hair
- visible or prominent bones (e.g. pointed chin in a baby)
- pale complexion (could suggest iron deficiency)
- poor sleep pattern

Clinical Paediatric Dietetics, Fourth Edition. Edited by Vanessa Shaw.
© 2015 John Wiley & Sons, Ltd. Published 2015 by John Wiley & Sons, Ltd.
Companion Website: www.wiley.com/go/shaw/paediatricdietetics

Table 28.1   Patterns of faltering weight.

- Sustained weight falling through two or more centiles
- A sawtooth pattern of fluctuating weights on lower centiles, where weights cross and re-cross centiles
- Plateauing and further centile weight loss
- Weight first noted to be below the 2nd centile
- Discrepancy between height and weight of more than two centiles

Table 28.2   Mid upper arm circumference of 1–5 year olds [6].

<14.0 cm	Very likely to be a significantly malnourished child
14.0–15.0 cm	May be malnourished (likelihood greater if age nearer to 5 years than 1 year)
>15.0 cm	Nutrition likely to be reasonable

- developmental delay (particularly in communication skills)
- emotional and behavioural issues (ranging from withdrawn/passive to active/chaotic with poor concentration)

Research has shown that health professionals do not always recognise faltering weight. Batchelor and Kerslake found that one in three children whose weight had fallen substantially were not identified [7]. There were various reasons for non-recognition: lack of awareness of the problem; well cared for children with no signs of physical neglect; no reported feeding difficulties; acceptance of children as small; under use of growth charts.

The incidence of faltering weight in the population depends very much on how faltering weight is defined. It is suggested that it affects 5% of infants in deprived inner city areas but also occurs across a wide social range [8].

Contributing factors

In the early years of life, energy and nutrient requirements are high to allow for rapid growth. Infants and young children are vulnerable at this time when there can be problems around feeding or, in a minority of cases, food is unavailable. For some children, medical conditions are clearly the principal reason for their undernutrition (Table 28.3) [1].

Table 28.3   Organic factors contributing to faltering weight.

- Inability to digest or absorb nutrients
  - coeliac disease
  - cystic fibrosis
- Excessive loss of nutrients
  - vomiting
  - chronic diarrhoea
  - protein-losing enteropathy
- Increased nutrient requirements due to underlying disease
  - chronic cardiac or respiratory failure
  - chronic infection
- Inability to fully utilise nutrients
  - metabolic disease
- Reduced intake of nutrients
  - functional problems
  - suck/swallow incoordination
  - oral hypersensitivity

Despite an often seemingly adequate intake, gastrointestinal disorders may lead to faltering weight because of malabsorption, e.g. coeliac disease. Children with congenital cardiac or respiratory defects may show poor growth due to the breathing problems, anorexia or increased energy requirements caused by their disease.

Children with neurological dysfunction may have problems with oromotor development which can affect the ability to suck and swallow. They may also suffer from oral hypersensitivity and therefore refuse to feed. Children with metabolic disorders can present with faltering weight as a result of poor feeding or inability to utilise energy correctly. Faltering weight is common in infants born prematurely; their special nutritional needs and oromotor problems are reviewed separately (p. 101).

For the children with poor weight gain and no apparent medical problem, an inadequate intake of energy is still the underlying cause. There is increasing recognition of various possible factors contributing to an inadequate intake (Table 28.4).

Early feeding problems

It is suggested that faltering weight is a result of chronic feeding difficulties [9] and feeding

Table 28.4   Factors contributing to inadequate intake.

- Delayed/problematic progression of solids
- Early feeding difficulties, e.g. tube feeding, gastro-oesophageal reflux
- Poor appetite following illness or dental problems
- Parental attitudes to food and feeding, including cultural practices
- Behavioural difficulties, e.g. coercive feeding
- Limited or rigid parenting skills
- Parental ill health, e.g. maternal depression
- Family characteristics, e.g. chaotic household and lack of routine, poor facilities, neglect

problems are the most commonly cited reason for faltering weight. For many infants, weight begins to falter around the time of weaning when a young infant's oromotor skills develop, allowing the acceptance of new tastes and textures. If this opportunity is missed, the progression through weaning and the acceptance of more solid textures can be difficult, leading to over-dependence on milk. Intake is then restricted and is inappropriate for age with insufficient energy for normal growth. Excessive consumption of fluids, whether milk or juice, can exacerbate the problem [10, 11].

A young infant, particularly as weaning progresses, will show increasing independence and want to self-feed. They must be given the opportunity to develop these self-feeding skills. Where parents are unable to read these cues and continue to feed the child, poor intake or food refusal may occur.

In a population based study, children with faltering weight had significantly more feeding problems. These infants were introduced to solids and finger foods later than the control group and were identified as variable eaters with low appetite and poor feeding skills. These factors could lead to the onset and persistence of faltering weight [12]. One study reported the experiences of parents with children with faltering weight who had severe feeding difficulties. Parents described stressful mealtimes, children crying, clamping their lips, turning away, pushing food away, spitting out food and being sick [13].

Behavioural feeding problems, including food refusal, can happen at an early age and there are many contributing factors [14]. One of the earliest forms of infant communication occurs during feeding with carer and infant responding and reacting

to each other. Parental feeding interaction, which might well be affected by worry, anxiety or concern about a child's intake, will influence how a child reacts to food. In turn, clear cues from the child might not be noticed by the carer. For young infants with gastro-oesophageal reflux, food might well be associated with vomiting and pain. Feeding can then be an unpleasant experience, leading to food refusal. There are many reasons for food refusal including dental caries, extreme temperatures of food, inappropriately sized pieces, insensitive feeding or reluctance of parents to allow the child to feed itself and make the inevitable 'mess'. Feeding problems often frustrate parents who will differ in their ways of dealing with it. This often causes great distress and disruption to family life. All this contributes to the persistence of faltering weight.

Family and maternal influences

Some studies have focused on psychosocial characteristics of the family and the environment of the child who has faltering weight. Parents' inability to provide emotional nurturing may well contribute to the problem. Family conflict before the age of 7 has also been shown to have a strong and significant association with slow growth [15].

Maternal attitudes towards food and feeding have been shown to have an influence on the eating habits of children. McCann *et al.* reported that mothers of children whose weight faltered showed greater dietary restraint both concerning what they ate themselves and what they were prepared to offer their children [16]. In another study, infants of mothers who were both depressed and deprived showed poorer weight gain [17].

Poverty

Poverty is not a factor in isolation and there is little evidence to suggest an increased risk of faltering weight in the poorest [17], but there is a strong suggestion that larger families constitute a risk [5].

Neglect and abuse

Two population studies found that between 5% and 10% of children who had faltering weight had been registered for abuse or neglect [12, 18]. It is suggested that children in abusive or neglecting families are at an increased risk of faltering weight, but these families only represent a small proportion of all cases.

Outcomes for children with poor weight gain

Nutrition in the early years of life is a major determinant of growth and development and it influences future adult health [19]. Evidence suggests that poor weight gain from birth to 6–8 weeks of life is a stronger predictor of developmental delay than poor weight gain over the remainder of the first year [20]. A meta-analysis found that infants with early onset faltering weight were likely to be shorter and thinner than age matched peers, but there was little evidence of damaging consequences for growth and intellectual development. However, it was acknowledged that poor growth can be an important marker for the need for intervention for children where there is neglect, a medical condition, developmental problems or feeding issues [21]. Early home intervention has been reported as mitigating the effects of faltering weight [22].

Assessment of faltering weight

Health visitors, with appropriate training, are ideally placed to identify children with faltering weight when they are undertaking routine child health surveillance. A holistic assessment, preferably undertaken at home, should look at a child's intake, feeding behaviour and family circumstances. The community paediatric dietitian will help to clarify any dietary concerns and assess nutritional adequacy. There might also be an oromotor skills assessment by a speech and language therapist.

When poor weight gain continues, a multidisciplinary team approach has been advocated where the medical and psychosocial aspects are combined into a clear focus on food and feeding [23, 24]. This will allow for a full paediatric assessment to be undertaken: medical assessment, taking a feeding history, assessment of current dietary intake, psychosocial and developmental aspects. Potential members of a multidisciplinary feeding team are

- community paediatrician
- community paediatric dietitian
- specialist health visitor
- clinical psychologist
- nurse/nursery nurse
- speech and language therapist (for some children)

Joint working enables discussion of individual cases and close cooperation between families and professionals. Clinical investigations only need to be undertaken if there are any suggestions of symptoms, in order to exclude organic disease and to reassure anxious parents.

Dietary assessment

It is important to construct a complete picture of all aspects of and influences on the child's feeding. Early feeding history, together with the start and progression of solids, will help to identify if there were problems in the first year of life. Dietary recall with further information on the variety and the frequency of foods offered and eaten, mealtime routines and drinks taken through the day will all help to assess the child's current intake. Information on the purchasing of food and its preparation within the home may also be revealing. Discussion with the parent will identify how long mealtimes last and whether they are stressful. Gathering background information will help to identify any difficulties experienced by the family.

There is little research on the dietary intake of children with faltering weight. One study raised the difficulties in collecting dietary information and suggested that only a minority of children with faltering weight will have dietary histories that are obviously inadequate, but that wider ranging nutritional assessment will be more revealing [25].

A food diary is a useful tool in nutritional assessments, revealing invaluable qualitative information as well as helping to establish the nature of dietary inadequacies [26]. Table 28.5 shows a food record of a 2-year-old child completed by the parent. This reveals the routine, frequency and limited range of foods as well as types and amounts of fluids. Immediate advice would be to ensure the child had an adequate intake of minerals and vitamins whilst urgent further assessment of feeding would need

Table 28.5 Three day food record of a 2-year-old child.

FOOD DIARY

NAME _ _ _ _ _ _ _ _ , _ _ _ _ _ _ _ DATE OF BIRTH _ _ _ _ _ _ _ _ _ _ _ _

DATE DIARY STARTED _ _ _ _ _ _ _ _ _ _ _ _ _ _ _

TIME	DAY 1	DAY 2	DAY 3
MIDNIGHT			
6.00 am	Milk (8 oz)		Milk (8 oz)
7.00 am			
8.00 am			
9.00 am			
10.00 am		1 cup (rice + fish cooking)	
11.00 am	1 cup (rice + meat cooking)		½ cup instant noodle
12.00 noon		Milk (8 oz)	
1.00 pm	Milk (8 oz)		Milk (8 oz)
2.00 pm		1 banana.	
3.00 pm	Milk (8 oz)		Yoghurt (100mg)
4.00 pm			
5.00 pm		1 cup (rice + fish)	
6.00 pm			Milk (8 oz)
7.00 pm	1 cup (rice + meat cooking)	Milk (8 oz)	
8.00 pm	Yoghurt (100mg)		Two eggs
MIDNIGHT	Milk (8 oz)	Milk (8 oz)	Milk (8 oz)

to be undertaken by a community dietitian and health visitor.

Table 28.6 shows a food record of an under-weight 18-month-old child completed by a parent. This shows that the child is predominantly offered meals, food is puréed or mashed to give mainly softer textures, and bottles of juice are offered as drinks. Although the quantities taken cannot be seen from this information, the parent can be helped to think about the amounts of drinks offered and the age appropriateness of the food. Further discussion with the parent will need to clarify if these are typical days.

Observing a child eating is crucial to obtain more information about

- the seating of the child and parent positioning
- the child's interest in its own food or food of other family members
- the quantity, texture and type of food offered and what is eaten
- the child's desire or ability to feed or drink by themselves

Table 28.6   Three day food record of an 18-month-old child.

Time	Day 1	Day 2	Day 3
.00 am			
8.30	1½ weetabix with full fat milk + small cup milk to drink	As day 1	As day 1, but no drink
.00 am			
0.00 am		Cup of Blackcurrant Juice + 1 custard cream biscuit	Bottle of juice
1.00 am			
12.30	Puréed stewing steak/potato/carrots/Broccoli (1 cup) 3 Tbs Thick + Creamy Yoghurt Small Cup of Blackcurrant Juice	Mashed Potato + Baked Beans (large cup) 2 Tbs yoghurt Small Piece Choc. Gateau	Puréed chicken in white sauce/Potato/Carrots/Peas/Broccoli (1 cup) 2 small fromage frais
1.00 pm			
2.00 pm	Small Packet White Choc. Buttons	Small Packet White Choc. Buttons	
3.00 pm			
4.00 pm	Puréed Fish in Parsley Sauce/Potato/Carrots/Broccoli (1 cup) 2 small fromage frais ½ cup of water	Fish - as day 1 1 small fromage frais	Mashed potato + Baked Beans (Med. Potato) 2 Biscuits 1 cup of Juice
5.00 pm			
6.00 pm			
7.00 pm			
8.00 pm			

- the child's oromotor and self-feeding skills
- the interaction between the child and parent, including parental response to child's cues
- communication between the child and parent, e.g. verbal encouragement
- the atmosphere and emotions at mealtime

Some specialist teams, with parental agreement, will video a mealtime. The mealtime observation, when shared with the family, can allow the parents to see the feeding from a different perspective. A comment from one parent having viewed a feeding session was: 'Well I'm not surprised she's not eating. I didn't realise I was so forceful. If someone tried to feed me like that, I wouldn't eat either.' When parents are able to suggest changes and contribute to the management plan, there is a greater chance of success.

Observation can also highlight ineffective ways of feeding an infant or young child (Table 28.7) and the issues can be sensitively raised with the parents.

It is important to listen to parental concerns and their view should be taken into account. It is also useful to know who else is involved in the care and feeding of the child. For some children, and again with parental agreement, it is useful to observe the child's behaviour around food in a setting other than home, e.g. nursery, children's centre or school. This can help in identifying differences in eating and feeding, adding further valuable information.

Assessment of oromotor function

For a small number of children who may have neurodevelopmental problems or continue to exhibit food refusal and faltering weight, it is important for a speech and language therapist (SLT) to assess oromotor function. Such assessments, often in conjunction with video-fluoroscopy, will identify infants who are unable to coordinate the suck/swallow reflex. These children are likely to aspirate feeds and may require nasogastric or gastrostomy feeding. The SLT will also detect oral hypersensitivity and be able to help with desensitisation programmes.

Nutritional management

Nutritional requirements

A dietary intake which provides energy and protein requirements for age [27] will usually allow for maintenance of growth along a particular centile. Additional protein and energy will be required to allow for weight to improve. Guidelines suggest that the percentage of energy supplied from protein should be between 8.9% and 11.5% to provide optimal improvement of lean and fat mass [28]. Supplementing the diet with glucose polymers to increase energy density, hence providing a lower percentage of energy from protein, has been associated with higher rates of fat deposition.

A formula for predicting energy requirements to improve weight gain in infants and young children has been suggested [29]:

$$\text{kcal (kJ)/kg} = \frac{120 \times \text{ideal weight for height (kg)}}{\text{actual weight (kg)}}$$

This may mean an intake of 1.5–2.0 times the normal recommended energy requirements for age.

Anaemia is common in children with faltering weight and in one study one-third of the sample had iron deficiency anaemia [30]. There is also evidence of zinc deficiency affecting growth [31]. Requirements for vitamins, minerals and trace elements are increased during periods of rapid growth and a suitable supplement should be included if the child's intake is thought to be inadequate. No guidelines exist, but intakes should be at least appropriate for the proposed energy intake.

Achieving nutritional requirements

Following feeding assessment, a strategy for catch-up growth needs to be planned. The main nutritional objectives are

Table 28.7 Poor feeding techniques.

- Infant fed with a bottle in a semi-lying position
- Infant fed with a bottle whilst asleep ('dream' feeding)
- Anxious parent following the child around with food or forcefully feeding a child
- Excessive cleaning of the child with every mouthful of solids
- Dummy (pacifier) or infant bottle available at any time
- Child discouraged from participating in feeding itself
- Child chastised with threats or punishment for not eating

- to improve protein and energy intake
- to promote weight gain enabling catch-up and allowing optimum growth
- to correct nutritional deficiencies and achieve an adequate nutritional intake

If a child is underweight for height and failing to gain weight at the expected rate, whatever they are consuming is not enough for their needs. Working in partnership with parents, engaging them in any decisions on nutritional intervention, is crucial.

In a young breast fed infant where weight is faltering, the maternal diet needs to be assessed and its quantity and quality improved. Supplementation of breast feeds may be necessary, but this should be done under dietetic supervision and with caution as it may suppress production of breast milk. For formula fed infants, one study showed the benefits of using a ready-to-feed nutrient dense formula (Table 1.18) rather than adding energy supplements to standard infant formula [32]. Full strength high energy formula has been shown to be tolerated well by infants under the age of 12 months with faltering weight, but some may benefit from a gradual introduction to avoid increased bowel frequency [33].

In general, young children have a high energy requirement relative to their size. In cases of poor weight gain, when catch-up growth is the aim, requirements are even higher. This is difficult to achieve as many children have small appetites, consuming small food portions at any one time. There are various ways of increasing energy intake:

- regular meals
- snacks in between meals
- use of energy dense foods
- fortification of foods
- supplements
- enteral feeding

Provision of regular feeding

Children need a good routine of regular meals, which include energy dense foods. It is advisable to start with small quantities and offer realistic portions of everyday family foods, with the opportunity for the child to be given more if they can manage. Emphasis needs to taken off mealtimes and the importance of total intake emphasised.

Frequent snacks

Meals alone will usually not enable the child to catch up. One study showed that when children with faltering weight were offered a high energy snack, they took more at the next meal than the control group where there were no concerns about growth [34]. In clinical practice, small regular snacks as well as meals are advised to encourage interest in food and improve appetite, so increasing overall energy intake. Excess juice consumption encountered in many young children should be discouraged and solids should be offered first.

Energy dense foods

Children still need to consume as wide a variety of foods as possible from the five food groups: bread, other cereals and potatoes; meat, fish and alternatives; full fat milk and dairy foods; fruit and vegetables; fatty and sugary foods (Table 26.8) with a greater emphasis on the energy dense foods. Foods high in fibre are bulky and may contain high phytate levels compromising both energy intake and the bioavailability of micronutrients.

Fortification of foods

Energy dense products, such as butter, margarine and cheese, can be added to popular foods. Dried full fat milk powder can be used to fortify puddings, soups and milk. If necessary, the iron status of young children can be improved initially by giving iron supplements and, in the longer term, encouraging children to consume iron containing foods.

Supplements

The use of dietary supplements is not recommended for children with no medical reason for poor weight gain. The use of these products can medicalise the problem and give the impression to parents or carers that they do not have a role in helping their child to improve nutritional intake.

However, for children who are unable to take an adequate intake from food alone, dietary supplements may be necessary and can be prescribed. Carbohydrate, fat or protein supplements can be used to enrich foods, or ready-to-feed

Table 28.8   Case study of a child with faltering weight.

A full term baby boy, birthweight 3.4 kg (above 25th centile)

- Breast fed exclusively for 26 weeks and reported by mother to be a hungry infant
- Between 8 and 12 weeks his weight dropped to the 9th centile and by 34 weeks to the 0.4th centile
- On referral his intake was assessed and feeding observed

Reported intake at 36 weeks of age:

8.00 am	40 mL formula milk
12.30 pm	6 teaspoons baby rice with vegetable purée
4.00 pm	2 × 60 g pots of fromage frais
7.00 pm	4 teaspoons of baby rice made up with vegetable purée
9.00 pm	Offered bottle but usually refused
	Breast feed

Breast feeding × 3 through the night

Observation of feeding at 9 months:

- food was puréed
- child was fed by mum on her knee
- child gave clear cues of not wanting to be fed by moving head from side to side
- child reached out for the food but was discouraged by mum
- mum was anxious and quite forceful in getting teaspoon into child's mouth
- meal took about 75 minutes

Dietary advice:

- thickening savoury food with mashed potato or sweet potato; mashed banana can be added to soft fruits
- chopping rather than purée food
- finger foods offered at mealtimes and as snacks in between meals
- extra energy added to meals using foods such as butter, cheese
- multivitamin and iron supplement following a blood check

Focus of work with the family:

- establishing a better mealtime setting
- mum helped to recognise cues from child
- play sessions encouraging the child to touch, lick, taste and enjoy exploring different textures
- food offered first followed by a drink
- mealtimes limited to 20–30 minutes

Outcomes:

- mum got a highchair for child
- child gradually participated more in feeding and making a mess
- mum offered meals and snacks
- mum ate with child and shared her food with him
- formula was added to foods and offered as a drink after meals during the day
- breast milk still offered at bedtime
- as the child developed self-feeding skills he began to eat more
- child gained weight and by 20 months of age he was above the 9th centile

nutrient and energy dense drinks (oral nutritional supplements) may be more suitable (Tables 1.19, 1.21, 11.3). The principle of frequent feeding, regular meals and snacks, use of energy dense foods and fortification of solids with extra energy still applies.

Enteral feeding

If the child has severe faltering weight and it is not possible to achieve a reasonable intake orally, enteral feeding (nasogastric or gastrostomy) may be required initially. The use of overnight feeds may be preferred as this allows oral feeding to be established during the daytime.

Behavioural management

For the child where there are negative associations with food, parents should be helped in a sensitive way, offering support and constructive advice, with no blame attached and no criticism of their parenting. Behavioural management includes

- no force feeding
- positive reinforcement of good feeding behaviour; aberrant behaviour should be ignored, e.g. by turning the face away from the child
- a time limit of 20–30 minutes for mealtimes
- small, frequent meals are a possibility, to maximise the opportunity for feeding practice and to reduce the pressure to eat at any one meal

Young children with feeding difficulties often benefit from messy play. In a relaxed and fun way, a child is encouraged to touch, feel, smell and possibly attempt different food tastes and textures. The case study in Table 28.8 illustrates the benefit from play experience which tackles fears around food, mess and delayed self-feeding skills.

Social care

In some families where there has been no improvement, or poor weight gain continues, with evidence of parental inability to address the child's physical, nutritional and emotional needs, a common assessment framework (CAF) may be initiated by a concerned professional which in many cases is the health visitor. A CAF is a shared assessment and planning framework to identify a child's additional needs and coordinated services to meet them. If the family still struggles to engage and no progress is made, a referral to social care services requesting input from a social worker under the category of a 'child in need' is necessary. This will enable a better assessment of the family dynamics and allows support from a wider range of services. Social work referral is very important whenever there are concerns about a child's care, safety or wellbeing [35].

Summary

To thrive, children need adequate nutrition and appropriate nurturing. The routine use and correct interpretation of growth charts, proactive health visiting and acknowledgement of poor weight gain will allow early intervention before poor nutrition and growth become firmly entrenched.

Many factors contribute to a child's poor weight gain and intervention benefits from a multidisciplinary team approach encompassing diagnosis of any underlying organic cause, assessment of nutritional intake, oromotor function and feeding, and behavioural difficulties. It is important that parental concerns are acknowledged, there is avoidance of blame, that strengths are built on and, wherever possible, there is partnership working between the team and the family.

29 Feeding Children with Neurodisabilities

Jennifer Douglas and Leanie Huxham

Introduction

Neurodisability is a term used to describe conditions affecting the brain and central nervous system (CNS) and includes muscular, developmental, motor, sensory, learning and neuropsychiatric disorders. CNS damage can be due to disease, genetics, oxygen deprivation or acquired brain injury, amongst other causes, and can occur at any stage in a child's life. The majority of research is on children with motor disorders and cerebral palsy, which are the two most common causes of neurodisability [1]. These children often have neurological involvement of other body systems as part of their condition [2]. In the past 10 years there has been a steady increase in the number of children with severe disability due to increased survival of preterm infants and better survival outcomes for children with brain injury. The EPICure study has shown that between 1995 and 2006 survival rate has improved for preterm infants born at or before 26 weeks. Survival rate in the UK for preterm infants born at 26 weeks is 78%, but many of these have neurodevelopmental disability [3, 4].

Many children with neurodisability have difficulties with eating and drinking, and they are likely to have nutritional concerns that need to be addressed [1]. Oromotor dysfunction is associated with poor health and nutritional outcomes, affecting up to 90% of children with moderate to severe cerebral palsy [5]. Those with motor, physical or sensory impairments are more likely to struggle [2] and the more severe the disability, the more likely the child is to be at nutritional risk [1,6]. The ability of infants, children and adolescents to achieve their potential for growth and development depends on the intervention provided at critical time periods. Many children with neurological impairment would benefit from individual nutritional assessment and management as part of their overall care [7]. It has been accepted in the past that children with neurodisability, especially those with CP, are small as part of their condition. With the evolution of enteral feeding it has become evident that children with neurodisability have the potential to grow if adequate nutrition is provided.

Cerebral palsy

Cerebral palsy (CP) is defined as 'a persistent (but not unchanging) disorder of movement and posture, as the result of one or more non progressive abnormalities in the brain, before its growth and development are complete. Other clinical

Clinical Paediatric Dietetics, Fourth Edition. Edited by Vanessa Shaw.
© 2015 John Wiley & Sons, Ltd. Published 2015 by John Wiley & Sons, Ltd.
Companion Website: www.wiley.com/go/shaw/paediatricdietetics

signs may be present as well' [8]. The children more severely affected are likely to have multiple comorbidities including sensory impairments (vision, hearing, touch), perceptual difficulties (resulting in impaired sensory interpretation), learning disabilities, limited communication and medical conditions such as respiratory difficulties, seizure disorders and gastro-oesophageal reflux (GOR). There is currently no test before birth to identify CP. The incidence in the UK is currently 1 in 400 children and 2.1 per 1000 live births [9].

CP is a condition where there may be abnormal brain development or brain injury during development. This can occur before, during or after birth, and even during early childhood. It is not unusual for children to be diagnosed at a later stage when the child's motor development is almost complete. Even before diagnosis is established children may already be experiencing oromotor problems.

Causes of CP may be complex with no obvious single cause. However, there are certain risk factors that may contribute: infection during early pregnancy; oxygen deprivation to the brain due to birth complications or cerebrovascular event in childhood; restricted intrauterine growth; blood disorder (very rare platelet abnormalities); twins or multiple birth; mother's age over 40; low birthweight (<1.5 kg); premature birth (<37 weeks); fertility treatments, severe jaundice and kernicterus, infections to the brain and brain injury during childhood [10–12].

There are four main types of CP, which correspond to injuries to different parts of the brain [13]. Children with:

- spastic CP have permanent increased muscle tone and impairment of voluntary movement or posture due to non progressive damage to the immature brain
- hypotonic CP have low muscle tone with little or no resistance to movement. These children frequently have feeding difficulties
- athetoid CP have some loss of control of their posture and they tend to make unwanted movements. They have a mixture of high and low muscle tone and often have a high requirement for energy
- ataxic CP usually have problems with balance. They may also have shaky hand movements and irregular speech. Their muscle tone tends to be low, but can fluctuate

A child with CP may have one distinct type or, more commonly, a mixture of these. The distribution of CP can be limited to one limb (monoplegia), diplegia with two limb involvement or quadriplegia with all four limbs affected.

Factors to consider when assessing patients with CP:

- type of CP and limb involvement
- mobility: include information about locomotion such as use of wheelchair or a walker
- gastrointestinal problems: GOR and chronic constipation are common in children with CP [14]
- dependence on feeding: ability to self-feed, dependent or partially dependent on assistance from parents/carers
- feeding dysfunction: detailed information regarding how the child manages food textures such as puréed, mashed or chopped foods [15]
- feeding skills: should be assessed at regular intervals in order to identify children at nutritional risk [16] (assessment of feeding skills in Down's syndrome are relevant for children with CP). Parents/carers should be asked about the presence of tongue thrust, drooling/dribbling causing fluid loss, lack of hand to mouth coordination, poor lip seal causing food or fluid loss, inability to communicate hunger, prolonged feeding times and dysphagia [17–19]
- environment: environmental factors can have an impact on growth and nutrition, e.g. the child's living situation, mealtime environment, lifestyle, involvement in therapy groups, school, respite care arrangements [20]. Information about the family and the child's experience with oral feeding should be sought as this may affect decisions about future oral or non oral feeding methods
- other medical conditions and respiratory health: these children are vulnerable to respiratory morbidity for several reasons so it is important to find out about frequency of chest infections and other respiratory problems that may have an effect on energy requirements [21]
- bone health: there is a higher risk of low bone mineral density, osteopenia and osteoporosis due to reduced weight bearing activity or being bed bound; lack of nutrition; medication limiting vitamin D metabolism; limited sun exposure

- anthropometry: there is no universally accepted method for measuring children with CP. Alternatives to measuring height are available and are discussed later (p. 780).

Improved nutritional status in children with CP is associated with improvements in general health, such as decreased irritability and spasticity, improved healing of pressure sores and improved circulation. In contrast, undernutrition is significantly associated with poor functional status, poor motor function, reduced communication ability as well as increased dependence on the carer for feeding [18]. A large multicentre study of 230 children and young people with moderate to severe CP living in the community showed that the level of feeding dysfunction was directly related to the degree of undernutrition and even those who had mild feeding dysfunction had poor growth and limited fat stores [8]. Therefore, a child requiring any modified consistency of food and fluids can be at risk of nutritional compromise. It has also been documented that 89% of children with CP need help with feeding and 56% regularly choke during mealtimes [1]. Almost a third of children with CP were found to have a height for age <25th centile in a study by Vik *et al.* whilst 7% were classified as being obese (weight >99.6th centile) [15].

Low micronutrient intake and low micronutrient serum concentrations are common in children with CP [22]. Nutritional status should be assessed frequently to ensure that micronutrient requirements are met. Tube feeding and the use of nutritional supplements are associated with higher micronutrient concentrations [23]. Improving nutritional status is important to improve motor function with weight gain, especially fat free mass gain, showing the most benefit [14]. It is important to take into account the type of CP the child is diagnosed with (including other comorbidities) as this has significant implications on the chosen nutritional management plan. Children with spastic quadriplegic CP, hypotonic patients and those having seizures often have significant feeding difficulties [24].

Improved nutritional status is associated with improved feeding ability and undernourished children may have poorer feeding skills. A study of 90 children with CP showed feeding competence was positively correlated to weight, triceps skinfold and mid arm circumference [25]. Findings

from a more recent study on feeding methods and health outcomes concluded that oral interventions for children with CP may promote oromotor function; however, they may not be effective in promoting feeding efficiency or weight gain. The author recommended gastrostomy feeding as an alternative for children with severe feeding and swallowing problems, as well as poor weight gain [26]. Parents/carers need to know that oral feeding competence may improve (depending on the patient's ability) by improving nutritional status and it is important to communicate this to them when making decisions about feeding methods, especially when considering artificial methods such as gastrostomy feeding.

Down's syndrome

The incidence of Down's syndrome in the UK is estimated at approximately 1 per 1000 live births, accounting for 725 births in 2011 [27]. Due to prenatal screening this figure has remained relatively constant, despite the rise in maternal age, with 92% of women receiving the diagnosis prenatally opting for a termination [28]. Median life expectancy has improved for people with Down's syndrome, rising from 25 years in 1983 to 49 years in 1997, with some people living into their 60s [16].

Down's syndrome (also called Trisomy 21) is the most common genetic cause of learning disabilities [16]. Many children with Down's syndrome are born with congenital abnormalities such as heart defects (44%–58%), gastrointestinal problems (4%–10%), recurrent respiratory infections, joint problems, endocrine dysfunction particularly hypothyroidism, constipation and GOR. A higher incidence of coeliac disease and haematological cancers has also been found [29]. Regular screening is recommended for children with Down's syndrome to enable early identification of the common comorbidities.

Down's syndrome is associated with anatomical facial abnormalities, which can have significant effects on feeding. Feeding skills should be assessed at regular intervals [16]. Dysfunction occurs due to poor neuromotor control, dental anomalies, orofacial dysmorphology and hypotonia particularly of the tongue and lips. Children with Down's syndrome are frequently mouth breathers due to narrowing of the nasal cavity and chronic inflammation of the tonsils as a result of an increased incidence of upper respiratory infections. The palate is often short and narrow, and this underdevelopment of the maxilla may alter the position of the muscles used for chewing. Infants with Down's syndrome may have difficulty in initiating a suck and have a weak lip seal, poor coordination of the suck/swallow/breathing sequence with early fatigue, as well as having jaw instability [30]. Breast feeding is possible for infants with Down's syndrome, but for many it will be more difficult to establish due to the associated oromotor difficulties. Adequate support is needed to achieve successful breast feeding [31]. Down's syndrome is associated with impaired immune function and higher incidence of obesity; therefore breast feeding may confer long term benefits. Comorbidities such as congenital heart disease and gastrointestinal dysmotility may further compromise feeding [32].

Parental surveys suggest that 60% of children are totally independent feeders by early childhood and the most common problems are slight oral hypotonia, tongue thrust, difficulties in chewing, poor lip seal, and choking and gagging on food [33]. However, it is noted that this feeding success may be partly as a direct result of feeding programmes and not simply a natural developmental step, thus reinforcing the need for assessment and management programmes. Hopman et al. noted that solids were introduced at a later stage compared with controls, possibly due to low parental expectations of developmental ability [34]. Foods requiring less chewing were given, further inhibiting oromotor development. Children with Down's syndrome often have increased oral sensitivity, interfering with the acceptance of new foods, and a high incidence of aspiration, which is possibly related to the high incidence of respiratory disease [35].

Anthropometric assessment of children with Down's syndrome is complicated because of the associated abnormalities related to growth such as short stature, decreased head circumference and altered growth patterns. Cronk suggests that while height in people with Down's syndrome is significantly lower than the norm, the period in which most significant growth failure occurs is during the first 5 years of life [36, 37]. Growth rate is reduced by a fifth between the ages of 3 and 36 months in

both sexes. Longitudinal studies corroborate this, but show that growth velocity of children aged 7–18 years was not significantly different to the norm [38]. There are specific charts for children with Down's syndrome [39]; they describe typical growth, not necessarily ideal growth.

Despite an energy intake below the normal requirement there is a high prevalence of obesity in children and adults with Down's syndrome [40–42]. A 10%–15% lower resting metabolic rate, but equivalent expenditure above resting, has been found in prepubescent children with Down's syndrome [37]. Crino et al. report that 66% of pubertal children with Down's syndrome were obese [43]. As obesity is prevalent in adolescence and adulthood it is recommended that growth charts are used in conjunction with body mass index (BMI), using the same cut-offs for obesity as are applied to the general paediatric population. With appropriate support around nutrition and exercise obesity can be managed successfully [44].

Some studies have shown deficiencies and/or risk of deficiency of vitamin A, vitamin C, vitamin E, zinc, calcium and other nutrients in children with Down's syndrome [41, 45–48]. It is important to note that the majority of these studies have small sample sizes and questionable study methods. The general consensus is that the majority of children with Down's syndrome can meet vitamin and mineral requirements, but monitoring may be needed for those who are unable to eat a healthy balanced diet [49].

Neuromuscular and progressive neurological disorders

There are approximately 60 different types of muscular dystrophy and related neuromuscular conditions. Congenital neuromuscular disorders in children include spinal muscular atrophy and muscle disorders such as Duchenne muscular dystrophy and congenital muscular dystrophies. These conditions are characterised by the loss of muscle strength as progressive muscle wasting or nerve deterioration occurs.

Progressive neurological disorders are extremely rare conditions where deterioration advances over time. There are a large number of different diagnoses, e.g. Batten's disease, leukodystrophies, Cockayne syndrome and Rett syndrome. Some conditions progress at a steady rate and others degenerate in phases.

Due to the vast number of different neuromuscular and progressive neurological disorders it is essential to conduct a literature search at the time of patient review for the most up to date information. Table 29.1 shows some of the more common disorders referred to the dietitian and some of the nutritional considerations associated with each disorder.

Nutritional requirements

Energy

Disabled children often have lower resting energy expenditures due to reduced mobility so their total energy requirements are often lower than the norm. Prediction equations and dietary reference values therefore tend to overestimate needs [50–52]. This has been shown by the Oxford Feeding Study research team, where disabled children tended to lay down stores of fat rather than muscle when gastrostomy fed beyond their requirements [53, 54]. Krick *et al.* have proposed a complicated formula using muscle tone, activity and growth to calculate nutritional requirements [55]. There is currently no universally accepted formula for predicting energy requirements in children with neurodisability. Requirements are based on individual clinical assessment and degree of mobility.

Children with neurodisability are smaller than their non disabled counterparts and until further research becomes available, dietetic consensus opinion is to use height age (a crude estimation of bone age) as a basis to estimate nutritional requirements. This should be adjusted depending on whether weight loss or weight gain is needed. A child entering their pubertal growth spurt will require more energy than one who is not. In practice energy requirements are often no more than 75% of the estimated average requirement (EAR) for height age and are often considerably less; a child receiving as little as 20–30 kcal/kg/day (85–125 kJ/kg/day) can still gain weight. The exceptions to this are those children with mixed CP which includes an athetoid component; excessive involuntary movements make their energy requirements higher and closer to the EAR for chronological age.

Protein and micronutrients

There are no studies informing the requirement for these nutrients. However, as disabled children tend to be smaller than their non disabled peers, reference nutrient intakes (RNI) for actual age are likely to be too high. Height age may be used as a basis for estimations and it is advisable to meet at least the lower reference nutrient intakes (LRNI).

Fluid

Actual body weight is used to calculate fluid requirements and can be based on general recommendations (p. 16). However, it is interesting to note that many children appear well hydrated on fluid intakes that are lower than those derived by calculation and 75% of estimated fluid requirements may be adequate to maintain hydration.

Fibre

Currently there are no UK recommendations for fibre intake in children. In the absence of these, dietitians may refer to American recommendations which suggest the calculation of fibre intake in grams: age (years) + 5 g–10 g [56].

Nutritional assessment

Anthropometry

There are no randomised controlled trials on dietetic assessment to ascertain nutritional status in children with neurodisability. Thus the following information has been developed as a consensus guideline of best practice based on the most current literature [57]. Most research has been conducted on children with CP; therefore, caution must be taken when extrapolating these recommendations to children with other neurodisabilities.

Weight

Weight should be measured routinely on the most appropriate weighing equipment for the individual child. These include hoist scales, wheelchair

Table 29.1 Neuromuscular and progressive neurological disorders and nutritional considerations.

Common conditions	Nutritional considerations	Useful websites
Lysosomal storage disease (Tay Sachs, Fabry, Pompe, metachromic leukodystrophy, Krabbe, Canavan, Zellweger)	Commonly have short stature, skeletal deformities, muscle weakness or lack of control (e.g. ataxia, seizures), neurological failure/decline and/or loss of gained development. Poor swallow may require tube feeding or texture modified diet. Can have both undernutrition and overnutrition. Frequent dietetic monitoring required due to progressive nature of the disease [1]	www.ninds.nih.gov www.lysosomallearning.com www.rarediseases.org www.ulf.org
Adrenoleukodystrophy (see Chapter 20)	Lorenzo's oil can be used in children who are asymptomatic and this may delay onset of symptoms. Symptom control is needed for all other children [1]	www.ninds.nih.gov www.rarediseases.org www.ulf.org
Rett syndrome	Growth failure, oromotor dysfunction, gastro-oesophageal reflux, constipation and low bone density are common. Often need assistance with feeding. May need gastrostomy feeding to improve growth [1]	www.rettuk.org www.reverserett.org.uk www.ninds.nih.gov www.rarediseases.org
Duchenne muscular dystrophy	Predominantly affects males. High prevalence of obesity related to lower resting energy expenditure, steroid use and reduced physical activity. Muscle wasting, poor feeding and poor swallow coordination can lead to malnutrition as they get older. Assistance is often needed with oral feeding and texture modification may improve intakes. Tube feeding may be required. Will need supplementary calcium and vitamin D if they are on steroids. Regular dietetic monitoring required [1]	www.ninds.nih.gov www.rarediseases.org www.muscular-dystrophy.org www.nlm.nih.gov www.dfsg.org.uk
Spinal muscular atrophy	Muscle weakness and bulbar dysfunction lead to swallowing difficulties. Respiratory problems are common including aspiration pneumonia. Undernutrition and overnutrition can occur and regular dietetic monitoring is essential. Undernutrition needs aggressive therapy to avoid exacerbation of pre-existing weaknesses. Gastro-oesophageal reflux is common and may require anti-reflux surgery or jejunal feeding. Constipation and delayed gastric emptying can commonly occur [1]	www.jtsma.org.uk www.smafoundation.org www.actsma.co.uk www.ninds.nih.gov www.lysosomallearning.com www.rarediseases.org
Prader–Willi syndrome (see Chapter 30)	At birth the infant typically has low birth weight for gestation, poor muscle tone ('floppy'), difficulty sucking and may require tube feeding to prevent faltering growth. Feeding difficulties resolve over time and at 2–5 years of age hyperphagia sets in and lasts throughout the lifetime, leading to obesity if not correctly managed [1]	www.pwsa.co.uk www.praderwillisyndrome.org.uk www.geneticdiseasefoundation.org www.fpwr.ca www.pwsausa.org www.fpwr.org
Cockayne syndrome	Premature ageing and short stature. Growth failure and likely to have feeding problems especially as an infant. Will need tube feeding to treat faltering growth and/or manage poor swallow coordination. Likely to have developmental delay and increased tone/spasticity. Regular dietetic monitoring needed due to progressive nature of the disease [1]	www.amyandfriends.org www.cockayne-syndrome.net www.cockaynesyndrome.net www.ncbi.nlm.nih.gov

(continued overleaf)

Table 29.1   *(continued)*

Common conditions	Nutritional considerations	Useful websites
Batten's disease	A neurodegenerative disease. Feeding becomes more difficult with resulting poor weight gain and frequent symptoms of aspiration or difficulty coordinating swallowing (due to progressing lack of coordination and progressive poor muscle tone). Most children will eventually need tube feeding. If they manage to feed orally they are likely to need assistance due to abnormal limb movement and poor muscle strength. Frequent dietetic monitoring is required to support child at various stages of disease progression	www.bdfa-uk.org.uk www.ninds.nih.gov www.bdsra.org www.nathansbattle.com www.hideandseek.org www.battens.org.au

scales and sitting scales for the child, as well as the carer holding the child on the scales and then their weight being subtracted. There is no evidence comparing the accuracy of the various weighing methods; thus all should be accepted as of equal value. The chosen method should be recorded and used when subsequently weighed. Weight measures should be plotted on growth charts, the frequency depending on local practice and the child's individual circumstances, but should be a minimum of every 6 months for older children and young people but more frequently for children under the age of 2 years.

Height

Accurate height measures are often difficult to obtain in disabled children and young people, due to scoliosis or kyphosis caused by a twisted posture or contractures of the spine. A standing height is preferable, but where this is not possible a supine length is an acceptable second choice. It is important to note, however, that a supine length will measure longer than a standing height and serial measures should not be confused.

Where a length or height is not possible there are three suggested alternatives; upper arm length, lower leg length and knee height all of which have been found to correlate with actual height [58]. The frequency of measurements will depend on local practice and individual circumstances; height should be taken a minimum of every 6 months and plotted on a growth chart.

Upper arm length

Upper arm length (UAL) is measured from the acromion to the head of the radius (Fig. 29.1). It should be measured on the right or the least affected side. Two measurements are taken and then averaged. Research suggests it can only be taken accurately using an anthropometer. The measurement can be converted into a height measure and plotted on a growth chart, using the following formula [58]:

$$stature = (4.36 \times UAL) + 21.8$$

The technical error is ± 1.7 cm

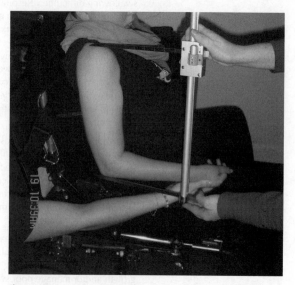

Figure 29.1   Upper arm length.

Lower leg length

The lower leg length, also known as the tibial length (TL), is measured from the tibia to the sphyrion. It requires the child to be sitting and is taken on the right side or the least affected side. This measurement can be taken accurately with an anthropometer or steel tape measure (Fig. 29.2). Two measurements should be taken and averaged. The measurement can be converted into a height measure and plotted on a growth chart, using the following formula [59]:

$$\text{stature} = (3.26 \times \text{TL}) + 30.8$$

The technical error is $\pm$ 1.4 cm

Knee height

Knee height (KH) is measured with the child sitting down and the knee and ankle bent to 90°. Using a sliding caliper the distance between the heel to the superior surface of the knee over the femoral condyle is measured on the left side or least affected side (Fig. 29.3). Two measurements should be taken and averaged. The measurement can be converted into a height measure and plotted on a growth chart, using the following formula [59]:

$$\text{stature} = (2.69 \times \text{KH}) + 24.2$$

The technical error is $\pm$ 1.1 cm

When an alternative length measurement is taken, note of the limb from which the measurement was taken should be made, and this should be consistently used for all subsequent measures. There are centiles specifically for each of the alternative measurements based on American data by Snyder *et al.* [59], but these tables are not widely available at present in the UK; thus conversion to a height measure and plotting on a growth chart is recommended.

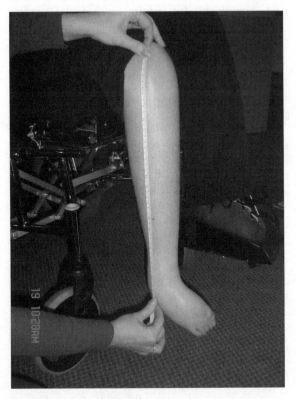

Figure 29.2   Lower leg length.

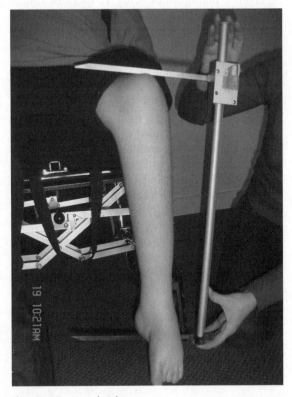

Figure 29.3   Knee height.

Body composition

There is good evidence that body composition of disabled children can be ascertained by measuring skinfold thickness. Triceps and subscapular skinfold thicknesses in particular correlate highly with true fat and fat free mass. However, in routine practice, it can be difficult to take accurate skinfold thickness measurements, e.g. subscapular skinfold thickness measurement may be impractical due to the need to remove clothing or spinal jackets. In practical terms annual serial measurements of mid arm circumference (MAC) and triceps skinfold thickness (TSF) can be a useful monitoring tool and can be used to estimate mid arm muscle circumference (MAMC) [60]:

$$\text{MAMC (cm)} = \text{MAC (cm)} - 0.314 \times \text{TSF (cm)}$$

Skinfold thicknesses and mid arm circumference can be compared with the WHO arm circumference and skinfold thickness charts and tables [61, 62] or Addo and Himes charts [63]. Measurements should be taken a minimum of every 12 months. Where possible other anthropometric measurements, such as subscapular skin fold thickness, should be taken.

Growth charts

The standard UK-WHO 2009 growth charts should be used for monitoring weight and height centiles for the majority of disabled children [58, 64]. There are specific charts for children with Down's syndrome that should be used instead of the standard UK-WHO 2009 charts [39].

Growth charts are available for children with CP aged 2–20 years, classifying children into groups according to the severity of their CP. The charts show observed growth patterns in these groups, but may not indicate optimal growth [65, 66]. The charts show that children with moderate to severe CP lack a significant pubertal growth spurt. These charts should not be used exclusively, but rather in combination with clinical assessment, UK growth charts and anthropometric measurements.

Biochemistry

Serum albumin and prealbumin levels do not reflect nutritional status in children with neurodisability. A recent study indicated that albumin and prealbumin levels were very rarely below normal reference values and did not correlate with anthropometric measurements or general health [67]. Annual blood tests may be useful for children who are at risk of nutritional deficiencies, such as those on texture modified diets due to dysphagia, or those with faltering growth due to poor oral intake. The 2007 Scottish enteral feeding guidelines suggest that tube fed children have annual blood samples taken that monitor electrolytes, full blood count (FBC), kidney and liver functions, bone health, specific minerals (zinc, copper, iron) and specific vitamins (A, D, E, B_{12}) [68].

Clinical

Clinical assessment requires knowledge of the type of neurodisability, level of disability and stage of disease (for progressive disorders). The following indices are useful to make an overall assessment of nutritional needs: neurological function (including seizure activity), respiratory function, cardiac function, muscle tone (including limb function), skin integrity, sensory difficulties, gastrointestinal function, urinary and/or faecal incontinence.

Dietary assessment

There are three common methods of assessment: food diaries, dietary recall and food frequency questionnaires. Evidence to support these methods of assessing food intake is poor and no method gives accurate information on food intake. Over-reporting is the main problem and can be as high as 54% more than the child's actual intake so it should be used with caution [69].

Dietary assessments, however, are useful for assessing meal patterns and the types of food offered and eaten, in relation to the food groups. Observation of a child at a mealtime may be more useful and can highlight other factors that affect dietary intake such as the child's posture and the mealtime environment [58].

Social context

Children with disabilities are more vulnerable to both physical and emotional abuse and child protection is a high priority. It is important that services work together to ensure there is a focus on safeguarding children [70, 71]. Individual needs assessments ensure that a child can achieve good health, safety, enjoyment/achieving, make a positive contribution and have economic wellbeing as laid out in *Every Child Matters* [72]. Specific standards for the health and social care of disabled children are described in the National Service Framework for Children, Young People and Maternity Services: *Disabled Children and Young People and those with Complex Health Needs* [73].

The social issues affecting a disabled child are far reaching and the pressure on parents/carers to provide for their child is immense as they cope with difficulties in all areas of life: housing, transport, finances, education, family dynamics and managing medical interventions. Consideration of all aspects of the child's life is important when giving recommendations for nutrition intervention. Ideally the dietitian should work within a multidisciplinary team to get an understanding of any social factors that could affect the child's ability to achieve nutritional goals.

Multidisciplinary assessment

Multidisciplinary and multi-agency working is vital in supporting and safeguarding children with complex needs. Disabled children are classified as in need in the Children's Act (1989) and as such it is the duty of care of every local authority to provide a range of services at the level appropriate to these children's needs [72]. Strong links within the professional team and effective communication are essential to ensure each child's potential is met and maintained [74]. Having an overview of all sources of information is important to ensure a holistic assessment and allows for practical interventions to optimise the child's potential. Often these children, with very complex health and social needs, have a large number of professionals and services involved (Fig. 29.4). If managed well, this can be a huge benefit to those involved and the families themselves.

Current literature highlights the importance of the multidisciplinary approach to nutritional assessment of children with neurodisabilities [61, 75, 76], drawing together the skills and

expertise of parent, carer and a range of healthcare professionals. In the absence of a validated nutrition screening tool, nutrition and feeding problems are identified by measuring children, observing mealtimes and questioning parents, carers and nursing staff.

Speech and language therapist

A feeding assessment by a speech and language therapist (SLT) should always be included in the nutritional assessment of a child with neurodisability [25]. Assessment of feeding competence provides important information for identifying children at risk of poor nutritional status. Feeding dysfunction is related to nutritional risk and it has been shown that even those who have mild dysfunction are still lighter and shorter than their peers [6, 77]. The assessment will also highlight any problems with drooling or excess salivation, which will need to be factored into calculation of fluid requirements.

Occupational therapist

The occupational therapist (OT) takes a particular interest in the child's position for eating and drinking, their level of independence and any special equipment that may aid the child. A child will need to have a secure base and symmetrical position to obtain optimum trunk, limb, head and oral control. The position may be either on the carer's lap for infants and small children or in adapted seating. The assessment should also involve the carer's needs so they adopt a position that is comfortable, safe for their back and facilitates the techniques necessary to help the child. Sometimes this will require the parent or carer experimenting with different positions until they have the best arrangement for them both.

The child's position during mealtimes can affect their ability to swallow safely. Young babies are usually fed in a reclined position. Children should eat and drink in an upright position to ensure a safe swallow. If a degree of tilt is required on their seating system a reassessment of their ability to swallow safely should be carried out.

There is a wide range of specialised equipment available to assist with eating and drinking for

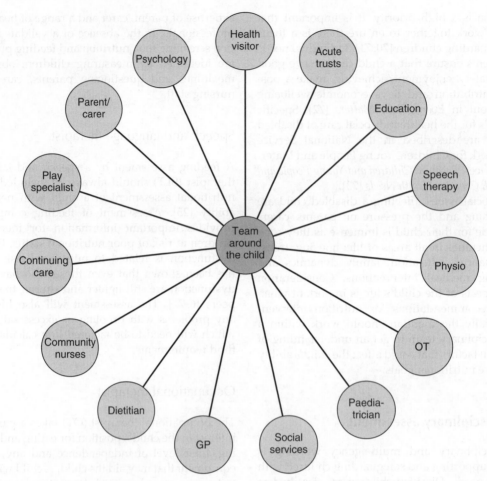

Figure 29.4   Professionals and services involved in the care of the disabled child. GP general practitioner, OT occupational therapist.

children with special needs. A joint assessment between the child's OT and SLT (and perhaps also a physiotherapist) is required to ensure the correct equipment is selected.

Clinical psychologist

The input of a clinical psychologist is necessary for the maximum benefit to be derived from a feeding assessment. A child's early feeding experiences may impact on how they currently feed, particularly those children who have experienced distress because of early feeding practices. This can sometimes result in learned aversive behaviour often mistaken for a dislike of food or a poor appetite, which can only be resolved with adequate psychological support. The psychologist will consider factors influencing feeding including:

- the environment where the child usually eats
- parents' eating history and attitude to food
- early attachment difficulties, especially with an ill child
- marital/family stress, life events, social support, family networks
- general parenting skills
- parent–child relationship and interaction
- past and present parental mental health
- parental level of anxiety and obsessions

Nutritional management

Nutritional management of children with neurodisabilities can be challenging and there is little supportive research. Nutritional care is determined by the individual child's needs and is often based on observations rather than set guidelines.

Oral nutrition

Food fortification

This should be based on the same principles as for other children whose growth is faltering. The energy content of food should be increased by using energy dense foods and monitoring the outcome. Energy dense foods need to be of the correct consistency for the child's oromotor skills. Carers familiar with prevailing healthy eating messages are often concerned about the use of high fat foods for their child and their re-education is important. Children with neurodisabilities often can only eat small portions and therefore adding fat/sugar into foods can increase energy density without appreciably increasing volume. Parents should choose high fat dairy products, such as whole milk, butter, cream, full fat yoghurt as additions to meals/snacks. Adding oil to foods can also increase energy density. Foods which can quickly be added to instant mashed potato, e.g. grated cheese, cream cheese, mashed tinned fish, corned beef, paté, avocado pear, all provide variety without too much preparation time. Protein foods, e.g. eggs, lentils, meat, nuts and cheese, can be added to meals to increase nutritional value as can skimmed milk powder added to foods or milkshakes. Adding sugar to puddings and milkshakes will increase the energy content.

Fluids

Inadequate consumption or excessive fluid loss is a feature common to many children with feeding difficulties. Advice should be based on assessment of why the child is not able to consume adequate fluids. Children with poor lip seal and who thus lose fluid from the mouth will need to be offered drinks more frequently. The OT and SLT can identify the best drinking method, allowing the child to drink enough fluid safely.

For some children thickened fluids can enable more successful drinking. Commercial pre-thickened drinks are available (Table 29.2). Other fluids can be thickened using food products such as thick yoghurts, ice cream, instant powdered desserts, instant sauce granules and smooth puréed fruit. A range of proprietary thickening agents is also available on prescription (Table 29.2). Many carers have fears about offering thick drinks as they perceive these as not as thirst quenching and their use should be fully discussed.

For children who manage food better than fluids offering foods with a high water content between meals, e.g. puréed fruit, thick yoghurts, fromage frais, ice cream and ice lollies, will increase their fluid intake. Jelly can be useful, but it dissolves immediately on entering the mouth resulting in the same problems as thin fluids.

Table 29.2   Prescribable thickeners and pre-thickened drinks.

	Manufacturer	Product	Suitable for*
Thickeners	Cow & Gate	Instant Carobel	Infants and small children
	Sutherland	Thixo-D original	Over 1 year
	Vitaflo	Vitaquick	Over 1 year
	Nestle	Resource ThickenUp	Over 1 year
	Nestle	Resource ThickenUp Clear	Over 3 years
	Fresenius Kabi	Thick and Easy	Over 3 years
	Nutricia	Nutilis Powder	Over 3 years
Thickened drinks	Nestle	Resource Thickened Juice Drinks	Over 1 year
	Fresenius Kabi	Fresubin Thickened Stage 1	Over 3 years
	Fresenius Kabi	Fresubin Thickened Stage 2	Over 3 years
	Nutricia	Nutilis Clear	Over 3 years
	Nutricia	Nutilis Complete Stage 1	Over 3 years
	Nutricia	Nutilis Complete Stage 2	Over 3 years
	Nutricia	Nutilis Complete Stage 3	Over 3 years
Semi-solid dessert	Nutricia	Fortini Creamy Fruit	Over 1 year
	Nutricia	Forticreme Complete	Over 3 years
	Fresenius Kabi	Fresubin Creme	Over 5 years
	Abbott	Ensure Plus Creme	Over 6 years

*Indicated by manufacturer.

To monitor an increase in fluid intake note whether there have been more wet nappies; fewer urinary tract infections; softer or more regular bowel movements. Despite all efforts some children still find it extremely difficult to achieve an acceptable fluid intake orally and may require tube feeding to meet fluid requirements.

Increasing fibre

Increasing dietary fibre may help with constipation; however, adequate fluid intake and medications are likely to be more effective [78]. Increasing the child's intake of fruit and vegetables increases soluble fibre intake. Puréed fruit can be added to breakfast foods and extra vegetables can be incorporated in gravy, mashed potato, casseroles and thick soups. Insoluble fibres such as wholegrain cereals and breads can help with constipation, but should only be considered if the child is consuming adequate fluids.

The use of prescribed soluble fibre supplements may be useful where it is difficult to increase dietary fibre or when children are tube fed, e.g. Resource Optifibre, based on partially hydrolysed guar gum. This supplement can be used for either constipation or diarrhoea.

Supplementation

Prescribed oral nutritional supplements, e.g. Paediasure, Frebini Energy, Fortini (Table 11.3), may be appropriate for some children. The child's current nutritional intake should be assessed first to ensure that the supplement with the desired composition is selected. The use of supplements should be reviewed regularly. Supplements can be thickened as recommended by the SLT, but can also be supplied ready thickened (Table 29.2). Energy modules based on fat and/or carbohydrate, e.g. Duocal, Calogen, Vitajoule, can be used to improve energy intakes and these can be added to food or enteral feeds. Protein supplements, e.g. Protifar, Vitapro, can be added to foods and drinks to increase protein intakes.

Communication

A child or young person with a severe neurodisability may not be able to verbalise or signal their wish for food. This inability to make their request leads to an increased risk of insufficient nutrition, as they are unable to make the same demands as their non disabled counterparts. As a child grows older or their condition progresses, oromotor abilities may also change which can result in new difficulties with managing food and drinks. Children with unrecognised feeding difficulties may be incorrectly interpreted at mealtimes. Often rejection of certain textures or consistencies can be mistaken for the child being fussy, lazy or badly behaved, or disliking the food. They may even display self-injurious behaviour or pica as a sign of distress. When a child is reported to be fussy or badly behaved at mealtimes, thorough investigation of exactly what is happening is needed, as the possibilities of misinterpreting intentions are very great. Special communication aids, also known as Augmentative and Alternative Communication (AAC), may be used such as communication boards, charts, books or electronic communication aids with voice output to help the child communicate their needs.

Presentation of food and drink

Mealtimes need to be enjoyable for the child; otherwise they are unlikely to eat and drink to their best ability. When the child is alert and healthy they will manage a more challenging consistency of food than if they are tired or unwell and the carer needs to be sensitive to the child's needs on each eating or drinking occasion. To reduce the risk of aspiration and improve swallow coordination a child should be offered a reasonable choice of food with a texture they can manage. If the child can feed assisted this should be encouraged as the hand to mouth action will help with anticipation of receiving food into the mouth.

The way food is presented to the child is important for success. Food should be given slowly and rhythmically, allowing time to finish each mouthful and anticipate the next one. Small mouthfuls are more likely to be successful; for some children the food needs to be heaped towards the tip of the spoon to provide sensory cues for the lips. The spoon should normally be presented horizontally from the front and, depending on the techniques being practised at the time, it could be centrally or towards the side of the mouth when encouraging chewing. Scraping food off the spoon with the top teeth should be avoided. The SLT or OT can suggest other methods to help the child to learn to take food from the bowl of the spoon and achieve lip closure.

Prompts

If the child is unable to feed themselves then the carer will need to use appropriate prompts to ensure the child is aware that food is coming and of what they are eating. Prompts can be:

- visual, e.g. an environment with other people eating; mirrors; seeing, smelling and hearing the food being prepared or arriving at the table
- physical, such as the smell of food; stroking the lower lip with the spoon; giving very small amounts so allowing time for the child to experience the taste, texture and temperature of the food
- verbal, to promote the awareness of the concepts of eating; asking the child how they would like to be fed; telling the child what is going to happen next; explaining what is being done as it occurs. Repetitive phrases throughout the meal help the child know what they are doing, e.g. 'bite', 'chew' and 'swallow'
- object recognition, such as a spoon being placed in the child's hand prior to each meal, helps the child to understand and anticipate that a food is on its way

Assessment will inform which combination the child will prefer; however, consistency by all helpers is important.

Assistance with feeding

All people who could possibly be involved with feeding the child should be identified. Total reliance on one main carer should be discouraged as this can make the child dependent on one person's feeding technique. Other members of the family, friends, respite carers, social service family support, students and volunteers can all give support at mealtimes. The carer should be encouraged to let another person help with at least one meal a week. Training and support should be offered to the helpers and they should be involved in the assessment and review process. Clear details of the

programme such as a 'mealtime guidance sheet' must be accessible to all involved with feeding. A model of how the task of feeding is best carried out provides the carer with a clear picture of what is expected. Also, this can increase the empathy of the demonstrator by briefly experiencing the difficulties experienced by the feeder at every meal.

Special feeding aids and equipment

Positioning of the child is important to ensure they can feed safely as even a slight change in the angle of the child's head or body can affect their ability to feed safely [19]. Children may need their seating adapted to ensure they are in the correct posture and the OT can help with this.

Special feeding aids and equipment are tailored to improve eating and drinking and promote independence. Examples of these are [79]

- eating systems
- special bowls and plate guards
- cutlery such as spoons with textured, contoured or curved handles, e.g. angled spoons and good grip spoons
- drinking equipment: cups, mugs and bottles with special features such as two handles, one way valves, weighted bases to reduce tipping, cup holders and straws. Specific special cups are the Doidy cup (slanted towards the child for easier drinking); the anyway drinking cup (designed to reduce spillage); special needs Medela teats, bottles, cups; Easyflow cups
- bibs and aprons to help keep children clean during mealtimes
- slip resistant tableware such as placemats

Eating with other people

Eating with other people is important for children with feeding difficulties. However, limitations may prevent this from happening; for instance the special chair may not fit under the family table. Such problems should be identified in a multidisciplinary mealtime assessment. In some cases the carer may find it easier to give the child their meal before everyone else. Practical ways in which the child can join in with family mealtimes need to be identified. Eating out may be a problem and familiarisation with popular commercial menus will provide ideas for the carer, e.g. many venues serve thick shakes which, if transferred to the appropriate cup, can provide a perfect consistency for some children requiring thickened drinks.

Enteral nutrition

Disabled children form the largest group of children requiring long term home enteral tube feeding (HETF) in the UK [80]. The British Artificial Nutrition Survey (BANS) report, 2010, found that 31% of children registered for HETF in 2009 had neurodisabilities [81].

The decision to initiate enteral feeding is an emotive one which has many ethical considerations. The decision must be in the best interests of the child from a medical point of view and in terms of quality of life and ensuring dignity is maintained. Parents are often reluctant to consent to placement of a gastrostomy tube for feeding, as it can be perceived as a failure on their part to nurture their child by providing food. Gastrostomy feeding may present another loss of normality and be a sign of disability for some parents [82]. Parents should be given all the information they need to reach an informed decision about the benefits and risks of gastrostomy placement and the process should not be rushed [83–86].

Enteral nutrition should be considered in children with

- malnutrition, or where they are unable to achieve catch-up growth with oral nutrition alone
- unsafe swallow
- severe oral aversion
- significant stress during mealtimes
- inadequate hydration
- inability to take medications orally

The choice of nasogastric versus gastrostomy feeding has to be carefully assessed for the child with feeding difficulties. Nasogastric feeding can be used as a short term method of feeding; however, this can cause oral/facial aversion if used for extended periods of time. Gastrostomy feeding is a longer term, safe and useful method to allow adequate nutritional intake and prevention of dystrophy in children with neurodisability and dysphagia [87]. Gastrostomy placement carries a surgical risk. Tube feeding does not prevent aspiration of oral secretions or of gastric contents unless the tube is placed in the jejunum.

Enteral feeding in children with neurodisabilities is well tolerated and can improve energy and protein intake, weight gain and nutritional status in addition to improving the parent's/carer's perceptions of their child's health and quality of life [88–94] .

Feeds

Sullivan *et al.* demonstrated that children with CP have relatively low energy expenditure and high body fat content, and caution should be taken not to overfeed patients [96]. Many children with neurodisability appear to grow adequately on very low energy intakes and it may not be possible to meet their macronutrient and micronutrient requirements (based on the child's height age) if standard 1 kcal/mL (4 kJ/mL) enteral feed volumes are simply reduced to provide less energy. In this case a low energy paediatric feed, such as Nutrini Low Energy Multifibre (0.75 kcal/mL, 3 kJ/mL), may be the best choice (Table 3.2). A vitamin and mineral supplement may be needed to complement any low energy feed, e.g. Paediatric Seravit or Phlexy-vits; additional sodium and potassium supplementation may be given from an oral rehydration solution, e.g. Dioralyte; protein modules may be added to the feed if required, e.g. Vitapro, Protifar. Feeds designed for older children or adults, including feeds that are complete in 1000–1200 mL (such as Fresubin 1000 Complete, Nutrison 1000 Complete, Jevity Promote) are worth considering in smaller volumes for children. However, the micronutrient levels must be checked and kept within safe intakes. Constipation is often an issue so it is worthwhile using a feed containing fibre.

Feed choices include

- energy dense infant formula (Table 1.18)
- standard paediatric feed with or without fibre
- high energy paediatric feed with or without fibre
- low energy paediatric feed with fibre
- adult feeds for older children/adolescents with energy density 1–2 kcal/mL (4–8 kJ/mL) with varying protein content
- adult feeds nutritionally complete in 1000–1200 mL volume

- specialised paediatric/adult feeds based on amino acids, peptides or soya (Tables 7.5, 7.6, 7.7, 7.11)

A case study to illustrate enteral tube feeding is given in Table 29.3.

Feeding regimens

The feeding regimen should be discussed with the child, their family and carers. Common choices are

- continuous
- bolus via syringe or gravity set
- slow bolus via pump

The choice of regimen will also be affected by whether the child is still allowed to eat and drink (safe swallow). The feed may be used merely as a top up after meals or it may replace all oral intake. Commonly, children who are at risk of aspiration may still be allowed to take small tastes of food for pleasure (as directed by the SLT) and this should be taken into account when calculating energy requirements.

If the enteral feed is to be the sole or major source of nutrition, it is common to give a small feed via bolus or pump at each mealtime to replace the psychological and physiological effects of a meal. Overnight feeding can accompany this type of regimen if a larger volume is required, but this should be used with caution if the child has a nasogastric tube due to the risk of displacement and aspiration, particularly as disabled children often have irregular postures when lying down. Overnight gastrostomy feeding can only be offered if the child can maintain a safe sleeping position, propped up to at least 30°. The use of a sleep system can help with safe positioning. The choice of feeding regimen may depend on the child's tolerance, particularly if gastro-oesophageal reflux is present.

Overweight

Gastrostomy feeding is beneficial for children with neurodisabilities who have oral or motor dysfunction and clinical signs of undernutrition. It aids weight gain; however, caution should be taken not to overfeed as children with CP have significantly higher body fat content and lower lean body mass [95,96]. Sometimes children become very overweight when enteral feeds have not been carefully monitored, or higher volumes (and hence higher energy) have been given to ensure a supply of minimum levels of protein and micronutrients. This can be a very difficult problem to rectify and has led to the precaution of underestimating energy requirements rather than overestimating these when feeds are initially started. A low energy paediatric feed or a reduced volume of an adult feed can be useful.

Monitoring and follow-up

Monitoring and follow-up will depend on the type of neurodisability, stage of progressive disorder and symptom control as it arises; therefore it is difficult to give guidance on frequency or method. There are often limited resources for regular review of these patients and dietitians may rely on other healthcare professionals, parents, or carers to highlight problems and monitor nutritional parameters for these children. Many of the children may be lost to follow-up due to non attendance at reviews. To minimise non attendance it is important to choose locations that are convenient for the child and their parents and carers, e.g. home, special school.

Weight gain is a crude guide to assessing whether the right amount of nutrition has been prescribed. Often the subjective opinion of the parent or carer on how well nourished their child appears is sought as a guide. However, these children tend to put on weight as fat rather than muscle and often do not grow taller no matter how much additional nutrition is provided [54]. Measuring body composition by taking skin fold thickness measurements can help clarify this quandary. The rate of growth and weight gain can be tracked using the child's growth chart. It is usual for many of these children to be tracking below the 0.4th centile for both height and weight and this is acceptable providing they are following the shape of the growth curve.

Children receiving tube feeds should be reviewed every 2–6 months, depending on their age, to monitor weight and height, assess clinical indices and alter feeds as necessary. These guidelines may be used for children feeding orally who are at risk of nutritional deficiencies or problems with growth. Monitoring nutritional parameters in blood tests for high risk children or those on tube feeds should be carried out every 6–12 months [69].

Table 29.3   Case study to illustrate enteral tube feeding.

A 2-year-old boy with quadriplegic cerebral palsy

Insertion of a gastrostomy tube and Nissen fundoplication procedure done simultaneously at the age of 18 months due to feeding difficulties, poor weight gain, constipation and severe GOR
Weight prior to gastrostomy placement 8 kg at the age of 17 months (0.4th centile)
Length measurement (using alternative measure) 77 cm (2nd centile)

He was established on full gastrostomy feeds of 800 mL Paediasure, 1 kcal/mL (4 kJ/mL) given as 130 mL × 4 boluses through the day (intermittent with feeding pump)
35 mL/hour over 8 hours continuously overnight (via feeding pump)
He was allowed tastes of puréed food 1–2 times per day as recommended by the SLT

He was not reviewed for 6 months post gastrostomy placement. The dietitian visited at home at age 2 years and on assessment his weight gain had been rapid: weight = 11 kg (9th–25th centile)

Clinically he appeared overweight, well hydrated with regular bowel movements, adequate absorption of feeds with no feed loss due to vomiting
Alternative length measurement was taken: tibial length = 15.4 cm
Using Stevenson's formula [55], this equates to standing height = 81 cm (2nd centile)

Plan at 2 years of age Feed changed to 800 mL Nutrini Low Energy Multifibre, 0.75 kcal/mL (3 kJ/mL) = 600 kcal (2510 kJ)/day
Although fluid requirement for 11 kg child was 1050 mL/day (p. 16) he was well hydrated on 800 mL total fluid volume (assessment of bowel movements, urine output and concentration, alertness and skin turgor)

Follow up at 2 years 3 months of age Further dietetic assessment undertaken
Weight 11.9 kg (>25th centile for age)
Rate of weight gain had slowed down; however, still too rapid when plotted on UK-WHO growth chart and CP [63] growth charts. He is not mobile therefore his requirements are much lower than originally estimated. He continued to gain weight on a low energy feed

Plan at 2 years 3 months of age Volume of Nutrini Low Energy Multifibre further reduced to 500 mL providing 375 kcal (1570 kJ)/day: 30% of EAR energy for actual age, equivalent to 32 kcal (135 kJ)/kg

Additional water flushes of 300 mL to be given to meet his fluid requirement of 800 mL/day. The reduced feed volume does not meet RNI for micronutrients. Consider the addition of Paediatric Seravit and Dioralyte to improve the nutritional profile:

Nutrient	RNI (1-3-year-old-boy)	Daily requirements based on 10.9 kg (using height age)	500 mL Nutrini Low Energy Multifibre	Addition of 5 g Paediatric Seravit	Addition of ½ sachet Dioralyte (dissolved in 100 mL water)	500 mL Nutrini Low Energy MF + 5 g Paed Seravit + ½ sachet Dioralyte
Energy	95 kcal (400 kJ)/kg/day (EAR)	1036 kcal (4330 kJ)	375 kcal (1570 kJ)	14 kcal (58 kJ)		389 kcal (1625 kJ) 36 kcal (150 kJ)/kg
Protein	1.1 g/kg/day	12 g	10.5 g	–	–	10.5 g (1 g/kg/day)
Sodium	1.7 mmol/kg/day	15.5 mmol	13 mmol	0.05 mmol	10.2 mmol	23.25 mmol (2.1 mmol/kg)
Potassium	1.6 mmol/kg/day	17.4 mmol	17 mmol	0.04 mmol	3.85 mmol	20.9 mmol (1.9 mmol/kg)
Calcium	350 mg/day	350 mg	300 mg	129 mg	–	429 mg
Iron	6.9 mg/day	6.9 mg	5 mg	3.50 mg	–	8.5 mg

Table 29.3   *(continued)*

Nutrient	RNI (1-3-year-old boy)	Daily requirements based on 10.9 kg (using height age)	500 mL Nutrini Low Energy Multifibre	Addition of 5 g Paediatric Seravit	Addition of 1/2 sachet Dioralyte (dissolved in 100 mL water)	500 mL Nutrini Low Energy MF + 5 g Paed Seravit + 1/2 sachet Dioralyte
Vitamin A	300 µg/day	300 µg/day	205 µg	210 µg	–	415 µg
Vitamin D	7 µg/day	7 µg/day	5 µg	2.80 µg	–	7.8 µg
Vitamin E	3.2 mg/day	3.2 mg/day	6.5 mg	1.10 mg	–	7.6 mg
Thiamin	0.36 mg/day	0.36 mg/day	0.75 mg	0.16 mg	–	0.91 mg
Riboflavin	0.5 mg/day	0.5 mg/day	0.8 mg	0.22 mg	–	1.02 mg
Vitamin B_6	0.7 mg/day	0.7 mg/day	0.6 mg	0.17 mg	–	0.77 mg

EAR, estimated average requirement; RNI, reference nutrient intake.

The addition of 1/2 sachet of Dioralyte in 100 mL water and 5 g of Paediatric Seravit makes up the requirements for vitamins and minerals. The GP and paediatrician were notified of the patient's feed plan and a request was made to monitor his bloods annually to ensure nutritional adequacy of the feed with electrolyte supplementation.

Complications

Faltering growth

Faltering growth, or low weight for height, has been well documented for children with neurodisabilities [97–100]. Studies show the positive impact of nutrition intervention for children with CP [101–104]. Sanders' prospective study demonstrated the importance of early intervention during the first year of CNS damage in order to prevent or reverse growth deficits [102]. Some studies have proposed that growth failure in children with CP is independent of nutrition [105, 106]. In addition, beliefs that it is 'normal' for children with severe disabilities, particularly children with CP, to have poor stature and low weights have often been ascribed to their underlying cerebral deficit or physical inactivity rather than to chronic malnutrition [102, 106, 107]. Normal parameters for identifying faltering growth may not be appropriate in this population. Many patients with neurodisabilities have malnutrition and growth failure as the result of inadequate energy intake [107]. There is evidence that the severity of feeding problems in children with neurodisability is directly related to the degree of faltering growth [6]. Resulting malnutrition is linked to poorer health status and reduced ability to participate in normal daily activities [70].

Gastro-oesophageal reflux disease

Gastro-oesophageal reflux (GOR) is the passage of stomach contents into the oesophagus. Gastro-oesophageal reflux disease (GORD) is GOR with secondary complications such as feeding difficulties, respiratory problems, faltering growth, abdominal pain and excessive regurgitation [108]. GORD affects 15%–75% of children with neurodisability [109]. The most important mechanism of GOR is the prolonged relaxation of the lower oesophageal sphincter. Other mechanisms are reflux and strain-induced reflux, when abdominal pressure exceeds the pressure of the lower oesophageal sphincter [110]. GOR differs from vomiting, the emetic reflex following ingested toxins which acts as a protective mechanism. Diagnosing GORD involves taking a thorough history and physical examinations. Oesophageal pH studies are used to diagnose GOR and involve insertion of a microelectrode probe into the lower oesophagus for 24 hours and measuring the duration and number of reflux episodes. Oesophageal pH studies will not show non acid reflux [111]. A barium swallow may be used to detect anatomical abnormalities. An endoscope and biopsies may identify oesophagitis, strictures and can help exclude Crohn's disease [111].

Treatment for GORD depends on the age of the child and the severity of GORD. Many symptoms of GORD may be indistinguishable from that of food allergy and therefore this will need exclusion with a trial of hypoallergenic formula [109]. In older children diet modification, weight loss (if overweight) and other lifestyle changes may help to improve reflux. Milk thickening agents do not improve reflux index scores but do decrease the episodes of vomiting. Elevating the cot or bed head when a child is sleeping may help, but drug therapy is mainly used to treat GORD. H_2 receptor antagonists, e.g. ranitidine, can help relieve symptoms and promote mucosal healing. Proton pump inhibitors, e.g. omeprazole, lansoprazole, are the most effective acid suppressants. Prokinetics agents, e.g. domperidone, are also used in combination with acid suppressants to accelerate gastric emptying.

Where drug therapy fails the child may be offered anti-reflux surgery as either a complete fundoplication or partial wrap [111]. Often a gastrostomy tube is placed at the same time. Complications such as dumping syndrome, gas bloating and retching can occur (p. 150). If underlying oesophageal dysmotility still remains and if retching or attempted vomiting are not controlled by continuing drug therapy, slippage or unwrapping of the fundoplication can occur [111]. An alternative to fundoplication for children on tube feeds is for a change to transpyloric feeding via nasojejunal (NJ) tube; percutaneous endoscopic jejunostomy (PEJ); or percutaneous endoscopic gastrostomy with jejunal tube (PEG-J). The latter two procedures have been shown to improve quality of life and to show decreases in aspiration pneumonia in children with neurological impairment, with similar rates of mortality [112, 113]. However, small amounts of reflux may still occur with transpyloric feeding [114].

Constipation

Constipation is a common problem for children with neurodevelopmental disabilities with an estimated prevalence of 26%–74% depending on the definition [1, 115, 116]. There is often a delay in recognising and treating the problem either because of the inability of the child to communicate effectively; or because constipation is accepted as inevitable; or because higher priority has been given to other aspects of the child's medical management [117]. There are multiple factors predisposing to constipation, both neurological and

lifestyle. Colonic transit times are prolonged and some children have problems with coordination in anal sphincter and pelvic floor muscles [118]. It is generally felt that constipation is related to poor ambulatory function with CNS damage being suggested as an important risk factor [118]. Constipation has also been linked with medications, particularly those known to slow intestinal motility [117].

Dietary fibre and fluid intakes in these children are often poor. One study found 41% of children took ≥6 g less than the recommended fibre intake and 87% did not meet the minimum recommended fluid intake. Despite this, no significant correlation between fibre or water intake and constipation was found [117]. Other studies have demonstrated a reduction in constipation when dietary fibre intake was increased and Evans et al. concluded that the use of fibre containing feeds should become standard practice in tube fed children, although they advised increasing the amount of fibre in these feeds as many children did not meet recommended intakes due to the small feed volumes taken [79, 119, 120].

National Institute for Health and Care Excellence (NICE) guidelines recommend a clear treatment for constipation, starting with disimpaction and then maintenance of regular and painless defaecation. Laxatives are recommended as first line treatment, starting with polyethylene glycol, e.g. Movicol, and then moving on to stimulant or osmotic laxatives as necessary. Dietary manipulations are recommended alongside laxatives but not as a first line treatment [79, 121]. There is no well studied treatment regimen for children with neurodevelopmental disabilities with constipation but a consistent approach with clear instructions for carers on how and when to adjust medications is recommended [117, 120]. A diary can be useful in assessing response to treatment.

Dietetic assessment and treatment is necessary in order to avoid further nutritional compromise and supplementation with dietary fibre from food, enteral feeds or commercial preparations may help to normalise bowel function [122–125]. However, often simply increasing the child's fluid intake can have the most success [126].

Micronutrient deficiency

Studies on vitamin and mineral intakes and deficiencies in children with feeding problems are not well documented. However, nutritional assessment often highlights inadequate intakes due to poor variety, small quantities of food eaten and potential vitamin losses through liquidising foods or long cooking methods. Sodium and potassium intakes tend to be low; however, current opinion is that a level between the RNI and LRNI for height age is acceptable provided urine and blood biochemical parameters are within normal ranges [22].

Osteopenia

Children with neurodisabilities are more susceptible to osteopenia (poor bone density) and increased risk of fractures because they are often non weight bearing and have limited exposure to sunlight. Many studies have found deficiencies in vitamin D status [118, 127, 128]. Long term use of anticonvulsant therapy has been associated with alterations in vitamin D and calcium metabolism [118]. NICE guidelines suggest that children are supplemented with vitamin D from 6 months to 4 years of age [129]. It is advisable that vitamin D and calcium intakes meet the RNI for age. It is thought that vitamin D deficiency can be prevented by taking an oral supplement of 10 µg (400 IU) of ergocalciferol or colecalciferol daily [130]. It is also important to ensure there is an adequate calcium intake.

For children at high risk of deficiency, a preparation with calcium and vitamin D may be indicated. There is limited evidence to show that routine supplementation of vitamin D and calcium is needed in children with neurodisabilities. Regular blood monitoring for bone indices should be done and supplementation given as indicated.

Dental caries

Boyd *et al.* conclude that 'Developmentally delayed children have the greatest diversity in nutritional and oral health needs' and that 'The special needs child will require early anticipatory guidance and intensive preventive dental therapy with frequent prophylaxis' [131]. Dental caries can be caused by a number of factors:

- poor dental hygiene due to hypersensitivity to teeth cleaning
- inability to clean teeth oneself and dependent on carers for support

- difficulty accessing oral cavity for children who have behavioural, structural or muscular conditions
- cariogenic effect of some medications due to sugar content or decreasing saliva production
- inability to clear the mouth of food after eating
- gastro-oesophageal reflux disease
- frequent consumption of energy dense meals and drinks
- children may be unable to communicate to carers that they have dental pain and therefore caries are not investigated promptly

There are some strategies to help prevent dental caries:

- teeth should be brushed twice daily with a small amount (a smear for children <2 years and a pea-sized amount for children >2 years) of fluoride toothpaste (1000 ppmF ± 10%). If the child is nil by mouth a cloth or suction catheter should be used to wipe away excess toothpaste
- Chlorohexidine mouthwash can be wiped over the teeth and gums using a pink sponge
- teeth should be flossed daily
- children should be seen by their local dentist biannually; they may advise topical fluoride application as a preventative measure
- children who cannot be treated by their local dentist should be referred to a specialist community or hospital dental team; they may also be able to arrange dental cleaning at hospital with sedation
- a dry mouth or decreased saliva production increases the risk of dental caries; Luborant artificial saliva sprays can be used for these children
- care should be taken when advising on diet and nutritional supplements for possible cariogenic effect on the teeth
- bottle feeding for prolonged periods of time should be avoided where possible and alternatives should be advised

Oral dysfunction and dysphagia

Oral dysfunction may result from either structural abnormalities such as high roof of the mouth, cleft, enlarged tongue, abnormal dentition or motor difficulties such as those seen in CP. Children with neurological impairment commonly have oromotor difficulties and these can occur in 30%–81% of children with neurodisability [118].

There are four stages of swallowing, all of which need to be functioning correctly for the safe and efficient passage of fluid or solids to the stomach (Table 29.4).

From infancy to childhood, as the CNS matures, certain reflexes usually disappear. Children with physical disabilities may keep some of these and, when coupled with abnormal movement patterns, they can make it difficult to coordinate the passage of food and fluids to the mouth. Table 29.5 summarises the effect of abnormal movement on eating.

Texture modification

In order to ensure a safe swallow and to allow for different structural, behavioural or reflexive movements the SLT may alter food and fluid consistencies to reduce the risk of aspiration and improve swallow. Dysphagia diet food texture descriptors are described [132]:

- normal diet
- texture B: thin purée dysphagia diet
- texture C: thick purée dysphagia diet
- texture D: pre mashed dysphagia diet
- texture E: fork mashable dysphagia diet

If fluid consistencies need to be altered the SLT may choose from

- normal fluids
- stage 1 thickened fluids (nectar like)
- stage 2 thickened fluids (honey like)
- stage 3 thickened fluids (spoon thick)

The required texture should be described to the carer, giving plenty of examples of ways of achieving the desired texture. The effect that cooling or warming the food may have on texture, the effect of stirring the food repeatedly and how saliva from the spoon will thin the consistency during a prolonged meal needs to be discussed.

Cleft lip and palate

Children with neurodisability may also have a cleft lip and/or palate. They are at risk of poor growth and nutrition because they may not be able to get an effective suck. Feeding adaptation may involve using different techniques when breast feeding, different shaped teats with enlarged or different positioned holes, soft squeezy bottles that may help the flow of milk, temporary maxillary plates, or if the child is unable to safely meet nutritional needs orally then they may be tube fed [133].

Table 29.4   Stages of swallowing.

Stage of swallow	What is happening	Difficulties that can occur at this stage
Oral preparatory	The process consists of head and jaw movements including voluntary opening of the mouth, lip closure around the utensil or biting food, transferring the food around the mouth including chewing, sorting and mixing to form a bolus and holding onto this bolus ready for swallowing	• Inability to open the mouth voluntarily • Inadequate lip closure • Overbite or tonic biting (biting down hard) • Tongue thrust • Oral hypersensitivity indicated by food refusal
Oral	This relates to the initiation of the swallow and involves elevation of the front of the tongue to seal the mouth, propulsion of the bolus by the tongue to the back of the mouth and raising the soft palate to provide a nasopharyngeal seal	• Lack of coordination of tongue movement • Incomplete nasopharyngeal seal
Pharyngeal	This is an involuntary stage triggered by the closure of the pharynx. The bolus of food is transported through the pharynx and into the oesophagus by peristalsis. Closure of the vocal fold prevents aspiration	• Ineffective function of peristalsis • Problems with pharyngeal anatomy
Oesophageal	This depends on the peristaltic action of oesophageal muscles to propel the bolus of food into the stomach and the contraction of the criopharyngeus muscle to prevent reflux	• Oesophageal obstruction • Gastro-oesophageal reflux

Table 29.5 Abnormal movements and reflexes affecting eating and drinking.

Name	Description	Effect on mealtimes
Asymmetrical tonic neck reflex	Caused by turning the head and triggers extension of the limbs on the side which the head is rotated and an increased flexion of the opposite side	Posture: the child can be difficult to position Feeding: the child may be unable to look at their hand and bring their hand to mouth Swallow: head turned severely to one side may prevent an effective swallow
Extensor thrust	Voluntary or involuntary strong push back of head and trunk	Posture: the child can be difficult to position Swallow: chin thrust inhibits effective swallow, may cause choking Oral: jaw thrust prevents mouth closure and can obstruct suckling and chewing
Startle reflex	Sudden extension of arms and opening of hands, stimulated by sudden noise or unexpected movements	Posture: the child can be difficult to position for self or assisted feeding Feeding: the sudden loss of posture may rouse feelings of insecurity Swallow: associated with a fast intake of breath which may cause choking
Rooting reflex	When cheek is touched, the head turns to that side	Oral: when head is out of midline, the configuration of the mouth changes including the jaw and lip positioning
Bite reflex	When mouth touched there is a sudden jaw closure	Oral: cannot coordinate jaw movement in order to introduce or withdraw utensil
Tongue thrust	Tongue moves in direction when touched	Oral: difficult to introduce food, retain food and deal with it in the mouth

Surgical repair of the lip and palate can occur any time from 4 to 12 months. Normal feeding can often resume if the cleft has been completely repaired [134].

Drug and nutrient interactions

Medications can have an impact on nutritional status by causing changes in taste, appetite, weight, alertness and/or gastrointestinal upset. This can be a problem when a new drug is being introduced and adjusted. Antiepileptic drugs (AED) can impact on bone health and are significantly associated with an increased risk of bone fractures and reduced bone mineralisation relating to lower availability of vitamin D. Supplementation with calcium and vitamin D can reduce the rate of bone loss and has been suggested as prophylactic treatment for all on long term AED treatment. Alterations in vitamin B and hyperhomocysteinaemia have been noted with long term AED treatment and B vitamin supplementation may be required [135].

Muscle relaxants such as Baclofen are commonly used for children with CP and other neurological conditions. If the dose is correct, posture for eating can be improved in children with spasticity. However, if the dose is too high then muscle weakness can lead to feeding difficulties.

Food can affect absorption of some medications making them more or less effective, e.g. phenytoin, which should be given 2 hours before or after a meal/feed.

Transition to adult care

The transition of children to adult care normally takes place when the child leaves full time education and this could be up to 19 years of age. Children are often very carefully monitored within a paediatric multidisciplinary team (MDT) and care should be taken to ensure that all relevant information is handed over to all the adult team such as dietitian, GP, hospital consultant, allied healthcare team and district nurses (where appropriate). There is often a transition period where a child will start getting used to daycare units and the MDT needs to support this transition. Parents and carers will need support as often adult services offer different facilities to children's services and they may find the change quite stressful.

Future research needs and unanswered questions

The following issues need to be addressed in children with neurodisability:

- long term use of adult enteral feeds and the effects of high micronutrient intakes over prolonged periods of time
- body composition, weight, height and BMI reference values
- the need for routine supplementation of vitamin D and calcium
- energy and protein requirements and whether the use of height age is a good estimator of requirements

Acknowledgements

Thanks to Sara Sabey, Sijbrigje Hood, Sue Williams, Eulalee Green and Caroline Culverwell for their help in reviewing this chapter.

Useful addresses

Down's Syndrome Association

Provides information and support for people with Down's syndrome, their families and carers, and the professionals who work with them
http://www.downs-syndrome.org.uk

The Down's Syndrome Medical Interest Group

An information and advisory service for health care professionals about issues concerning the medical care of people with Down's syndrome. Growth charts can be accessed through this site
http://www.dsmig.org.uk

SCOPE

A charity supporting disabled people and their families
www.scope.org.uk

The Bobath Centre for Children with Cerebral Palsy

Specialist treatment centre in London for children with CP and other neurological conditions
www.bobath.org.uk

Cerebra

A charity to help improve the lives of children with brain related conditions through research, education and directly supporting the children and their carers
www.cerebra.org.uk

National Institute of Conductive Education

A charity working to improve the lives of children and adults with motor disorders.
www.conductive-education.org.uk
www.redboots.org.uk

Capability Scotland

An organisation providing support for disabled people and their families in Scotland
http://www.capability-scotland.org.uk/

The Scottish Centre for Children with Motor Impairments

The centre provides educational and therapy services for children, young people and their families affected by cerebral palsy and related conditions
http://www.craighalbert.co.uk/

Norah Fry Research Centre – University of Bristol

The centre aims to make a positive difference to the lives of disabled children, young people and adults, with a particular emphasis on issues for people with learning disabilities and their families
http://www.bristol.ac.uk/norahfry/

Rett Syndrome Association UK

A charity supporting families affected by Rett syndrome
http://www.rettuk.org

Rainbow Trust

A charity providing emotional and practical support for families who have children with a life threatening or terminal illness
http://www.rainbowtrust.org.uk

The Jennifer Trust for Spinal Muscular Atrophy

Provides a range of information and support to families and health professionals as well as promoting and supporting research
http://www.jtsma.org.uk

Muscular Dystrophy Campaign

Funds research, provides practical and emotional support and awards grants for specialised equipment
www.muscular-dystrophy.org

Prader–Willi Syndrome Association UK

Provides information, training and support to improve the lives of people with PWS and all who are affected or work with them
www.pwsa.co.uk

30

Obesity

Laura Stewart

Introduction

Obesity is the most common childhood nutritional disorder in the world and is widely acknowledged as being a global epidemic [1,2]. In the UK the importance of implementing effective strategies for the prevention and treatment of childhood obesity has national significance with the publication of government policy documents [3,4] as well as evidence based guidelines [5,6]. The role of the specialist dietitian in the management of childhood obesity has now gained prominence. Dietitians may work with obese children and their families in primary or secondary care, utilising group or individual sessions [7,8]. Background information, lifestyle advice and the use of behaviour change tools that a specialist paediatric dietitian will require to manage childhood obesity in any combination of these settings are discussed.

Definition

The definition of childhood overweight and obesity associates excess body fatness with the clinical relevance of such excess body fat. Body mass index (BMI) is generally recognised as the most appropriate proxy measure for body fat to define and diagnose childhood obesity and overweight [2,5,9]. BMI in childhood changes with age and differs between the sexes; therefore it must be plotted correctly on age and sex specific centile charts (UK 1990 data). UK BMI centile charts are available from Harlow Printing Ltd (see Useful addresses) and all dietitians working in the UK with obese children and adolescents should use these charts [10,11].

There is a debate over the most appropriate centile cut-off points for defining childhood overweight and obesity; however, both the National Institute for Health and Care Excellence (NICE) and Scottish Intercollegiate Guideline Network (SIGN) clinical guidelines recommended ≥98th centile (UK 1990 data) for obesity and ≥91st centile (UK 1990 data) for overweight. For epidemiological studies ≥95th centile (UK 1990 data) defines obesity and ≥85th centile (UK 1990 data) defines overweight [5,6].

Data on waist circumference centiles for British children [12] are available on the reverse side of the UK BMI centile charts. Currently, with no agreement on the relevant clinical cut-off points for the waist centile charts, they are not recommended for diagnosis of childhood obesity [2,6,9] although they have a use in monitoring progress.

Clinical Paediatric Dietetics, Fourth Edition. Edited by Vanessa Shaw.
© 2015 John Wiley & Sons, Ltd. Published 2015 by John Wiley & Sons, Ltd.
Companion Website: www.wiley.com/go/shaw/paediatricdietetics

Aetiology

Obesity is the accumulation of excess body fat associated with medical consequences (p. 800). The aetiology of all obesity is both complex and multifactorial [13]. It is well recognised that the development of childhood obesity is an interaction between the modern obesogenic environment and family lifestyle choices. Increases in the amount of energy dense foods eaten combined with large portion sizes, more time spent watching television, using computers and playing video games (screen time) with a simultaneous decrease in the amount of physical activity undertaken by children have all been mooted as causes of the current epidemic [2, 14, 15].

Genetics

The polygenetic theory of obesity suggests that the most common genetic cause will be found to involve a number of genes which could 'predispose' a person to gaining excess fat, which in turn would lead to obesity if or when that person is then exposed to an environment which encourages the necessary behaviours, i.e. a high energy diet and low levels of activity [16–18]. It has been suggested that by identifying common gene variants that predispose individuals to obesity subgroups of obese people could be targeted for particular interventions such as specific diets, behavioural approaches or drugs [19, 20]. The Human Obesity Gene Map is an interesting resource to look for information in this area [19]. Research into polygenetics and obesity is complex and it may be some years before any findings can be of use in day to day clinical practice [17].

Although described as rare, monogenetic causes of obesity in humans have been found [16, 21, 22] with much of the research being carried out by the Genetics of Obesity Study (GOOS) group. The GOOS project recruited children from across the world who have severe obesity (BMI >3.0 SD), a strong family history of obesity and from consanguineous families. The GOOS has identified seven monogenetic causes of obesity [18]. Most of these have involved mutations in leptin production, leptin receptors, propeptide pro-opiomelanocortin (POMC) and the melanocortin 4 receptor (MC4R) [16–18].

Mutations in MC4R are believed to be found in approximately 3%–5% of people with a BMI >40. Mutations in MC4R appear to result in a range of phenotypes ranging from those showing no obesity to individuals with severe obesity (particularly at an early age), hyperphagia, increased lean body mass, increased linear growth and hyperinsulinaemia [16, 21]. Deficiencies in the hormone leptin are reported to produce morbid obesity (usually from a young age), increased appetite, hyperphagia and hypogonadotropic hypogonadism. Injections of leptin in these individuals have been shown to reverse the hyperphagia and morbid obesity [16]. Individuals with POMC mutations are reported as having severe obesity (from an early age), hyperphagia, altered pigmentation, usually red hair and adrenal insufficiency [16, 22].

Inheritable disorders

A number of known inheritable disorders have obesity as a clinical feature of the syndrome. Lobstein *et al.* [2] noted around 30 such inherited disorders; most are associated with learning disabilities and dysmorphic features. The most common inherited disorders associated with childhood obesity seen in routine clinical practice are

- Down's syndrome
- Prader–Willi syndrome
- Duchenne muscular dystrophy
- Fragile X

Endocrine causes

The endocrine glands produce hormones that are important in the regulation and maintenance of a stable body environment. In childhood they are important in ensuring normal growth and puberty. Dysfunction of these hormones can lead to hypothyroidism, growth hormone insufficiency, hypopituitarism, hypogonadotropic hypogonadism, hypogonadism, excessive corticosteroid administration, pseudohypoparathyroidism and craniopharyngioma, all of which are associated with rare causes of childhood obesity [23, 24].

Many of these endocrine disorders and the inheritable syndromes present with short stature as a clinical feature [23, 25]. There is strong agreement in clinical guidelines and practice that obese children who present with short stature for their age and weight should be referred to a paediatric endocrinologist for further investigation of possible underlying medical reasons for their obesity [2, 5, 6].

Consequences

There are a number of consequences of childhood obesity that are seen both in childhood and adolescence, and indeed later life. Clustering of cardiovascular risk factors has been reported in children and adolescents including high blood pressure; dyslipidaemia; abnormalities in left ventricular mass and/or function; abnormalities in endothelial function; hyperinsulinaemia and/or insulin resistance. There is evidence that these cardiovascular risk factors are seen in adults who were obese children or adolescents [26, 27]. Hyperinsulinaemia, the metabolic syndrome and type 2 diabetes are also seen in adolescents [28, 29]. Psychological problems, particularly in girls, have been reported in relation to low self-esteem and behavioural problems. There are also long term consequences of social and economic effects, particularly in women achieving a lower income [26, 27].

An important reason why tackling childhood and adolescent obesity is government policy is the evidence that obesity in childhood and adolescence tracks in to adulthood. Risk factors for persistence into adulthood include

- parental obesity (high risk if one parent is obese, higher if both are obese)
- level of obesity (increasing risk with increasing level of obesity)
- obesity in adolescence [26, 27]

Management

The role of the dietitian, either as a sole professional or as part of a multidisciplinary team, is to educate the child and family on the necessary lifestyle changes while facilitating behavioural change. A dietitian should be positive, non judgemental and empathetic while developing a rapport with the child and parents [30, 31].

For group sessions it is common practice to include some separate child and parents sessions.

Practice shows that parents value the opportunity to discuss situations and solutions with other parents without the child being present. For dietitians working with individual children and their families consideration should also be given to seeing the parents alone, as information is often revealed by parents that would otherwise not be discussed in front of their child [7].

Good practice suggests that different age groups require different engagement:

- for preschool and lower primary school age children the intervention, including ownership and responsibility, engagement directly with the parent/carer
- for upper primary aged children engagement jointly with the child and parent/carer
- for teenagers engagement directly with the adolescent, with the parent in a supporting role

Assessment

At the first session weight and height should be measured and plotted on child growth centile charts. BMI should be calculated [weight $(kg) \div height\ (m)^2$] and plotted at the correct age on the appropriate centile chart for sex (UK 1990 data). Although used regularly in research in clinical practice, arm anthropometry such as triceps skinfold measurement and mid upper arm circumference are rarely used. Taking the waist measurement can be difficult in obese children, but can be a useful tool in monitoring progress in weight management.

Lifestyle changes

Establishing current lifestyle

A 'typical day' scenario or a lifestyle diary is useful for establishing current lifestyle and is more child friendly for developing rapport [30, 31].

Behavioural change tools

Both NICE 43 and SIGN 115 guidelines concur that behavioural change tools in particular stimulus control, goal setting, self-monitoring, problem solving and use of rewards should be utilised in the management of childhood obesity [5, 6, 31].

Goal setting

Goal setting is used to help the child (and parents) to identify small and reasonable behavioural changes towards the long term target of positive lifestyle changes. Goal setting allows the child (and parents) to take responsibility and ownership for identifying the lifestyle changes they feel able to make and subsequently keep to these agreed goals [32,33]. The dietitian should facilitate goal setting by ensuring that the goals are SMART: Specific, Measurable, Achievable, Recorded and Timed [7,34]. Typically goals are written down to help with the continuing progress [35].

Rewards for reaching goals

Some programmes use 'rewards' for achieving the agreed lifestyle goal as these can be a positive reinforcement to both the setting and attainment of goals [33,36,37]. Rewards should be inexpensive, non food or screen time items such as a book, football or a family excursion. It should be remembered that praise can be a very powerful reward and should be utilised by the dietitian [35].

Self-monitoring of lifestyle

The recording of specific lifestyle elements by the child and/or parents is a key component of behavioural change tools which enhances motivation to change lifestyle by increasing self-awareness [33,36,38]. Monitoring the child's food and drink intake, physical activity levels and screen time in a diary/journal helps raise awareness of current lifestyle, helps to identify potential goals for changes and then monitors progress towards their goals [35].

Problem solving

Problem solving is used to help the child and their parents to identify barriers and then to explore ways to overcome these barriers [33,37]. A patient centred approach would recommend that the child and/or parent identify their own solutions to barriers and difficult situations [32,35].

It is also used in relapse prevention by identifying 'high risk' situations where keeping to goals could be difficult, e.g. holidays, parties and wet weather, and then exploring strategies to cope with these situations such as participating in an indoor activity during wet weather. Relapse prevention is particularly important at the end of the programme to ensure that the child and family maintain behaviour/lifestyle changes in the long term [35,37].

Stimulus control

Environmental/stimulus control involves identifying and then changing/removing stimuli or cues which encourage or sustain the 'unhealthy behaviour' and substituting cues that support/promote the new necessary lifestyle changes [37]. Examples include parents reducing the purchase of high sugar/high fat snacks in their shopping; or the child avoiding walking home from school past a local sweet shop; or a football being left at the front door to encourage physical activity after school [35].

Guidelines also recommend that parents should be encouraged to be role models for the positive behavioural changes required, i.e. they need to change their eating habits, physical activity and screen time behaviours and let their child see them undertaking these positive activities. Giving positive, concrete praise to the child when they undertake positive changes is also important to reinforce behavioural change [5,6].

Implementing lifestyle changes

As discussed, the aetiology of childhood overweight and obesity is multifactorial and management requires both energy in and energy out to be tackled. A Cochrane review of the treatment of childhood obesity showed that the most effective treatments were those which combined diet and lifestyle changes [39]. Therefore, the dietitian must facilitate changes in total energy intake, physical activity levels and screen time (sedentary behaviours) while using the behavioural change tools outlined above.

Dietary advice

A review concluded that no one particular type of dietary manipulation in childhood obesity was more effective than any other [40]. The child (and the whole family) needs to reduce the total energy intake in their diet while balancing essential nutrients. Collins *et al.* found that the traffic lights type scheme was the most commonly used [7, 36, 40–42]. Calorie counting is not normally used with children.

Children and their families should be encouraged to reduce the amount of foods and drinks in their diet that are high in sugar and fat and replace them with foods with lower energy content such as fruits and vegetables. Very importantly the dietitian needs to explore that age appropriate portions are being taken by all the family. This can often be the main area of education for the child and family. There should also be consideration of

- the number of takeaway meals taken
- the amount and types of snacks the child eats
- the amount of pocket money the child has
- school lunches

It is important to ensure that normal growth occurs when dietary intake is restricted and that age appropriate quantities of protein, vitamins and minerals are taken. There are some children who dislike certain foods and do not consume a nutritionally adequate diet and they may require a supplement of vitamins or minerals (particularly iron and calcium). Some children may therefore require regular assessment to compare their intake with recommended nutrient requirements [43]. Regular plotting of weight, height and BMI on approved growth and BMI centile charts is important.

Physical activity

NICE and SIGN obesity guidelines recommended that overweight and obese children undertake at least 60 minutes of moderate to vigorous activity per day [5, 6]. Recent physical activity guidelines recommend that children under 5 years who can walk unaided should take up to 180 hours of activity each day [44].

Many overweight and obese children dislike team sports and physical education (PE) at school. It is therefore important to help the child and family find local activities that they enjoy and are not embarrassed to take part in. In practice this can be done by working in partnership with local leisure/physical activity organisations. Increasing everyday 'lifestyle activities', such as walking, taking the stairs rather than lifts, has been demonstrated to be effective in controlling weight in the long term [36].

Sedentary behaviours

NICE and SIGN guidelines recommend that children reduce their screen time (watching television, using computers, playing video/computer games) to no more than 2 hours daily or an average of 14 hours over a week [5, 6, 45, 46]. For some children and parents this is the most difficult change to make and there needs to be a discussion how this reduction can be attained over time.

Infants and preschool children

The management outlined above covers all age groups; however, infants and preschool children may require particular consideration.

It is difficult to overfeed a breast fed infant, but bottle fed infants can be persuaded to consume a greater volume than they require; in addition feeds can be made more concentrated than recommended or items such as cereal can be added to the bottle [47]. In general there should no need to restrict an infant's diet, but for those gaining weight too quickly, or those who are already obese, specific advice on feeding and weaning practices and lifestyle will be necessary. The following advice may be helpful:

- make sure that parents react appropriately to the infant's crying; often crying is perceived as indicating hunger, when in fact the baby may be bored, tired or uncomfortable
- avoid any additions to the infant's bottle, e.g. sugar or cereal
- make certain that the feed dilution is correct and that the volume is appropriate for age
- solids should not be introduced before the age of 6 months
- weaning solids should initially have a low energy density, e.g. vegetables and unsweetened fruits
- reduced fat products can be used in the weaning diet, e.g. low fat yoghurts, reduced fat cheese
- when a greater variety of foods is being consumed, e.g. lean meat, white fish and cereals, the quantity of milk should be decreased

- infants should be introduced to a cup or teacher beaker from about 7–8 months of age and bottles omitted by 1 year of age; more milk is generally consumed when feeding from a bottle
- semi-skimmed and skimmed milk should not usually be used before the ages of 2 and 5 years respectively; however, these lower fat milks are a useful way of decreasing energy intake in the overweight toddler; it is important that a supplement of vitamins A and D are given with these milks
- drinks of water should be offered with and in between meals; if the child is reluctant to drink water, then pure unsweetened fruit juice (well diluted) can be given once or twice daily with meals

Adolescents

Adolescents present dietitians with their greatest challenge. Normal adolescent behaviours and peer pressure for the consumption of snack foods dense in fat and sugar can lead to resistance towards lifestyle changes. The lifestyle advice outlined above should be given, but with careful consideration of how to approach the adolescent to ensure that they feel ownership of goal setting and all stages towards behavioural change.

Slimming foods and medications

'Slimming foods' and drinks as a replacement for a meal are not appropriate as they generally contain insufficient protein, minerals and micronutrients to meet the requirements for this age group.

Drugs for the treatment of obesity are used in adults, although these have not been licensed for use in children or adolescents in the UK. NICE and SIGN guidelines both recommend that they could be used in obese adolescents with comorbidities under strict supervision [5, 6].

Written advice

Written information should be provided to support any advice that has been given. It is usual to record goals and rewards (if used). Nutrition and Diet Resources UK (NDRUK) has resources for dietitians and other health professionals to use.

The Caroline Walker Trust has very useful pictorial information on portion sizes. Written information on reading food labelling can be helpful, e.g. that produced by the British Heart Foundation.

Treatment success criteria

Current guidelines agree that the goal of childhood weight management for most children is weight maintenance, with height growth leading to a natural decrease in BMI. For some older children, and particularly those with very severe and extreme obesity, a weight loss of around 0.5–1.0 kg per month is acceptable [5, 6].

When reporting outcomes on programmes it is standard practice to report on BMI standard deviation (SD) scores, also known as z scores. There is a limited but mounting evidence base on the impact of BMI SD scores on reducing cardiovascular disease risk factors. The studies suggest that a reduction of between 0.1 and 0.5 BMI SD score after 1–2 year follow-up is significant enough to show changes in cardiovascular risk factors [48, 49].

Prevention

Promotion of a healthy lifestyle must start in childhood if the present trend in childhood obesity is to be reversed. Current government initiatives around healthy eating and increasing physical activities at schools may be helpful in the future. Dietitians, particularly those working in the area of public health nutrition, have a key role to play in prevention strategies.

Growth in infancy and the early years is an important period in relation to the risk of obesity later in childhood and adulthood. It appears that infants at the upper end of weight and BMI for their age, and also those who gain weight rapidly as infants, are at a higher risk of excess body fat and obesity later [50–53]. The Avon Longitudinal Study of Parents and Children (ALSPAC) has noted eight particular risk factors in early childhood that were significantly related to later childhood obesity [51]. These are

- parental obesity
- very early BMI or adiposity rebound
- more than 8 hours watching television per week at age 3 years

- weight at 8 and 18 months
- catch-up growth
- weight gain in the first year
- birthweight
- short sleeping duration at age 3 years

Prevention programmes which take place in schools and also target parents would appear to be an effective route. Prevention strategies need

to focus on the complex issues around childhood obesity involving diet, physical activity, sedentary behaviour, family lifestyle and environment. These interventions must therefore engage complex behavioural changes. An example of such an intervention is the school based Planet Health project, although this appeared to be more effective for girls than boys [54].

Prader–Willi syndrome

Introduction

Prader–Willi syndrome (PWS) is a rare genetic disorder in which genes on chromosome 7 are either deleted or unexpressed. PWS occurs equally in males and females and affects all ethnic groups. The main characteristics are hypotonia, short stature, hypogonadism, varying degrees of mental retardation (most patients with PWS score between 60 to 80 on intelligence quotient, IQ, tests) [55], short stature and poor emotional and social development. Children with PWS have an insatiable appetite leading to gross obesity, if not controlled, as the result of a chronic imbalance between energy intake and energy expenditure [56] due to hyperphagia, decreased physical activity and reduced metabolic rate. The prevalence has been estimated at 1 in 10 000 to 20 000 births [57] making PWS the most common genetic cause of obesity.

Historically two distinct phases are characteristic of this syndrome. At birth infants present with hypotonia and feeding difficulties and subsequently fail to thrive (Fig. 30.1). Tube feeding is often required during this period [58], which is typically from birth to approximately 2 years of age. It is from around 2–3 years onwards [59] that the second phase is seen with weight escalating as a switch from poor feeding to hyperphagia occurs. However, more recently a large US study has proposed a more gradual and complex range of phases. In total seven different nutritional phases are described (five main phases and two sub-phases) each with distinct characteristics [59].

The combination of behavioural and nutrition problems requires a multidisciplinary team

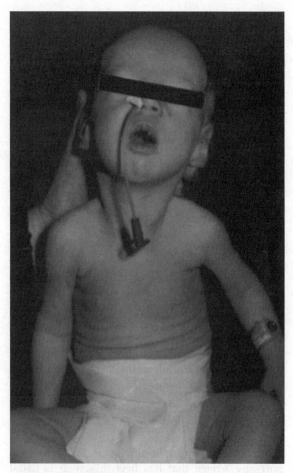

Figure 30.1 Infant with Prader-Willi syndrome.

approach to the management of individuals with PWS [55, 60]. It is important that dietary intervention and advice is given before the onset of weight gain in order that excessive weight gain is curtailed. Consistent dietary advice from all professionals must be given to parents and carers and the need to adhere to this explained. This can prove very difficult because of the hyperphagia associated with this syndrome. Gross obesity often occurs during adolescence (Fig. 30.2) and behavioural problems encountered during this period can add to the difficulties of treatment [61–63]. Weight can be controlled with comprehensive management.

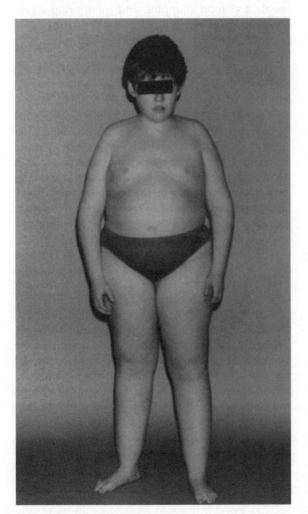

Figure 30.2   Adolescent with Prader-Willi syndrome (same boy as Fig. 30.1). With kind permission of Dr J.K. Brown.

Growth assessment

The inherent growth pattern of PWS children varies from that of healthy children (early childhood obesity, absent pubertal growth spurt and adolescent short stature) and subsequently plotting on normal growth charts may make growth interpretation difficult. PWS specific charts are therefore recommended for evaluating growth for comparison purposes, monitoring growth patterns, nutritional assessment and recording responses to growth hormone therapy. Several PWS specific growth charts have been proposed and produced from groups in Japan [64], Germany [65] and the USA [66] although there are no charts from UK data. More recent data from the USA [67] give detailed percentiles from birth up to 36 months, which were lacking in earlier charts. These are particularly useful for monitoring growth and nutritional status during the time of initiation and treatment with growth hormone, which is commonly beginning at a younger age.

There are thought to be no racial differences in growth patterns but interestingly on comparison the data suggest the degree of overweight is milder in Japanese children compared with Caucasian, with the same pattern reflected in adults [64].

Skin fold (infants with PWS show excessive fat as early as 6 months [68]) and electrical body composition measurements are useful in the long term monitoring of PWS children and are particularly useful for those on growth hormone where the often inevitable weight gain can be shown to be due to increased muscle mass.

Nutritional requirements

Due to low muscle tone and abnormal body composition the child with PWS requires a considerably lower energy intake than his or her normal peers. Limited studies have evaluated energy requirements and calculating specific energy requirements for PWS children is controversial. There is particular uncertainty on energy requirements for small children. There are several proposals for basing energy intake on kcal/cm (6–8 kcal (25–35 kJ)/cm height for weight loss and 10–12 kcal (40–50 kJ)/cm height for maintenance) which can be useful but most of the literature agrees that requirements are around 60% of normal energy requirements for age [68]. The US PWS association has proposed sample energy guidelines [69] but these are not based on prospective data and caution is recommended if using them. As with all children, the precise energy intake required will depend on BMI and level of physical activity. Micronutrient requirements do not appear to be different than age matched healthy controls.

Dietary treatment

Care is needed to provide sufficient energy and nutrients for growth without excess energy intake leading to unwanted weight gain. Prevention of over restriction, particularly in the younger more vulnerable infant, is of particular importance. Surprisingly, for a condition with fundamental links to dietary intake, there are very few systematic studies published on the actual nutritional intake in people with PWS. A Norwegian study, however, highlighted iron, vitamin D and calcium as particular nutrients that commonly fell below recommendations [70]; iron and calcium were also highlighted as commonly low in a similar UK based pilot study [71]. Low bone mineral density is frequently reported in PWS and therefore vitamin D and calcium are of particular importance.

In addition to awareness of likely low micronutrient intakes care must also be taken in ensuring balanced macronutrients and in particular fat. Historically a low fat intake was the diet of choice for management but several studies have suggested that over restriction of fat (<20% of total energy intake) can occur [70–73]. This is associated with polyunsaturated fatty acid deficiency, increasing the risk of associated negative consequences on development.

Several dietary modifications have been proposed for treating adults: simple energy restriction (6–7 kcal (25–30 kJ)/cm height per day); the 'red, yellow, green' diet that limits foods with higher energy density, sugar or fat; and general fat restriction [74, 75]. However, evidence based approaches in children with PWS are more scarce. A recent study proposed the principle of altering the proportion of energy from macronutrients in the diet (30% fat, 45% carbohydrates and 25% protein).

When compared with a simple energy restricted diet encouraging results were shown in both weight and body composition [72].

As a low energy diet may be lacking in some nutrients it is widely recommended that children have a daily vitamin and mineral supplement [68]. In addition ensuring sufficient essential fatty acid intake in the form of small quantities of polyunsaturated and mono-unsaturated fats is advised. Nutritional supplements such as coenzyme Q10 are widely used but there is no evidence for their benefit.

In addition to specific nutrient advice several practical restrictive interventions have been proposed including locking refrigerators, supervising meals and food shopping and monitoring access to spending money [76]. Maintaining strict control of portion sizes through standardised weights or measurements can also be very useful.

The preconception that PWS children will eat indiscriminately has been challenged by several studies. Joseph et al. conducted a small experiment offering PWS children and obese controls the option of a larger quantity of food delivered after a delay (15, 30 or 60 seconds) or a small quantity of food delivered immediately. Individuals with PWS selected the larger food quantity suggesting perceived differences in food quantity may be an important determinant of food choice [77]. Work has also suggested PWS children have food preferences with the same consistency over time as non PWS controls. One study showed PWS children consistently choosing to eat a small amount of a sweet tasting preferred food rather than a larger amount of a non preferred food [78, 79].

Attempts should be made to check any potential sources of food, e.g. from neighbours or friends. There are reports of children getting up during the night to eat, and inappropriate foods such as bread for the birds or dog and cat food are commonly eaten. The majority of the data on food behaviours supports the common theme that restricted but predictable food availability is an ideal model utilising the inherent behaviours of this group to the child's benefit.

Constipation is common in PWS children and usual dietary treatments and prevention strategies can be applied.

Regardless of the type of dietary treatment it is widely agreed that proactively starting on a consistent approach to mealtimes and intake before the child becomes hyperphaghic is a key recommendation for the long term successful management of the PWS child. In addition to this, understanding and appreciation of the psychological aspects are important. PWS children are preoccupied with thoughts of food and ensuring food security (such as the use of visual menus) is important in managing the difficult anger behaviours and limiting food seeking behaviours.

Communication with other health professionals is essential to ensure a consistent message and therefore consistent approach to management. Equally important is the emphasis of communication by the parents to the extended family. This should include family, friends, teachers and other carers to prevent them from undermining established and agreed management principles.

Growth hormone

Best practice in early intervention management in PWS now includes recommendations for growth hormone (GH) therapy. It is widely recognised that GH will aid height growth, promote leaner body composition, improve weight management, increase energy and physical activity, improve strength and agility endurance and respiratory function [80–82]. A Swiss study also showed it increases energy expenditure as a result of an increase in lean mass by an estimated 25% [83]. Work from the 1980s first suggested a link between maintenance of a lower body weight and improved intellectual performance [84]. A more recent 4 year longitudinal randomised controlled trial of 50 PWS children (aged 3.5–14 years) on GH treatment suggested it prevented deterioration in cognition function with the most benefit being seen in those with the greater deficit [85].

In a small study GH treatment showed improved body composition to be variable and suggested it increases total energy and fat intakes (although effects appear to vary depending on the developmental status of the child). It should also be noted that in this study the children on GH still had raised BMIs and the authors concluded that the treated children should have been on a tighter calorie controlled intake [73].

Activity

It is very easy for people with PWS to gain weight due to the combination of the overriding desire to eat coupled with the low muscle tone (if GH has not been used) which makes exercising difficult, slow and therefore no fun. However, activity is a key element of treatment. Increasing physical activity levels can increase energy expenditure and overall feeling of wellbeing. Some activities are physically difficult for the PWS child due to poor muscle strength, but walking and swimming can be accomplished by most and should be encouraged to increase energy expenditure. Contrary to some views it has been shown that during exercise individuals with PWS require as much energy as others with simple obesity for the same level of work [86].

Summary

The diet presents tremendous difficulty for the child, family, carers and school due to the insatiable appetite; food is uppermost in the thoughts of most children with PWS. Weight control and even weight loss, however, are achievable and are often associated with improved behaviour (due to the establishment of routines and rules that are clear), and importantly a sense of pride and achievement for the individual with PWS.

Dietitians must be aware that medical and other health workers may not have encountered PWS previously and may lack the understanding necessary to give proper support to the family. However, with a good multidisciplinary approach, agreed early interventions and careful appropriate monitoring, quality of life can be greatly improved for people with PWS and their families; individuals need support to ensure they reach their maximum potential.

Parents are encouraged to join the UK PWS Association charity for support and information.

Acknowledgement

Laura Stewart would like to thank Chris Smith, Senior Paediatric Dietitian, Royal Alexandra Children's Hospital, Brighton, for his significant contribution to the section on Prader–Willi syndrome.

Useful addresses

Harlow Printing Ltd

UK BMI charts
www.healthforallchildren.co.uk

Nutrition and Diet Resource UK

www.ndr-uk.org

Caroline Walker Trust

www.cwt.org.uk

British Heart Foundation

www.bhf.org.uk

Prader-Willi Syndrome Association PWSA (UK)

www.pwsa.co.uk

31

Prevention of Food Allergy

Kate Grimshaw

Introduction

Allergic diseases, such as asthma, rhinitis, eczema and food allergies, are increasing worldwide [1–4] and the increasing prevalence of allergic disease is becoming a major public health concern, particularly in urbanised countries [5]. In the UK, allergic disease accounts for 6% of general practice consultations and 10% of the prescribing budget [6]. Add to this the impact allergic disease has on quality of life of both sufferers and carers [7–9] and that there is currently no cure, it is natural that attention turns to possible prevention strategies.

It is evident that allergic disorders change and progress from eczema and food allergy in infancy and early childhood to asthma, rhinitis and inhalant allergy in older childhood, adolescence and adulthood. This is referred to as the 'allergic march' [10]. Food allergy, let alone other manifestations of allergy, has significant individual, household and societal costs [11, 12].

Prevention of the first stage of the allergic march where the body reacts to a food protein after being exposed to it for the first time (known as allergic sensitisation) is the obvious course of action when trying to reduce the prevalence of all allergic disease. The infant's immune system which first comes into contact with food allergens *in*

utero [13] continues to be exposed after birth via breast milk [14], and then again when solids are introduced into the diet. It is unclear which, if not all, of these exposure time points are important in initiating the allergic march. This is why prevention strategies tend to focus on pregnancy and the first year of life [15].

It is reported that infants born to families with a history of atopy are more at risk of developing allergic diseases than those born to non-atopic families [16], with genetic influences definitely playing a role [17–19]. This means that some infants are more likely to develop allergic disease compared with others and are described as 'high risk'. Much research into the development of food allergy is carried out in these high risk populations and it needs to be remembered that findings from such studies may not be applicable to the general population.

Strategies during pregnancy

It is well established that early life factors influence the development of all atopic disease, including food allergy [20], with research showing that events taking place during pregnancy and foetal development play a key role in determining whether an infant will develop allergic disease [13, 15, 21–23].

Nutritional factors affect the development and function of the immune system [24] and since the foetus is solely dependent on the mother for its nutrition, it stands to reason that the maternal diet during pregnancy will affect the immune development of the foetus and therefore the likelihood of it developing food allergy.

Dietary antigens

It has been known for many years that cord blood contains immunological factors which demonstrate that the foetus has been responding immunologically to its *in utero* environment [25]. Consequently, it was hypothesised that if mothers eliminate dietary antigens from their diet whilst pregnant it would reduce the risk of the child developing an allergic disease. The first randomised controlled trial to investigate this hypothesis was carried out by Falth-Magnusson and Kjellman [26], with a number of similar trials being carried out subsequently [27–29]. None of these studies demonstrated a reduction in allergy risk associated with maternal allergen avoidance.

Due to the inconclusive results of these intervention studies, and concerns that allergen avoidance diets may adversely affect maternal nutrient status, allergen avoidance during pregnancy is no longer recommended as an allergy prevention measure [15, 30, 31]. In 2009 the UK Department of Health (DH) altered its previous advice (1998) concerning avoidance of peanuts during pregnancy, stating avoidance was no longer recommended [32].

Polyunsaturated fatty acids

Intake of long chain polyunsaturated fatty acids (LCPUFA) increased over the latter part of the twentieth century as a result of health concerns regarding the consumption of saturated fats [33] and this increase has been causally linked to the increase in allergic diseases [34, 35]. This possible link is backed up by epidemiological observations [36–38] and is mechanistically explained by the fact that LCPUFA are precursors for eicosanoid inflammatory factors including prostaglandins (PG) and leukotrienes (LT). These inflammatory factors are involved in modulating and controlling immune responses. Prostaglandins and leukotrienes such as PGE_2 and LTB_4 which are derived from n-6 LCPUFA (e.g. sunflower oil) via arachidonic acid (AA) strongly promote inflammatory responses and play a role in allergic sensitisation, whereas n-3 LCPUFA lead to the production of the less biologically active prostaglandins and leukotrienes such as PGE_3 and LTB_5 via eicosapentaenoic acid (EPA) and docosahexaenoic acid (DHA) [39].

There are intervention studies where the maternal diet has been supplemented with fish oils [40, 41] and whilst they demonstrated immunological changes in cord blood, they can only suggest at improved clinical outcome [39]. A recent intervention study of salmon supplementation during pregnancy showed no difference in total IgE sensitisation and atopic dermatitis in infants at 6 months of age [42]. Further intervention studies are being carried out, but in the meantime encouraging mothers to eat the recommended two portions of oily fish a week [43] appears sensible.

Probiotics

Intestinal microbiota play an important role in the development of the mucosal and systemic immune system [44]. Observational studies show differences in gut microbiota composition between atopic and non-atopic infants and, since they already exist in the first few weeks of life, a causal relationship is suggested [45–47]. Consequently, manipulating the intestinal microflora of atopic children, using probiotics, towards a more 'non-atopic flora' could be a way to prevent allergic diseases. There have been a number of trials to investigate the ability of probiotics to prevent allergic disease in high risk infants, but these studies have mainly focused on atopic dermatitis and not on food allergy and have conflicting results [48–52]. These findings need to be repeated in similar studies using more readily available probiotics before mothers are advised to take probiotics during pregnancy.

Vitamins and minerals

A number of vitamins and minerals are thought to have a role in the development of allergic disease including vitamins C, D and E and folic acid. The role of vitamin D in the development of allergy was first proposed in 1999 [53]. Since then its role has been strongly debated and, whilst the first papers advocated that increased vitamin D supplementation was the cause of rising allergy prevalence [54–56], others have since argued the protective effect of vitamin D [57–61]. There are currently intervention studies taking place, looking particularly at the role of maternal vitamin D exposure and food allergy in their offspring, to try and clarify the role of vitamin D in allergy development.

Other vitamins suggested to have a role in allergy prevention are vitamins C and E. A recent review stated that, although the studies that had found a positive relationship between these vitamins and allergy outcome were methodologically weak, the possible relationships warranted further work [62].

There are studies looking at the relationship between folate and allergic disease. Two studies have shown a positive relationship between increased folate intake and subsequent allergic disease [63,64]. A third study looked at serum folate and total immunoglobulin E (IgE) levels and demonstrated an inverse association [65]. Since folate supplementation is widely advocated for pregnant women to protect against neural tube defects, further research studies have been urgently called for to investigate the relationship between maternal folate intake and allergy development [66].

'Healthy' diet

A change in diet to one that could be considered to be less healthy has been hypothesised as a reason for the observed increase in the prevalence of asthma and allergic disease since the 1970s [34,67]. However, the studies considering the 'healthfulness' of the diet, by looking at different dietary constituents, have used different outcome measures and different methodologies. This makes it difficult to interpret the findings in relation to the 'healthfulness' of maternal diet and allergy outcome. Three studies found an association between constituents of the maternal diet and wheeze in their offspring [37,68,69]; however, another found no association [70]. A meta-analysis [62] concluded that there was a (weak) protective effect of fruit and vegetable intake in the development of asthma

and allergy and also a weak protective effect of a 'Mediterranean' diet for asthma outcome. More research in this field is required.

Additional evidence pointing to the importance of a 'full' maternal diet in allergy prevention is emerging [71]. Consequently, recommending a healthy balanced maternal diet with sufficient portions of fruit, vegetable and n-3 fatty acids with no avoidance of any foods seems the sensible way forward.

Infant feeding strategies

In 2001 the World Health Organization (WHO) recommended exclusive breast feeding for the first 6 months of an infant's life and the nutrient adequacy of exclusive breast feeding for the term infant during this period is documented [72]. The UK Scientific Advisory Committee on Nutrition (SACN) states there is sufficient evidence to suggest that exclusive breast feeding for 6 months is nutritionally adequate [73]. Exclusive breast feeding provides both passive and active support of the infant's gut function during the first 6 months of life and should therefore be recommended for general health [74]. It is unclear at present whether this is applicable for allergy prevention *per se*.

Breast feeding and the development of allergic disease

Breast milk is thought to play an important role in the development of oral tolerance as there are a number of components in breast milk that are important in protecting the infant from microbial/antigen attack [75]. Some of these factors initiate the innate immune response, but some are closely involved in the development of the infant's adaptive immune system (p. 335). Immunological factors in breast milk consist of maternal immunoglobulins, oligosaccharides, cytokines, glycoproteins, LCPUFA, lysozyme, nucleotides and complement. Many of these are thought to have a role in the development of oral tolerance, in particular transforming growth factor beta (TGF-β) [76,77], interleukin-12 (IL-12) [78] and soluble cluster of differentiation 14 (CD14) [79]. Additionally, secretory IgA in breast milk is thought to shield the breast fed infant's gut-associated lymphoid tissue from dietary allergens, thereby reducing local immunostimulation and contributing to the establishment of oral tolerance [14].

However, the role of breast milk in allergy development remains unclear with studies showing protection, no effect and even increased risk. This has been explained by the fact that the levels of nutritive and bioactive factors in breast milk vary according to the nutritional and atopic status of the mother [75, 80, 81]. When levels of cytokines in the milk are taken into account then a relationship is seen [82]. Due to these findings, and that a number of randomised controlled trials in high risk infants investigating the effect of different dietary allergy prevention programmes during breast feeding [83, 84] or pregnancy and breast feeding [29, 85, 86] found no real benefit, maternal dietary intervention during lactation to reduce allergy risk is no longer recommended [15, 30, 31].

Another explanation for the apparently conflicting findings of the role of breast milk on allergy development is that the immunomodulatory effect of breast milk is only apparent when the infant's immune system is exposed to a food at the same time as breast milk [87–89]. This possible relationship requires further investigation.

Despite these conflicting findings, breast feeding is recommended for all infants due to its nutritional, immunological and psychological benefits, and it should ideally be continued whilst allergenic solids are introduced to the infant's diet [90–92].

Infant formula and allergy prevention

It has long been agreed that feeding with a whole protein infant formula compared with breast feeding increases the risk of the child developing allergic disease [93]. However, there will always be a demand for alternative feeding for mothers who cannot or choose not to breast feed so it is important that the risk of allergy development associated with infant formula use should be reduced. This has been achieved by using alternative protein sources to whole cow's milk such as soya or hydrolysed cow's milk protein.

Soya infant formula

The use of soya based infant formula differs throughout the world and there has been a debate around its use and whether it leads to

an increased likelihood of allergy to soya [94–96]. A meta-analysis in 2006 [97] concluded that soya formula should not be recommended for the treatment of cow's milk allergy in infants and, more recently, the American Academy of Pediatrics and EAACI have stated that soya formula should not be used for the prevention of food allergy [15, 30].

Hydrolysed protein infant formulas

There have been a number of studies examining the merits of hydrolysed protein infant formulas as a primary prevention for allergic disease. Intervention studies in high risk infants who are not breast fed have compared both partially and extensively hydrolysed cow's milk formulas with formulas based on intact (whole) cow's milk protein. In two studies, a protective effect of hydrolysed infant formulas was found [98, 99] while in three other studies no difference was seen [100–102]. The German Infant Nutritional Intervention (GINI) study examined three different hydrolysed infant formulas and standard infant formula, comparing different allergy outcomes between the groups. Both the extensively hydrolysed casein formula and partially hydrolysed whey formula were shown to have a preventative effect on both physician diagnosis of allergic manifestation and atopic dermatitis. Inexplicably, this was not found for the extensively hydrolysed whey formula [103]. It is because of these somewhat contradictory findings that recommendations regarding prevention may not specify whether an extensively or partially hydrolysed formula should be used, but that the formula should be of 'proven reduced allergenicity' [31]. Both extensively hydrolysed (e.g. Nutramigen Lipil, casein based; Aptamil Pepti, whey based) and partially hydrolysed formulas (e.g. SMA HA) have shown an allergy preventative effect [104].

A Cochrane review in 2006 [105] concluded that 'there is no evidence to support feeding with a hydrolysed formula for the prevention of allergy compared to exclusive breast feeding. In high risk infants who are unable to be exclusively breast fed, there is limited evidence that prolonged feeding with a hydrolysed formula compared to a cow's milk formula reduces infant and childhood allergy and infant cow's milk allergy'.

The European Academy of Allergy and Clinical Immunology (EAACI) therefore recommends that if a mother is not breast feeding she should use an infant formula with 'documented reduced allergenicity'. This advice applies only to infants born into high risk families, i.e. mother, father or sibling suffers from documented allergic disease [15].

The introduction of solids and the development of allergic disease

In 2001 WHO advised exclusive breast feeding for at least 26 weeks of age [106] and this recommendation was supported by the DH in 2003 [107]; prior to this the advice in the UK was for solids to be introduced between 4 and 6 months (but not before 17 weeks) [108]. The necessity for exclusive breast feeding for 26 weeks has recently been called into question [109]. The ideal age for the introduction of foods in the context of the prevention of allergy is controversial and is currently being considered by SACN.

The first studies in this field in the 1980s were observational. Fergusson *et al.* looked at both the timing and rate of introduction of solids into an infant diet with the later development of eczema at 2 years of age [110] and found that solid food introduction before 4 months of age and the number of foods introduced was associated with an increased incidence of physician reported eczema. This association persisted to 10 years of age [111]. Kajosaari and Saarinen compared the early introduction of allergenic foods with introduction after 6 months of age and showed no differences in the prevalence of food allergy, either in the first year of life [112] or at age 5 years [113]. A number of similar studies followed and a systematic review looking at complementary feeding before 4 months of age could find few data linking early solid feeding and allergic conditions other than an association with early solids introduction and persistent eczema [114]. However, a recent study using data collected from prospective food diaries has shown solid introduction before 17 weeks of age to be associated with an increased risk of food allergy development [89].

From 2004 infant feeding data collected as part of birth cohort studies have been analysed to investigate the relationship between solid food introduction and the later development of atopy [115–118]. No study found any benefit on allergic outcome by delaying the introduction of solids and two found an association

between the delayed introduction of milk [117] and egg [116, 118] and increased incidence of eczema and atopic sensitisation. More recently it has been suggested that children exposed to cereal grains before 6 months of age (as opposed to after 6 months of age) are protected from the development of wheat specific IgE [119]. However, all studies collected feeding data retrospectively which makes the findings vulnerable to both recall bias and reverse causality. Nevertheless, these studies have raised the possibility that delaying the introduction of foods into an infant's diet (particularly delaying the introduction of allergenic foods) is not beneficial and may actually increase the risk of the child developing allergic diseases, as suggested recently by a number of authors [115–120].

A different way of looking at these findings is that delayed introduction may lead to a nutrient difference in the infant diet which has an effect on allergy development. For example, two papers have reported an association between the delayed introduction of egg into an infant's diet and increased allergy risk [115, 121]; this association may not be due to the timing of egg into the diet *per se*, but the fact that delaying the introduction of egg may lead to a diet with lower levels of immunologically active nutrients, namely vitamins A and D, zinc and selenium. Additionally, there have been reports of an association between fish introduction into an infant's diet and allergy outcome with early introduction reducing the risk of allergic disease [122, 123]. Again, this association may not be due to delaying the introduction of the allergenic food (fish) into the diet, but to a reduced intake of LCPUFA, selenium, zinc and vitamin D, all of which have a potential role in the aetiology of food allergy [62, 66, 124, 125]. New research looking at infant dietary patterns and allergy development supports the theory that a full infant diet that meets current feeding recommendations is protective against allergy [126].

Whether weaning at 4 months as opposed to 6 months poses a higher risk for developing allergic disease remains largely unanswered. Until there is any research that definitely answers this question advice should continue to recommend exclusive breast feeding for 4-6 months [15], but that if it is necessary to introduce solids into an infant's diet before the age of 6 months then that food should be of low allergenicity (i.e. it should not contain milk, egg, wheat, fish, shellfish, soy, peanut, tree nuts and sesame) [127]. After 6 months there is no reason to further delay the introduction of allergenic foods since delaying the introduction of solids into the diet to prevent the development of allergic disease has not been shown to be beneficial [15, 30, 31, 90]. However, where there is a family history of allergy it is prudent to introduce allergenic foods one at a time, and in the case of egg to give it initially in a well-cooked form such as an ingredient in a biscuit [90]. In the case of peanuts the revised advice from the DH is that peanuts can be given after the age of 6 months, but if the infant already has another kind of allergy or is at a higher risk of developing a food allergy then mothers should talk to their GP, health visitor or medical allergy specialist before giving peanut to the child for the first time [32].

Other strategies (not food related)

An association has been shown between passive smoking (tobacco smoke exposure) and asthma [128] and also other allergic diseases [129]. An important allergy prevention measure is to avoid smoking during pregnancy and to ensure the baby is not exposed to tobacco smoke.

Exposure to high levels of house dust mite should also be avoided. Following anti-dust mite procedures, such as covering the mattress, ventilation of the infant's room, regular vacuuming and cleaning with a damp cloth, have been shown by one study centre to reduce sensitisation to house dust mite at 1 year of age and atopy at 8 years of age [130, 131]. However, these results need to be replicated elsewhere before such stringent avoidance advice is recommended.

Intake of anti-reflux medication during pregnancy has been linked to the development of allergic disease in the child [89, 132, 133] as has non-steroidal anti-inflammatory drug (NSAID) intake during lactation [89, 134, 135]. Further work is needed in both areas to substantiate any possible associations.

Recommendations

Although more research needs to be carried out in order to offer definitive allergy prevention advice, a number of recommendations can be made from the evidence base at this time. The following recommendations are taken from the consensus statement of the Food Allergy and Intolerance Specialist Group of the British Dietetic Association [90].

For all infants

- Mothers should eat a healthy, balanced diet during pregnancy and lactation, including all major allergens
- Ideally, breast feeding should be the sole source of nutrition until around the age of 6 months
- Standard cow's milk formula should not be given for the first 4–6 months unless the child has other forms of cow's milk in their diet
- Other milks, including soya and goat milk formulas, or non-formula off-the-shelf cow, goat, sheep, soya or rice milks, must not be given
- Weaning should never commence before the age of 17 weeks and any solids introduced between 4 and 6 months should be low allergenic foods
- Once weaning has become established with traditional weaning foods, then the introduction of high allergenic foods can begin
- Weaning foods should ideally be introduced whilst an infant is still being breast fed
- By the age of 12 months all the major allergenic foods, which would normally be suitable for a child of this age, should have been introduced into the diet
- Delayed weaning, beyond 6 months, could adversely affect the normal dietary and developmental milestones essential to establishing a good varied diet and may increase the risk of allergy development
- Avoid exposure to cigarette smoke during pregnancy as well as to the infant after birth
- The use of anti-reflux medication and NSAID should be kept to a minimum

Additionally, for high risk infants

- There is no evidence that delaying the introduction of allergenic foods beyond the age of 6 months is beneficial to at risk infants, but parents of high risk infants are advised to seek medical approval before introducing nuts into their infant's diet
- Recommended alternatives to breast milk are partially or extensively hydrolysed infant formulas with infants at highest risk being given extensively hydrolysed casein formula.

These hydrolysed formulas should be used for 4–6 months or until the time that cow's milk in any form has been introduced into the infant's diet

- When allergenic foods such as wheat, egg and milk are commenced, each food category*

should be introduced singly, starting with a small amount, e.g. ¹⁄₂ teaspoon (2.5 mL). No more than one new allergenic food group should be introduced at a time

- Avoid exposure to high levels of house dust mite

---

*Food category: for example, introduce wheat as one category by giving pasta, bread and other suitable wheat-based products, over a 2–3 day period [136].

Appendix I

L-amino acid supplements for phenylketonuria (data compiled February 2013).

Nutrient	Unit	PKU Anamix Infant	PKU Start	PKU Anamix First Spoon	PKU Squeezie	PKU Gel*	PKU Anamix Junior*	PKU Anamix Junior LQ*	PKU Cooler 10	PKU Cooler 15	PKU Cooler 20
		Nutricia	Vitaflo	Nutricia	Vitaflo	Vitaflo	Nutricia	Nutricia	Vitaflo	Vitaflo	Vitaflo
		Per 100 mL	Per 100 mL	Per 12.5 g	Per 85 g	Per 24 g	Per 29 g	Per 125 mL	Per 87 mL	130 mL	174 mL
Energy	kJ/kcal	287/69	286/68	168/41	565/135	339/81	474/113	497/118	261/62	393/92	526/124
Protein equivalents	g	2	2	5	10	10	8.4	10	10	15	20
Total amino acids equivalents	g	2.3					10				
Carbohydrate	g	7.4	8.3	4.8	22.5	10.3	11	8.8	4.7	7	9.4
Fat	g	3.5	2.9	0.15	0.5	0.02	3.9	4.8	0.3	0.5	0.7
Fibre	g	0.8	0	0	0.26	0	0	0.31			0
Vitamin A	µg	58.8	100	150	144	144	165	196	139	208	278
Vitamin D	µg	1.3	1.7	3.3	3.5	3.5	4.1	4.9	5	7.5	10
Vitamin E	mg	0.69	0.7	1.8	2.2	2.2	1.7	2.1	2.6	3.9	5.2
Vitamin C	mg	7.4	17	18.8	15	15	16	19	18	27	36
Vitamin K	µg	5.6	6	14.3	9.8	9.8	7.3	8.6	17	25	34
Thiamin	mg	0.08	0.05	0.19	0.24	0.24	0.27	0.33	0.4	0.5	0.7
Riboflavin	mg	0.08	0.1	0.19	0.29	0.29	0.32	0.38	0.38	0.57	0.77
Niacin	mg	0.33	0.9	0.85	3.4	3.4	4.4	5.1	4.2	6.2	8.4
Niacin equivalents	mg	1.1	1.7	2.9	7.4	7.4	7.7	8.7	8.4	12.5	16.8
Vitamin B_6	mg	0.08	0.04	0.19	0.26	0.26	0.38	0.44	0.4	0.7	0.9
Folic acid	µg	8.3	8	21	50	50	29	34.5	67	100	134
Vitamin B_{12}	µg	0.18	0.2	0.46	0.48	0.48	0.38	0.45	0.8	1.2	1.6
Biotin	µg	2.7	1.7	7	6	6	10.2	12.1	31	47	63
Pantothenic acid	mg	0.42	0.4	1.1	1.2	1.2	1.1	1.4	1.3	2	2.6
Choline	mg	13.7	5.2	34.8	67	67	23.2	27.6	100	150	201
Myo-inositol	mg	14.7	10	37.4	0	0	10.2	12.1			
Sodium	mmol	1.2	1	2.3	3.9	3.9	8.7	10.1	3.7	5.5	7.3
Potassium	mmol	1.9	1.5	3.4	5.6	5.6	7.3	8.6	4	5.9	7.9
Chloride	mmol	1.5	1	2.3	3.9	3.9	4.3	5.1	3.4	5.1	6.8
Calcium	mg	61.5	60	157	260	260	274	326	200	299	400
Phosphorus	mg	45	45	115	198	198	139	165	178	267	357
Magnesium	mg	8.7	6	22	40	40	47.9	56.9	63	94	125
Iron	mg	1.2	0.8	3.1	3.4	3.4	4.1	4.9	3.7	5.4	7.3
Copper	mg	0.065	0.05	0.16	0.19	0.19	0.32	0.36	0.37	0.55	0.73
Zinc	mg	0.86	0.9	2.2	2.6	2.6	2.9	3.5	3.7	5.4	7.3
Manganese	mg	0.06	0.07	0.16	0.41	0.41	0.23	0.28	0.5	0.8	1
Iodine	µg	12.5	10	31.8	33.1	33.1	29	34.5	42	63	84
Molybdenum	µg	1.8	4	4.6	12	12	12.5	14.9	24	36	48
Selenium	µg	2.3	2	5.9	8.4	8.4	16.2	19.3	14	22	29
Chromium	µg	2.1	2.0	5.3	17	17	8.1	9.6	14	22	29
Package size		400 g (Scoop 5 g)	500 mL	12.5 g sachet	85 g pouch	24 g sachet	29 g sachet	125mL	87 mL	130 mL	174 mL

(continued overleaf)

(continued)

Nutrient	Unit	PKU Anamix Infant	PKU Start	PKU Anamix First Spoon	PKU Squeezie	PKU Gel*	PKU Anamix Junior*	PKU Anamix Junior LQ*	PKU Cooler 10	PKU Cooler 15	PKU Cooler 20
Flavours/other		Contains prebiotics			Apple and banana	Raspberry, orange, unflavoured	Unflavoured, pineapple and vanilla, chocolate	Unflavoured, orange, berry	Red, orange, purple, white	Red, orange, purple, white	Red, orange, purple, white
Linoleic acid	mg	615	350	7			673	448			
α-Linolenic acid	mg	99	40	3			175	48			
Arachidonic acid	mg	21	30	26	126						
DHA	mg	10	15	26	63			60	67	100	134
EPA	mg								15	23	31
Dilution		15%		12.5 g to 10 mL		24 g plus 30 mL or 24 g plus 80 mL	29%				
Osmolality	mOsm/kg water	380	483		2240	3000 or 1540	1110	1320	1900	1900	1900

*Analysis unflavoured. DHA, docosahexaenoic acid; EPA, eicosapentaenoic acid.

Nutrient	Unit	PKU Lophlex LQ10 Nutricia Per 62.5 mL	PKU Lophlex LQ20 Nutricia Per 125 mL	PKU Lophlex LQ10 Juicy Orange/Berry Nutricia Per 62.5 mL	PKU Lophlex LQ20 Juicy Orange/Berry Nutricia Per 125 mL	PKU Lophlex Advance Nutricia Per 27.8 g	XP Maxamaid* Nutricia Per 100 g	XP Maxamum* Nutricia Per 100 g	XP Maxamum* Nutricia Per 50 g
Energy	kJ / kcal	245 / 58	490 / 115	246 / 58	493 / 116	385 / 91	1311 / 309	1260 / 297	630 / 149
Protein equivalents	g	10	20	10	20	20	25	39	19.5
Total amino acids	g					24	30	47	23.5
Carbohydrate	g	4.4	8.8	4.4	8.8	2.5	51	34	17
Fat	g	0	0	0	0	0.06	<0.5	<0.5	<0.25
Fibre	g	0.25	0.5	0.25	0.5	0.22	0	0	0
Vitamin A	µg	143	285	143	285	285	525	710	355
Vitamin D	µg	1.8	3.6	4	8	3.6	12	7.8	3.9
Vitamin E	mg	1.6	3.2	1.6	3.2	3.2	4.35	5.2	2.6
Vitamin C	mg	8.9	17.8	8.9	17.8	17.8	135	90	45
Vitamin K	µg	12.5	24.9	12.5	24.9	24.9	30	70	35
Thiamin	mg	0.21	0.42	0.21	0.42	0.4	1.08	1.4	0.7
Riboflavin	mg	0.25	0.50	0.25	0.50	0.5	1.2	1.4	0.7
Niacin	mg	3.6	7.1	3.6	7.1	7.1	12	13.6	6.8
Niacin equivalents	mg	7	14	7	14	15	22	28.6	14.3
Vitamin B_6	mg	0.29	0.58	0.29	0.58	0.6	1.4	2.1	1.1
Folic acid	µg	125	249	60	120	249	240	500	250
Vitamin B_{12}	µg	0.9	1.8	0.9	1.8	1.8	3.9	3.6	1.8
Biotin	µg	26.7	53.4	26.7	53.4	53.4	120	140	70
Pantothenic acid	mg	0.9	1.8	0.9	1.8	1.8	3.7	5	2.5
Choline	mg	76	152	76	152	152	110	321	161
Myo-inositol	mg	20.3	40.6	20.3	40.6	40.6	55.5	85.7	42.9
Sodium	mmol	<5	<10	<5	<10	<0.24	25.2	24.3	12.2
Potassium	mmol	<5	<10	1.3	2.6	<0.07	21.5	17.9	9
Chloride	mmol	<5	<10	<5	<10	<0.04	12.7	15.8	7.9
Calcium	mg	178	356	178	356	356	810	670	335
Phosphorus	mg	138	276	138	276	276	810	670	335
Magnesium	mg	53.5	107	53.5	107	107	200	285	143
Iron	mg	2.7	5.3	2.7	5.3	5.3	12	23.5	11.8
Copper	mg	0.26	0.53	0.26	0.53	0.53	1.8	1.4	0.7
Zinc	mg	2	3.9	2	3.9	3.9	13	13.6	6.8
Manganese	mg	0.27	0.53	0.27	0.53	0.53	1.6	2.1	1.1
Iodine	µg	29.2	58	29.2	58	58.4	100	107	53.5
Molybdenum	µg	12.5	25	12.5	25	25	100	107	53.5
Selenium	µg	13.4	26.7	13.4	26.7	26.7	40	50	25
Chromium	µg	5.3	10.6	5.3	10.6	10.6	40	50	25
Package size		62.5 mL	125 mL	62.5 mL	125 mL	27.8 g sachets	500 g	500 g	50 g sachets

(continued overleaf)

(continued)

Nutrient	Unit	PKU Lophlex LQ 10	PKU Lophlex LQ 20	PKU Lophlex LQ 10 Juicy Orange/Berry	PKU Lophlex LQ 20 Juicy Orange/Berry	PKU Lophlex Advance	XP Maxamaid*	XP Maxamum*	XP Maxamum*
Flavours /other		Citrus, orange, berry, tropical	Citrus, orange, berry, tropical	Juicy orange, juicy berry	Juicy orange, juicy berry	Unflavoured, berry, orange	Orange/ unflavoured	Orange/ unflavoured	Orange/ unflavoured
Linoleic acid	mg								
α-Linolenic acid	mg								
Arachidonic acid	mg								
DHA	mg								
EPA	mg								
Dilution %						27.8 g to 65 mL	1 to 7 / 1 to 5	1 to 7 / 1 to 5	1 to 7 / 1 to 5
Osmolality	mOsm/kg water	2400, 2240, 2390, 2460	2400, 2240, 2390, 2460	2460	2460	2710	690 (1 to 5)	1000 (1 to 5)	1000 (1 to 5)

*Analysis unflavoured. DHA, docosahexaenoic acid; EPA eicosapentaenoic acid.

Nutrient	Unit	Easiphen	PKU Express 15*	PKU Express 20*	Add Ins	Phlexy 10 Drink Mix	PK-Aid 4	Phlexy 10 Tablets	Phlexy 10 Capsules
		Nutricia Per 250 mL	Vitaflo Per 25 g	Vitaflo Per 34 g	Nutricia Per 18.2 g	Nutricia Per 20 g	Nutricia Per 100 g	Nutricia Per 100 tablets	Nutricia Per 200 capsules
Energy	kJ / kcal	688 / 163	310 / 74	416 / 99	359 / 86	291 / 69	1420 / 334	1601 / 377	1552 / 365
Protein equivalents	g	16.8	15	20	10	8.3	79	83.3	83.3
Total amino acids	g	20			11.1	10	95	100	100
Carbohydrate	g	12.8	3.4	4.7	0	8.8	4.5	6.5	0
Fat	g	5	0.05	0.07	5.1	0	0	2	0
Fibre	g	0.3	0	0	0	0	0	30	16
Vitamin A	µg	303	208	283	143				
Vitamin D	µg	3.3	3.3	4.5	1.8				
Vitamin E	mg	2.2	3.9	5.3	1.6				
Vitamin C	mg	37.5	27	36.7	8.9				
Vitamin K	µg	29.8	25	34	12.4				
Thiamin	mg	0.58	0.5	0.68	0.22				
Riboflavin	mg	0.58	0.57	0.78	0.25				
Niacin	mg	5.8	6.2	8.4	3.6				
Niacin equivalents	mg	13.3	12	16.3	7.2				
Vitamin B_6	mg	0.9	0.70	1.0	0.29				
Folic acid	µg	213	100	136	124				
Vitamin B_{12}	µg	1.6	1.2	1.6	0.87				
Biotin	µg	60	47	63.9	26.8				
Pantothenic acid	mg	2.1	2	2.7	0.87				
Choline	mg	135	150	204	76.3				
Myo-inositol	mg	36.5	0	0	20.4				
Sodium	mmol	10.3	5.5	7.5	0	<0.04			
Potassium	mmol	7.8	5.9	8.0	0	0.2			
Chloride	mmol	6.8	5.1	6.9	0			50	
Calcium	mg	400	299	407	178				
Phosphorus	mg	288	267	363	138				
Magnesium	mg	121	94	128	53.5			1.5	
Iron	mg	10	5.4	7.3	2.6				
Copper	mg	0.58	0.55	0.75	0.27				
Zinc	mg	5.8	5.4	7.3	1.9				
Manganese	mg	0.88	0.8	1.1	0.25				
Iodine	µg	45.5	63	85.7	29.3				
Molybdenum	µg	45.5	36	49	12.5				
Selenium	µg	21.3	22	29.9	13.4				
Chromium	µg	21.3	22	29.9	5.3				

(continued overleaf)

(continued)

Nutrient	Unit	Easiphen	PKU Express 15*	PKU Express 20*	Add Ins	Phlexy 10 Drink Mix	PK-Aid 4	Phlexy 10 Tablets	Phlexy 10 Capsules
Package size		250 ml	25 g sachet	34 g sachet	18.2 g	20 g sachet	500 g (with 5 g scoop)	75 tablets per tub	200 capsules per tub
Flavours / other		Forrest berries, tropical	Orange, lemon, tropical, unflavoured	Orange, lemon, tropical, unflavoured	Unflavoured powder added to food/drinks	Apple and blackcurrant, tropical surprise, citrus burst	Unflavoured		
Linoleic acid	mg	750							
α-Linolenic acid	mg	210							
Arachidonic acid	mg								
DHA	mg								
Dilution			25 g plus 80 mL	34 g plus 80 mL		1 to 5	1 to 20		
Osmolality	mOsm/kg water	1130	1896	2380		1172, 1140, 1180	349		

*Analysis unflavoured. DHA, docosahexaenoic acid; EPA eicosapentaenoic acid.

L-amino acid supplements for MSUD.

Nutrient	Unit	MSUD Anamix Infant (Nutricia, Per 100 mL)	MSUD Gel (Vitaflo, Per 24 g)	MSUD Anamix Junior (Nutricia, Per 29 g)	MSUD Anamix Junior LQ (Nutricia, Per 125 mL)	MSUD Cooler 10 (Vitaflo, Per 87 mL)	MSUD Cooler 15 (Vitaflo, Per 130 mL)	MSUD Cooler 20 (Vitaflo, Per 174 mL)	MSUD Lophlex LQ (Nutricia, Per 125 mL)	MSUD Express 15 (Vitaflo, Per 25 g)	MSUD Express 20 (Vitaflo, Per 34 g)
Energy	kJ / kcal	287 / 69	339 / 81	474 / 113	497 / 118	263 / 62	386 / 92	526 / 124	509 / 120	310 / 74	416 / 99
Protein equivalents	g	2	10	8.4	10	10	15	20	20	15	20
Total amino acids	g	2.3		10							
Carbohydrate	g	7.4	10.3	11	8.8	4.7	7	9.4	8.8	3.4	4.7
Fat	g	3.5	0.02	3.9	4.8	0.3	0.5	0.7	0.44	0.05	0.07
Fibre	g	0.8	0	0	0.31	0	0	0	0.5	0	0
Vitamin A	µg	58.8	144	165	196	139	208	278	285	208	283
Vitamin D	µg	1.3	3.5	4.1	4.9	5	7.5	10.1	8	3.3	4.5
Vitamin E	mg	0.69	2.2	1.7	2.1	2.6	3.9	5.2	3.2	3.9	5.3
Vitamin C	mg	7.4	15	16	19	18.3	27	36	17.8	27	36.7
Vitamin K	µg	5.6	9.8	7.3	8.6	16.5	25	34	24.9	25	34
Thiamin	mg	0.08	0.24	0.27	0.33	0.35	0.5	0.7	0.43	0.5	0.68
Riboflavin	mg	0.08	0.29	0.32	0.38	0.38	0.57	0.77	0.5	0.57	0.78
Niacin	mg	0.33	3.4	4.4	5.1				7.1	6.2	8.4
Niacin equivalents	mg	1.4	9.2	8.9	9.5	10.7	14	21.4	15.9	14.7	20
Vitamin B$_6$	mg	0.08	0.26	0.38	0.44	0.44	0.7	0.87	0.58	0.70	1.0
Folic acid	µg	8.3	50	29	34.5	67	100	134	120	100	136
Vitamin B$_{12}$	µg	0.18	0.48	0.38	0.45	0.78	1.2	1.6	1.8	1.2	1.6
Biotin	µg	2.7	6	10.2	12.1	31.3	47	62.6	53.4	47	63.9
Pantothenic acid	mg	0.42	1.2	1.1	1.4	1.3	2	2.6	1.8	2	2.7
Choline	mg	13.7	67	23.2	27.6	100	150	201	153	150	204
Myo-inositol	mg	14.7	0	10.2	12.1	0	0	0	40.6	0	0
Sodium	mmol	1.2	3.9	8.7	10.1	3.7	5.5	7.3	<10	5.5	7.5
Potassium	mmol	1.9	5.6	7.3	8.6	3.9	5.9	7.9	2.6	5.9	8.0
Chloride	mmol	1.5	3.9	4.4	5.1	3.4	5.1	6.8	<10	5.1	6.9
Calcium	mg	61.5	260	274	326	200	299	400	356	299	407
Phosphorus	mg	45	198	139	165	178	267	357	276	267	363
Magnesium	mg	8.7	40	47.9	56.9	62.6	94	125	107	94	128
Iron	mg	1.2	3.4	4.1	4.9	3.7	5.4	7.3	5.3	5.4	7.3
Copper	mg	0.065	0.19	0.32	0.36	0.37	0.55	0.73	0.53	0.55	0.75
Zinc	mg	0.86	2.6	2.9	3.5	3.7	5.4	7.3	3.9	5.4	7.3
Manganese	mg	0.06	0.41	0.23	0.28	0.52	0.8	1	0.53	0.8	1.1
Iodine	µg	12.5	33.1	29	34.5	42.6	63	84	58.4	63	85.7
Molybdenum	µg	1.8	12	12.5	14.9	24.4	36	48	25	36	49
Selenium	µg	2.3	8.4	16.2	19.3	14.8	22	29	26.8	22	29.9
Chromium	µg	2.1	17	8.1	9.6	14.8	22	29	10.6	22	29.9
Package size		400 g (Scoop 5 g)	24 g sachet	29 g sachet	125 mL	87 mL	130 mL	174 mL	125 mL	25 g sachet	34 g sachet

(continued overleaf)

(continued)

Nutrient	Unit	MSUD Anamix Infant	MSUD Gel	MSUD Anamix Junior	MSUD Anamix Junior LQ	MSUD Cooler 10	MSUD Cooler 15	MSUD Cooler 20	MSUD Lophlex LQ	MSUD Express 15	MSUD Express 20
Flavours / other		Contains prebiotics			Orange	Red	Orange, red	Red	Juicy berries		
Linoleic acid	mg	620		38							
α-Linolenic acid	mg	100									
Arachidonic acid	mg	20		48							
DHA	mg	10			60	67	100	134			
EPA	mg					16	23	31			
Dilution		15%	24 g plus 30 mL, 24 g plus 80 mL	29 g plus 100 mL						25 g plus 80 mL	34 g plus 80 mL
Osmolality	mOsmol/kg water	380	3000 or 1540	1130	1430	1900	1900	1900	2460	1896	2380

[a]DHA, docosahexaenoic acid; EPA, eicosapentaenoic acid.

Nutrient	Unit	MSUD Maxamaid	MSUD Maxamum	MSUD Aid 111	MSUD Five	MSUD Five
		Nutricia	Nutricia	Nutricia	Vitaflo	Vitaflo
		Per 100 g	Per 100 g	Per 100 g	Per 100 g	Per 6 g
Energy	kJ / kcal	1311 / 309	1260 / 297	1386 / 326	1411 / 332	85 / 20
Protein equivalents	g	25	39	77	83	5
Total amino acids	g	30	47	93	100	6
Carbohydrate	g	51	34	4.5	0	0
Fat	g	<0.5	<0.5	0	0	0
Fibre	g	0	0	0	0	0
Vitamin A	µg	525	710			
Vitamin D	µg	12	7.8			
Vitamin E	mg	4.35	5.2			
Vitamin C	mg	135	90			
Vitamin K	µg	30	70			
Thiamin	mg	1.08	1.4			
Riboflavin	mg	1.2	1.4			
Niacin	mg	12	13.6			
Niacin equivalents	mg	25.7	35.3			
Vitamin B_6	mg	1.4	2.1			
Folic acid	µg	240	500			
Vitamin B_{12}	µg	3.9	3.6			
Biotin	µg	120	140			
Pantothenic acid	mg	3.7	5			
Choline	mg	110	321			
Myo-inositol	mg	55.5	85.7	Trace		
Sodium	mmol	25.2	24.3			
Potassium	mmol	21.5	17.9			
Chloride	mmol	12.7	15.8			
Calcium	mg	810	670	145		
Phosphorus	mg	810	670	75		
Magnesium	mg	200	285			
Iron	mg	12	23.5			
Copper	mg	1.8	1.4			
Zinc	mg	13	13.6			
Manganese	mg	1.6	2.1			
Iodine	µg	100	107			
Molybdenum	µg	100	107			
Selenium	µg	40	50			
Chromium	µg	40	50			
Package size		500 g	500 g	500 g	30 × 6 g sachets	
Flavours / other			Unflavoured, orange		unflavoured	
Linoleic acid	mg					
α-Linolenic acid	mg					
Arachidonic acid	mg					
Docosahexaenoic acid	mg					
Eicosapentaenoic acid	mg					
Dilution		1 to 7 / 1 to 5	1 to 7 / 1 to 5	1 to 20		
Osmolality	mOsm/kg water	690 (1 to 5)	1000 (1 to 5)	330		

L-amino acid supplements for homocystinuria

Nutrient	Unit	HCU Anamix Infant Nutricia Per 100 mL	HCU Gel Vitaflo Per 24 g	XMet Maxamaid Nutricia Per 100 g	XMet Maxamum Nutricia Per 100 g	HCU Cooler 10 Vitaflo Per 87 mL	HCU Cooler 15 Vitaflo Per 130 mL	HCU Cooler 20 Vitaflo Per 174 mL	HCU Lophlex LQ Nutricia Per 125 mL	HCU Express 15 Vitaflo Per 25 g	HCU Express 20 Vitaflo Per 34 g	XMet Homidon Nutricia Per 100 g	HCU LV Nutricia Per 27.8 g
Energy	kJ / kcal	287 / 69	339 / 81	1311 / 309	1260 / 297	258 / 62	386 / 92	517 / 124	509 / 120	310 / 74	416 / 99	1386 / 326	390 / 92
Protein equivalents	g	2	10	25	39	10	15	20	20	15	20	77	20
Total amino acids	g	2.3		30	47							93	
Carbohydrate	g	7.4	10.3	51	34	4.7	7	9.4	8.8	3.4	4.7	4.5	2.5
Fat	g	3.5	0.02	<0.5	<0.5	0.3	0.5	0.7	0.44	0.05	0.07	0	0.19
Fibre	g	0.8	0	0	0	0	0	0	0.5	0	0	0	0.04
Vitamin A	µg	58.8	144	525	710	139	208	278	285	208	283		228
Vitamin D	µg	1.3	3.5	12	7.8	5	7.5	10	8	3.3	4.5		2.8
Vitamin E	mg	0.69	2.2	4.35	5.2	2.6	3.9	5.2	3.2	3.9	5.3		2.6
Vitamin C	mg	7.4	15	135	90	18	27	36	17.8	27	36.7		14.2
Vitamin K	µg	5.6	9.8	30	70	17	25	34	24.9	25	34		20
Thiamin	mg	0.08	0.24	1.08	1.4	0.3	0.5	0.7	0.43	0.5	0.68		0.3
Riboflavin	mg	0.08	0.29	1.2	1.4	0.38	0.57	0.77	0.5	0.57	0.78		0.4
Niacin	mg	0.33	3.4	12	13.6	4.2	6.2	8.4	7.1	6.2	8.4		5.7
Niacin equivalents	mg	1.2	7.7	22.7	30.3	8.8	12.5	17.6	14.6	12.5	17		13.6
Vitamin B$_6$	mg	0.08	0.26	1.4	2.1	0.4	0.7	0.9	0.58	0.70	1.0		0.5
Folic acid	µg	8.3	50	240	500	67	100	134	120	100	136		199
Vitamin B$_{12}$	µg	0.18	0.48	3.9	3.6	0.8	1.2	1.6	1.8	1.2	1.6		1.4
Biotin	µg	2.7	6	120	140	31	47	63	53.4	47	63.9		42.8
Pantothenic acid	mg	0.42	1.2	3.7	5	1.3	2	2.6	1.8	2	2.7		1.4
Choline	mg	13.7	67	110	321	100	150	201	153	150	204		121
Myo-inositol	mg	14.7	0	55.5	85.7	0	0	0	40.6	0	0		32.5
Sodium	mmol	1.2	3.9	25.2	24.3	3.7	5.5	7.3	<10	5.5	7.5		<1
Potassium	mmol	1.9	5.6	21.5	17.9	3.9	5.9	7.9	2.6	5.9	8.0		<1
Chloride	mmol	1.5	3.9	12.7	15.8	3.4	5.1	6.8	<10	5.1	6.9		<1
Calcium	mg	61.5	260	810	670	200	299	400	356	299	407	110	316
Phosphorus	mg	45	198	810	670	178	267	357	276	267	363	60	245
Magnesium	mg	8.7	40	200	285	63	94	125	107	94	128		85
Iron	mg	1.2	3.4	12	23.5	3.7	5.4	7.3	5.3	5.4	7.3		4.3
Copper	mg	0.065	0.19	1.8	1.4	0.37	0.55	0.73	0.53	0.55	0.75		0.42
Zinc	mg	0.86	2.6	13	13.6	3.7	5.4	7.3	3.9	5.4	7.3		3.1
Manganese	mg	0.06	0.41	1.6	2.1	0.5	0.8	1.0	0.53	0.8	1.1		0.42
Iodine	µg	12.5	33.1	100	107	43	63	84	58.4	63	85.7		46.7
Molybdenum	µg	1.8	12	100	107	24	36	48	25	36	49		19.9
Selenium	µg	2.3	8.4	40	50	15	22	29	26.8	22	29.9		21.4
Chromium	µg	2.1	17	40	50	15	22	29	10.6	22	29.9		8.5

(continued overleaf)

(continued)

Nutrient	Unit	HCU Anamix Infant	HCU Gel	XMet Maxamaid	XMet Maxamum	HCU Cooler 10	HCU Cooler 15	HCU Cooler 20	HCU Lophlex LQ	HCU Express 15	HCU Express 20	XMet Homidon	HCU LV*
Package size		400 g (Scoop 5 g)	24 g sachet	500 g	500 g	87 mL	130 mL	174 mL	125 mL	25 g sachet	34 g sachet	500 g	27.8 g sachet
Flavours/other		Contains prebiotics				Red	Orange, red	Red	Juicy berries				Un-flavoured, tropical
Linoleic acid	mg	620											
α-Linolenic acid	mg	100											
Arachidonic acid	mg	20											
DHA	mg	10				67	100	134	150				
EPA	mg					16	23	31					
Dilution		15%	24 g plus 30 ml or 24 g plus 80 mL	1 to 7 or 1 to 5	1 to 7 or 1 to 5					25 g plus 80 mL	34 g plus 80 mL	1 to 20	27.8 g to 65 mL
Osmolality	mOsm/kg water	380	3000 or 1540	690 (1 to 5)	1000 (1 to 5)	1900	1900	1900	2460	1896	2380	350	

* Analysis unflavoured. DHA, docosahexaenoic acid; EPA, eicosapentaenoic acid..

L-amino acid supplements for tyrosinaemia.

Nutrient	Unit	Tyr Anamix Infant (Nutricia Per 100 mL)	Tyr Gel (Vitaflo Per 24 g)	Tyr Anamix Junior (Nutricia Per 29 g)	Tyr Anamix Junior LQ (Nutricia Per 125 mL)	TYR Cooler 10 (Vitaflo Per 87 mL)	Tyr Cooler 15 (Vitaflo Per 130 mL)	TYR Cooler 20 (Vitaflo Per 174 mL)	Tyr Lophlex LQ (Nutricia Per 125 mL)	Tyr Express 15 (Vitaflo Per 25 g)	Tyr Express 20 (Vitaflo Per 34 g)	XPhen, Tyr Maxamaid (Nutricia Per 100 g)	XPhen, Tyr Maxamum (Nutricia Per 100 g)	XPhen, Tyr Tyrosidon (Nutricia Per 100 g)
Energy	kJ / kcal	287 / 69	339 / 81	475 / 113	500 / 119	263 / 62	386 / 92	526 / 124	509 / 120	310 / 74	416 / 99	1311 / 309	1260 / 297	1386 / 326
Protein equivalents	g	2	10	8.4	10	10	15	20	20	15	20	25	39	77
Total amino acids	g	2.3		10								30	47	93
Carbohydrate	g	7.4	10.3	11	8.8	4.7	7	9.4	8.8	3.4	4.7	51	34	4.5
Fat	g	3.5	0.02	3.9	4.8	0.3	0.5	0.7	0.44	0.05	0.07	<0.5	<0.5	0
Fibre	g	0.8	0	0	0.31	0	0	0	0.5	0	0	0	0	0
Vitamin A	µg	58.8	144	165	196	139	208	278	285	208	283	525	710	
Vitamin D	µg	1.3	3.5	4.1	4.9	5	7.5	10	8	3.3	4.5	12	7.8	
Vitamin E	mg	0.69	2.2	1.7	2.1	2.6	3.9	5.2	3.2	3.9	5.3	4.35	5.2	
Vitamin C	mg	7.4	15	16	19	18	27	36	17.8	27	36.7	135	90	
Vitamin K	µg	5.6	9.8	7.3	8.6	17	25	34	24.9	25	34	30	70	
Thiamin	mg	0.08	0.24	0.27	0.33	0.35	0.5	0.7	0.43	0.5	0.68	1.08	1.4	
Riboflavin	mg	0.08	0.29	0.32	0.38	0.38	0.57	0.77	0.5	0.57	0.78	1.2	1.4	
Niacin	mg	0.33	3.4	4.4	5.1	4.2	6.2	8.4	7.1	6.2	8.4	12	13.6	
Niacin equivalents	mg	1.2	7.9	7.7	9.3	9	12.5	17.9	15.5	12.9	17.5	23.5	30.3	
Vitamin B$_6$	mg	0.08	0.26	0.38	0.44	0.44	0.7	0.87	0.58	0.70	1.0	1.4	2.1	
Folic acid	µg	8.3	50	29	34.5	67	100	134	120	100	136	240	500	
Vitamin B$_{12}$	µg	0.18	0.48	0.38	0.45	0.78	1.2	1.6	1.8	1.2	1.6	3.9	3.6	
Biotin	µg	2.7	6	10.2	12.1	31	47	63	53.4	47	63.9	120	140	
Pantothenic acid	mg	0.42	1.2	1.1	1.4	1.3	2	2.6	1.8	2	2.7	3.7	5	
Choline	mg	13.7	67	23.2	27.6	100	150	201	153	150	204	110	321	
Myo-inositol	mg	14.7	0	10.2	12.1	0	0	0	40.6	0	0	55.5	85.7	<0.2
Sodium	mmol	1.2	3.9	8.6	10.1	3.7	5.5	7.3	<10	5.5	7.5	25.2	24.3	
Potassium	mmol	1.9	5.6	7.3	8.6	3.9	5.9	7.9	2.6	5.9	8.0	21.5	17.9	
Chloride	mmol	1.5	3.9	4.4	5.1	3.4	5.1	6.8	<10	5.1	6.9	12.7	15.8	
Calcium	mg	61.5	260	274	326	200	299	400	356	299	407	810	670	126
Phosphorus	mg	45	198	139	165	178	267	357	276	267	363	810	670	65
Magnesium	mg	8.7	40	47.9	56.9	63	94	125	107	94	128	200	285	
Iron	mg	1.2	3.4	4.1	4.9	3.7	5.4	7.3	5.3	5.4	7.3	12	23.5	
Copper	mg	0.065	0.19	0.32	0.36	0.37	0.55	0.73	0.53	0.55	0.75	1.8	1.4	
Zinc	mg	0.86	2.6	2.9	3.5	3.7	5.4	7.3	3.9	5.4	7.3	13	13.6	
Manganese	mg	0.06	0.41	0.23	0.28	0.52	0.8	1	0.53	0.8	1.1	1.6	2.1	
Iodine	µg	12.5	33.1	29	34.5	43	63	84	58.4	63	85.7	100	107	
Molybdenum	µg	1.8	12	12.5	14.9	24	36	48	25	36	49	100	107	
Selenium	µg	2.3	8.4	16.2	19.3	15	22	29	26.8	22	29.9	40	50	
Chromium	µg	2.1	17	8.1	9.6	15	22	29	10.6	22	29.9	40	50	

(continued overleaf)

(continued)

Nutrient	Unit	Tyr Anamix Infant	Tyr Gel	Tyr Anamix Junior	Tyr Anamix Junior LQ	TYR Cooler 10	Tyr Cooler 15	TYR Cooler 20	Tyr Lophlex LQ	Tyr Express 15	Tyr Express 20	XPhen, Tyr Maxamaid	XPhen, Tyr Maxamum	XPhen, Tyr Tyrosidon
Package size		400 g (Scoop 5 g)	24 g sachet	29 g sachet	125 mL	87 mL	130 mL	174 mL	125 mL	25 g sachet	34 g sachet	500 g	500 g	500 g
Flavours / other		Contains prebiotics			Orange	Red	Orange, red	Red	Juicy berries					
Linoleic acid	mg	620		673	359									
α-Linolenic acid	mg	100		175	38									
Arachidonic acid	mg	20												
DHA	mg	10			60	67	100	134	150					
EPA	mg					16	23	31						
Dilution		15%	24 g plus 30 mL or 24 g plus 80 mL	29 g to 100 mL						25 g plus 80 mL	34 g plus 80 mL	1 to 7 or 1 to 5	1 to 7 or 1 to 5	1 to 20
Osmolality	mOsm/kg water	380	3000 or 1540	1110	1520	1900	1900	1900	2460	1896	2380	690 (1 to 5)	1000 (1 to 5)	370

*DHA, docosahexaenoic acid; EPA, eicosapentaenoic acid.

Appendix II

Dietetic Products

The following dietetic products are mentioned in this book. A full list of Borderline Substances and vitamin preparations may be found in the *BNF (British National Formulary) for Children* (www.bnf.org)

Manufacturers of low protein foods are given at the end of Chapter 17. L-amino acid supplements for phenylketonuria, maple syrup urine disease, homocystinuria and tyrosinaemia are given in Appendix I.

Abidec	Chefaro UK
Adamin G	SHS
Additrace	Fresenius Kabi
Alicalm	Nutricia
Althera	Vitaflo
Aminoplasmal	B Braun
Aptamil AR	Milupa
Aptamil Pepti 1	Milupa
Aptamil Pepti 2	Milupa
Aptamil Preterm	Milupa
Babiven Maintenance	Fresenius Kabi
Babiven Term	Fresenius Kabi
Calogen	SHS

Caloreen	Nestle
Calshake	Fresenius Kabi
Caprilon	SHS
ClinOleic	Baxter
Clinutren Junior	Nestle
Complete Amino Acid Mix (Code 0124)	SHS
Cow & Gate anti-reflux	Cow & Gate
Cow & Gate Nutriprem 1	Cow & Gate
Cow & Gate Nutriprem 2	Cow & Gate
Cow & Gate Nutriprem breast milk fortifier	Cow & Gate
Dalivit	LPC
Decan	Baxter
Dialamine	Nutricia
Dialyvit Paediatric	Vitaline
Dioralyte	Sanofi-Aventis
Dioralyte Relief	Sanofi-Aventis
DocOmega	Vitaflo
Duocal Liquid	SHS
EAA supplement	Vitaflo
Electrolade	Actavis
Elemental 028 Extra	SHS
Emsogen	SHS
Energivit	SHS

Clinical Paediatric Dietetics, Fourth Edition. Edited by Vanessa Shaw.
© 2015 John Wiley & Sons, Ltd. Published 2015 by John Wiley & Sons, Ltd.
Companion Website: www.wiley.com/go/shaw/paediatricdietetics

Enfamil AR	Mead Johnson	Hydrolysed Nutriprem	Cow & Gate
Enfamil O-Lac	Mead Johnson	InfaSoy	Cow & Gate
Enshake	Abbott	Infatrini	Nutricia
Ensure	Abbott	Infatrini Peptisorb	Nutricia
Ensure Plus	Abbott	Instant Carobel	Cow & Gate
Ensure Plus Creme	Abbott	Intralipid	Fresenius Kabi
Ensure Plus Juce	Abbott	Isosource Junior	Novartis
Ensure TwoCal	Abbott	Jevity Promote	Abbott
Essential Amino Acid	Nutricia	Kabiven	Fresenius Kabi
Mix		KetoCal 3:1	SHS
Forceval Junior Capsule	Alliance	KetoCal 4:1	SHS
Forceval Tablet	Alliance	KetoCal 4:1 LQ	SHS
Forticreme Complete	Nutricia	Ketovite	Paines & Byrne
Fortijuce	Nutricia	KeyOmega	Vitaflo
Fortini	Nutricia	Kindergen	SHS
Fortini Creamy Fruit	Nutricia	Lipidem	B Braun
Fortini Energy	Nutricia	Lipofundin MCT/LCT	B Braun
Fortini Multi Fibre	Nutricia	Liquigen	SHS
Fortini Smoothie	Nutricia	Locasol	SHS
Fortisip	Nutricia	Loprofin Drink	SHS
Fortisip Compact	Nutricia	Lorenzo's Oil	SHS
Fortisip Fruit Dessert	Nutricia	Maxijul	SHS
Fortisip Multi Fibre	Nutricia	Maxijul Liquid	SHS
Fortisip Yoghurt Style	Nutricia	MCT Duocal	SHS
Frebini	Fresenius Kabi	MCT Oil	SHS
Frebini Energy	Fresenius Kabi	MCT Pepdite	SHS
Frebini Energy Fibre	Fresenius Kabi	MCT Pepdite 1+	SHS
Fresubin	Fresenius Kabi	MCT Procal	Vitaflo
Fresubin 5kcal Shot	Fresenius Kabi	MMA/PA Anamix Infant	SHS
Fresubin Creme	Fresenius Kabi	MMA/PA Cooler	Vitaflo
Fresubin Energy Fibre	Fresenius Kabi	MMA/PA Gel	Vitaflo
Fresubin Jucy	Fresenius Kabi	Modulen IBD	Nestle
Fresubin Thickened	Fresenius Kabi	Monogen	SHS
Stage 1 Drink		Multi-thick	Abbott
Fresubin Thickened	Fresenius Kabi	Neocate LCP	SHS
Stage 2 Drink		Neocate Active	SHS
Fresubin 1000 Complete	Fresenius Kabi	Neocate Advance	SHS
Fruitivits	Vitaflo	Nepro HP	Abbott
GA amino5	Vitaflo	Numeta G13%	Baxter
GA Gel	Vitaflo	Numeta G15%	Baxter
GA Express	SHS	Nutilis	Nutricia
GA1 Anamix Infant	SHS	Nutilis Clear	Nutricia
Galactomin 17	SHS	Nutilis Complete	Nutricia
Galactomin 19	SHS	Stage 1 Drink	
Generaid Plus	SHS	Nutramigen Lipil 1	Mead Johnson
Glycerol Trioleate Oil	SHS	Nutramigen Lipil 2	Mead Johnson
Glycerol Trierucate Oil	SHS	Nutramigen AA	Mead Johnson
Glycosade	Vitaflo	Nutrini	Nutricia
Heparon Junior	SHS	Nutrini Energy	Nutricia

Nutrini Energy Multi Fibre	Nutricia
Nutrini Low Energy Multifibre	Nutricia
Nutrini Multi Fibre	Nutricia
Nutrini Peptisorb	Nutricia
Nutriprem 1	Cow & Gate
Nutriprem 2	Cow& Gate
Nutriprem breast milk Fortifier	Cow & Gate
Nutrison 1000 Complete	Nutricia
Nutrison Energy	Nutricia
Nutrison Energy Multi Fibre	Nutricia
Nutrison MCT	Nutricia
Nutrison Peptisorb	Nutricia
Nutrison Standard	Nutricia
Oliclinomel	Baxter
Omegaven	Fresenius Kabi
Osmolite	Abbott
Osmolite 1.5	Abbott
Paediasure	Abbott
Paediasure Fibre	Abbott
Paediasure Peptide	Abbott
Paediasure Plus	Abbott
Paediasure Plus Fibre	Abbott
Paediasure Plus Juce	Abbott
Paediatric Seravit	SHS
Pectigel	Vitaflo
Peditrace	Fresenius Kabi
Pepdite	SHS
Pepdite 1+	SHS
Peptamen	Nestle
Peptamen AF	Nestle
Peptamen Junior	Nestle
Peptamen Junior Advance	Nestle
Pepdite Module (Code 0767)	SHS
Pepti-Junior	Cow & Gate
Perative	Abbott
Phlexy-Vits	SHS
Polycal	Nutricia
Polycal Liquid	Nutricia
Pregestimil Lipil	Mead Johnson
Primene	Baxter
Pro-Cal Shot	Vitaflo
ProMod	Abbott
Protifar	Nutricia
Prozero	Vitaflo
QuickCal	Vitaflo
Renamil	KoRa
Renastart	Vitaflo
Renilon	Nutricia
Renapro	KoRa
Resource Optifibre	Novartis
Resource Dessert Energy	Novartis
Resource Junior	Novartis
Resource Thickened Juice Drink	Novartis
Resource ThickenUp	Novartis
Scandishake	SHS
Similac High Energy	Abbott
SMA breast milk fortifier	SMA Nutrition
SMA Gold Prem 1	SMA Nutrition
SMA Gold Prem 2	SMA Nutrition
SMA HA	SMA Nutrition
SMA High Energy	SMA Nutrition
SMA LF	SMA Nutrition
SMA Staydown	SMA Nutrition
SMOF	Fresenius Kabi
Sno-Pro	SHS
Solvil	Vitaflo
Solivito	Fresenius Kabi
Sucraid	BS Orphan
Tentrini	Nutricia
Tentrini Energy	Nutricia
Tentrini Energy Multi Fibre	Nutricia
Tentrini Multi Fibre	Nutricia
Thick and Easy	Fresenius Kabi
Thixo-D	Sutherland
Tracutil	B Braun
Vamin 9 Glucose	Fresenius Kabi
Vaminolact	Fresenius Kabi
Vita-Bite	Vitaflo
Vitajoule	Vitaflo
Vitapro	Vitaflo
Vitaquick	Vitaflo
Vitlipid Infant	Fresenius Kabi
Wysoy	SMA Nutrition
XLYS LOW TRY Maxamaid	SHS
XLYS LOW TRY Maxamum	SHS
XLYS TRY Glutaridon	SHS
XMTVI Maxamaid	SHS
XMTVI Maxamum	SHS
Wysoy	SMA Nutrition

Index